Terry 1982

Second Edition

NEUROLOGICAL SURGERY *Volume 4*

A Comprehensive Reference Guide to the Diagnosis and Management of Neurosurgical Problems

Edited by

JULIAN R. YOUMANS, M.D., Ph.D.

Professor, Department of Neurological Surgery,
School of Medicine, University of California
Davis, California

1982 W. B. SAUNDERS COMPANY
Philadelphia • London • Toronto • Mexico City • Sydney • Tokyo

W. B. Saunders Company: West Washington Square
Philadelphia, PA 19105

1 St. Anne's Road
Eastbourne, East Sussex BN 21 3UN, England

1 Goldthorne Avenue
Toronto, Ontario M8Z 5T9, Canada

Cedro 512
Mexico 4, D.F. Mexico

9 Waltham Street
Artarmon, N.S.W. 2064, Australia

Ichibancho, Central Bldg., 22-I
Chiyoda-ku, Tokyo 102, Japan

Library of Congress Cataloging in Publication Data

Youmans, Julian Ray, 1928–
　　Neurological surgery.

　　1. Nervous system—Surgery.　I. Title.
[DNLM:　1. Neurosurgery.　WL368 N4945]
RD593.Y68　　1980　　617'.48
ISBN 0-7216-9665-1 (v. 4)　　　　80-21368

Volume 1　ISBN　0-7216-9662-7
Volume 2　ISBN　0-7216-9663-5
Volume 3　ISBN　0-7216-9664-3
Volume 4　ISBN　0-7216-9665-1
Volume 5　ISBN　0-7216-9666-X
Volume 6　ISBN　0-7216-9667-8
Six Volume Set　ISBN　0-7216-9658-9

Neurological Surgery—Volume Four

Last digit is the print number:　　9　　8　　7　　6　　5　　4　　3　　2　　1

Contributors

EHUD ARBIT, M.D.

Extradural Dorsal Spinal Lesions

Instructor in Neurological Surgery, Cornell University Medical College. Neurological Surgeon, The New York Hospital Cornell Medical Center, New York.

DONALD P. BECKER, M.D., F.A.C.S.

Pathophysiology, Diagnosis, Treatment, and Outcome of Head Injury in Adults

Professor of Neurological Surgery, Chairman of Division of Neurological Surgery, Virginia Commonwealth University, Medical College of Virginia. Chief of Neurological Surgery, Medical College of Virginia Hospitals; Consultant, McGuire Veterans Administration Hospital and St. Mary's Hospital, Richmond, Virginia.

HENRY BERRY, M.D., M.R.C.P.(U.K.), F.R.C.P.(C.)

Peripheral Nerve Entrapment

Associate Professor of Medicine (Neurology), University of Toronto School of Medicine. Director, Clinical Neurophysiology Laboratory, St. Michael's Hospital, Toronto, Ontario.

ROGER BOLES, M.D., F.A.C.S.

Cranial Nerve Injury in Basilar Skull Fractures

Professor of Otolaryngology, Chairman of Department of Otolaryngology, School of Medicine, University of California at San Francisco. Chief of Otolaryngology Services, University of California at San Francisco General Hospital; Attending Staff, San Francisco General Hospital and Veterans Administration Hospital; Consultant, Letterman Army Hospital, San Francisco, California; Consultant in Otolaryngology to Surgeon General of the United States Air Force, San Francisco, California; Consultant, United States Naval Hospital, Oakland, California.

CHARLES E. BRACKETT, M.D., F.A.C.S.

Pulmonary Care and Complications, Arachnoid Cysts, Subarachnoid Hemorrhage, Post-Traumatic Arachnoid Cysts, Cordotomy

Professor of Neurological Surgery, Chairman of Department of Neurological Surgery, University of Kansas Medical Center, College of Health Sciences and Hospital. Chief of Neurological Surgery Service, University of Kansas Medical Center; Attending Staff, Kansas City Veterans Administration Hospital, Kansas City, Missouri.

SHELLEY N. CHOU, M.D., Ph.D., F.A.C.S.

Urological Problems; Scoliosis, Kyphosis, and Lordosis; Tumors of Skull

Professor of Neurological Surgery, Head of Department of Neurological Surgery, University of Minnesota Medical School. Chief of Neurological Surgery Service, University of Minnesota Hospitals; Consultant, Minneapolis Veterans Administration Hospital, Minneapolis, Minnesota.

KEMP CLARK, M.D., F.A.C.S.

Cervical, Thoracic, and Lumbar Spinal Injury; Anterior Operative Approach to Cervical Spine

Professor of Neurological Surgery, Chairman of Division of Neurological Surgery, University of Texas Health Science Center at Dallas. Director of Neurological Surgery Service, Parkland Memorial Hospital; Chief of Neurological Surgery Service, Children's Medical Center, Dallas, Texas.

WILLIAM M. COCKE, JR., M.D., F.A.C.S.

Scalp Injuries, Tumors of Scalp

Professor of Surgery, Chief of Plastic and Reconstructive Surgery, School of Medicine, Texas Technical University. Chief of Plastic Surgery, Health Sciences Center; Attending Staff, St. Mary's of the Plains, Lubbock, Texas; Consultant, Veterans Administration Hospital, Big Springs, Texas.

COURTLAND H. DAVIS, JR., M.D., F.A.C.S.

Extradural Lumbar Spinal Lesions

Professor of Surgery (Neurological Surgery), Bowman Gray School of Medicine, Wake Forest University. Staff Neurological Surgeon, North Carolina Baptist Hospital, Winston-Salem, North Carolina.

STEWART B. DUNSKER, M.D.

Hyperextension-Hyperflexion Injuries

Adjunct Associate Professor of Anatomy, University of Cincinnati College of Medicine. Assistant Attending Neurological Surgeon, University of Cincinnati Hospital; Attending Neurological Surgeon, Good Samaritan Hospital and Christ Hospital, Cincinnati, Ohio.

GEORGE EHNI, M.D., M.S., F.A.C.S.

Extradural Cervical Spinal Injuries

Professor of Neurological Surgery, Baylor College of Medicine. Senior Attending Staff, Methodist, St. Luke's, Ben Taub, and Veterans Administration Hospitals, Houston, Texas.

ANDREW J. GABOR, M.D., Ph.D.

Post-Traumatic Epilepsy

Associate Professor of Neurology, University of California, School of Medicine at Davis, Davis, California. Director, Laboratory of Electroencephalography and Clinical Neurophysiology, University of California Davis Medical Center at Sacramento, Sacramento, California.

RICHARD PAUL GREENBERG, M.D., Ph.D.

Diagnosis, Treatment, and Outcome of Head Injury in Adults

Assistant Professor of Neurological Surgery, Medical College of Virginia, Virginia Commonwealth University. Attending in Neurological Surgery, Medical College of Virginia Hospitals, Richmond, Virginia.

ALAN R. HUDSON, M.D., Ch.B., F.R.C.S.(Ed.), F.R.C.S.(C.)

Peripheral Nerve Entrapment

Professor of Neurological Surgery, Chairman of Division of Neurological Surgery, University of Toronto. Neurological Surgeon-in-Chief, St. Michael's Hospital, Toronto, Ontario.

PULLA R. S. KISHORE, M.D.

Head Injury in Adults

Professor of Radiology, Medical College of Virginia, Virginia Commonwealth University, Richmond, Virginia. Director of Neuroradiology, Medical College of Virginia Hospitals; Consultant in Radiology, McGuire Veterans Administration Hospital, Richmond, Virginia.

DAVID G. KLINE, M.D., F.A.C.S.

Peripheral Nerve Injuries

Professor of Neurological Surgery, Head of Department of Neurological Surgery, Louisiana State University School of Medicine; Chief of Louisiana State University Neurological Surgery Service. Attending Staff, Touro and Hotel Dieu Hospitals; Academic Staff, Ochsner Clinic; Consultant, United States Public Health, Veterans Administration Hospital, New Orleans, Louisiana, and Biloxi Air Force Base Hospital, Biloxi, Mississippi.

JOHN E. LONSTEIN, M.D., F.A.C.S.

Scoliosis, Kyphosis, and Lordosis

Assistant Professor of Orthopedic Surgery, University of Minnesota Medical School. Attending Surgeon, Minneapolis Fairview Hospital, Minneapolis, Minnesota; Gillette Children's Hospital, St. Paul, Minnesota.

FRANK H. MAYFIELD, M.D., F.A.C.S.

Peripheral Nerve Entrapment

Clinical Professor of Neurological Surgery, Emeritus, University of Cincinnati School of Medicine. Director, Department of Neurological Surgery, Christ Hospital; Senior Attending Staff, Good Samaritan Hospital, Cincinnati, Ohio.

ROBERT L. McLAURIN, M.D., F.A.C.S.

Head Injury in Children, Post-Traumatic Syndrome

Professor of Surgery and Neurological Surgery, University of Cincinnati College of Medicine. Chief of Neurological Surgery, University of Cincinnati Medical Center, University Hospital, and Children's Hospital Medical Center; Consultant, Veterans Administration Hospital, Jewish Hospital, and Christ Hospital; Attending Neurological Surgeon, Good Samaritan Hospital, and Bethesda Hospital, Cincinnati, Ohio.

JAMES E. McLENNAN, M.D., F.A.C.S.

Head Injury in Children

Assistant Professor of Surgery and Neurological Surgery, University of Cincinnati School of Medicine. Attending Neurological Surgeon, University of Cincinnati Hospital and Children's Hospital, Cincinnati, Ohio.

JAMES DOUGLAS MILLER, M.D., M.B., Ch.B., Ph.D., F.R.C.S. (Ed.), F.A.C.S.

Diagnosis, Treatment, and Outcome of Head Injury in Adults

Forbes Professor of Surgical Neurology and Chairman of Department of Surgical Neurology, University of Edinburgh School of Medicine. Chairman of Department of Surgical Neurology, Royal Infirmary and Western General Hospital, Edinburgh, Scotland.

THOMAS J. MIMS, JR., M.D.

Trauma to Carotid Arteries

Resident in Neurological Surgery, Baylor College of Medicine Affiliated Hospitals, Houston, Texas.

FRANK E. NULSEN, M.D., F.A.C.S.

Peripheral Nerve Injuries

Professor of Neurological Surgery, Chairman of Neurological Surgery, Case Western Reserve University. Director of Neurological Surgery Division, University Hospitals of Cleveland; Consulting Neurological Surgeon, Veterans Administration Hospital and Cleveland Metropolitan General Hospital, Cleveland, Ohio.

AYUB K. OMMAYA, M.D., F.R.C.S., F.A.C.S.

Mechanisms of Cerebral Trauma

Clinical Professor of Neurological Surgery, George Washington University School of Medicine. Attending Neurological Surgeon, George Washington University Medical Center, Washington, District of Columbia. Chief Medical Adviser, National Highway Traffic Safety Administration, Department of Transportation; Former Chief of Applied Research in Neurological Surgery, Clinical Center, National Institutes of Health, Bethesda, Maryland.

RUSSELL H. PATTERSON, JR., M.D., F.A.C.S.

Extradural Dorsal Spinal Lesions, Metastatic Brain Tumors, Hypophysectomy by Craniotomy

Professor of Neurological Surgery, Cornell University Medical College. Attending Surgeon-in-Charge, Department of Neurological Surgery, The New York Hospital, New York, New York.

MORRIS W. PULLIAM, M.D., F.A.C.S.

Problems with Multiple Trauma

Assistant Clinical Professor of Neurological Surgery, University of North Dakota School of Medicine. Staff Neurological Surgeon, Department of Neurosciences, Quain and Ramstad Clinic; Attending Neurological Surgeon, Bismarck Hospital and St. Alexius Hospital, Bismarck, North Dakota.

RALPH M. REITAN, Ph.D.

Psychological Testing After Craniocerebral Injury

Professor of Psychology, University of Arizona, Tucson, Arizona.

SETTI S. RENGACHARY, M.D.

Arachnoid Cysts, Post-Traumatic Arachnoid Cysts

Associate Professor of Neurological Surgery, The University of Kansas Medical Center, College of Health Sciences. Chief, Neurological Surgery Service at Kansas City Veterans Administration Hospital, Kansas City, Kansas.

MICHAEL JOHN ROSNER, M.D.

Head Injury in Adults

Assistant Professor of Neurological Surgery, Medical College of Virginia, Virginia Commonwealth University. Attending Neurological Surgeon, Medical College of Virginia Hospitals; Assistant Chief of Neurological Surgery, McGuire Veterans Administration Hospital, Richmond, Virginia.

RICHARD CARLTON SCHULTZ, M.D., F.A.C.S.

Maxillofacial Injuries

Professor of Surgery, Head of Division of Plastic Surgery, University of Illinois Abraham Lincoln College of Medicine. Chief of Division of Plastic Surgery and President of Medical Staff, Lutheran General Hospital; Attending Staff, University of Illinois Hospital, Chicago, Illinois.

JOHN BERNARD SELHORST, M.D.

Head Injury in Adults

Associate Professor of Neurology, Medical College of Virginia, Virginia Commonwealth University. Attending Neurologist, Richmond Eye Hospital and Medical College of Virginia Hospital; Consultant Neurologist, McGuire Veterans Administration Hospital, Richmond, Virginia, and Central State Hospital, Petersburg, Virginia; Eastern State Hospital, Williamsburg, Virginia.

ROBERT F. SPETZLER, M.D., F.A.C.S.

Dural Fistulae

Associate Professor of Neurological Surgery, Case Western Reserve University. Attending Neurological Surgeon, University Hospitals, Case Western Reserve University, Cleveland, Ohio; Veterans Administration; Consultant, Lakewood Hospital, Lakewood, Ohio.

ROBERT L. TIMMONS, M.D., F.A.C.S.

Cranial Defects

Clinical Professor of Surgery, East Carolina University School of Medicine, Attending Neurological Surgeon, Pitt County Memorial Hospital, Greenville, North Carolina.

JAMES L. TITCHENER, M.D.

Post-Traumatic Syndrome

Professor of Psychiatry, University of Cincinnati Medical Center. Attending Staff, Cincinnati General Hospital; Consultant, Veterans Administration Hospital, Cincinnati, Ohio.

JOHN D. WARD, M.D.

Head Injury in Adults

Assistant Professor of Neurological Surgery, Medical College of Virginia Hospital, Virginia Commonwealth University. Chief, Pediatric Neurological Surgery, Medical College of Virginia Hospital, Richmond, Virginia.

CLARK C. WATTS, M.D., F.A.C.S.

Problems with Multiple Trauma

Professor of Neurological Surgery, University of Missouri School of Medicine. Chief of Neurological Surgery, University Hospital, University of Missouri/Columbia Health Sciences Center; Consultant, Harry S Truman Memorial Veterans Administration Hospital, Columbia, Missouri.

CHARLES B. WILSON, M.D., F.A.C.S.

Dural Fistulae, Chemotherapy, Sellar and Parasellar Tumors, Indications for and Results of Hypophysectomy, Stereotaxic Hypophysectomy

Professor of Neurological Surgery, Chairman of Department of Neurological Surgery, University of California. School of Medicine at San Francisco. Chief of Neurological Surgery, University Hospital, San Francisco, California.

ROBERT B. WINTER, M.D., F.A.C.S.

Scoliosis, Kyphosis, and Lordosis

Professor of Orthopedic Surgery, University of Minnesota School of Medicine. Attending Staff, University of Minnesota Hospitals, Fairview Hospital, St. Mary's Hospital, Minneapolis Children's Hospital, Minneapolis, Minnesota; Gillette Children's Hospital, St. Paul Children's Hospital, and St. Paul Ramsey Hospital, St. Paul, Minnesota.

JULIAN R. YOUMANS, M.D., Ph.D., F.A.C.S.

Diagnostic Biopsy, Cerebral Death, Cerebral Blood Flow, Trauma to Carotid Arteries, Glial and Neuronal Tumors, Lymphomas, Sarcomas and Vascular Tumors, Tumors of Disordered Embryogenesis, Peripheral and Sympathetic Nerve Tumors, Parasitic and Fungal Infections.

Professor of Neurological Surgery, University of California, School of Medicine at Davis, Davis, California. Attending Neurological Surgeon, University of California Davis Medical Center at Sacramento, Sacramento, California; Consultant in Neurological Surgery, United States Air Force Medical Center, Travis Air Force Base, California; Veterans Administration Hospital, Martinez, California.

HAROLD FRANCIS YOUNG, M.D.

Head Injury in Adults

Professor of Neurological Surgery, Vice-Chairman of Department of Neurological Surgery, Medical College of Virginia, Commonwealth University. Chief of Neurological Surgery, McGuire Veterans Administration Hospital, Richmond, Virginia; Attending Neurological Surgeon, Medical College of Virginia Hospitals, Richmond, Virginia.

Contents

VIII

TRAUMA

MECHANISMS OF CEREBRAL CONCUSSION, CONTUSIONS, AND OTHER EFFECTS OF HEAD INJURY

The word "concussion" is derived from the Latin "concutere," which means to shake, and is commonly used to describe a very common physical effect of mechanical input to the nervous system as well as the physiological response to it. The input is in the dynamic range of impacts, i.e., within a frequency range of about 1000 Hz to approximately 10 kHz, with the duration of loading being from a few milliseconds upward to a cut-off at about 200 msec. Mechanical loading beyond this range results in crushing of the head as a result of applying a static load, an input that produces effects very different from those of true impacts.

It is now well established that to define cerebral concussion as a reversible phenomenon in every case is a simplistic and erroneous idealization. The concept of concussion as a reversible loss of function in the nervous system in response to trauma is inexact.[31] In an earlier review of the experimental, pathological, and clinical data on concussion, Symonds has stated:

Concussion should not be confined to cases in which there is immediate loss of consciousness with rapid and complete recovery, but should include the many cases in which the initial symptoms are the same but with subsequent, long-continued disturbances of consciousness, often followed by residual symptoms.[27]

There are valid reasons for such a more comprehensive definition because a study of the known facts would support the concept of cerebral concussion as a spectrum or set of syndromes ranging from the apparently reversible to the irreversible.

In a general sense, it can be said that the basic phenomenon of head injury is cerebral concussion, or commotio cerebri. The other primary phenomena that occur—skull fracture, contusions, hemorrhages—plus all the secondary phenomena such as brain swelling that are initiated by the primary damage are epiphenomena in the sense that in themselves they are not the major determinant of the final outcome in the majority of cases. This is not to say that the epiphenomena are not critical modulators of that outcome. This thesis is further developed in what follows, wherein it is shown that the diffuse effects of cerebral concussion and the focal effects of the epiphenomena interact to produce the final outcome.

CONCUSSION AT THE LEVEL OF A NERVE

The term "concussion" by itself, unqualified by the word "cerebral," can be illustrated at the simplest levels of the nervous system, for example, in a peripheral nerve,

A. K. OMMAYA

or at more complex levels in the spinal cord or even higher levels of the nervous system. Figure 56–1A shows an experimental set-up wherein controlled mechanical loading can be applied to a frog sciatic nerve.[28] A pyrex column is filled with fluid containing the nerve. A piston at the base of the column is applied to the fluid. Piston impacts to the system can produce either acoustic waves through the fluid medium or bulk movements of the fluid (if the column is opened to allow such movement). In this way, a combination of loads can be applied under controlled conditions to the sciatic nerve of the frog. The effects of this complex normal loading (a combination of tensile, compressive, and shear loading) can be tested by measuring the electrophysiological properties of the nerve in response to stimulation. Shear loading occurs only when the fluid is allowed to move, and when this is prevented, only tension and compression affect the nerve. The apparatus is calibrated to allow a range of loads from slight shock waves to high-level impacts. In this way it is possible to modulate the compound action potential recorded

from the nerve obtained before, during, and after actual loading. At an impact pressure equal to 0.8 atm with a duration of load of approximately 10 msec, the amplitude of the compound action potential is reduced and then gradually restored (Fig. 56–1B). Within 10 minutes after this impact, the compound action potential is restored and the loss of function is reversible.

Keeping all the conditions the same but increasing the load to 1.5 atm for the same duration of loading produces essentially an irreversible phenomenon.[28] Histological examination of such permanently "paralyzed" nerves has revealed no significant structural damage to the nerve that could be detected by light microscopy. In other words, by simply varying the amplitude of the impact it has been possible to show a range of disturbances of nerve function, from the reversible to the irreversible, the nature of which could not be correlated to the microscopic structure. This lack of correlation between functional changes and structural changes seen under the light microscope in neural tissues is a key element in the phenomena of concussion.

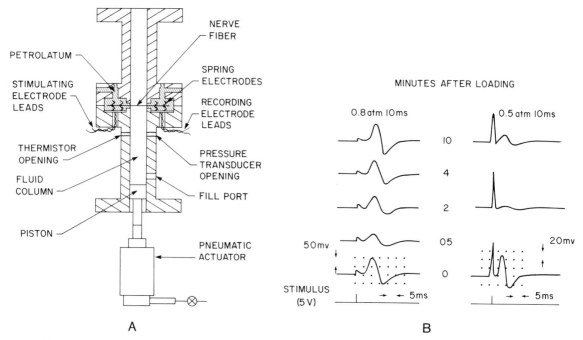

Figure 56–1 *A.* Apparatus for controlled mechanical loading of peripheral nerve in the dynamic range. *B.* Results of two experiments on frog sciatic nerve at 0.8 and 1.5 atm pressure for durations shown. Note reversible loss of compound action potential at 0.8 atm and essentially irreversible change after impact at 1.5 atm. (Developed by L. Thibault.)

CEREBRAL CONCUSSION

Cerebral concussion may be regarded as a graded phenomenon. It includes the classic concussion in which the patient suffers from what is a sensorimotor paralysis (traumatic unconsciousness). It is important that when concussion with unconsciousness occurs, there is always a period of retrograde amnesia, and when recovery occurs, the patient has a period of post-traumatic amnesia. In other words, there is always an association between the loss of sensorimotor control and coordination, i.e., the *paralytic* phenomena, and the memory disturbance, i.e., the *amnesic* phenomena. Therefore, the association of the two kinds of phenomena, the paralytic and the amnesic, have to be explained in any theory of cerebral concussion. Cerebral concussion also includes, however, both *lesser* and more severe grades of concussion. Lesser grades (which are common) are not associated with sensorimotor paralysis, i.e., the amnesic phenomena are dissociated from the paralytic phenomena. More severe grades of concussion, in addition to sharing both amnesic and paralytic phenomena, also result in varying degrees of irreversible sequelae. How can one explain such a range of phenomena? The retrograde amnesia of most cerebral concussions usually is short-term, lasting less than one day, and the patient's future learning capacity remains intact in most cases. Retrograde amnesia extending for many days to months is usually only a transient phenomenon. In other words, most patients who are recovering from significant head injury (loss of consciousness over an hour) will have a fairly long period of retrograde amnesia but one that invariably shrinks down to a short span of retrograde amnesia of a few minutes in duration. When retrograde amnesia is long-term, i.e., a matter of many months to years, it is inevitable in such cases that there has been significant structural damage, most often in the medial aspects of the temporal lobes. It is also important to note that as patients recover from traumatic unconsciousness they pass through a series of behavioral stages—coma, stupor, confusion, automatisms, and the like. In patients who have had a lesser degree of injury, these stages occur rapidly and are therefore not seen as clearly as in the patient who has been unconscious for many days. Close study of the recovery process discloses a remarkable similarity in the behavioral nature of the stages of such recovery, however. It appears that the reintegration of the nervous system after trauma follows certain rules (probably genetic) that are laid down in the brain structure and may well be key determinants in the recovery of the nervous system after trauma.[17]

MECHANICS OF CONCUSSION AND CONTUSION

In order to understand the relation between the mechanical input and the neural response to trauma the following paradigm is a convenient idealization of the phenomena of mechanical injury to the brain (Fig. 56–2). Mechanical input applied for longer than 200 msec is essentially static, i.e., causes slow crushing of the head. The forces can be very great, but a critical fact to note is that patients subjected to such loads do not lose consciousness. Russell and Schiller, in a classic report describing 12 such cases, clearly brought out the relationship between such essentially crushing injuries and the related severe *local* lesions without significant *diffuse* damage to the brain.[26a] Patients with this type of head injury have severe skull fractures, spinal fluid otorrhea and rhinorrhea, but no primary loss of consciousness. It therefore appears to be important conceptually to understand the separation of focal effects from diffuse effects in both functional and structural terms. A focal effect is that which arises from a discrete area as opposed to diffuse effects, which are distributed throughout most of or significantly large areas of the brain on both sides. Most impact head injuries are dynamic events, i.e., occurring in a time domain of less than 200 msec. Although most head injuries are caused by direct impact, indirect loading of the head can also produce significant brain injuries. Thus, falls on the buttocks, severe hyperflexion-hyperextension injuries produced by violent shaking of the head, especially in children, and severe "whiplash" types of head movement of sufficient magnitude can cause visible brain injuries as well as other effects of neural trauma that result in definitive sequelae.[20,21,29,30]

Two types of phenomena occur in direct impacts: *contact phenomena* and *inertial*

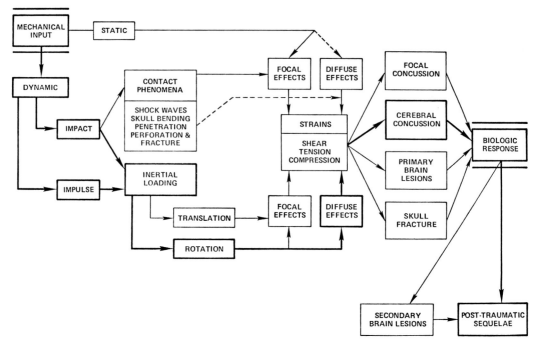

Figure 56–2 A flow chart for critical factors in the mechanics of head injury. The traumatic mechanical input is shown at the top left. Heavy lines are used to indicate areas where our experimental data are adequate to test the hypothesis proposed. Lighter lines connect areas where work remains to be done, and dotted lines are used to indicate predicted causal relationships that are least supported by available data.

loading. Contact phenomena include shock waves, which are probably not injurious, skull bending, or fracture, and may produce primarily focal injuries. Such injuries can be trivial or significant, depending on the severity of the impact and the location of the focal lesion. The same is also true for "cavitation"-induced focal lesions due to compressive-rarefactive strains.

Inertial loading occurs in all kinds of dynamic impact resulting in head movements consisting of two components, translation and rotation. Movement of the head in a linear fashion is called translation, whereas movement through any angle is rotational. In real life, of course, both motions are always associated in various proportions. Theoretically and experimentally, it is important to separate the two. The brain as a structure is a soft viscoelastic material that is very easily deformed under shear or tension but is relatively resistant to pure compression strains, partly because of its high-bulk modulus, i.e., its almost incompressible nature, and partly because of its viscosity. A simple mechanical analogy is seen in how it is difficult to distort water or gelatin in a container if it is merely pushed along a flat smooth surface. Sudden jostling or angulation of the container, e.g., by a small bump on the counter, will, however, always cause the contents to spill or swirl around. It is the author's theory that rotation is the key determinant of diffuse injuries and that translation produces only focal injuries. The effects of rotation and translation together with the focal effects of contact phenomena produce brain damage as a result of shear, tensile, and compressive strains that in turn cause the variety of effects seen in the patient.[3]

Since cerebral concussion is the result of diffuse effects caused by shear strains, it is important to review where these strains occur, i.e., where they have their maximum and minimum effects. From theoretical physics it would be predicted that the effect would be maximal on the surface and would diminish toward the center of a spherical mass of viscoelastic material such as the brain. Moreover, specific injury would be intensified wherever there are junctional boundaries or sudden transition between tissues, for example, a bony or dural partition or protrusion into the brain. An increase in the tensile and shear strains will always occur at that point. Thus, a general principle can be stated: impacts to the mo-

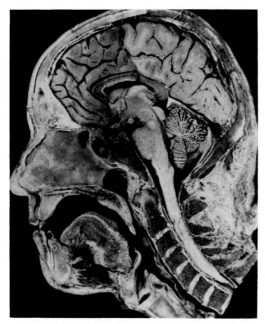

Figure 56–3 Cross section of human head to show central location of rostral brain stem with reference to surfaces of the cerebral-cerebellar mass. Note that rotation-induced strains will be initially maximal at the surfaces and minimal at the center. Note also the significant intrusion of the skull base into the frontal and temporal zones of the brain mass.

bile head cause effects that will be maximal at the surface, minimal at the center of the brain, and intensified at specific locations of tissue transitions, especially when these transitions are caused by a bony or dural protrusion (Fig. 56–3). Conversely, surface injuries to the brain will be minimized where the skull interior is smooth and there are no venous attachments, as over the occipital lobes.

CLINICAL–PATHOLOGICAL CORRELATIONS

A review of anatomical, physiological, and pathological data will test the theoretical predictions given earlier. Figure 56–3 illustrates how the critical area for sensorimotor integration, the reticular formation in the rostral brain stem, is located approximately in the center of the mass of the brain including the cerebellum. If the theory is correct, in this location the reticular activating system would be the last area to be affected in head impacts involving inertial loading. The first effects would be at the

cortical surfaces and especially at those surfaces where there are irregular protrusions such as the frontotemporal areas in relation to the anterior and middle cranial fossae. These predictions fit the known clinicopathological and experimental data on which the hypothesis for cerebral concussion and contusions is developed.

The amnesic component of concussion is a more sensitive witness to injury than are the paralytic phenomena. For example, when a patient receives a blow to the head that does not produce unconsciousness, he does not fall down and is still able to walk, albeit in a slightly erratic manner, i.e., sensorimotor integration is not completely lost. He will, however, always have a significant memory disturbance that can be of varying duration. Typical examples of this type are boxing and football injuries in which almost pure amnesic loss with no sensorimotor disturbance have been reported.[2] The opposite situation, i.e., traumatic unconsciousness with sensorimotor paralysis but no amnesia has not been reported. Thus, there are no cases in which a paralytic phenomenon is produced separate from the amnesic phenomenon, although the reverse is possible. It appears that there is a one-way dissociation between the amnesic and paralytic components of cerebral concussion, with the strength of the association increasing with increasing severity of head injury. This concept is summarized in Figure 56–4, which depicts a set of syndromes of cerebral concussion graded from I to VI.

Cerebral concussion with very mild confusion and restoration of normal consciousness without amnesia (i.e., transient disturbance of memory and disturbance of highest cognitive cerebral function without sensorimotor paralysis) constitutes a grade I cerebral concussion. Grades II and III show increasing confusion plus amnesia with decreasing speed and capacity of return to normal consciousness. As impact levels increase, the resultant shear strains progressively affect deeper parts of the brain. When the diencephalic-mesencephalic core is affected, a grade IV syndrome is produced, i.e., the classic cerebral concussion of a "knock-out" blow with coma, paralysis, subsequent confusion, amnesia, and finally restoration of most brain functions but with persisting retrograde amnesia. In the same way higher

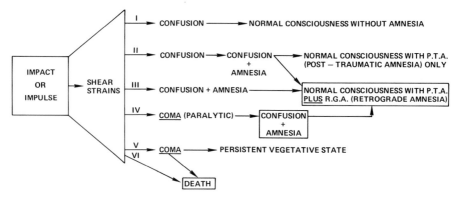

Figure 56–4 Diagrammatic description of the author's hypothesis for the syndromes of cerebral concussion with increasing severity of primary injury causing more extensive disconnections between the cortex and the mesencephalic-diencephalic "core" of the brain. Grades I and II represent cortical-subcortical disconnection: II and III, cortical-subcortical-diencephalic disconnection; and IV to VI, cortical-subcortical-diencephalic disconnection. Note that grade IV cerebral concussion is that state of traumatic unconsciousness that may be further subdivided according to duration of coma or severity of neurological sequelae.

levels of impact can cause irreversible coma and even death. This classification of cerebral concussion has the advantage of displaying the common mechanism and showing how and why the more severe cases as well as the minor ones can be included. At the severe end of the spectrum severe disconnection of outer brain layers from the *recovering* brain stem can result in the so-called persistent vegetative state, a condition wherein restored brain stem function is about all that survives.[8] The term "vegetative state" does not specify the site of the injuries precisely, which is correct because as yet there is no precise correlation between the structural and the functional aspects of the mechanically induced disconnective disturbances. It is also obvious why, if the impact is sufficiently severe, death can ensue rapidly because of the irreversible paralysis of brain stem control over vital functions. One of the earliest cases of cerebral concussion described in the literature, by Littré, was of this type of fatal "commotio cerebri." A French prisoner threw himself at a prison wall in trying to escape, smashed his head against the wall, fell down, and died almost immediately. Postmortem examination revealed no visible brain lesions. It is obvious that death occurred in this case before primary lesions could form. Such early cases formed the basis of descriptions of concussion as a phenomenon of paralysis without concomitant structural damage, a simplification that does not accurately represent the facts.[1,13,22]

Are there alternative explanations of the mechanisms of cerebral concussion and contusions that can better explain the facts and refute the proposed hypothesis that effects would be greatest at the surface, least at the center, and intensified at junctional boundaries? One way of examining this issue is to consider whether there are any observations that if shown to be true would clearly refute the theory. The following four possibilities must be considered. First of all, is it possible to have a severe head injury with documented *primary* brain stem injury without associated diffuse damage? Such a case would refute the theory and the classification of cerebral concussion and its relationship to brain injuries. The second possibility that could refute the hypothesis would be a patient with a grade I to III concussion who recovered but then died of an unrelated cause in whom autopsy revealed brain stem lesions. Because the theory states that in grades I to III of concussion the level of strain has not been severe enough to reach the mesencephalic core, the finding of structural damage here would not be explicable. The third test would be to find a grade IV concussion, i.e., a patient who had sustained a classic "knock-out" without subsequent traumatic amnesia. Finally, the demonstration of no correlation between increasing severity of anatomical head injury and severity of impairment of higher cerebral functions would also tend to refute the hypothesis, which predicts that there should be a graded correlation between increasing severity of head injury and increasing neuropsychological deficits. After a detailed review of the literature and extensive discussions with other workers in the field, the author is convinced that none of the foregoing four possibilities are valid. Review of some of the supportive data follows.

Neuropathological Data

Hume-Adams and Graham and their co-workers studied the primary brain stem damage in cases of severe head injury.[11,26] They were unable to find a single case of *primary* brain stem damage without associated diffuse damage, thus providing strong support to the centripetal theory of cerebral concussion and the genesis of diffuse versus focal lesions as described earlier. Oppenheimer has described cases of cerebral concussion in patients who, having recovered from their head injuries, then died of unrelated causes. Neuropathological studies of these cases revealed evidence of small microglial "stars" distributed in a fairly diffuse pattern through the brain but not in the brain stem.[24] It is possible that these lesions of cerebral concussion are the final signatures of the petechial hemorrhages that the author found in experimental animals.[18]

Detailed histopathological studies of primary and secondary lesions of head injury in the human provide a basis for correlating the clinical effect with the neuropathological effect.[6,17,18] Furthermore, computed tomography offers in vivo clinicopathological correlations in patients with head injuries, and the data obtained have been of significant diagnostic and prognostic value.[1,15,23,32]

Review of these human neuropathological data in conjunction with the experimental data to be described clearly supports the view that cerebral concussion is a graded phenomenon that must be defined in terms that include progressively less reversible cases as well as cases of fatality as a primary effect of head injury. Functional reversibility is not linearly correlated with structural changes as seen at the light microscopic level. The precise mechanism of concussion at the cellular level remains to be uncovered.[16,18]

Experimental Data

Clinical and Pathological Indices

Earlier work showed that rotational head movement was critical for cerebral concussion, but it was not possible to discern the relative effects of rotation, translation, and the contact phenomena of impact.[13,22] By achieving almost pure inertial loading, the apparatus shown diagrammatically in Figure 56–5 permits the separation of some of these effects.[18] Using a restraining helmet and a set of linkages, it has made possible clear-cut comparisons of translation and rotation. Thus, the effects of translation in which the center of gravity of the head moves approximately 1 inch and of rotation

Figure 56–5 Experimental layout for evaluating effects of rotation, translation, and impact. Note that both the observational and input variables were recorded and controlled by the PDP-12 computer. The motions of the head controlled by the head accelerating device (HAD-II and subsequent improved version for rhesus monkeys, HAD-III) are shown in Figure 56–6. (HAD-III designed by L. Thibault.)

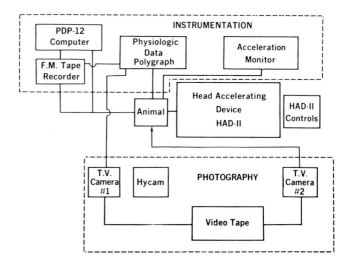

in which it moves through 45 degrees while simultaneously translating approximately 1 inch can be directly evaluated (Fig. 56–6).

Measuring uncontrolled head movements during head impact and "whiplash"-type inertial loading experiments in three subhuman primate species has made possible the prediction of levels of rotation that would be injurious to man (Fig. 56–7).[19] All experiments with the controlled head injury apparatus shown in Figure 56–5 have been done with squirrel and rhesus monkeys at the predicted acceleration levels at which paralytic, or grade IV, concussion associated with some degree of focal damage and visible lesions in the brain would occur.[19,21] The data show that restricting the animal's head from rotating in any vector prevented the occurrence of cerebral concussion even though head acceleration

in translation exceeded 1000 g. In contrast when rotation was allowed while acceleration was kept at approximately the same levels as in translation, concussion occurred in every case (Fig. 56–8). These data established for the first time that inertial loading must include a rotational component if a head injury is to produce the diffuse effect on the brain that is necessary for the production of cerebral concussion.[18]

Additional support for the proposed theory was obtained from autopsy performed on the animals within 24 hours of impact. In those that were rotated, subdural hematomas and subarachnoid hemorrhages were found diffusely over both hemispheres. In cross sections, all of the brain also showed small petechial hemorrhages, distributed bilaterally in a symmetrical manner. In contrast to these diffuse cerebral hemorrhages

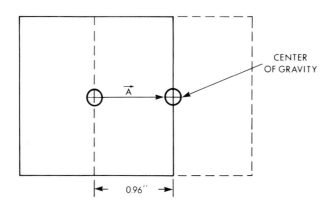

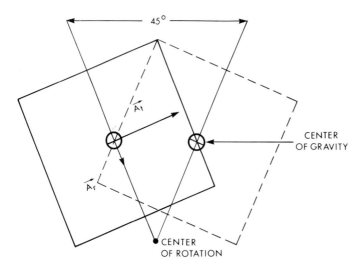

Figure 56–6 Motions of animal head as constrained by a form-fitting helmet. Note that in both rotational and translational motions, the center of gravity of the head-helmet mass is moved an equal 0.96 inch. $\vec{A}$, translational acceleration; $\vec{A}_t$, tangential acceleration; $\vec{A}_r$, radial acceleration.

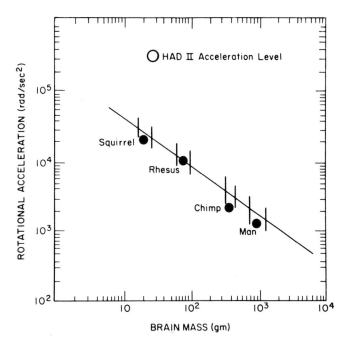

Figure 56–7 Tolerance levels (at 50 per cent probability level) for cerebral concussion obtained from experimental data on three subhuman primate species and scaled to man. Note that the head accelerating device (HAD-II) acceleration level was deliberately chosen to be well above that required. The scaling relationship is based on an inverse proportionate relationship to brain mass that was theoretically derived.

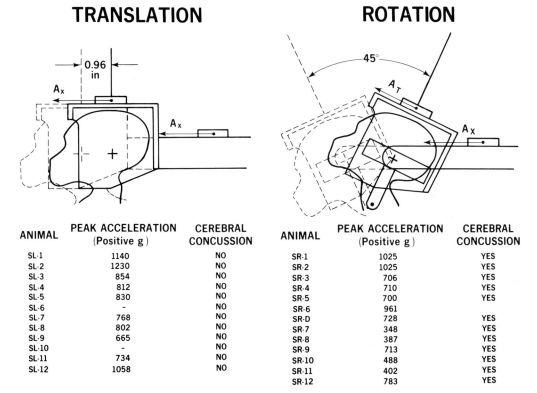

ANIMAL	PEAK ACCELERATION (Positive g)	CEREBRAL CONCUSSION
SL-1	1140	NO
SL-2	1230	NO
SL-3	854	NO
SL-4	812	NO
SL-5	830	NO
SL-6	-	NO
SL-7	768	NO
SL-8	802	NO
SL-9	665	NO
SL-10	-	NO
SL-11	734	NO
SL-12	1058	NO

ANIMAL	PEAK ACCELERATION (Positive g)	CEREBRAL CONCUSSION
SR-1	1025	YES
SR-2	1025	YES
SR-3	706	YES
SR-4	710	YES
SR-5	700	YES
SR-6	961	
SR-D	728	YES
SR-7	348	YES
SR-8	387	YES
SR-9	713	YES
SR-10	488	YES
SR-11	402	YES
SR-12	783	YES

Figure 56–8 Summary of data relating input accelerations in rotation and in pure translation to the genesis of cerebral concussion. Note inability to produce traumatic unconsciousness in the translated animals with accelerations up to 1230 g.

associated with concussion, the surface lesions that were produced in translated animals (in which concussion could not be produced) were consistently found to be focal small patches of subdural and subarachnoid hemorrhage. No petechial hemorrhages were seen in cross section, but in two animals significant intracerebral hemorrhagic cavities restricted to an asymetrical focal pattern in the occipital lobe were noted. Figure 56–9 is a line diagram summarizing the distribution of the lesions in two groups. Note the subdural, subarachnoid, and petechial hemorrhages. The latter lesions are notable for their symmetry and bilaterality and also for their tendency to occur at the junction between white and

gray matter. Note also the more focal, patchy nature of the lesions produced when the head is accelerated in pure translation without rotation. Figure 56–10 is a photomicrograph of the type of petechial hemorrage that is produced in the rotated animals. It should be emphasized that it was very difficult to produce such hemorrhages in the brain stem and impossible to do so without associated diffuse surface lesions. It is possible to produce brain stem hemorrhages only with high levels of rotational loading and only in very severe head injuries from which the animal subsequently dies without regaining consciousness as a direct result of the rotational injury. In other words, it was not possible to obtain

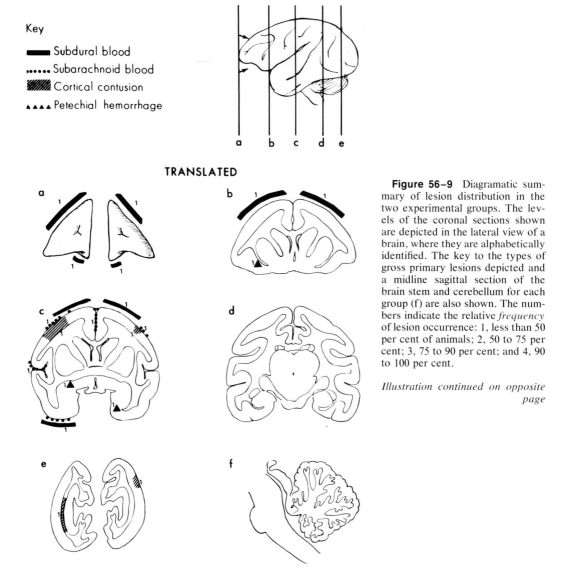

Figure 56–9 Diagramatic summary of lesion distribution in the two experimental groups. The levels of the coronal sections shown are depicted in the lateral view of a brain, where they are alphabetically identified. The key to the types of gross primary lesions depicted and a midline sagittal section of the brain stem and cerebellum for each group (f) are also shown. The numbers indicate the relative *frequency* of lesion occurrence: 1, less than 50 per cent of animals; 2, 50 to 75 per cent; 3, 75 to 90 per cent; and 4, 90 to 100 per cent.

Illustration continued on opposite page

primary brain stem hemorrhages with the animal surviving or without associated diffuse, very severe bilateral lesions, including bilateral subdural and subarachnoid hemorrhage.

Experimentally, therefore, in terms of the distribution of the lesions, the basic hypothesis could not be refuted. It is important, however, to examine the focal lesions of pure translation. Their location and nature strongly suggest the role of an additional mechanism for focal brain injury, i.e., the mechanism of cavitation. Such focal contusions may be quite small at the surface and involve only the cortex or extend into a large interior cavity (Fig. 56–11). It appears that a cavitation-induced effect, most probably by formation of cavi-

tation bubbles in the blood or cerebrospinal fluid rather than primarily in the brain, could be the mechanism responsible for such lesions in animals. Recent experiments by Lubock and Goldsmith in a physical model would support this hypothesis.[10] Cavitation is explicable in terms of linear acceleration that results in areas of negative pressure. These areas can be quite localized and cause rarefactive strains that cause the focal lesions. Whether this type of injury mechanism was operative in the author's experiments is difficult to prove, but in two animals the focal destructive intracerebral and cortical lesions were certainly suggestive. Theory would also suggest, however, that "cavitation" lesions would be related to implosive bubble-in-

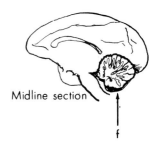

Midline section

f

ROTATED

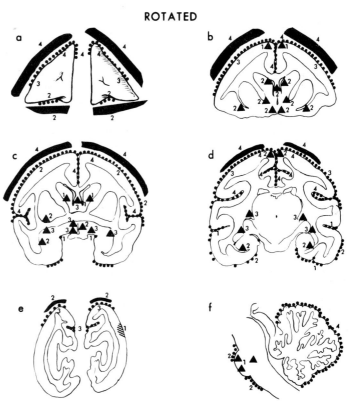

Figure 56–9 (*continued*) Note the bilateral symmetry and greater severity of all lesions except intracerebral hemorrhages in the rotated group as compared with the scanty, asymmetrical lesion distribution in the translated group. This figure should be studied in conjunction with Figure 56–8.

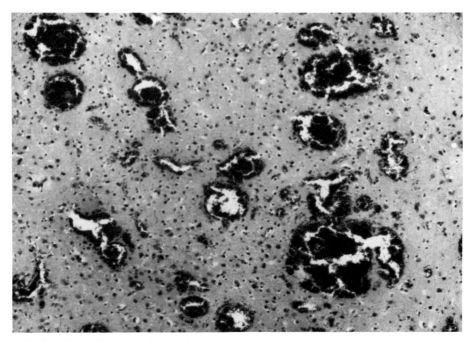

Figure 56–10 Photomicrograph of petechial hemorrhages that were noted only in the concussed brains of rotated animals. Note that these lesions were distributed symmetrically and bilaterally as shown in Figure 56–9.

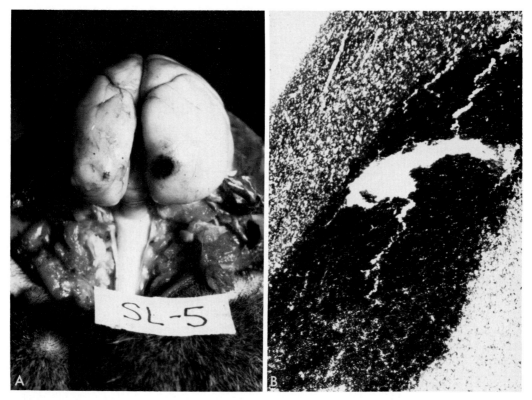

Figure 56–11 An occipital lobe hemorrhagic cavity found in one translated animal. *A.* Such focal contusions may be quite small at the surface. *B.* Cross section through the cavity. This unique lesion suggests a cavitation mechanism, as discussed in the text.

duced strains in blood and cerebrospinal fluid primarily rather than in the gel-like structure of the brain per se.[14] Therefore, it is possible that some of the focal contusions in head injuries are caused by cavitation.

Physiological and Neuropsychological Indices

The relatively slow event-related potentials or sensory evoked potentials have provided a useful tool for measuring the conduction and processing of stimuli through the nervous system after trauma.[16,18] In an animal model it was possible to analyze somatosensory potentials that sampled activity in both the specific and nonspecific input systems. It is established that the specific, or lemniscal, relay is an oligosynaptic pathway destined primarily for the opposite cortex, whereas the nonspecific system is multisynaptic and more diffusely projected bilaterally. The stimulus was applied to the median nerve at the wrist, and extradural electrodes recorded the evoked potentials bilaterally over the somatosensory cortex (Fig. 56–12). Data were obtained before and at varying intervals after the controlled head injury loading was produced as described earlier in the animal model. Further observations were also made by using somatosensory as well as photic flash–in-duced visual evoked potentials in patients at varying intervals after closed head injuries. In animals that sustained a cerebral concussion, all components of the evoked potentials were obliterated; as the animal recovered consciousness the P-2 wave correlated well with the return of sensorimotor responsiveness in the animal's behavior (Figs. 56–13 and 56–14). It is important to note that this index of sensory signal processing and conduction through the brain stem appears to correlate precisely with the animal's first recovery of response to external stimuli (i.e., "coming out of coma"), but the shape and amplitude of the waveforms always retained some abnormality for a longer time. This delay in full restoration of the evoked potential signals was temporally correlated with the delay in full return to normal behavior of the concussed animal. In the nonconcussed translated animal to which equivalent accelerations were given, some distortion of the potential amplitude but no loss of signal was seen (Fig. 56–15).

Examination of the latency of arrival at the contralateral cortex of the P-2 component in the translated animal (no concussion) revealed essentially no change in latency. In the rotated animal, however, there was a marked increase in latency of this signal. This latency prolongation per-

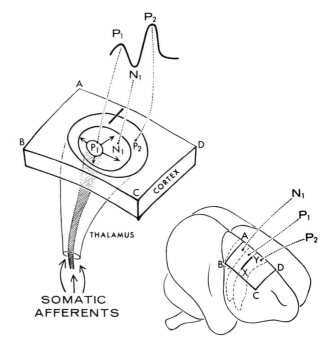

Figure 56–12 Diagram of the origin and spatial distribution of cortically recorded somatosensory evoked response in the squirrel monkey. ABCD, block of cortex; X = Y, central dimple; P_1, specific thalamocortical response; P_2 nonspecific thalamocortical response; N_1, corticocortical response.

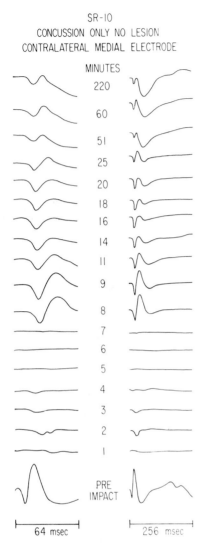

nels to the opposite cortex (Fig. 56–16). This electrophysiological evidence clearly supports the hypothesis that at the time of a paralytic concussion and inhibition of rostral brain stem function there is always an associated severe disturbance of subcortical and cortical mechanisms that is diffuse and bilateral and that should recover last after a concussive head injury. Examination of the visual evoked responses in head injury patients provides further insight. In Figure 56–17, data from a case of cortical blindness after cerebral concussion are shown. Note that as vision recovers from blindness to light perception and through finger counting to normal vision, concomitantly there is a restoration of the visual evoked potentials, and the simultaneously recorded electroretinogram also recovers in

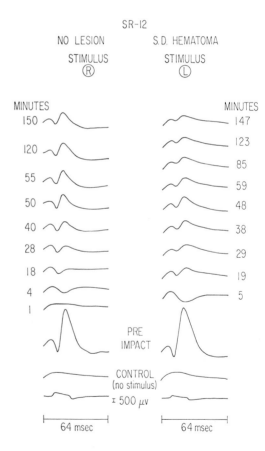

Figure 56–13 Serial display of the somatosensory evoked response to median nerve stimulation in a rotated animal. Note the preimpact components, all of which are obliterated at impact. This animal remained unconscious for seven minutes, and the return of the second positive wave (P-2, representing conduction in the nonspecific pathways) coincided precisely with the arousal of the animal from unresponsive coma. The animal remained somnolent for more than six hours after impact, and at 220 minutes the somatosensory evoked response component had not yet returned to normal. The response display in this and in Figures 56–14 and 56–15 is shown in two time scales, with the longer duration display on the right.

Figure 56–14 Bilateral somatosensory evoked response in a concussed monkey that subsequently developed a subdural hematoma unilaterally. The response is absent for the four minutes of unconsciousness and then progressively recovers in the left hemisphere (left traces with contralateral (R) stimulus). On the right, recovery ceases at 48 minutes and subsequently the response is diminished over the hematoma.

sisted much beyond the time at which the P-2 waveform itself had been restored to normal. In other words, neural processing and conduction through the brain stem reticular formation was restored well before transmission and integration of the signal through the cortex via corticocortical chan-

SL-II
NO CONCUSSION NO LESION
RIGHT MEDIAN NERVE STIMULATION
LEFT LATERAL ELECTRODE

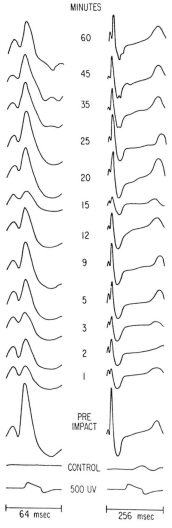

Figure 56–15 The somatosensory evoked response in a translated animal. Note that in comparison with Figure 56–13, only decreases in amplitude with no loss of the signal components are seen. This animal, like all those in the translated group, showed no clinical impairment of the preimpact alert state of awareness.

a graded series. A most interesting aspect of the recovery process was that the best type of signal response was reliably evoked only at low frequencies (1 to 5 Hz) and that if the light flashes were given at a higher frequency a marked degradation of the response was noted and the patient could not produce a good following response until the recovery of full vision. In other words, recovery of the ability to process visual information in the nervous system at different rates and especially at the faster rates after cerebral concussion seemed to correlate with the ability of the patient to see normally. This recovery, which is gradual and correlated with symptomatic visual recovery, is most probably analogous to recovery of cognitive functions after minor, moderate, and severe head injuries. Such recovery data on cerebral concussion in the human separate from the epiphenomena are difficult to isolate and study. Clinical data available from studies of large series of head injuries such as those of Jennett and Overgaard and their associates are available and worthy of detailed examination from this aspect.[9,25] Those of Becker and his group are discussed in Chapter 60.

Assuming that the outcome of a head injury was determined to a critical extent by the primary damage, it would then be expected that the outcome could be predicted in the majority of cases from the initial clinical examination. If later events, i.e., the secondary phenomena, were more critical than the primary event in determining the outcome, then correlation of outcome with the initial clinical condition of the patient would be poor. Examination of the evidence suggests that in 75 to 80 per cent of cases, the outcome *is* predictable from the first examination, thus emphasizing the importance of the primary damage as a key determinant of the final outcome.[9,25]

The neuropsychological data of Gronwall and Wrightson are particularly relevant.[5] These workers studied two series of patients who had sustained grade II to IV concussions with no significant epiphenomena. One group had recovered except for the so-called post-traumatic or postconcussion syndrome. This syndrome is a puzzling and difficult condition to treat because it is seldom associated with objective clinical deficits. Yet, such patients suffer for prolonged periods of time and constitute difficult problems in management and a major source of economic loss. The second group consisted of patients who had suffered an approximately equivalent duration of loss of consciousness after head injury but without the subsequent difficulties in memory, inability to concentrate, dizziness, headaches, and other subjective complaints of the postconcussion syndrome. Both groups were given a simple test of serial addition of

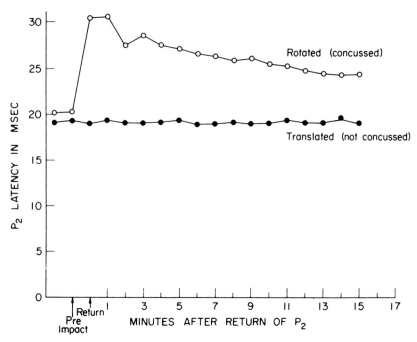

Figure 56–16 Latency of contralateral to ipsilateral conduction of P-2 wave (P_2) plotted as a function of time after impact for the two groups of animals. This reflects interhemispheric cortical functional integrity. The data clearly show the marked increase in per cent delay of P-2 conduction in the rotated group as compared with the unimpaired translated group. Moreover, this increased latency persists far longer than either the P-2 conduction deficit noted in Figure 56–4 or the duration of loss of consciousness. These data suggest that cortical injury is more significant than brain stem injury at this level of traumatic input and also that pure translation does not produce any significant diffuse effects at either brain stem or cortical levels at the levels of acceleration tested (up to 1230 g).

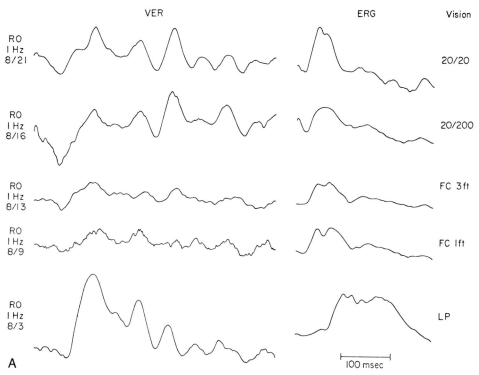

Figure 56–17 *A.* Serial visual evoked response (VER) and electroretinographic (ERG) recordings in a patient who incurred a brief cerebral concussion and transient cortical blindness. Both the electroretinogram and the visual evoked response are abnormal until visual recovery is complete. Dates are shown on the left, the injury having occurred on 8/3. By 8/21, the vision was 20/20 and the visual evoked and electroretinographic waveforms were restored.

Illustration continued on opposite page

two numbers with recall of the first number. This test was given at four rates ranging from slow to fast and thus provided a simple test for short-term memory as well as for evaluating the processing efficiency of the brain. Only those patients who had persistent symptoms of the post-traumatic syndrome had difficulty in doing the test at the faster rates. In other words, although capable of functioning in this cognitive test at the slow rate of information processing, patients in the first group began making mistakes as soon as the rates increased. The second group of patients who had no postconcussive symptoms performed as well as normal unconcussed subjects with no performance decrement at the increasing rates.[5]

These data are analogous to the electro-physiological evidence found with visual evoked potentials in the author's patients with postconcussive cortical blindness. As the visual system and related cortical function returned, the ability to follow signals at a higher frequency was also re-established. Thus it appears that one of the significant functional effects of the diffuse strains of cerebral concussion is difficulty in *rate* of information processing. It should be noted that symptoms very similar to the postconcussive syndrome also are found after certain so-called whiplash injuries. As explained earlier, these symptoms may also be due to the same mechanism.[20,29,30] Whether these effects are caused by membrane distortions in axons, synapses, neuronal soma, or porportions of all three, or whether the cognitive deficit is best un-

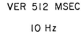

VER 512 MSEC

10 Hz

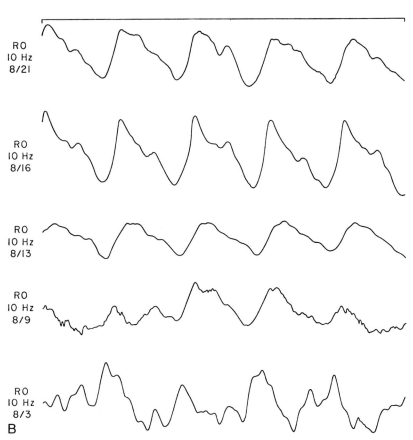

Figure 56-17 (*continued*)   *B*. Visual evoked response (VER) in the same patient in response to rapid (10 Hz) stimulus. Progressive restoration of amplitude and waveform correlates with restoration of visual acuity. These data support the concept that postconcussive syndrome symptoms are due to difficulty in processing neural information at higher rates.

derstood in terms of the organization of neural cell assemblies remains to be solved by experiments at both the cellular and the organismic level.[16,18] It should be stressed that future studies of what may be called the effects of "microtrauma" must be supplemented by neuropsychological data. These latter data are essential because the problem of post-traumatic amnesic and similar high-level cognitive disorders after head injury may well be due to disorganization at the level of neural cell assemblies rather than only at the cellular level. Because such correlations were found in patients who had made good recoveries from coma and had normal brain stem functions, it is reasonable to suggest that the cause was a persisting disconnection effect that was diffuse and primarily at the cortical level. These data also support the theory that in significant head injuries there is always persisting diffuse impairment at higher levels whenever brain stem function is temporarily lost at the time of cerebral concussion.

REFERENCES

1. Ambrose, J., Gooding, M. R., and Uttley, D.: EMI scan in the management of head injuries. Lancet, *1*:847–848, 1976.
2. Fisher, C. M.: Concussion amnesia. Neurology (Minneap.), *16*:826–830, 1966.
3. Goldsmith, W.: Biomechanics of head injury. M. Fung, Y. C., Perrone, N., and Anliker, M., eds.: Biomechanics, Its Foundations and Objectives. New York, Prentice-Hall, 1970.
4. Goldsmith, W.: Some aspects of head and neck injury and protection. *In* Nuri Akkas, ed.: Progress in Biomechanics. Leiden, Netherlands, Sijthoff & Noordhoff, 1979, pp. 33–377.
5. Gronwall, D., and Wrightson, P.: Delayed recovery of intellectual function after minor head injury. Lancet, *2*:605–609, 1974.
6. Hardman, J. M.: Pathology of traumatic brain injuries. Advances Neurol., *22*:15–50, 1979.
7. Hume-Adams, J.: The neuropathology of head injuries. *In* Vinken, P. J., and Bruyn, G. W., eds.: Handbook of Clinical Neurology. Vol. 23, Part I. 1975, pp. 35–36.
8. Jennett, B., and Plum, R., Persistent vegetative state after head injury. Lancet, *1*:734–737, 1972.
9. Jennett, B., Teasdale, G., Braakman, R., Minderhoud, J., and Knill-Jones, R.: Predicting outcome in individual patients after severe head injury. Lancet, *1*:1031–1034, 1976.
10. Lubock, G., and Goldsmith, W.: Cavitation in a head injury model. J. Biomech., in press.
11. Mitchell, D. E., and Hume-Adams, J.: Primary focal impact damage to the brain stem in blunt head injuries. Does it exist? Lancet, *1*:215–218, 1973.
12. Nelson, L. R., Bourke, R. S., Popp, A. J., Cragoe, E. J., Signorelli, A., Foster, V. V., and Creel, W.: Evaluation of treatment modalities in severe head injuries using an animal model. In Popp, J. A., ed.: Neural Trauma. New York, Raven Press, 1979, pp. 297–311.
13. Ommaya, A. K.: Trauma to the nervous system. A clinical and experimental study. (Hunterian Lecture.) Ann. Roy. Coll. Surg. Eng., *39*:317–347, 1966.
14. Ommaya, A. K.: The mechanical properties of tissues of the nervous system. J. Biomech., *2*:1–12, 1968.
15. Ommaya, A. K.: Computerized axial tomography: The EMI scanner, a new device for direct examination of the brain "in-vivo." Surg. Neurol., *1*:217–222, 1973.
16. Ommaya, A. K.: A physiopathologic basis for non-invasive diagnosis and prognosis of head injury severity. *In* McLaurin, R., ed.: Head Injury. New York, Grune & Stratton, Inc., 1976.
17. Ommaya, A. K.: Reintegrative action of the nervous system after trauma. *In* Popp, A. J., et al., eds.: Neural Trauma. New York, Raven Press, 1979.
18. Ommaya, A. K., and Genarelli, T.: Cerebral concussion and traumatic unconsciousness. Brain, *97*:633–654, 1974.
19. Ommaya, A. K., and Hirsch, A. E.: Tolerances of cerebral concussion from head impact and whiplash in primates. J. Biomech., *4*:13–22, 1971.
20. Ommaya, A. K., and Yarnell, P. R.: Subdural haematoma after whiplash injury. Lancet, *2*:237–239, 1969.
21. Ommaya, R. K., Faas, F., and Yarnell, P. R.: Whiplash injury and brain damage: An experimental study. J.A.M.A., *204*:285–289, 1968.
22. Ommaya, A. K., Hirsch, A. E., Flamm, E. S., and Mahone, R. M.: Cerebral concussion in the monkey: An experimental model. Science, *153*:211–212, 1966.
23. Ommaya, A. K., Murray, G., Ambrose, J., Richardson, A., and Hounsfield, G.: Computerized axial tomography: Estimation of spatial and density resolution capacity. Brit. J. Radiol., *49*:604–611, 1976.
24. Oppenheimer, D. R.: Microscopic lesions in the brain following head injury. J. Neurol. Neurosurg. Psychiat., *31*:299–306, 1968.
25. Overgaard, J., Christiansen, S., Haase, J., Hein, O., Hvid-Hansen, O., Land, A. M., Pedersen, K. K., and Tweed, W. A.: Prognosis after head injury based on early clinical examination. Lancet, *2*:631–635, 1973.
26. Reilly, P. L., Graham, D. I., Hume-Adams, J., and Jennett, B.: Patients with head injury who talk and die. Lancet, *2*:375–381, 1975.
26a. Russell, W. R., and Schiller, F.: crushing injuries of the skull: Clinical and experimental observations. J. Neurol. Neurosurg. Psychiat., *12*:52–60, 1949.
27. Symonds, C. P.: Concussion and its sequelae. Lancet, *1*:5, 1962.
28. Thilbault, L. E., Genarelli, T. A., and Ommaya, A. K.: Effect of dynamic mechanical loading on frog sciatic nerve. Proceedings: Society for Neuroscience, Oct. 1974. Unpublished data.

29. Torres, F., and Shapiro, S. K.: Electroencephalograms in whiplash injury. A comparison of electroencephalographic abnormalities with those present in closed head injury. Arch. Neurol. (Chicago), 5:28–35, 1961.

30. Unterharnschiedt, F., and Higgins, L. S.: Neuropathologic effects of translational and rotational acceleration of the head in animal experiments. *In* Walker, A. E., Caveness, W. F., and Critchley, MacD., eds.: The Late Effects of Head Injury. Springfield, Ill., Charles C Thomas, 1969, pp. 158–167.

31. Ward, A. A.: The physiology of concussion. Clin. Neurosurg., *12*:95–111, 1966.

32. Zimmerman, R., and Bilaniuk, L.: Computed tomography in diffuse traumatic cerebral injury. *In* Popp, A. J., et al., eds.: Neural Trauma. New York, Raven Press, 1979.

57

GENERAL
PRINCIPLES AND
PATHOPHYSIOLOGY
OF HEAD INJURY

Many factors interact to determine the disability caused by a head injury. After the primary injury many secondary processes, both cerebral and systemic, take place that can serve either to ameliorate or, more often, to worsen the initial effects of impact to the head.

These secondary processes are of particular importance to the neurosurgeon for two main reasons: unlike the primary damage, they often occur while the patient is under neurosurgical care, and they may be influenced for good or ill by the form of management that is chosen. Research in this area is extending the understanding of many of the secondary mechanisms that impair brain function.[196,210,239] As a result the phenomena that affect the brain after injury can be assembled in a logical order to indicate the cause and effect relationships and interactions that occur.[24,52,69,185]

In formulating therapeutic approaches to patients with head injury, it is important to emphasize the role of the *secondary insult* in adversely modifying the clinical course. In Chapters 58 and 59 emphasis is placed on avoidance of the secondary insult by early diagnosis of mass lesions and the use of surgical and medical measures; in this chapter the ways in which secondary injury from intracranial hypertension, brain shift, cerebral ischemia and hypoxia, and other insults produces ill effects on brain function are described. Before these adverse effects can be understood, the primary effects of trauma on the brain and related structures

have to be considered, since in many cases they set in motion mechanisms that produce secondary insults. In addition, the preinjury status of the patient must be considered, since it will affect the results of the trauma.

PREINJURY STATUS

Many pre-existing factors serve to modify subsequent events (Table 57–1). Clearly, variations in the thickness of the scalp and skull and in the shape of the head modify the forces transmitted to the contents from an external impact.[75] The thinness and degree of adhesion of the dura to the skull, greater in the elderly, will modify the readiness with which the dura tears in relation to an overlying skull fracture. In turn these tears affect the frequency with which the patient is exposed to the risk of meningitis after injury. These factors also influence the incidence and the extent of epidural hematoma formation after a blow to the head. That epidural hematoma without skull fracture is a phenomenon confined largely to children and young adults probably is because of the flexibility of the skull and the readiness with which the dura strips off the bone.[63]

The type and incidence of transtentorial herniation depends on the location and size of expanding intracranial lesions and on the configuration of the tentorium cerebelli and the size of the tentorial notch, both of

---

J. D. MILLER AND D. P. BECKER

TABLE 57-1 PRE-EXISTENT FACTORS THAT MODIFY THE EFFECTS OF HEAD INJURY

FACTOR	COMMENT
Scalp	
Thickness	Dissipation of force
Mobility	Concealment of underlying fracture
Skull	
Shape, thickness, pliability (age)	Determinants of fracture type, location, and extent
Dura	
Thickness, adhesion to skull	Tendency to tear with fracture and to strip off the skull (epidural hematoma)
Tentorial hiatus	
Size, shape	Extent of tentorial herniation and related signs
Brain	
Volumes of tissue, blood, cerebrospinal fluid	Relationship of mass, brain shift, and intracranial pressure
Neurons	
Degenerative disease, previous injury	Extent of intellectual and psychosocial recovery after injury

which have considerable variation.[38,110,240] Also the relationship between the size and rate of expansion of an intracranial mass lesion and intracranial pressure and brain shift is modified by pre-existing brain atrophy. Thus a patient with advanced brain atrophy may harbor a large epidural or subdural hematoma with no clinical neurological manifestation.

The level of function before the injury clearly sets the limits of recovery of mental and somatic neurological function. In addition, in patients with pre-existing mild dementia or those who have made an apparently good recovery from previous head trauma or stroke, even a mild head injury may produce devastating disability. This factor can assume immense importance in medicolegal judgments. The cumulative effect of repeated minor head injury is seen most obviously in the traumatic encephalopathy ("punch-drunk" syndrome) of boxers but may also be a problem in participants in other sports that engender blows to the head.[209,221]

PRIMARY DAMAGE TO THE BRAIN IN HEAD INJURY

One of the main factors that have hindered understanding of the pathophysiology of brain trauma has been the difficulty of discriminating between primary brain damage (the pathological processes that arise as an immediate, direct result of trauma), and secondary lesions that are due to raised intracranial pressure, brain shift, post-traumatic biochemical processes, cerebral ischemia, and hypoxia. In this section, the cellular basis of primary brain damage is considered first; the concept of primary brain stem injury is examined critically and then contrasted with the concept of diffuse brain injury; and finally, polar and severe penetrating injuries of the brain are described.

The Cellular Basis of Brain Injury

This is a rather elusive entity, for taken alone, none of the changes are caused exclusively by injury. Furthermore, some of these changes are essentially reactive in nature. Damage to axons in the brain as elsewhere in the nervous system produces two sets of changes. In the cell body there are swelling, dissolution of the Nissl bodies, and displacement of the nucleus to the periphery of the cell. This process of chromatolysis, which can be identified soon after injury, may be followed by complete dissolution of the cell, or if the damage is less it may be arrested, then reversed over a period of months.

A modern concept of "chromatolysis" is that it represents evidence of increased cellular metabolism working toward repair of cell damage.[49] The fact that cells in the central nervous system may undergo these histological alterations and then go on to recover or die suggests that after injury many cells may be in a precarious and marginal state. If the internal environment remains ideal for recovery of partially damaged cells, more may go on to recover and fewer may die. This is not to suggest that complete axonal disruption in the central nervous system will go on to regeneration.

Rather, cells with their subcellular components may be damaged but not disrupted. If disruption does occur in the distal part of the axon, wallerian degeneration takes place, with absorption of the axon cylinder, breakdown of the myelin sheath, and phagocytosis of fatty droplets. Histopathological evidence of these processes can be seen in several different ways, depending on the time that has elapsed from the original injury. An early sign of axonal damage is the appearance of retraction balls, formed from axoplasm extruded from torn axons. If special stains are used, axon discontinuity may be identifiable. Within a few days reactive changes are taking place—reactive astrocytes, hypertrophied microglial cells, form microglial stars around small tissue tears.[199] Later changes include demyelination and gliosis, as described later.

The effects of injury on glial cells are not known with certainty, nor are the effects of glial injury on surrounding neurons. In virtually all accounts of the neuropathology of head injury, glial changes are viewed uniformly as reactive in response to neuronal (axon) or vascular damage.[2] The earliest effect of both ischemic and cold injury of the brain appears to be glial swelling, which has been detected both microscopically and by inference from intracellular membrane potential studies.[72,73] Grossman and Seregin have postulated that the glial swelling following trauma may reflect uptake of potassium or even of neurotransmitters released from damaged neurons into the extracellular space.[73]

The most obvious effect of trauma on cerebral blood vessels is disruption, producing visible or microscopic hemorrhages. A question remains, however, concerning the effects of lesser degrees of trauma. Local injury to the exposed cortical surface can, without altering resting blood flow, alter the response of these vessels to changes in arterial blood pressure so that flow becomes pressure passive.[19,217] After autoregulation has been lost in this way, arterial hypertension produces brain swelling, extracellular edema, and extravasation of Evans blue into the damaged area.[163,225] Presumably this type of response to injury also occurs at the poles of the brain and in the track of a penetrating injury. It is not yet clear what happens within the brain subjected to blunt injury of the type that produces temporary concussion in the human.

In a model of temporary concussion in the mouse, a significant increase in the penetration of intravascular radioactive tracer into brain has been found in the 24 hours after injury.[34] In the cat and monkey subjected to blunt trauma, specific areas of blood-brain barrier breakdown have been identified by using fluorescein as a tracer, but questions still exist about the duration after injury of such "leakiness," the precise route by which the tracers leave the vascular system, and its clinical relevance.[198,220]

Since the demonstration of the tight junction between cerebral capillary endothelial cells, theories of causation of blood-brain barrier breakdown and brain edema have focused on mechanisms that open the tight junction. Such barrier opening can be demonstrated in vessels around brain tumors, after intracarotid administration of hyperosmotic substances, with arterial hypertension and capillary distention, and after cold injury to the cerebral cortex.[17,122-124]

In a fluid percussion model of head injury in the cat and light microscopy and ultrastructural studies with horseradish peroxidase as a tracer, Povlishock and associates have shown that at injury levels above 2 atmospheres (1500 mm of mercury) considerable vascular leakage occurred in the midline of the brain stem from arterioles and capillaries and veins (Fig. 57–1A and B).[210,239] Opening of the tight junction in capillary endothelium was not observed, however, and the transport of horseradish peroxidase from the vascular system was vesicular in the form of pinocytotic vesicles that deposited the reaction product on the basal lamina, from where it migrated freely in the extracellular space and into pericytes and glial cells. This process was seen within five minutes of injury and appeared to be diminished after two hours from injury. A similar increase in micropinocytosis has recently been demonstrated in the brains of rats after experimental seizures.[204] It is important to point out, however, that no evidence of cerebral edema has been seen in these areas of blood-brain barrier alteration. Similarly, Rapaport and his colleagues did not observe brain edema after induction of reversible opening of the blood-brain barrier in the Rhesus monkey.[215] Thus vascular leakage should not be thought of solely as a potential source of brain edema.

A further interesting finding in Povlishock's study was that both at lower levels of brain injury than those associated with leakage of intravascular tracer and at comparable levels of injury force, distinct ultrastructural changes were seen in nerve terminals where synaptic vesicles formed paracrystalline arrays (Fig. 57–1C). In another study it was found that there is a greater uptake of tritiated norepinephrine into synaptosomes isolated from the rat brain shortly after blunt head trauma than in synaptosomes obtained from the brains of control animals.[6] It is tempting to make a speculative link between these two findings, and they are mentioned here to indicate some of the directions that must be taken to explain neurological dysfunction after head injury at the cellular level. The hypothesis developed from this work is that transient coma and other temporary neurological dysfunction after head injury may be due to malfunction of the neurotransmitter system, or at least to reversible biochemical dysfunction in the neuron.

Brain Stem Injury

In experimental studies on head injury dating from the 1940's, considerable emphasis was laid on the occurrence of cellular changes in the brain stem affecting larger interneurons and cell groups such as the nucleus giganto-cellularis.[71,77] These observations were made at a time when the importance of the brain stem reticular activating system in the regulation of consciousness was being established.[190] It was proposed also that concussion or transient loss of consciousness must be due to a reversible disturbance of these same central gray areas. Therefore, marked clinical emphasis was placed on the importance of brain stem lesions in patients with head injury as an explanation for prolonged unconsciousness and decerebrate rigidity, particularly in cases in which there was no complicating intracranial mass lesion. Thus, the term "brain stem injury" evolved, with the implication that primary damage elsewhere in the brain is less important. This view of the neuropathology of head injury is still current in recent articles.[26,39,249]

The problem with this viewpoint is that the crucial support from neuropathological studies is lacking. It is true that in patients who have been unconscious for considerable periods after injury, pathological changes are found in the brain stem: retraction balls, microglial stars, ischemic areas, and microhemorrhages.[40] It has been proposed that these small infarcts and microhemorrhages in the brain stem constitute primary brain damage.[39,249] Since tissue can be examined only after the death of the patient, however, it may be hard to distinguish brain stem hemorrhage as a manifestation of primary damage from the secondary brain stem hemorrhage that is related to brain shift.[111,112] In a small number of cases of fatal head injury that were carefully screened to exclude any with evidence of secondary brain compression, such primary brain stem hemorrhages were not found by Adams and Graham.[2]

While it is not in dispute that pathological changes do occur in the brain stem in patients who sustain severe head injuries, what is in doubt is whether such structural lesions ever occur exclusively in the brain stem without evidence of primary damage elsewhere in the brain. If only the brain stem is examined in detail this question cannot be settled. The strongest position on this topic to date has been taken by Mitchell and Adams, who did a meticulous survey of the entire brain of patients who died after head injury and in whom raised intracranial pressure and brain shift were not factors. They state: "The principal reason for the difficulty in defining localized brain stem damage due to a blunt head injury is that it does not exist as a pathological entity. What clinicians refer to as the syndrome of primary brain stem damage is more accurately defined as the clinical manifestations of brain stem dysfunction occurring soon after."[186] Dysfunction may represent deafferentation rather than damage, because all brains in which brain stem lesions were seen also showed widespread evidence of damage in the cerebral hemispheres. These findings have recently been confirmed by Adams and his colleagues in their study of an expanded series of 152 fatal head injuries.[5]

Thus, the hypotheses developed from animal models, which proposed that the primary effects of blunt head injury were localized to the brain stem and were in turn exclusively responsible for the loss of consciousness, have not been substantiated by careful examinations of autopsy material. The more comprehensive and detailed the examination made of the brain, the more extensive the lesions that have been identi-

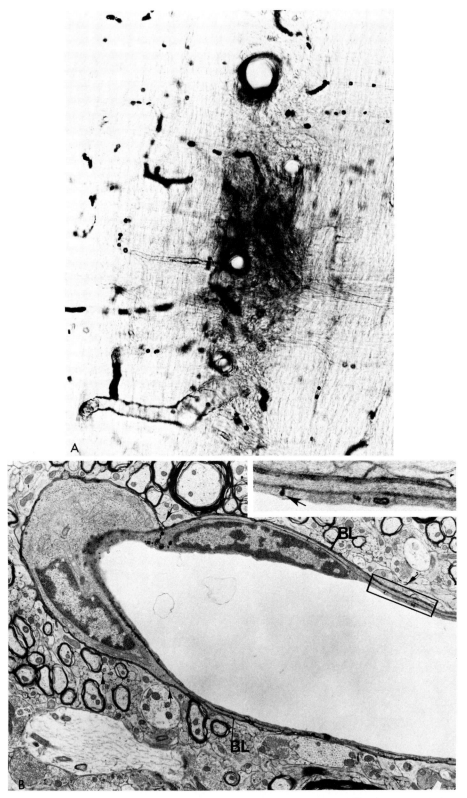

Figure 57–1 *A*. In this light micrograph the peroxidase reaction product is readily visualized within both the vessels and the parenchyma of the medullary raphe region. 200×. *B*. This vessel displays numerous peroxidase-containing endothelial vesicles and pits. The perivascular basal lamina (BL) is flooded with the peroxidase reaction product, and the peroxidase within the basal lamina is continuous with that found in the parenchymal extracellular space (*arrows*). The inset is an enlargement of the blocked out endothelial segment. In the inset note that the peroxidase in one pit (*arrow*) is directly confluent with that in the underlying basal lamina. 12,000×: inset, 30,000×.

1900

Illustration continued on opposite page

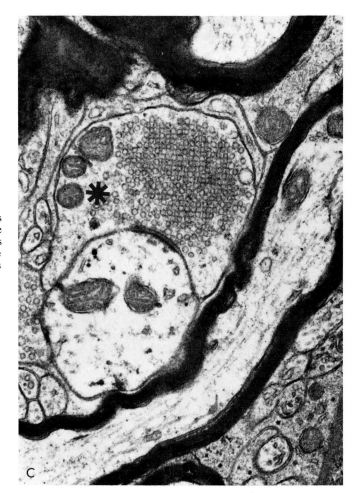

Figure 57–1 (*continued*) *C.* This electron micrograph displays a nerve terminal* containing clumped vesicles that form a linear, paracrystalline array. 51,000×. (Electron micrographs by courtesy of Dr. John Povlishock.)

fied.[1] It does remain entirely possible, however, that functional disturbances occur in the brain stem following blunt head trauma that are not associated with pathological damage and that may relate to temporary loss of consciousness. The leakage of intravascular tracer restricted to the midline of the brain stem, which has already been alluded to, may be an example of such a functional disturbance.

Diffuse Brain Injury

It is well established that considerable movement of the entire brain takes place within, and relative to, the cranium after impact to the head.[211] Corresponding with such tissue movements, it has been proposed, widespread tearing of axons and myelin sheaths in the white matter of the cerebral hemispheres occurs.[95] This diffuse brain damage is thought to be responsible for the prolonged unconsciousness in those patients with severe head injury uncomplicated by the formation of intracranial mass lesions.[47,243] The brains of such patients may look normal macroscopically. If survival after injury is longer than two months, widespread degeneration of white matter tracts can be demonstrated by stains that are specific for myelin breakdown products, e.g., Marchi technique. Demyelination is more evident in the brain stem, but this may merely reflect the convergence of many degenerating fibers in the long tracts. In patients dying earlier, microscopically visible damage is limited to retraction balls and microglial stars spread diffusely in white matter and in the brain.[194,203,233–236]

Inability to define clearly the extent and severity of diffuse brain injury in patients who die before sufficient time has elapsed for demyelination to act as a "tracer" presents major problems in following the pathophysiology of head injury. Techniques that stain selectively for degenerating axons can, however, be used to show the location of brain damage at an earlier stage after head injury (Fig. 57–2).[58,192]

It can therefore be proposed that retraction balls, neuronophagia and microglial stars, and axonal degeneration and demyelination form elements in a temporal continuum of reaction to primary impact damage to the brain, and that such changes are also widely spread throughout the brain. Ommaya and Gennarelli have proposed that in blunt head injury, neuronal damage occurs from the cortex inward toward the brain stem as the injuring force increases.[196,197] The corollary of this hypothesis is that

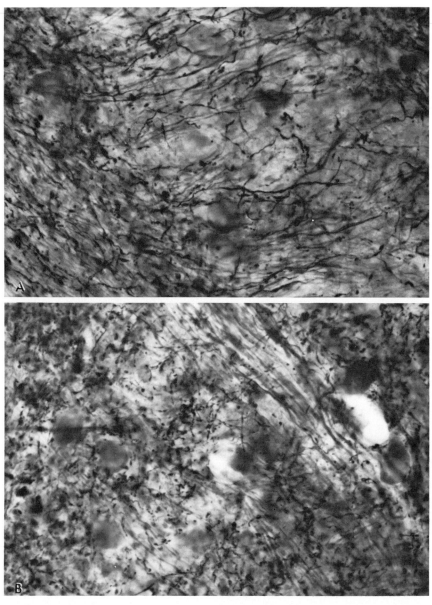

Figure 57–2 *A*. Nauta preparation showing axonal degeneration in the region of the inferior olive in a patient who remained decerebrate and died three weeks after injury with normal intracranial pressure and no mass lesions. The distribution of damaged fibers indicates that the responsible lesion is not local in the brain stem but located at a higher, e.g., cortical or subcortical, level. *B*. Section taken at the nucleus gigantocellularis in the same patient. (Photomicrographs by courtesy of Dr. Juan Astruc.)

structural brain stem damage can *never* occur without damage to the cerebral hemispheres. The pathological studies of Strich, Oppenheimer, and Adams would all support this view.[199,236] As is described in the following chapter, neurophysiological studies during life in patients with head injury also demonstrate that diffuse hemispheric damage rather than brain stem damage is the best correlate with decerebrate rigidity and with prolonged coma.[70]

Polar and Focal Brain Injury

Although this form of damage is the most obvious to the pathologist at autopsy, it has more importance for the sequelae of head injury than as a determinant of the immediate effects of impact. Consequent on the brain's mobility within the cranium, its poles sustain the greatest deformation. Holbourn has postulated that the poles are particularly stressed during rotational injuries, and that shearing forces especially at the frontal and temporal tips cause most of the damage (Fig. 57–3).[95] The more popular view is that the brain's poles forcibly impinge on the interior of the skull with sudden deceleration or acceleration; the frontal poles against the anterior fossa, the temporal tips against the sphenoid bones, and less commonly, the occipital poles against the smoother internal surface of the occipital bone. Since most forces applied to the head contain a lateral rotational element, there is usually more damage on one side than on the other, but it is common to have damage on both sides of the brain. This bilateral damage is an important factor in the determination of outcome.[241] Demonstration of midline brain shift may only be an indication of which is the more severely damaged side.

The resulting injuries of the brain are similar to those that occur underneath a severe and localized impact to the skull, namely surface contusion and laceration of the brain. It is the location of the damage that characterizes polar lesions. In brain contusion there is subpial extravasation of blood and swelling of the affected area; if the lesion is severe much of the damaged area may be necrotic, soft, and hemorrhagic. When the pia mater is torn, cerebral laceration is present by definition, but the borderline between contusion and laceration may not be very clear. When laceration is severe at the temporal lobe tip and when subdural and intracerebral hemorrhage occurs and merges with brain swelling, the descriptive term "burst temporal lobe" is a useful one.

Contusion and laceration of the brain both produce appropriate signs of neurological dysfunction when located in eloquent areas of the brain, e.g., the motor area, and are important in the differential diagnosis of hemiparesis after head injury (versus intracranial hematoma). There are not any immediate specific neurological signs to indicate the more common lesions of the frontal or temporal tips, and old scars in these areas may be seen as incidental findings at autopsy in patients who made excellent recoveries from head injuries years earlier and had no focal neurological signs. The clinical importance of polar lesions in the immediate or early postinjury period derives from their propensity to swell or to bleed, or both, and thereby to act as intracranial expanding lesions potentially responsible for secondary brain dysfunction. This process, which is at its peak in the first three days after injury, is discussed in more detail in the following section.

Severe Intracerebral Injury

Penetrating injuries of the head produce deep lacerations of the brain that may communicate with the ventricular system. The neurological deficit resulting from such injuries depends entirely on the site if they are of very low velocity, e.g., stab wound, since brain damage is limited to the track of entry, and consciousness is normally retained. In such cases the main concern is for complicating intracerebral hemorrhage or infection. In higher-velocity wounds brain damage is much more extensive because of three factors. The inward carriage of multiple bone fragments at the site of entry may produce more widespread brain damage. The missile may spin irregularly after smashing through the skull and cut a wide swathe of brain damage, then ricochet off the opposite inner table, causing still more brain laceration and contusion. Finally, ultra-high-velocity missiles (rifle bullets), even in passing cleanly through the head, will produce an enormous amount of brain disruption due to shock waves ex-

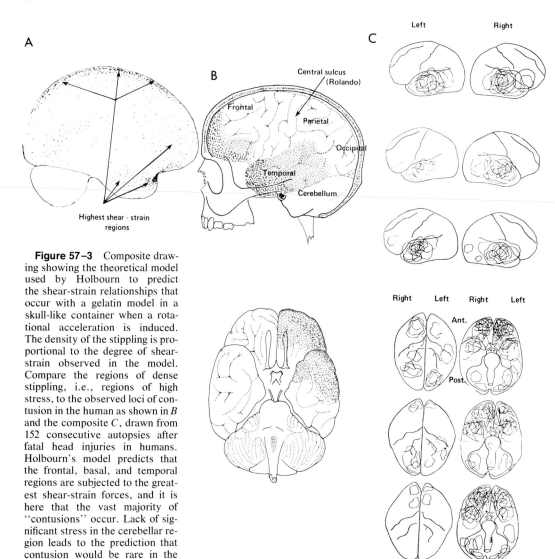

Figure 57-3 Composite drawing showing the theoretical model used by Holbourn to predict the shear-strain relationships that occur with a gelatin model in a skull-like container when a rotational acceleration is induced. The density of the stippling is proportional to the degree of shear-strain observed in the model. Compare the regions of dense stippling, i.e., regions of high stress, to the observed loci of contusion in the human as shown in B and the composite C, drawn from 152 consecutive autopsies after fatal head injuries in humans. Holbourn's model predicts that the frontal, basal, and temporal regions are subjected to the greatest shear-strain forces, and it is here that the vast majority of "contusions" occur. Lack of significant stress in the cerebellar region leads to the prediction that contusion would be rare in the posterior fossa, which in fact is true. This is somewhat modified by the frequent occurrence of microscopic hemorrhage at the medullary spinal junction due to the concentration of stress in this region (Holbourn did not address this aspect of injury in his original work). Holbourn also predicted a narrow band of severe strain along the superior margin of the hemisphere, which correlates well with the frequently observed avulsion of cortical-sinus anastomotic veins. (From Holbourn, A. H. S.: The mechanics of brain injuries. Brit. Med. Bull., *3*:147–149, 1945, and Gurdjian, E. S.: Recent advances in the study of impact injury of the head. Clin. Neurosurg., *19*:1–42, 1972. Reprinted by permission.)

tending laterally from the missile track. In such cases brain damage is so extensive that consciousness is usually lost. Death is usually due, however, to the swelling and hemorrhage that ensue.

PRIMARY DAMAGE TO RELATED STRUCTURES

Scalp

Although this subject is covered in more detail in another chapter, scalp injuries are

worthy of mention here because of their importance as a potential source of secondary insult to the brain after head injury. The position was stated clearly during the First World War by Cushing: ". . . though many scalp wounds which appear serious prove to be trifling, more which appear trifling prove to be serious."[42] What Cushing was referring to was the danger of overlooking the possibility that a small scalp wound may be the only external manifestation of a penetrating brain wound via fractured skull and torn dura. Failure to recognize this and to provide proper exploration, debridement, and closure of the wound can lead to infection (meningitis, brain abscess) or to overlooking a developing intracerebral hematoma. This situation is as true today as it was in Cushing's day, and one of the principal reasons for failure to treat scalp wounds with the respect they deserve is that in cases of low-velocity penetrating injury of the head the damage to the brain may be so localized and involve so little acceleration and deceleration of the whole head that many patients have never or have only briefly been unconscious.[107,177] The conclusion that follows from this is that all patients with a scalp laceration ought to have an x-ray of the skull, whether or not they have been or are unconscious.

Scalp contusion may be a valuable clue to the side of the skull fracture seen only on lateral skull x-rays. If neurological deterioration is proceeding so rapidly as to preclude the performance of localizing studies (e.g., computed tomography or angiography), this clue may be lifesaving in determining which side to explore first. Bruising of the periorbital areas (raccoon eyes) or behind the ears (Battle's sign) is an indication of basal skull fracture in the anterior or middle fossa, respectively. Its appearance should alert the neurosurgeon to look for cerebrospinal fluid rhinorrhea or otorrhea, to do brow-up lateral skull x-rays looking for intracranial air and sinus air-fluid levels, and to be alert for the possibility of postinjury meningitis (remembering that these sequelae depend on the tearing of dura mater in association with the fracture). Scalp laceration must always be considered a potential route for intracranial infection and meningitis until proved otherwise. The scalp is quite vascular, and extensive blood loss from a scalp laceration can occur. Arterial hypotension from this cause is a rare problem in adults but may occur in young children.

Trauma to the Skull

There is a tendency for nonmedical persons to overemphasize the importance of a skull fracture relative to the associated brain damage; but the surgeon caring for patients with head injury must be careful not to underestimate the importance of skull fracture. Damage to the skull in patients with head injury has two main connotations. To a limited extent the type of skull damage gives some indication of the site and type of impact. Of more importance, the nature of the skull injury, visible on clinical examination and on x-ray, should signal potential underlying brain injury and alert one to the likelihood of the different complications that may occur. These complications, particularly hemorrhage and infection, which may devastate a patient who would otherwise have made a good recovery from his initial brain injury, can occur entirely as a result of the skull fracture. Three broad categories of skull fracture can be recognized: linear fractures, depressed fractures, and penetrating or perforating injuries of the skull.

Linear (Fissure) Fracture of the Vault

Linear or fissure fractures of the skull vault imply a considerable degree of force deforming the cranium but spread over a wide surface area. There is a variable degree of brain perturbation, depending on whether the responsible blow is associated with acceleration or deceleration of the head. One situation in which very severe fissure fractures of the skull can be seen without such movements of the head and in which there is little evident brain dysfunction is in crushing injuries of the head. A good example of this, a coal miner who was pinned by the head in a roof fall and could remember hearing his own skull crack, was seen by one of the authors. It must be emphasized, however, that absence of a skull fracture following injury does not imply that brain damage will be trivial. In only one of eight fatal cases of head injury with severe diffuse primary impact brain damage but no evidence of increased intracranial pressure reported by Adams and his colleagues had there been a skull fracture.[5]

The development of serious infective complications related to fissure fractures of the vault depends mainly on associated tearing of the dura and overlying laceration of the scalp.

The most dramatic complication of a linear fracture of the skull vault is epidural hematoma. This is discussed in detail later, but at this point it is worth emphasizing that formation of the hematoma is a complication of the skull injury. The extent of brain injury and the neurological status of the patient prior to the point at which the hematoma itself influences matters are largely independent of the skull damage. Thus patients who develop epidural hematomas may be alert, drowsy, or deeply comatose prior to the onset of brain compression.

Fissure Fracture of the Skull Base

Linear fractures of the cranial vault frequently extend down to and across the base of the skull. Depending on the site of the basal skull fracture, any of several complications may result. Fractures that involve the paranasal air sinuses may, if the dura mater is also torn, expose the patient to the risk of meningitis sooner or later after injury. The presence of this cranionasal fistula may or may not be signaled by the occurrence of cerebrospinal fluid rhinorrhea or intracranial air on plain skull x-rays, or both. Similarly, with fractures and dural tears that run across the floor of the middle cranial fossa through the middle ear, there may also be a risk of meningitis, which again may or may not be accompanied by cerebrospinal fliud otorrhea (via a torn tympanic membrane) or, rarely, cerebrospinal fluid rhinorrhea (via the eustachian tube).

Basal fractures that involve the temporal bone not infrequently cause complete facial palsy on the ipsilateral side, usually accompanied by deafness. Other cranial nerves may be injured also: the optic nerve by fractures that run into the optic foramen, and the oculomotor and abducens nerves by fractures that run into the petrous apex or superior orbital fissure. The main branches of the trigeminal nerve, which ought to be equally vulnerable to trauma, seem to be less commonly involved.

Depressed Skull Fracture

When one part of the skull has been driven inward so that its outer table is at or below the level of the surrounding inner table, this is a depressed fracture. This type of fracture results when the impact responsible for the head injury makes contact over a relatively small area of the skull. Depending on the total force involved in the blow, there may be only a small dent in the skull, an intact dura, and only minimal underlying brain contusion; a more severe local injury with dural tearing, indriven bone fragments, and signs of focal brain damage; or a much more widespread and

severe injury with an unconscious patient in whom the depressed fracture is merely a focal addition to severe diffuse brain damage. In general, most patients have never or only briefly been unconscious (Table 57–2). Because of the "sandwich" configuration of the skull, the inbending involved in depressed fracture usually produces a much more extensive fracture of the inner table than of the outer table. Also the edge of the inner table fragments may be sharp and lacerate dura at some distance from the visible outer table fracture.

The principal problems arising from depressed skull fracture relate to the presence of an overlying scalp laceration, whether dural penetration has occurred, the extent of indriven contamination, the extent of hemorrhage in the damaged area under the fracture, and finally, the location of the fracture relative to the major dural venous sinuses. In a series of 400 civilian cases of depressed skull fracture the three principal complicating factors were intracranial infection, intracranial hemorrhage, and actual or potential hemorrhage from dural venous sinuses at operation (Table 57–3). These complications affected 25 per cent of the patients in this series and were associated with significant increases in mortality and morbidity rates (Table 57–4).[177] Depressed fractures that involve the frontal air sinuses are particularly prone to infection even after debridement of the injury site.[138]

Penetrating Injuries of the Skull

In this type of injury, the differences already mentioned between linear and depressed fractures are amplified. The scalp is always breached in this type of wound, and the dura is always torn. Skull fragments may be driven deep into the brain, and the

TABLE 57–2 CLINICAL FEATURES OF 400 PATIENTS WITH DEPRESSED SKULL FRACTURE*

FEATURES	INCIDENCE (PER CENT)
Males	84
Aged 0–15 yr.	51
Never unconscious	25
Amnesia	53
Compound fracture	90
Dura penetrated	60

* From Miller, J. D., and Jennett, W., B.: Complications of depressed skull fracture. Lancet, 2:991–995, 1968. Reprinted by permission.

TABLE 57–3   COMPLICATIONS OCCURRING IN 104 OF 400 PATIENTS WITH DEPRESSED SKULL FRACTURE*

COMPLICATION	NUMBER OF PATIENTS	PER CENT OF SERIES
Infections	38	9.5
Brain abscess	15	3.8
Meningitis	9	2.2
Wound infection	17	4.2
Cerebral fungus	3	0.8
Intracranial hematomas	28	7.0
Intracerebral	17	4.3
Epidural	8	2.0
Subdural	3	0.8
Venous sinus involved	46	11.5
Sagittal sinus torn	16	4.0
Transverse sinus torn	6	1.5
Bridging vein at sinus torn	6	1.5
Overlying fracture not elevated	18	4.5

* From Miller, J. D., and Jennett, W. B.: Complications of depressed skull fracture. Lancet, 2:991–995, 1968. Reprinted by permission.

extent of brain damage is a function of this and the energy still possessed by the agent that caused the penetration. In most centers "penetrating" wound of the head is taken as synonymous with a missile injury. These may be divided into high- and low-velocity injuries, depending on the kinetic energy of the missile, a rifle bullet being an example of the former and a grenade fragment or pistol bullet fired from a distance, an example of the latter.

The complications of these types of skull damage are very similar to those of depressed skull fracture, namely infection, intracranial hemorrhage, and bleeding from dural venous sinuses at operation. Additional problems relate to deeply placed bone fragments and distant hemorrhages caused by ricochet of the missile within the skull. Finally, in tangential injuries in which the bone is scored but not penetrated by the missile, there may be extensive underlying intracranial hematomas.

Perforating Injury of the Skull

Because of the common association of the term "penetrating injury" with missile wounds of the head, it is necessary to use a different term for those injuries of the head caused by stab or puncture wounds of the head, and in this chapter the term "perforating injury" is used for this category. The cranial cavity may be entered from the vault via the scalp or from below via the orbit and thin orbital roof or, more rarely, through the nose or face—an injury to which children rather than adults seem to be prone.

Infection is the principal danger from such injuries and not infrequently is the mode of presentation.[78] Primary brain damage is so focal that there are rarely any neurological signs, and patients are seldom unconscious. If the wounding instrument has been removed, diagnosis may be a difficult problem, as the hole in the skull may be very small and obscured by overlying bone on x-ray, e.g., perforation of the thin temporal bone under the zygomatic arch. Also some perforating implements may be radiolucent, e.g., wooden sticks or slivers of glass. Finally, in cases in which the entry wound is in the sclera of the eye, it is usually completely obscured by subsequent swelling of the conjunctiva and eyelids.

Dura Mater and Brain Surface Blood Vessels

The role of dural tears in the formation of routes of infection of the brain after injury

TABLE 57–4   RELATIONSHIP OF INCIDENCE OF ADVERSE SEQUELAE OF DEPRESSED SKULL FRACTURES TO PRESENCE OF COMPLICATIONS*

SEQUELAE	WITH COMPLICATIONS		NO COMPLICATION		P
	No. of Patients	Per Cent	No. of Patients	Per Cent	
	104		296		—
Mortality	8	8	4	1	<0.005
Persistent neurological deficit	24	23	32	11	<0.005
Late post-traumatic epilepsy	16	15	22	7	<0.05

* From Miller, J. D., and Jennett, W. B.: Complications of depressed skull fracture. Lancet, 2:991–995, 1968. Reprinted by permission.

has been mentioned. Tearing of the dura over or near the dural venous sinuses has obvious repercussions in the formation of acute subdural hematoma, or in producing severe hemorrhage when indriven bone fragments are prematurely pulled out (a maneuver mentioned only to be condemned). An acute subdural hematoma, with little associated brain damage, can also occur when brain movement, particularly of a shrunken atrophic brain, is sufficiently great to avulse a bridging vein from the venous sinus. This often involves a vein linking the vein of Labbé with the sigmoid sinus or veins communicating with the superior sagittal sinus, as well as the veins from the temporal poles that drain into the petrosal sinuses. In patients who have cerebral arteriosclerosis, an injury may "fracture" a small artery on the cortical surface, and this may also be a source of the "pure" acute subdural hematoma, that is, one not associated with laceration of the brain. Injury to a small dural or cortical artery or to the carotid artery as it traverses the skull base may result in a traumatic aneurysm.

Pituitary and Hypothalamic Injury

Damage to the hypothalamopituitary axis probably occurs frequently in cases of severe injury. Its incidence is uncertain because evidence of damage is not always searched for and the relationship between clinical manifestations and observed pathological damage has not been well documented, as reports in the literature tend to focus on either one or the other aspect exclusively.[250]

Hypothalamic damage takes the form of petechial hemorrhages in the supraoptic and paraventricular nuclei and mamillary body with little neuronal loss, infarction in the infundibulum, and subependymal hemorrhage in the wall of the third ventricle.

Pituitary damage consists of petechial hemorrhage and retraction balls in the pituitary stalk and posterior lobe of the pituitary, while in the anterior lobe of the gland early acute infarctions involving up to 90 per cent of the lobe have been reported in 10 per cent of patients with severe head injury.[46] It is likely that these ischemic changes are due to interruption of the portal blood supply as it runs through the pituitary stalk, which is vulnerable to damage during deformation of the brain at impact.[127]

Clinical manifestations of pituitary damage appear to be much less frequent and severe than might be expected from the pathological damage. Diabetes insipidus occurs in less than 1 per cent of patients with head injury.[208] Panhypopituitarism following trauma is rare and has never been recorded in the first few days following head injury. Thus, acute hypocorticoid states cannot be invoked to explain low blood pressure in the early stages after head injury. Labile body temperature with a tendency to poikilothermia may indicate damage in the hypothalamus.

In summary, damage to the pituitary gland and associated hypothalamus can occur in patients with head injury because of direct trauma, or because of ischemia distal to vascular damage. Despite the abundant evidence of pathological lesions in those patients who die, abnormalities of the endocrine system that can be firmly attributed to this damage are rare.[155]

Associated Spinal Injuries

Considerable stress is appropriately laid on the possibility that head and spinal trauma may coexist—with resultant diagnostic pitfalls and possibilities for therapeutic disaster. In 206 consecutive cases of spinal injury, Harris noted 95 patients (41 per cent) with an associated head injury. The spinal injuries were distributed fairly evenly along the vertebral column in patients with concomitant head injury, but many of these head injuries were minor. If only major head injury was considered, then cervical spine injuries were predominant.[83] Similar conclusions have been reached by Sevitt, who found that of 250 road accident fatalities 9 per cent had combined head and spinal injuries, of which 60 per cent were cervical spine injuries.[227] Maloney and Whatmore analyzed 173 fatal head injuries and found 5 per cent that were associated with spinal injuries.[158] The authors have encountered only two cases of spinal (cervical) injury in the last 100 patients who were comatose on admission. In neither case was there spinal cord damage.

The combination of spinal and head trauma must always be searched for, even though it is infrequent. Examination of the spine ought not to be confined to the neck. In addition to posing diagnostic problems in the early assessment of acute head trauma, concomitant high spinal cord trauma may be responsible for respiratory insufficiency or a fall in arterial pressure resulting in anoxic or ischemic cerebral hypoxia. These are severe secondary insults to the already traumatized brain.

Systemic Injuries and Brain Dysfunction

The problems of the patient with multiple injuries are discussed separately in Chapter 77, but in the present context systemic injury is important as a potential source of secondary insult to the already injured brain. The mediators of such insults are cerebral ischemia due to arterial hypotension, cerebral anoxia as part of systemic anoxia, cerebral fat embolism, and increased cerebral venous pressure due to mediastinal block impeding venous return.

Although transient arterial hypotension is thought to be an immediate sequel of concussion, low arterial pressure, persisting at the time of admission to hospital, is seldom the result of head injury alone. When seen, this must prompt the search for a source of hemorrhage. Illingworth and Jennett found only 14 instances of shock in 470 head injuries seen within six hours of injury, and in 11 of these cases a source of substantial blood loss, usually in the chest, abdomen, or pelvis, could be identified. In only three instances was scalp wound blood loss contributory. Unsuspected high cervical (atlantoaxial) spinal trauma was the cause of hypotension in one case.[98] The authors encountered 12 patients with arterial hypotension in their last 100 cases of severe head injury, and in all 12 the low blood pressure was associated with substantial injuries to the trunk or limbs.

Later causes of arterial hypotension are gastric, duodenal, or jejunal hemorrhage from acute erosions or ulceration, perforation of the esophagus, and gram-negative septicemic shock from infective complications of prolonged coma.[44,152]

SECONDARY DAMAGE BY BRAIN COMPRESSION IN HEAD INJURY

Intracranial Expanding Lesions

Following head injury several different processes can occur, each of which has the common result of producing an expanding intracranial lesion. These lesions may be extracerebral or intracerebral, and produce dysfunction in a combination of ways, by brain shift and distortion, by increased intracranial pressure, and by focal disorders of the involved or adjacent brain. The different forms of secondary mass lesions are described here, and the relevant mechanisms of brain dysfunction they produce are discussed in the following sections.

Epidural Hematoma

Acute epidural hematoma, formation of a solid mass of clotted blood between the skull and the dura mater, is probably the best-known intracranial complication of head injury, yet the mortality rate remains high, the diagnosis is often suspected too late to prevent severe brain distortion and damage, and it is not particularly common, occurring in 1 per cent of patients with head injury admitted to the hospital, i.e., about half as often as acute subdural hematoma.[139,144,245] The well-publicized concept of acute epidural hematoma is of an arterial hemorrhage into the epidural space produced by tearing of the middle meningeal artery due to a temporoparietal fracture of the skull. As the blood clot enlarges, stripping off the dura, it produces, in a patient who was not or was only briefly rendered unconscious by the blow to the head, a syndrome of progressive brain compression. This leads to gradual obtundation, contralateral hemiparesis, and ipsilateral oculomotor nerve paresis, followed by decerebrate rigidity, arterial hypertension, cardiorespiratory irregularity, apnea, and death. This, then, is the "textbook description" of acute epidural hematoma.

This presentation occurs, in fact, in less than 10 per cent of patients with epidural hematoma.[100] In many cases an "unusual" presentation of epidural hematoma is the explanation for delay in diagnosis or referral for neurosurgical care. For this reason the emphasis in this section is placed on deviations of the clinical presentation from the so-called "classic" presentation.

Most cases of epidural hematoma are associated with a linear fracture, usually in the temporoparietal area. Depressed skull fracture may rarely be associated with epidural hematoma (2 per cent of 400 cases), and occasional cases without skull fracture, virtually all in persons under the age of 30 years, have been reported.[63,177] It is usually assumed, with hematomas associated with a temporal bone fracture, that it is invariably the meningeal artery that is torn as it runs in its groove. Gallagher and Browder have pointed out that it is the middle meningeal vein that causes the groove in the bone and cite cases in which the epidural hematoma was evidently produced by bleeding from this vein and not from the artery.[64] If this is the case it would suggest that dura mater is stripped from the inner table of the skull by the force of injury and not by a build-up of pressure in the hematoma.

Although in textbooks, illustrations of acute epidural hematoma almost invariably show the clot to lie over the lateral aspect of the hemisphere centered at the pterions, this is the site of the clot in only 70 per cent of cases. Epidural hematomas may also

occur in frontal, occipital, and posterior fossa locations—each in 5 to 10 per cent of cases (Fig. 57–4).[100]

In up to 60 per cent of cases the epidural hematoma forms against a background of minor underlying brain damage with little or no loss of consciousness: in about 20 per cent of cases the patient has never been more than drowsy prior to the advent of brain compression, and in a further 20 per cent, patients have been unconscious from the start.[64] In this latter group with more severe primary brain injury, if epidural hematoma is associated with an intradural lesion (cerebral contusion, subdural or intracerebral hematoma) the mortality rate greatly increases, from 6 to 27 per cent in one series.[96,100,154]

In the clinical presentation of epidural hematoma the classic "lucid interval" in which the patient is stunned by the blow, recovers consciousness, then lapses into unconsciousness as the clot expands, is present in only 20 per cent of cases.[100,154] Furthermore, a "lucid interval" may also be seen in the development of certain types of acute subdural hematoma and in mild head injuries complicated by meningitis.

The contralateral hemiparesis, which is thought to be due to direct pressure on the underlying motor cortex, is of course a sign

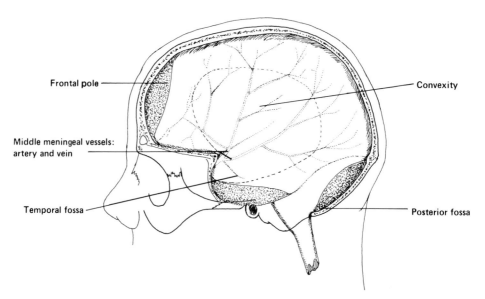

Frontal pole

Convexity

Middle meningeal vessels:
artery and vein

Temporal fossa

Posterior fossa

Figure 57–4 Typical sites of epidural hemorrhage are primarily over the lateral aspect of the hemisphere (within the dotted region) in 70 to 75 per cent of cases of epidural hematoma. Usually they result from laceration of the middle meningeal vein (40 to 45 per cent) or middle meningeal artery (40 to 45 per cent) or from bleeding originating at a dural venous sinus (10 per cent). More unusual loci are the frontal poles (5 to 10 per cent), temporal fossa (5 to 10 per cent), and posterior fossa (5 to 10 per cent)—all indicated by stippling.

limited to those epidural collections that occur in that site. Patients with frontal or occipital clots may present with drowsiness followed directly by bilateral decerebrate rigidity. Hemiparesis may even be ipsilateral to the hematoma, owing to pressure of the opposite peduncle on the edge of the tentorium, although less often than is seen with chronic subdural hematoma. Dilatation of the ipsilateral pupil, one of the "classic" signs of epidural hematoma, occurs in only just over 50 per cent of cases.

The clinical picture of progressive brain compression usually evolves over several hours, but may extend for days or, rarely, weeks with a fluctuating course suggestive of chronic subdural hematoma. The prognosis is better for those cases in which the evolution is slower (>12 hours).[144]

The pathological effects of epidural hemorrhage, which always remains a solid mass, are mediated by compression of underlying brain, and later by swelling of this compressed area together with brain distortion and herniation and raised intracranial pressure.[36,99] These factors, and the time over which they occur, act against the state of the brain prior to injury, the space available for an expanding process within the cranium, and any primary brain damage produced by the injury that initiated the epidural hematoma.

Subdural Hematoma

Of the distinct clinicopathological conditions that fall under this heading, about the only factor they have in common is that the hematoma collects in the subdural space. Most clinicians recognize acute subdural hematoma, chronic subdural hematoma, and infantile subdural effusion as separate entities, and some also classify separately as subacute subdural hematoma those collections that present 4 to 14 days after injury.[141] In this section the argument is made that subacute subdural hematoma should not be regarded separately, but that two varieties of acute subdural hematoma should be recognized.

Acute Subdural Hematoma

Just as in most cases of severe head injury some subarachnoid blood is present, so also is subdural blood common after major injury. This subdural bleeding may, however, become extensive enough to act as an extra-axial compressive lesion and pose a threat to life. Sizeable subdural hematomas can develop under two circumstances, each of which may have different implications for the patient.

Bleeding may accumulate around a brain laceration, often a polar laceration of the temporal or frontal lobe. Frequently, such patients have also sustained severe diffuse primary brain injury and have been unconscious from the start. The subdural hematoma forms adjacent to damaged and necrotic brain and is often continuous with intracerebral hematoma, formed in the depths of the brain laceration. This complex of hematoma and lacerated necrotic and swollen brain is aptly termed "burst temporal (or frontal) lobe." Patients with this lesion may show delayed neurological deterioration around the third or fourth day after injury, and some such cases may be labeled subacute subdural hematoma. This term probably is erroneous, because computed tomography (CT) or other studies performed on admission in such patients show that the hematoma is present soon after the injury in nearly all cases. Probably the reason for the later deterioration is delayed swelling of the damaged brain—a case of the brain compressing the clot rather than the clot compressing the brain. The advent of computed tomographic x-ray scanning has shed new light on this area by revealing developing areas of lucency in the temporal lobe of such cases over a period of days following injury (see Fig. 57–3). It should be added that routine CT scanning also shows anterior temporal subdural and intracerebral hematomas in some patients who have been only briefly unconscious and have no clinical indications whatsoever of an intracranial space-occupying lesion. These findings suggest that it would be unwise to make a simple causal link between polar damage with intracerebral or subdural hematoma and neurological deterioration.

The second circumstance in which subdural hematoma may rapidly form is when a surface or bridging vessel (usually a vein) is torn during the movement of the brain that accompanies head acceleration or deceleration at impact. In some cases the actual brain damage is mild, so a dramatic clinical picture results in which there is a brief lucid interval following injury, followed by an extremely rapid neurological deterioration. The same picture may develop after a direct blow to the skull in which a surface artery is ruptured by the blow. In these cases the threat to the patient's life is entirely due to the hematoma, as in the "typical" case of epidural hematoma. Unfortunately, the speed of the neurological deterioration is such that, in the main, these patients fare no better than those in whom the hematoma is merely an extension of severe primary brain damage.

Reports in which both forms of hematoma are included show a very high mortality rate ranging from 25 per cent to over 90 per cent.* This high mortality rate relates to the major underlying diffuse brain injury that many of these patients have sustained, which is then compounded by rapid brain compression as a result of the subdural or intracerebral hematoma. Because many of these patients are unconscious when first seen in hospital, further neurological deterioration, which prompts the search for an intracranial mass lesion, all too often takes the patient to the point at which operative decompression cannot reverse the secondary brain stem damage. In such cases, decompression is often followed by brain stem hemorrhage.[126]

Chronic Subdural Hematoma in the Adult

In contrast to the acute hematoma, of which the effects of secondary brain compression are so often inextricably mixed with the effects of the primary brain damage, chronic subdural hematoma represents pure brain compression occurring weeks after injury. The injury itself is often mild and in some cases is denied altogether.

The exact cause of the fluid collection in the subdural space is unknown. As the hematoma becomes older, it is bounded by a membrane attached to the dura and arachnoid that gradually thickens. Also the contents gradually change from dark, thick, tarry blood to an orange-tinged protein-rich fluid.

Intracranial pressure is usually low, but brain shift is often severe.[25,191] This apparently paradoxical phenomenon relates to the prominent brain atrophy most of

these patients had prior to development of the hematoma. An atrophic brain appears to permit the development and growth of subdural hematoma without the development of intracranial hypertension. In regard to this phenomenon, it should be noted that chronic subdural hematoma in the adult is limited almost exclusively to geriatric patients or alcoholics with brain atrophy.[25,76] It is almost never seen past early childhood in younger people with full resilient brains, and is almost impossible to produce experimentally in healthy animals whose brains are not atrophic.[8]

When coning occurs with unilateral subdural hematoma the signs of lateral tentorial herniation usually predominate. A notable finding in these cases is that in about 30 per cent hemiparesis is ipsilateral to the hematoma.[153] When chronic subdural hematomas are bilateral, the signs are of posterior tentorial herniation, as described later. Brain distortion is often so severe that even when the hematoma is evacuated the brain remains depressed from the dura and rapid expansion of the brain to fill the cavity may be difficult to achieve. Thus chronic subdural hematoma differs from acute subdural hematoma in several respects: associated brain damage is usually severe with acute hematoma, mild with chronic; intracranial pressure is high in acute subdural hematoma, often low in chronic; the blood is clotted in acute hematomas, liquid in chronic collections; brain distortion tends to be more pronounced relative to conscious level in chronic hematomas.

Subdural Effusion of Infancy

The major difference between the chronic subdural hematoma seen in the adult and the subdural effusion in a child with an expansile calvarium is that the latter can lead to a significant degree of craniocerebral disproportion. Subdural effusions may, therefore, reach a relatively larger size in children than in adults, and because of the disproportion between brain size and skull size, therapy may be more difficult than in adults.

The pathophysiology of infantile subdural effusions and chronic subdural hematomas of adults has not been established. Membrane formation is thought to be an irritative desmoplastic response to the pres-

---

* See references 37, 56, 84, 101, 129, 139, 144, 153, 187, 213, 219, 244.

ence of blood in the subdural space, but it is extremely difficult to create a subdural hematoma experimentally.[8,65,67,128] Why these lesions enlarge also remains a mystery. Gardner proposed that an osmotic pressure gradient between the contents of the effusion and the cerebrospinal fluid or blood causes progressive enlargement of chronic subdural hematomas, but Weir did simultaneous measurements of serum, cerebrospinal fluid, and subdural fluid osmolarity in 23 patients and could find no osmotic difference between subdural fluids and either the serum or the cerebrospinal fluid.[65,258] An old theory explaining growth of subdural effusions is that of recurrent hemorrhage into the subdural space from the membranes themselves, but this theory cannot explain why some patients have a history of recent neurological deterioration but the subdural fluid does not contain fresh blood.

Acute Subdural Hygroma

Occasionally, a patient with a head injury will have a small extra-axial collection of fluid shown on angiography or computed tomography that is composed of clear cerebrospinal fluid and that often spurts forth under pressure when the dura is opened. This condition is quite different from a watery subdural effusion or hematoma in which the fluid is yellow or orange in color. The mechanism of formation of this fluid, which is indistinguishable from cerebrospinal fluid, is not certain, but it has been proposed that a small tear in the arachnoid occurs and, coupled with a one-way valvular action of the thin membrane, is enough to open up the subdural space as the pulsations of the brain propel fluid outward from the subarachnoid space.[76] This theory has never been proved.[94] It is not clear either whether this collection really can act as an intracranial space-occupying lesion to the extent of producing herniation of the brain. Clinical improvement is often noted in patients after the fluid is released, but this may be no more than would have occurred had the lateral ventricle been tapped. Some authors have suggested that acute subdural hygroma per se is associated with a high mortality rate, and this finding of this clear fluid in the subdural space carries an ominous prognostic significance.[76] It appears more likely that the prognosis of these patients is related to the extent of the primary brain damage and not to the pressure exerted by the (usually) small mass lesion. High pressure in such collections may be due entirely to the influence of swollen underlying brain. Furthermore, with the advent of routine tomographic scanning this "lesion" is being seen quite often in patients with no neurological indications of brain compression, and it has even been suggested that in some instances, in children at least, it represents part of the normal sequence of events of recovery following blunt injury.[22]

Intracerebral Hematoma

This lesion is seen more commonly in those head injuries in which force is applied to the head over a small area, that is, missile injuries, perforating wounds, or depressed skull fractures. This is in contrast to injuries in which the entire head is subjected to accleration and deceleration, when hematomas are more likely to be subdural or epidural. Intracerebral hematomas, however, do occur in blunt head injury. Usually they are found to be associated with frontal or temporal lobe lacerations and some element of subdural hematoma. With the advent of computed tomography, patients who clinically would not have been suspected of harboring an intracerebral mass lesion are being found to have small deeply placed intracerebral densities suggestive of hematoma. Intracerebral hemorrhage in the brain stem is most commonly related to axial displacement of the brain secondary to brain compression, as discussed later. Patients who are receiving long-term anticoagulant therapy can be at great risk from developing substantial intracerebral hematoma after even mild head injury.

Schorstein found 83 substantial intracranial hematomas in 2000 consecutive missile wounds of the head during World War II, of which 69 per cent were intracerebral.[224] As evacuation of the wounded has become faster, correspondingly higher proportions of intracerebral hematomas have been reported.[141,167,168,212] In 400 consecutive cases of civilian depressed skull fracture, Miller and Jennett noted 28 patients with intracranial hematomas, of which 61 per cent were intracerebral (see Table 57–3).[177] In all these cases of intracerebral hematoma, dural tearing was associated with the fracture, confirming the association with penetrating injuries.

Only in a minority of cases is the source of the intracerebral hemorrhage a division of a major vessel such as a middle cerebral branch. In most cases the source of the hemorrhage is small vessels in the parenchyma. As is the case in spontaneous intracerebral hematoma, usually no specific bleeding vessel is visible in the hematoma cavity when it is evacuated operatively.

The clinical presentation of traumatic intracerebral hematoma is a result of the severity of initial impact, the size and rate of increase of the hematoma, and its site. Of particular importance is an intracerebral hematoma that complicates a perforating wound of the head, such as a stab injury. In these cases consciousness is usually not lost, and when the patient presents in the emergency room with a small laceration of the scalp the significance of the lesion may not be appreciated. If the onset of brain compression is slow or delayed, the patient may be sent home or to police custody, only to deteriorate outside the hospital with disastrous consequences.

Brain Swelling

In the first seven days after injury a sequence of events may occur in which intracranial pressure increases, signs of brain compression develop, and radiological studies show that brain shift or ventricular compression has developed since the first day after injury. Computed tomography in-

dicates that the mass effect is not due to hematoma formation, and it is usually considered that the patient is suffering from post-traumatic brain edema. This process may occur as a focal or as a diffuse phenomenon.

Extensive focal brain swelling may complicate frontal or temporal polar contusion and hematoma. In these patients the CT scan shows decreased density radiating outward from the affected area, and at operative decompression the brain is soft and necrotic. This process, which is maximal around the third postinjury day, often is responsible for the clinical presentation of the "subacute" subdural hematoma (Fig. 57–5).

The process appears to represent the outward spread from the polar injury of true brain edema (increased brain water content) and to be a similar process to the spread of edema around tumors or infarcts.[122,123] In these situations the edema fluid is extracellular, mainly in white matter, and issues from blood vessels across a defective blood-brain barrier. The factors regulating the rate at which edema fluid flows in the tissues are hydrostatic in nature and related to the extent of the blood-brain barrier defect, the level of blood pressure, and the degree of local cerebral vasodilatation, which will increase arteriolar and capillary pressure.[124] Factors that impede the outward flow of fluid are those that decrease tissue compliance, that is, swelling of the cellular elements, reduction of the extracellular space, and raised intracranial

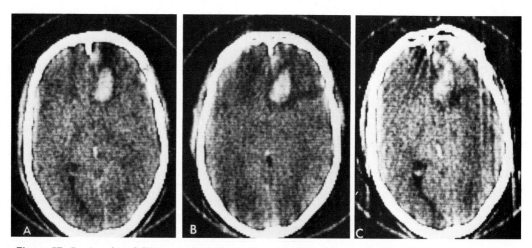

Figure 57–5 A series of CT scans of a patient with a right frontal hemorrhagic contusion show the development over time of edema spreading posteriorly in the right hemisphere. *A*. Scan taken on the day of admission. *B*. Four days later. *C*. One week after admission.

pressure. Once the fluid is in the extracellular space it is itself a source of increased intracranial and tissue pressure. The fluid is believed to permeate toward the ventricles, and the passage of the edema front into the ventricular system, and its dissolution thereby, is aided by factors that increase tissue compliance, that is, reduction of intracranial pressure and shrinkage of cellular elements.[92,214,218]

After head injury, brain swelling may also occur as a generalized phenomenon that is manifested by disappearance of the ventricles on the CT scan and elevation of intracranial pressure. In 1945 Evans and Scheinker proposed that the initial event following severe head trauma was a functional cerebrovascular disturbance with capillary dilatation, producing true edema later.[53,54] An immediate increase in cerebral blood volume following head trauma has been shown in experimental animals, and Bruce and his colleagues have reported this phenomenon after relatively mild injury in children, pointing out that computed tomography does not show decreased density at an early stage and that regional cerebral blood flow and blood volume are increased.[22,142] They have proposed that the increase in intracranial pressure is not due initially to brain edema but to swelling due to vascular engorgement, and in these cases the course is usually benign. In other cases, however, progressive intracranial hypertension follows, then true edema certainly develops, to be verified at autopsy when a diffusely swollen brain with an increase in white matter volume is observed. Diffuse, extensive white matter edema after head injury is rather uncommon, tends to occur mostly in young adults, and is invariably preceded by unstable and severe fluctuations in intracranial pressure caused by variations in cerebral vasomotor tone and cerebral blood volume.

Infective Intracranial Mass Lesions

Epidural Abscess

A sizeable collection of pus in the epidural space is a rare complication of head injury. It was found in 1 of 400 cases of depressed fractures reported by Miller and Jennett, and in 1 postoperative case of 226 reported by Meirowsky.[167,177] In these cases the mass lesions were not large

enough to threaten the life of the patient, although the potential for dangerous brain compression did exist. If a localized infection is going to complicate a head injury, it is more likely to produce a subdural or intracerebral abscess or meningitis because the dura is so often torn by the type of localized penetrating injury that tends to drive contaminated material into the wound. In epidural abscess the intact dura makes an efficient barrier, and signs of meningitis are often absent.

Subdural Empyema

Although subdural abscess is usually caused by severe sinusitis and seldom results from head injury, when it does occur, it is devastating for the patient. Fortunately it is an uncommon complication of infection; Miller and Jennett encountered only three cases among 400 depressed fractures, although the dura was torn in half of the patients.[177] It presents a severe problem for several reasons. Unlike epidural abscess, subdural empyemas spread widely, with pus dipping into the sulci. Concurrent meningitis is usual, and associated intracerebral abscesses are not uncommon. The underlying brain is profoundly affected, and focal neurological deficits related to the site of the collection and focal seizures are frequent occurrences. Most patients have evident systemic signs of infection, toxemia, leukocytosis, and pyrexia in addition to the signs of meningeal irritation. This situation is in contrast to that of patients with epidural or intracerebral abscesses, in whom signs of systemic upset or meningitis are often lacking.

Although subdural pus usually forms only a thin layer, this is not always so, and substantial collections may form over the convexity, on the floor of the anterior or middle fossa, or even on the medial side of the hemisphere.[120] Swelling of the underlying brain greatly compounds the problem, producing raised intracranial pressure and brain displacement and making it difficult to drain pus through multiple burr holes.

Thus, the patient with a head injury (usually a penetrating wound but occasionally a fracture through infected paranasal sinuses) who develops this complication is exposed simultaneously to the risks of brain compression, epilepsy, and meningitis.[120,177] Moreover, the responsible organisms are usually anaerobic streptococci or gram-negative rods, and antibiotic treatment alone is never effective. The mortality rate for subdural empyema is over 30 per cent, and for those who survive, the risk of continuing epilepsy is also 30 per cent.[13,91,195] The tragedy of these rare cases is that the patient has often recovered fully from the effects of the initial head injury when the infective complication supervenes.[175,177]

Intracerebral Abscess

Brain abscess is the feared complication of all penetrating head wounds, particularly missile injuries. The nature of these injuries, in which hair and bone fragments are driven deep into the brain and much localized necrosis of brain tissue occurs, favors the establishment of infection if complete and prompt debridement is not performed. The literature from World War II and the Korean and Vietnam wars abounds with reports emphasizing the importance of early operation, complete removal of hair and bone fragments and foreign bodies, debridement of necrotic and contaminated tissue, tight dural closure, and skin closure without excessive tension.*

Despite these many reports suggesting that the principles of head wound treatment were uniformly well known and adhered to, Jefferson pointed out that, although Cushing had clearly laid down these same principles many years before in the First World War, in the Second World War many surgeons learned about the problems of post-traumatic brain abscess only by bitter personal experience.[42,103] The need for continued attention to the dangers of intracerebral abscess formation remains unchanged today and applies equally to civilian and military injuries.

When intracerebral abscess formation occurs, the mass effect of the collection of pus is greatly compounded by edema and expansion of the surrounding white matter. This produces increased intracranial pressure, brain shift, and herniation, as well as increasing focal neurological deficit related to the site of the abscess. If wound debridement and closure is inadequate or long delayed, herniation of swollen edematous brain occurs through the wound, leading to

_____

* See references 29, 30, 51, 80, 85, 87, 159, 164, 169, 223, 231, 255–257.

necrosis and further swelling and extrusion of tissue, the so-called "cerebral fungus."

It is generally considered that the source of infection in brain abscess is retained bone fragments, but some investigators have emphasized the more important role of infection from indriven skin, hair, and foreign material, the risk of which increases by the hour following injury until debridement.[33,80,205] Retained metallic fragments are not usually considered a serious source of infection. Though brain abscess formation usually occurs within days or weeks of injury, much longer delays, up to seven years from injury, have been reported.[48] In these cases it is possible that the infection is blood borne, maturing to an abscess in a vulnerable area of the brain.

Although post-traumatic intracerebral brain abscess is mentioned most often in the context of missile injuries of warfare, it occurs sufficiently often in civilian series of head injuries to merit close attention. It was the single most common type of intracranial infection in Miller and Jennett's series of 400 depressed fractures (15 cases, or 4 per cent).[177] Now that chronic middle ear infection is decreasing, head injury is becoming a more significant causative factor in recent cases of brain abscess, 9 per cent of the series reported by Carey and co-workers, and 12 per cent of those cases reported by Morgan and his colleagues.[32,189] Like missile injuries, however, this type of brain abscess tends to be associated with dural tearing and penetration of the brain by hair, dirt, and bone fragments. Jennett and Miller emphasized that most of these patients were fully conscious when first seen at the hospital, or never sought medical help at all, so the full significance of the injury was not appreciated and appropriate treatment was therefore delayed.[107]

Secondary Displacement of the Brain

Any discrete expanding intracranial mass, whatever its nature, be it hematoma, abscess, or edematous brain, and its site, epidural, subdural or intracerebral, supra- or infratentorial, will usually produce brain shift and distortion together with increased intracranial pressure, which will ultimately lead to herniation of brain out of the bony-dural compartment in which the mass originates.[176] The relationship between the volume of the mass, the rate at which it expands, the intracranial pressure, the degree of distortion and herniation of the brain, and the neurological dysfunction that results therefrom is subtle and influenced by antecedent factors referred to earlier, such as the cerebrospinal fluid volume and the shape of the tentorial hiatus.[38,176] Broadly speaking, the faster a mass expands, the higher is the intracranial pressure relative to the degree of brain distortion produced. This is clearly illustrated by comparison of acute and chronic subdural hematoma. In the former case the intracranial pressure is often over 50 mm of mercury on admission to the hospital in patients who have 10 mm of midline shift, whereas in a patient with chronic subdural hematoma that has developed over a longer time interval, a midline shift of 20 mm may be associated with normal pressure.[185]

There is, however, a close intertwining of brain shift and increased intracranial pressure. Many of the neurological signs that occur with major mass lesions and are attributed to raised pressure are more probably due to brain displacement (Table 57–5). In a similar vein, increases in pressure, particularly differential changes in pressure across the tentorium and foramen magnum, are often related to the process of brain shift and herniation from one compartment to another.

In head injury the great majority of expanding mass lesions are supratentorial. The infratentorial lesions, posterior fossa epidural hematoma, cerebellar hematoma, or contusion, are rarities. Supratentorial lesions, which in patients with head injury may not infrequently be bilateral, produce characteristic types of brain displacement, distortion, and herniation according to the site or sites of the mass lesions.

General Features

An extra-axial mass depresses underlying brain, flattening the gyri and compressing surface vessels.[228] Elsewhere the subarachnoid space becomes obliterated, and the gyri flatten against the dura. The subarachnoid cisterns decrease in size, and the lateral ventricle on the side of the lesion also becomes narrowed. When the mass is intra-axial, gyri are also flattened, and the subarachnoid space and cisterns become obliterated.

The decrease in intracranial cerebrospinal fluid volume is important in relation to the regulation and transmission of intracranial pressure. Displacement of the fluid is one factor responsible for spatial compensation in which intracranial pressure can remain close to normal despite expansion of the mass lesion.[130] As the fluid spaces around the midbrain at the tentorial hiatus become occluded, however, the mechanisms for bulk flow and absorption of cerebrospinal fluid are interfered with, and transmission of pressure across the tentorium becomes progressively impaired so that the true level of supratentorial pressure is no longer reflected in measurements taken from the spinal subarachnoid space (cisternal or lumbar). As the block becomes more complete, lumbar pressure deviates more from supratentorial pressure until lumbar subarachnoid pressure may return to normal at a time when intraventricular

TABLE 57–5 SITES OF BRAIN HERNIATION, STRUCTURES INVOLVED, AND RESULTING CLINICAL SIGNS

SITE OF HERNIATION	STRUCTURES INVOLVED	SIGNS
Lateral tentorial (uncal)	Oculomotor nerve	Ptosis, mydriasis, lateral deviation
	Cerebral peduncle	Hemiparesis
	Posterior cerebral artery	Hemianopsia
Posterior tentorial (tectal)	Tectal plate	Bilateral ptosis, failure of upward gaze
Central tentorial (axial–brain stem)	Reticular formation	Depression of consciousness
	Corticospinal tracts	Decerebrate rigidity
	Midbrain and pons	Impairment or absence of eye movement reflexes
		Irregular respiration
	Medulla	Arterial hypertension and bradycardia
		Irregular respiration, apnea
Foraminal (tonsillar)	Medulla	Apnea
Subfalcine (cingulate)	Cingulate gyrus	Leg weakness
	Anterior cerebral arteries	

pressure is over 50 mm of mercury.[119,134,135] When this stage has been reached, the outlook for the patient is poor unless decompression is immediately effected.

Midline Shift

When the expanding mass lesion is predominantly unilateral, the midline structures are shifted to the opposite side. The interventricular septum and the third ventricle, which are detectable by echoencephalography, ventriculography, or computed tomography, and the pineal gland, which, if calcified, will be visible on plain x-rays, can define the degree of midline shift. The internal cerebral vein and anterior cerebral–pericallosal artery complex also shift and can be visualized by angiography.

As this shifting process proceeds, the cingulate gyrus herniates under the free edge of the falx cerebri, pressing the corpus callosum downward on the side of the mass lesion; this produces the characteristic "tilted gull-wing" appearance on angiography (in the anteroposterior view). The falx, contrary to earlier belief, may also be tilted or shifted away from the mass. If the process is extensive and severe, subfalcine herniation may compromise one or both pericallosal arteries with infarction in their territory of distribution and result in paresis of one or both legs. This is a rare occurrence, however, and tends to be overshadowed by the other processes of brain herniation that occur simultaneously. Even lesser degrees of supracallosal hernia do, however, leave detectable pathological damage in the form of sclerotic or hemorrhagic lesions of the cingulate gyrus.[1,3]

The medial portion of the temporal lobe on the side of the lesion (uncus and hippocampal gyrus) becomes pressed against the side of the midbrain; this is part of the process of obliteration of the cisterna ambiens, and the whole process of midline brain shift can be viewed as a prelude to tentorial herniation, which has more important physiological consequences for the patient. Nonetheless, in patients with head injury there is a correlation between the occurrence of significant midline shift and the incidence of signs of severe neurological dysfunction (Table 57–6).

Tentorial Herniation

A major landmark in neurological surgery was the recognition of the clinical features of tentorial herniation and the identification of the pathological processes leading to it. In patients with head injury it allowed the differentiation of primary and secondary lesions of the brain. The primary lesions are due to impact forces at the time of injury, and the secondary lesions are due to the effects of a secondary space-occupying lesion such as a hematoma, swollen contusion, or even an abscess.[171,240]

After the clinical descriptions of the tentorial pressure cone by Vincent and coworkers and Jefferson, it was firmly linked with ipsilateral oculomotor palsy and medial occipital (posterior cerebral artery) infarction.[102,188,216,274] Later the link between disturbances of consciousness and tentorial herniation was elucidated.[28,156] Detailed experimental studies further explained the link between tentorial coning, pupillary dil-

TABLE 57–6   RELATIONSHIP BETWEEN PRONOUNCED MIDLINE SHIFT AND NEUROLOGICAL DYSFUNCTION IN 160 PATIENTS WITH SEVERE HEAD INJURY*

NEUROLOGICAL DYSFUNCTION	MIDLINE SHIFT (mm)				P
	0–9		10–30		
	Number of Patients	Per Cent	Number of Patients	Per Cent	
	130		30		
Best motor response decorticate, decerebrate, or flaccid	51	39	23	77	<0.001
Bilateral absence of pupillary light response	20	15	14	47	<0.001
Impairment or absence of oculocephalic response	44	34	20	66	<0.001

* Data from Miller, J. D., Becker, D. P., Ward, J. D., et al.: Significance of intracranial hypertension in severe head injury. J. Neurosurg., 47:503–516, 1977.

atation, changes in pulse and blood pressure, and brain stem hemorrhages.[93,108,125,126,247] Finally came the recognition of the different, though overlapping, syndromes of tentorial herniation.[110–112,206]

Lateral (Uncal) Tentorial Herniation

This process, the best-known form of tentorial herniation, consists of the bulging and herniation of the uncus and medial portion of the hippocampal gyrus between the free edge of the tentorium and the midbrain (Fig. 57–6A). In consequence, the midbrain is compressed from side to side and thus elongated in its anterior-posterior diameter, and the opposite cerebral peduncle may be compressed against the tentorial edge on the other side sufficiently hard to create a detectable lesion. This mechanism is invoked to explain ipsilateral hemiparesis in chronic subdural hematoma.[76] It must be said, however, that this lesion can be seen in patients who did not have ipsilateral motor signs prior to death. The herniating brain also causes distortion of the oculomotor nerve by compression between the posterior cerebral artery and the petroclinoid ligament, and the posterior cerebral artery itself may be so compromised as to produce infarction in its territory of distribution. The late pathological sequelae of lateral tentorial herniation that has been reversed and from which the patient has recovered are sclerotic pressure lesions in the parahippocampal gyrus. In the acute stage visible grooving of the under surface of the temporal lobe can be seen at autopsy. In certain patients, hemorrhage occurs into the ipsilateral oculomotor nerve where it crosses the posterior cerebral artery and may be easily seen after death. Infarction of the ipsilateral medial occipital cortex due to occlusion of the posterior cerebral artery is also easily recognized at autopsy.

The clinical correlates of this process are depression of consciousness, possibly due to distortion or deafferentation of the upper part of the reticular activating system; contralateral (or sometimes ipsilateral) hemiparesis progressing to decerebrate rigidity; and ipsilateral pupillary dilatation with loss in the affected eye of the direct and consensual light response and external movements other than abduction. By the time occipital infarction occurs, the patient is not sufficiently conscious to be tested for visual field deficits. This clinical and pathological picture of lateral tentorial herniation is seen in its purest form in patients with expanding lesions in the temporal lobe.

Posterior (Tectal) Tentorial Herniation

In patients who have purely frontal or occipital lesions, or bilateral lesions such as bilateral chronic subdural hematoma, an important clinical variant of tentorial herniation occurs that has been described by Johnson.[110] In this situation, the herniation of medial temporal structures occurs posteriorly or on both sides so that the herniating brain impinges not upon the third nerve and posterior cerebral artery but upon the quadrigeminal plate at the level of the superior colliculi (Fig. 57–6B). This produces findings similar to Parinaud's syndrome—a characteristic clinical appearance of a drowsy patient with a wrinkled forehead and closed or half-closed eyes due to the bilateral ptosis; on elevation of the eyelids it can be seen that upward gaze is defective. Pupillary light responses are, however, usually preserved until a late stage in the process of herniation.

Central or Axial Herniation of the Brain Stem

Occurring at the same time as the lateral or posterior herniation of the temporal lobe, there is a downward shift of the entire brain stem toward the foramen magnum, and much of the disturbance of consciousness mentioned under lateral tentorial herniation may in fact be due to this axial displacement. It has been clearly shown that during this process stretching and elongation of the central perforating brain stem branches of the basilar artery occur, both because the brain stem migrates downward more than does the parent basilar artery and because the brain stem is enlarged in its anteroposterior diameter.[86,112] This stretching and narrowing of the vessels produces ischemia and hemorrhage, or hemorrhage can occur when the displacement is reversed by operative decompression.[125,126] It appears most likely that the brain stem lesions are arterial in origin rather than venous as was thought earlier.[188]

The cardiorespiratory features of brain

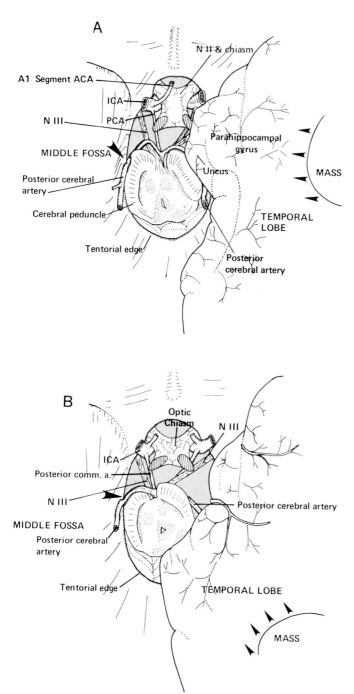

Figure 57–6 *A.* Anterior lateral herniation. Uncus and parahippocampal gyrus are compressing the right cerebral peduncle, and the third cranial nerve (N III) is kinked and stretched, giving rise to ipsilateral (to mass) dilated pupil and contralateral hemiparesis. If process occurs with the proper vectors, the contralateral peduncle ("Kernohan's notch") will be compressed or the contralateral third nerve will be stretched, or there may be any combination of these. These clinical signs will therefore be unreliable indicators of the laterality of a mass lesion, though the dilated pupil will be ipsilateral to the mass in about 85 per cent of cases. The posterior cerebral artery may be kinked or compressed (*arrow*) on either side (though usually this will be ipsilateral to the mass as well), giving rise to ischemic infarction in the area of the posterior communicating artery (PCA). *B.* Posterior lateral herniation. Essentially same type of phenomena may occur when the mass imposes a more posterior vector and the temporal lobe herniates against the collicular plate. This may result in Parinaud's syndrome with paralysis of upward gaze. Peduncular compression is not usually as marked, but this may also occur as well as posterior cerebral artery compression. N II, second cranial nerve; ACA, anterior cerebral artery; ICA, internal carotid artery.

compression, arterial hypertension, bradycardia, and respiratory irregularity are also linked to lesions or disorders in the brain stem, and it is tempting to postulate that the Cushing response is always mediated through local brain stem ischemia as originally proposed by Cushing.[41] The work of Hoff and Reis and of Thompson and Malina, however, suggests that mechanical distortion of the lower brain stem can also be invoked as an explanation.[93,247] Furthermore, Rowan and Teasdale have shown during experimental brain compression that at the point at which the Cushing response occurs, brain stem blood flow, which they measured directly, is not decreased.[222]

Downward displacement of the brain stem also produces traction on the oculomotor nerves, so attempts to delineate completely the clinical features of lateral, posterior, and central tentorial herniation cannot be pursued too far.

Tonsillar Herniation

When supratentorial compression continues unchecked or when the expanding mass is situated below the tentorium, tonsillar herniation follows, in which the cerebellar tonsils prolapse through the foramen magnum, obliterating the cisterna magna and compressing the medulla oblongata, with resultant apnea (Fig. 57–7). The readiness with which tonsillar herniation follows a supratentorial lesion is related to the shape and size of the tentorial opening. When the tentorial opening is small, signs of tentorial herniation predominate, and the patient may in a sense be protected against tonsillar herniation. When the tentorial opening is large and when the tentorium itself can be displaced downward, tonsillar herniation may occur with little warning sign of tentorial herniation. This possibility is one reason why section of the tentorium is not recommended in cases of expanding supratentorial lesions, as any subsequent temporal lobe swelling may result in apnea with little or no warning.[106]

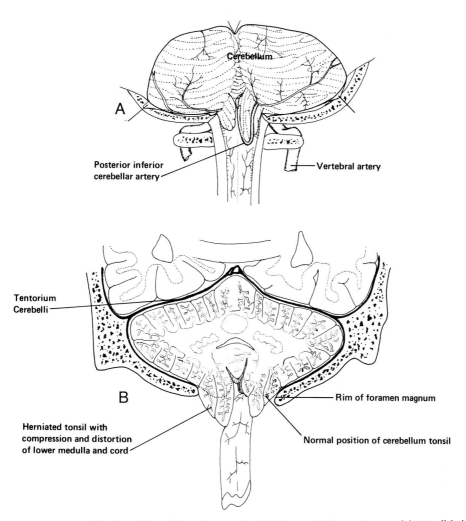

Figure 57–7 *A.* Tonsillar herniation. Note the posterior inferior cerebellar artery on right tonsil being depressed to level of C1. Angiographically, appearance of the posterior inferior cerebellar artery at this level is *abnormal* in 80 to 90 per cent of cases, and when accompanied by tonsillar branches is always abnormal and indicative of tonsillar herniation. *B.* Cross section showing normal position of tonsils and compression of lower medulla and upper cervical cord.

Raised Intracranial Pressure

It has been widely held for many years that cerebral trauma was associated with high intracranial pressure, despite some opinions to the contrary.[21,31,45,50] With the introduction of continuous monitoring of intraventricular pressure and other techniques for measuring supratentorial pressure continuously over periods of hours or days, many reports attest to the frequency with which considerable elevations of intracranial pressure occur and also clearly indicate some patients with severe brain dysfunction in whom increased intracranial pressure is not a factor.* In the course of these and of many experimental studies, the subtleties involved in the phenomena of intracranial hypertension as related to many different aspects of brain injury and the mechanisms by which intracranial hypertension interferes with brain function have become recognized.[130,132,173] Discussion of this topic is dealt with under three broad headings: causes of intracranial hypertension in head injury, relationships between intracranial pressure and brain shift and herniation, and relationships between intracranial pressure, cerebral blood flow, and neurological function in brain trauma.

Causes of Intracranial Hypertension in Head Injury

Raised intracranial pressure is the rule in patients with acute mass lesions complicating head injury (epidural and subdural hematoma or contusion and swelling), and as many as 30 per cent of patients with diffuse brain damage also have unequivocal intracranial hypertension (Fig. 57–8). Even after artificial ventilation or operative decompression or both, elevated intracranial pressure still remains a problem in many patients, requiring further therapy—in 50 per cent of those with mass lesions and in 33 per cent of those with diffuse brain injury.[185] It has long been customary to think of the possible causes of intracranial hypertension in head injury in terms of volume perturbations of the craniospinal axis—the volume of blood in a hematoma or

* See references 113, 116, 150, 185, 201, 248, 251, 253.

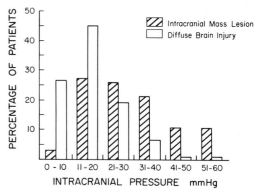

Figure 57–8 Distribution of intracranial pressure levels recorded on admission in 160 patients with severe head injury (62 patients with intracranial mass lesions requiring operative removal or decompression and 98 patients with diffuse brain injury). (From Miller, J. D., Becker, D. P., Ward, J. D., Sullivan, H. G., Adams, W. E., and Rosner, M. J.: Significance of intracranial hypertension in severe head injury. J. Neurosurg., 47:503–516, 1977. Reprinted by permission.)

contained in distended veins in the congested swollen brain, the volume of extracellular fluid in brain edema around a contusion, or the volume of swollen cells in areas of ischemic or traumatic necrosis. In this scheme, based on the modified Monro-Kellie doctrine, a certain amount of accommodating volume can be displaced—in the form of cerebrospinal fluid into the spinal compartment and venous blood to the extracranial space and away from the spinal epidural veins—to accommodate the increase in spinal intradural cerebrospinal fluid volume. Pathological volume increases should not at first cause any increase in intracranial pressure, but as the fluid available for compensatory displacement of volume becomes exhausted, intracranial pressure would begin to rise, slowly at first, then more and more rapidly as decompensation continues.[130] As pressure increases, however, the extent to which it rises depends not only on volume changes but also on the elastic properties of the brain, which transduce changes in volume into changes in pressure. Some of the factors that produce relative alterations in intracranial volumes also influence the elastic properties of the brain. Changes in the elastic properties of the brain have the effect of altering the gradient of the steeply ascending portion of the pressure-volume curve. When intracranial pressure is already increased, a rise in blood pressure makes the brain "stiffer" and the pressure-volume curve even steeper, while a fall in blood pressure at this stage will flatten the curve by making the brain less stiff. Under favorable circumstances (e.g., peritumoral edema) steroids and mannitol flatten the curve so that alterations in cerebrospinal fluid volume now produce smaller changes in its pressure.[173]

This concept of intracranial pressure-volume dynamics is still insufficient to explain certain observations, notably the fact that when intracranial pressure is extremely high, changes in cerebrospinal fluid volume may cause little change in pressure, while volume added to an intracranial mass lesion may still cause a sharp elevation in pressure.[135,178,237,238]

It is important to recognize that the pressure-volume characteristics of the cerebrospinal fluid space are likely to be different from those of other compartments or of the craniospinal axis as a whole. In the cerebrospinal fluid space, pressure-volume relationships must take into account the inflow, outflow, and total volume of the fluid as well as the properties of the boundaries of its space. The second major consideration is that the starting point for the cerebrospinal fluid pressure-volume curve is not fixed but depends at any time on the equilibrium volume of the fluid, that volume at which inflow and outflow precisely match when intracranial pressure is at "resting" level. To explain intracranial pressure-volume relationships one must therefore envisage a cerebrospinal fluid pressure-volume curve that not only may alter in gradient but may also shift in its entirety, moving to the left on the volume axis as cerebrospinal fluid equilibrium volume decreases, as for example during the steady expansion of an intracranial mass lesion when ventricles and subarachnoid space diminish in size (Fig. 57–9). Thus, a mass lesion with surrounding edema will present a challenge to the craniospinal axis and the regulation of the pressure within it, in several ways. The eventual intracranial pressure will be determined by many factors. Among them are the volume of the mass lesion, changes in the outflow resistance of the cerebrospinal fluid and the volume, and distribution of its intracranial spaces (ventricular and subarachnoid), and the change in the stress-strain properties of brain tissue itself, which is compacted in some areas and expanded by extracellular fluid or distended cells in others. Also influencing the intracranial pressure are the effects of changes in arterial and intracranial pressure on the intravascular pressures within the cerebral vascular network, which can be considered as a scaffolding within the brain, which may greatly modify its elastic properties (Fig. 57–10).[135–137,238]

There are many potential causes of altered intracranial pressure in patients with head injury. Mass lesions (hematoma, swollen contusion) decrease equilibrium cerebrospinal fluid volume, increase brain stiffness, and may impede outflow of cerebrospinal fluid. Several factors act by their effect on the cerebral vascular bed: alterations in blood gases, local cerebral metabolism, blood pressure, intrathoracic pressure, body and neck position, arousal of consciousness, and changes in body temperature. These factors also will alter both cerebrospinal fluid equilibrium volume and brain stiffness. When it is considered that the size of the stimulus will vary, that the

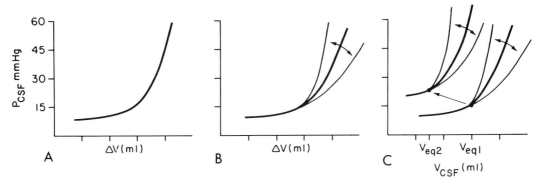

Figure 57–9 Evolving concepts of intracranial pressure-volume relationships. *A.* Single fixed pressure-volume curve. *B.* Inflection in the curve as produced by changes in blood pressure, steroids, mannitol. *C.* A series of possible curves, each originating at a set cerebrospinal fluid equilibrium volume and each capable of inflection.

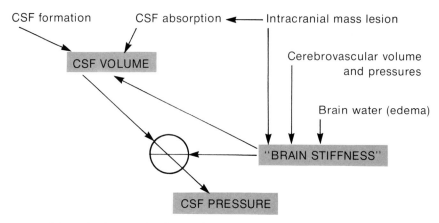

Figure 57–10 Schematic diagram showing the interaction between cerebrospinal fluid (CSF) volume and "brain stiffness" in determining intracranial pressure.

response in terms of change in intravascular pressure or volume will vary, and that the change in stiffness of the brain will also vary, then it is clear that a wide range of changes in intracranial pressure can be expected in patients with head injury. Indeed, this proves to be the case. It is believed that the most rapid variations in intracranial pressure, the various types of pressure wave and particularly the brief, sharply peaked B waves, are due to vascular phenomena.[149] Slower trends of increasing intracranial pressure, on which such rapid variations may be superimposed, are more often due to hematoma formation or re-collection, to increasing brain edema, or to developing hydrocephalus.[173]

As the systems by which normal intracranial pressure is maintained come under stress from the protean changes set in motion by the brain injury, it becomes important to try to assess the capacity of the craniospinal system to tolerate further stress. Approaches to this issue have been made by Shulman and Marmarou and by Miller and his colleagues in which low-volume bolus injections are made into the ventricular system and measurements made of the immediate change in cerebrospinal fluid pressure and its return to resting levels.[160, 161,178,179,229] In this way it is possible to assess the elastic properties of the brain surrounding the lateral ventricles. In addition, Marmarou has developed equations for deriving cerebrospinal fluid outflow resistance from the rate of the fall in pressure. It has been shown that intracranial mass lesions affect the cerebrospinal fluid pres-

sure-volume relationship, but that alterations in arterial pressure affect it only when intracranial pressure is elevated, confirming experimental data on intracranial pressure-volume relationships reported by Löfgren and his colleagues.[145–148] This field of investigation is continuing and promises to yield more information on the relative roles of alterations in cerebrospinal fluid dynamics versus cerebrovascular changes in the genesis of intracranial hypertension in patients with head injury.

Intracranial Pressure and Brain Herniation

As has been implied earlier, many of the neurological signs attributed to increased intracranial pressure—headache, vomiting, drowsiness, bradycardia, arterial hypertension, and irregular respiration—are likely to be due to brain stem shift or distortion. Thus, it is important to try to relate increased intracranial pressure to brain distortion and herniation rather than to any particular neurological symptom or sign.

Brain herniation at the tentorial or foramen magnum level clearly has an influence on intracranial pressure in that there is loss of the free transmission of pressure between the cranial and spinal compartments.[119,133,134] In addition, since the distribution of the compliance of the entire craniospinal axis is 50 per cent supratentorial, 20 per cent infratentorial, and 30 per cent spinal, it may be expected that when tentorial herniation occurs secondary to a supratentorial mass lesion, compliance would decrease and the pressure-volume curve in the supratentorial compartment would become much steeper.[146,160,200]

The next question to consider is the role of intracranial pressure in the genesis or augmentation of brain shift. It has generally been assumed that shift and distortion of the brain result from pressure gradients in which the pressure in the expanding mass is higher than the pressure in the yielding brain.[20,27] Similarly, the factor responsible for the spread of edema through the brain has been thought of as a gradient of tissue pressure down which the edema front moves.[162,218] In practice, however, it has been difficult to demonstrate these differences in tissue pressure in adjacent areas of brain; they tend to be small (<10 mm of mercury) and present *only* when there is a constant generation of volume expansion in the mass lesion.[115,218,230] There is no doubt, however, about the establishment of large pressure gradients across the tentorium and foramen magnum. Fitch and McDowall have shown that when this pressure gradient has developed, but before telltale pupillary changes have occurred, halothane-induced cerebral vasodilatation produces a much greater increase in intracranial pressure above the tentorium than below it, with increase in the magnitude of the gradient and onset of pupillary dilatation presumably indicating increased tentorial herniation.[60] This has also been seen during hypercapnia.[174] It appears, therefore, that changes in neurological status that are apparently associated with alterations in intracranial pressure are in fact mediated by the influence of intracranial pressure on brain shift. This relationship would explain the paucity of neurological signs despite severely elevated pressures that are seen in patients with benign intracranial hypertension, a condition in which brain shift does not occur.[114]

Intracranial Pressure and Cerebral Blood Flow

Another way in which intracranial pressure may affect neurological function is by increasing to the extent that it becomes a factor limiting cerebral blood flow. This is most obvious in those critically ill patients in whom angiography shows nonfilling of the intracranial portion of the internal carotid artery.[10,88,97,131,252] In such patients, it is thought that the intracranial pressure has attained the level of arterial pressure, with the result that cerebral perfusion pressure has fallen to zero. In some cases of angiographic nonfilling, however, measurement of intracranial pressure has shown it to be below the level of arterial pressure.[176] In these cases, it is possible that intracranial pressure has previously been sufficiently high to arrest the cerebral circulation and that blood flow has subsequently failed to restart despite the re-establishment of adequate perfusion pressure.[7,89,165]

These are extreme problems, however, and in most patients with head injury neurological and neurophysiological dysfunction becomes markedly more frequent when the intracranial pressure is persistently over 40 mm of mercury.[69] It is clear now that an important link between intracranial pressure and brain function is the level of cerebral blood flow. Under controlled experimental conditions, if cerebral blood flow can be maintained, intracranial hypertension causes no impairment of cortical neurophysiological function up to intracranial pressure levels of 50 mm of mercury and more. If the cerebral blood flow decreases, then lesser degrees of intracranial hypertension impair cortical electrical activity and it fails altogether when the flow falls below 40 per cent of normal.[74,246] This relationship of neuronal function and perfusion pressure may form the basis for the sudden neurological deterioration that can occur precipitately in patients with no brain shift or mass lesion when intracranial pressure rises over 30 or 40 mm of mercury.[12]

The extent to which increases in intracranial pressure will decrease cerebral blood flow depends on several factors: local and general levels of the cerebral rate of oxygen metabolism ($CMRO_2$), arterial pressure, impairment of autoregulation on a general or focal basis, and the presence of brain edema (Fig. 57–11). Any or all of these factors may operate in head injury. In experimental models of intracranial hypertension, a progressive pattern of disordered function can be discerned, in which cerebral blood flow first remains relatively constant despite rising intracranial pressure until the difference between arterial and intracranial pressures is reduced to 40 mm of mercury. Further increases in intracranial pressure then cause a sharp decrease in cerebral

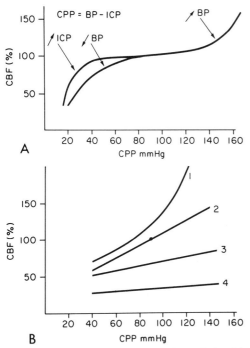

Figure 57-11 A concept of the relationship between cerebral perfusion pressure (CPP) and cerebral blood flow (CBF) in which cerebral perfusion pressure is the difference between mean arterial (BP) and mean intracranial pressures (ICP). *A*. The normal autoregulatory curve. *B*. A series of abnormalities associated with impaired autoregulatory function. 1, Hyperemia with complete absence of autoregulatory function; 2, impaired autoregulation but normal cerebral blood flow at a normal perfusion pressure; 3 and 4, impaired autoregulation in addition to moderately and severely reduced cerebral blood flow.

blood flow.[79,117,118,242] This maintenance of cerebral blood flow despite rising intracranial pressure is a form of autoregulation, since when autoregulation in response to changing arterial pressure is impaired, increases in intracranial pressure then cause a perfusion pressure–passive reduction in blood flow.[180,181] If arterial pressure is deliberately increased, then cerebral blood flow should increase under these circumstances because cerebral perfusion pressure rises. Impaired autoregulation is commonly observed in many forms of brain insult, including local trauma and hypoxia, both of which occur in patients with head injury. Sometimes an increase in arterial pressure is accompanied by a parallel increase in intracranial pressure. In such a case cerebral perfusion pressure does not change and cerebral blood flow would not be expected to change either.

When cerebral edema is present the picture becomes more complex; cerebral blood flow decreases as brain water content rises even before intracranial pressure is increased, and any subsequent reduction in cerebral perfusion pressure will further reduce the already low blood flow.[166] In this circumstance it has been observed that induced increases in cerebral perfusion pressure produced either by elevating arterial pressure or reducing intracranial pressure fail to restore the reduced cerebral blood flow.[24,183,184] Furthermore, even when cerebral edema is unilateral there may be reduction of cerebral blood flow in the opposite, and nonedematous hemisphere.[61,162,184]

As an accompaniment of dysregulation of cerebral blood flow response to changes in blood pressure and intracranial pressure, it is common to find a decrease in the cerebral vasodilator response to carbon dioxide, although complete absence of this response is found only in severe intracranial hypertension when intracranial pressure is near the level of arterial pressure.[81,182] When vasoreactivity to carbon dioxide changes is impaired, the vascular responses to hypoxia and hyperoxia are similarly affected. Finally, any or all of these disorders of cerebral blood flow and its regulation may be present throughout the brain or limited to a defined region, depending on the location, extent, and nature of the insult inflicted on the brain.[24,52,184,217]

Only in experimental animals is it possible to dissect and control variables so as to shed light on the disorders of cerebral blood flow that may follow head injury and to determine which are attributable to increased intracranial pressure and which result from other factors. In patients with head injury, many important factors may be operating simultaneously, and most of the understanding and interpretation of cerebral blood flow studies in patients has come from controlled animal studies in which one component of head injury at a time, e.g., raised intracranial pressure or brain edema, has been studied.

It should come as no surprise, therefore, that a wide range of cerebral blood flow levels should have been found in clinical studies of head injury together with a variety of disorders of its regulation, and that the relationship between cerebral blood flow and intracranial pressure should have appeared somewhat capricious.[24,52] Despite the variety of abnormalities seen, certain common themes occur. In deeply comatose patients cerebral blood flow and the rate of oxygen metabolism are both low because the cerebral arteriovenous oxygen content difference does not increase as flow decreases. When intracranial pressure is over 40 mm of mercury, cerebral blood flow is below normal in virtually all cases.[24] It usually does not increase generally, however, when intracranial pressure is abruptly lowered by drainage of cerebrospinal fluid. Administration of intravenous mannitol tends to increase cerebral blood flow, even if intracranial pressure is not much reduced. If arterial pressure is reduced blood flow reductions are common, especially in the frontal and temporal areas. Elevation of arterial pressure increases blood flow in some areas and produces no change in flow in others in a most variable way. Impairment of the cerebrovascular response to elevation of arterial carbon dioxide tension is common, but complete absence of this response is very rare, even in isolated regions of the brain. The occurrence of both low (<25 ml per 100 gm per minute) and high (>70 ml per 100 gm per minute) levels of mean flow in the brain is associated with a poor outcome from the head injury.[9,24,52,66,121]

ISCHEMIC BRAIN DAMAGE AFTER HEAD INJURY

Areas of ischemic necrosis are a common finding in the brains of patients who die from head injury.* In the foregoing sections several pathological processes have been alluded to, each of which may produce well-defined focal cerebral ischemia: brain shift producing lesions in the anterior or posterior cerebral artery territories by distortion of those vessels during supracallosal and lateral tentorial herniation respectively, brain stem ischemic lesions and hemorrhages resulting from traction on central perforating arteries, extensive cerebral ischemia produced by severe intracranial hypertension or by failure of arterial pressure to maintain an adequate pressure differential between itself and increased intracranial pressure, and ischemia produced by brain edema.

---

* See references 1, 62, 68, 90, 140, 143, 260.

Even this variety of possible mechanisms is unable to explain all forms of cerebral ischemia found after fatal head injury. Jellinger and Seitelberger have emphasized the occurrence of brain ischemia in those patients who remain severely disabled or vegetative for long periods after head injury, but Graham and Adams have placed the incidence of post-traumatic brain ischemia in better perspective by their detailed study of 100 consecutive fatal head injuries.[1,68,104,109] In these cases ischemic foci were seen in the cerebral cortex in 46 per cent of cases. These cortical lesions were seen in boundary zones between arterial territories of distribution (usually only between anterior and middle cerebral areas) in more than half these cases, and in the remainder the cortical ischemia was squarely situated in the territory of supply of a major intracranial artery. Ischemic foci were even more common in the basal ganglia and in the hippocampus (80 per cent). In the cerebellum the most striking changes seen consisted of loss of Purkinje cells and were, like some of the pathological hippocampal changes, identical with the changes produced by hypoxemia. Boundary zone infarction was rarely seen in the cerebella of patients with head injury.

After an extensive search for causal factors these authors were unable to incriminate proximal carotid artery stenosis or occlusion or changes in arterial oxygen tension or blood pressure.[68,109] Raised intracranial pressure had been present in many of these patients, but in contrast to the close association between raised intracranial pressure and the neuropathological telltales of brain shift and herniation (scars in the cingulate and hippocampal gyri), the link between intracranial pressure and brain ischemia was not close.[3] Other factors have to be searched for, and in the end, the determinants of focal brain ischemia may be a complex multifactor interaction.

Lindenberg has proposed that focal cerebral ischemia is due to compression of small arteries by raised intracranial pressure, but such an explanation does not account for ischemic lesions in patients who have not suffered intracranial hypertension and runs counter to present theories on the relationships between cerebral perfusion pressure and cerebral blood flow.[143] Boundary zone infarction has been clearly linked to severe arterial hypotension and profound cerebral ischemia—as seen in the person who faints in the upright position.[4,16] At these low levels of blood pressure, cerebral blood flow falls below the 40 per cent level required to maintain consciousness, neurophysiological function, and cellular integrity.[59] What is not clear is whether increased intracranial pressure in the patient with head injury can be regarded in exactly the same way as reduced arterial pressure as a factor reducing perfusion pressure. In simple animal models intracranial hypertension causes less reduction in cerebral blood flow than do equivalent decreases in blood pressure.[180,181] One explanation has been that the sympathetic vasoconstriction of larger vessels leading to the brain that accompanies hemorrhagic hypotension is absent during intracranial hypertension.[82] When the brain is damaged, impairment of autoregulation of cerebral blood flow in response to reduced arterial pressure is common.[24,52] Since this autoregulatory mechanism also preserves blood flow in the face of rising intracranial pressure, failure of this mechanism may explain reduced flow in damaged brain with only modest increases in intracranial pressure. The occurrence of brain edema will further reduce blood flow in these affected areas even before intracranial pressure is elevated and even in distant areas.[162,166,184]

A further mechanism for the production of focal brain ischemia in patients with head injury is arterial spasm.[259] In the context of subarachnoid hemorrhage, close correlation between neurological status, cerebral blood flow, and the presence of vascular spasm has been found only in cases of very severe spasm.[57] In a survey of carotid arteriograms performed in a group of 33 patients with head injury who were subsequently demonstrated at autopsy to have ischemic brain damage to the cortex in 42 per cent of cases and in basal ganglia and white matter in 90 per cent, Macpherson and Graham found a 57 per cent incidence of cerebral arterial spasm. There was a positive correlation between cortical ischemia and angiographic spasm. There was no correlation between spasm and other ischemic damage, nor was there a relationship between angiographic slowing, seen also in 57 per cent of cases, and ischemic damage.[157] Farrar and Roach have proposed that the crucial linking factor between vas-

cular spasm and symptomatic ischemia is the extravascular pressure in the brain, intracranial pressure that reduces cerebral arterial transmural pressure.[55] This pressure, combined with spasm, can dramatically reduce flow in affected vessels.

When such changes are considered together with reduced arterial pressure and hypoxemia, which can also threaten the patient with head injury, there clearly are many ways in which head trauma may be followed by brain ischemia. Several of these can, however, be favorably influenced by optimal management of the patient after injury, so it is crucial for the care of the patient that these mechanisms be understood and their effects anticipated.

OTHER CAUSES OF SECONDARY CEREBRAL DAMAGE

Hypoxemia, Hypoglycemia, Epilepsy

There is a considerable overlap in the neuropathological consequences of hypoxemia, hypoglycemia, epilepsy, and profound systemic arterial hypotension, even in animal models in which the physiological conditions have been rigorously controlled.[14,15,170] Detectable damage occurs in the neocortex, involving primarily the small pyramidal neurons in the third, fifth, and sixth layers, and it is concentrated at the boundary zones between adjacent arterial territories of distribution. Damage is also detectable in the basal ganglia, the hippocampus, in the Sommer sector of Ammon's horn, and in the Purkinje cells of the cerebellar cortex, again being most pronounced in the watershed between the superior cerebellar and posterior inferior cerebellar arterial distribution. This differs from the neuropathological sequelae of total cerebral circulatory arrest in the boundary zone, as opposed to diffuse, distribution of lesions. These areas of predilection are probably based as much on the greater metabolic demands of the cells in question as on physiological or anatomical factors related to blood supply; epilepsy produces general increases in cerebral metabolic rate and blood flow, and hypoxia increases cerebral blood flow also, but presumably not enough in the areas of damage.[151,172,207] At the cellular level, all these insults produce a progressive sequence of neuronal damage starting with cytoplasmic microvacuolation as mitochondria disintegrate and proceeding through loss of cellular detail, increasing density of the nucleus with loss of cytoplasm, microglial proliferation, and neuronophagia.[16,232] Ultrastructural studies suggest that the very earliest changes may affect the nucleus and nucleolus.[105]

Any or all of these insults can easily be visualized as adding to the degree and extent of cerebral cellular dysfunction and damage that follows head injury. In addition, hypoxemia and epilepsy, especially when accompanied by paroxysmal arterial hypertension, may increase intracranial pressure and may lead to worsening of brain swelling and brain shift.

Hyperpyrexia

Initial enthusiasm for hypothermia as a method for managing brain damage and intracranial hypertension has become much more cautious, but it has become clear that increases in body temperature, even before they reach the stage of severe hyperpyrexia, are deleterious. Increases in body temperature increase the rate and extent of spread of edema, probably by increasing cerebral metabolic rate with vasodilatation, which will also increase intracranial pressure.[35,193] At levels over 40°C neuronal damage begins to occur in the cerebellum, Purkinje cells drop out, and it may well be that cerebral blood flow is unable to increase sufficiently to meet increased cellular demand so that a relative hypoxia is produced.

Meningitis

One of the most devastating secondary insults that can affect the patient with a severe head injury is the development of meningitis.[175] It is not exactly clear why the brain damage and dysfunction should be so severe in such a short time. Even severe vascular damage on the surface of the brain does not seem adequate to explain the profound neurological deterioration that can occur. Cerebral blood flow and oxygen metabolism are both reduced, more in pneumococcal meningitis and encephalitis than in meningococcal meningitis, while focal variations in cerebral blood flow are more common in encephalitis.[202] Again, the final basis may be hypoxic damage.

Meningitis following head injury may be a consequence of basal skull fracture with tearing of the dura and can supervene even in cases in which there has been neither an aerocele nor cerebrospinal fluid rhinorrhea, or in which this has occurred and then resolved. Infection may also result from penetrating injury and following craniotomy or ventricular puncture for intracranial pressure monitoring or cerebrospinal fluid drainage.[175] In unconscious patients the diagnosis is often not made until the patient is already moribund, so the mortality rate continues to be high, despite the use of antibiotics.

Later consequences of meningitis, discussed elsewhere, are epilepsy and impairment of cerebrospinal fluid absorption resulting in post-traumatic hydrocephalus.

CONCLUSION

In this chapter emphasis has been placed on the concept that in those patients who reach the hospital alive after head injury, a considerable degree of recovery usually is possible; it is, however, influenced by the degree and extent of primary brain damage and pre-existing brain function. Also several different pathological processes are set in motion from the time of injury, any and all of which can increase brain damage and dysfunction and reduce the extent of functional recovery.

Much of the understanding of the secondary pathological processes that follow head injury has been gathered from experimental models and from study of the brains of those patients who die. This poses certain problems; for example, is ischemic brain damage equally common in patients who survive severe brain trauma? The solution to questions like these is to study patients with head injury in depth, using appropriate diagnostic aids that are now available. Only in this way will the understanding of these vitally important secondary processes during life improve.

Acknowledgment. This work was supported in part by NIH Grant No. 1 P50 NS 12587.

REFERENCES

1. Adams, J. H.: The neuropathology of head injuries. *In* Vinken, P. J., and Bruyn, G. W., eds.: Handbook of Clinical Neurology. Vol. 23, Injuries of the Brain and Skull Part I. Amsterdam, Elsevier–North Holland Publishing Co., 1975, pp. 35–65.

2. Adams, H., and Graham, D. I.: The pathology of blunt head injuries. *In* Critchley, M., O'Leary, J. L., and Jennett, B., eds.: Scientific Foundations of Neurology. London, William Heinemann, Ltd., 1972, pp. 478–491.

3. Adams, J. H., and Graham, D. I.: The relationship between ventricular fluid pressure and neuropathology of raised intracranial pressure. Neuropath. Appl. Neurobiol., 2:323–332, 1976.

4. Adams, J. H., Brierley, J. B., Connor, R. C. R., and Treip, C. S.: The effects of systemic hypotension on the human brain. Brain, 89:235–268, 1966.

5. Adams, J. H., Mitchell, D. E., Graham, D. I., and Doyle, D.: Diffuse brain damage of immediate impact type. Its relationship to "primary brain stem damage" in head injury. Brain, 100:489–502, 1977.

6. Adams, W. E., Hadfield, M. G., Becker, D. P., and Rigby, W. F. C.: Functional alterations of traumatized synaptosomes. *In* McLaurin, R. L., ed.: Head Injuries: Proceedings of the Second Chicago Symposium on Neural Trauma. New York, Grune & Stratton Inc., 1976, pp. 225–228.

7. Ames, A., Wright, F. L., Kowada, M., Thurston, J. M., and Majno, G.: Cerebral ischemia. II. The no-reflow phenomenon. Amer. J. Path., 52:437–453, 1968.

8. Apfelbaum, R. I., Guthkelch, A. N., and Shulman, K.: Experimental production of subdural hematomas. J. Neurosurg., 40:336–346, 1974.

9. Baldy-Moulinier, M., and Frerebeau, P.: Cerebral blood flow in cases of coma following severe head injury. *In* Brock, M., Fieschi, C., Ingvar, D. H., Lassen, N. A., and Schürmann, K., eds.: Cerebral Blood Flow. Berlin, Springer-Verlag, 1969, pp. 216–218.

10. Balslev-Jorgensen, P., Heilbrun, M. P., Boysen, G., Rosenklint, A., and Jorgensen, E. O.: Cerebral perfusion pressure correlated with regional cerebral blood flow, and aorto-cervical arteriography in patients with severe brain disorders progressing to death. Europ. Neurol., 8:207–212, 1972.

11. Barnett, J. C., and Mierowsky, A. M.: Intracranial haematomas associated with penetrating wounds of the brain. J. Neurosurg., 12:34–38, 1955.

12. Becker, D. P., in discussion of Miller, J. D.: Clinical aspects of intracranial pressure-volume relationships. *In* McLaurin, R. L., ed.: Head Injuries: Second Chicago Symposium on Neural Trauma. New York, Grune & Stratton Inc., 1976, pp. 247–248.

13. Bhandari, Y. S., and Sarkari, N. B. S.: Subdural empyema. A review of 37 cases. J. Neurosurg., 32:35–39, 1970.

14. Brierley, J. B.: Comparison between effects of profound arterial hypotension, hypoxia and cyanide on the brain of Macaca mulatta. Advances Neurol., 10:213–221, 1975.

15. Brierley, J. B., Brown, A. W., and Meldrum, B. J.: The nature and time course of the neuronal alterations resulting from oligaemia and hypoglycaemia in the brain of Macaca mulatta. Brain Res., 25:483–499, 1971.

16. Brierley, J. B., Brown, A. W., Excell, B. J., and Meldrum, B. S.: Brain damage in the rhesus monkey resulting from profound arterial hypotension. Brain Res., 13:68–100, 1969.

17. Brightman, M. W., and Reece, T. S.: Junctions between intimately opposed cell membranes in the vertebral brain. J. Cell Biol., 40:648–677, 1969.

18. Brightman, M. W., and Robinson, J. S.: Some attempts to open the blood-brain barrier to protein. *In* McLaurin, R. L., ed.: Head Injuries: Second Chicago Symposium on Neural Trauma. New York, Grune & Stratton Inc., 1976, pp. 107–113.

19. Brock, M.: Regional cerebral blood flow changes following local brain compression in the cat. Scand. J. Clin. Lab. Invest., 22:suppl. 102: 14:A, 1968.

20. Brock, M., Beck, J., Markakis, E., and Dietz, H.: Intracranial pressure gradients associated with experimental cerebral embolism. Stroke, 3:123–130, 1972.

21. Browder, J., and Meyers, R.: Observations on behavior of the systemic blood pressure, pulse and spinal fluid pressure following craniocerebral injury. Amer. J. Surg., 31:403–427, 1936.

22. Bruce, D. A., Schut, L., and Bruno, L. A.: The role of intracranial pressure monitoring in a pediatric intensive care unit. *In* Beks, J. W. F., Bosch, D. A., and Brock, M., eds.: Intracranial Pressure III. Berlin, Springer-Verlag, 1976, pp. 323–326.

23. Bruce, D. A., TerWeeme, C., Kaiser, G., and Langfitt, T. W.: The dynamics of small and large molecules in the extracellular space and cerebrospinal fluid following local cold injury of the cortex. *In* Pappius, H. M., and Feindel, W., eds.: Dynamics of Brain Edema. Berlin, Springer-Verlag, 1976, pp. 122–128.

24. Bruce, D. A., Langfitt, T. W., Miller, J. D., Shuz, H., Vapalahti, M. P., Stanek, A., and Goldberg, H. I.: Regional cerebral blood flow, intracranial pressure and brain metabolism in comatose patients. J. Neurosurg., 38:131–144, 1973.

25. Bucy, P. C., and Oberhill, H. R.: Subdural hematoma in adults. Arizona Med., 25:186–189, 1968.

26. Budzilovich, G. N.: On pathogenesis of primary lesions in blunt head trauma with special reference to the brain stem injuries. *In* McLaurin, R. L., ed.: Head Injuries: Second Chicago Symposium on Neural Trauma. New York, Grune & Stratton, Inc., 1976, pp. 39–43.

27. Cairns, H.: Raised intracranial pressure: hydrocephalic and vascular factors. Brit. J. Surg., 27:275–294, 1939.

28. Cairns, H.: Disturbances of consciousness with lesions of the brain stem and diencephalon. Brain, 75:109–146, 1952.

29. Cairns, H., Calvert, C. A., Daniel, P., and Northcroft, C. B.: Complications of head wounds with special reference to infection. Brit. J. Surg., War Surg. suppl. 1:198–243, 1947.

30. Campbell, E. H., Jr.: Compound comminuted skull fractures produced by missiles: Report of 100 cases. Ann. Surg., 122:375–397, 1945.

31. Cannon, W. B.: Cerebral pressure following trauma. Amer. J. Physiol., 6:91–121, 1901.

32. Carey, M. E., Chou, S. N., and French, L. S.: Experience with brain abscesses. J. Neurosurg., 36:1–9, 1972.

33. Carey, M. E., Young, H. F., Mathis, J. L., and Forsythe, J.: A bacteriological study of craniocerebral missile wounds from Vietnam. J. Neurosurg., 34:145–154, 1971.

34. Cassen, B., and Neff, R.: Blood brain barrier behavior during temporary concussion. Amer. J. Physiol., 198:1296–1298, 1960.

35. Clasen, R. A., Pandolfi, S., Laing, I., and Casey, D.: Experimental study of relation of fever to cerebral edema. J. Neurosurg., 41:576–581, 1974.

36. Cook, A. W., Browder, J. E., and Carter, W. B.: Cerebral swelling and ventricular alterations following evacuation of intracranial extracerebral hematoma. J. Neurosurg., 19:419–423, 1962.

37. Cooper, P. R., Rovit, R. L., and Ransohoff, J.: Hemicraniectomy in the treatment of acute subdural hematoma: A re-appraisal. Surg. Neurol., 5:25–29, 1976.

38. Corsellis, J. A. N.: Individual variation in the size of the tentorial opening. J. Neurol. Neurosurg. Psychiat., 21:279–283, 1958.

39. Crompton, M. R.: Brain stem lesions due to closed head injury. Lancet, 1:669–673, 1971.

40. Crompton, R. M., Teare, R. D., and Bowen, D. A. L.: Prolonged coma after head injury. Lancet, 2:938–940, 1966.

41. Cushing, H.: Concerning a definite regulatory mechanism of the vasomotor center which controls blood pressure during cerebral compression. Johns Hopkins Hosp. Bull., 12:290–292, 1901.

42. Cushing, H.: Notes on penetrating wounds of the brain. Brit. Med. J., 1:221–226, 1918.

43. Cushing, H.: A study of a series of wounds involving the brain and its enveloping structures. Brit. J. Surg., 5:558–684, 1918.

44. Cushing, H.: Peptic ulcers and the interbrain. Surg. Gynec. Obstet., 55:1, 1918.

45. Dandy, W. E.: Diagnosis and treatment of injuries of the head. J.A.M.A., 101:772–775, 1933.

46. Daniel, P. M., and Treip, C. S.: Lesions of the pituitary gland associated with head injuries. In Harris, G. W., and Donovan, B. T., eds.: The Pituitary Gland. Vol. 2. London, Butterworth & Co., Ltd., 1966, pp. 519–534.

47. Denny-Brown, D., and Russell, W. R.: Experimental cerebral concussion. Brain, 64:93–164, 1941.

48. Drew, J. H., and Fager, C. A.: Delayed brain abscess in relation to intracranial foreign bodies. J. Neurosurg., 11:386–393, 1954.

49. Ducker, T. B., Kempe, L. G., and Hayes, G. J.: The metabolic background for peripheral nerve surgery. J. Neurosurg., 30:270–280, 1969.

50. Duret, H.: Etudes expérimentales et cliniques sur les traumatismes cérébraux. Paris, 1878.

51. Ecker, A. D.: Tight dural closure with pedicled graft in wounds of the brain. J. Neurosurg., 2:384–390, 1945.

52. Enevoldsen, E. M., Cold, G., Jensen, F. T., and Malmros, R.: Dynamic changes in regional CBF, intraventricular pressure, CSF pH and lactate levels during the acute phase of head injury. J. Neurosurg., 44:191–214, 1976.

53. Evans, J. P., and Scheinker, I. M.: Histologic studies of brain following head trauma: Post-traumatic cerebral swelling and oedema. J. Neurosurg., 2:306–314, 1945.

54. Evans, J. P., and Scheinker, I. M.: Histologic studies of the brain following head trauma. VI. Post-traumatic central nervous system changes interpreted in terms of circulatory disturbances. Res. Publ. Ass. Res. Nerv. Ment. Dis., 24:254–273, 1945.

55. Farrar, J. K., and Roach, M. R.: The effects of raised intracranial pressure on flow through major cerebral arteries in vitro. Stroke, 4:795–806, 1973.

56. Fell, D. A., Fitzgerald, S., Moiel, R. H., and Caram, P.: Acute subdural hematomas: A review of 144 cases. J. Neurosurg., 42:27–42, 1975.

57. Ferguson, G. G., Harper, A. M., Fitch, W., Rowan, J. O., and Jennett, W. B.: Cerebral blood flow measurements after spontaneous subarachnoid haemorrhage. Europ. Neurol., 8:15–22, 1972.

58. Fink, R. P., and Heimer, L.: Two methods for selective silver impregnation of degenerating axons and their synaptic endings in the cerebral nervous system. Brain Res., 4:369–374, 1967.

59. Finnerty, F. A., Wilkin, L., and Fazekas, J. F.: Cerebral hemodynamics during cerebral ischemia induced by acute hypotension. J. Clin. Invest., 33:1227–1232, 1954.

60. Fitch, W., and McDowall, D. G.: Effect of halothane on intracranial pressure gradients in the presence of intracranial space-occupying lesions. Brit. J. Anaesth., 43:904–912, 1971.

61. Frei, H. J., Wallenfang, T., Pöll, W. Reulen, H. J., Schubert, R., and Brock, M.: Regional cerebral blood flow and regional metabolism in cold-induced edema. Acta Neurochir. (Wien), 29:15–28, 1973.

62. Freitag, E.: Autopsy findings in head injuries from blunt forces. Arch. Path. (Chicago), 75:402–413, 1963.

63. Galbraith, S. L.: Age distribution of extradural haemorrhage without skull fracture. Lancet, 1:1217–1218, 1973.

64. Gallagher, J. P., and Browder, E. J.: Extradural hematoma: Experience with 167 patients. J. Neurosurg., 29:1–12, 1968.

65. Gardner, J. W.: Traumatic subdural hematoma with particular reference to the latent interval. Arch. Neurol. Psychiat., 27:847–858, 1932.

66. Gobiet, W., Bock, W. J., Grote, W., and Bettag, M.: Cerebral blood flow in patients with traumatic cerebral edema. In Lundberg, N., Pon-

ten, V., and Brock, M., eds.: Intracranial Pressure II. Berlin, Springer-Verlag, 1975, pp. 508–511.

67. Goodel, C. L., and Mealey, J.: Pathogenesis of chronic subdural hematoma. Experimental studies. Arch. Neurol. (Chicago), 8:429–437, 1963.

68. Graham, D. I., and Adams, J. H.: Ischaemic brain damage in fatal head injuries. Lancet, 1:265–266, 1971.

69. Greenberg, R. P., Mayer, D. J., and Becker, D. P.: Correlation in man of intracranial pressure and neuroelectric activity determined by multimodality evoked potentials. In Beks, J. W. F., Bosch, D. A., and Brock, M., eds.: Intracranial Pressure III. Berlin, Springer-Verlag, 1976, pp. 58–62.

70. Greenberg, R. P., Becker, D. P., Miller, J. D., and Mayer, D. J.: Evaluation of brain function in severe human head trauma with multi-modality evoked potentials. Part II. Localization of brain dysfunction and correlation with posttraumatic neurological conditions. J. Neurosurg., 47:163–177, 1977.

71. Groat, R. A., Windle, W. F., and Magoun, H. W.: Functional and structural changes in the monkey's brain during and after concussion. J. Neurosurg., 2:26–35, 1945.

72. Grossman, R. G.: Alterations in the microphysiology of glial cells and neurones and the environment in the injured brain. Clin. Neurosurg., 19:69–83, 1972.

73. Grossman, R. G., and Seregin, A. I.: Effects of traumatically induced edema on membrane potentials of cortical glial cells and neurones. In McLaurin, R. L., ed.: Head Injuries: Second Chicago Symposium on Neural Trauma. New York, Grune & Stratton Inc., 1976, pp. 273–275.

74. Grossman, R. G., Turner, J. W., Miller, J. D., and Rowan, J. O.: The relationship between cortical electrical activity, cerebral perfusion pressure and cerebral blood flow during increased intracranial pressure. In Langfitt, T. W., McHenry, L. C., Reivich, M., and Wollman, H., eds.: Cerebral Circulation and Metabolism. Berlin, Springer-Verlag, 1975, pp. 232–234.

75. Gurdjian, E. S.: Recent advances in the study of the mechanism of impact injury of the head. A summary. Clin. Neurosurg., 19:1–42, 1972.

76. Gurdjian, E. S., and Thomas, L. M.: Traumatic intracranial hemorrhage. In Feiring, E. H., ed.: Brock's Injuries of the Brain and Spinal Cord and Their Coverings. 5th Ed. New York, Springer Publishing Co., 1974, pp. 203–267.

77. Gurdjian, E. S., Webster, J. E., and Lissner, H. R.: Observations on the mechanism of brain concussion, contusion and laceration. Surg. Gynec. Obstet., 101:680–690, 1955.

78. Guthkelch, A. N.: Apparently trivial wounds of the eyelids with intracranial damage. Brit. Med. J., 2:842–844, 1960.

79. Häggendal, E., Löfgren, J., Nilsson, N. J., and Zwetnow, N. N.: Effects of varied cerebrospinal fluid pressure on cerebral blood flow in dogs. Acta Physiol. Scand., 79:262–271, 1970.

80. Hammon, W. M.: Early complications following penetrating wounds of the brain from Vietnam. J. Neurosurg., 34:132–141, 1971.

81. Harper, A. M.: Autoregulation of cerebral blood flow: influence of arterial blood pressure on the blood flow through the cerebral cortex. J. Neurol. Neurosurg. Psychiat., 29:398–403, 1966.

82. Harper, A. M., Deshmukh, V. D., Rowan, J. O., and Jennett, W. B.: The influence of sympathetic nervous activity on cerebral blood flow. Arch. Neurol. (Chicago), 27:1–6, 1972.

83. Harris, P.: Craniospinal injuries. In Head Injuries: Proceedings of an International Symposium. Baltimore, Williams & Wilkins Co., 1971, pp. 42–46.

84. Harris, P.: Acute traumatic subdural hematomas: Results of neurosurgical care. In Head Injuries: Proceedings of an International Symposium. Baltimore, Williams & Wilkins Co., 1971, pp. 321–326.

85. Harsh, G. R.: Infection complicating penetrating craniocerebral trauma. In Coates, J. B., and Meirowsky, A. M., eds.: Neurological Surgery of Trauma. Washington, D.C., U.S. Govt. Printing Office, 1965, p. 135.

86. Hassler, O.: Arterial pattern of human brain stem normal appearance and deformation in expanding supratentorial conditions. Neurology (Minneap.), 17:368–375, 1967.

87. Haynes, W. G.: Penetrating brain wounds: Analysis of 342 cases. J. Neurosurg., 2:365–378, 1945.

88. Heiskanen, O.: Cerebral acute arrest caused by acute increase of intracranial pressure. Acta Neurol. Scand., 40:suppl. 7, 1964.

89. Hekmatpanah, J.: Cerebral circulation and perfusion in experimental increased intracranial pressure. J. Neurosurg., 32:21–29, 1970.

90. Helfand, M.: Cerebral lesions due to vasomotor disturbances following brain trauma. J. Nerv. Ment. Dis., 90:157–179, 1939.

91. Hitchcock, E., and Andreadis, A.: Subdural empyema: A review of 29 cases. J. Neurol. Neurosurg. Psychiat., 27:422–434, 1964.

92. Hochwald, G. M., Martin, A. E., Wald, A., and Malhan, C.: Movement of water between blood, brain and CSF in cerebral edema. In Pappius, H. M., and Feindel, W., eds.: Dynamics of Brain Edema. Berlin, Springer-Verlag, 1976, pp. 129–137.

93. Hoff, J. T., and Reis, D. J.: Localization of regions mediating the Cushing response in the central nervous system of the cat. Arch. Neurol. (Chicago), 22:228–240, 1970.

94. Hoff, J., Bates, E., Barnes, B., Glickman, M., and Margolis, T.: Traumatic subdural hygroma. J. Trauma, 13:870–876, 1973.

95. Holbourn, A. H. S.: Mechanisms of brain injuries. Lancet, 2:438–441, 1943.

96. Hooper, R.: Observations on extradural hemorrhage. Brit. J. Surg., 47:71–87, 1959.

97. Hunt, W. E., Meagher, J. N., Friemanis, A., and Rossel, C. W.: Angiographic studies of experimental intracranial hypertension. J. Neurosurg., 19:1023–1030, 1962.

98. Illingworth, G., and Jennett, W. B.: The shocked head injury. Lancet, 2:511–514, 1965.

99. Ishii, S., Hayner, R., Kelly, W. A., and Evans, J.

P.: Studies of cerebral swelling II: Experimental cerebral swelling produced by supratentorial extradural compression. J. Neurosurg., *16*:152–166, 1959.

100. Jamieson, K. G., and Yelland, J. D. N.: Extradural hematoma: Report of 167 cases. J. Neurosurg., *29*:13–23, 1968.

101. Jamieson, K. G., and Yelland, J. D. N.: Surgically treated traumatic subdural hematoma. J. Neurosurg., *37*:137–149, 1972.

102. Jefferson, G.: The tentorial pressure cone. Arch. Neurol. Psychiat., *40*:857–876, 1938.

103. Jefferson, G.: Head wounds and infections in two wars. Brit. J. Surg., War Surg. suppl. 1:3–8, 1947.

104. Jellinger, K., and Seitelberger, F.: Protracted post-traumatic encephalopathy. *In* Walker, A. E., Caveness, W. F., and Critchley, M., eds.: The Late Effects of Head Injury. Springfield, Ill., Charles C Thomas, 1969, pp. 168–181.

105. Jenkins, L. W., Povlishock, J. T., Becker, D. P., Miller, J. D., and Sullivan, H. G.: Complete cerebral ischemia: An Ultrastructural study. Acta Neuropathol., *48*:113–125, 1979.

106. Jennett, W. B.: Experimental brain compression. Arch. Neurol. (Chicago), *4*:599–607, 1961.

107. Jennett, B., and Miller, J. D.: Infection after depressed fractures of skull: Implications for management of non-missile injuries. J. Neurosurg., *36*:333–339, 1972.

108. Jennett, W. B., and Stern, W. E.: Tentorial herniation, the midbrain and the pupil. J. Neurosurg., *17*:598–609, 1960.

109. Jennett, W. B., Graham, D. I., Adams, J. H., and Johnston, I. H.: Ischaemic brain damage after fatal blunt head injuries. *In* McDowell, F. H., and Brennan, R. W., eds.: Cerebral Vascular Diseases: Eighth Conference. New York, Grune & Stratton Inc., 1973, pp. 163–170.

110. Johnson, R. T.: Pattern of midbrain deformity in expanding intracranial lesions. *In* Williams, D., ed.: Modern Trends in Neurology: 2nd Series. London, Butterworth & Co., Ltd., 1957.

111. Johnson, R. T., and Yates, P. O.: A clinico-pathological aspect of pressure changes in the tentorium. Acta Radiol. (Stockholm), *46*:241–249, 1956.

112. Johnson, R. T., and Yates, P. O.: Brain stem haemorrhages in expanding supratentorial conditions. Acta Radiol. (Stockholm), *46*:250–256, 1956.

113. Johnston, I. H., and Jennett, W. B.: The place of continuous intracranial pressure monitoring in neurosurgical practice. Acta Neurochir. (Wien), *29*:53–63, 1973.

114. Johnston, I., and Paterson, A.: Benign intracranial hypertension. II. CSF pressure and circulation. Brain, *97*:301–312, 1974.

115. Johnston, I. H., and Rowan, J. O.: Raised intracranial pressure and cerebral blood flow. 4: Intracranial pressure gradients and regional cerebral blood flow. J. Neurol. Neurosurg. Psychiat., *37*:585–592, 1974.

116. Johnston, I. H., Johnston, J. J., and Jennett, W. B.: Intracranial pressures following head injury. Lancet, *2*:433–436, 1970.

117. Johnston, I. H., Rowan, J. O., Harper, A. M., and Jennett, W. B.: Raised intracranial pressure and cerebral blood flow. I. Cisterna magna infusion in primates. J. Neurol. Neurosurg. Psychiat., *35*:285–296, 1972.

118. Johnston, I. H., Rowan, J. O., Harper, A. M., and Jennett, W. B.: Raised intracranial pressure and cerebral blood flow. 2. Supratentorial and infratentorial mass lesions in primates. J. Neurol. Neurosurg. Psychiat., *36*:161–170, 1973.

119. Kaufmann, G. E., and Clark, K.: Continuous simultaneous monitoring of intraventricular and cervical subarachnoid cerebrospinal fluid pressure to indicate the development of cerebral or tonsillar herniation. J. Neurosurg., *33*:145–150, 1970.

120. Keith, W. S.: Subdural empyema. J. Neurosurg., *6*:127–139, 1949.

121. Kelly, P. J., Iwata, K., McGraw, C. P., and Tindall, G. T.: Intracranial pressure, cerebral blood flow and prognosis in patients with severe head injuries. *In* Langfitt, T. W., McHenry, L. C., Reivich, M., and Wollman, W., eds.: Cerebral Circulation and Metabolism. Berlin, Springer-Verlag, 1975, pp. 241–244.

122. Klatzo, I.: Pathophysiological aspects of brain edema. *In* Reulen, H. J., Schürmann, K., eds.: Steroids and Brain Edema. Berlin, Springer-Verlag, 1972, pp. 1–8.

123. Klatzo, I., Piraux, A., and Laskowski, E. J.: The relationship between edema, blood brain barrier and tissue elements in a local brain injury. J. Neuropath. Exp. Neurol., *17*:548–564, 1958.

124. Klatzo, I., Wisniewski, H., Steinwall, O., and Streicher, E.: Dynamics of cold injury edema. *In* Klatzo, I., and Seitelberger, F., eds.: Brain Edema. Berlin, Springer-Verlag, 1967, pp. 554–563.

125. Klintworth, G. K.: The pathogenesis of secondary brain stem hemorrhage as studied with an experimental model. Amer. J. Path., *47*:525–536, 1965.

126. Klintworth, G. K.: Secondary brain stem haemorrhage. J. Neurol. Neurosurg. Psychiat., *29*:423–425, 1966.

127. Kornblum, R. N., and Fisher, R. S.: Pituitary lesions in craniocerebral injuries. Arch. Path. (Chicago), *88*:242–248, 1969.

128. Labadie, E. L., and Glover, D.: Physiopathogenesis of subdural hematomas: Part 1—Histological and biochemical comparisons of subcutaneous hematoma in rats with subdural hematoma in man. J. Neurosurg., *45*:382–392, 1976.

129. Landig, G. H., Browder, E. J., and Watson, R. A.: Subdural hematoma: A study of one hundred and forty-three cases encountered during a five year period. Ann. Surg., *133*:170–188, 1941.

130. Langfitt, T. W.: Increased intracranial pressure. Clin. Neurosurg., *16*:436–471, 1969.

131. Langfitt, T. W., and Kassell, N. F.: Non-filling of cerebral vessels during angiography: Correlation with intracranial pressure. Acta Neurochir. (Wien), *14*:96–104, 1966.

132. Langfitt, T. W., Weinstein, J. D., and Kassell, N. F.: Vascular factors in head injury. *In* Caveness, W. F., and Walker, A. E., eds.: Head In-

jury. Philadelphia, J. B. Lippincott Co., 1966, pp. 172–194.

133. Langfitt, T. W., Weinstein, J. D., Kassell, N. F., and Gagliardi, L. J.: Transmission of increased intracranial pressure. II. Within the supratentorial space. J. Neurosurg., 21:998–1005, 1964.

134. Langfitt, T. W., Weinstein, J. D., Kassell, N. F., and Simeone, F. A.: Transmission of increased intracranial pressure: I. Within the craniospinal axis. J. Neurosurg., 21:989–997, 1964.

135. Leech, P. J., and Miller, J. D.: Intracranial volume/pressure relationships during experimental brain compression in primates. I. Pressure responses to changes in ventricular volume. J. Neurol. Neurosurg. Psychiat., 37:1093–1098, 1974.

136. Leech, P. J., and Miller, J. D.: Intracranial volume/pressure relationships during experimental brain compression in primates. II. Effects of induced changes in arterial pressure. J. Neurol. Neurosurg. Psychiat., 37:1099–1104, 1974.

137. Leech, P. J., and Miller, J. D.: Intracranial volume/pressure relationships during experimental brain compression in primates. III. The effect of mannitol and hypocapnia. J. Neurol. Neurosurg. Psychiat., 37:1105–1111, 1974.

138. Leech, P. J., and Paterson, A.: Conservative and operative management for cerebrospinal fluid leakage after closed head injury. Lancet, 1:1013–1015, 1973.

139. Lewin, W.: Acute subdural and extradural hematoma in closed head injuries. Ann. Roy. Coll. Surg. Engl., 5:240–274, 1949.

140. Lewin, W.: Vascular lesions in head injuries. Brit. J. Surg., 55:321–331, 1968.

141. Lewin, W., and Gibson, R. M.: Missile head wounds in the Korean campaign. Brit. J. Surg., 43:628–632, 1956.

142. Lewis, P., Ramirez, R., and McLaurin, R.: Intracranial blood volume after head injury. Surg. Forum, 19:433–435, 1968.

143. Lindenberg, R.: Compression of brain arteries as pathogenetic factor for tissue necroses and their areas of predilection. J. Neuropath. Exp. Neurol., 14:223–243, 1955.

144. Loew, F., and Wüstner, S.: Diagnose, Behandlung und Prognose der traumatischen Hämatome ses Schädelinneren. Acta Neurochir. (Wien) suppl., 8:1–158, 1960.

145. Löfgren, J.: Effects of variations in arterial pressure and arterial carbon dioxide tension on the cerebrospinal fluid pressure-volume relationships. Acta Neurol. Scandinav., 49:586–598, 1973.

146. Löfgren, J., and Zwetnow, N. N.: Cranial and spinal components of the cerebrospinal fluid pressure-volume curve. Acta Neurol Scand., 49:575–585, 1973.

147. Löfgren, J., and Zwetnow, N. N.: Influence of a supratentorial expanding mass on intracranial pressure-volume relationships. Acta Neurol. Scand., 49:599–612, 1973.

148. Löfgren, J., Von Essen, C., and Zwetnow, N. N.: The pressure-volume curve of the cerebrospinal fluid space on dogs. Acta Neurol. Scand., 49:557–574, 1973.

149. Lundberg, N.: Continuous recording and control of ventricular fluid pressure in neurosurgical practice. Acta Psychiat. Neurol. Scand., 36:suppl. 149:1–193, 1960.

150. Lundberg, N., Troupp, H., and Lorin, H.: Continuous recording of the ventricular fluid pressure in patients with severe acute traumatic brain injury. J. Neurosurg., 22:581–590, 1965.

151. McDowell, D. G.: Interrelationships between blood oxygen tensions and cerebral blood flow. In Payne, J. P., and Hill, D. W., eds.: Oxygen Measurements in Blood and Tissues. London, J. & A. Churchill Ltd., 1966. pp. 205–214.

152. MacIver, I. N., Smith, B. J., Tomlinson, B. E., and Whitby, J. D.: Rupture of the eosophagus associated with lesions of the central nervous system. Brit. J. Surg., 181:505–512, 1956.

153. McKissock, W., Richardson, A., and Bloom, W. H.: Subdural haematoma—a review of 389 cases. Lancet, 1:1365–1370, 1960.

154. McKissock, W., Taylor, J. C., Bloom, W. H., and Till, K.: Extradural hematoma. Observation on 125 cases. Lancet, 2:167–172, 1960.

155. McLaurin, R. L., and King, L. R.: Metabolic effects of head injury. In Vinken, P. J., and Bruyn, G. W., eds.: Handbook of Clinical Neurology. Vol. 23, Injuries of the Brain and Skull Part I. Amsterdam, Elsevier–North Holland Publishing Co., 1975, pp. 109–131.

156. McNealy, D. E., and Plum, F.: Brain stem dysfunction with supratentorial mass lesions. Arch. Neurol. (Chicago), 7:10–32, 1962.

157. Macpherson, P., and Graham, D. I.: Arterial spasm and slowing of the cerebral circulation in the ischaemia of head injury. J. Neurol. Neurosurg. Psychiat., 36:1069–1072, 1973.

158. Maloney, S. F. J., and Whatmore, W. J.: Clinical and pathological observations in fatal head injuries—a 5 year survey of 173 cases. Brit. J. Surg., 56:23–31, 1969.

159. Maltby, G. L.: Penetrating craniocerebral injuries. Evaluation of late results in a group of 200 consecutive penetrating cranial war wounds. J. Neurosurg., 3:239–249, 1946.

160. Marmarou, A., and Shulman, K.: Pressure-volume relationships—basic aspects. In McLaurin, R. L., ed.: Head Injuries: Second Chicago Symposium on Neural Trauma. New York, Grune & Stratton Inc., 1976, pp. 233–236.

161. Marmarou, A., Shulman, K., and Lamorgese, J.: Compartmental analysis of compliance and outflow resistance of the cerebrospinal fluid system. J. Neurosurg., 43:523–534, 1975.

162. Marmarou, A., Pöll, W., Shapiro, K., and Shulman, K.: The influence of brain tissue pressure upon local cerebral blood flow in vasogenic edema. In Beks, J. W. F., Bosch, D. A., and Brock, M., eds.: Intracranial Pressure III. Berlin, Springer-Verlag, 1976, pp. 10–13.

163. Marshall, W. J. S., Jackson, J. L. F., and Langfitt, T. W.: Brain swelling caused by trauma and arterial hypertension. Arch. Neurol. (Chicago), 21:545–553, 1969.

164. Martin, J., and Campbell, E. H., Jr.: Early complications following penetrating wounds of the skull. J. Neurosurg., 3:58–73, 1946.

165. Matakas, F., Cervos-Navarro, J., and Schneider,

H.: Experimental brain death: I. Morphology and fine structure of the brain. J. Neurol. Neurosurg. Psychiat., *36*:497–508, 1973.

166. Meinig, G., Reulen, H. J., and Magavly, C.: Regional cerebral blood flow and cerebral perfusion pressure in global brain edema induced by water intoxication. Acta Neurochir. (Wien), *29*:1–13, 1973.

167. Meirowsky, A. M.: Penetrating wounds of the brain. *In* Coates, J. B., and Meirowsky, A. M., eds.: Neurological Surgery of Trauma. Washington, D.C., U.S. Govt. Printing Office, 1965, pp. 103–104.

168. Meirowsky, A. M.: Penetrating cranicerebral trauma. *In* Caveness, W. F., and Walker, A. E., eds.: Head Injuries: Conference Proceedings. Philadelphia, J. B. Lippincott Co., 1966, pp. 195–202.

169. Meirowsky, A. M., and Harsh, G. E., III: The surgical management of cerebritis complicating penetrating wounds of the brain. J. Neurosurg., *10*:373–379, 1953.

170. Meldrum, B. S., Papy, J. J., Toure, M. F., and Brierley, J. B.: Four models for studying cerebral lesions secondary to epileptic seizures. Advances Neurol., *10*:147–161. 1975.

171. Meyer, A.: Herniation of the brain. Arch. Neurol. Psychiat., *4*:387–400, 1920.

172. Meyer, J. S., Gotoh, F., and Favale, E.: Cerebral metabolism during epileptic seizures in man. Electroenceph. Clin. Neurophysiol., *21*:10–22, 1966.

173. Miller, J. D.: Volume and pressure in the craniospinal axis. Clin. Neurosurg., *22*:76–105, 1975.

174. Miller, J. D.: Effects of hypercapnia on pupillary size, intracranial pressure and cerebral venous PO_2 during experimental brain compression. *In* Lundberg, N., Ponten, U., and Brock, M., eds.: Intracranial Pressure II. Berlin, Springer-Verlag, 1975, pp. 444–446.

175. Miller, J. D.: Infection after head injury. *In* Vinken, P. J., and Bruyn, C. W., eds.: Vol. 24, Injuries of the Brain and Skull Part II. Amsterdam, Elsevier–North Holland Publishing Co., 1976, pp. 215–230.

176. Miller, J. D., and Adams, H.: Physiopathology and management of increased intracranial pressure. *In* Critchley, M., O'Leary, J. L., and Jennett, B., eds.: Scientific Foundations of Neurology. London, William Heinemann Ltd., 1972, pp. 308–324.

177. Miller, J. D., and Jennett, W. B.: Complications of depressed skull fracture. Lancet, *2*:991–995, 1968.

178. Miller, J. D., and Pickard, J. D.: Intracranial volume/pressure studies in patients with head injury. Injury, *5*:265–269, 1974.

179. Miller, J. D., Garibi, J., and Pickard, J. D.: Induced changes of cerebrospinal fluid volume: Effects during continuous monitoring of ventricular fluid pressure. Arch. Neurol. (Chicago), *28*:265–269, 1973.

180. Miller, J. D., Stanek, A., and Langfitt, T. W.: Concepts of cerebral perfusion pressure and vascular compression during intracranial hypertension. Prog. Brain Res., *35*:411–432, 1972.

181. Miller, J. D., Stanek, A. E., and Langfitt, T. W.: Cerebral blood flow regulation during experimental brain compression. J. Neurosurg., *39*:186–196, 1973.

182. Miller, J. D., Fitch, W., Ledingham, I. M. C. A., and Jennett, W. B.: The effect of hyperbaric oxygen on experimentally increased intracranial pressure. J. Neurosurg., *33*:287–296, 1970.

183. Miller, J. D., Garibi, J., North, J. B., and Teasdale, G. M.: Effects of increased arterial pressure on blood flow in the damaged brain. J. Neurol. Neurosurg. Psychiat., *38*:657–665, 1975.

184. Miller, J. D., Reilly, P. L., Farrar, J. R., and Rowan, J. O.: Cerebrovascular reactivity related to focal brain edema in the primate. *In* Pappius, H. M., and Feindel, W., eds.: Dynamics of Brain Edema. Berlin, Springer-Verlag, 1976, pp. 68–76.

185. Miller, J. D., Becker, D. P., Ward, J. D., Sullivan, H. G., Adams, W. E., and Rosner, M. J.: Significance of intracranial hypertension in severe head injury. J. Neurosurg., *47*:503–516, 1977.

186. Mitchell, D. E., and Adams, J. H.: Primary focal impact damage to the brain stem in blunt head injuries, does it exist? Lancet, *2*:215–218, 1973.

187. Moiel, R. H., and Caram, P. E.: Acute subdural hematomas: A review of eighty-four cases—a six year evaluation. J. Trauma, *7*:660–666, 1967.

188. Moore, M. T., and Stern, K.: Vascular lesions of the brain stem and occipital lobe occurring in association with brain tumors. Brain, *61*:70–81, 1938.

189. Morgan, H., Wood, M. W., and Murphey, F.: Experience with 88 consecutive cases of brain abscess. J. Neurosurg., *38*:698–704, 1973.

190. Moruzzi, G., and Magoun, H. W.: Brainstem reticular function and activation of the EEG. Electroenceph. Clin. Neurophysiol., *1*:455–473, 1949.

191. Munro, D.: Cerebral subdural hematomas. A study of 310 verified cases. New Eng. J. Med., *227*:87–95, 1942.

192. Nauta, W. J. H.: Silver impregnation of degenerating axons. *In* Windle, W. F., ed.: New Research Techniques of Neuroanatomy. Springfield, Ill., Charles C Thomas, 1957, pp. 17–26.

193. Nemoto, E. M., and Frankel, H. M.: Cerebral oxygenation and metabolism during progressive hyperthermia. Amer. J. Physiol., *219*:1784–1788, 1970.

194. Nevin, N. C.: Neuropathological changes in the white matter following head injury. J. Neuropath. Exp. Neurol., *26*:77–84, 1967.

195. Northcroft, G. B., and Wyke, B. D.: Seizures following treatment of intracranial abscesses. J. Neurosurg., *14*:249–263, 1957.

196. Ommaya, A. K., and Gennarelli, T. A.: Cerebral concussion and traumatic unconsciousness: Correlation of experimental and clinical observations on blunt head injuries. Brain, *97*:633–654, 1974.

197. Ommaya, A. K., and Gennarelli, T. A.: A physiopathologic basis for noninvasive diagnosis and prognosis of head injury severity. *In* McLaurin, R. L., ed.: Head Injuries: Second

Chicago Symposium on Neural Trauma. New York, Grune & Stratton Inc., 1976, pp. 46–75.

198. Ommaya, A. K., Rockoff, S. D., Baldwin, M., and Friauf, W. S.: Experimental concussion. J. Neurosurg., *21*:249–265, 1964.

199. Oppenheimer, D. R.: Microscopic lesions in the brain following head injury. J. Neurol. Neurosurg. Psychiat., *31*:299–306, 1968.

200. Pasztor, E., Pasztor, A., Bodo, M., and Bogsch, S.: The role of spinal arachnoidal spaces in compensation of intracranial hypertension. *In* Lundberg, N., Ponten, U., and Brock, M., eds.: Intracranial Pressure II. Berlin, Springer-Verlag, 1975, pp. 82–85.

201. Paul, R. L., Polaneo, O., Tunney, S. Z., McAlsam, T. C., and Cowley, R. A.: Intracranial pressure responses to alterations in arterial carbon dioxide pressure in patients with head injuries. J. Neurosurg., *36*:714–720, 1972.

202. Paulson, O. B., Brodersen, P., Hansen, E. L., and Kristensen, H. S.: Regional cerebral blood flow, cerebral metabolic rate of oxygen, and cerebrospinal fluid acid-base findings in patients with acute pyogenic meningitis and with acute encephalitis. *In* Langfitt, T. W., McHenry, L. C., Reivich, M., and Wollman, H., eds.: Cerebral Circulation and Metabolism. Berlin, Springer-Verlag, 1975, pp. 306–309.

203. Peerless, S. J., and Rewcastle, N. B.: Shear injuries of the brain. Canad. Med. Ass. J., *96*:577–582, 1967.

204. Petito, C. K., Schaefer, J. A., and Plum, F.: The blood brain barrier in experimental seizures. *In* Pappius, H. M., and Feindel, W., eds.: Dynamics of Brain Edema. Berlin, Springer-Verlag, 1976, pp. 38–42.

205. Pitlyk, P. J., Tolchin, S., and Stewart, W.: The experimental significance of retained bone fragments. J. Neurosurg., *33*:19–24, 1970.

206. Plum, F., and Posner, J. B.: The Diagnosis of Stupor and Coma. Philadelphia, F. A. Davis Co., 1966.

207. Plum, F., Posner, J. B., and Troy, B.: Cerebral metabolic and circulatory responses to drug-induced convulsions in animals. Arch. Neurol. (Chicago), *18*:1–13, 1968.

208. Porter, R. J., and Miller, R. A.: Diabetes insipidus following closed head injury. J. Neurol. Neurosurg. Psychiat., *11*:258–262, 1948.

209. Potter, J.: Footballer's amnesia. J. Neurol. Neurosurg. Psychiat., *21*:67–68, 1958.

210. Povlishock, J. T., Becker, D. P., Sullivan, H. G., and Miller, J. D.: Vascular permeability alterations to horseradish peroxidase in experimental brain injury. Brain Res., *153*:223–239,1978.

211. Pudenz, R. H., and Shelden, R. H.: The Lucite calvarium—a method for direct observation of the brain II. Cranial trauma and brain movement. J. Neurosurg., *3*:487–505, 1946.

212. Purvis, J. T.: Craniocerebral injuries due to missiles and fragments. *In* Caveness, W. F., and Walker, A. E., eds.: Head Injury—Conference Proceedings. Philadelphia, J. B. Lippincott Co., 1966, pp. 133–141.

213. Ransohoff, J., Vallo, B., Gage, E. J., and Epstein, F.: Hemicraniectomy in the management of acute subdural hematomas. J. Neurosurg., *34*:70–76, 1971.

214. Rapaport, S. I.: Blood-brain barrier permeability, autoregulation of cerebral blood flow and brain edema. *In* McLaurin, R. L., ed.: Head Injuries: Second Chicago Symposium on Neural Trauma. New York, Grune & Stratton Inc., 1976, pp. 115–121.

215. Rapaport, S. I., Matthews, K., and Thompson, H. K.: Absence of brain edema after reversible osmotic opening of the blood-brain barrier. *In* Pappius, H. M., and Feindel, W., eds.: Dynamics of Brain Edema. Berlin, Springer-Verlag, 1976, pp. 18–22.

216. Reid, W. L., and Cone, W. V.: The mechanism of fixed dilatation of the pupil resulting from ipsilateral cerebral compression. J.A.M.A., *112*:2030–2034, 1939.

217. Reivich, M., Marshall, W. J. S., and Kassell, N.: Loss of autoregulation produced by cerebral trauma. *In* Brock, M., Fieschi, C., Ingram, D. H., Lasser, V. A., and Schurmann, K., eds.: Cerebral Blood Flow. Berlin, Springer-Verlag, 1969, pp. 205–208.

218. Reulen, H. J., Graham, R., Fenske, A., Tsuymu, M., and Klatzo, I.: The role of tissue pressure and bulk flow in the formation and resolution of cold-induced edema. *In* Pappius, H. M., and Feindel, W., eds.: Dynamics of Brain Edema. Berlin, Springer-Verlag, 1976, pp. 103–112.

219. Richards, T., and Hoff, J. T.: Factors affecting survival from acute subdural hematoma. Surgery, *75*:253–258, 1974.

220. Rinder, L., and Olsson, Y.: Studies on vascular permeability in experimental brain concussion. I. Distribution of circulating fluorescent indicators in the brain and cervical cord after sudden mechanical loading of the brain. Acta Neuropath. (Berlin), *11*:183–200, 1968.

221. Roberts, A. H.: Brain Damage in Boxers: A Study of the Prevalence of Traumatic Encephalopathy Among Professional Boxers. London, Pitman Publishing Ltd., 1969.

222. Rowan, J. O., and Teasdale, G.: Brain stem blood flow during raised intracranial pressure. *In* Ingvar, D. H., and Lassen, N. A., eds.: Cerebral Function, Metabolism and Circulation. Copenhagen, Munksgaard Ltd., 1977, pp. 520–521.

223. Rowe, S. N., and Turner, O. A.: Observations on infection in penetrating wounds of the head. J. Neurosurg., *2*:391–401, 1945.

224. Schorstein, J.: Intracranial haematoma in missile wounds. Brit. J. Surg., War Surg. suppl. 1:96–111, 1947.

225. Schutta, H. S., Kassell, N. F., and Langfitt, T. W.: Brain swelling produced by injury and aggravated by arterial hypertension—a light and electron microscopic study. Brain, *91*:281–294, 1968.

226. Schwartz, H. G., and Roulhac, G. E.: Craniocerebral war wounds: Observations on delayed treatment. Ann. Surg., *121*:129–151, 1945.

227. Sevitt, S.: Fatal road accidents. Brit. J. Surg., *55*:481–505, 1968.

228. Shapiro, H. M., Langfitt, T. W., and Weinstein, J. D.: Compression of cerebral vessels by intracranial hypertension. II. Morphological evidence for collapse of vessels. Acta Neurochir. (Wien), *15*:223–233, 1966.

229. Shulman, K., and Marmarou, A.: Pressure-vol-

ume considerations in infantile hydrocephalus. Dev. Med. Child Neurol., *13*:suppl. 25:90–95, 1971.

230. Shulman, K. Marmarou, A., and Shapiro, K.: Brain tissue pressure and focal pressure gradients. *In* McLaurin, R. L., ed.: Head Injuries: Second Chicago Symposium on Neural Trauma. New York, Grune & Stratton Inc., 1976, pp. 279–285.

231. Small, J. M., and Turner, E. A.: A surgical experience of 1200 cases of penetrating brain wounds in battle, N.W. Europe, 1944–45. Brit. J. Surg., War Surg. suppl. 1:62–74, 1947.

232. Spielmayer, W.: Histopathologie des Nervensystems. Berlin, Springer-Verlag, 1922.

233. Strich, S. J.: Diffuse degeneration of the cerebral white matter in severe dementia following head injury. J. Neurol. Neurosurg. Psychiat., *19*:163–185, 1956.

234. Strich, S. J.: Shearing of nerve fibres as a cause of brain damage due to head injury. A pathological study of 20 cases. Lancet, *2*:443–448, 1961.

235. Strich, S. J.: The pathology of brain damage due to blunt head injury. *In* Walker, A. E., Caveness, W. F., and Critchley, M., eds.: The Late Effects of Head Injury. Springfield, Ill., Charles C Thomas, 1969, pp. 501–524.

236. Strich, S. J.: Lesions in the cerebral hemispheres after blunt head injury. J. Clin. Path., *23*:suppl. (Roy. Coll. Path.) 4:166–171, 1970.

237. Sullivan, H. G., Miller, J. D., Griffith, R. L., and Becker, D. P.: CSF pressure transients in response to epidural and ventricular volume loading. Amer. J. Physiol., *234*:R167–R171, 1978.

238. Sullivan, H. G., Miller, J. D., Becker, D. P., Flora, R. E., and Allen, G. A.: The physiological basis of ICP change with progressive epidural brain compression. An experimental evaluation in cats. J. Neurosurg., *47*:532–550, 1977.

239. Sullivan, H. G., Martinez, J., Becker, D. P., Miller, J. D., Griffith, R., and Wist, A. O.: Fluid-percussion model of mechanical brain injury in the cat. J. Neurosurg., *45*:520–534, 1976.

240. Sunderland, S.: The tentorial notch and complications produced by herniation through that aperture. Brit. J. Surg., *45*:422–438, 1958.

241. Sweet, R. C., Miller, J. D., Lipper, M., Kishore, P., and Becker, D. P.: The significance of bilateral abnormalities on the CT scan in patients with severe head injury. Neurosurgery, *3*:16–21, 1978.

242. Symon, L., Pasztor, E., Branston, N. M., and Dorsch, N. W. C.: Effects of supratentorial space-occupying lesions on regional intracranial pressure and local cerebral blood flow. An experimental study in baboons. J. Neurol. Neurosurg. Psychiat., *37*:616–626, 1974.

243. Symonds, C. P.: Concussion and its sequelae. Lancet, *1*:1–6, 1962.

244. Tallala, A., and Morin, M. A.: Acute traumatic subdural hematoma: A review of one hundred consecutive cases. J. Trauma, *11*:771–777, 1971.

245. Teasdale, G., Galbraith, S., and Jennett, W. B.: Traumatical intracranial hematomas: Detection, prognosis and management. J. Neurol. Neurosurg. Psychiat., *39*:918, 1976.

246. Teasdale, G., Rowan, J. O., Turner, J., Grossman, R., and Miller, J. D.: Cerebral perfusion failure and cortical electrical activity. *In* Ingvar, D. H., and Lassen, N. A., eds.: Cerebral Function, Metabolism and Circulation. Copenhagen, Munksgaard Ltd., 1977, pp. 430–431.

247. Thompson, R. K., and Malina, S.: Dynamic axial brain-stem distortion as a mechanism explaining the cardio-respiratory changes in increased intracranial pressure. J. Neurosurg., *16*:664–675, 1959.

248. Tindall, G. T., McGraw, C. P., Vanderveer, R. W., and Iwata, K.: Cardiorespiratory changes associated with plateau waves in patients with head injury. *In* Brock, M., and Dietz, H., eds.: Intracranial Pressure. Berlin, Springer-Verlag, 1972.

249. Tomlinson, B. E.: Brain stem lesions after head injury. J. Clin. Path., *23*:suppl. (Roy. Coll. Path.), 4:154–165, 1970.

250. Treip, C. S.: Hypothalamic and pituitary injury. J. Clin. Path., *23*:suppl. (Roy. Coll. Path.) 4:178–186, 1970.

251. Troupp, H.: Intraventricular pressure in patients with severe brain injuries. J. Trauma, *5*:373–378, 1965.

252. Troupp, H., and Heiskanen, O.: Cerebral angiography in cases of extremely high intracranial pressure. Acta. Neurol. Scand., *39*:213–223, 1963.

253. Vapalahti, M., and Troupp, H.: Prognosis for patients with severe brain injuries. Brit. Med. J., *3*:404–407, 1971.

254. Vincent, C., David, M., and Thiebaud, F.: Le cône de pression temporal dans les tumeurs des hémisphères cérébraux. Sa symptomatologie; sa gravité; les traitements qu'il convient de lui opposer. Rev. Neurol. (Paris), *65*:536–545, 1936.

255. Wallace, P. B., and Meirowsky, A. M.: The repair of dural defects by graft. An analysis of 540 penetrating wounds of the brain incurred in the Korean war. Ann. Surg., *151*:174–180, 1960.

256. Wannamaker, G. T., and Pulaski, E. J.: Pyrogenic neurosurgical infections in Korean battle casualties. J. Neurosurg., *15*:512–518, 1958.

257. Webster, J. E., Schneider, R. C., and Loftrom, J. E.: Observations on early types of brain abscess following penetrating wounds of the brain. J. Neurosurg., *3*:7–14, 1946.

258. Weir, B.: The osmolarity of subdural hematoma fluid. J. Neurosurg., *34*:528–533, 1971.

259. Wilkins, R. H.: Intracranial vascular spasm in head injuries. *In* Vinken, P. J., and Bruyn, G. W., eds.: Handbook of Clinical Neurology. Vol. 23, Injuries of the Brain and Skull, Part I. Amsterdam, Elsevier–North Holland Publishing Co., 1975, pp. 163–197.

260. Winkelman, N. W., and Eckel, J. L.: Brain trauma: Histopathology during the early stages. Arch. Neurol. Psychiat., *31*:956–986, 1934.

58

DIAGNOSIS AND TREATMENT OF HEAD INJURY IN ADULTS

> Follow-up of many patients with severe head injuries . . . does not allow us to conclude that we have reached the limit in the management of these patients . . . the advances will come from the meld of the basic disciplines of physiological experiment, pathology and clinical observation.
>
> Walpole Lewin, 1975

These words, delivered by Lewin in the Victor Horsley Memorial Lectures in 1975, anticipate the theme of this discussion of head injury.[200] The essence is that attentive modern neurosurgical care for victims of head injury, guided by a detailed understanding of the pathophysiology and therapeutic principles involved, will improve care for the individual patient and achieve better overall results.

The last two decades have witnessed great advances in the diagnostic, therapeutic, and technical aspects of applied neurological surgery. It is fair to say, however, that application of improved methods to management of head injury has lagged behind other areas of neurosurgery. The reasons for this are not clear, but what is clear to those actively involved in the study of clinical head injury is that application of high-quality modern neurosurgical principles will yield appropriate rewards for the patient, his family, and the neurosurgeon.[25,156,218] This chapter deals with the present state of the art in the area of head trauma, and attempts to place mechanical brain injury in perspective so that it gets the attention it deserves from the neurosurgical and general medical community.

One important misconception must be cleared up at the outset. The idea that an operation is rarely necessary in head injury is false. While it is true that in an unselected series of all patients with concussion (at least transient loss of consciousness) the incidence of intracranial hematomas is only 6 to 7 per cent, in patients with severe head injury the incidence is far higher.[200] In virtually every reported large series of patients with severe head injury, i.e., patients unable to speak or follow commands, the incidence of intracranial mass lesions treated operatively is in the range of 40 to 60 per cent.[25,159,263,267,296] This figure is a striking one and must be kept in mind; that is, approximately *half* of all patients who arrive at the hospital unconscious from a head injury will be harboring a major intracranial mass. Untreated, these lesions give rise to an extremely high mortality rate. It follows that, ideally, neurological surgeons should be actively involved in the critical management of these patients, or at least readily available. Since an emergency operation is often required in the care of a patient with severe brain injury, the surgeon should have a working knowledge of all as-

D. P. BECKER, J. D. MILLER, H. F. YOUNG,

J. B. SELHORST, P. R. S. KISHORE,

R. P. GREENBERG, M. J. ROSNER, AND J. D. WARD

pects of the operative techniques required for treating head injury.

Head trauma with brain injury is one of the most common medical conditions the neurosurgeon is confronted with. An understanding of the causes of death and morbidity in head injury is a prerequisite for providing proper patient care. After a head injury, patients who die usually do so for one of three reasons: prolonged apnea at the scene of the accident; severe uncontrolled intracranial hypertension; or an undesirable systemic medical event (myocardial infarction, respiratory arrest, blood loss, or the like). Morbidity also is the result of these secondary concomitants of trauma.[27]

The classic textbooks on head injury by Lewin and Rowbotham, and the contributions by Gurdjian, Ommaya and Gennarelli, and others provide the foundation for understanding the physics, pathobiology, and management of mechanical brain injury as described herein.[126,200,259,297] In this chapter, the emphasis is on the severe brain injury. The problems of mild concussion and the effects of repeated "minor" brain injury are, however, also discussed.

An understanding of the morphological substrate and pathophysiological alterations that occur intracranially and systemically at the moment of impact and in the minutes, hours, and days following the initial damage provide the basis for sound management. Three broad concepts are important in comprehending the nature of head injury. The first concept is that in a severe injury many brain cells are functionally impaired but not disrupted by the initial impact, and if conditions are favorable, the cells can recover after minutes, or even after hours or days. The next concept is that secondary pathophysiological processes, both biochemical and structural (mass lesions), may result in further major cellular damage, both to the previously injured neurons and even to uninjured cells; a major goal of therapy is to avert these secondary processes. Finally, an understanding of the loci, extent, and types of brain injury in each patient is necessary because the entire management program should and will center on an understanding of the patient's intracranial disorder in structural and functional terms.

Chapter 60 is devoted to outcome following head injury. This is a topic that has attracted more attention in recent years. In severe brain injury, an enormous effort often goes into the patient's initial therapy. With improvements in intensive care support systems as well as in the treatment of more severely injured patients, it appears that more patients survive. With this intensive effort in early treatment, and the potential for improved results, it is imperative for the neurosurgeon to understand, on the one hand, the final psychosocial and neurological result that may be expected for a given patient, and on the other, the types of, usefulness of, and indications for various late rehabilitative programs. Such knowledge is important, since the vast majority of patients who suffer severe brain injuries will end up with some residual neurological, psychological, mental, or adaptive handicap. This may be barely detectable, but is usually present even in patients whose ultimate results are classified as excellent or good. The recognition and management of these problems remain to challenge the neurosurgeon. Better evaluation of rehabilitation methods and refinement of late therapeutic measures are certain to receive much needed attention from the medical community in the near future.

In describing the clinical effects of head injury on neurological function and outcome, an objective and uniform terminology is required. Terms such as concussion, contusion, coma, posturing, and the like are often used to mean different things among clinicians. The attempt here is to use universally acceptable terminology, and in the hope of improving communication on head injury, an acceptable system of terminology is described wherever indicated. Neurosurgeons need to be rigorous in adhering to accepted definitions, and thus the emphasis on strict terminology for the neurological description of patients, their pathological conditions, and the pathophysiology of those conditions.

EPIDEMIOLOGY OF CRANIOCEREBRAL TRAUMA

Head injury is of paramount interest to the neurological surgeon because quality care can make an important difference in outcome. Both minor and major head injuries occur in epidemic proportions in industrialized nations. One need only consider that, in the United States, trauma is the leading cause of death in the age group 1 to 44 years. Further, in men aged 45 to 64, trauma exceeds even stroke as a cause of death.[345] In over half of trauma-related deaths, the head injury contributes significantly to the outcome. In patients with multiple injuries, the head is the most commonly injured part, and in fatal road accidents, injury to the brain is found in nearly 75 per cent of the victims at autopsy.[110]

In the United States the National Safety Council reported 100,000 deaths from accidental injuries in 1976 in a population of 211 million.[251] How many of these deaths were directly due to the head injury is not known, but from what is known of the incidence of brain injury in accidental trauma, head trauma was probably the leading injury causing death. These figures provide incidence information for the extreme effect of injury, namely death, and give insight into the magnitude of the problem. But the total figures on the overall incidence of general trauma, and of head injury in particular, are even more remarkable.

Caveness recently presented the incidence figures for craniocerebral trauma in the United States in 1976, which were obtained from the National Center for Health Statistics, United States Department of Health, Education, and Welfare.[53] According to these figures, there were 7,560,000 head injuries in 1976. Of these, 6,305,000 were superficial and arbitrarily classified as minor. A staggering 1,255,000, however, were classified as major head injuries, which included concussion, intracranial hemorrhage, cerebral laceration, cerebral contusion, and crushing of the head. Thus, there is no doubt that serious head injury is a problem of major medical, social, and epidemiological significance.

In summary, trauma is the leading cause of death in youth and early middle age, and death is often associated with major head trauma. Trauma is the third most common cause of death in the United States, exceeded only by cardiocerebral vascular disease and cancer.[345] Because most of the serious head injuries occur in people under age 30, the long-term morbidity is tremendous. The recent rejuvenation of interest in the clinical and scientific problems of head injury is certainly justified.

PREVENTION OF HEAD INJURY

The importance of protecting the head from injury is gaining wider recognition. Serious preventive efforts can clearly be effective in reducing the incidence of serious head injuries. Caveness reported that the number of major head injuries occurring at work almost halved from 1970 to 1975, and this is the area that has received the most constructive thought regarding protection against accidental head injury.[53] Rules regarding mandatory wearing of protective devices remain controversial, but it is clear that such devices can reduce the incidence and degree of serious injury. There is statistical evidence that the use of automatic shoulder belts in cars is associated with a threefold reduction in the mortality rate from automobile crashes.[346] The United States Department of Transportation reported that Volkswagen Rabbits equipped with automatic crash protection seat belts had a rate of 0.5 fatalities per 100 million miles, whereas Volkswagen Rabbits with regular seat belts carried a rate of 1.7 fatalities per 100 million miles. The Department of Transportation has also estimated that passive restraints such as automatic air bags could save 9000 to 12,000 lives and prevent 100,000 to 200,000 serious injuries per year.[346] Mandatory wearing of helmets for motorcycle riders has reduced the incidence of death and severe head injury in those states that have passed such laws. In two states that had mandatory helmet laws, Rhode Island and Connecticut, the motorcycle fatality rate per accident doubled after repeal of the helmet requirement.[209] The value of a satisfactorily designed helmet in reducing the ill effects of injury is established.[51] The helmet spreads the impact energy of the blow over a wider area of the skull. Also, by reducing the speed of impact (rotational forces) and absorbing some of the energy itself, the helmet provides for a reduction in the degree and extent of brain injury.

Some knowledge of the social habits, backgrounds, and personalities of people who suffer accidental injury is revealing.

The National Safety Council reported in 1970 that alcohol is a factor in at least half of all fatal road traffic accidents.[250] Recently, it has been emphasized that psychological factors may play a role in trauma in the "accident prone" individual.[94] The aggressive-hostile personality of the auto driver, and even suicidal intent may be at the bottom of some vehicular accidents.[134]

The neurological surgeon, as the physician called upon to treat the devastating results of accidental injury, is an ideal spokesman and advocate for the application of effective protective and preventive measures.

DIAGNOSTIC EVALUATION IN HEAD INJURY

Diagnostic procedures should be used to define the total intracranial damage, in vivo, in as detailed a manner as possible. Only with such knowledge can the best treatment be provided for each patient. This is especially true of the patient with severe brain injury, but is just as desirable for patients with mild head injuries. The term "closed head injury," while useful in categorizing head injuries involving nonpenetrating wounds, oversimplifies the consequences of trauma to the head. Physicians attempting to improve the classification of brain injuries have usually described the most obvious and immediate clinical complication, i.e., epidural or subdural hematoma, intracerebral hemorrhage, and cerebral contusion. As appropriate as these terms are, they do not mention either the functional state of adjacent brain or additional brain injuries. "Brain stem contusion," "severe concussion," "minor contusion syndrome" are similar examples of attempts to describe the pathophysiological state of the patient that fail to define the true pathological or physiological disruptions that are present. The widespread cerebral and systemic effects of trauma compounded by the protean degrees of severity of head injury observed from patient to patient cast an air of uncertainty over the prognosis and management of each patient. The only apparent solution to these difficulties is the precise definition of all intracranial pathological states.

Fortunately, the past 15 years have witnessed a number of important advances that serve to clarify the nature and variations of brain damage and dysfunction that may be seen in human head trauma. The recent neuropathological studies of Graham and Adams and the introduction of computed tomography have provided new insight into the pathology of trauma.[119] Recent interest in prognosis in head injury has assisted in the development of norms for management of the patient with head injury.[28,339] These contributions are leading to improved treatment and to a better understanding of the likely outcome from mild, moderate, and severe primary brain injuries and their secondary intracranial complications.[25]

A prompt and orderly analysis of the nature and magnitude of all damage sustained by patients with head injury is necessary for appropriate and definitive emergency management. While this assessment includes superficial examination of scalp and skull, the most immediate requirement is to determine the intracranial damage. The physician must define the presence or absence of intracranial hematomas, contusions, and major zones of diffuse or focal edema. These processes are the direct cause, or potentially the cause, of dangerous elevations in intracranial pressure and cerebral herniations. The urgency of a given situation can be quickly determined by testing the ability of the patient to follow a simple single-stage command, which serves as a measure of a considerable degree of cerebral function. Although inability to follow such a command is not necessarily associated with impending neurological deterioration, should deterioration occur in such a patient, he will immediately be in a critical neurological state. For this reason *loss of this ability should initiate prompt diagnostic testing.* This principle must be adhered to in all patients, since successful therapy must take place *before* herniation syndromes occur or are permitted to progress. Criteria for operative intervention need to be established in each patient promptly, *before* clinical signs of herniation (deepening coma, dilating pupil, progressive paresis, posturing limbs, and the Cushing response) appear. Intracranial pressure associated with impending herniation syndromes is usually above 40 to 50 mm of mercury. These high levels of pressure and accompanying brain shifts result in secondary tissue necrosis. While delayed but technically satisfactory operations performed after these signs occur may salvage the patient, the final outcome is always less satisfactory. A better recovery for the patient can be achieved by earlier recognition and evacuation of mass lesions.[25]

While the first priority is the identification of major mass lesions and elevated intracranial pressures, it is important that diagnostic procedures be directed toward defining the type and severity of the brain damage in anatomical, pathological, and physiological terms. This information guides therapy and should aid in establishing a more accurate prognosis. An example illustrates the value of comprehensive diagnostic studies performed immediately following the initial neurological examination:

Three young individuals are involved in a high-speed auto accident and arrive simultaneously at the hospital. In the emergency room they have comparable neurological examinations. Each patient is unable to follow a simple command. Bilateral decerebrate posturing occurs with noxious stimulation. Oculocephalic responses are impaired but oculovestibular responses, tested by caloric stimulation, are intact. Pupillary light reflexes are normal. In the past, such responses were categorized under the term "brain stem injury" because the coma and motor posturing were thought to result primarily from the direct effect of trauma to the upper brain stem. In each patient, further diagnostic evaluation demonstrates different intracranial abnormalities. The first patient has severe bilateral hemispheral injury evidenced by a CT scan with midline slit ventricles and diffuse low densities, increased intracranial pressure at 40 mm of mercury, and markedly abnormal visual evoked potentials. The second patient has normal CT scan, intracranial pressure, and evoked potentials. In the third patient, with the same signs as the others, the CT scan shows a large extra-axial mass, ventriculography reveals a 1-cm shift of the midline, intracranial pressure is 50 mm of mercury, and flash-evoked potentials average into slow, reduced amplitudes. Thus, while the clinical neurological appearances of the three patients are similar, definitive diagnostic procedures demonstrate distinct differences in intracranial damage that re-

quire separate therapeutic approaches. Therapy in the first patient is directed toward reduction of brain swelling and elevated intracranial pressure. The second patient, who shows minimal structural or physiological evidence of hemispheral injury, requires no direct therapeutic measures but needs close medical management, including respiratory assistance and careful attention to fluid balance. Outcome for the third patient with the acute subdural hematoma depends upon the timeliness of operative intervention.

This simplified example shows that ideal emergency management requires complete identification of the number and nature of intracranial mass lesions and assessment of disordered intracranial function. With detailed information at the outset, patient care in the days and weeks following head injury can be based on scientific grounds. The physician is better able to direct medical and surgical therapy and to anticipate delayed complications of the head injury.

While management priorities are directed toward identification of major mass lesions and elevated intracranial pressure, diagnostic procedures also assist in determining the prognosis of individual patients on the basis of brain damage described in anatomical, pathological, and physiological terms. If based solely on the neurological examination, an accurate prognosis in the first hours after injury is limited. Improved predictions of neurological and intellectual deficit have resulted with the addition of information concerning intracranial structure and function.[26,121] These factors are discussed more fully in Chapter 60, but detailed diagnostic information is important for accurate prognostic determinations because many patients with severe brain injury ultimately have some residual neurological impairment, including those whose recovery is finally classified as "excellent" or "good."

In summary, the major goals in the diagnosis of intracranial damage in patients with head injury are: (1) to define as quickly as possible the presence of major mass lesions that require operative removal, preferably and ideally before herniation syndromes are evident; (2) to determine abnormal intracranial function in order to guide and direct appropriate operative and nonoperative therapy; (3) to localize the number, size, and nature of all brain injuries to clarify obstacles to ongoing management and to provide accuracy in predicting outcome; and (4) to identify all scalp and skull injuries, for these may be a source of both immediate and delayed brain insults.

Clinical Neurological Evaluation

Available diagnostic procedures include plain x-rays, computed tomography, echoencephalography, angiography, ventriculography, measurements of intracranial pressure, estimations of cerebral blood flow and cerebral metabolism, electroencephalography, and averaged evoked potentials. The indications for, timing of, and order in which each is performed depend upon the clinical status of the patient and the diagnostic tools readily available. The first procedure is always the neurological examination, which is necessary to determine the neurological state of the patient and the diagnostic tests that are required, their sequence, and their urgency.

Despite its limitations, the neurological examination remains the single most comprehensive process in the diagnostic evaluation of the patient with head injury, providing a rapidly available index of generalized and focal dysfunction of the nervous system. The speed, safety, and ease with which an appropriately thorough examination can be performed permits serial examinations that generate data indicating progress or deterioration of the patient.

The depth of the neurological examination will vary according to the type and degree of brain injury that the patient has suffered. In patients who are alert the initial examination is as thorough as possible, while the scope of the first examination in patients with impaired consciousness is limited. Therefore, in patients with altered consciousness, emphasis is given to certain critical aspects of the examination. Subsequent examinations are appropriately expanded to include those functions that involve full cooperation, subjective interpretation, or higher cognitive capacities of the patient.

History

The physician should seek as much information as possible concerning the precise time and mechanism of injury. Information regarding the mode of injury is important if the type and consequences of various brain injuries are to be understood. For example, the sudden deceleration of vehicular accidents and falls is usually associated with diffuse brain damage and polar contusions. Blows to the cranial vault usually result in underlying focal brain damage with a lesser component of diffuse brain injury. Crush injuries of the skull, trauma in which the head is usually in a fixed position, often produce focal injury without loss of consciousness but with extensive brain injury directly under the site of impact.

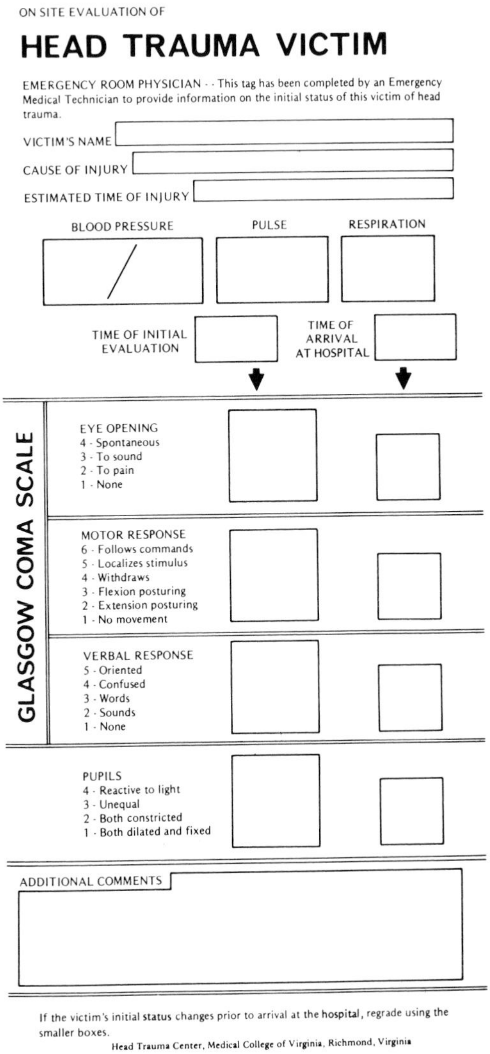
ON SITE EVALUATION OF

HEAD TRAUMA VICTIM

EMERGENCY ROOM PHYSICIAN - - This tag has been completed by an Emergency Medical Technician to provide information on the initial status of this victim of head trauma.

VICTIM'S NAME

CAUSE OF INJURY

ESTIMATED TIME OF INJURY

BLOOD PRESSURE | PULSE | RESPIRATION

TIME OF INITIAL EVALUATION | TIME OF ARRIVAL AT HOSPITAL

GLASGOW COMA SCALE

EYE OPENING
4 - Spontaneous
3 - To sound
2 - To pain
1 - None

MOTOR RESPONSE
6 - Follows commands
5 - Localizes stimulus
4 - Withdraws
3 - Flexion posturing
2 - Extension posturing
1 - No movement

VERBAL RESPONSE
5 - Oriented
4 - Confused
3 - Words
2 - Sounds
1 - None

PUPILS
4 - Reactive to light
3 - Unequal
2 - Both constricted
1 - Both dilated and fixed

ADDITIONAL COMMENTS

If the victim's initial status changes prior to arrival at the hospital, regrade using the smaller boxes.

Head Trauma Center, Medical College of Virginia, Richmond, Virginia

Figure 58–1 Head trauma card used by emergency service personnel in Richmond, Virginia. This simple card can be distributed to local emergency medical technicians and ambulance services. With minimal instruction, rescue squad workers are able to fill in the information with a high degree of accuracy.

HEAD INJURY PROGRAM

                                                                    -2-

I. PERSONAL DATA

First name:_____ Last name:_____ Hosp number:_____
Sex: M F_____ Age:_____ Race: B W O
Address:_____
                                    Tel.No.:_____

II. INJURY

Date:__/__/__ Time:_____ Place:_____
Type of accident: Auto/Pedestrian/Cycle/Sport/Work/Gun/Assault/Other_____
Details:_____

Lucid interval: Unknown/None/Duration _____
Seizures: Unknown/None/Describe _____

III. CONDITION AT SITE OF ACCIDENT

1.Pulse_____ , BP_____ , Temp____C or _____ F, Resp rate_____
2.Respiration: Regular/Irregular/Spasmodic/Absent
               Normal/Hyperventilation/Hypoventilation
               Hypoxia: Absent/ Present. Approx duration _____
                        Apparent cause_____
3.Consciousness: Alert/Obtunded/Stuporose/Comatose
4.Eye opening : Not tested/Spontaneous/To call/To pain/None
5.Orientation : Not tested/Oriented/Semi-oriented/Not oriented
6.Verbal respon: Not tested/Appropriate/Inapprop/Incomprehensible/None
7.Motor respon : Not tested/Normal/Impaired
8.Pupil size   : O-NT,1-Normal,2-Miotic,3-Mydriatic   R____ L____
9.Pupil respon : O-NT,1-Normal,2-Sluggish,3-Absent   R____ L____

IV. FIRST AID

_____
_____

V. COURSE

Distance of accident site from MCVH:
Transport to hospital: Private auto/ Ambulance (Name & Address) _____
Direct to MCVH/ Via other hospital(s). Time spent there: from_____ to_____
Name of other hospital:_____

VI. CONDITION AT EXAMINATION AT OTHER HOSPITAL

1.Consciousness: Alert/Obtunded/Stuporose/Comatose
2.Eye opening : NT/Spontaneous/To call/To pain/None
3.Orientation : NT/Oriented/Semi-oriented/Not oriented
4.Verbal respon: NT/Appropriate/Inapprop/Incomprehensible/None
5.Motor respon : O-NT,1-Obeys commands,2-Semipurposeful withdrawal,3-Decorticate,
                 4-Decerebrate, 5-Flaccid
6.Oculocephalic: O-NT,1-Normal,2-Impaired,3-Absent   R____ L____
7.Pupil size   : O-NT,1-Normal,2-Miotic,3-Mydriatic   R____ L____
8.Pupil respon : O-NT,1-Normal,2-Sluggish,3-Absent   R____ L____

9.VIIth n. function: O-NT,1-Normal,2-UMN,3-LMN,4-Either 2 or 3 R___ L___
10.Fundus   : O-NT,1-Normal,2-Borderline,3-Abnormal   R___ L___
11.Reflexes   : O-NT,1-Normal,2-Hypo,3-Hyper,4-Clonic   R___ L___
12.Babinski   : O-NT,1-Absent,2-Present,3-Equivocal   R___ L___

VII. GENERAL CONDITION ON ARRIVAL AT MCVH

Pulse_____ , BP_____ ,Temp____C or _____F, Resp rate_____
Respiratory status:
   Normal/Airway/Tube   Spontaneous/Assisted   Air/Enriched air/Oxygen
   Blood gases: Art pO$_2$ _____ , pCO$_2$_____, O$_2$ saturation_____%
Arterial pH __.___ , Alcohol level _____ , Hb/PCV _____
Clinical evidence of hypoxia: _____
Other injuries:_____

VIII. NEUROLOGICAL STATUS:

1.Consciousness: Alert / Obtunded / Stuporose / Comatose
2.Eye opening : NT / Spontaneous / To call / To pain / None
3.Orientation : NT / Oriented / Semi-oriented / Not oriented
4.Verbal respon: NT/ Appropriate / Inappropriate / incomprehensible / None
5.Motor respon : O-NT, 1-Obeys commands, 2-Semipurposeful withdrawal,
                 3-Decorticate, 4-Decerebrate, 5-Flaccid
6.Oculocephalic: O-NT, 1-Normal, 2- Impaired, 3-Absent   R___ L___
7.Pupil size   : O-NT, 1-Normal, 2-Miotic, 3-Mydriatic   R___ L___
8.Pupil respon : O-NT, 1-Normal, 2-Sluggish, 3-Absent   R___ L___
9.VIIn function: O-NT, 1-Normal, 2-UMN, 3-LMN, 4-Either 2 or 3 R___ L___
10.Fundus   : O-NT, 1-Normal, 2-Borderline, 3-Abnormal   R___ L___
11.Reflexes   : O-NT, 1-Normal, 2-Hypoactive, 3-Hyper, 4-Clonic R___ L___
12.Babinski   : O-NT, 1-Normal, 2-Absent, 3-Present, 4-Equivocal R___ L___

IX. PRELIMINARY INVESTIGATIVE FINDINGS

1.Initial ICP _____ cm H$_2$O
2.Midline shift _____ mm
3.EMI/Angio:_____
_____
_____

                                    ****

SUMMARY OF EVENTS:

   Time of accident   _____
   Arrival of ambulance _____
   Departure from site   _____
   Arrival at Hosp X   _____
   Departure from Hosp X _____
   Arrival at MCVH   _____
   Time seen by NS   _____
   Surgery commenced   _____

                        PATIENT ADMITTED ON: _____
                        DATA COMPILED ON: _____

Figure 58–2 Following injury, many patients are initially seen in receiving rooms or small primary care hospitals. Critical aspects of the patient's condition during the interval from injury to evaluation by the neurosurgeon should be systematically obtained. Forms such as the one shown here can be completed quickly and provide valuable information for the overall evaluation of patients.

A history of the patient's vital signs and neurological deficits obtained at the scene of the accident and during transport to the hospital should always be sought. Most emergency rescue squads are capable of providing some, if not all, of this information. The Glasgow coma scale has been designed so that it can be used by emergency medical technicians. This simple examination is seen on the check sheet in Figure 58–1. This information, along with data concerning pupils and vital signs, has proved to be practically obtainable.[339] The rescue squads can also provide helpful information concerning the type of accident. A report of the patient's condition from a referring hospital should also be sought and recorded as in Figure 58–2.

Initial Examination

A continuum of altered consciousness is recognized between the fully alert and the deeply comatose patient.[272] An objective measure of this continuum is a major difficulty in the evaluation of patients with head injury. Various terminology has been suggested to reduce these altered states into simplified stages. "Neurosurgical watch sheets" on which one records independent components of the neurological examination are in common use. Recently, the need for widely applicable, clearly defined terminology and methods to describe the neurological state of the patient was realized. Only with precise definition of terms and techniques can physicians communicate about and compare patients. Without this understanding, proper evaluation of the efficacy of new forms of therapy or prognosis in head injury is unlikely to occur.

In recent years Teasdale and Jennett have carefully studied patients with head injuries and impaired consciousness. As a result of these studies, they developed and described the Glasgow coma scale in 1974.[338] This method of grading the level of consciousness is particularly useful because arbitrary staging or grading of patients and ambiguous terms are carefully avoided. Teasdale and Jennett's studies confirm that the simplicity of the chosen

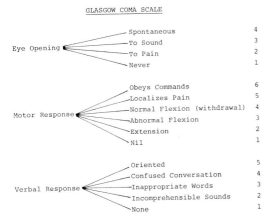

GLASGOW COMA SCALE

Eye Opening	Spontaneous	4
	To Sound	3
	To Pain	2
	Never	1

Motor Response	Obeys Commands	6
	Localizes Pain	5
	Normal Flexion (withdrawal)	4
	Abnormal Flexion	3
	Extension	2
	Nil	1

Verbal Response	Oriented	5
	Confused Conversation	4
	Inappropriate Words	3
	Incomprehensible Sounds	2
	None	1

Figure 58–3 The Glasgow coma scale for evaluating level of consciousness has come into widespread use. Studies by Teasdale and Jennett have confirmed its reliability and the consistency of grading performed by various medical personnel (nurses, junior physicians, attending physicians).

terms affords a consistent and accurate assessment when performed by nurses or junior physicians. Because the Glasgow scale is widely applicable, accurate, and straightforward, Langfitt has recommended that all evaluations of coma in head injury include it (Fig. 58–3).[190]

If, during a short interval, several different responses occur, Teasdale and Jennett recommend that the best response in each category be used in grading the patient's reaction. To follow trends in an individual patient's progress, however, it is better to report both the best and the worst responses. Right and left motor responses should be recorded separately. In the patient who obeys commands, motor responses to single-stage commands can be divisible into brisk and sluggish responses. This distinction separates the patient who is quite lethargic but follows commands after much stimulation from the patient who is nearly alert and requires little prompting to respond to verbal orders. The pain stimulus applied by different examiners is often quite variable, but deep nail bed pressure should be used as the standard stimulus.

The physician, however, should not limit the examination to the parameters of unconsciousness in the Glasgow coma scale, which are eye opening and motor and verbal responses. Of equal importance in the initial examination of the patient with impaired consciousness are vital signs, pupils, eye movements, and motor power. When these features are coupled with the

TABLE 58–1 INITIAL NEUROLOGICAL EXAMINATION IN HEAD INJURY*

Glasgow coma scale (level of consciousness)
Pupillary examination
Eye movements
  Oculocephalic
  Oculovestibular
Motor power

* The basic parts of the neurological examination that all patients with head injuries should have are particularly pertinent for patients who are unresponsive to verbal commands. The examination can be expanded when patients are more responsive.

Glasgow coma scale, a dependable and rapid clinical assessment of the patient's overall neurological status is obtained. The Glasgow coma scale provides a simple grading of the arousal and functional capacity of the cerebral cortex. Because of the widespread nature of brain injuries, in addition to cortical function, brain stem function must also be assessed. This assessment is best done by observation of the pupil and ocular motility. The limitations in localizing brain dysfunction on the basis of only decorticate and decerebrate postures was clarified recently; posturing does not necessarily imply brain stem damage. Alert patients with decerebrate rigidity have also been described.[39] In summary, the initial neurological examination in all patients with severe head injury should include, in addition to the Glasgow coma scale, examination of the pupils, eye movements, and motor power (Table 58–1) (see also Fig. 58–92).

Pupils

Careful notation of pupil size and response to light is of utmost importance at the initial examination. A well-known early sign of temporal lobe herniation is mild dilation of the pupil and a sluggish pupillary light response. Either compression or distortion of the oculomotor nerve during herniation impairs the function of parasympathetic axons transmitting efferent signals for pupillary constriction.[171] According to McNealy and Plum, bilateral miotic pupils (1 to 3 mm) occur in the early stages of central-cephalic herniation.[229] Bilateral compromise of pupillomotor sympathetic pathways originating in the hypothalamus permits predominance of parasympathetic tone and pupillary constriction. In either instance continued herniation causes wider dilation of the pupil and paralysis of its light response. With full mydriasis (8 to 9-mm pupil), ptosis and paresis of the medial rectus and other ocular muscles innervated by the oculomotor nerve appear. A bright light is always necessary to determine pupillary light responses. To distinguish between a weak pupillary light reaction and absence of a reaction, especially if the pupil is small, a magnifying lens such as the plus-20-diopter lens on standard ophthalmoscopes is helpful.

Recognition of additional pupillary disorders that occur in unconscious patients is useful in the examination of the patient with head trauma. Hippus is an unexplained phenomenon consisting of spontaneous dilation and contraction of the pupil that is often observed in patients with Cheyne-Stokes respirations. Rather than indicating disordered function, however, it suggests functional integrity of sympathetic and parasympathetic pupillary pathways. Disruption of the afferent arc of the pupillary light reflex within the optic nerve is detected by employing the swinging flashlight test.[316] As the flashlight is swung from the normal to the injured eye, deafferentation of the optic nerve is indicated by the first and paradoxical response of the pupil: dilation rather than constriction of the light-adapted pupil. Apparently, light signals transmitted to the Edinger-Westphal nucleus in the midbrain through the injured optic nerve are insufficient to maintain the constriction brought about by illumination of the first or normal eye. The paradoxical pupillary dilation observed as the light is moved from the normal to the abnormal eye is termed an afferent pupillary defect; in the absence of opacification of the ocular media it is unequivocal evidence of optic nerve injury.

The ciliospinal reflex is often mentioned as being useful in the examination of unconscious patients. However, because of the evidence for direct activation of intermediate sympathetic neurons for pupillomotor dilation in C8 and T1 spinal cord segments by painful stimuli to the limbs, the ciliospinal test is not recommended by Reeves and Posner in the evaluation of central nervous system function above the foramen magnum.[283] Bilateral small pupils suggest that the patient has used certain drugs, particularly opiates, or has one of several metabolic encephalopathies or de-

structive lesions of the pons.[96] In these conditions pupillary light responses usually can be seen if examined with a magnifying lens. The miosis that occurs with pontine lesions apparently results from structural or physiological inactivation of sympathetic pathways descending from the hypothalamus through the reticular activating system to the spinal cord. Unilateral Horner's pupil is seen occasionally with brain stem lesions, but in the trauma patient attention should be given to the possibility of a disrupted efferent sympathetic pathway at the apex of the lung, base of the neck, or ipsilateral carotid sheath. Midposition pupils with variable light responses are observed in all stages of coma. Traumatic oculomotor nerve injury is the diagnosis in patients with a history of a dilated pupil from the onset of injury, an improving level of consciousness, and appropriate ocular muscle weakness.[235] A mydriatic pupil (6 mm or more) occurs occasionally with direct trauma to the globe of the eye. This traumatic mydriasis is usually unilateral and is not accompanied by ocular muscle paresis. Rarely recognized is the corectopic pupil associated with midbrain disorders. In this sign, the pupillary aperture appears to migrate within the iris stroma as various sectors of the iris musculature contract and expand asynchronously.[305]

Finally, bilateral dilated and fixed pupils in patients with head injury may be the result of inadequate cerebral vascular perfusion. This situation can be due to hypotension secondary to blood loss, or to elevation of intracranial pressure to a degree that impairs cerebral blood flow. Return of the pupillary response may occur promptly after the restoration of blood flow, if the time of inadequate perfusion has not been too long.

Eye Movements

Ocular movements are an important index of the functional activity that is present within the brain stem reticular formation. If the patient is sufficiently alert to follow simple commands, a full range of eye movements is easily obtained and the integrity of the entire ocular motor system within the brain stem is affirmed. In states of depressed consciousness, voluntary eye movement is lost and there may be dysfunction of the neural structures activating eye movements. In these instances oculocephalic or oculovestibular responses are used to determine the presence or absence of an eye movement disorder. To employ these tests, an understanding of the anatomical connections involved in the normal response is necessary.

Clinicians have long realized that a conjugate gaze center controlling ipsilateral horizontal fast eye movements (saccades) and vestibular responses lies within the lower paramedian pontine reticular formation.[308] This region includes a pulse generator for fast eye movements and a neural integrator that determines the ultimate resting position of the eye. Recent studies in cats show that the caudal portion of the horizontal gaze center extends into the nucleus prepositus hypoglossi in rostral medulla and significantly participates in saccadic vestibular and voluntary slow eye movements.[18] Thus, clinical and animal investigation indicates that the final common pathway for all ipsilateral conjugate horizontal eye movements is located within the tegmentum of the paramedian pontomedullary junction. From here signals for horizontal eye movements are transmitted to the nearby ipsilateral abducens nucleus and cross the midline in the para-abducens region to ascend in the contralateral medial longitudinal fasciculus to medial rectus neurons in the oculomotor nucleus.[289]

In the unconscious patient with trauma to the head, loss of horizontal eye movement indicates the need for urgent diagnostic study. If a neck fracture has been excluded, function of the pontine gaze center is quickly ascertained by the oculocephalic maneuver. The head is raised 30 degrees from the supine position and briskly rotated to and fro in the horizontal plane. In the normal doll's-eyes response both eyes tend to maintain their position in space by moving opposite to the rotation of the head and horizontally toward their respective lateral and medial positions in the orbit. As this maneuver is performed, the eyelids may be manually retracted to better observe movements of the globe. Afferent impulses from cervical nerve roots and the semicircular canals contribute to the normal compensatory reflexes that shift the eyes in the direction opposite to rotation of the head. Impairment or absence of the oculocephalic response may be due to malpositioning or inadequate head rotation. Some patients whose oculocephalic responses are impaired or absent will have normal caloric responses. Therefore, all patients with at least impaired oculocephalic responses, in addition to those in whom neck fracture has not been ruled out, should have caloric stimulation of oculovestibular pathways. This stimulation can be accomplished with ice water and only a small expenditure of time. Obstructions within the external auditory canal of blood or cerumen need to be removed.

Movement of endolymph within the horizontal semicircular canal acts primarily upon conjugate movement of the medial and lateral rectus muscles.[334] To produce maximal shift of this fluid during caloric stimulation, the horizontal canal is positioned in the vertical plane by lifting the patient's head 30 degrees from the supine position. Conduction of the temperature gradient between the irrigating fluid and the endolymph produces movement of the latter within the semicircular canal. Normally this occurs in between 20 and 60 seconds and lasts several minutes. Warm water irrigation of the external canal causes endolymphatic fluid to rise, which causes contralateral tonic deviation of the eyes. Irrigation with cold water causes the endolymph to fall, and this causes ipsilateral tonic gaze deviation. Although direct connections between vestibular and ocular neurons are known, tonic eye deviation following caloric stimulation is likely to be the result of complex interactions within the eye movement control systems of the pontomedullary reticular system. In alert patients caloric stimulation causes fast-phase nystagmus in the direction opposite the tonic eye deviation. As a rule, nystagmus reflects functional activity for complex eye movement control within the reticular system. Functional suppression of the reticular activating system is reflected, in comatose patients, by the absence of nystagmus in response to caloric stimulation, so that only the tonic eye deviation is seen. Use of 20 ml of ice water suffices, but if no response occurs within one minute, it is best to repeat the test with larger volumes. If the second irrigation does not elicit eye movement, simultaneous oculocephalic maneuvers can be used to enhance the stimulus. To eliminate semicircular canal or vestibular nerve injury as the cause of absence of cold caloric responses, normal warm water caloric responses of the opposite ear should be obtained.

Full oculocephalic responses in the unconscious patient indicate that the process producing the coma spares the paramedian pontine reticular formation, the medial longitudinal fasciculus, and the oculomotor and abducens nuclei and their nerve roots. Moreover, the suppression of the reticular activating system responsible for the loss of consciousness is assumed to be operant rostral to these pontine and midbrain structures. An intermediate vestibulo-ocular response, i.e., absence of oculocephalic responses but intact caloric responses, has been reported to occur with supratentorial lesions.[249] Absence of both oculocephalic and caloric responses indicates a severe pathological process extending to the lower pons.

Limitation of ocular muscle movement occurs in patients with orbital edema. Intraorbital swelling is usually obvious to the examiner but should not discourage use of oculocephalic or caloric testing. Much information can still be gained.

While oculocephalic and caloric testing is being performed, infranuclear, internuclear, and supranuclear ocular motility disorders are recognizable. A destructive lesion of either a frontal or pontine gaze center results in tonic overaction of the opposite frontal-pontine axis for horizontal eye movement. Tonic deviation of the eyes occurs from the action of the spared frontal pontine system. This overaction results in ipsilateral deviation of the eyes with frontal lobe lesions and contralateral gaze deviation with pontine lesions. In deep coma, gaze deviation due to this overbalance is not necessarily present. To distinguish frontal or pontine lesions in patients with or without gaze deviations, oculocephalic and caloric testing is needed. In gaze deviations due to frontal lobe lesions, oculocephalic and caloric reflexes remain intact because vestibular input into the paramedian pontine reticular formation is preserved. Pontine lesions interrupt oculocephalic and oculovestibular–paramedian pontine reticular formation interaction so that rotation of the head toward the deviated eyes or cold water irrigation of the ear contralateral to the gaze deviation does not overcome the gaze deviation. Incomplete or paretic conjugate horizontal gaze following appropriate caloric stimulation suggests a partially damaged pontine gaze center. Dysconjugate oculocephalic and oculovestibular responses are due to either a third or sixth cranial nerve palsy or internuclear ophthalmoplegia if only one horizontal muscle is paretic. If both horizontal muscles for conjugate gaze are paretic, but one more than the other, a perverted form of a pontine gaze palsy is present.

Skew deviation is divergence of the eyes in the vertical plane and is a sign of a lesion within the brain stem. An explanation for the tonic and vertical deviation of one or both eyes is not known. In skew deviations neuroanatomical localization within the brain stem is not ordinarily possible either by notation of the downward or hypometric eye nor of its fellow upward or hypermetric eye.

Generally third and sixth nerve palsies are not difficult to recognize in patients with head injury. Fourth nerve palsies cannot ordinarily be identified in coma because of the select action of the superior oblique muscle. In the alert and recovering patient, however, superior oblique paresis causes troublesome double vision, especially with downward gaze. With a trochlear nerve injury, the greatest amount of diplopia occurs as the patient looks down and inward. Head tilt opposite the side of the paretic muscle lessens the double vision, while ipsilateral tilt of the head increases diplopia. Internuclear ophthalmoplegia is suggested by select adduction paresis without additional involvement of the pupil, lid, or vertical muscles innervated by the third nerve. The ophthalmoplegia results from disruption of the ipsilateral medial longitudinal fasciculus that connects the oculomotor subnucleus for medial rectus neurons to the contralateral horizontal gaze center. Either bilateral or unilateral internuclear ophthalmoplegia may be seen, depending upon the extent of the brain stem trauma.

Little is known about the incidence of vertical gaze palsies in coma states. Downward eye deviation is rare in head injury but may be associated with posterior thalamic hemorrhage.[316] Failure of upward gaze is, however, seen occasionally in patients with bilateral subdural hematoma or hydrocephalus, and is thought to represent compression of the tectal plate. With unilateral cold caloric testing, downward deviation of the eyes has been reported in coma caused by drug intoxication.[96,343] Vertical gaze is tested by manually rotating the head in the vertical plane. This maneuver results in compensatory up-and-down gaze. Simultaneous irrigation of both ears activates the semicircular canals to cause vertical response; bilateral cold water tests produce tonic upward movement of the eyes, and bilateral warm water tests produce tonic down gaze.

Motor Function

The basic examination is completed by a test of motor strength in those patients who are sufficiently responsive for such a determination to be made. Each extremity is examined and graded on the internationally used five-level scale as follows:

Normal power	5
Moderate weakness	4
Severe weakness (antigravity)	3
Trace movement	2
Paralysis	1

Responses to painful stimulus are recorded under the level of consciousness, as described previously.

Expanded Examination in Acute and Chronic Phases of Head Injury

As soon as the patient is alert and able to follow simple commands, a more complete neurological examination should be performed. This effort potentially identifies additional focal neurological deficits and makes the accumulated laboratory data more comprehensible. Serial examinations should be performed because recovery from brain trauma proceeds by stages that vary according to age, severity of impact, and secondary systemic and intracranial complications. These repeated examinations are necessary to guide and judge the effectiveness of management and to establish, as early as possible, evidence of fixed neurological dysfunction.

External examination of the head sometimes discloses evidence of a basilar skull fracture: ecchymosis over the mastoid eminence (Battle's sign) or hemorrhage behind the tympanic membrane. Periorbital hemorrhage of the upper and lower eyelid occurs either with skull fractures of the anterior fossa or direct orbital trauma.

Cranial nerves traversing a fractured middle and anterior fossa are often contused or lacerated. Therefore, in the patient with head trauma, special attention is given to cranial nerves subserving olfaction, vision, ocular motility, facial sensation and movements, and equilibrium and hearing. In alert patients, determination of central visual acuity is helpful in screening for optic nerve or intraocular injuries. Monocular altitudinal visual field defects, especially those involving the lower field owing to impingement of the superior optic nerve fibers on the falciform process at the proximal end of the optic canal, can be seen with optic nerve injuries. Confrontation visual field tests are useful in searching for a homonymous visual field defect from trauma affecting intracranial pathways.

Most often the ocular fundus is normal, even with severe head injury. Small or large intraretinal hemorrhages are sometimes seen but are of little consequence to the overall neurological condition. Although swollen optic discs are occasionally reported to occur within minutes of raised intracranial pressure, papilledema is seen in a minority of patients with serious head injuries. Moreover, swelling of the optic discs is usually not seen until the third to fifth day, often after decompression of an intracranial mass and relief of elevated intracranial pressure. This delay is curious, since the bulk of the elevated papilla occurring in papilledema is attributed to axons dilated as a result of mechanical impediment to axoplasmic flow.[343,344] Severely attenuated retinal arteries are occasionally due to very high intraocular pressure from massive swelling of traumatized orbital tissue. Retinal and optic nerve infarction follow. This situation is potentially reversible, if recognized early, by a simple lateral canthotomy. Various types of traumatic retinopathies have been reported.[352] One type is Purtscher's disease, which consists of multiple scattered hemorrhages in superficial layers of the retina and deep white areas in the posterior poles. This injury is associated with sudden elevations in systemic venous pressure, as occurs with crush injuries or forceful impacts on the chest or abdomen.[215]

In comatose patients the prognostic significance of a sluggish corneal response or its absence has yet to be fully determined. Corneal sensation is tested by placing a twist of cotton at the limbus and passing it over the cornea. The corneomandibular reflex, contralateral deviation of the jaw with corneal stimulation, occurs with dysfunction of corticobulbar pathways to the trigeminal motor nucleus. It occurs in patients with severe brain stem lesions. The seventh and eighth cranial nerves are often injured in petrous bone fractures. Facial nerve injury is apparent in a widened palpebral fissure and sagging facial muscles. Coherent mentation is needed to evaluate auditory function unless auditory evoked potentials are obtained. Delayed onset of ocular palsies can be seen with fractures of the clivus.[301]

Loss of memory is very common in patients with head injury and often persists long after consciousness is regained.[333] Commonly memory is separated into three categories: immediate, recent, and remote. Immediate or instant memory applies to those brief memories retained for no more than 30 to 60 seconds, such as occurs in repeating an address or telephone number. Immediate recall is tested by repetition of forward and backward digit spans (seven digits forward and backward suffice for average intelligence). Coding for storage and retrieval of engrams beyond one minute involves a complex process termed recent memory. Recent memory can be determined at the bedside by careful instruction and presentation of four unrelated words or simple geometric designs.[320] Following initial presentation the patient is distracted for up to 10 minutes by further history taking or examination. Then the patient is requested to recall or draw from memory the four original pieces of data. Alternatively, the patient observes four objects being hidden, is distracted, and locates the objects upon command 10 minutes later. Known anatomical substrates for recent memory are in hippocampal-diencephalic regions.[348] The precise pathophysiological alteration that accounts for the frequence of memory dysfunction in head trauma, if it occurs in these regions, is now known. Remote memories are made from recent memories following a consolidation period that takes years. By ascertaining scholastic, occupa-

tional, or family facts from early life, function of remote memory is determined. Remote memories are thought to be retained in cerebral cortex.

Memory loss for events prior to injury is termed retrograde amnesia. As recovery ensues, retrograde amnesia often contracts from several hours or days to several minutes or seconds.[32] This shrinkage indicates that the pathological alteration is not in the maintenance of stored memories but in their retrieval. Inability to form new memories after injury is termed antegrade amnesia. In severe head injuries, antegrade amnesia may persist indefinitely. In studies to determine the significance of amnesia surrounding a head injury, the term "post-traumatic amnesia" is used and refers to the time from injury until the return of continuous memory. Thus, post-traumatic amnesia is a defined class of antegrade amnesia.

In the serial examination of patients with head trauma, post-traumatic amnesia should be clearly distinguished from observed impairment of consciousness. The amnesia always is longer in duration. Usually the post-traumatic amnesia also is longer than the retrograde amnesia. Russell and collaborators have established the significance of post-traumatic amnesia by collating its duration with the severity and the outcome of head injury. They used the following scale for the amnesia: mild head injury, 0 to 1 hour; moderate injury, 1 to 24 hours; severe injury, 1 to 7 days; very severe injury, 7 days or longer.[299,300] Deficient memory following head trauma is associated with duration of the post-traumatic amnesia, especially in patients over age 30.[41] When determining post-traumatic amnesia, caution must be exercised to avoid mistaking an occasional island of memory from true termination of antegrade amnesia. Such misconceptions arise partly from the observation of normal behavior during the post-traumatic amnesia, e.g., a stunned football player who performs throughout a game, none of which he subsequently recollects. Correct post-traumatic amnesia intervals are best determined retrospectively or by repeated and discriminate testing of recent memory function.

The significance of retrograde amnesia, a failure in retrieval of stored memories, is not well established in head trauma patients. Russell and Nathan reported that retrograde amnesia was not found in one third of patients who had post-traumatic amnesia after gunshot wounds of the head.[299] Nevertheless, a prolonged retrograde amnesia is often concomitant with protracted post-traumatic amnesia. Conversely, shorter retrograde amnesia often identifies lesser head injuries as well as stabilization of the post-traumatic period following head injury. The tendency for retrograde amnesia to shrink with recovery, the frequency of alcohol intoxication at the time of injury, and the lack of precise determination of the time of impact have hampered investigation into the significance of retrograde amnesia.

Trauma to the surface of the dominant cerebral cortex may result in disturbed speech. Disorders of speech are occasionally misconstrued as the confused state that occurs in the early stages of post-traumatic amnesia. Recent investigations have shown that careful attention to the language examination is helpful in neuroanatomical localization of many common forms of aphasia.[33] By employing a brief practical examination of the major components of speech, it is possible to characterize many of these forms of aphasia.

Attention to fluency or rate of speech and its articulation determines the presence of a motor, or nonfluent, aphasia. This type of aphasia results from a lesion about Broca's area in the frontal operculum, anterior to the precentral gyrus region for discrete control of oral, pharyngeal, and laryngeal musculature. Auditory comprehension of speech is quickly determined by asking the patient to carry out a series of motor commands such as "close your eyes," "raise your left hand," and "stick out your tongue." If hand or facial apraxia is not present, this three-stage command is rapidly performed. Deficient auditory comprehension indicates a pathological disruption of Wernicke's area in the posterior superior temporal gyrus. The arcuate fasciculus connecting Wenicke's area and Broca's area serves the neural requirements of speech repetition.[106] Assessment of the ability to repeat short series of words, phrases, or simple sentences is important in separating types of speech disturbances, particularly division of the fluent aphasias into comprehension (Wernicke's), conduction, isola-

tion, and anomic forms.[107] In Wernicke's aphasia the ability to follow commands and to repeat is impaired. In conduction aphasia the arcuate fasciculus is damaged and repetition, principally, is compromised. In isolation aphasia, repetition is the only expression of language that is performed by the patient. A pure anomic aphasia is rare. Nonetheless, naming of objects, particularly their parts, is a function wholly separate from amnestic states. It rarely occurs alone in aphasic conditions but commonly accompanies the various aphasias.

The capacity to read is located about the posterior edge of the superior temporal sulcus in the angular gyrus. Dysfunction of this area results in acquired alexia. The capacity to read is tested by reading both aloud and silently. Some degree of agraphia, loss of the ability to employ linguistic symbols, occurs with many of the aphasias. Determination of these seven components of language—fluency, articulation, repetition, naming, auditory comprehension, reading, and writing—is obtainable within a short period at the bedside. The information so gained provides a practical guide for localization within the dominant hemisphere.

Evaluation of power, tone, and fine coordination of the limbs; primary and integrated (parietal) sensory modalities; deep tendon and pathological reflexes; and cerebellar functions is all part of the first complete examination and subsequent examinations. Careful attention is given to patients with psychological complaints and poor concentration, and in this case, special testing of intelligence and behavior is useful (see Chapter 63).

Computed Tomography

Prior to the advent of computed tomography in 1972, radiological investigation in acute head injury consisted primarily of radiography of the skull, cerebral angiography, and encephalography. The radiographs of the skull were helpful in the detection of fractures, scalp injury, foreign bodies, and pneumocephalus. Evaluation of intracranial lesions was limited to the detection of mass effect as shown by displacement of the pineal body or choroid plexus if they were calcified. Contrast procedures such as angiography and to a lesser degree encephalography were necessary to localize the traumatic intracranial lesions as shown by the displacement of either vascular structures or the ventricular system. The contrast procedures, in addition to being time-consuming, are associated with morbidity. Angiography provides a specific diagnosis only in the case of extracerebral lesions or vascular injury. It is difficult, if not impossible, to distinguish intracerebral lesions such as focal swelling and edema from hematomas.

Introduced by Hounsfield and Ambrose in 1972, computed axial tomography, or computed tomography (CT), has revolutionized the diagnostic evaluation of intracranial disorders in general and traumatic intracranial lesions in particular.[9,142] Computed tomography is a noninvasive technique and requires only 30 minutes to study the entire intracranial cavity with the first-generation scanner manufactured by EMI Medical, Inc. With its unique ability to detect the subtle differences in soft-tissue density, computed tomography proved valuable in detecting various traumatic intracranial lesions: intra- and extracerebral hematomas, infarctions, edema, contusions, and the like. These features prompted the early investigators to state that "The accuracy of diagnosis is such that emergency cerebral angiography has been virtually eliminated."[266] Although this view has been somewhat tempered by further experience, computed tomography has nevertheless replaced cerebral angiography as the primary radiological method of investigation in head injury.

When computed tomography is used as the primary radiological technique in the evaluation of acute head injury, the patient should be handled with caution to avoid further injury during the procedure. Associated injuries, especially those involving the cervical spine, should be considered before the patient is moved or manipulated. It is essential that a transtable lateral radiograph of the cervical spine be obtained to detect the presence of a fracture before the patient is transferred for computed tomographic examination. If a fracture is present, depending upon its severity and extent, the cervical spine should be adequately immobilized before the scan is performed. If necessary, a physician should be with the patient throughout the scanning to assure immobilization.

Procedure and Technique of CT Examination in Brain Injury

Four conventional cuts covering approximately 10 cm of intracranial contents are performed, care being taken to include the uppermost surface of the cerebral hemispheres, visualizing the sulci in the parasagittal region. Whenever possible, the examination should include the posterior fossa structures. Demonstration of these structures can be accomplished by flexing the patient's neck and angling the x-ray beam between 15 and 20 degrees caudally to the orbitomeatal line (Reid's baseline). The flexion of the neck is not necessary with the newer scanners on which the gantry can be tilted to varying degrees. The patient is moved 2.5 cm at the end of each scan. Each scan produces two images, each of which represents a reconstructed section of the brain of approximately 1.3 cm thickness based upon the attenuation coefficients of structures in that plane. Eight images resulting from four sequential scans should adequately cover the brain, including the posterior fossa.

The quality of the computed tomographic image can be markedly compromised by patient motion during the scanning period. This problem has been somewhat minimized by the development of faster scanners. Nevertheless, any movement can produce artifacts and obscure significant intracranial lesions. Therefore, immobilization should be accomplished by the use of adequate restraining devices. It may be advantageous to intubate the patient and paralyze him during scanning. Most patients with severe brain injuries are best studied in this manner.

In patients with multiple injuries and in whom hemorrhage is suspected in other parts of the body that may require an immediate operative procedure, the cranial CT examination can be modified to save time. In such instances only a single scan through the level of the lateral ventricles should be obtained. This view is adequate to evaluate the supratentorial structures and will reveal the presence of midline displacement or a large extra- or intracerebral hematoma that would require immediate craniotomy (Fig.

Figure 58–4 A single scan at the level of the lateral ventricles revealing a large subdural hematoma on the left side with appropriate left-to-right midline displacement. The patient was immediately taken to the operating room for craniotomy without performing a complete computed tomographic examination, thus saving time. A subsequent examination revealed the full extent of the right-sided intracerebral hematoma, which did not require operative removal.

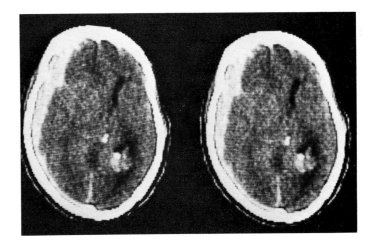

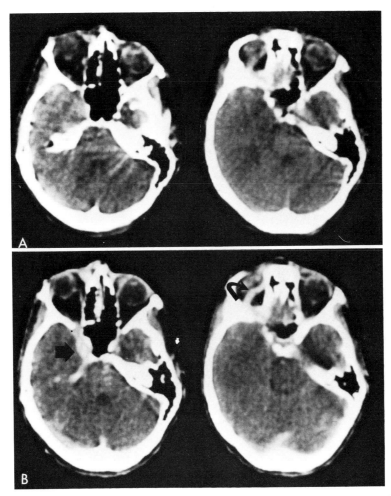

Figure 58–5 *A.* The precontrast CT image reveals no significant abnormality. *B.* Following intravenous administration of contrast material an area of increased density is seen in the left parasellar region and the orbit, indicating the presence of a carotid cavernous fistula, with visualization of the superior ophthalmic vein (*arrows*). (Courtesy of M. S. Huckman, M.D., Rush Presbyterian Medical College, Chicago, Ill.)

58–4). A complete examination can be performed subsequently for the detection of additional intracranial lesions. It should be noted, however, that a significant hematoma may be present over the high convexity bilaterally and still escape detection if only a single scan is obtained. The need to obtain complete computed tomographic examination should be based upon the guidelines discussed in the section on the management of patients with head injury.

If the patient's condition is stable clinically and a complete and accurate history is not available, in addition to conventional CT scanning, repeat scanning following intravenous administration of iodinated contrast material (Renografin or Hypaque) should be performed. Contrast helps to enhance lesions not clearly discernible on conventional computed tomography. Lesions such as arteriovenous fistulae, arteriovenous malformations, and highly vascular membranes around chronic subdural hematomas are detected because of the intravascular pooling of iodine (Figs. 58–5 and 58–6). Double scanning (scanning both before and after contrast administration) is also beneficial in demonstrating traumatic infarctions (Fig. 58–7). Enhancement in the latter condition is probably secondary to the breakdown of the blood-brain barrier and leakage of iodine into the diseased part of the brain. Contrast enhancement is helpful in the detection of abscess formation and extracerebral empyemas (Figs. 58–8 and 58–9). Some of the isodense hematomas may be detected by contrast enhancement, thus obviating the need for angiography, as discussed later. Finally, contrast enhancement can help to differentiate an apparent hematoma on the unenhanced image from a tumor by bringing out additional abnormal areas (Fig. 58–10).

Although computed tomography is a very sensitive examination for the evaluation of most lesions resulting from acute head trauma, patients with focal neurological deficit may not show any abnormality on

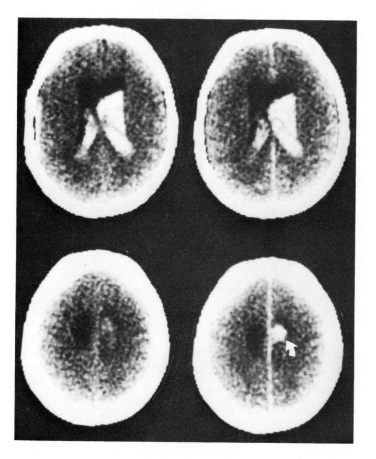

Figure 58–6 Precontrast computed tomography reveals intracerebral and intraventricular hemorrhage in a 68-year-old woman, apparently following a fall (*left*). Following contrast administration (*right*) a small area of increased density is seen in the right parasagittal region (*arrow*) because of intravascular pooling of iodine in an arteriovenous malformation. The diagnosis was confirmed at autopsy.

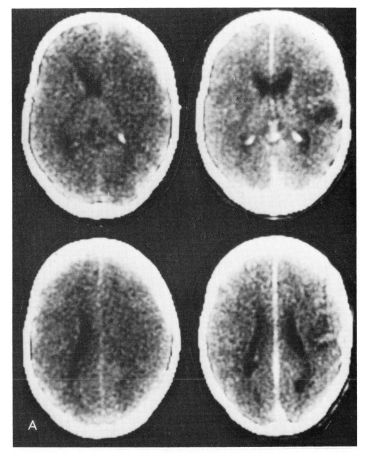

Figure 58–7 *A*. Precontrast CT scan in a 36-year-old woman who underwent right craniotomy for the evacuation of a subdural hematoma following head injury reveals no abnormality (*left*). Following intravenous contrast administration (*right*) areas of increased density indicative of infarction are seen. *B*. Right carotid angiogram revealing occlusion of multiple branches of the middle cerebral artery (*arrows*).

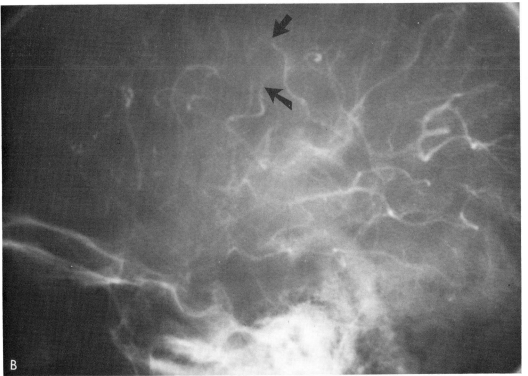

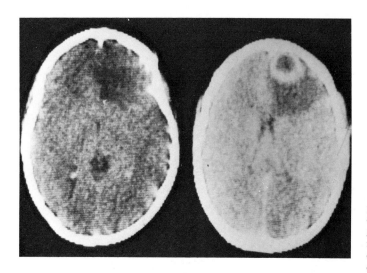

Figure 58-8 Precontrast computed tomography revealing an area of low density in the right frontal region in a patient with a fracture of the right frontal bone (*left*). Following contrast administration a well-circumscribed peripheral rim of enhancement consistent with an abscess is seen (*right*). The abscess was excised. (Courtesy of C. V. G. Krishna Rao, M.D., University of Maryland Hospital, Baltimore, Md.)

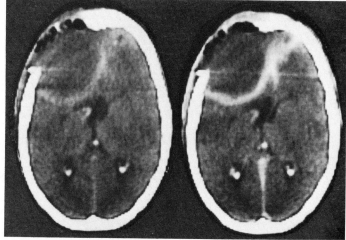

Figure 58-9 Precontrast computed tomography in a patient who underwent left frontal craniectomy for evacuation of an epidural hematoma shows an area of low density consistent with an extra-axial collection (*left*). Following administration of contrast the periphery of the lesion is enhanced, indicating inflammatory changes (*right*). At operation this was found to be an epidural empyema. (Courtesy of C. V. G. Krishna Rao, M.D., University of Maryland Hospital, Baltimore, Md.)

the *initial* examination. Merino-de-Villa-sante and Taveras showed that in 6 of 20 patients with lateralizing findings following head injury, the CT scan was entirely normal.[236] Similar experiences have been reported by other investigators.[87,100,173] Four of ten patients who developed subdural collections, or "hygromas," as reported by French and Dublin, had normal scans in the immediate post-traumatic period.[100] Sweet and his colleagues showed that 13 of the 52 patients (25 per cent) with bilateral lesions revealed on repeat scans during the first week had had only unilateral lesions on the initial scan.[332] These reports indicate the need for *repeat* computed tomography during the first week to detect additional lesions. Detection of edema and infarctions is also facilitated by following this routine.

If the CT scan is normal in the presence of a focal neurological deficit or if the abnormal findings on computed tomography do not correlate with the patient's clinical findings, one should consider proceeding to cerebral angiography. It is the only way to detect vascular injury in the acute stage. In such cases both the extra- and intracranial vascular tree should be evaluated.

The general principles of computed tomography are discussed in Chapter 5; the special requirements and principles necessary for evaluation of patients with head trauma are discussed here.

In computed tomography (or reconstructive tomography) the x-rays enter only the plane of the desired area and do not enter other layers, thus eliminating the blurred image. By its ability to reconstruct the image of intracranial structures, depending upon the attenuation characteristics of the

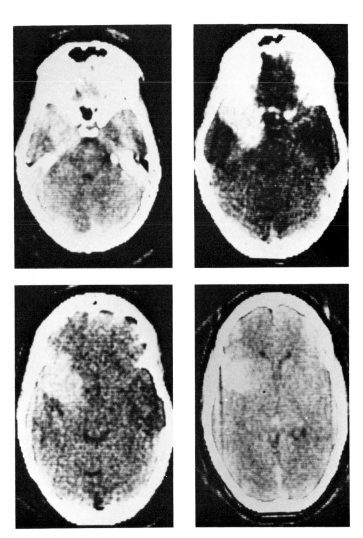

Figure 58–10 A. 34-year-old woman presenting with a history of injury during skiing 15 days prior to examination. Precontrast examination reveals a well-circumscribed area of increased density in the left temporal region with attenuation values in the range of 65, consistent with a hematoma (*left*). Following intravenous contrast administration there is increased density with an additional area of enhancement (*right*). At operation this was a meningioma.

x-ray beam, computed tomography is capable of revealing subtle differences in soft-tissue density of approximately 0.5 per cent.[142,223,260] The sensitivity of this method required a new description of attenuation coefficients. The first scale introduced by Hounsfield referred to the absorption coefficient of water as 0, that of air as −500, and that of bone as +500.[142] This scale has been expanded by a factor of 2, making air −1000 and bone +1000. Absorption values are described in Hounsfield (H) numbers.[42]

Hounsfield numbers can be defined by the following:

$$H = \frac{\mu \text{ tissue} - \mu \text{ water}}{\mu \text{ water}} \times 1000$$

where μ is the linear attenuation coefficient.

Because of the difference in absorption coefficients, various structures are clearly seen on images reconstructed with the assistance of the computer.

The H numbers for intracranial structures are approximately as follows:

Fat	−100
Cerebrospinal fluid	4–10
White matter	22–36
Gray matter	32–46
Extravasated blood	50–90
Bone or calcification	80–1000

To be able to evaluate traumatic intracranial lesions, one must be aware of the limitations of the resolution on computed tomography and the degradation of the images secondary to artifacts.

Partial Volume Effect

A structure that only partially fills the slice of a tissue does not contribute its full density to the image. The reason for this is that the density at any point of the image is the result of an average of attenuation over the entire beam height or slice thickness (Fig. 58–11). Thus, if half of the slice thickness is occupied by a blood clot with an attenuation value of 80 and the other half by bone with an attenuation value of 1000 the resultant density of the entire slice thickness would be 540 H and will be shown on the reconstructed image as bone. Therefore, a 6-mm (half of the usual slice thickness of 1.3 cm) deep subdural hematoma located over the high convexity may appear

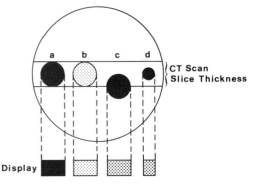

Figure 58–11 Schematic diagram of partial volume effect. Lesions with low attenuation such as cystic cavities (a) and high attenuation such as hematomas (b), when they occupy the entire thickness of the slice of a tissue, are displayed accordingly on the computed tomographic image. If they contribute only partially to the slice (c,d), the image displays the result of averaged attenuation, including the values of adjacent tissues, with varying degrees of density.

as a part of the bony calvarium and go undetected on a conventional CT image. In one series of 21 extracerebral lesions in 15 patients, four hematomas were not detected on computed tomography.[331] Two of these four were 4 mm in thickness on the angiogram and were confirmed at operation. These 2 hematomas and 2 of the 10 hematomas not seen on computed tomography by Levander and his associates were considered to be acute.[196] The nonvisualization of these hematomas may, in part, be secondary to the partial volume effect. A small intracerebral hematoma also may not be detected for this reason. In such cases a scanning technique that allows overlapping of adjacent sections of brain would help in detecting lesions (Fig. 58–12). Partial volume effect would also partly explain the discrepancy in the size of a hematoma as seen on the CT scan and that at operation, where it is usually found to be larger. The reverse of this situation is also true. In the region of the inferior frontal lobe the bony irregularity of the orbital roof may give rise to an artifactual high density mimicking a hemorrhagic contusion. This problem can be resolved by scanning the area at a different angle (Fig. 58–13).

Movement of the patient's head during scanning causes artifacts, thus degrading the image. These motion artifacts are particularly severe in the vicinity of bone, where the extracerebral hematomas are located. Thus, in the case of a patient with a

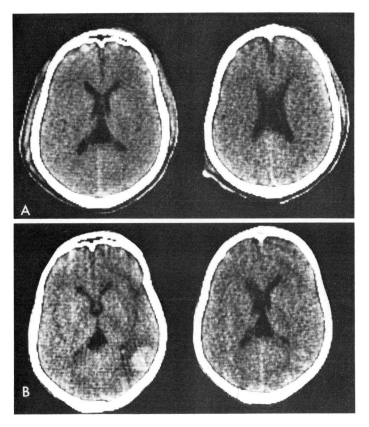

Figure 58–12 *A*. Initial examination of a 50-year-old man with acute head injury. No abnormality is noted. *B*. Because of clinical findings referable to the right hemisphere, a repeat examination was performed with overlapping cuts (the patient was moved only 2 cm at the end of each scan to offset the partial volume effect). A right paraventricular hematoma measuring approximately 2.5 cm is now clearly seen.

Figure 58–13 An area of increased density is seen in the right inferior frontal region (*arrow*), suggesting a hemorrhagic contusion because of the partial volume effect from the irregular floor of the anterior fossa (*left*). The same area is found to be normal following scanning in a slightly different angle of x-ray beam (*right*).

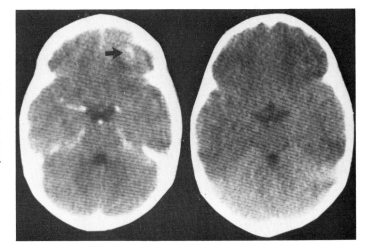

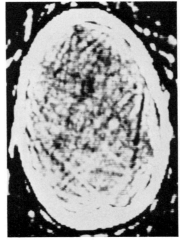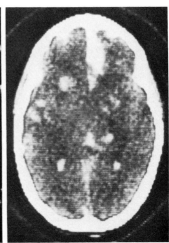

Figure 58–14 Severe motion artifacts make the scan uninterpretable (*left*). Repeat examination following adequate sedation reveals multiple intracerebral hematomas that were totally obscured by motion artifacts (*right*).

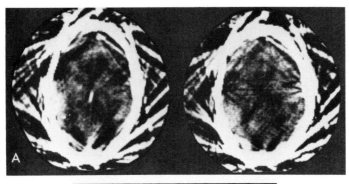

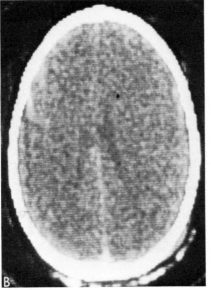

Figure 58–15 *A*. Motion artifacts causing "apparent hematomas." *B*. Repeat examination without motion artifacts reveals no evidence of hematomas.

head injury who is unable to cooperate by holding his head still during scanning, artifacts can totally obscure significant intracranial hematomas or produce "apparent" hematomas in normal patients (Figs. 58–14 and 58–15).

Traumatic Craniocerebral Lesions Demonstrable on Computed Tomography

The incidence of abnormal findings on computed tomography in patients with head injury has varied considerably in reports in the literature, from 37 per cent in the series reported by Baker and co-workers to 73 per cent in that of Paxton and Ambrose.* The incidence of abnormalities reported will depend upon the accessibility of the scanner, the patient population selected, and the severity of the head injuries included in the study. In one of the largest series published so far, by French and Dublin, consisting of 316 patients with head injury, 51 per cent showed abnormal CT findings and 38 per cent had more than one abnormality. Only 13 per cent of patients who were alert and neurologically intact had abnormalities on the CT scan as compared with 50 per cent with focal neurological deficit who showed such abnormalities.[100] In another retrospective study by Merino de Villasante and Taveras, 75 per cent of the patients with lateralizing findings showed CT scan abnormalities.[236] Sweet and his associates in their review of 140 patients with severe head injury (patients unable to give a verbal response and unable to follow a simple command at the time) who were managed by a standardized protocol, found 114, or 82 per cent, to have abnormalities on the initial CT scan. Of these 114 patients, 37 had a unilateral extracerebral mass, 32 had unilateral intracerebral hematoma or hemorrhagic contusion, 6 had edema or necrotic contusion, and the remaining 39 showed bilateral intra- and extracerebral lesions.[332] Fifty-eight patients (41 per cent) were considered to have lesions requiring operative decompression and went on to have craniotomy. An accurate and meaningful assessment of computed tomographic abnormalities can only be made by studies that separate the vari-

ous clinical categories of patients with head injury rather than lumping mild and severe injuries together.

Evolution of Hematoma

In order to evaluate the CT findings in head injury it is necessary to understand the pathophysiology of the evolution of an intracranial hematoma. Recently extravasated blood has higher attenuation values than brain tissue and ranges from 50 to 90 H units. The high attenuation value of a recent hematoma is attributed to the clot retraction and high degree of absorption in the hemoglobin, particularly the globin molecule.[35,253] The attenuation value of a hematoma decreases gradually over a period of weeks and is dependent upon its initial size and whether fluids of low attenuation value, such as cerebrospinal fluid, are mixed with the clot, as is usually the case with subdural lesions. The exact location of the hematoma, whether extradural, subdural, or intracerebral, also may influence the attenuation value. As the clot disintegrates, a decrease in attenuation occurs. During this resolution, at a certain time (usually two to four weeks in the case of an intracerebral hematoma), the attenuation is similar to that of the adjacent brain and the hematoma is not detectable by the naked eye.[82] These hematomas may be termed "isodense." Bergstrom and coworkers have shown a similar evolution in subdural hematomas.[35]

Changes in the appearance of a hematoma over time probably occur by different mechanisms for intracerebral and extracerebral hematomas. In the case of a subdural hematoma some absorption of fluid probably takes place across the membrane into the hematoma, and the attenuation value gradually decreases toward that of cerebrospinal fluid. The membrane that is formed around the subdural hematoma has a rich vascularity, and this may be detected following contrast enhancement (Fig. 58–16). Scotti and his associates reported enhancement of this membrane in two of their five patients with isodense hematomas. The remaining three had no evidence of membrane at operation.[304]

Occasionally, one may be able to see a low-attenuation collection in the supernatant area with increased density in the dependent portion in the case of a subdural

---

* See references 17, 87, 100, 173, 180, 196, 236, 266.

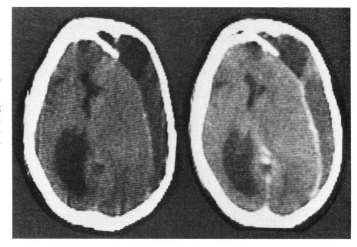

Figure 58-16 Precontrast CT scan revealing extracerebral collection on the right side (*left*). Following intravenous contrast administration there is enhancement of the membrane (*right*). The lesion was confirmed at operation.

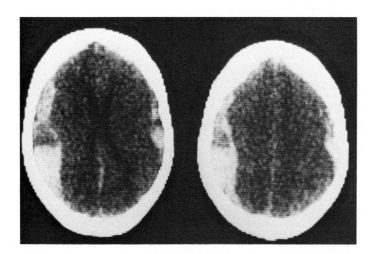

Figure 58-17 Large left subdural hematoma showing increased density in the dependent portion with supernatant clear zone.

Figure 58-18 Several areas of low density are seen in the right hemisphere. Compression and displacement of the right lateral ventricle are seen on the examination performed on the fifth day following head injury. These areas probably represent "edema."

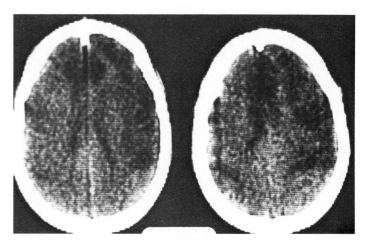

hematoma (Fig. 58–17). This is probably secondary to the sedimentation of corpuscular elements in the dependent part of the hematoma. A similar phenomenon can also be seen with hemorrhage into the ventricular system. The CT scan shows increased density in the dependent portion of the ventricles and relatively decreased density due to the cerebrospinal fluid in the uppermost portion (see Fig. 58–6). The initial high attenuation value of a fresh hematoma may go on to a "hypodense" stage or even drop to the cerebrospinal fluid range by three weeks.[304]

Edema

On computed tomography edema is seen as a zone of low density with attenuation values ranging between 16 and 24 H as compared with white matter (22 to 36 H). Associated with this low density, a mass effect on the adjacent ventricles may be seen, reflected as compression, distortion, and displacement of the ventricular system (Fig. 58–18). The edema may be mild and focal, or may be multifocal, bilateral, or diffuse, With diffuse cerebral edema, one may not be able to appreciate an area of low density, as no area of normal brain density is evident for comparison. Generalized edema may be apparent only as generalized compression and decrease in ventricular size, which may be so gross as to result in nonvisualization of the ventricular system (Fig. 58–19). In such cases the attenuation value of the hemisphere should be measured by using the devices available on the display units. These devices vary from the "measure" mode available on the first-generation EMI scanners to a "joy stick" by which the mean attenuation value of any region is measured instantly.

While computed tomography provides the opportunity to detect brain edema, it is important to recognize that not all areas of low density on the CT scan represent edema. Each picture point of a CT image represents the average of the attenuation coefficients of all histological elements in that volume of tissue, i.e., $1.5 \times 1.5 \times 13$ mm (using 160×160 matrix). Predominance of low-attenuation components such as lipids, cavitation, and necrosis in a block of tissue may obscure the presence of small hemorrhages and appear as areas of low density similar to that of edema.

Similarly, as shown by Lanksch and coworkers, edema may not be apparent on computed tomography as an area of low density if there is a concurrent decrease in the lipid content, offsetting the decreased attenuation of increased cerebral water content.[191]

Contusion

Cerebral contusions are seen as nonhomogeneous areas of high density often interspersed with areas of low density with attenuation values in the range of 50 to 60 H (Fig. 58–20A). The CT appearance results from multiple small, scattered areas of hemorrhage within the brain substance associated with areas of edema and tissue necrosis. Depending upon the extent of hemorrhage, the degree of edema, and the time elapsed since injury, contusion may appear predominantly dense or lucent. Usually, on scans performed within 24 hours after injury contusions appear as an area of predominantly increased density. As the hemorrhage resolves, they appear to have a lower density and may look similar to "edema" (Fig. 58–20B). This phenomenon was evident in the series reported by French and Dublin.[100] They described 54 patients with contusion or edema. In the 33 patients said to have contusion, 24, or 72 per cent, of the scans had been performed early, during the first day after injury. On the other hand, in 21 of the 54 patients said to have edema, 17, or 81 per cent, had their scans performed more than 24 hours after injury.

The margin of the contusion is usually poorly defined. Contusions are often surrounded by a low-density zone, probably representing true edema. Occasionally, contusions may be difficult to differentiate from an extracerebral hematoma with intracerebral extension, particularly in the frontal area. Contusions may be single or multiple. A cerebral contusion may also demonstrate a mass effect with ventricular distortion and displacement. Serial scanning can detect the progression in the size of a contusion and the development of new hemorrhagic lesions not present in the immediate post-traumatic period (Figs. 58–21 and 58–22). The contusion may ultimately resolve completely over several days and

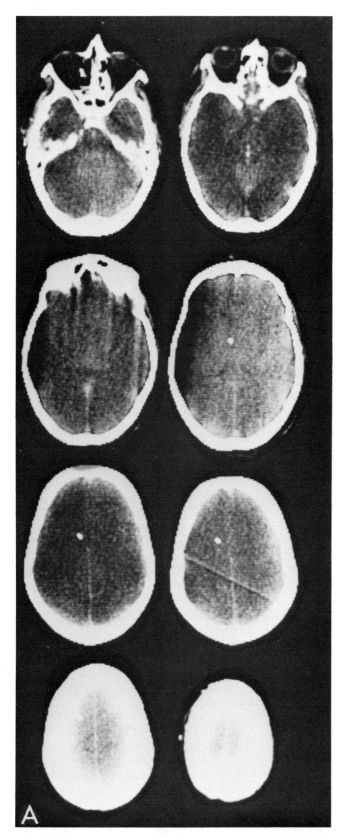

Figure 58–19 *A*. Three days after the patient's injury, nonvisualization of both lateral ventricles is presumably secondary to edema. Attenuation values measured in the range of 20.

Illustration continued on opposite page

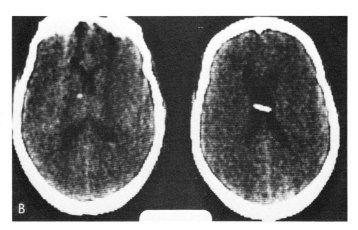

Figure 58–19 (*continued*) *B.* Computed tomography on the day of admission reveals normal-sized ventricles.

leave residual changes similar to porencephaly or focal atrophy, shown on computed tomography as areas of cerebrospinal fluid density (Fig. 58–23).

Intracerebral Hematoma

Intracerebral hematomas are seen as well-circumscribed areas of homogeneous high density with attenuation values in the range of 70 to 90. These are also usually surrounded by areas of low density due to edema (Fig. 58–24). Because of the high attenuation value of a recent hematoma, which is surrounded by the low density of brain, even a 0.5-cm lesion can be detected on computed tomography (Fig. 58–25). This markedly increased density of an acute hematoma diminishes gradually with time, owing to the disintegration of blood components. In the isodense stage, a hema-

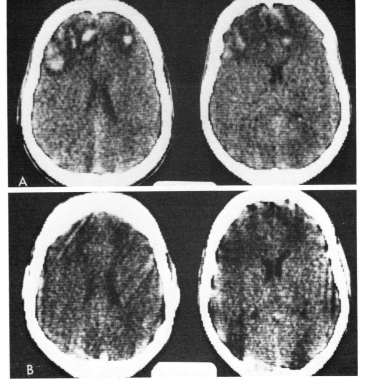

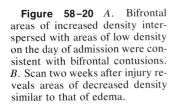

Figure 58–20 *A.* Bifrontal areas of increased density interspersed with areas of low density on the day of admission were consistent with bifrontal contusions. *B.* Scan two weeks after injury reveals areas of decreased density similar to that of edema.

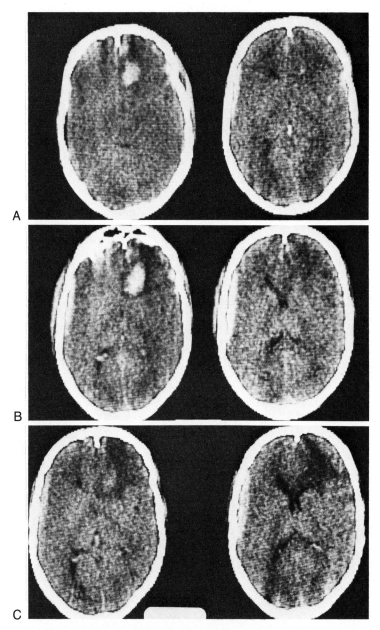

Figure 58–21 Serial computed tomography. *A.* The patient presented with right frontal contusion. *B.* On the third day, a slight increase is seen in the size of the contusion, which went on to apparent resolution. *C.* Increased density gradually decreased, reaching the isodense stage by 14 days.

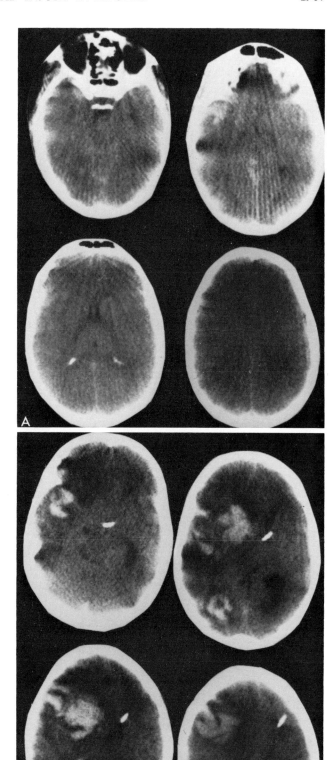

Figure 58–22 *A*. Initial CT scan on day 1 revealing small areas of increased density in the left temporal region with surrounding areas of decreased density. *B*. Scan performed within 48 hours following the first examination reveals large left temporofrontal homorrhagic areas causing marked left-to-right midline displacement.

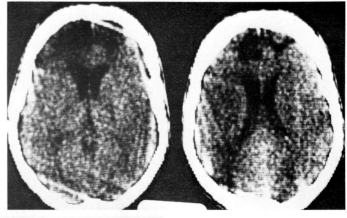

Figure 58-23 The patient shown in Figure 58–21 went on to show residual changes (areas of decreased density similar to that of cerebrospinal fluid) similar to those of focal atrophy.

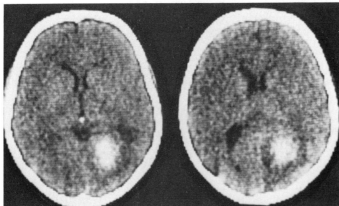

Figure 58–24 Intracerebral hematoma with well-defined margins in surrounding zone of low density presumably secondary to edema.

Figure 58–25 A small hematoma measuring less than 1 cm in diameter is seen in the left temporal region following trauma (*left*). Repeat computed tomography five weeks following injury reveals no discernible residual parenchymal change (*right*).

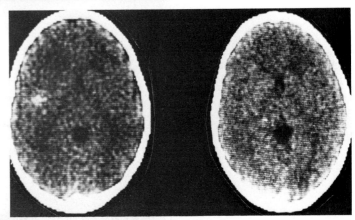

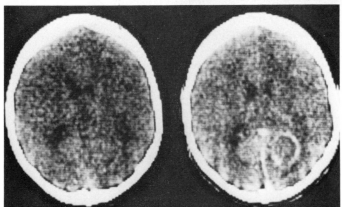

Figure 58–26 Precontrast CT scan reveals no abnormality in the right hemisphere of a patient with a four-week-old hematoma (*left*). Peripheral enhancement in the post-contrast scan reveals the presence of a hematoma (*right*).

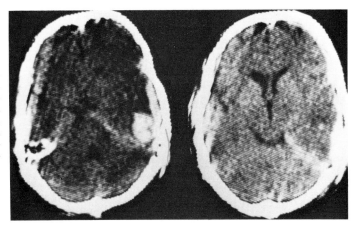

Figure 58–27 Hematoma located near the surface of the right hemisphere simulates an extra-axial collection. The medial margin of the hematoma forms an acute angle with the inner table of the skull, however, suggesting the intracerebral location of hemorrhage. A small subdural hematoma is also associated with the intracerebral hematoma.

toma may be completely missed unless close attention is paid to the presence of a mass effect as shown by midline displacement or distortion of the ventricular system.[238] Contrast-enhanced computed tomography may help to visualize these isodense lesions (Fig. 58–26). As the resolution of the intracerebral hematoma progresses further, it leaves an area of low density that appears similar to porencephaly (cf. Fig. 58–23). As shown in Figure 58–26, a discernible residual change may not be seen in the case of a hematoma less than 2 cm in its initial size.[82]

Traumatic intracerebral hematomas may be multiple, in contradistinction to the hematomas usually resulting from hypertension, aneurysms, or arteriovenous malformations (cf. Fig. 58–14). Traumatic hematomas are usually located in the frontal and the anterior temporal lobes, although they may be seen in other intracranial areas. The majority of the intracerebral hematomas develop immediately after head injury. They may, however, develop after a certain delay in time ranging from hours to three weeks after injury. The most common time for delayed occurrence is reported to be during the first week after injury.[19,288,332]

An intra-axial hematoma located near the surface of the brain may occasionally mimic an extracerebral hematoma. Koo and LaRoque pointed out that they can be distinguished by the relationship of the medial margin of the hematoma to the inner table.[180] The medial margin of an intracerebral clot tends to form an acute angle with the inner table, whereas the angle is obtuse in the case of an extracerebral hematoma (Fig. 58–27).

Subdural Hematoma

The majority of acute subdural hematomas are seen as zones of increased density following the surface of the brain, thus

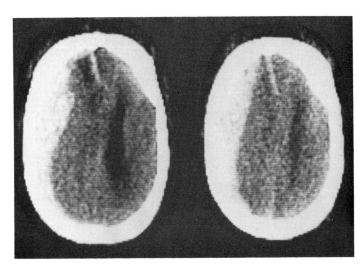

Figure 58–28 Acute subdural hematoma follows the surface of the brain, thus having a concave inner margin.

having a concave inner margin and a convex outer margin adjacent to the inner table of the skull (Fig. 58–28). The typical subdural hematoma tends to be more diffuse than an epidural hematoma, the peripheral expansion of which is limited by firm dural attachment to the inner table.

A subdural hematoma measuring 5 to 6 mm in depth is usually clearly seen on computed tomography. Smaller lesions, however, may not be seen because of the close proximity of the hematoma to the bony calvarium, and even a significant hematoma along the high convexity and displacing the ventricle may be missed on the scan because of the partial volume artifact described earlier. Often some of these high lesions can be detected if the scanning is performed with the x-ray beam perpendicular to the region of interest, as shown by Svendsen (Fig. 58–29).[331] This view is easily accomplished by either tilting the head or positioning the patient in a lateral decubitus position.

Attempts to classify subdural hematomas as acute, subacute, and chronic on the basis of the density seen on computed tomography created considerable confusion. Scotti and his associates evaluated the age of a subdural hematoma on the basis of its density and found a high degree of correlation between the density and the age.[304] Forty-two patients with subdural hematomas were divided into three groups: acute cases (duration of symptoms 0 to 7 days), subacute (7 to 22 days), and chronic (>22 days). One hundred per cent of patients whose hematomas were in the acute category had lesions that appeared hyperdense on computed tomography. Seventy per cent of lesions in the subacute category were isodense, and 76 per cent of the chronic hematomas were hypodense. Absolute reliance on classification of hematomas as acute or chronic based on CT density, however, can lead to inaccuracies. For example, recent hemorrhage into a chronic subdural hematoma causing compression of the brain with midline displacement may be isodense on the CT scan because of the mixture of blood and clear fluid. This would be referred to as a "subacute" hematoma according to the foregoing classification. An example of this is illustrated in Figure 58–30. The density of an acute subdural hygroma would look similar to a chronic sub-

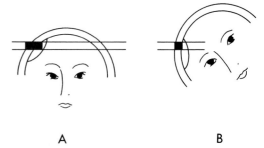

A   B

Figure 58–29 Schematic representation of an extracerebral hematoma along the high convexity. *A.* Conventional CT section. A large part of the hematoma is masked by the high degree of attenuation of bone. *B.* With the head tilted in relation to the tomographic plane, the partial volume effect is minimized, enabling better visualization of the hematoma, since the x-ray beam is at 90 degrees to the bone and lesion. (After Svendsen, P.: Computer tomography of traumatic extracerebral lesions. *Brit. J. Radiol. 49*:1004–1012, 1976.)

dural hematoma on the computed tomogram (Fig. 58–31). Additionally, because of a low hemoglobin concentration, the hematoma of a patient with a low hematocrit at the time of hemorrhage may demonstrate relatively low density, even in the acute stage.[253] An accurate clinical history would help in determining the nature of these lesions, but such information is often not available in patients with acute head injury.

Compression of the brain and midline displacement is often seen with a subdural hematoma. If an appropriate midline displacement is not seen in the presence of a subdural mass lesion, one should look for lesions on the contralateral side, particularly in the subtemporal and temporal regions where, because of artifacts, the hematomas are often difficult to visualize. It is also useful to remember that approximately 45 per cent of subdural hematomas are associated with other abnormalities such as cerebral contusions and hematomas.[87,288]

The hematomas in the "isodense" stage, if not associated with a significant mass effect, may not be seen on computed tomography. There are certain clues present in such cases that should alert the clinician to the necessity of evaluating such a patient further by other techniques. Usually there is effacement of cerebral sulci over the convexity on the side of the subdural hematoma (Fig. 58–32). Distortion of the ipsilateral lateral ventricle may also be evident.

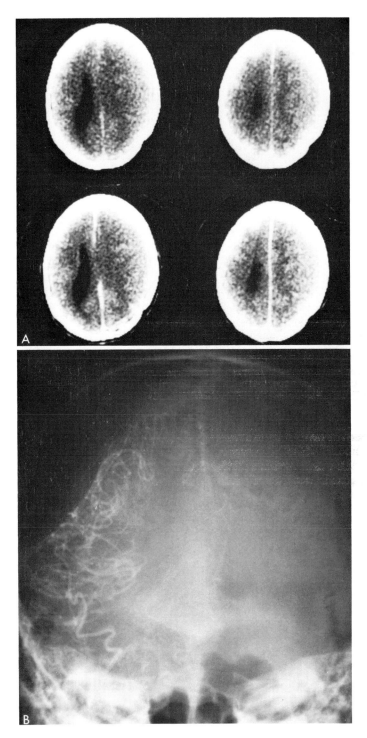

Figure 58–30   Sixty-year-old man with altered mental status and left-sided weakness of recent onset. There was no history of recent trauma. *A*. Precontrast (*top*) and postcontrast (*bottom*) CT scans demonstrate right-to-left midline displacement and distortion of right lateral ventricle without evidence of an extra-axial mass lesion. *B*. Right carotid angiogram in anteroposterior projection reveals a localized subdural hematoma. At operation the extracerebral collection was shown to be a chronic subdural hematoma. Evidence of recent hemorrhage accounted for the "isodense" appearance on computed tomography.

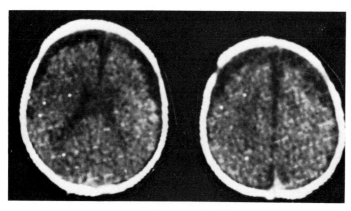

Figure 58–31 CT scan of a patient with history of head injury two days prior to the examination shows bilateral extracerebral low-density collections. At operation they were found to be subdural hygromas.

If contrast enhancement does not show significant focal alteration in density within the hemisphere, the mass is probably extra-axial in location. Exceptions are seen, however, for occasionally an intra-axial lesion may not show a discernible focal alteration in density on a contrast-enhanced CT scan (Fig. 58–33). Contrast enhancement may enable the visualization of the membrane around the subdural hematoma, or the contrast material may seep into the subdural collection itself and show as an area of increased density. If may also enhance the brain tissue enough to show some

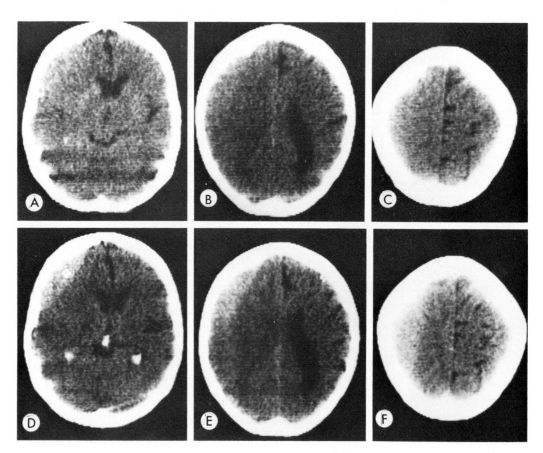

Figure 58–32 *A*, *B*, and *C*. There is minimal left-to-right midline displacement and effacement of the sulci over the left convexity on the precontrast CT scan, secondary to a subdural hematoma. *D*, *E*, and *F*. The hematoma is shown on the delayed postcontrast scan. (From Amendola, M. A., and Ostrum, R. J.: Diagnosis of isodense subdural hematomas by computed tomography. Amer. J. Roentgen., *129*:693–697, 1977. Reprinted by permission.)

increased density, making the isodense hematoma appear as a relatively lucent area. Amendola and Ostrum have shown that 40 per cent of isodense subdural hematomas can be enhanced and visualized by scanning the patient four to six hours after intravenous administration of iodinated contrast material (Fig. 58–34).[11] Digital filtering techniques as well as subtraction techniques may also help in demonstrating these lesions.[42,192]

The CT image of hemiatrophy can simulate an isodense hematoma. A relatively small lateral ventricle, absence of sulci or normal sulci over the convexity, and midline shift to the atrophic side harboring a large ventricle could easily suggest the presence of an isodense lesion on the normal side.

A subdural hematoma with decreased attenuation is shown in Figure 58–35. Usually hematomas in their chronic stages have a biconvex appearance and do not pose a diagnostic problem. In patients with atrophy, particularly atrophy that is focal in nature, the dilated subarachnoid space may resemble a chronic subdural hematoma, but observation of the cerebrospinal fluid den-

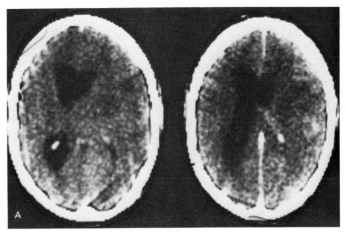

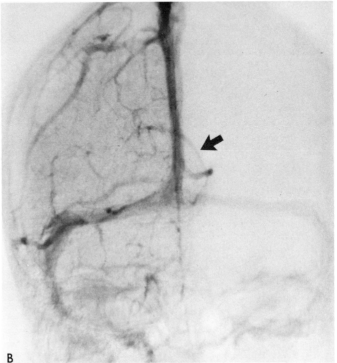

Figure 58–33 *A.* Pre- and postcontrast computed tomography does not reveal an alteration in parenchymal density indicative of an extracerebral mass effect. *B.* Angiography reveals no extracerebral mass. Instead there is superior and medial displacement of the thalamostriate vein consistent with a thalamic mass lesion (*arrow*).

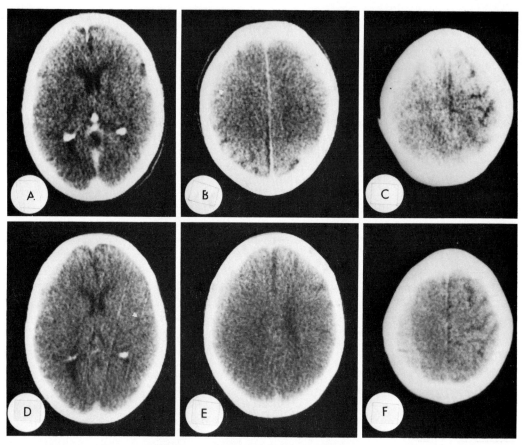

Figure 58–34 *A, B,* and *C.* Immediate postcontrast infusion examination fails to reveal the presence of extracerebral hematoma. *D, E,* and *F.* Scanning performed six hours following intravenous administration of contrast material brings out the well-localized subdural hematoma. (From Amendola, M. A., and Ostrum, R. J.: Diagnosis of isodense subdural hematomas by computed tomography. Amer. J. Roentgen., *129*:693–697, 1977. Reprinted by permission.)

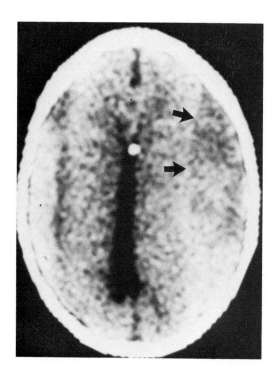

Figure 58–35 Bilateral chronic subdural hematomas with decreased attenuation and biconvex configuration (*arrows*).

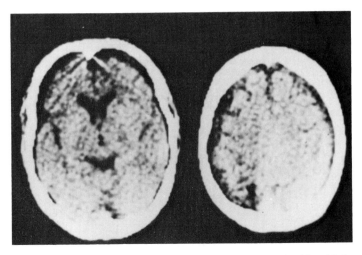

Figure 58–36 The bifrontal extracerebral areas of decreased density have the appearance of a chronic subdural hematoma or an acute subdural hygroma (*left*). On the subsequent scan at a higher level (*right*) the low-density zones are seen to extend into the sulci, indicating that they are dilated subarachnoid spaces and not subdural hematomas (Courtesy of M. S. Huckman, M.D., Rush Presbyterian Medical College, Chicago, Ill.)

sity extending into the enlarged sulci rules out a chronic hematoma (Fig. 58–36). An acute subdural hygroma may resemble a chronic subdural hematoma in density but does not have the biconvex appearance of the latter.

Subdural hygromas may also develop after a delay following head injury. They are usually located in the frontal and temporal areas and are frequently bilateral (Fig. 58–37A and B). They are reported to occur between 6 and 46 days following head injury.[100] Subdural and intracerebral hematomas may develop on the contralateral side following operative evacuation of an extracerebral hematoma (Fig. 58–37C, D, and E).[288]

Epidural Hematoma

Epidural hematomas are usually biconvex in configuration and are seen as high-density lesions in the acute stage. Since the hemorrhage occurs into the epidural space, and the dura is closely adherent to the inner table, the dura prevents the hematoma from spreading and causes the lenticular appearance (Fig. 58–38). Unless there is an associated parenchymal injury, the midline displacement will be disproportionately smaller than with a subdural hematoma. Unlike a subdural hematoma, in which mixing of cerebrospinal fluid with blood occurs, thus decreasing the attenuation value of blood, an epidural hematoma usually appears as a uniformly dense lesion. An epidural hematoma may develop in a delayed fashion. Occasionally, a small epidural hematoma may not be seen initially when associated with a large subdural

hematoma on the contralateral side. Following evacuation of the subdural hematoma and decompression, the contralateral epidural hematoma may enlarge rapidly (Fig. 58–39). A postoperative CT scan is helpful in detecting these lesions at an early stage.[288] The chances of development of an acute isodense epidural hematoma are considerably less than with a subdural hematoma. This is particularly true in case of an isolated epidural hematoma because there is less chance for admixture of other fluids. Exact localization of the hematomas to the epidural or subdural space may not always be possible on computed tomography. Approximately 20 per cent of patients with extracerebral hematomas show blood in both the epidural and subdural spaces at operation or autopsy.[148]

Intraventricular Hemorrhage

Traumatic intraventricular hemorrhage is being recognized increasingly because of computed tomography. Ventricular hemorrhage is frequently associated with parenchymal hemorrhage (Fig. 58–40).[100] The high density of blood in the ventricles changes to cerebrospinal fluid density, usually in three to four days, and disappears completely by a week, a relatively short period when compared with the density diminution associated with extraventricular hematoma.

Intraventricular hemorrhage does not carry as grave a prognosis as it implied in the past. Four of nine patients with intraventricular hemorrhage made good recovery following drainage in the series reported by

Text continued on page 1980

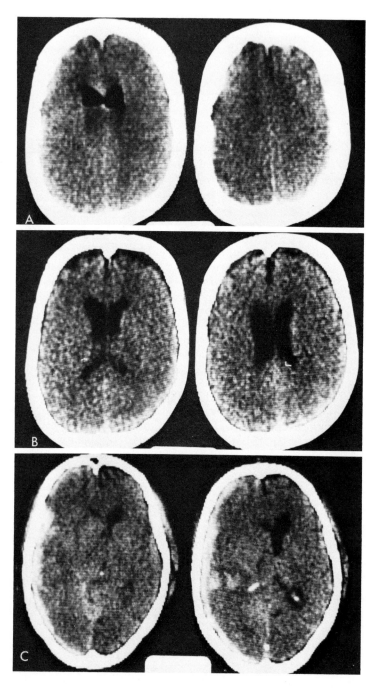

Figure 58–37 *A* and *B*. Bifrontal subdural hygromas developing in a patient 14 days after severe head injury. *C*. Preoperative computed tomogram on admission shows a left subdural hematoma.

Illustration continued on opposite page

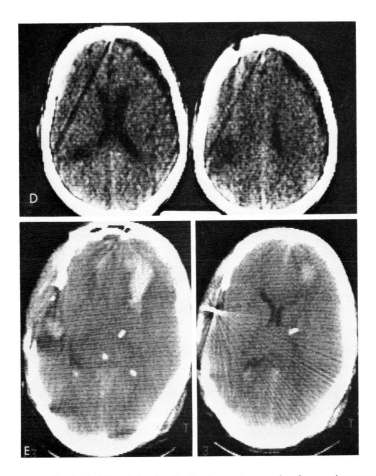

Figure 58–37 (*continued*)   *D.* A right subdural collection is seen two weeks after craniotomy and evacuation of the left subdural hematoma. *E.* Delayed development of right frontal intracerebral hematoma seen on the CT scan three days after head injury and evacuation of a left subdural hematoma.

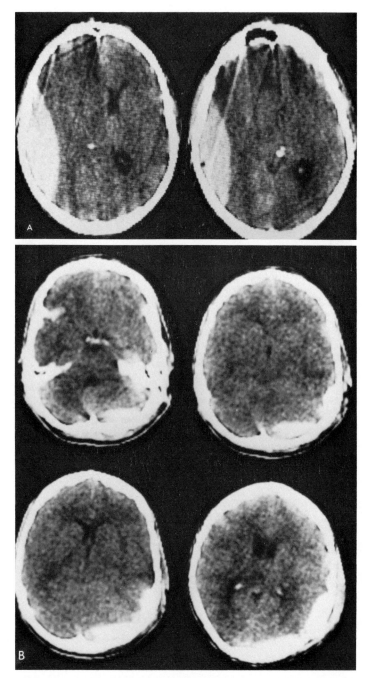

Figure 58–38   *A*. Typical appearance of an acute epidural hematoma with convex medial margin. *B*. Extension of hematoma above and below the tentorium, indicating its epidural location.

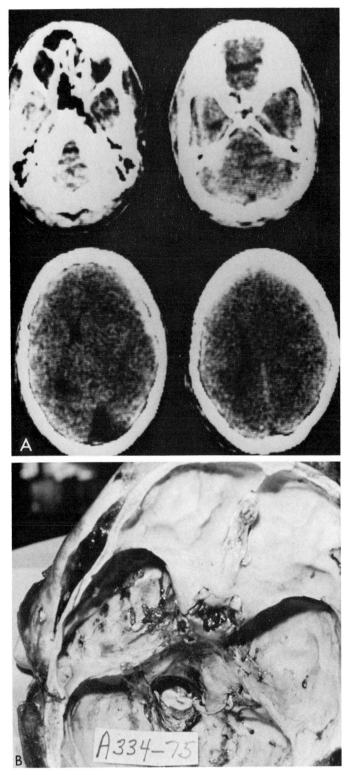

Figure 58–39 *A*. CT scan of a patient presenting with history of severe head injury. A large right-sided sub-dural hematoma with appropriate right-to-left midline displacement is seen. The patient died 36 hours after craniotomy and evacuation of the subdural hematoma. *B*. At autopsy he was found to have a large epidural hematoma measuring approximately 120 cc in the left temporal region.

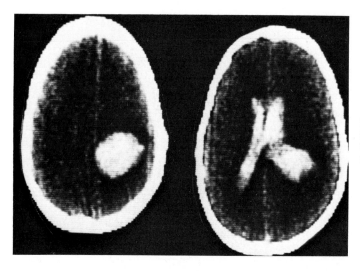

Figure 58–40 Intraventricular hemorrhage outlining the lateral ventricles is seen extending from the traumatic right intracerebral hematoma.

French and Dublin.[100] Administration of prompt therapeutic measures such as ventricular drainage has been aided by computed tomography.

Subarachnoid Hemorrhage

The presence of blood in the subarachnoid space is a frequent phenomenon in patients with head injury. It is seen as linear zones of high density in the basal cisterns, sylvian fissures, or interhemispheric fissure (Fig. 58–41). The appearance of subarachnoid hemorrhage is frequently associated with an intracerebral or extracerebral hematoma.

Hydrocephalus

Acute obstructive hydrocephalus may develop secondary to a posterior fossa hematoma that obstructs the ventricular pathways. Development of communicating hydrocephalus, however, is believed to be a more frequent phenomenon as a delayed sequel to head trauma. In one report of 95 patients with severe head injuries, 48 of whom were studied by serial computed tomography for up to three months, 3 patients developed communicating hydrocephalus.[174] In all three cases, hydrocephalus was evident by the fourteenth day. The communicating hydrocephalus results from blood in the subarachnoid space that causes obstruction of the bulk flow of cerebrospinal fluid. The ventricles enlarge, usually by one and one half to two weeks following trauma.[100,174,223] Periventricular decreased density indicative of edema may be seen with hydrocephalus (Fig. 58–42). Atrophy can be distinguished from hydrocephalus by visualization of enlarged sulci, present in the former.

The lateral ventricles may appear slitlike

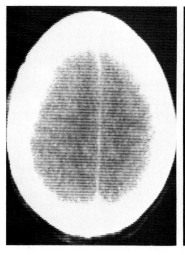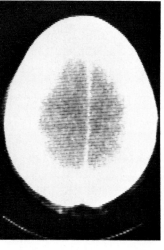

Figure 58–41 Linear zones of increased density outline the interhemispheric fissure because of blood in the subarachnoid space.

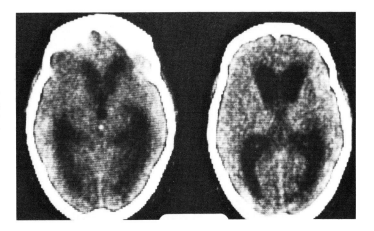

Figure 58–42 Moderate enlargement of the lateral ventricles with periventricular decreased density is seen by 15 days after head injury.

or small in size in the immediate post-traumatic period as a result of swelling of the brain or hematomas. The subsequent return of the ventricles to normal size should not be mistaken for hydrocephalus secondary to trauma.

Post-Traumatic Infarction

Acute ischemic infarction appears as a low-density area compared with the adjacent brain. This is believed to be due to edema.[4] The time required for the alteration of density depends upon the size of the infarction, and a lesion less than 2 cm in size may not be seen on computed tomography.[4,74] The infarction may be detectable on the CT scan within 24 hours of onset, and over 60 per cent are clearly seen by seven days.[74,363] Pre- and postcontrast-infusion scanning improves the diagnostic yield by nearly 15 per cent (see Fig. 58–7).[361] Contrast enhancement of infarcted tissue occurs most frequently between one and four weeks, but may be seen within a day after the onset.[254,361]

Abscess Formation, Post-Traumatic Atrophy, and Leptomeningeal Cyst

Abscess development is one of the delayed sequelae usually resulting from a penetrating injury or a fracture in the region of the petrous bone, or as a complication of operation. It takes the form of a low-density zone surrounded by a ring of enhancement following intravenous injection of a contrast agent (see Fig. 58–8). Ventricular compression and displacement may be present, depending upon the location. Abscesses are usually surrounded by low-density areas secondary to edema.

Another delayed sequela is post-traumatic atrophy, which may occur a few months to a year after the trauma. This is seen as ventricular dilatation with increase in the width of the cortical sulci. Leptomeningeal cysts are seen on the CT scan as a localized low-density zone on the periphery of the cortex, usually associated with a clearly identified fracture overlying this area. Progressive widening of the fracture may be noted on serial scanning and is thought to be due to the herniation of the cerebrospinal fluid–containing subarachnoid space through a dural tear.

Current Role of Angiography in Head Injury

The limitations of computed tomography in visualizing traumatic isodense lesions have been discussed. Its major limitation, however, is its inability to demonstrate adequately the vascular damage resulting from head injury. While one may see the result of vascular injury on computed tomography, the exact location and nature of the vascular injury itself can be evaluated only by angiography.

The internal carotid artery may be injured extracranially, with resulting intimal tear, thrombus formation, and subsequent embolization (Fig. 58–43). But for the clinical suspicion of vascular injury and performance of angiography, the case shown in Figure 58–43 could have been mistaken for a resolving contusion (see Chapter 9).

Although any segment of the vascular tree may be damaged in head injury, meningeal arteries are reported to be the most commonly involved.[34] Injury may result in an extracerebral hematoma, traumatic aneurysm, and arteriovenous fistula (Fig. 58–44). Post-traumatic arteriovenous fistulae may occur extracranially, involving the scalp vessels, or at the base of the skull (Figs. 58–45 and 58–46). If an arteriovenous fistula is suspected, selective angiography of the various arteries in the region may be needed to determine its extent, as shown in Figure 58–46.

The presence of an aneurysm may be suspected on computed tomography fol-

lowing contrast infusion. Small traumatic aneurysms of the cortical arteries are difficult to visualize, however, and if they are associated with extracerebral hematomas, it may be impossible to detect the aneurysm without angiography (Fig. 58–47).

Subfalcial herniations are generally well seen on CT scan, but transtentorial herniation, a well-known secondary complication of head injury, may not be detected. As shown by Osborn, if there is narrowing of the subarachnoid space around the brain stem on one side with evidence of brain stem distortion and in the presence of su-

Text continued on page 1987

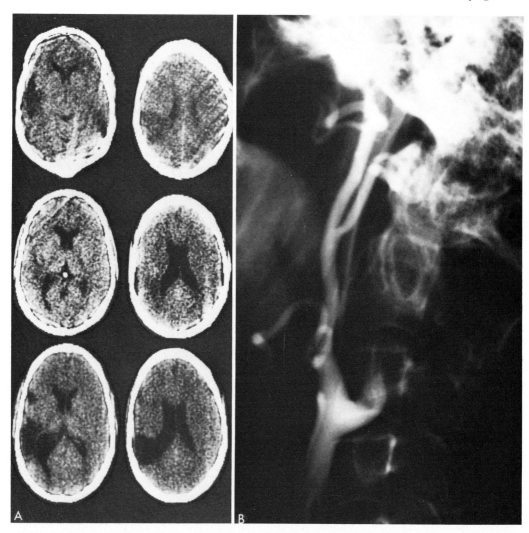

Figure 58–43 *A.* An area of decreased density is seen in the left posterior temporal and parietal regions two days after head injury (*top*). These areas appear similar to resolving contusion. *B.* Because of the clinical suspicion of vascular injury, a left carotid angiogram was performed, which reveals traumatic occlusion of the left internal carotid artery just distal to its origin. The infarcted area is not discernible on the scan 10 weeks following injury (*A, middle*). One year after the initial examination, computed tomography (*A, bottom*) reveals the infarcted area, showing densities similar to that of cerebrospinal fluid with focal enlargement of the left lateral ventricle.

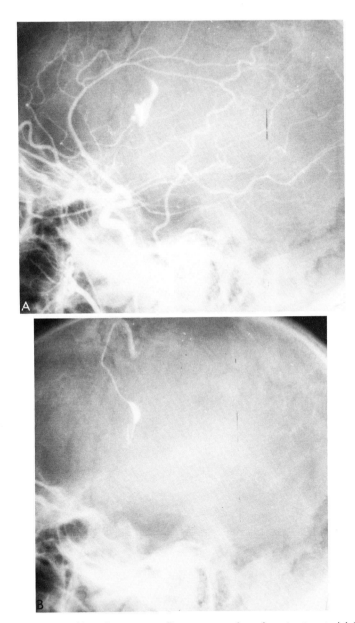

Figure 58–44   *A*. Right carotid angiogram revealing extravasation of contrast material from the meningeal artery. *B*. Same angiogram in the later phase reveals the meningeal arteriovenous fistula. (Courtesy of F. S. Vines, M.D., Medical College of Virginia, Richmond, Va.)

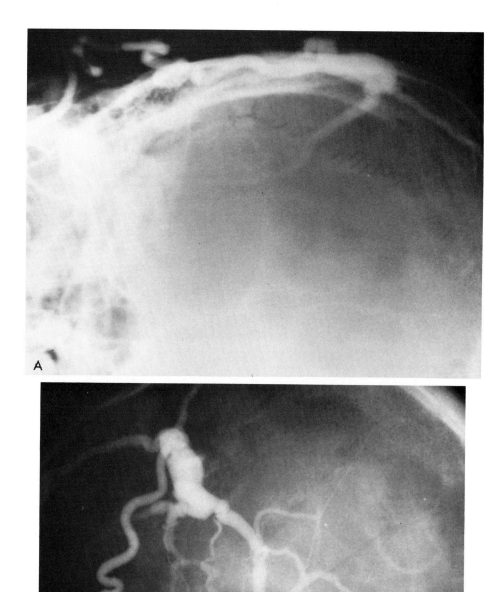

Figure 58–45   Right external carotid angiogram of a 28-year-old man who sustained head injury from a severe blow three months prior to the examination reveals a markedly enlarged superficial temporal artery supplying the extracranial arteriovenous fistula.

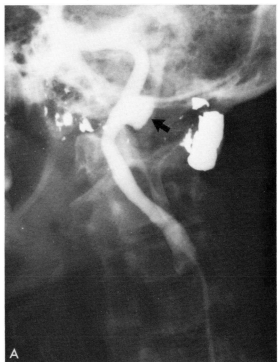

Figure 58–46 *A*. Large traumatic aneurysm of the right internal carotid artery just before it enters the petrous bone in a patient who sustained a gunshot wound in the face and base of the skull (*arrow*). *B*. Selective arteriography of the external occipital artery reveals a large arteriovenous fistula being supplied by that artery. (Courtesy of Dr. F. S. Vines, Medical College of Virginia, Richmond, Va.)

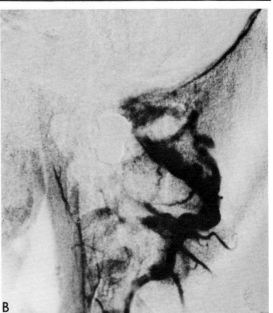

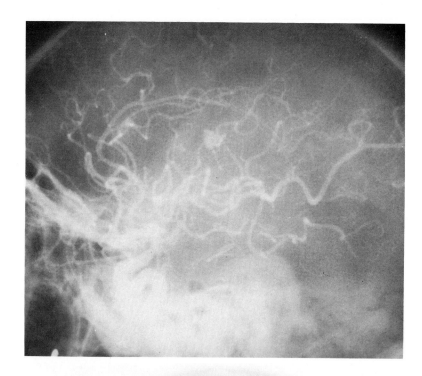

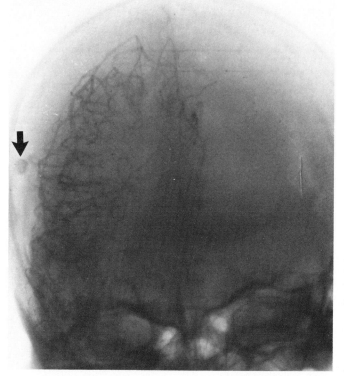

Figure 58–47 Traumatic aneurysm of the cortical branch of the middle cerebral artery projecting into a large subdural hematoma (*arrow*). This aneurysm may not be seen on computed tomography because of the adjacent clot. (Courtesy of Dr. F. S. Vines, Medical College of Virginia, Richmond, Va.)

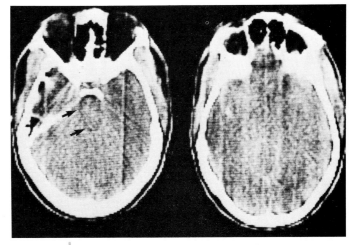

Figure 58-48 Narrowing and distortion of the subarachnoid space around the brain stem on the left side is suggestive of transtentorial herniation (*arrows*) in a patient with temporal lobe clot and swelling.

pratentorial mass, the diagnosis of transtentorial herniation may be suggested (Fig. 58–48).[261] Angiography may be required to detect the displacement of such vascular structures as the anterior choroidal artery, posterior communicating and cerebral arteries, and basilar vein of Rosenthal to make the radiological diagnosis of impending transtentorial herniation. Vertebral angiography can detect the presence of upward herniation, but marked distortion of the quadrigeminal plate cistern associated with a posterior fossa mass may be evident on computed tomography. Vertebral angiography is also valuable in the detection of tonsillar herniation.

In summary, angiography should be considered in situations when: (1) vascular injury is suspected, (2) the findings on computed tomography are not consistent with the patient's neurological status, and (3) isodense lesions are suspected either clinically or because of mass effect seen on the CT scan.

Plain Skull Radiography

Plain radiographs of the skull, although not as helpful as computed tomography, still play an important role in the management of patients with head injury. They should be obtained as soon as the patient's clinical status permits. Even if a complete skull series is not possible, a single lateral radiograph of the skull in supine position should be performed. Pneumocephalus secondary to basal skull fracture is seen clearly on the CT scan, as shown in Figure 58–49, but evidence of a basal skull fracture, which is not seen by any other means, may be recognized by the presence of air fluid levels in the sphenoid sinus on the lateral

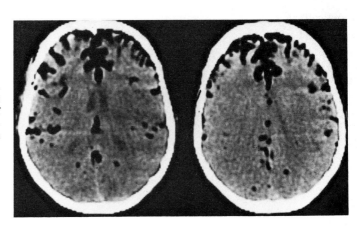

Figure 58-49 Traumatic pneumoencephalus. Markedly decreased density secondary to the presence of air in the subarachnoid spaces and interhemispheric fissure is seen on computed tomography.

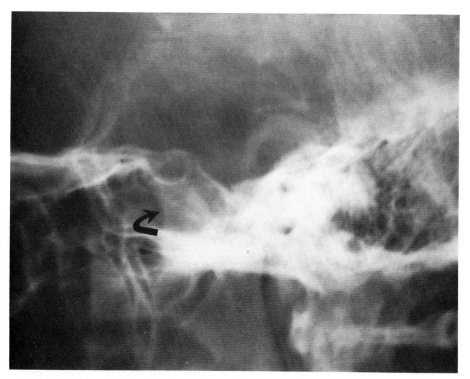

Figure 58–50 Radiograph of the skull in the lateral projection with the patient supine reveals the air-fluid level in the sphenoid sinus secondary to a basal skull fracture (*arrow*).

film (Fig. 58–50). These fractures may be present without evidence of cerebrospinal fluid rhinorrhea or cranial nerve dysfunction.

Linear fractures are demonstrated best on plain skull films. Although computed tomography may provide additional informa-

tion in depressed fractures, exactly localizing intracranial fragments as shown in Figure 58–51, skull films are necessary to define the margins of the fracture. These films, taken immediately after injury or operation, provide baseline information helpful in the early detection of osteomyelitis

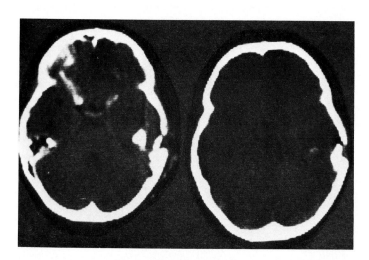

Figure 58–51 CT scan of a patient with depressed skull fracture involving the right petrous bone shows the exact location of the bone fragments displaced intracranially.

subsequently. Finally, for the repair of fractures of the facial bones and cerebrospinal fluid rhinorrhea, conventional tomography is often necessary to identify the exact sites of fractures.

Skull Films for Pineal Position and Echoencephalography

One should inspect the skull x-rays for position of a calcified pineal gland. Since acute head injury is more of a problem in younger people, however, a pineal gland adequately calcified for determination of the midline is rarely seen. Echoencephalography for midline determination has never been widely applied. This is because an accurate study requires a person skilled and experienced with the technique, and even then false results can occur. Now that computed tomography is becoming more widely available, there is little place for this test in acute head injury.

Ventriculography and Intracranial Pressure Measurement in Diagnosis

Ventriculography with intracranial pressure measurement in acute head injury provides information that will effectively guide appropriate early management. This test can be done rapidly and in experienced hands carries minimal risk to the patient.[28,168] It provides two critical bits of information for the treating physician: the degree of supratentorial brain shift and the level of intracranial pressure. Prior to the advent of computed tomography, this test and angiography were the most useful emergency radiological studies for patients who were not following commands after head injury. In a few clinics, ventriculography and intracranial pressure measurement was the emergency procedure of choice because of the speed with which it could be obtained.[29] In comparison with ventriculography, computed tomography and angiography both define the degree of brain shift at least as well and are certainly better for determining locations of injury. But knowledge of the patient's intracranial pressure soon after injury is of great benefit in overall diagnosis and management.

The test still has an important role in emergency diagnosis. If the hospital has no computed tomography available, and angiography cannot be obtained quickly, this test should be used in patients who are unable to speak or follow commands. Other indications include conditions in which patients with severe brain injuries have other extracranial injuries that require immediate operation or that prevent transfer for computed tomography or angiography. Approximately 50 per cent of patients who are not speaking or following commands on admission will harbor major intracranial mass lesions. A delay in diagnosis of intracranial damage until after the patient has had operative treatment for an extracranial lesion should not be permitted.

Methods

If the procedure is performed in a methodical and standardized fashion, the ventricle can almost always be cannulated to provide a satisfactory intracranial pressure measurement and air study, even when there is a major ventricular shift or the ventricles are tiny, or both. If there are no focal signs that favor a unilateral mass lesion, the right side should be chosen for the study. If the clinical examination suggests the presence of a right-sided intracranial mass lesion, the left side of the skull is entered, for it is easier to cannulate the ventricle on the side opposite the lesion.

The entry site can be either in the forehead, as favored by Kaufmann and Clark, just behind the hairline, or at the more standard precoronal suture level (Fig. 58–52).[168] The technique described here has been used by the authors in well over 500 patients, many with acute brain injury, with a morbidity rate of less than 0.5 per cent and a failure rate of 3 per cent (Fig. 58–53).[21]

The scalp is shaved in the region of the coronal suture, and a twist drill hole is made with a small drill, 4 cm off the midline and approximately 1.5 cm anterior to the coronal suture. The hole is directed toward the nasion and in the sagittal plane 2 cm anterior to the external auditory canal. The dura is penetrated with a No. 18 needle. A No. 16 brain cannula is directed first toward the nasion. If the ventricle is not hit, the cannula is next directed toward the ipsilateral pupil, and if this fails, a third pass is made toward the contralateral pupil. If

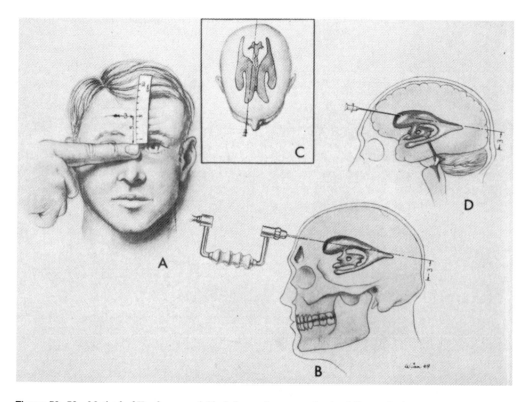

Figure 58–52   Method of Kaufmann and Clark for performance of twist drill ventriculostomy. A limited ventriculogram or single intracranial pressure measurement can be performed or a catheter can be placed for long-term intracranial pressure measurement. (From Kaufmann, G. E., and Clark, K.: Emergency frontal twist drill ventriculostomy. J. Neurosurg., *33*:226–227, 1970. Reprinted by permission.)

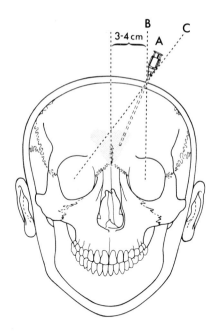

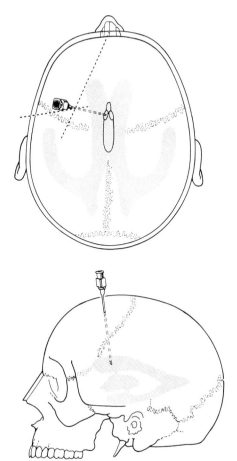

Figure 58–53 Precoronal suture method for performance of twist drill ventriculostomy. The hole is directed toward the nasion and in the sagittal plane 2 cm anterior to the external auditory canal. No more than three passes per side should be made (the first toward the nasion, A; the second toward the ipsilateral pupil, B; and the third toward the contralateral pupil, C. If three passes on the opposite side also fail, the procedure should be abandoned. With this method, the ventricle can almost always be cannulated, even when it is compressed or shifted.

three passes fail, the procedure is repeated in a similar fashion on the other side. If three passes on the second side also fail, the procedure should be abandoned. When the ventricle is entered, care must be taken to lose as little cerebrospinal fluid as possible. A manometer previously filled with sterile saline to a level of 300 mm of water and extended by flexible tubing is then connected via a stopcock on the end of the tubing to the ventricular cannula. A resting intracranial pressure value is obtained from the level of the foramen of Monro with the patient lying flat. At the time of measurement, the arterial blood pressure should not be below normal and any hypercarbia or hypoxia should have been corrected. With these abnormalities, intracranial pressure readings can be misleading, for arterial hypotension may falsely lower the pressure, and hypercarbia and hypoxia may raise it.

After measuring the pressure, approximately 7 cc of air is carefully exchanged for cerebrospinal fluid, the head is tilted from side to side, and a brow-up anteroposterior Towne's position skull x-ray is obtained after the cannula is removed (Fig. 58–54).

Interpretation

Normal intracranial pressure in the relaxed patient who is neither hypotensive, hypercarbic, nor hypoxic is 10 mm of mercury or less.[207] Elevations above this level are abnormal. While pressure in the range of 10 to 15 mm of mercury may occur with only minor shifts of intracranial volume, when pressures are over 15 mm of mercury a major intracranial alteration has

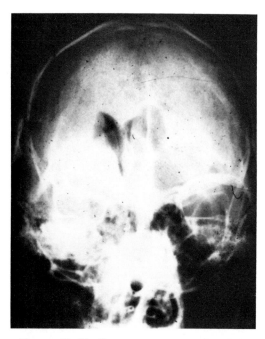

Figure 58–54 Brow-up anteroposterior limited ventriculogram performed in the emergency room via a precoronal twist drill ventriculostomy. The combination of information on intracranial pressure level and degree of supratentorial midline brain shift and ventricular compression greatly aids in defining the type of immediate management that is indicated.

occurred.[241] When pressures are recorded in the range of 20 mm of mercury or more, this implies either a major intracranial hematoma, a serious diffuse brain injury, or both.[29] A sizeable change in intracranial volume and pressure-volume dynamics is required to raise intracranial pressures to this level.

Most dangerous acute traumatic unilateral intracranial mass lesions will shift the midline 5 mm or more. This will invariably be associated with an elevated intracranial pressure unless a cerebrospinal fluid leak is present.[29] Serious temporal lobe lesions may cause only minimal shift of the midline, but in this case the intracranial pressure will be elevated, and if the third ventricle is seen on the air study, it will often be shifted more than the lateral ventricles. If there is little or no midline shift, the pressure is elevated, and the patient is not hypercarbic, then there are either bilateral mass lesions or a serious diffuse brain injury. In this case, if the pressure is above 20 mm of mercury, the patient should have angiography or computed tomography promptly to rule out bilateral hematomas or contusions that might require operative intervention.

If there are no focal intracranial hematomas or contusions, and the intracranial pressure is over 20 mm of mercury with little midline shift, and there is neither hypoxia, hypercarbia, nor impairment of cerebral venous return, the diffuse brain injury is usually severe. The pressure may be elevated here from either diffuse cerebral vasodilation and hyperemia, diffuse bilateral edema, or a combination of both. If this syndrome is combined with abnormal motor responses on neurological examination (decorticate or decerebrate posturing), the ultimate outcome for the patient will be poor despite an uncomplicated course. This is because the original diffuse brain insult has been so extensive.[29]

Diagnostic or Exploratory Burr Holes in Deteriorating Patients

Prior to the availability of angiography and computed tomography, diagnostic or exploratory burr holes were a useful initial procedure, but they now have a limited role in the modern diagnosis and management of acute head injury. If a patient shows a progressive deficit that can be temporarily arrested or reversed with osmotic agents such as mannitol, operative treatment should be preceded by computed tomography, ventriculography, or angiography to define the location of the intracranial lesions. If a particularly urgent operation is required, one can get a single-level CT cut across the midsupratentorial space, a rapid ventriculogram, or a single-injection, single-x-ray, anteroposterior carotid angiogram in the emergency room or on the operating table.

An exploratory burr hole should be considered as the primary diagnostic procedure only if computed tomography and angiography are not promptly available, the ventricle cannot be cannulated, and the patient is rapidly deteriorating with the signs of unilateral progressive brain shift and tentorial herniation. If this rapid deterioration occurs, the side to be explored first should be determined by the following signs in order to importance: (1) the side of the dilating pupil, (2) the side of any unilateral skull fracture, and (3) the side contralateral to any progressive motor sign such as weakness or posturing. Almost all major *acute hematomas* causing tentorial herniation will be on the side of the dilating pupil.[170] Similarly, if there is a unilateral skull fracture, most progressively growing acute intracranial hematomas will be on the side of the fracture.[200] False localizing signs, such as pupillary dilation developing contralateral to the clot, are seen more often in association with chronic subdural hematoma, a disorder quite distinct from acute traumatic intracranial mass development.[43,329] Rarely, the pupil ipsilateral to an acute developing hematoma may initially constrict because of impending medial temporal lobe herniation.[128,329] In this case, even though the contralateral pupil is larger, both pupils usually will remain reactive, and the observer should not be misled into thinking that this represents contralateral pupillary dilation from brain stem shift and opposite third nerve compression.

In acute closed head injury, the burr hole should be in the temporal region. It should be enlarged to a small craniectomy so the area under the dura is clearly visible and can be inspected and an initial decompression can be performed (see Fig. 58–81). If an acute extradural or subdural clot is not identified and *the patient has clearly shown the clinical signs of unilateral supratentorial mass development,* further multiple ipsilateral or contralateral burr holes should *not* be done, as this will delay diagnosis and treatment. Rather, one should proceed with the trauma craniotomy shown in Figure 58–80, as this will most rapidly provide for an accurate intraoperative diagnosis and permit adequate therapy.

Only in the rare situation in which one might be operating upon a patient who is showing progressive deterioration without focal signs, such as from a frontal or occipital hematoma, and no other diagnostic test could be performed, might the use of multiple diagnostic holes be useful. Similarly, exploratory burr holes contralateral to a completed craniotomy are indicated only if the surgeon strongly suspects a contralateral previously undiagnosed mass, for example, when there is acute intraoperative swelling of a normal-looking hemisphere that might be due to an enlarging contralateral hematoma.

In summary, in acute brain trauma, exploratory diagnostic burr holes are no longer considered the first order of treatment. Rather, the burr hole–craniectomy is to be used only to provide initial rapid decompression in a patient who is suffering rapid progressive brain compression or shift or both.

Brain Electrical Activity

Both spontaneous and stimulated brain electrical activity, as shown by the electroencephalogram and evoked potential respectively, can be of considerable value in the diagnosis and management of brain injury. While electroencephalographic abnormalities obtained from a single study may be nonspecific and of little localizing value, serial recordings can yield important information concerning both global and regional brain compromise. Once the strengths and limitations of the electroencephalogram in head trauma are defined and understood, it becomes clear that this test is an important, safe, and inexpensive aid to diagnosis in both the early and later periods after head trauma.

The brain evoked potential is a relatively new but useful method whereby electrical activity can be used in diagnosis of brain injury. It can localize regional brain dysfunction even in neural pathways coursing deep in the brain stem. Not only is the evoked potential useful in diagnosis, but it also has important prognostic applications. Moreover, it promises to become a sensitive noninvasive continuous monitoring tool for the evaluation of comatose patients.

Most diagnostic studies used to evaluate the patient with head injury yield information concerning the anatomical condition, i.e., the presence or absence of hematomas, brain displacements, and the like, not the functional condition of the brain. A normal cerebral angiogram or computed tomogram may be obtained in patients who survive with neurological deficits never detected by these studies. Brain electrical activity, on the other hand, like the patients' neurological examination, depends upon neuronal vitality for its realization and is, therefore, an important method of assessing the functional state of the brain irrespective of the presence or absence of anatomical alterations.

The study of brain electrical activity is particularly useful in patients confused or comatose from head injury because it offers an objective evaluation of central nervous system function that can both complement and supplement that obtained from the clinical examination. Computer analysis of brain electrical activity enables diagnostic evaluations to be made that define areas of brain dysfunction not obvious from the clinical examination. Studies of brain electrical activity can potentially make distinctions, not always possible with the neurological examination, between dysfunction of the cerebral hemispheres and of the brain stem, and can help evaluate dysfunction of localized brain areas or individual neural systems and pathways (visual, auditory, motor, somesthetic). The techniques utilized clinically to record neuroelectrical potentials are noninvasive and allow frequent serial studies to be obtained at little risk to the patient. They provide a safe and simple method for indirectly evaluating the functional and metabolic state of the brain.

The two techniques currently available with which to study neuroelectric phenomena in patients with head injury are: (1) spontaneous electrical activity, the electroencephalogram, and (2) event-related computer-averaged potentials, evoked potentials.

The Electroencephalogram

Recorded from the scalp, the electroencephalogram represents an amalgamation of large numbers of postsynaptic potentials generated in neuronal cell membranes.[64,65,89] The recording electrode detects electrical signals from cortical cells directly underlying it as well as from cells in more distant areas.[181] Evidence suggests that the rhythmicity of the electroencephalogram may be partly under the control of brain stem neurons.[175] The electroencephalogram reflects both cortical and subcortical neuronal function.[36]

Clinical Interpretation

Three features are used to characterize encephalographic records—the rhythm (cycles per second, Hz), the amplitude (μv), and the waveform (sinusoidal, spike and wave).[175,181] While there is general agreement on the parameters constituting a normal record (8 to 13 Hz, as shown in Figure 58–55B), about 10 to 15 per cent of the so-called normal population may have variations of their electroencephalograms that could be mistakenly considered abnormal in a patient with head injury.[36,175,322] Thus, a major problem in the interpretation of a single record from a patient with suspected head trauma is the lack of a preinjury record with which to compare it.[36,175,239,291]

With the exception of epileptiform discharges, the electroencephalographic abnormalities associated with central nervous system dysfunction after head trauma are the loss of "normal" rhythms and amplitudes and the appearance, commonly, of slower rhythms with or without amplitude changes—theta, from 4Hz to less than 8Hz (Fig. 58–55E); delta, less than 4Hz (Fig. 58–55C).[36,85,322,360] Clinical and laboratory studies of electroencephalography following head trauma have, however, demonstrated rather variable associations of patterns with brain dysfunction.[291,350] Discrepancies between the electroencephalographic data and the clinical findings are frequent.[273] While lack of preinjury records, variability of "normal" records, absence of serial studies following head injury, and difficulty in sampling more basal areas of the cortex located subfrontally or subtemporally are manageable sources of error, there remain encephalographic realities that make clinical interpretation of electroencephalograms problematic. For example, focal areas of dysfunction that occur as a result of brain contusion or a collection of blood might not be detectable on the electroencephalogram because surrounding healthy brain activity could mask them (Fig. 58–56A).[273,291] Localized cortical injury can also be masked by widespread changes in brain electrical activity (slowing perhaps) caused by such things as intracranial hypertension or brain stem dysfunction.[217,239] White matter damage may not be detectable, although it occurs frequently following head trauma.[273,324,325]

Altered Level of Consciousness

Generally a relationship exists between the patient's level of consciousness and the appearance of abnormalities on the electro-

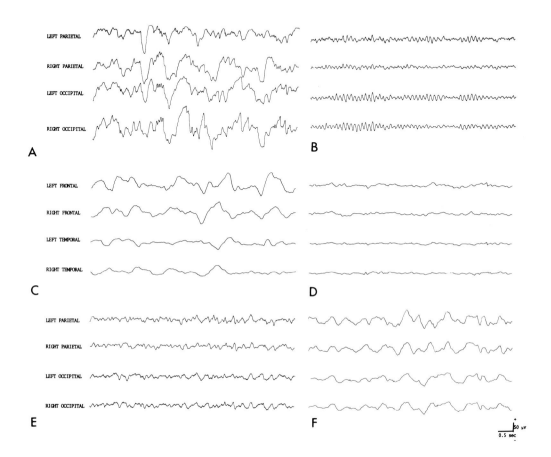

Figure 58–55 *A.* Abnormal electroencephalogram demonstrating delta frequencies (less than 3 Hz). This record was obtained three days after head injury from a patient who regained consciousness and was alert less than 24 hours following the trauma. *B.* Three months later the same patient had a normal electroencephalogram (8 to 13 Hz). *C.* The electroencephalogram from a patient with severe head trauma demonstrates 1 to 2 Hz delta frequencies and suppressed background electrical activity. *D.* Two weeks later the same patient's electroencephalogram revealed generalized suppression of amplitude for all frequencies. The patient died one week after this study. *E.* An adult patient whose electroencephalogram, recorded two days after head injury while the patient was unresponsive, had theta range frequencies (4 to 8 Hz) with little delta activity. This patient became alert by the sixth day postinjury and made an excellent recovery. *F.* The electroencephalogram of an 8-year-old who regained consciousness within 36 hours of head injury. The record during the first day posttrauma demonstrated high-amplitude delta frequencies with background suppression.

encephalogram.[85,360] Slowing of electroencephalographic frequencies will often be obtained in records done while a patient is unconscious and may resolve after consciousness is regained (see Fig. 58–55A and B).[273,291,360] Likewise, the closer in time to the head trauma that the study is performed, the more likely that abnormalities will be seen. Studies on patients with mild head injuries reveal that transient slowing may occur and resolve within minutes of the trauma.[85] Often these patients have post-traumatic amnesia or are confused, yet their electroencephalograms are normal (Fig. 58–56C). Frequencies below 8Hz commonly occur in patients who have lost consciousness; however, frank delta activity (less than 3Hz) also can be found even in

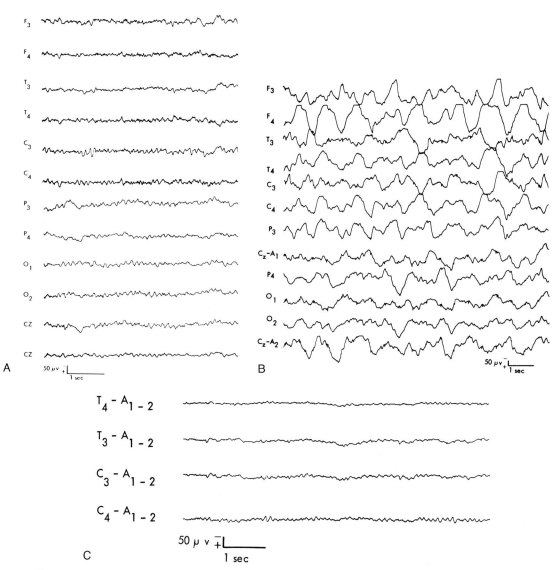

Figure 58–56 A. Electroencephalogram from a 28-year-old patient who had an acute subdural hematoma that was removed operatively. Contusion of the left frontal lobe was noted during the procedure. The patient's electroencephalogram three months later did not indicate a lateralized or focal lesion, although the patient had residual right hemiparesis at that time. B. Electroencephalogram of a 58-year-old man recorded four days after head injury. The record revealed generalized delta frequencies as well as faster background activity without focal or lateralized electrical abnormalities. The patient had left hemiparesis and intracranial hypertension at the time the study was obtained. C. Representative sample of an electroencephalogram recorded from a confused patient 24 hours after injury. The patient was conscious but not oriented to time or place.

patients whose symptoms resolve rapidly (cf. Fig. 58–55F).[175,273]

A difficult medicolegal situation can arise if one is asked to document the occurrence of head injury on the basis of a single electroencephalogram obtained after alleged trauma. Neither the presence nor the absence of abnormalities on one record is an indication of the occurrence of actual head injury.[85,291] If a normal electroencephalogram is recorded, the abnormality may have already cleared, while an abnormal record may be unrelated to the head trauma. Serial studies that show resolution of an abnormal electroencephalogram over days or weeks point to the diagnosis of mild brain trauma.[36,322]

The presence of coma in patients sustaining head injuries may be the result of barbiturate poisoning, postictal epileptic states, tumors, and the like, with head trauma occurring as a secondary phenomenon.[36] Electroencephalography may be useful in singling out the underlying cause of coma, which may not be the head injury.[273] For example, the appearance of a barbiturate pattern with fast frequencies in the electroencephalogram, or spike and wave activity in cases of epilepsy, might raise the question of pre-existing central nervous system compromise. In this way the electroencephalogram may help to define the cause of the coma or point to other factors affecting the patient.

Evidence that the degree of frequency or amplitude abnormalities of an electroencephalogram can be correlated in a meaningful way with the severity of coma is conflicting. Patients in whom the duration of coma following head trauma is longer than 48 hours generally have records showing frequencies of less than 4Hz and suppression of background alpha rhythms.[85,292,360] These patients are considered to have had substantial generalized central nervous system dysfunction (see Fig. 58–55C and D).[77,273] There remains the possibility, however, that a strategically located brain stem lesion can cause diffuse slowing of the rhythm.[36,273,322] To further confound the interpretation in comatose patients, slowing below 4Hz may continue for several days after the patient has regained consciousness and appears perfectly normal. The record shown in Figure 58–55A was obtained three days after head injury from an individual who regained full consciousness less than 24 hours after being traumatized.

A paradoxical phenomenon may exist in which the electroencephalogram appears quite normal while the patient is decerebrate and unresponsive following head injury. There are a number of reports with neuropathological documentation that reveal pontomesencephalic-tegmental lesions in such patients, accounting for the clinical and electroencephalographic findings.[55,204] Apparently, there can be profound dissociation between the "normal" electroencephalogram and the grave clinical condition of the patient when this brain stem area is injured.[359]

Shearing and disruption of subcortical white matter can also be associated with normal, awake-like patterns even though the patients have sustained severe central nervous system injury. Both early after injury and months later the electroencephalogram can maintain a normal appearance in spite of the patient's vegetative state.[273,324,325]

Focal or Lateralizing Hemispheric Lesions

Cerebral contusions and intracranial hematomas that are unilateral can be associated with reduced amplitude or slowing of the electroencephalogram, or both, either on the side of injury alone or less often on both sides.[36,175,181] Frequencies ipsilateral to the cerebral injury, for example, may be 6 to 8Hz or less, while the contralateral side may generate normal (8 to 13Hz) frequencies. Considerable difficulty exists in distinguishing cerebral contusion from unilateral subdural hematoma by employing the electroencephalographic criteria alone. If, during serial studies on the same patient who has had a head injury, a lateralized abnormality appears where there previously was none, a subdural hematoma may be suspected. On the other hand, abnormalities from contused cortex often resolve over time.[273,322]

Both unilateral subdural hematoma and cerebral contusion can be masked by projected slow-wave activity (less than 4Hz) emanating from brain stem structures if the intracranial pressure is high or if a stem injury has occurred (see Fig. 58–56B). In these situations diffuse delta activity or bilateral triphasic waves, especially in the anterior electrode (frontal) placements, may be associated with preservation of faster background frequencies over both hemispheres.[36,273,322] Bilateral cerebral contusions, or bilateral subdural hematomas may also present with generalized slowing, the electroencephalogram thus being similar to that seen with diffuse central nervous system injury or brain stem dysfunction.[291]

Another problem in interpretation of the electroencephalogram in focal cortical injury may occur if a limited zone of traumatized brain is rendered electrically silent. Electrical activity from surrounding normal cortex will be recorded by the electrodes and mask the area of damage.[239]

Penetrating Intracranial Injuries

Dramatic changes in the electroencephalogram can be associated with brain injury produced by objects penetrating the calvarium because of the neural damage and, additionally, because of defects in the brain investments, especially the skull. Under normal conditions electrical potentials recorded from the scalp have had their amplitudes markedly reduced by the resistance of the dura, skull, and scalp. Electrical potentials from electrodes overlying a traumatic defect or a craniectomy site can have greatly augmented amplitudes compared with potentials recorded through bone and other tissues. Thus, care must be taken in interpretation of these studies.[175,181]

Approximately 50 per cent of patients with hemiparesis or hemiplegia following penetrating brain injury have normal electroencephalograms. Only 43 per cent of World War II soldiers who survived penetrating head injury had electroencephalographic abnormalities detectable in follow-up studies. The number of studies that were abnormal did, however, increase in proportion to the severity of the injury.[350]

Following a penetrating brain injury, the electroencephalogram may signal the onset of intracranial infection. If meningitis occurs, the rhythms may become diffusely slowed. Background activity could still be present and might look similar to that on the preinfection recordings.[322] Encephalitis generally presents with widespread delta activity and suppressed background activity.[175] Cerebral abscess formation could be difficult to detect if the preabscess record manifests focal delta rhythms over the area of brain damage. Focal delta rhythms that appear over time, however, can be extremely helpful in the diagnosis of brain abscess or other progressive lesions.[181,322]

Brain Evoked Potentials

Physiology and Anatomy

While the electroencephalogram represents spontaneous or intrinsic brain electrical activity, event-related neuroelectrical activity such as the sensory evoked potential represents the brain's response to the application of a specific extrinsic stimulus.[64,65] Theoretically, any sensory stimulus sufficient to cause depolarization of a peripheral or cranial nerve can be used to evoke neuroelectrical potentials in the central nervous system.[84,113] In practice the visual (flash of light), auditory (tone pip), and somesthetic (peripheral nerve depolarization) systems have been most often utilized for clinical evoked potential studies.*

Application of a brief sensory stimulus to a peripheral receptor can initiate a depolarization wave that travels toward the central nervous system at velocities determined by fiber diameter. The time interval from stimulation to arrival of the depolarization wave at the primary sensory receiving area in the cortex depends upon the patient's body size and the site of stimulation, the presence or absence of neuronal abnormality, the conduction velocity of the axons, and the number of synapses in the respective neural pathways (Fig. 58–57). Groups of cortical neurons can then process this afferent impulse for variable time periods after its arrival, thereby generating potentials that may be recorded for seconds after stimulation.[84] Evoked potentials are recorded for variable epochs after stimulation, generally between 100 and 1000 msec, as this time period allows the primary cortical response and the associated neural activity to be studied.[113]

For an evoked potential to be recorded from the scalp, the neural pathway stimulated from the periphery and cortical neurons elaborating afferent information must be functional (Fig. 58–58).[193,323] It is some-

---

* See references 7, 8, 57, 114, 182, 270.

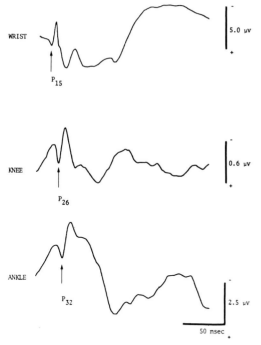

Figure 58–57 Somatosensory evoked potentials recorded from parietal scalp after peripheral nerve stimulation at the wrist (median nerve), knee (common peroneal nerve), and ankle (posterior tibial nerve) in an adult. The initial positive wave (positivity down) can be recorded 15 msec after peripheral nerve stimulation at the wrist, but it requires 32 msec to arrive and be recorded when the posterior tibial nerve is stimulated at the ankle.

times possible to differentiate the location in a neural pathway of structures that generate components of complex evoked po-

tentials by measuring the period of time elapsed from stimulation to the evoked potential component of interest. Evoked potentials arising from brain stem elements of the auditory and somesthetic system occur within the first 10 to 15 msec after stimulation, while the potentials that follow those early electrical events are generated by more rostral structures such as the cortex.[63,122,160,162,319]

Jewett and Williston introduced the concept of near-field and far-field (brain stem) recording of electrical potentials from the auditory system.[161] They demonstrated that electrical potentials seen in the first 6 to 7 msec after stimulation are generated by elements of the auditory system located in the brain stem. These were called auditory far-field potentials (Fig. 58–59). Jewett and Williston distinguished auditory far-field potentials from the auditory near-field potentials generated in more rostral elements of the auditory system located nearer to the recording scalp electrode in the cerebral cortex. It is thought that the first five early latency potentials (far-field) arise from the eighth nerve, cochlear nucleus, superior olivary complex, nucleus of the lateral lemniscus, and inferior colliculus successively (Fig. 58–60).[319] Cracco and Cracco demonstrated that early latency brain stem (far-field) somatosensory evoked potentials could be recorded in man and that these occur at approximately 10 msec and 12 msec after stimulation.[63]

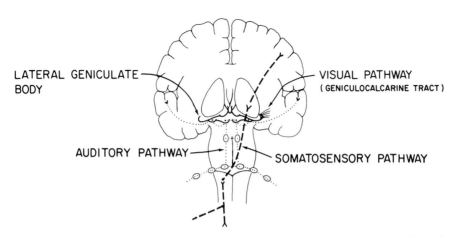

Figure 58–58 Schematic view of sensory pathways involved in the generation of multimodality evoked potentials. The sensory input generating somatosensory and auditory evoked potentials traverses more caudal regions of brain stem than does sensory input for visual evoked potentials. (From Greenberg, R. P., Becker, D. P., Miller, J. D., et al.: Evaluation of brain function in severe human head trauma with multimodality evoked potentials. J. Neurosurg., 47:150–177, 1977. Reprinted by permission.)

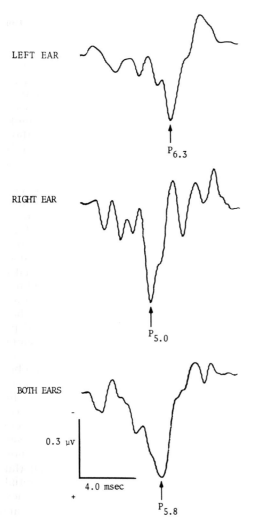

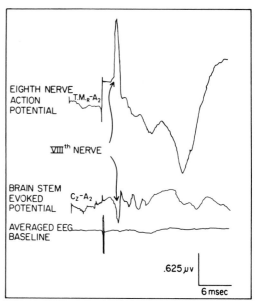

Figure 58–60 Simultaneous eighth nerve action potential and brain stem evoked potential showing the normal appearance of the electrical wave produced by the eighth nerve. The eighth nerve action potential (*upper tracing*) was recorded from a cotton wick electrode near the tympanic membrane. The auditory brain stem evoked potential (*lower tracing*) was recorded at the vertex. Their electrical polarities are opposite because the electrical dipole is between the electrodes. T. M.$_{-R}$, tympanic membrane; A$_2$, right ear; C$_Z$, vertex. (From Greenberg, R. P., Mayer, D. J., Becker, D. P., et al.: Evaluation of brain function in severe human head trauma with multimodality evoked potentials. J. Neurosurg., *47*:150–177, 1977. (Reprinted by permission.)

Figure 58–59 Auditory brain stem potentials (far-field) recorded after left, right, and both ears were stimulated by 75-db tone pips in a patient with decreased hearing in the left ear subsequent to head trauma. The brain stem potentials generated by stimulating the right ear alone are normal with a 5.0-msec latency (normal) from time of stimulation to the fourth positive component (positivity down). Stimulation of the left ear alone, on the other hand, generated an abnormal brain stem response with a significant latency delay to the fourth positive component (P 6.3). Stimulation of both ears simultaneously produced an average of the potentials generated by each ear with a latency delay to the fourth positive component of 5.8 msec.

Electroencephalogram Versus Evoked Potential

Central nervous system neurons that respond to applied sensory stimuli and generate evoked potentials also generate the electroencephalogram.[64,65] Any mode of in-jury sufficient to cause neuronal dysfunction will stop or alter the electroencephalogram and the evoked potential activity as well.[16,234] Potentials generated following brain damage originate from surviving neurons. Since both the electroencephalogram and the evoked potentials depend upon neuronal functional integrity, what benefit can be derived from recording evoked potentials that cannot be gotten with the electroencephalogram alone? The technique of evoked potential recording offers diagnostic advantages that depend upon specificity in defining the location of functional loss in afferent neural pathways and cerebral cortex.[122,132,133,203,323]

Signal Averaging

It is not feasible to record evoked potentials from scalp electrodes without signal averaging because the amplitude of an

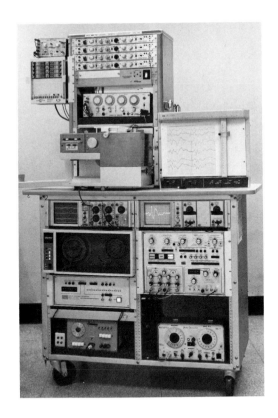

Figure 58–61   A computer and evoked potential stimulating and recording equipment mounted on a single cart that can be moved to a patient's intensive care unit bed or into the operating room. Data have been plotted on an x-y plotter as well as stored on magnetic tape. (From Greenberg, R. P., et al.: Evaluation of brain function in severe human head trauma with multimodality evoked potentials. J. Neurosurg., *47*:150–177, 1977. Reprinted by permission.)

EEG 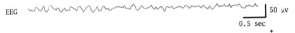 50 µV
0.5 sec

SOMATOSENSORY EVOKED POTENTIALS

Figure 58–62   An example of computed signal averaging. The electroencephalogram (EEG) has not been averaged. The somatosensory evoked potential is displayed after 1, 8, 128, and 512 epochs of the time-locked electroencephalogram have been averaged.

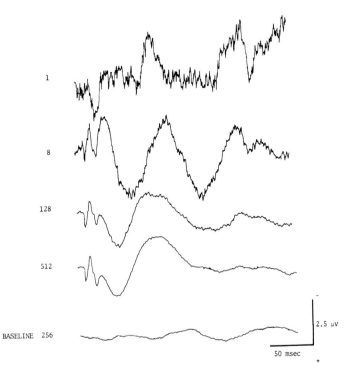

1

8

128

512

BASELINE 256

2.5 µV

50 msec

evoked potential is one to three orders of magnitude less than the amplitude of an electroencephalogram.[84,89,113] Various techniques have been used to extract the low-amplitude evoked potential signal from the larger-amplitude background electrical "noise" composed mainly of the electroencephalographic but also of the nonneural electrical activity. Computers are now available at relatively low cost that can store and display the final average on an oscilloscope screen for photographic records of the evoked potential or can plot the evoked potential on graph paper (Fig. 58–61). An example of computer signal averaging is shown in Figure 58–62, where the intrinsic, spontaneous electroencephalogram is progressively replaced by the completed evoked potential after 512 time-locked electroencephalographic epochs have been averaged.

Technical Problems

In head injury diagnosis, artifacts from potentials generated in muscle, 60-cycle alternating current, the electrocardiograph, and the like are common and frustrating to deal with.[84] Stimulating difficulties can be caused by things such as blood and wax in the external auditory meatus, gaze preferences and eye movements, swollen eyelids, and infiltrated intravenous fluid in the subcutaneous tissue over the nerve to be depolarized. These problems must be noted and corrected, but with attention to detail and careful technique, good-quality evoked potentials can be recorded from most patients with head injury even in an active intensive care unit (Fig. 58–63).[123]

Evoked Potential Analysis

A suitable method with which to categorize the complex abnormal evoked re-

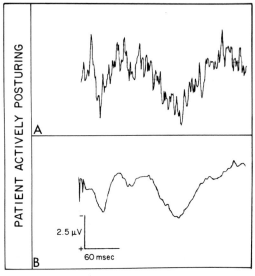

Figure 58–63 Artifact rejection. *A.* Myogenic contamination of the auditory evoked potential from a decerebrate patient makes meaningful data analysis difficult. *B.* A clean auditory evoked potential was obtained from the same patient after high-frequency muscle potentials were eliminated by artifact rejection techniques. (From Greenberg, R. P., et al.: Evaluation of brain function in severe human head trauma with multimodality evoked potentials. J. Neurosurg., *47*:150–177, 1977. Reprinted by permission.)

sponses produced by neuronal embarrassment is required.[113] Analyses of evoked potential wave latency, amplitude, duration, and morphology have been done. Latency to each wave is the most commonly used clinical parameter. Typical latency data from 20 normal subjects are given in Table 58–2. By convention the waves, regardless of modality, can be labeled as either positive or negative (P or N), and the latency from time of stimulation to wave peak is expressed in milliseconds (Fig. 58–64). Computer programs that detect positive or negative evoked potential peaks and print out latency and amplitude data are

TABLE 58–2 MULTIMODALITY EVOKED POTENTIAL NORMATIVE DATA*

MODALITY	POTENTIAL								
Somatosensory	[P]15 ± 1	[N]20 ± 1	[P]29 ± 2	[N]35 ± 2	[P]50 ± 3	[N]78 ± 2	[P]98 ± 2	[N]138 ± 3	[P]188 ± 5
Visual	[P]53 ± 4	[N]70 ± 2	[P]98 ± 3	[N]148 ± 4	[P]192 ± 5	[N]235 ± 5	[P]290 ± 10		
Auditory	[P]26 ± 1	[N]42 ± 2	[P]50 ± 3	[N]98 ± 5	[P]170 ± 10	[N]270 ± 10	[P]340 ± 10		
Brain stem	[P]1.5 ± 0.1	[P]2.5 ± 0.1	[P]3.6 ± 0.2	[P]4.7 ± 0.2	[P]5.6 ± 0.2	[P]6.7 ± 0.1	[P]7.2 ± 0.1	[P]10 ± 0.4	

* Wave latencies were obtained from a normal volunteer group. Similar wave latencies for each modality can be recorded from different normal subjects. Wave amplitudes differ greatly in a normal population. Latencies are given in milliseconds. P, positive; N, negative; ±, range. (From Greenberg, R. P., Mayer, D. J. Becker, D. P., and Miller, J. D.: Evaluation of brain function in severe human head trauma with multimodality evoked potentials. J. Neurosurg., *47*:150–162, 1977. Reprinted by permission.)

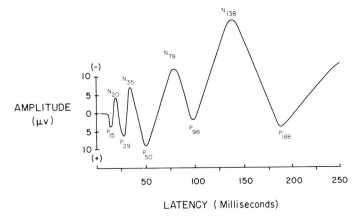

Figure 58–64 Schematic somatosensory evoked potential illustrates a method of labeling waveforms. All waves, regardless of modality, are labeled as either positive (P) or negative (N) followed by the latency from time of stimulation to wave peak in milliseconds. Positive waves are down by convention. (From Greenberg, R. P., et al.: Evaluation of brain function in severe human head trauma with multimodality evoked potentials. J. Neurosurg., *47*:150–177, 1977. Reprinted by permission.)

available (Fig. 58–65). Greenberg and co-workers presented a system of grading sensory evoked potentials obtained from patients with head injuries that categorizes the abnormal evoked potentials by grouping them into four distinct patterns according to similarity of wave latencies and waveform.[123] The patterns that emerge are arranged into an ordered system of functional grades from I through IV (Fig. 58–66, Table 58–3). Grade I and II evoked potentials are mildly to moderately abnormal, whereas grade III and IV evoked potentials are severely abnormal to absent.

Evoked Potential Diagnosis of Focal Neurological Deficits in Head Injury

Clinical evaluation of visual, auditory, or somesthetic system dysfunction in confused or comatose patients with head injury

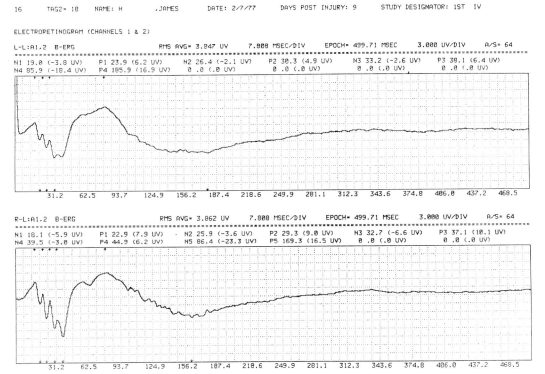

Figure 58–65 Electroretinograms printed by computer in analog form with the amplitudes and latencies of each positive or negative peak calculated automatically. This program allows a significant saving in time to be made by providing quick, accurate data analyses.

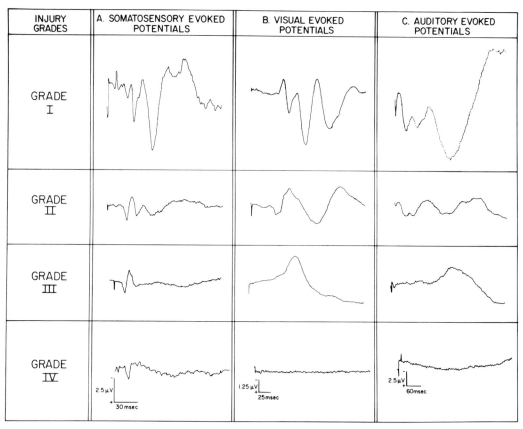

Figure 58–66 Graded injury potentials. Four distinct injury patterns can be recognized in each modality and are arranged in a system of functional grades from I to IV according to increasing abnormality. Each evoked potential trace depicted represents the average of at least 15 evoked potentials. (From Greenberg, R. P., et al.: Evaluation of brain function in severe human head trauma with multimodality evoked potentials. J. Neurosurg., 47:150–177, 1977. Reprinted by permission.)

TABLE 58–3 GRADED INJURY POTENTIALS IN HEAD INJURY*

MODALITY	GRADE								NUMBER STUDIES
Somatosensory	I	^{P}15	^{N}20	^{P}29	^{N}35	^{P}50	^{N}78	^{P}98	55
	II	^{P}15	^{N}20	^{P}29	^{N}35	$(^P$50$)^a$	—	—	27
	III	^{P}15	^{N}23	—	—	—	—	—	19
	IV	^{P}15	—	—	—	—	—	—	21
									$\overline{122}$
Visual	I	^{P}66	^{N}75	^{P}98	^{N}110	^{P}129	^{N}150	^{P}187 ^{N}420	62
	II	$(^P$65$)$**	—	^{N}90	—	—	^{P}150	— ^{N}220	29
	III	—	—	^{N}95	—	—	—	—	15
	IV	No activity		—	—	—	—	—	16
									$\overline{122}$
Auditory	I	^{P}45	^{N}63	^{P}87	^{N}143	^{P}232	^{N}370		43
	II	^{P}45	^{N}62	^{P}85	^{N}143	^{P}230	$(^N$260$)$†		38
	III	—	—	—	—	—	^{N}250		17
	IV	No activity		—	—	—	—		24
									$\overline{122}$
Brain stem	I	^{P}1.5	^{P}2.5	^{P}3.6	^{P}4.7	^{P}5.6	^{P}6.7	^{P}7.2 ^{P}10	65
	II	^{P}1.5	^{P}2.5	^{P}3.6	—	^{P}6.1	—	—	21
	III	^{P}1.5	—	—	—	^{P}6.0	—	—	5
	IV	^{P}1.5	—	—	—	—	—	—	6
									$\overline{97}$

^{a} Not always present—see text.

* Grading of sensory evoked potentials is based on similarity of wave latencies. Grade I and II evoked potentials are mildly to moderately abnormal; grade III and IV evoked potentials are severely abnormal to absent. See text for exact latency ranges in specific disorders. (From Greenberg, R. P., Mayer, D. J., Becker, D. P., and Miller, J. D.: Evaluation of brain function in severe human head trauma with multimodality evoked potentials. J. Neurosurg., 47:150–162, 1977. Reprinted by permission.)

may sometimes be difficult. In the same patients, however, evaluation of these neural systems with evoked potential techniques can contribute much to the early diagnosis of neurological deficits such as retrobulbar visual dysfunction, deafness, somesthetic deficits, or hemiparesis.*

RETROBULAR VISUAL DYSFUNCTION. Electrophysiological diagnosis of visual system dysfunction with evoked potentials requires first a careful consideration of retinal function, as the retina may be damaged by local trauma.[93,120,122] Electroretinograms assess retinal function and should be performed and analyzed prior to evaluation of visual evoked potential data.[13] For example, a patient's visual evoked potential

study may appear isoelectric (grade IV), suggesting intracranial visual system dysfunction when, in fact, a severely traumatized retina may be inhibiting generation or transmission of visual information to the occipital lobes (Fig. 58–67). Stimulation of each eye separately can also enhance the diagnostic value of visual potentials because each optic nerve can be individually assessed in this manner.[347] Visual evoked potentials recorded a few days after injury in comatose patients correlate well with dysfunction noted by neuro-opthalmological examination done months later when the patients are responsive (Table 58–4). In one study early clinical evaluation of visual dysfunction performed soon after injury correlated with the patient's final visual function in only 30 per cent of cases, while the visual evoked potential data recorded a

---

* See references 57, 93, 109, 132, 133, 318, 347.

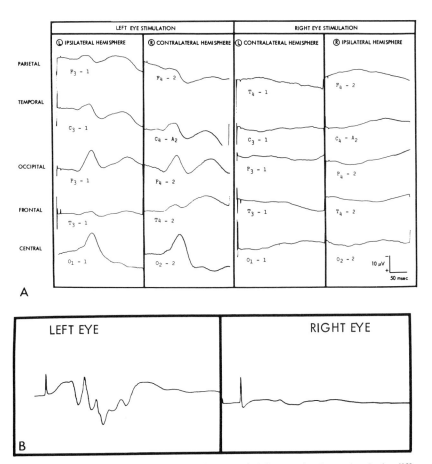

Figure 58–67 *A.* The visual evoked potential study, recorded from scalp electrodes, had a different outcome depending on which eye was stimulated. Left eye photic stimulation (*left*) generated severely abnormal but detectable visual evoked potentials (grade III), while right eye photic stimulation produced apparent electrically silent visual evoked potentials (grade IV). *B.* The electroretinogram of each eye, however, revealed right eye retinal dysfunction that had caused the apparent grade IV (electrically silent) visual potentials. (From Greenberg, R. P., et al.: Evaluation of brain function in severe human head trauma with multimodality evoked potentials. J. Neurosurg., *47*:150–177, 1977. Reprinted by permission.)

TABLE 58–4 CORRELATION BETWEEN EVOKED POTENTIALS FOLLOWING HEAD INJURY AND FINAL NEUROLOGICAL OUTCOME*

| FOCAL DEFICIT | OUTCOME[a] | EVOKED POTENTIALS[b] | | NUMBER OF PATIENTS |
		GRADE I–II	GRADE III–IV	
Hemiparesis	Acute (resolved) hemiparesis	6	0	6
	Residual (permanent) hemiparesis	0	9	9
		(P < .001)[d]		15
Retrobular visual dysfunction	Visual dysfunction	1	9	10
	No visual dysfunction	20	3	23
		(P < .001)[d]		33[c]
Auditory dysfunction	Deafness	1	5	6
	No deafness	24	3	27
		(P < .001)[d]		33[c]

[a] Outcome determined from 3 months to 30 months.
[b] Mean study performed on day 3.
[c] Eighteen of 51 patients died or could not be evaluated.
[d] Based on Fisher's exact test for 2 × 2 table.

* From Greenberg, R. P., Mayer, D. J., Becker, D. P., and Miller, J. D.: Evaluation of brain function in severe human head trauma with multimodality evoked potentials. J. Neurosurg., 47:150–162, 1977. Reprinted by permission.

few days after injury (mean day 3) correctly evaluated ultimate visual function in 90 per cent of cases.[122]

AUDITORY DYSFUNCTION. Deafness due to head trauma is difficult to evaluate clinically in children and confused or comatose adult patients.[57] Auditory evoked potentials permit early diagnosis of deafness in these patients, although it can be difficult to distinguish pre-existing auditory disease from that due to the head injury. Nevertheless, eighth nerve, brain stem, and hemispheric auditory dysfunction can be correctly evaluated electrically in most cases. Damage to the eighth nerve can be detected with brain stem auditory potentials.[317] The first potential seen in these records reflects eighth nerve function and is delayed or absent with peripheral auditory system damage.[319] Each ear should be stimulated separately to distinguish unilateral auditory dysfunction. Binaural stimulation will often mask a unilateral deficit, as the evoked response obtained will be an average of the activity generated from each ear (see Fig. 58–59). Auditory dysfunction, defined by audiometric examination months after trauma, has been compared with auditory evoked potential data recorded within days of head injury, as given in Table 58–4. In the initial few days following trauma (mean day 3) clinical evaluation of auditory dysfunction was shown in this study to be accurate in 17 per cent of cases when compared with the audiometric data gathered months later. Auditory evoked potential

data obtained at the same time correctly diagnosed auditory dysfunction in 83 per cent of cases.[122]

HEMIPARESIS OR HEMIPLEGIA. Owing to the close topographical association of the somesthetic and motor systems, associations between the presence or absence of hemiparesis and somatosensory evoked potential abnormalities have proved helpful in the diagnosis of motor deficits (Fig. 58–68B). Abnormalities in somatosensory evoked potential data obtained in the first week after injury correlate well with the presence of residual lateralized motor deficits.[122] Mildly or moderately abnormal somatosensory evoked potentials (grade I or II) recorded in the period immediately following head injury in patients with hemiparesis indicate the probable resolution of the hemiparesis some months later, while a severely abnormal or isoelectric somatosensory evoked potential indicates the likelihood of a persistent motor deficit (see Table 58–4).[123]

Localization of Focal Hemispheric Neuroanatomical Lesions

Efforts to correlate evoked potential data with central nervous system anatomical lesions verified by either computed tomograms, angiograms, intraoperative findings, or autopsy material have proved to be rewarding. The presence of a lesion such as a brain contusion does not necessarily imply a clinically detectable functional deficit;

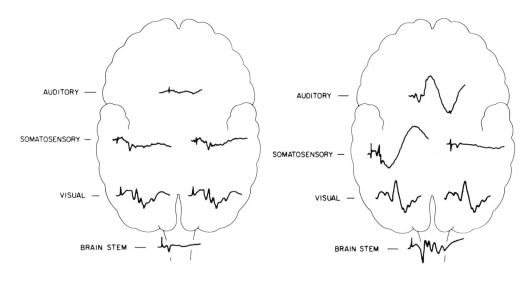

A   B

Figure 58–68   Brain images with the approximate location of sites of generation of multimodality evoked potentials superimposed. *A.* The visual evoked potential in this comatose patient is normal, while the somatosensory and auditory near- and far-field evoked potentials are absent, suggesting brain stem dysfunction. *B.* The right parietal lobe response to left median nerve depolorization is absent in a patient with dense left hemiparesis. All other multimodality evoked potentials were normal in this patient. (From Greenberg, R. P., et al.: Evaluation of brain function in severe human head trauma with multimodality evoked potentials. J. Neurosurg., *47:*150–177, 1977. Reprinted by permission.)

therefore, the evoked potential will not reflect all anatomical lesions. When electrically detectable anatomical lesions are present, however, positive correlations with evoked potential data verify the accuracy with which this electrophysiological technique can localize brain injury. Although the data are scant, it appears possible to localize focal brain lesions in all but the frontal lobes.

FRONTAL LOBE LESIONS.   Because of the lack of a technically suitable sensory stimulus with which to challenge them directly, these lesions are poorly localized by present evoked potential techniques.[122] Direct cortical stimulation and response recording as applied by Grossman can provide some information about the frontal lobes. This technique, however, requires the invasive placement of an electrode on the cortex.[125] Further refinements and the development of noninvasive means of stimulating the large frontal brain regions will help considerably.

PARIETAL LOBE LESIONS.   Somatosensory evoked potentials alone can accurately localize parietal lobe lesions.[122,323] The extent of a lesion necessary to alter the

evoked response is not known. Damaged areas detected by abnormal somatosensory evoked potentials may include the prerolandic frontal lobe as well as the parietal lobe, since clinical correlations with hemiparesis and aphasia have been made.[122,203] It can be seen in Figure 58–68*B* that the right parietal lobe response to left median nerve depolarization is quite depressed in a patient with a left hemiparesis in whom an acute subdural hematoma with severe right parietal lobe contusion was noted intraoperatively. The left parietal lobe response to right median nerve stimulation as well as the visual and auditory near- and far-field responses is normal in this patient?

TEMPORAL LOBE LESIONS.   Both the auditory and visual evoked potentials must be evaluated to determine temporal lobe lesions. Obtaining and evaluating data for one of these modalities alone is insufficient to detect the majority of temporal lobe lesions.[122] As can be seen in Figure 58–69, both the right visual and right auditory evoked responses were depressed in a patient who sustained a severe right temporal lobe hemorrhagic contusion that was treated by excision of the mass. The CT

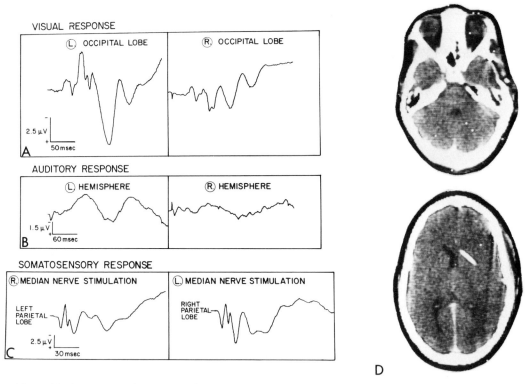

Figure 58–69 *A, B,* and *C.* The multimodality evoked potential study recorded postoperatively in a patient with a right temporal lobe lesion for which a partial right temporal lobectomy was required. *D.* The CT scan was also done postoperatively on the same day as the evoked potential study. (From Greenberg, R. P., et al.: Evaluation of brain function in severe human head trauma with multimodality evoked potentials. J. Neurosurg., *47*:150–177, 1977. Reprinted by permission.)

scan was obtained postoperatively and was done on the same day as the evoked potential study.

OCCIPITAL LOBE LESIONS. The visual evoked potentials correlate very well with occipital lobe lesions as long as electroretinograms are performed to avoid confusion with retinal dysfunction (cf. Fig. 58–67).

Diagnosis of Brain Stem and Hemispheric Dysfunction

Localization of dysfunction in brain regions (differentiating brain stem from hemispheric dysfunction) is best accomplished by utilizing the wider scope afforded by multimodality evoked potentials (visual, auditory, and somatosensory) as opposed to one modality alone.[121–123] The sensory imput producing somatosensory and auditory near-field and far-field evoked potentials traverses regions of the medulla, pons, midbrain, and part of the diencephalon located caudal to the lateral

geniculate body, which is the most caudal region traversed by sensory input producing visual evoked potentials (cf. Fig. 58–58).* Visual sensory input leaves its caudal position in the lateral geniculate body and turns rostrally into the cerebrum, passing through the temporal and parietal lobes into the occipital lobe. Therefore, abnormal somatosensory and auditory near- and far-field (brain stem) evoked potentials recorded from comatose patients with head trauma who have normal visual evoked potentials implicate dysfunctional brain stem more than dysfunctional cerebral hemispheres (compare Figures 58–16 and 58–68A).[121,122,359] On the other hand, an electrophysiological cerebral hemispheric dysfunction may exist if the data indicate normal auditory and somatosensory brain stem potentials (far-field) and abnormal auditory near-field evoked potentials coupled with

_____

* See references 63, 109, 270, 319, 323, 347.

abnormal visual and somatosensory near-field potentials.[40,121,122]

BRAIN STEM DYSFUNCTION. Except at autopsy, brain stem lesions are difficult to verify. Therefore, relatively few cases are available with which to correlate human evoked potential data. Starr and Hamilton compared auditory brain stem potentials with autopsy material and intraoperative observations in 10 patients to determine the brain stem structural correlates of far-field auditory response. They concluded that lesions of different regions of the brain stem can be associated with abnormalities of the auditory brain stem response.[319] Wilkus and co-workers could not obtain auditory evoked potentials in a patient with an extensive infarct of the pons. They were, however, able to obtain normal visual evoked responses and electroencephalograms.[359]

Greenberg and associates correlated multimodality evoked potentials of three patients whose brain stem lesions secondary to head injury were confirmed at autopsy. The gross autopsy examination of one patient, who died 10 days after head trauma, revealed a cerebrum that was moderately edematous, especially on the side of a partial left temporal lobectomy that had been done on the day of admission. The brain stem was grossly normal except for two small agonal hemorrhages, but microscopically, clusters of microglial cells were seen to be scattered throughout the midbrain, pons, and medulla (del Rio Hortega silver carbonate stain). Somatosensory and auditory near-field potentials were severely depressed, grade IV, in this patient, and the auditory brain stem potentials were grade III (Fig. 58–70). A normal simultaneous eighth nerve action potential ruled out eighth nerve focal damage as a cause of the severely abnormal auditory responses (Fig. 58–70D).[69] Visual evoked potentials were nearly normal bilaterally, grade I (Fig. 58–70C). Thus, the results for both modalities whose pathways traverse the medulla, pons, midbrain, and part of the diencephalon (i.e., somatosensory and auditory near- and far-field potentials) were severely abnormal. The visual evoked potentials were unaffected by the brain stem lesion because the optic pathways did not traverse the damaged caudal regions of the brain stem.[122]

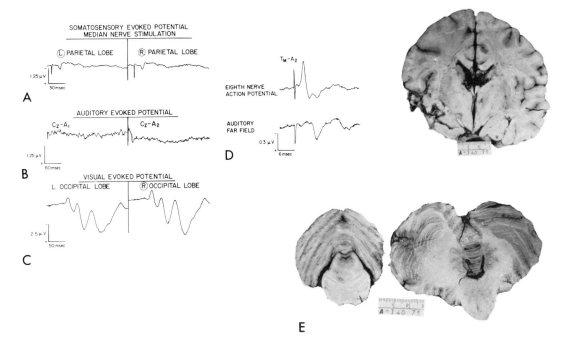

Figure 58–70 *A,B,C,* and *D.* The multimodality evoked potential study recorded in a patient with a brain stem lesion, in vivo, who subsequently died. *E.* Autopsy revealed, in the brain stem, many small hemorrhages and, on microscopic examination, clusters of microglial cells. (From Greenberg, R. P., et al.: Evaluation of brain function in severe human head trauma with multimodality evoked potentials. J. Neurosurg., *47*:150–177. 1977. Reprinted by permission.)

It is clear that evoked potentials, especially in comatose patients, can localize central nervous system dysfunction better than has heretofore been possible. This sensitive measure of brain function, along with the electroencephalogram, can be particularly useful in improving diagnosis and, thus, management in brain injury.

MANAGEMENT

Closed Head Injury

General Principles of Modern Management

Chapter 57 emphasized the separate but interrelated phenomena of primary brain damage due to the impact and secondary brain damage that occurs following the injury. The secondary injuries may be caused by obvious physiological abnormalities such as hypoxia, ischemia, hyperthermia, and brain shift. Further brain injury may occur as a result of new metabolic processes set up in already damaged brain; they may include an altered blood-brain barrier, lysosomal breakdown with release of proteolytic enzymes, release of free radicals, and excessive release of neurotransmitter substances. The exact role of such mechanisms of secondary brain damage is the subject of much investigation. Secondary brain damage is, however, a recognized, serious, and common problem.[29,293] The principles and specific maneuvers involved in treating patients with head injury should be based on an understanding of the phenomena of primary and secondary brain injury.

The first principle to be followed is *to anticipate and prevent an additional brain insult resulting from an abnormal physiological event.* In patients with severe brain injury, there is a *surprisingly high incidence* of these secondary insults occurring both before and after the patient arrives at the hospital.[29,284,293] These "second accidents" are often overlooked unless one carefully reviews the patient's course. They occur at the site of the accident, during emergency transportation, at receiving hospitals, in the emergency room, during transportation in the hospital, in the operating room during anesthetic induction, intraoperatively prior

to opening the dura, and even in the intensive care unit. These harmful physiological events further damage the already traumatized brain and predispose to further morbidity and death. An example is a severe generalized convulsion that causes a combination of hypoxia and hypercarbia secondary to inadequate ventilation with raised intracranial pressure and excessive neuronal energy demand. This combination of insults can seriously injure the brain and leave the patient much worse neurologically. Other examples include acute upper airway obstruction and delayed recognition of insidious respiratory insufficiency. Sepsis with high fever and septic shock frequently causes a dramatic neurological setback. Perhaps the most obvious second brain insult is that which occurs from an intracranial mass lesion that causes progressively increasing intracranial pressure and brain shift. This is most clearly seen in a patient with a "mild concussion" who becomes progressively more restless and disoriented in the hospital and then abruptly comatose and decerebrate from a combination of brain shift and high intracranial pressure resulting from an epidural clot. The patient's life may be saved by evacuation of the clot, but he will have suffered brain damage and have a permanent residual disability.

The second principle is *to provide an ideal internal milieu for the recovery of partially injured but potentially recoverable brain cells.*[184] With respect to the brain, the concept that *certain traumatized cells* may be *subtotally damaged* and go on to recover and function normally again has yet to be proved but is probably accurate.[24] Consider that patients may be in profound coma for days following a brain injury, perhaps with a focal neurological deficit. Within weeks or months such patients may go on to make a good recovery. It is not clear whether such recovery is due to central nervous system plasticity, with uninjured neurons taking on the functions of the destroyed neurons. More likely, brain cells that were rendered dysfunctional by the injury go on to recover normal function.[99] Possibly, certain inhibitory brain centers become hyperactive as a result of the injury and this perpetuates the comatose state, but this also seems less likely. Given an optimal internal milieu, it would seem reasonable to expect maximal recovery of the partially damaged neurons. The treating surgeon must strive to avoid those environments that are hostile to the recovery of the injured nervous system and could lead to progressive neuronal loss, brain edema, and further injury beyond the initial irreversible disruption and destruction of brain tissue.

The method for treating patients with acute brain injuries should utilize an intensive approach based on the principles just defined. There is evidence that such treatment can reduce the mortality rate.[25,47,130,218,357] A criticism leveled against such an intensive approach to the management of severe brain injury is that while more lives may be saved, a greater number of totally dependent vegetative survivors will result.[154] In fact, the number of severely disabled or vegetative patients who ultimately survive has not increased. Rather, the results from these studies show that some patients with potential for good recovery, who might otherwise have died of a secondary brain insult while in the hospital, have been allowed to make a good recovery. Most patients whose primary brain injury is so extensive that they can never become independent will die when intensive care is discontinued (Table 58–5). The incidence of true vegetative survival from

severe brain injury is about 2 per cent, even with intensive treatment.[25,263,267]

A practical and effective treatment protocol is centered on hospital care because this is where the neurosurgeon first gains control. Since secondary processes and insults may follow rapidly on the heels of the initial injury, however, therapy and management are discussed from the scene of the accident through rehabilitation. Major emphasis is placed on the care of patients with severe brain injury.

Immediate Management

Scene of the Injury and Emergency Transportation

It has been estimated that up to 20 per cent of injured victims die after accidents because of inadequate or inappropriate treatment prior to hospitalization.[286] Serious systemic abnormalities resulting from major trauma and including shock, hypoxemia, hypercarbia, and anemia are common. Any of these can lead to a second damaging brain injury. Miller and co-workers reported that of 100 consecutive patients with severe brain injury evaluated on arrival in the emergency room, 30 per cent were hypoxemic ($Pa_{O_2} < 65$ mm of mercury), 13 per cent were hypotensive (systolic

TABLE 58–5 **COMPARISON OF CLINICAL FEATURES AND OUTCOME IN SIX REPORTED SERIES OF SEVERE HEAD INJURIES**

FACTOR	RICHMOND	GLASGOW*	HOLLAND*	ROSSANDA†	PAZZAGLIA‡	PAGNI§
No. of patients	148[a]	428	172	223	282	1091
Clinical features						
Average age (yr)	27	34	33	—	38	—
Mass lesion (%)	40	57	27	39	41	61
Decerebrate/flaccid (%)	36	33	33	34	—	43
Hemiparesis (%)	20	19	21	—	—	—
Bilateral fixed pupils (%)	23	19	29	16	—	<21
Impaired/absent oculocephalic responses (%)	43	46	42	—	—	21
Outcome						
Good recovery/moderate disability (%)	57	39	42	—	40	—
Severe disability/vegative state (%)	11	10	6	—	11	—
Dead (%)	32	52	52	52	49	52

[a] For comparison purposes, 12 patients who gave a vocal response to stimuli on admission have been omitted.

* Jennett, B., et al: Predicting outcome in individual patients after head injury. Lancet, 1:1031–1034, 1976.

† Rossanda, M., et al.: Role of automatic ventilation in treatment of severe head injuries. J. Neurol. Sci., 17:265–270, 1973.

‡ Pazzaglia, P., et al.: Clinical course and prognosis of acute post-traumatic coma. J. Neurol. Neurosurg. Psychiat., 38:149–154, 1975.

§ Pagni, C. A.: The prognosis of head injured patients in a state of coma with decerebrated posture. J. Neurosurg. Sci., 17:289–295, 1973.

TABLE 58–6 PRE-HOSPITAL SYSTEMIC INSULT*

TYPE OF INSULT	NUMBER	ASSOCIATED WITH MULTIPLE INJURY	
		Number	Per cent
Hypotension (B.P. < 95)	13	13	100
Anemia (Hct. < 30)	12	11	92
Hyp (Pa_{O_2} < 65)	30	20	67
Hypercarbia (Pa_{CO_2} > 45)	4	4	100
Total insults	59		
Total patients	44	31	70

*Type and numbers of systemic insults noted in 100 patients with severe head injuries on arrival at a major trauma center.

blood pressure <95 mm of mercury), and 12 per cent were anemic (hematocrit <30 per cent) (Table 58–6).[244] These abnormalities all can further injure the already damaged brain. In the same study, the average time from accident to hospital entry (excluding secondary transfers) was 30 minutes. This early period is critical to the patient's outcome and should not be a "therapeutic vacuum."[24]

OXYGENATION. The most pressing immediate requirement is *to establish adequate oxygenation*. In addition to being certain that there is no upper airway obstruction, one must evaluate the total respiratory system. A patient may have respiratory insufficiency from upper airway obstruction or hypoventilation (inadequate tidal volume or respiratory rate), but patients may be hypoxemic even with a clear upper airway, a normal or rapid respiratory rate, and a normal or increased minute volume.

A fundamental component of a concussion is transient respiratory arrest.[258] The more severe the concussion, the longer the period of apnea. With severe brain injury and more marked brain stem deformation resulting from the impact, apnea may last over a minute or even longer.[21] Prolonged apnea may be the cause of "immediate" death at the scene of the accident, and if artificial respiration can be promptly instituted, a good salvage rate can result.[183] This phenomenon, although rarely documented in humans, has been defined in cattle in the abbatoir by Patterson and Hardy, who found that prompt artificial ventilation could keep animals alive after the type of blow to the head that ordinarily caused death.[265] Others have noted the same in experimental animals.[21] The following case was observed by a neurosurgical resident at the Medical College of Virginia and documents prolonged postconcussion apnea.[198]

The physician came upon a car that had turned over three times and landed on its hood. A man had been thrown from the car. A girl was pinned on her back under it and was presumed to be dead. From the midchest down she was in the passenger compartment; her upper chest and head were through the windshield under the hood—with her head pinned to the right. She was immobile, flaccid, without respiration, and no femoral pulse was obtainable. The head was too remote to be examined. A group lifted the car while the girl was dragged free. Closer examination then disclosed: (1) no carotid pulse, (2) no respiration, (3) no response to deep pain, (4) no corneal reflex, (5) pupils fixed to light and maximally dilated. Since at least five minutes had passed prior to the arrival of the physician and several minutes had passed prior to her examination, she was presumed to be dead. A sheet was pulled over the "body"—only to be thrown back when the girl took a gasping breath. Her pulse was now present at 100 per minute, and blood pressure was 160/90. The pupils were still dilated and fixed, and there was still no response to pain. At this point, an esophageal airway was placed. The respirations became rapid, and little ventilatory assistance was necessary. The total apneic period was in excess of 10 minutes. The time from placement of the airway to arrival in the emergency room was approximately 15 minutes. At that time the pupils were down to midposition and sluggishly reactive. Motor responses to pain were decerebrate. She was then intubated. A CT scan was normal, and intracranial pressure was normal. In two days she was awake and talking. In three weeks, she was back at work and apparently normal in every respect.

Emergency respiratory care at the scene of the accident begins with the suctioning of blood and vomitus from the airway as well as the removal of other foreign obstructing objects such as loose or false teeth. At a minimum, an oral airway should be placed. After clearing of the airway, artificial respiration, if necessary, should be begun by mouth-to-mouth, Ambu bag, or other means.

Additional oxygen by nasal catheter, bag, or mask should be given *without hesitation*. Even with a clear airway, the presence of tracheal aspirate, atelectasis, or pulmonary contusion may cause hypoxemia despite adequate ventilation; i.e., normocapnia. At high flow rates, a nasal catheter delivers no more than 35 to 50 per cent concentration of inspired oxygen (FI_{O_2}). To obtain higher concentrations, rebreathing masks can be used, but they function only if the patient is ventilating spontaneously. Likewise, special tubing is required on most "Ambu" bags to delivery 100 per cent oxygen. There is no danger of oxygen toxication if 100 per cent oxygen is used during the transport of the comatose patient because 100 per cent oxygen is toxic only if used for over 48 to 72 hours.[118]

Even after spontaneous respiration returns, and with no airway obstruction, the patient may remain hypoxemic. The respiratory rate and volume may be hypoventilatory or hyperventilatory, but still the arterial oxygen tension (Pa_{O_2}) may be below acceptable levels. Blood gas determinations on comatose patients with head injury done at admission to the emergency room show a surprisingly high incidence of low Pa_{O_2} even in the presence of hyperventilation.[244] The precise etiology of the low oxygen tension with a clear airway is unknown. It probably represents, in part, ventilation-perfusion abnormality in the lung secondary to atelectasis from the apneic period, since the hypoxemia can often be reversed with positive-pressure ventilation, provided that there is no primary pulmonary or thoracic injury.

All patients not responsive to verbal commands, even those who are tachypneic, should receive nasal oxygen, if available, at the scene and during transportation. This alone will often raise the arterial oxygen to acceptable levels, even if the patient has a slow respiratory rate. Endotracheal intubation, though preferable for hypoxemic patients, should be done only by experts, otherwise the esophagus may be intubated inadvertently and the patient rendered unsalvageable from hypoxemia. The esophageal occlusive airway may be useful here. It is inserted directly into the esophagus and can provide indirect access to positive-pressure pulmonary ventilation. It can be placed with relative ease and is already in use by some rescue squads (see Fig. 58–71). The emergency medical team should be capable of instituting assisted or artificial respiration at the very first suggestion that the patient's own respiratory system may

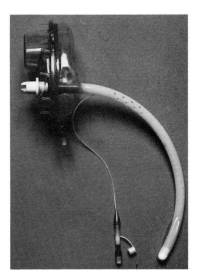

Figure 58–71 The assembled esophageal airway is shown as it would be used by the emergency medical technician. The mouth and nose are sealed by the mask and the esophagus is sealed by the distal tube. Air (oxygen) under positive pressure passes out through the exit holes and is able to enter only the trachea and inflate the lungs.

be failing. Progressive respiratory failure may be due to the presence of a progressing intracranial lesion, a pulmonary lesion, or these factors combined with depressant drugs such as alcohol, barbiturates, and narcotics. Even though a patient breathes well when he is placed in the ambulance, there is no guarantee that he will continue to do so.

TRANSPORT. After emergency ventilatory care has been provided at the scene, the patient should be rapidly moved to the hospital facility that can provide complete hospital care. Distance traveled is not the primary consideration. The only indication for transportation to a local receiving hospital is that the patient is in shock. If the patient is not hypotensive, ideally he should be transported directly to an optimal care hospital, where computed tomography and comprehensive neurosurgical care is immediately available. Prolonged delays at intermediate care hospitals should be avoided. All too often, major physiological secondary brain insults occur in this situation that could have been prevented with a proper transportation and emergency medical service system.[24,244] Each community and state should have a well-trained emergency medical service and a transfer system defined and developed to provide transport to a comprehensive optimal care hospital in less than one hour. During transport the patient should be maintained with nasal oxygen or, if intubated, on 100 per cent oxygen until it is *proved*, by blood gas analysis, that a lower inspired oxygen concentration is sufficient. Emergency squad personnel should be trained to administer intravenous fluids and to provide crystalloids or volume expanders if hypotension occurs. This can be lifesaving.

The patient should be transported in the neutral supine position. In this position the airway is easily attended to, emesis can be quickly cleared with suction, the patient can be observed clinically, vital signs can be taken and intravenous administration started, and the spinal cord can be better protected. This is emphasized because many emergency manuals still recommend transporting the patient in the three quarter prone position to avoid "tongue swallowing" or aspiration of vomitus. This principle of transport in the prone position was developed before oral airways and good vacuum suction devices became available.

The question is often raised whether rescue squad personnel or receiving hospital physicians should administer corticosteroids and osmotic agents such as mannitol during the period of transfer to the ultimate treatment facility. Some neurosurgeons recommend that steroids in dosages equivalent to 50 mg dexamethasone be administered as promptly as possible. At present, it is impossible to state whether this is beneficial, but the authors favor this policy because of preliminary evidence that large doses of steroids may reduce the mortality rate.[70,112] Osmotic agents such as mannitol should be given only under direction of a physician, when there is progressive neurological deterioration consistent with tentorial herniation; i.e., progressive loss of consciousness, a pupil changing from reactive to fixed and dilated. Two-way radio communication with the hospital physician may make possible supervision of this therapy during transport, and in certain selected situations it can be lifesaving.

Emergency Room Care

The emergency room management and responsibility for patients with head injury falls into five categories: (1) restitution and maintenance of respiratory and cardiovascular function; (2) performance and documentation of an appropriate clinical neurological and general physical examination; (3) planning and execution of appropriate diagnostic procedures; (4) determination of patient triage; i.e., to operating room, intensive care unit, or observation ward or home; and (5) certain limited types of therapy. The routine that is described as follows is for patients with severe brain injuries and must be modified appropriately for patients with less severe injuries. These modifications are commented upon where pertinent and particularly important.

URGENT MANAGEMENT. All patients who are not verbalizing *and* cannot follow any commands should be intubated promptly.[211,293] If endotracheal intubation cannot be performed easily by emergency room personnel, an anesthetist or anesthesiologist should be called to do it. The recommendation for early and prompt endotracheal intubation of the patient with a severe brain injury is, in part, based on observation of the high incidence of hypoxemia occurring in these patients. While the arterial oxygen tension can often be brought into a normal range with oxygen delivered by nasal catheter or mask, endotracheal intubation and positive-pressure ventilation usually are required to reverse atelectasis, and normoxemia can then be maintained with an inspired oxygen concentration of less than 40 per cent, which is in the nontoxic range. There are other reasons why prompt intubation is wise. Aspiration prior to arrival at the hospital and even after arrival is common. Aspiration of saliva or gastric contents may occur unobserved in patients with depressed pharyngeal and laryngeal reflexes. Even though frank clinical pulmonary edema with frothy fluid coming from the trachea is unusual after head trauma, there may be subclinical pulmonary edema that may, along with the atelectasis, account for early hypoxemia in these patients. In any event, intubation and positive-pressure ventilation are effective therapy for both conditions. Positive-pressure ventilation, particularly by means of a *volume* ventilator, is an important therapeutic maneuver in the treatment of pulmonary edema or the progressive respiratory distress syndrome following severe head injury.[313] When positive-pressure ventilation is initiated early, progressive respiratory failure is seen only rarely, though the ventilation frequently must be maintained for several days.[27] Additionally, respiratory insufficiency in the comatose patient can occur suddenly owing to upper airway obstruction, generalized seizure activity, or soft-tissue swelling in the neck, and intubation will prevent the problem. Acute respiratory insufficiency is especially important as a potential problem during in-hospital transportation or during computed tomography, angiography, or other diagnostic procedures. CT scanning is improved by keeping the patient immobile, and an intubated ventilated patient can easily be temporarily paralyzed with pancuronium (Pavulon).

Along with hypoxemia, low arterial pH on admission indicating a systemic acidosis is not uncommon. If the patient has been in shock, this is usually lactic acidosis. If the arterial carbon dioxide tension (Pa_{CO_2}) is high, the acidosis will be of mixed type, respiratory and metabolic. The acidosis should be corrected, and bicarbonate in a dosage of 1 mEq per kilogram every 10 to 15 minutes may be given until it is resolved. It should, however, be remembered that reversal of acidosis can occur quickly and spontaneously when ventilation and perfusion are restored by intubation and restoration of systemic arterial pressure.

The arterial blood pressure should be measured promptly in the emergency room. If the patient is hypotensive, the pressure should, of course, be brought to a normal range. The neurological examination is misleading in the hypotensive patient following head injury, and the patient who is "comatose" when his arterial blood pressure is 40 to 50 mm of mercury may become responsive, even to verbal stimuli, when the arterial blood pressure is brought to a normal range. Likewise, intracranial pressure measurements are invalid during arterial hypotension; low or mildly elevated intracranial pressure can be observed in a hypotensive patient, but as soon as arterial blood pressure is brought up to normal, the intracranial pressure can rise dramatically.[21]

In adults, shock usually is not due to primary brain injury.[244] Prolonged hypotension from the brain injury itself is seen only when medullary failure is occurring, and such patients will have other signs of impending brain death.[364] Acute transient hypotension may result from the primary brain insult, but by the time the patient arrives at the hospital, this should be over or should promptly reverse with administration of intravenous fluids. If a patient is hypotensive but has intact brain function, the shock state is almost always due to blood loss and hypovolemia, and this can be confirmed by noting a low central venous pressure. The blood volume must be expanded rapidly with appropriate crystalloid and colloid agents and blood if necessary. This is important because the brain of the patient with acute head injury is more vulnerable to hypotension and reduced cerebral perfusion pressure than the normal brain, owing to impairment of cerebrovascular autoregulation.[90] Additionally, cerebral vasospasm can be present in severe head injury.[219] The spasm can increase cerebral vascular resistance, with a concomitant profound reduction in cerebral blood flow due to low arterial blood pressure, leading to ischemia and infarction.[2,358]

Patients with severe brain injury with or without multiple trauma should have a central venous pressure line inserted, venous blood drawn for coagulation screening, blood count, blood typing and matching, electrolyte and alcohol assay, and, if available, a multichannel analyzer analysis such as the SMA 12 or SMAC 20. Screening of serum and urine for toxic agents may be indicated if drug overdose or abuse is suspected.

EXAMINATION. Immediately following evaluation and restitution of the vital signs, a general and neurological examination is undertaken. The immediate general examination must define those problems requiring prompt therapy. In victims with multiple injuries, which in the United States will be half the patients with severe head injuries, long-bone fractures must be recognized and stabilized, and any source of internal bleeding must be identified and managed appropriately.[244] Triage of the patient with major abdominal or thoracic injury and a potential intracranial hematoma can be vexing and is dealt with later. All patients with major head injury must have at least a lateral cervical spine film, and those with body trauma should have a chest x-ray, abdominal x-ray, and such other x-rays as are indicated by the general examination. The neurological examination in the patient with acute head injury should be limited to those crucial factors that will guide immediate treatment and triage. The key items are (1) level of consciousness as determined by eye opening, verbal response, and motor response; (2) motor strength; (3) pupillary size and responses to light; and (4) eye movements assessed as oculovestibular or oculocephalic reflexes. These same categories of neurological tests are the basic tests ordinarily done by the nurses in the intensive care unit for serial neurological testing and graphing.

The managing physician must decide which diagnostic procedures are to be performed in the individual patient. This decision will be based on the severity of the patient's brain injury as judged by his clinical picture. In order to separate patients simply and rapidly into broad groups for the purpose of planning immediate management, four simple categories suffice. More complex admission grading categories may be helpful for prognosis, but a simple categorization works best in a programmed management plan. Thus, this simple categorization is *solely* for the purpose of defining which management protocol the patient is to be assigned to.

CATEGORIZATION OF PATIENTS. The categories are defined primarily on level of consciousness and motor strength or response (Table 58–7).

Grade I applies to the patient who has had transient loss of consciousness but is now alert, oriented, and without neurologi-

TABLE 58–7 CATEGORIZATION OF PATIENTS*

Grade I	Transient loss of consciousness
	Now alert and oriented without neurological deficit
	May have headache, nausea, or vomiting
Grade II	Impaired consciousness but able to follow at least a simple command
	May be alert but with a focal neurological deficit
Grade III	Unable to follow even a single simple command because of disordered level of consciousness
	May use words, but inappropriately
	Motor response varies from localizing pain to posturing or nil
Grade IV	No evidence of brain function (brain death)

* Categories are based on initial presentation and provide a simple system for triage of patients into a management program appropriate to the degree of their brain injury.

cal deficit. He may have headache, nausea, or vomiting. Grade II comprises impaired consciousness with ability to follow at least a simple command. The patient may be alert but with a focal neurological deficit. The grade III patient is unable to follow even a single simple command because of a disordered level of consciousness. He may use words, but inappropriately. The motor response varies from localized pain to posturing or nil. Patients in grade IV show no evidence of brain function (brain death).

On the basis of this grading system, and if (and how) the patient's condition is changing, appropriate diagnostic procedures are planned, triage then follows, and certain forms of therapy are instituted.

TRIAGE BASED ON GRADE

Grade I. Skull x-rays should be obtained to define and document any linear or depressed skull fracture and to note the position of the pineal gland if it is calcified. Such patients are ordinarily observed in the hospital for 12 to 24 hours if circumstances permit. While the observation need not be in an intensive care unit or necessarily by specially trained neurological nurses, certain requirements should be met: the neurosurgeon should be rapidly available by phone, and physically able to reach the hospital in 15 to 20 minutes. The nurses should be carefully instructed in how to perform a simple evaluation of level of consciousness and motor examination, and should be told when to call the neurosurgeon in the particular case. The neurological checks should be repeated every 30 minutes for the first twelve hours. These basic points are belabored here because potentially curable patients with growing intracranial subdural or epidural clots can deteriorate to an unsalvageable state in the hospital environment while under supposed "observation." This has been documented even in staffed neurosurgical units.[284,293] The delay in diagnosis, resulting in death in patients who originally could talk on admission, usually results from an underestimation of the degree and rate of deterioration.[284]

An alternative to hospital admission for grade I patients is to perform skull x-rays and a CT scan from the emergency room. If the ventricles are midline, there is no extra-axial increased density (clot), no brain lesion, and no skull fracture it may be safe to send the patient home. This course of action would appear to be preferable, as it

INSTRUCTIONS FOR A PATIENT WHO HAS HAD A HEAD INJURY

AT PRESENT, WE FIND NO EVIDENCE OF SERIOUS INJURY. HOWEVER, ANY INDIVIDUAL WHO HAS RECEIVED A BLOW OR INJURY TO THE HEAD MAY DEVELOP SYMTOMS DUE TO THIS INJURY HOURS OR DAYS LATER.

THE FIRST TWENTY-FOUR (24) HOURS FOLLOWING INJURY ARE THE MOST IMPORTANT HOURS THAT THE INJURED PERSON NEEDS TO BE WATCHED. IF ANY OF THE FOLLOWING DEVELOP, YOUR DOCTOR SHOULD BE CALLED OR THE PATIENT SHOULD BE BROUGHT BACK TO THE HOSPITAL.

1) DROWSINESS OR DIFFICULTY IN AWAKENING. (WAKE THE PATIENT UP EVERY TWO (2) HOURS DURING PERIODS OF SLEEP)
2) NAUSEA OR VOMITING.
3) CONVULSIONS ("FITS")
4) ONE PUPIL (THE BLACK PART OF THE EYE) MUCH LARGER THAN THE OTHER, PECULIAR MOVEMENTS OF THE EYES, DIFFICULTY IN FOCUSING, OR OTHER VISUAL DISTURBANCE.
5) INABILITY TO MOVE ARMS OR LEGS ON ONE SIDE OF THE BODY OR THE OTHER, NUMBNESS OF ARMS OR LEGS, STUMBLING, OR PECULIAR WALKING.
6) SEVERE HEADACHES
7) CONFUSION, INABILITY TO CONCENTRATE, OR CHANGE IN PERSON-ALITY. (PATIENT DOESN'T ACT AS HE USUALLY DOES)
8) UNUSUAL RESTLESSNESS
9) A VERY SLOW OR VERY RAPID PULSE OR UNUSUAL CHANGE IN PATIENT'S BREATHING.
10) DIZZINESS.

IF THERE IS SWELLING AT SITE OF INJURY, APPLY AN ICE PACK, MAKING SURE THAT THERE IS SOME MATERIAL (SUCH AS A WASH CLOTH, PIECE OF CLOTH, ETC.) BETWEEN ICE PACK AND THE SKIN. IF THE SWELLING IN-CREASES MARKEDLY IN SPITE OF ICE PACK APPLICATION, CONTACT YOUR DOCTOR OR BRING PATIENT BACK TO THE HOSPITAL

NOTE: THE PATIENT SHOULD NOT HAVE ANY ALCOHOLIC BEVERAGES FOR 2-3 DAYS FOLLOWING THE INJURY. DO NOT LET PATIENT TAKE ANY PAIN MEDICATION THAT IS STRONGER THAN ASPRIN, BUFFERIN, EXCEDRINE OR TYLENOL, UNLESS PRESCRIBED BY THE DOCTOR.

Figure 58–72 A typical warning sheet for patients with mild head injuries who are to be sent home.

would save the cost of a hospital bed, the time of many hospital employees, and discomfort for the patient. While consideration should be given to this form of management, it should, perhaps, be tempered by the fact that it is not yet known how often the grade I patient with a normal CT scan will develop an intracranial mass. Ideal management of grade I patients would be to perform CT scans and skull films, and if these are normal, discharge the patient with a warning to return if increasing headache, lethargy, or vomiting develops (Fig. 58–72). If a lesion is noted on computed tomography, the patient must be admitted, and further management will depend on his course, as outlined next.

Grade II. These patients have had a serious brain injury and should be admitted to a full-service hospital. If available, a computed tomographic scan should be obtained within six hours. If there is no CT scanner and if the patient's level of consciousness or neurological deficit is not clearly improving, an angiogram should be performed in 12 to 24 hours. In the meantime, it is preferable that the patient be cared for in an intensive care unit by specially trained neurological nurses, where neurological checks can be done at 30-minute intervals initially. If no "operative mass lesion" as defined later in the text is present, management is continued in the short-term care unit, where the patient should be carefully maintained in metabolic balance. Because of the tentative evidence that large deses of corticosteroids are beneficial in mechanical brain injury, their use is favored for these patients.[92,112] Since intracranial pressure monitoring is at present an invasive technique, it is usually avoided in grade II patients because the large majority of patients in this group make uneventful recoveries as long as they have good general medical care and no secondary complications. Unless patients in this group have a clear respiratory problem or respiratory insufficiency, they need not be intubated routinely. Intracranial pressure monitoring should, however, be considered for those patients who have small "nonoperative" brain lesions but who are going to the

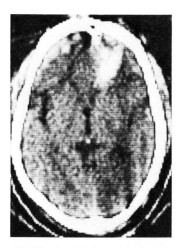

Figure 58–73 A right frontal high-density lesion consistent with a hemorrhagic contusion is present in this patient who was following one-stage commands on admission. The patient was followed with neurological examination and intracranial pressure monitoring and made a good recovery.

operating room and will be anesthetized for other nonneurosurgical problems, or for patients with multiple or borderline intracranial lesions upon which the surgeon decides not to operate (Fig. 58–73).

Grade III. Immediate endotracheal intubation and controlled positive-pressure ventilation are recommended for all these patients because they so commonly have respiratory insufficiency. These patients have had a major brain injury and they should all have an immediate CT scan. If computed tomography is unavailable, angiography or ventriculography should be performed promptly. Computed tomography is clearly the procedure of choice, and this or one of the contrast procedures should be done as an emergency because: (1) grade III patients may harbor mass lesions of major size with little evidence of focal neurological deficit, signs of tentorial herniation, or a Cushing cardiovascular response, and (2) they may, with little warning, suddenly deteriorate further and irreversibly from an intracranial mass. Patients who are deteriorating neurologically but do not yet show signs of brain stem compression from progressive tentorial herniation may · be considered for a CT scan prior to an emergency operation. But this course of action is to be used only if the scan is immediately available and the neurological picture improves with a large bolus of intravenous mannitol (1 gm per kilogram). In this situa-

tion, a single CT cut across the supratentorial space need take only an additional 5 to 10 minutes and provides valuable information that guides the operation. In no case should an operation be delayed more than 10 to 15 minutes in the deteriorating patient in the hospital with early signs of tentorial herniation, and in *every* case, mannitol (at least 1 gm per kilogram) should be given rapidly without fail. Finally, all patients in grade III who have an "operative mass lesion" as defined in the following text should receive the same large intravenous bolus of mannitol while on the way to the operating room.

Frequently grade III patients have a major intra-abdominal or thoracic injury that requires an emergency operation, and a quandary arises when the general surgical team wishes to take the patient to the operating room immediately. The following principles should be followed: If the systemic blood pressure is stable, computed tomography should be performed on the way to the operating room and may be limited to only one or two scans across the supratentorial space. This should delay an operation no more than 15 to 20 minutes. If the blood pressure is unstable, and the patient requires continuous intravenous infusions to maintain his blood pressure, either a twist drill ventriculogram with intracranial pressure measurement or an anteroposterior carotid angiogram can be done in the emergency room, or perhaps on the operating table, as a single arterial phase x-ray. With any of these tests, a major mass lesion can be identified, and, if it is, then the patient can undergo a craniotomy simultaneously with the other operative procedure.

All other grade III patients with no major mass lesions should go directly to an intensive care unit for management, which includes intracranial pressure monitoring, controlled ventilation, and maintenance of metabolic balance. Prompt administration of large doses of corticosteroids and an anticonvulsant is recommended.

Operative Treatment of Acute Closed Head Injuries

Indications for Operation

Two sets of factors define whether a patient with an acute closed head injury requires an operation: the clinical status of the patient, and the findings on x-ray studies of the head. Throughout these chapters on head injury, emphasis is placed on the importance of defining and evacuating intracranial mass lesions *before* they cause a secondary irreversible brain insult due to brain shift or intracranial hypertension and inadequate cerebral vascular perfusion. The operative indications and methods must be crisply defined by utilizing both clinical neurological and radiological information. Previous treatises on the management of patients with head injury have usually emphasized only the clinical signs of progressive neurological deterioration as an indication for operation, and have not addressed radiological criteria for operative treatment. Since an operation is advocated herein when a major intracranial mass is identified, whether or not signs of tentorial herniation have yet emerged, the criteria for considering a mass as "operative" are dealt with in detail.

CLINICAL STATUS AS AN INDICATION FOR OPERATION. A patient who *progressively* deteriorates from being able to talk to showing signs of tentorial herniation should have prompt operative therapy. Every basic neurosurgical textbook emphasizes that progressively diminishing responsiveness, development of unilateral pupillary dilation, associated flexor or extensor posturing, and increasing arterial hypertension and bradycardia associated with periodic breathing mean third nerve and brain stem compression from tentorial herniation. While such clinical pictures will inevitably occur and require an immediate operation, progressive deterioration should ideally be recognized earlier and the masses should be evacuated. It is incumbent, then, upon nurses and physicians evaluating such patients to be able to recognize the more subtle changes that develop while intracranial pressure is rising and brain shift is occurring. Even today, in some of the finest neurosurgical units, early subtle signs of deterioration escape recognition, and signs of brain compression and shift are discovered too late for reasonable salvage of the patient.[284,293]

RATIONALE FOR EARLY OPERATION FOR MASS LESIONS. Just as the shape of the pressure-volume intracranial pressure curve shows that the intracranial pressure may suddenly rise enormously with only a small increment of additional mass, so in the clinical situation patients may be doing reasonably well, only to deteriorate very suddenly and develop decerebrate posturing and a unilateral fixed and dilated pupil. This course is easily recognized in patients with a "lucid interval" who harbor an epidural hematoma, but may also be seen in patients with a large unilateral frontal or temporal contusion and hematoma. Three recent cases reviewed in depth by the authors emphasize this problem area:

Case 1

A 31-year-old fireman fell off the back of the fire truck during an alarm and was rendered unconscious. Upon arrival at the hospital he was lethargic and confused, but able to speak and follow simple commands. There was no focal neurological deficit. An angiogram was performed, which revealed a right frontal avascular mass and a shift of 4 mm of the anterior cerebral artery to the left. Because of his stable neurological condition and lack of focal signs he was treated with corticosteroids and general medical therapy in an intensive care unit. The following day, 24 hours after the injury, he was less responsive, no longer following commands. It was elected to operate on him and remove the frontal mass. When the patient was in the operating room, just prior to anesthesia induction, he rapidly developed a dilated and fixed right pupil and demonstrated spontaneous decerebrate motor activity bilaterally. He was given a large bolus of mannitol, and the contused right frontal lobe was then removed. There were no untoward intraoperative problems. Postoperatively, the patient remained decerebrate, had bilaterally fixed pupils, and died of medical complications several weeks later without ever regaining consciousness.

Case 2

A 14-year-old boy was struck in the left temple by another player during a school soccer game. He lost consciousness briefly, then became alert again, but with headache, and he vomited twice. In the hospital emergency room, the consulting neurosurgeon found him neurologically normal, but admitted him for observation and ordered vital signs and a neurological check every hour. The nursing notes revealed no change in his condition for seven hours. Then, over a period of one hour, the patient became more restless but still followed commands, verbalized well, and appeared oriented. Suddenly, his mother, who had been observing him all this time, noticed abnormal movements, and a nurse confirmed bilateral extensor posturing and unreactive pupils, although his vital signs remained unchanged. Two and one half hours later, after delay for an angiogram, a diagnosis of epidural hematoma was made and the clot was evacuated. Today the boy is severely handicapped.

Case 3

A 9-year-old girl was struck in the head by a swing at school, did not lose consciousness, but had severe headache when she came home. At the community hospital emergency room she was complaining of headache, had vomited once, but was neurologically normal. She was admitted for observation. Six hours later, the house resident was called by the nurses because the patient had become increasingly restless. The resident found her responsive, talking, and with normal vital signs, no pupillary changes, and a normal motor examination. Less than 30 minutes later the patient, in rapid succession, became decerebrate, developed unreactive pupils, had a cardiac arrest, and died. A large epidural hematoma was discovered at autopsy.

Several important points are to be made from the foregoing tragedies. First, brain function may remain surprisingly *good* in the face of a growing mass lesion and then *rapidly* deteriorate as intracranial spatial compensation is exceeded. In this situation, intracranial pressure rises suddenly and rapidly, impairing cerebral perfusion, and brain shift reaches a critical point at which signs of major upper brain stem compression suddenly appear. Progressive swelling in a frontal or temporal lobe around a contusion and hematoma can be as disastrous as the extra-axial clot. These cases emphasize the importance of defining trouble *early,* for when overt signs of herniation appear, the march of events is so rapid that irreversible brain damage occurs. The more subtle signs of neurological impairment must be attended to. Not only progressive depression in wakeful state, but a slight increase in disorientation and especially increasing restlessness demand a repeat diagnostic procedure. If it is already known that a mass exists, and profound disorientation, marked sleepiness, or increasing restlessness is occurring, serious consideration should be given to prompt evacuation of the mass. The development of mild or moderate contralateral weakness may be another early sign resulting from the cortex being compressed, but decorticate or decerebrate posturing is a late and

advanced sign of brain compression. Hypertension and bradycardia associated with periodic breathing are *very late* signs of severe brain stem compression or torque or both.

Theoretically, unilateral pupillary dilation should occur before the signs of upper brain stem compression, early enough to allow time for orderly diagnosis and treatment. Unfortunately, in acute head injury, development of a unilateral dilated and unreactive pupil from temporal lobe herniation is usually followed shortly by motor posturing.[116] In fact, decerebrate posturing may occur simultaneously with or even precede the pupillary abnormality.[21]

RADIOGRAPHIC INDICATIONS OF A MASS REQUIRING OPERATIVE TREATMENT

Computed tomography. In grade III patients with acute head injury, five variations of lesions seen in the CT scan are considered as potential operative mass lesions:

1. *Extra-axial mass with a definite shift of the midline.* If there is a clearly identifiable extra-axial lesion of increased or decreased density and the midline is seen with the naked eye to be shifted on the CT scan, the lesion should be evacuated. Any shift of the midline evident on computed tomography

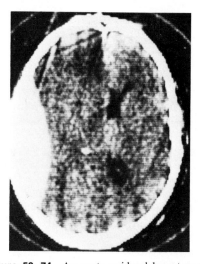

Figure 58–74 An acute epidural hematoma in a patient who was not following commands or speaking on admission. A marked midline shift is present. Such patients have markedly elevated intracranial pressure. Prompt evacuation of the clot is indicated, even if there are no signs of tentorial herniation or progressive neurological deterioration.

(1 mm on the print) is equivalent to a 4-mm true shift seen on ventriculography, and these lesions are almost always associated with high intracranial pressure in the early state after injury (Fig. 58–74).[243] If a small extra-axial lesion is seen, but there is no midline shift and no contralateral balancing lesion, the patient may be managed initially without operation.

2. *Midline shift with no extra- or intra-axial clot seen on CT scan.* If the midline is clearly shifted in an amount consistent with an actual shift of 5 mm or more and one ventricle is compressed, the patient should have a craniotomy even if no high-density masses are seen on the CT scan. At operation, the patient will often be found to have an acute subdural hematoma. Even if the shift is not due to an acute extra-axial clot, then a contusion will usually be discovered in the frontal or temporal lobe that, perhaps surprisingly, was not seen on the CT scan (Fig. 58–75). More often, a small extra-axial or intracerebral dense lesion is seen on the scan, with a large midline shift, and at operation one finds that the extra-axial

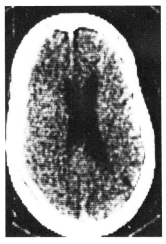

Figure 58–76   CT scan of a grade III patient injured in a fall following a seizure. The scan shows a left-to-right shift of the ventricular system with what appears to be a small subdural hematoma on the left. As is usual in cases like this, a large acute subdural hematoma was found at operation. The patient made a good recovery.

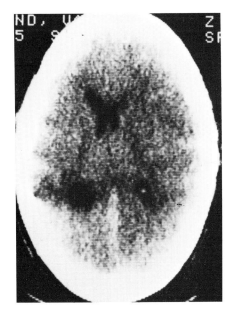

Figure 58–75   This grade III patient had a sizable midline shift on computed tomography but no obvious high-density lesion. At craniotomy a large right acute subdural hematoma was found. Evacuation relieved the elevated intracranial pressure. Patients in coma following head injury who have a CT scan showing major lateral ventricular shift or compression will usually be harboring an extra- or intra-axial clot or contusion that is contributing significantly to the shift. Craniotomy is recommended for this condition.

mass is much larger than expected from the CT scan (Fig. 58–76).

3. *Intra-axial mass with midline shift.* The same principles hold true here, and if there is a supratentorial intracerebral dense lesion with midline shift equivalent to 5 mm or more true shift, then the patient should have the contusion and hematoma evacuated. This is particularly important with intracerebral lesions because they almost always develop more surrounding edema and increased mass effect over several days, and if an initial midline shift of 5 mm or more is seen, any further brain swelling can be devastating (Fig. 58–77). Even if the lesion is in the anterior portion of the dominant hemisphere, operative evacuation should be done if the mass or the shift or both are large. Without operation death will almost certainly occur, and with operative evacuation of the mass an occasional good result can be obtained, depending on the location and extent of the irreversible damage. The indications for operation when there is less than 5 mm of midline shift are not clear as yet. In these situations, it is best to individualize treatment on the basis of the patient's clinical course and intracranial pressure.

4. *Multiple intra-axial lesions with midline shift.* Even when multiple unilateral or bilateral intracerebral lesions are present, if

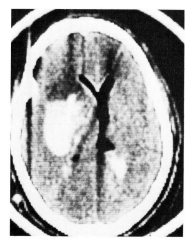

Figure 58–77 CT scan following twist drill ventriculography in a grade III patient. A large left temporal-parietal intracerebral hemorrhage is seen with a smaller hemorrhage on the right. The shift on the twist drill ventriculogram was 1 cm. Operation was done immediately, but the patient died. The morbidity and mortality rates for patients with acute intracerebral lesions are very high. When there is a sizable shift of the midline and the lesion is anterior, evacuation is recommended for grade III patients. An occasional good result will occur, although it is as yet not always possible to predict who will do well or poorly even with evacuation of clot and contusion.

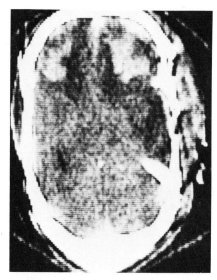

Figure 58–78 CT scan in a grade III patient following a right craniotomy for temporal contusion and acute subdural hematoma. At this point his intracranial pressure was 40 mm of mercury and he was deteriorating neurologically. Bifrontal hemorrhagic contusions not seen on initial computed tomography were confirmed at operation. The patient ultimately died of medical complications.

there is a major shift of the midline, the major shift-producing lesion or lesions should be evacuated. It is not advisable to extend the operation across the midline except very rarely for large bifrontal contusions (Fig. 58–78). Bilateral temporal lobe operation for intracerebral contusion and hematoma is also not advisable.

If there is no shift of the midline, the patients can often be managed successfully without operative intervention. But intracranial pressure monitoring and frequent neurological examinations must be performed in order to guide therapy and determine whether operative mass evacuation is ultimately required (Fig. 58–79).

5. *Bilateral extra-axial dense lesions without shift.* Small bilateral extra-axial hematomas may often be managed satisfactorily without operation. Large lesions, especially if they are causing clear brain compression with ventricular impingement, should be evacuated. While even the larger lesions may occasionally disappear without operation, the evidence of brain compression on computed tomography suggests the possibility of real or potential second-

ary brain injury, and this is best handled by evacuating the mass.

The foregoing indications for operation on computed tomographic criteria are de-

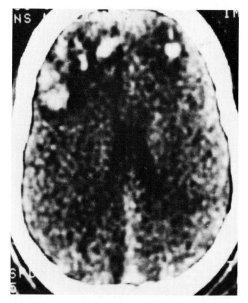

Figure 58–79 Bifrontal contusions are present in this grade III patient injured in a motorcycle accident. He was treated without operation and made a good recovery.

fined for grade III patients. Patients who are in better neurological condition, i.e., grade II, can more often be safely watched without operation, even with an intra-axial mass and some shift. These patients must be monitored very closely neurologically, and if their condition deteriorates to grade III status, then the mass should be evacuated.

The absolute criteria for operation based on the CT scan need better refinement. As methods for preventing or reversing brain edema (especially around a contusion) improve, the preceding recommendations may be modified and more patients may be adequately managed without operation. As improved prognostic criteria are defined concerning locations and extents of the lesions seen on computed tomography in relation to ultimate quality of outcome, certain patients may be better defined as inappropriate candidates for operation. At present, however, all grade III patients with a definite operative mass lesion, regardless of how neurologically impaired they may appear, are candidates for operation. This recommendation comes from the documented evidence that some patients with bilateral nonreactive pupils, impaired oculocephalic responses, and decerebrate posturing can make good recoveries if the mass is evacuated early. In one series, 3 of 19 patients treated with operative removal of the mass ended up in the good recovery–moderate disability category despite this foreboding constellation of signs.[25]

Ventriculogram. If immediate access to computed tomography is not available, a satisfactory diagnostic procedure for all grade III patients is a ventriculogram with intracranial pressure measurement performed in the emergency room. This quickly provides information on the presence and degree of midline shift and the level of intracranial pressure. The ventriculogram is valuable if the patient is deteriorating very rapidly or if he has other injuries that require immediate treatment, such as intra-abdominal hemorrhage. In these situations ventriculography with intracranial pressure measurement will make possible rapid general intracranial diagnosis. If the midline is shifted 5 mm or more, this is considered an indication for craniotomy. If the midline is shifted, but less than 4 mm, and the patient is not de-

teriorating, then the patient should have an angiogram or CT scan, or both, at an early convenient time. If there is no midline shift but the intracranial pressure is elevated above 15 mm of mercury, then angiography should be performed promptly, especially to rule out bilateral lesions.

According to the guidelines of operation, if the midline shift exceeds 4 mm, major extra-axial clots or sizeable surface intra-axial clots or contusions will almost always be found at operation. Only rarely will diffuse hemispheral brain swelling be the only operative finding. If the midline is shifted 5 mm or more, the intracranial pressure can be expected to be 30 or more millimeters of mercury, unless there is a cerebrospinal fluid leak or the patient has quite marked pre-existing brain atrophy.[243]

Angiographic indications for operation. It is not a simple matter to define absolute indications for operative therapy based on the angiogram, but it is still surprising that little has been done to define criteria, since angiography has been a commonly used radiological procedure for evaluating head injury. In general, the angiographic guidelines used are the degree of midline shift and the estimated size and location of any intra-axial or extra-axial mass lesion.[137] If the patient is not obeying commands (grade III), the following findings should be considered as indications for management by operation.

1. Extra-axial mass lesions more than 5 mm from the inner table, *if* they are associated with any degree of middle or anterior cerebral artery displacement. If there is associated major vessel displacement, this is a sign of brain compression, which should be relieved.

2. Bilateral extra-axial mass lesions more than 5 mm from the inner table. Except for patients who have prominent brain atrophy, intracranial masses of this size will usually summate to cause a major elevation of intracranial pressure.

3. Temporal lobe intra-axial mass lesions causing a major elevation of the middle cerebral artery or any degree of midline shift. These patients are in a most precarious position, as only slight swelling can cause a tentorial herniation syndrome that progresses very rapidly.

4. Intra-axial mass lesions causing shift of the midline vessels of 5 mm or more.

If patients are grade II, and any of the preceding criteria are present, nonoperative management may suffice. But very close neurological monitoring, perhaps coupled with intracranial pressure monitoring, is in order.

Preparations for Operation and Anesthesia

Once operative therapy is decided upon, the surgeon should proceed with dispatch. Blood should be sent for cross-matching, and two units of blood should be brought to the operating room as soon as available. Prior to anesthesia, the patient should virtually always be given intravenous mannitol in a dose that will elevate serum osmolarity by 10 to 12 mOsm. This requires at least 1 gm per kilogram; in an adult 500 ml of a 20 per cent solution will suffice. Some have advocated smaller doses of mannitol to bring down intracranial pressure, but smaller amounts should be used only if the pressure is being monitored so that the effectiveness of these smaller doses can be verified.[216] Furosemide (Lasix) has also been recommended, but there is no clear evidence yet that this agent directly dehydrates the brain or reduces intracranial pressure through other than indirect systemic diuresis and thus generalized dehydration. It is not recommended for this urgent situation.

Mannitol should be given *before* anesthesia is begun. The rationale for this maneuver is that the intracranial pressure is already dangerously high in almost all patients with large mass lesions, and serious further brain injury can occur in the 15 to 30 minutes prior to evacuation of the mass lesion.[26] Even if the patient appears reasonably stable on the way to the operation, mannitol should be given before or during endotracheal intubation and induction of anesthesia, as during these maneuvers the brain may be further insulted by increasing brain shift or increase in intracranial pressure, and some time must elapse before the dura can be opened.[30] Objections can be raised to the use of preoperative mannitol in that it might (1) cause increased intracranial bleeding because of increased overall cerebral blood flow and volume or diminished intracranial pressure tamponade of damaged vessels, (2) shrink the normal brain so much that the surgeon cannot determine whether he had indeed performed an adequate decompression, or (3) cause an immediate dangerous, but transient, elevation in intracranial pressure before it reduced the pressure to safe levels. While there may be some truth to each of these comments, the priority of overall brain protection afforded by immediate mannitol administration far outweighs these potential disadvantages.

Volatile anesthetics such as halothane should *not* be used because of their well-known cerebral vasodilator effect.[30] This will cause increased intracranial blood volume and, in a patient with a mass lesion, a dangerous rise in intracranial pressure toward blood pressure levels together with a reduction in blood pressure. Various combinations of nitrous oxide, barbiturates, narcotics, and tranquilizers are favored because of their minimal effect on intracranial pressure. Blood gases should be measured during the operation and arterial oxygen tension maintained above 80 mm of mercury. Arterial carbon dioxide tension should be quickly brought to levels between 25 and 30, but intraoperative ranges as low as 15 to 20 mm of mercury are usually well tolerated clinically.[21] Intraoperative hyperventilation should be accomplished with a large tidal volume and a slow to normal respiratory rate, rather than by increasing ventilatory rate much above normal levels, to allow time for good venous return.[27]

Operative Technique for Traumatic Intracranial Mass Lesions

The most skillful operative technique and the best surgical judgment should be brought to bear on traumatic intracranial mass lesions. Just as neurosurgeons accept that superior surgical skill and judgment will yield improved results in aneurysm, arteriovenous malformation, and benign brain tumor operations, these same efforts will also improve results in the operative treatment of trauma. In performing the "decompression," gentle handling of the brain is imperative, and firm brain retraction should *not* be done, as acutely injured brain tissue is quite vulnerable to this type of insult. The immediate goals of operation are reduction of intracranial pressure and brain shift, control of hemorrhage, and prevention of secondary delayed elevation in intracranial pressure and brain shift from brain swelling, inadequately evacuated clot or contusion, or recurrent clot. Judgment regarding extent of brain contusion excision may be a critical determinant of ultimate outcome. Likewise, meticulous hemostasis and maneuvers to prevent postoperative intracranial hematoma or brain herniation through bony defects can be expected to reduce the ultimate morbidity.

OPERATIVE APPROACH IN CLOSED HEAD INJURY. The past and recent literature on operative treatment of acute traumatic intracranial lesions presents a potpourri of operative approaches.[141] For epidural hematomas, most authorities have utilized a large subtemporal craniectomy or an osteoplastic bone flap. Indeed, Cushing was one of the earliest to use a large subtemporal craniectomy routinely for acute epidural hematoma, and he commented that Krause had recommended a formal craniotomy for epidural clots. Interestingly, Cushing reported in 1910 that 67 per cent of cases on which he operated recovered, and he stated that more would have recovered had the diagnosis been made earlier.[70] In the series of epidural hematomas reported by McKissock and co-workers and by Jamieson and Yelland, most cases were managed by large subtemporal craniectomies or craniotomies enlarged from local burr holes, but osteoplastic flaps were also utilized in some patients. The need for adequate exposure was stressed.[148,225] Gibbs, in 1960, came out strongly in favor of using an osteoplastic flap for epidural hematomas, while Hooper felt it was sometimes necessary, and Loyal Davis favored it.[76,108,140]

The recommendations for the operative management of acute and subacute hematomas have been far more varied. In the first half of this century the favored treatment was bilateral multiple burr hole drainage.[45,200,297,336,341] Cushing felt that the bleeding sites might not be controllable, and recommended only bilateral subtemporal decompressions.[70] Much fatalistic nihilism developed over this problem as mortality rates in the 80 to 90 per cent range were reported.[43,127,227,279] There was concern that, in this situation, a craniotomy was dangerous, possibly permitting further brain swelling, and that control of bleeding would be very difficult if not impossible.[341] It was not until 1948 that Whaley published an article describing acute subdural hematoma as being amenable to operative treatment by craniotomy.[356] In 1951 Chambers came out strongly in favor of craniotomy and radical clot evacuation for acute subdural hematoma.[54] Since then others have come to favor craniotomy, and with this form of operation, mortality figures have dropped to an average of 50 to 60 per cent.[25,95,279,285] Still today, the idea that the acute clotted subdural hematoma can be satisfactorily managed by multiple burr holes and irrigation lingers on and is occasionally recommended in modern texts.[302] Similar discrepancies have also existed regarding operative therapy for traumatic cerebral contusions and intracerebral hematomas.[24,73,297,302,341] As with the acute subdural hematoma problem, some of the more recent literature tends to favor excision of large intracerebral lesions that are causing elevated intracranial pressure and major brain shift.[24]

RATIONALE FOR USE OF THE BASIC LARGE CRANIOTOMY TRAUMA FLAP. Most closed head injuries cause a ''rotational brain injury.'' In this injury, as Holbourn has shown, the brain moves out of phase with the skull. During acceleration or deceleration injuries, the rotation causes brain deformation, with the major shear strains being at the frontal and temporal poles *as well as along the midline*.[139] Holbourn and Ommaya and Gennarelli have documented this experimentally, and clinical and autopsy observations have confirmed the predisposition of these sites to injury as illustrated in chapter 57 (see Fig. 57–3).[139,257,258] There is a high incidence of temporal and frontal contusions and tearing of midline bridging veins in severe brain injury associated with mass lesions requiring operation. The frontal and temporal contusions may not be demonstrable on angiography, and will of course not be seen on ventriculography. Likewise, smaller multifocal contusions may not be seen on computed tomography, particularly soon after injury, before progressive edema develops around the contusion. Since adequate decompressive operations may require debridement of these lesions, the frontal and temporal poles should be accessible in the field of exposure. While the temporal tip and pole are the sites usually involved in temporal lobe contusion, the frontal lesions commonly begin at the tips and extend over the inferior surface, involving the orbital gyri and inferior frontal lobe. Thus, the inferior frontal lobe should be accessible down the floor of the anterior fossa.

Similarly, with severe rotational brain injuries, one or more midline bridging veins may have been torn. This is a common cause of the acute subdural hematoma, and when the hematoma is evacuated, major intraoperative hemorrhage can occur from these vessels when the pressure tamponade is released.[24,128] In addition, patients with major temporal or frontal lobe contusions may also have torn bridging veins that are associated with little if any acute subdural hematoma because of tamponade from high intracranial pressure. When the intracranial mass effect is reduced by operative excision and mannitol, these vessels may bleed profusely. If only a limited temporal craniotomy is done for temporal lobe swelling and contusion, severe bleeding from these midline vessels may develop after the internal decompression, and great difficulty can be encountered in controlling the hemorrhage that is coming from a distance away from the bone flap.[54] To anticipate this potential problem, the craniotomy flap should also expose the area close to the midline. This exposure should be done even in the absence of an acute subdural hematoma when contrast studies reveal a shift of midline structures and an intracerebral lesion or only the latter. The basic craniotomy flap, therefore, should be generous enough and placed so as to permit one to deal quickly with the most frequently found disorder without further operative extension for additional exposure.[95] To accomplish this the exposure should provide adequate access: (1) to decompress the epidural and subdural space; (2) to debride contused cerebral tissue (anterior temporal and frontal lobes and orbital gyri) and remove associated intracerebral hematomas as necessary; (3) to control hemorrhage from avulsed bridging veins to the sagittal sinus and from temporal lobe to transverse sinus and petrosal sinuses; (4) to control hemorrhage from the skull base, to pack sinuses as necessary, and to repair potential cerebrospinal fluid fistulae; and (5) to explore and manage lesions of vascular and neural elements at the base as necessary.

Technique of Basic
Large Trauma Craniotomy

Scalp incision outline. The skin incision is outlined as shown in Figure 58–80. It is begun 1 cm anterior to the tragus at the temporal portion of the zygomatic arch, carried superiorly and posteriorly over the ear, posteriorly around the parietal bone to the midline, where it is brought anteriorly on the midline down to the midforehead. The forehead incision, which comes below the hairline, can be closed by using plastic surgical techniques, and the minimal visible scar is small sacrifice for the added exposure of the frontal lobe gained by this flap.

Immediate temporal decompression. If the patient has been deteriorating rapidly prior to operation, a quick decompression is the immediate goal. In this situation the portion of the incision just anterior to and above the ear should be opened first down through the temporalis muscle to bone (Fig. 58–81). A burr hole and small craniectomy should be accomplished quickly, and the dura opened in cruciate fashion. Most often this maneuver will afford some immediate relief of elevated intracranial pressure when a small amount of extra-axial clot or contused temporal lobe herniates out through the craniectomy site. One should then proceed to perform the formal craniotomy, and not be satisfied with this small decompression.[54,76,95,108,224]

Bone flap. Either a free bone flap or one based on the temporalis muscle can be raised. The medial portion of the craniotomy should be approximately 2 to 3 cm from the midline. The bone flap should be brought low across the frontal bone, across the sphenoid wing, below the pterion to the temporal bone. The opening is further enlarged by resection of the lateral portion of the sphenoid wing (Fig. 58–82).

Dural opening. The incision is begun in the temporal region, a continuation of the dural temporal opening if an initial temporal craniectomy and dural incision have been made or the anterior frontal region (Fig. 58–83). With this approach, if the brain herniates through the dura because of mass effect, the herniated cerebral tissue will be part of a relatively silent lobe. This herniation usually occurs only when the temporal or frontal tip is severely contused. Then the remainder of the dural opening can be completed with little further herniation of tis-

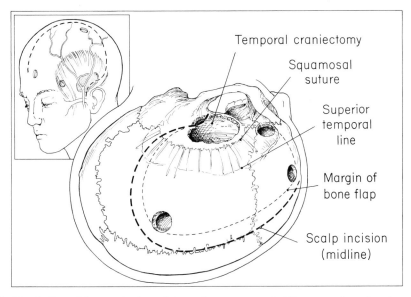

Figure 58-80 Outline of the standard craniotomy flap recommended for evacuation of acute epidural, subdural, and intracerebral hematomas and contusions. This exposure will provide access to the critical areas commonly injured in acute acceleration or deceleration "rotational" injuries. Through this flap the surgeon will be able to decompress the epidural and subdural spaces, debride contused anterior temporal and frontal lobes and orbital gyri, and control hemorrhage from midline avulsed bridging veins or the basal dural or skull areas.

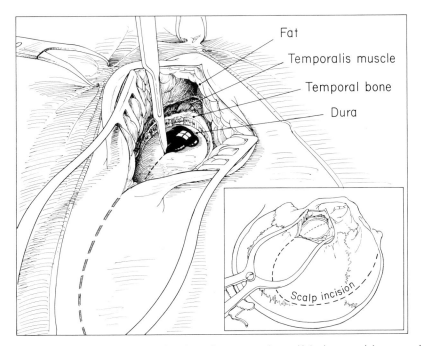

Figure 58-81 If the patient has been deteriorating prior to operation or if the intracranial pressure is known to be very high and there is a major shift, an initial quick subtemporal decompression should be done. One should then proceed with the formal craniotomy.

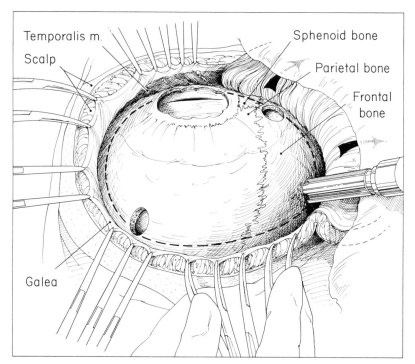

Figure 58–82   Either a free bone flap or one based on the temporal muscle can be raised. The medial portion of the bone flap should be 2 to 3 cm from the midline. Far anterior placement of the forward holes permits easy access to anterior temporal and orbital gyri zones.

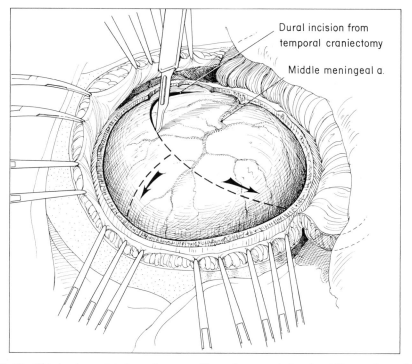

Figure 58–83   The dural opening shown here provides safe access to basal, midline, and anterior regions.

sue. If intact cortex begins to herniate, then further maneuvers to reduce brain swelling should be instituted immediately: additional mannitol, increased hyperventilation, and perhaps even transient reduction of arterial blood pressure to reduce and relieve cerebrovascular engorgement. The dural opening should be curved gently as it is carried anteriorly, up to the anterior medial border of the bone flap. An incision from the center of this dural flap, directed posteromedially, will complete the opening. This dural opening provides access to the frontal and temporal lobes and the anterior and middle fossae (Fig. 58–84).

The vast majority of unilateral intracranial hemorrhages and contusions can now be dealt with. The lateral parietal and occipital cortex may be inspected, but is not fully exposed. The orbital gyri (where most frontal lobe contusions occur) are readily accessible, as are the inferior temporal gyrus and more basal structures. Inspection of the basal structures, if necessary, is facil-

itated. Hemorrhage from the middle meningeal artery is readily controlled, even down to the foramen spinosum. The intracranial surface of the sagittal sinus is exposed, and hemorrhage from avulsed emissary cortical veins can be controlled without further bone resection or undue retraction on the brain.

The basic trauma flap should be used for a prediagnosed acute subdural hematoma because the clot is usually extensive and exposure of the bridging veins may be critically important. It should also be used when operating on a patient who has not had contrast studies or has had only a ventriculogram or angiogram for diagnosis. In these situations the extent of the lesion or lesions is not totally known ahead of time, and the large flap permits the surgeon to deal with unexpected intraoperative problems.

A temporal craniectomy might be adequate in cases in which a CT scan prior to operation clearly reveals only a temporal

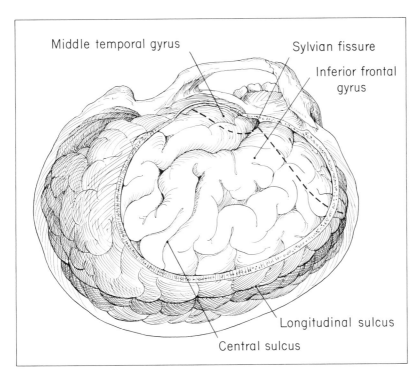

Figure 58–84 The extent of exposure is demonstrated here. The areas of common anterior contusion sites are accessible. Midline and basal hemorrhage can be managed. The posterior exposure permits easy safe extraction of extra-axial clots.

lobe contusion with major mass effect or an absolutely clear preoperative diagnosis is made of simple epidural hematoma uncomplicated by other intracranial lesions. Even in these situations, however, the intracranial injury often is more extensive than seen on computed tomography. Thus, even here wider exposure offers the patient greater benefits in that the operable mass lesions are more adequately exposed for excision. Further support for this approach of wide exposure, even with epidural hematoma, comes from Jamieson and Yelland's 1968 study of 167 patients with epidural hematoma. In this group, in addition to the epidural clot, 79 had major intradural lesions, which included 35 simple subdural hematomas and 30 cerebral lacerations with subdural hematomas, 5 with intracerebral hematomas, and 9 with mixed hematomas.[148]

While this basic flap will be adequate for over 95 per cent of unilateral operative exposures for closed head injury, occasional modifications are necessary. Rarely, an extra-axial clot or intracerebral contusion and clot may be seen to extend into the parietal and occipital regions, or be limited to those zones. In that case, the exposure should still be large and carried close to the midline, but should, of course, be placed more posteriorly. A "question mark" scalp incision is still favored here, but the inferior aspect of the incision may begin behind the ear rather than anterior to the tragus.

Traumatic posterior fossa hematomas or cerebellar contusions that require evacuation are rare, but if encountered, should be dealt with by a large posterior fossa exposure.[128] A midline incision with wide bilateral craniectomy and initial dural opening on the side of the offending lesion is recommended.

Operative Management of Specific Lesions in Trauma

EPIDURAL HEMATOMA. Complete exposure of the lesion is important, and in addition to the standard craniotomy flap, the craniectomy may need to be extended, although much initial decompression can be accomplished through such a small opening. It is important to visualize the peripheral margin of the clot and to remove it all, up to intact dura. The culprit bleeding vessel or vessels can usually be managed

with bipolar coagulation, but occasionally the middle meningeal artery must be occluded with bone wax or bone wax and cotton wool mixed and plugged into the foramen spinosum with a blunt nerve hook, especially when a basal skull fracture has lacerated the vessel. The epidural hematoma itself can usually be exposed adequately through a large temporal craniectomy or with a small bone flap.[108,225] But only if the patient has had a clear and definite lucid interval and shows no additional lesions on CT scan may one safely limit the exposure to a craniectomy or small bone flap. Even here, the dura should be opened over 2 to 3 cm to look underneath.[148]

If the patient has not had a lucid interval (he has been mentally depressed since the injury), the large trauma flap should be performed and the subdural space, temporal lobe, inferior frontal lobe, and orbital gyri directly inspected following evacuation of the epidural clot.[148] Any intradural lesions should be dealt with, and the dura should be closed and tacked up circumferentially and to the center of the bone flap. These maneuvers will help prevent clot recurrence (Fig. 58–85). Epidural hematoma that has been present for more than 24 hours often presents a particular problem at this stage, as the original bleeding point may not be evident and the entire underlying dural surface is extremely vascular, oozing blood at multiple points. Meticulous hemostasis cannot be too strongly stressed, as the clinical consequences of recurrent brain compression are disastrously severe even in a patient who tolerated the first episode remarkably well, as is often the case with the tardily diagnosed epidural clot.

ACUTE SUBDURAL HEMATOMA. This is the most common mass lesion requiring operative treatment in acute head injury.[25] It should always be dealt with via the large craniotomy, never through burr holes or a limited temporal craniectomy.[285,356] In fact, a rule to follow in all subdural hematomas, regardless of the age of the lesion, is that if any clotted blood is present, a craniotomy flap should be turned down.[48]

Once the dura is opened, the clot should be gently removed from the cortical surface (Fig. 58–86). Removal of the clot is best done with a combination of irrigation, cup forceps evacuation, and gentle suction. Large fragments of clot that are over the

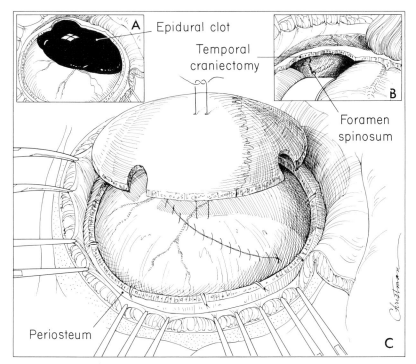

Figure 58–85 *A*. Adequate exposure of epidural hematomas is important, and acute major extradural clots usually cover an extensive area. *B*. Troublesome extradural bleeding from a basal skull fracture can be exposed if necessary. *C*. This large flap should be performed in patients who have not had a clear lucid interval, even though a preoperative diagnosis of epidural clot has been made, and the dura should be opened to permit adequate intradural exploration. Meticulous hemostasis with dural tacking as shown should reduce postoperative clot reaccumulation.

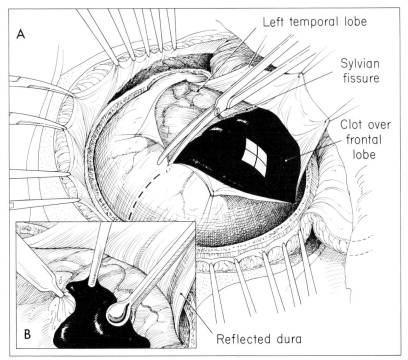

Figure 58–86 *A*. A typical acute subdural hematoma is shown here. *B*. After the dura is open the clot should be gently removed by means of irrigation, forceps extraction, and careful suctioning.

occipital lobe or on the floor of the anterior or middle fossae can be gently washed and teased out. These large fragments can be exposed by placing a brain retractor over the appropriate lobe and allowing the clot to extrude slowly to be extracted with forceps. While large clot fragments should be removed, tiny bits of clot under the dura and bone should not be vigorously pursued. If the brain remains full after removal of the surface clot and is bulging out at the craniotomy edges, more mannitol should be given, along with increased hyperventilation, to provide better exposure. This full brain may be due to extracerebral clot that is either in the anterior or middle fossa or over the occipital lobe, or due to an intracerebral contusion. Occasionally this full brain is due to increased cerebral blood volume, a developing contralateral hematoma, or acute brain edema.[178]

A bleeding major surface artery or vein will often be identified after the clot is removed.[54] It can usually be sealed by bipolar coagulation. If the bleeding is coming from a midline bridging vein, a middle fossa vessel, or a vessel that is located under the intact dura and bone, great care must be taken in exposing and controlling the bleeding vessel. In the management of an avulsed bridging vein, the cortical open end is usually easily controlled with bipolar coagulation. The sinus side of the vessel may be troublesome, and if bipolar coagulation or Gelfoam or operative packing fails, a small piece of beaten muscle carefully placed directly over the venous opening will usually produce satisfactory hemostasis (Fig. 58–87). The practice of expanding the brain by injection of saline into the lumbar theca or ventricle to control this bleeding by tamponade should *never* be done, as the increased pressure created by the injection is likely to further damage the brain.[341]

Similarly, in acute subdural hematoma, lumbar saline injections to expand the brain or disimpact a herniated temporal lobe should not be done, as it serves no useful purpose. The brain will shortly come to fill up the defect created by the clot. No attempt need be made to disimpact a herniated temporal lobe by tentorial section or medial temporal lobectomy. Evidence that these maneuvers benefit the patient is inconclusive.[200] Simple supratentorial de-

compression alone will almost always disimpact a herniated temporal mass, and the strangulated, swollen, and impacted medial temporal hernia occasionally seen at au-

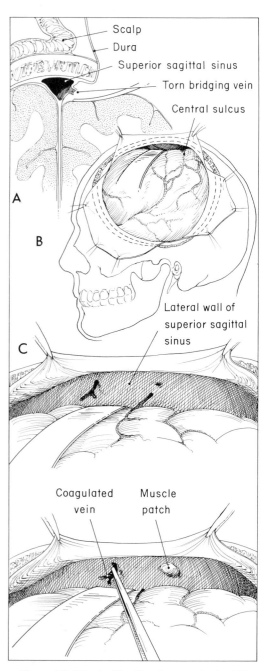

Figure 58–87 *A.* Bleeding from avulsed midline bridging veins commonly occurs after evacuation of the hematoma or contusion. *B,C,* and *D.* Simple coagulation will often suffice, but a patch of beaten muscle is still the finest hemostatic agent when sinus bleeding from an avulsed draining vein is not easily controlled with coagulation or synthetic hemostatic agents.

topsy occurs only in cases with such overwhelming brain damage and swelling that a salvage could not have been considered feasible.[2]

CEREBRAL CONTUSION, LACERATION, AND HEMATOMA. Contusions usually appear on the surface of the anterior and inferior frontal lobes and the temporal lobes (Fig. 58–88). They are composed of necrotic brain tissue that is infiltrated with blood. The brain tissue in a confluent contusion is irreversibly and irreparably destroyed and not only serves as a primary mass lesion but may go on to cause further major brain swelling in and around itself; for this reason necrotic contusions should be removed when exposed at operations. As a general rule, surface contusions larger than 1 to 2 cm in diameter should be removed.[24] Often a surface contusion 2 cm in diameter will extend several centimeters or more deep into the hemisphere, and the cortical edge of the contusion is only the "tip of the iceberg."[21]

Once the contusion is exposed it should be gently sucked out. The soft, friable, wet, purple-blue necrotic tissue can be easily aspirated. Suction should continue until a circumferential margin of healthy brain tissue is reached, as in debridement of a cerebral missile wound. One should not hesitate to aspirate *all* necrotic tissue, even in multiple sites, over the anterior temporal and frontal lobes.

Contusions over the more posterior-superior temporal lobe, or in the region of the central sulcus or the parietal or occipital lobes, should be evaluated carefully, and if they are clearly large necrotic contusions, they should also be removed following the same principles as used for the more common anterior contusions. Removing contusions in these areas will not increase the neurological deficit if one works entirely within the contusion, and ultimate postoperative neurological function may be surprisingly good even when contusions are removed from areas near the primary motor cortex and surface speech centers. The secondary brain edema that occurs around the contusions can be reduced by operative removal, and the postoperative clinical status and ultimate result improved.[24,138]

Traumatic intracerebral hematomas, in which the major component of the lesion is blood rather than mixed brain and blood, is

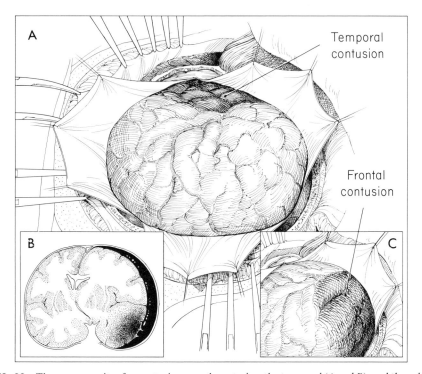

Figure 58–88 The common sites for contusions are the anterior, the temporal (*A* and *B*), and the subfrontal (*C*) regions. Frank contusions in these areas seen at operation should be removed to a margin of healthy brain tissue.

less common than contusion in closed head injury. Intracerebral hematomas tend to present deeper in brain tissue than contusions, but are still seen most commonly in frontal and temporal regions.[2] They may also appear directly on the cortical surface, and often the pathological characteristics are actually those of a combined hematoma and contusion. While pure hematomas also have a tendency to be associated with secondary circumferential brain edema, this is not nearly as marked as the edema that develops around the usual contusion. Hematomas should be dealt with in the same way as contusions. If they present on or near the surface and are greater than 1 to 2 cm in size, they should be aspirated. The deep intracerebral hematoma should be exposed and evacuated *only* if it is causing a major mass lesion effect with shift and with marked elevation of intracranial pressure, or if it is associated with neurological deterioration.[78]

ACUTE BRAIN SWELLING DURING OPERATION. Occasionally, sudden and rapid massive brain swelling will occur during an operation. The swelling may occur immediately after dural opening, or sometimes moments or even many minutes after a large clot or contusion has been excised and the brain has initially appeared to be relaxed. This brain swelling is probably the result of defective cerebral autoregulation. With the sudden decrease of extravascular pressure that occurs at dural opening or mass lesion evacuation, the cerebrovascular bed distends passively from the arterial blood pressure head, and a sizeable increase in cerebral blood volume results.[178] The other less common cause is from new acute intraoperative hemorrhage and the rapid accumulation of a clot contralateral to the craniotomy or in an ipsilateral area hidden from the operative exposure. True brain edema occurring as rapidly as this is only rarely the cause of such intraoperative swelling, and even then is probably associated with cerebral vasodilatation.

Intraoperative brain swelling must be dealt with promptly and aggressively. If it is caused by the more common cerebral vasodilation, the most effective short-term treatment is induced arterial hypotension.[29] Prompt reduction of systolic arterial blood pressure to 60 to 90 mm of mercury will almost always cause detumescence of the brain and return to its normal position. Simultaneously, the anesthesiologist should rapidly administer even more mannitol and increase the tidal volume to further lower the carbon dioxide tension. After two to four minutes the blood pressure should be allowed to seek its own level naturally again. Often, this combination of maneuvers will capture and reverse the acute swelling. The induced hypotension may have to be repeated until the mannitol further shrinks the brain or while autoregulation improves, but prolonged induced hypotension must be avoided or severe brain ischemia will ensue. Sodium nitroprusside should *not* be used to lower the blood pressure because this drug not only causes cerebral vasodilation but can directly disturb the integrity of cerebral autoregulation. Other agents such as trimethaphan (Arfonad) should be used for rapid induction of transient hypotension.[61] Recently the authors have noted that an intravenous bolus of thiopental (500 mg. in an adult) will often produce dramatic detumescence of the swollen brain and permit brain relocation.[21]

If the preceding maneuvers fail to relocate the brain within the skull, a frontal or temporal lobectomy may be necessary for internal decompression. An internal decompression by a frontal or temporal lobectomy should ordinarily be done only if one of these lobes shows some evidence of contusion or hemorrhage. All reasonable maneuvers should be considered to get the brain back into place to permit bone flap replacement.[60]

CLOSURE OF THE CRANIOTOMY FLAP. Complete closure of the dura and replacement of the bone flap should always be done, if possible, and may require a periosteal graft (Fig. 58–89). Dural closure is recommended because: (1) postoperative extradural bleeding is kept out of the subarachnoid space; (2) cortical adhesions to soft tissues are less likely; (3) cerebrospinal fluid wound leak or fistulae may be reduced; (4) any wound infection that may occur will more likely be isolated to the extradural space; and (5) dural closure, even with a graft, helps keep the brain from herniating through the craniectomy site across the bony edges (Fig. 58–90).

Unless brain swelling is massive and cannot be controlled, the bone flap should be replaced and fixed in place with non-

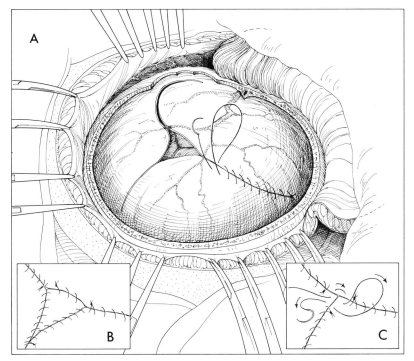

Figure 58–89 *A.* Complete closure of the dura, using a graft if necessary, is recommended for a number of reasons, the most important being that this will help keep the brain from herniating through the craniotomy site over bony edges. The bone flap is also replaced, if at all possible, and fixed in place with nonmetallic sutures. *B.* The graft. *C.* Detail of suture pattern.

metallic suture material so as not to interfere with postoperative CT scanning. Brain that herniates through a bony defect usually undergoes infarction and dies, and large craniectomies have not apparently reduced the mortality rate or morbidity.[56,60,176,279] In fact, this "herniated" brain that extends out over bony edges tends to develop progressively increasing edema that extends deep into white matter and may go on to in-

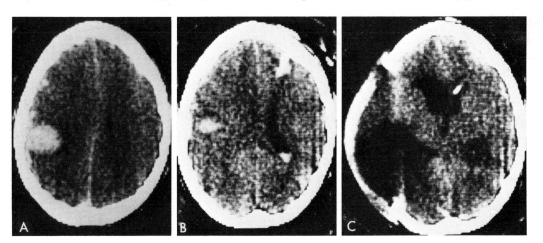

Figure 58–90 It is usually preferable after operation to keep the brain within the cranial vault and manage elevated intracranial pressure or brain swelling by medical means. *A.* The first of sequential scans of a patient with a traumatic intracerebral hematoma. *B.* He was treated with hyperventilation and barbiturates, but when these were stopped at seven days he developed severe intracranial hypertension, even as the lesion was becoming less dense. *C.* A craniotomy was performed, but the flap was not secured. Marked edema spread through the dominant hemisphere and is seen on a postoperative scan. (Courtesy of Dr. Lawrence Marshall, University of California, San Diego.)

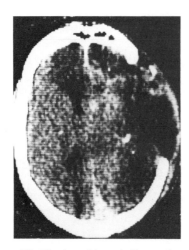

Figure 58–91 A problem similar to the one depicted in Figure 58–90. Here the bone flap was left out and the dura left open. Brain herniated over bony edges. Edema spread to involve most of the right hemisphere.

volve the entire hemisphere (Fig. 58–91). Brain swelling and elevated intracranial pressure in the postoperative period are best managed by medical means in the intensive care unit as described in the following section, and the bone flap should not be left out because the surgeon anticipates delayed brain swelling.[29]

Immediate Postoperative Care

The patient should not be extubated, but should be taken to the recovery room or intensive care unit and immediately connected to a volume respirator. This prevents early postanesthesia bucking and straining, and permits smooth continuation of controlled ventilation and total care of the helpless patient.

Intensive Care and Medical Management

General Principles

It is generally believed that high-quality intensive medical management will reduce mortality and morbidity after a major head injury.[25,190,218,302,357] This intuitively makes sense because a careful analysis of deaths in patients with head injuries who arrive at the hospital with neurological function reveals that about half die of general systemic medical complications, while the other half die from progressively increasing intracranial pressure that finally reaches blood pressure levels.[26] If medical problems such as pulmonary insufficiency, renal failure, hyperosmolar states, and progressively rising intracranial pressure are prevented or controlled, the number of deaths should be reduced and some reduction in morbidity should also be expected. A certain number of patients with only limited brain injuries consistent with good recovery die or are neurologically downgraded from a medical complication or elevated intracranial pressure. Quality intensive care may prevent or reverse these complications and improve morbidity and mortality rates.[25,216,218]

The overall goals of nonoperative care of the patient with head injury are: (1) to prevent or recognize early and treat systemic medical complications, (2) to maintain intracranial pressure in a safe range, (3) to anticipate and prevent additional brain insults from an abnormal physiological event such as hypoxemia or arterial hypotension, and (4) to maintain the patient in an environment that is physiologically and metabolically as normal or desirable as possible.

In order to accomplish these goals, patients should be carefully monitored in relation to their general neurological, physiological, and metabolic state, and managed with the aforementioned goals in mind.[124,361]

Monitoring in the Intensive Care Unit

There is nothing new about closely watching and evaluating patients with head injury in an intensive care environment. Careful and frequent neurological examinations have been performed for decades, along with serial studies of the patient's metabolic state.[44,212,226,302] However, the technological addition of electronic equipment that can continuously display physiological information has drawn new attention to patient monitoring. Additionally, the continuous monitoring of intracranial pressure, a critical parameter in brain injury, has further focused the neurosurgeon's attention on closer monitoring in the intensive care unit.[124]

Intensive care unit monitoring should serve the following two purposes: (1) it should provide continuous evaluation of the neurological status of the patient to define progressive recovery, deterioration, or a static condition, and thus to allow for timely and informed decisions regarding therapy, and (2) it should provide information that will permit the physician to recognize and correct abnormal physiological and metabolic states.[124,184,280]

NEUROLOGICAL MONITORING AND GENERAL GRAPHIC DISPLAY. Teasdale and Jennett have demonstrated the efficacy of a programmed neurological examination for patients with brain injury that can be performed repeatedly and reproducibly by nursing, medical, and paramedical personnel.[339] This examination can be used effectively to monitor the patient's neurological coma level continuously and includes eye opening, verbal response, and motor responses.

A clinical graph, which also includes a measure of voluntary motor strength, size and reactivity of the pupils, and a measure of oculocephalic reflexes, provides an excellent definition and graphic description of the patient's general neurological status (Fig. 58–92). A 24-hour record of the patient is thus available on one sheet. It provides a concise descriptive record of the patient's overall condition, and is useful for graphic display. The experienced clinician can glance at this record and obtain a clear picture of what the patient looked like neurologically at any given moment or judge the patient's progress over time.

The same side of the graphic neurological examination sheet shown in Figure 58–92 contains graphs or spaces for hourly recording of pulse rate, arterial blood pressure, intracranial pressure, body temperature, respiratory state and rate, and central venous pressure. The other side of the same sheet contains a record of the patient's 24-hour intake and output by 8-hour nursing shifts as well as space for the recording of special nursing treatments (Fig. 58–92B).

INTRACRANIAL PRESSURE MONITORING. The most accurate, reproducible, and simple methods employ a subarachnoid bolt or screw, or a ventricular catheter (Figs. 58–93 and 58–94).[30,207] In both these systems the pressure transducer is mounted outside the patient, preferably on a bedside pole with a manifold of stopcocks (Fig. 58–95). Mounting of the transducer in this way avoids patient movement artifact in recordings, and with the system so arranged, the transducer can be recalibrated, the line

flushed, and pressure-volume studies performed under sterile conditions without difficulty.

Both the subarachnoid hollow metal cannula and the ventricular catheter work on a fluid-coupled principle, the subarachnoid screw being filled with saline, and the ventricular catheter in direct communication with the ventricular cerebrospinal fluid. The fluid in the catheter or cannula is coupled directly to the pressure transducer sensor via fluid-filled extension tubing. Both will give accurate readings and yield a good waveform. If the waveform damps out, it usually means there is a leak somewhere in the connections of the system or at the pressure transducer dome, which permits tissue to enter and occlude the catheter or cannula. If the system is watertight, good waveforms can be achieved for days with little or no flushing with either system (Fig. 58–96).[30]

The ventricular catheter method is usually preferable because ventricular drainage can be used as one method for treating increases in intracranial pressure. When the ventricular catheter technique is employed, the catheter should be tunneled subcutaneously for several centimeters, and the duration of monitoring limited to four days at one site in order to minimize the likelihood of infection.[294] It may also be desirable to administer antistaphylococcal antibiotics prior to monitor insertion and for 6 to 12 hours following the procedure.

The subarachnoid cannula should be used when the ventricles are too small to cannulate or when the surgeon does not wish to transgress the brain. When using this method, it is important to *excise* the dura at the site of the twist drill hole and to be certain the system is totally leak-free (Fig. 58–97). Continuous monitoring here should also be limited to less than five days at one site.[30,294]

Epidural pressure monitoring may give readings that differ from intracranial cerebrospinal fluid pressure, and as the dura will quickly scar down over hours to a few days, the readings may become progressively more inaccurate.[22,197] The discrepancies seen between epidural and intradural recordings relate to technical difficulties with recording epidural pressure, because true epidural and intradural pressure should be close over the commonly seen pressure

Text continued on page 2042

VIRGINIA COMMONWEALTH UNIVERSITY
MEDICAL COLLEGE OF VIRGINIA HOSPITALS
Richmond, Virginia 23298

NEURO SCIENCE GRAPH

PATIENT IDENTIFICATION (PATIENT PLATE)

DATE		TIME	1 2 3 4 5 6 7 8 9 10 11 12 13 14 15 16 17 18 19 20 21 22 23 24	
RESPONSE LEVEL	Eyes Open	Spontaneously		C = Eyes closed by swelling
		To Speech		
		To Pain		
		None		
	Best Verbal Response	Oriented		T = Endotracheal tube or tracheostomy
		Confused		
		Words		
		Sounds		
		None		
	Best Motor Response	Obey Commands		Record Right (R) and Left (L) separately if there is a difference
		Localise Pain		B = Brisk
		Normal Flexor		S = Sluggish
		Abnormal Flexor		
		Extension to Pain		
		None		
PUPILS	Right	Size		+ Reacts
		Reaction		− No reaction
	Left	Size		
		Reaction		
O.C.R.		Right		4-Supp 2-Impair
		Left		3-Intact 1-None
LIMB MOVEMENT	Arms	Normal Power		Record Right (R) and Left (L) separately if there is a difference
		Moderate Weakness		
		Severe Weakness		
		Trace		
		None		
	Legs	Normal Power		
		Moderate Weakness		
		Severe Weakness		
		Trace		
		None		

Pupil Scale (mm): 1 2 3 4 5 6 7 8

BP ∨ ∧ : 240 230 220 210 200 190 180 170 160
Pulse ●—● : 150 140 130 120 110 100 90 80 70 60 50 40 30 20 10 0
ICP x—x : 40 30 20 10 0

Temperature ○—○ : 104 102 100 98 96

DRUGS	(M) Mannitol		RESPIRATIONS
	(P) Pavulon		(C) Controlled
	(O) Other		(A) Assisted
			(S) Spontaneous

A

Figure 58–92 *A.* A comprehensive 24-hour graphic monitoring sheet to be completed by the nursing service. From this sheet the experienced clinician can quickly gain a clear picture of the patient's neurological status and progress over time. O.C.R. oculocephalic reflex.

Illustration continued on opposite page

VIRGINIA COMMONWEALTH UNIVERSITY
MEDICAL COLLEGE OF VIRIGINIA HOSPITALS
RICHMOND, VIRGINIA 23298

PATIENT IDENTIFICATION (PATIENT PLATE)

INTAKE AND OUTPUT RECORD

FROM · · · · · 2200   TO · · · · · 2200

TIME	DESCRIPTION	INTAKE						OUTPUT					
		INTRAVENOUS			ORAL OR N.G.	8 HR. Totals	URINE			N.G.	Stool		8 HR. Totals
				Blood Prod.			VOL.	S.G.					
2300													
2400													
0100													
0200													
0300													
0400													
0500													
0600													
	8 HOUR TOTALS												
0700													
0800													
0900													
1000													
1100													
1200													
1300													
1400													
	8 HOUR TOTALS												
1500													
1600													
1700													
1800													
1900													
2000													
2100													
2200													
	8 HOUR TOTALS												
	24 HOUR TOTALS												

TREATMENT RECORD

INITIALS
7-3   3-11 11-7

DESCRIPTION	TIMES COMPLETED	WEIGHT	

B

Figure 58–92 (*continued*)   *B.* The other side of the clinical graphic sheet contains a matching 24-hour record of intake and output and space for recording special nursing treatments.

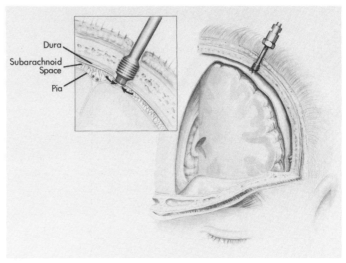

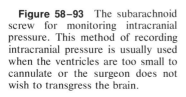

Figure 58–93 The subarachnoid screw for monitoring intracranial pressure. This method of recording intracranial pressure is usually used when the ventricles are too small to cannulate or the surgeon does not wish to transgress the brain.

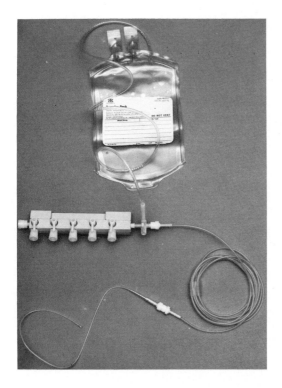

Figure 58–94 A complete ventricular monitoring and drainage unit, exclusive of the pressure transducer. An infant feeding tube serves as a satisfactory ventricular catheter. The catheter should be tunneled several centimeters in the hope of minimizing infection.

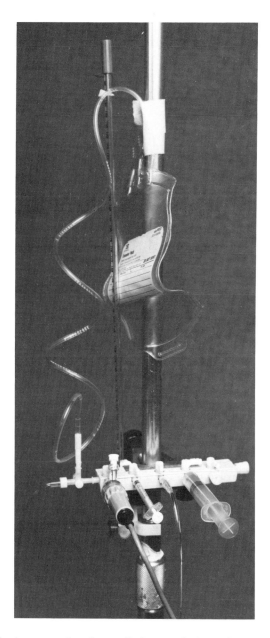

Figure 58–95 The monitoring system functions well when attached to an intravenous pole at the bedside. The manifold of stopcocks holds the pressure transducer, a saline-filled syringe for flushing the system, a drainage bag for ventricular drainage, and a catheter for calibration of the transducer. The manifold is placed at the level of the foramen of Monro and adjusted as the patient's head level is changed.

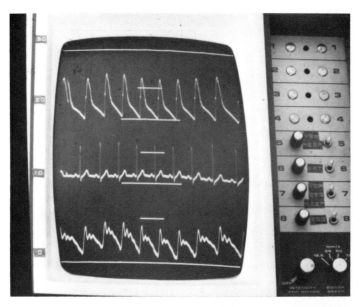

Figure 58–96 The monitoring system should be watertight and leak-free. This is especially important when the subarachnoid screw is being used because leaks can allow the cannula to become occluded. If the system is watertight, isovolumetric recordings will provide good waveforms, as seen in the bottom trace, with little or no flushing. In this figure the upper trace is the arterial blood pressure and the middle trace the intracranial pressure.

range. With meticulous technique and defined methods, accurate epidural pressure readings can be obtained for a limited time.[197] Epidural recording is certainly safer than intradural recording, but techni-

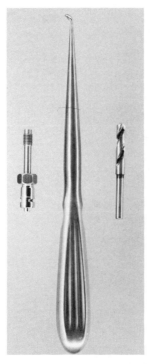

Figure 58–97 When the subarachnoid screw is used to monitor the intracranial pressure, it is important to *excise* the dura at the site of the twist drill hole. After the dura is incised with a pointed no. 11 blade, a curved curet, as shown here, is inserted through the incision, and the dura is curetted out.

cal improvements are needed before wide application can be recommended.

OTHER MONITORING PARAMETERS. Other parameters to be monitored at intervals, the frequency of which will depend on the patient's specific condition, include hemoglobin and hematocrit levels, white blood counts, arterial blood gases, serum electrolytes, and other pertinent metabolic measurements. Modern monitoring may also include serial CT scans and evoked potential studies. An arterial indwelling catheter can be used to monitor arterial blood pressure continuously and to obtain blood samples for blood gas and other measurements. The dorsal pedal artery is convenient and safe, with the radial artery being an alternative site. A mini heparin infusion via the transducer will keep the system patent, and this method can usually be used for three to five days.[124,226,340] If the patient has an indwelling bladder catheter, urine specimens should be sent for bacterial culture at least twice a week. Similarly, tracheal aspirate obtained via endotracheal tube or tracheostomy should be cultured for bacteria two or three times a week during the acute period.[5]

Intensive Medical Management of the Patient With Head Injury

Patients with severe brain injuries who have not been operated on and postoperative patients who had intracranial masses should both be cared for according to a similar protocol involving management of ventilation, the cardiovascular system, intracranial pressure, and general metabolism.[357] It is generally best for patients who have not had operations and who are not following commands to be intubated in the emergency room before transfer to the nursing unit, and patients who have had an operation to be transferred directly to the nursing unit *without extubation.*[24]

STEROIDS. While corticosteroids have not been proved to be beneficial in head injury, most neurosurgeons use them in severe cases. This probably is appropriate for several reasons. Two recent studies suggest that very large doses of steroids reduce the mortality rate of severe head injury.[92,112] Arrest and reversal of delayed pericontusion edema in head injury with progressively rising intracranial pressure has been observed with very high steroid dosage.[21] Experimental cerebral edema induced by cold lesion is reduced with steroid administration.[205,206] There are no animal studies that satisfactorily support or militate against the case for steroids in acute mechanical trauma because the models used have not been satisfactory for the task. There appears to be *no* good evidence that the administration of steroids per se increases the incidence of acute gastrointestinal ulceration and hemorrhage.

ANTICONVULSANTS. The question concerning the administration of prophylactic anticonvulsants in head injury remains controversial.[153] Some prefer to give anticonvulsants in closed head injury only if delayed epilepsy clearly develops and do not administer anticonvulsants even for seizure activity occurring during the first week after injury.[282] Because early seizures are not uncommon and can cause secondary hypoxic brain insults and severe intracranial pressure elevation, the prompt administration of anticonvulsants has been recommended.[281]

It seems wise to begin all grade III patients on a standard anticonvulsant regimen of phenobarbital. Adults are given diphenylhydantoin in addition to phenobarbital, starting with a loading dose to achieve adequate anticonvulsant blood levels as soon as possible. Patients continue to take the drugs for at least one year. By using this regimen in nonpenetrating brain injury, both early and delayed seizure activity may be reduced; but there is no definite evidence for this concept.[5,21,281,282] The side effects from these drugs, even when they are used in combination, have been negligible compared with the protection this regimen may afford in reducing the occurrence of early and delayed seizures, either of which can have disastrous physical as well as socioeconomic effects. The usefulness of prophylactic anticonvulsants for grade II head injury patients is even less clear, but the same anticonvulsant therapy is favored for them as for grade III patients, patients with missile or stab wounds, and patients with depressed fractures requiring operation.[281] Controlled trials to assess the efficacy of prophylactic anticonvulsants are being conducted.[268] It is hoped that these studies will define specific indications for individual patients more precisely than is possible at present.

RESPIRATORY CARE. It is clear that careful and continued attention to the patient's ventilatory status is imperative. What is less clear is the ideal way to manage the patient's airway. The application of controlled ventilation has received strong support, and there is clinical evidence that prolonged controlled hyperventilation in patients with severe brain injuries gives favorable results.* The use of controlled ventilation is based on the principles that (1) sudden unexpected hypoxic events can be avoided, (2) an important treatment of pulmonary edema and the adult respiratory distress syndrome is positive-pressure ventilation, (3) controlled hyperventilation will help reduce elevated intracranial pressure by maintaining a low arterial carbon dioxide tension and a normal arterial oxygen tension.[27]

Prolonged controlled positive-pressure hyperventilation, when begun shortly after severe brain injury, does seem to reduce the incidence of secondary hypoxic brain insults, will reduce the incidence of progressive pulmonary insufficiency, and will reduce intracranial pressure from levels seen on admission.[29] Controlled ventilation is best done with a volume respirator initially set in adults at a slow rate of 12 per minute with a tidal volume varying between 750 and 1000 cc (15 cc per kilo-

---

* See references 66, 117, 118, 211, 295, 296.

gram of body weight). This slow rate and high tidal volume are desirable because they provide for adequate venous blood return to the heart, and also the large volume helps re-expand collapsed alveolae. Minute volume is adjusted to bring the Pa_{CO_2} into a range of 25 to 30 mm of mercury, and oxygen flow (FI_{O_2}) to maintain Pa_{O_2} above 70 mm of mercury. In order to "phase" the patient onto the ventilator, one may administer intramuscular chlorpromazine or intravenous morphine or both. Neuromuscular blocking agents such as pancuronium (Pavulon) can smooth ventilation, but their use interferes with the neurological examination. Ventilator control is usually continued until the patient begins following commands or his condition remains stable with a normal intracranial pressure for several days. While initial ventilation is via an endotracheal tube, if controlled ventilation is to be used after 72 hours, a tracheostomy should be performed. In practice, patients are usually maintained on this regimen for three or four days, but the regimen can be used successfully for as long as two to three weeks.[295,313]

Positive end-expiratory pressure (PEEP) added to the system may be helpful when pulmonary insufficiency is advanced and arterial oxygen values do not come to normal levels with standard positive-pressure ventilation. Used properly, positive end-expiratory pressure usually does not have an adverse effect on intracranial pressure. When it is to be used, however, and the intracranial pressure is above the normal range of 10 to 11 mm of mercury, the patient should be nursed in the 30-degree upright position. Positive end-expiratory pressure values in excess of 10 cm of water should be avoided.[101] Weaning patients from mechanical to spontaneous ventilation must be individualized for each patient, should be done by gradually increasing the dead space, and should be done only after demonstrating that vital capacity and alveolar to arterial oxygen tension gradients are adequate.[49,313]

The use of prolonged controlled mechanical ventilation requires that the medical, nursing, and allied health staff caring for the patient have a working knowledge of pulmonary physiology and pathophysiology. Because pulmonary care is so critical in severe head injury, this level of care and knowledge is appropriate in any modern intensive neurological-neurosurgical unit.

As a general rule, the patients are nursed initially in the supine position with the bed flat or elevated approximately 10 degrees. Even with the use of controlled positive-pressure ventilation, it is still important to turn the patient every one to two hours. Also, tracheal suction must be performed as necessary to keep the airway clear and to avoid the presence of loose exudate, which may be driven distally to the bronchi with the positive-pressure ventilator. Pulmonary physical therapy should begin promptly.

FLUID AND ELECTROLYTE ADMINISTRATION. Since virtually every therapeutic maneuver can potentially harm as well as help the patient, abnormal metabolic or physiological states should be avoided unless or until they are definitely shown to be beneficial.

A good example of the application of this principle of homeostasis relates to fluid balance. Generalized dehydration may reduce brain swelling and intracranial pressure in the patient with head injury, but this maneuver predisposes the patient to hypotension, intravascular clotting, and other metabolic abnormalities, all of which can cause serious harm. Normal serum electrolyte levels should be maintained, and potential or actual brain swelling should be managed by methods other than generalized systemic dehydration. While generalized dehydration is not recommended, the patient must not be overhydrated. Thus, patients are best slightly underhydrated initially, but the practice of administering only 25 to 50 ml of fluid per hour to adults should be avoided.

To be certain that patients are not overhydrated, fluid administration in patients with acute head injury should be started at three fourths of the usual maintenance volume in both adults and children. Intravenous fluid administration is therefore recommended for adults, a volume of 1500 to 1800 ml a day being administered in fluids nearly isosmotic with serum, usually as either 5 per cent dextrose in 0.25 per cent saline or 2.5 per cent dextrose in 0.45 per cent saline. Adult patients should initially receive approximately 75 ml per hour, and subsequently the volume and electrolyte make-up of the fluids are adjusted as necessary, following basic principles of fluid and electrolyte administration for traumatized patients. A central venous pressure line is desirable, and the pressure should be maintained at 2 to 5 cm of water. Urinary output via the indwelling bladder catheter should be approximately 30 ml per hour. A urinary output rate much more or less than this means either too much or too little fluid administration or that there is some other specific medical abnormality.

It is critical to avoid hyponatremia. Even if patients are inadvertently overhydrated, brain edema will usually not occur if the serum sodium is maintained in a normal range. If, however, the patient is overhydrated, and serum sodium falls below 130 mEq per liter, edema will likely develop in the region of the brain injury. Usually, the rapid development of hyponatremia is due to inappropriate secretion of antidiuretic hormone. This syndrome may occur as early as the second or third day after injury, and if any drop in serum sodium is observed, both urinary and serum osmolarities should be checked to determine whether there is inappropriate secretion of antidiuretic hormone. The treatment is fluid restriction and very slow administration of 5 per cent dextrose and normal saline. In severe situations, hypertonic intravenous saline may be required, and sometimes steroid hormones that cause sodium retention may be necessary for control.

There should be no great rush to convert the patient to nasogastric feeding, because of the danger of aspiration and the possibility of cryptic abdominal injury. If the patient still cannot eat after five days, feeding via nasogastric tube can usually begin at that point.

BODY TEMPERATURE. Temperature control is important. While hypothermia has had its proponents, its usefulness and the specific indications for its use in acute head injury remain to be clarified. Induced chronic hypothermia creates a host of new medical problems. What is clear, however, is that hyperthermia can be detrimental and can cause elevated intracranial pressure and increase brain and body metabolism, or can predispose to seizure activity. It is probably best to keep the patient in a normothermic range until and unless specific indications for hypothermia are defined. This can almost always be accomplished with the use of rectal acetaminophen or as-

pirin and a cooling blanket or mattress. If these measures do not bring the temperature down, the administration of chlorpromazine can help by abolishing the shivering response to the cooling blanket.[195]

OTHER GENERAL MEDICAL FACTORS. Patients in an intensive care unit who are being actively maintained at normothermia must also be carefully monitored for the possible development of infection. Intermittent, but regular, bacterial cultures should be obtained from urine and sputum as well as regular urinalyses and blood counts.[5,184] It must be recognized that a sudden drop in arterial blood pressure often means generalized septicemia with septic shock, which should be promptly treated with antibiotics, corticosteroids, and vasopressors or volume expanders or both as indicated.

The hemoglobin should be kept above 10 gm per 100 ml (hematocrit 30 per cent), as lower levels cause impaired oxygen carrying capacity of the blood, increased cerebral blood flow, and impaired wound healing. Transfusions should be given as required. The use of anticholinergics to decrease gastrointestinal bleeding has been recommended, as well as the administration of vitamin A (50,000 units per day) and antacids (Maalox, 30 ml every 2 to 4 hours).[143,354] While few major gastrointestinal hemorrhages are seen with this regimen, it is not clear that the use of Maalox and vitamin A is the sole reason for the low incidence of bleeding. Cimetidine has been shown to reduce acid secretion by gastric parietal cells significantly.[315] This drug is now being evaluated for its effectiveness in preventing gastrointestinal hemorrhage after head injury, and initially it shows promise in accomplishing reduction in bleeding.

Elevated Intracranial Pressure in Head Injury

Before describing the specific therapeutic maneuvers recommended for treating elevated intracranial pressure, two questions concerning the significance of intracranial pressure levels in head injury must be addressed:

Does intracranial pressure monitoring warn the physician of impending neurological deterioration? The answer to this question is a definite yes, but the time interval between the beginning of serious progressive elevation of pressure and clear-cut neurological deterioration may be quite short, sometimes only a matter of minutes. At other times, progressively elevating intracranial pressure may begin an hour or more before neurological deterioration is seen. If neurological deterioration is noted in the absence of a medical complication or very advanced age, the intracranial pressure will usually be quite high and increasing. This association between high intracranial pressure and neurological deterioration is important for two reasons. First, if progressively rising intracranial pressure is recognized and aborted, then secondary neurological deterioration may be prevented. Second, when patients are restless or agitated, and controlled ventilation or nursing care requires sedation or paralyzing agents, the intracranial pressure can be used to monitor, indirectly, the stability of the neurological status. If the intracranial pressure begins to rise while the patient is paralyzed, this must be considered a perilous situation that demands prompt further evaluation to define the cause and determine therapy.[27,163,164]

What level of intracranial pressure is dangerous in the patient with head injury? Another way to state this question is to ask, at what level of intracranial pressure should specific measures be made to reduce it? Careful observation of the pressure in relation to neurological deterioration in head injury dictates that levels in the range of 25 to 30 mm of mercury should be treated and lowered.[21] In addition, any progressive elevation of pressure, if associated with neurological deterioration, should be treated.

Several clinical observations and principles form the basis for these recommendations: In acute head injury, it is common to see neurological deterioration follow elevations in pressure to levels of 25 to 30 mm of mercury even the absence of brain shift. While patients with brain tumors or benign intracranial hypertension may tolerate intracranial pressure as high as 60 to 70 mm of mercury, such tolerance of high pressure is almost never the case with the acutely injured brain. Moderate intracranial pressure elevations are particularly critical in the patient who has bilateral decerebrate posturing but reactive pupils. In this situation any

neurological deterioration may bring the patient close to brain death. Such patients have been observed to go suddenly from this state to motor flaccidity associated with unreactive pupils when the intracranial pressure reached levels of 30 to 40 mm of mercury. But even patients who are restless without focal motor weakness may show neurological deterioration with pressure rises to levels as low as 20 mm of mercury.[21] Why the injured brain tolerates elevations in intracranial pressure so poorly is not known, but it may be that associated vasospasm, increased cerebrovascular resistance, and impaired autoregulation predispose the injured brain to ischemia when the cerebral perfusion pressure is reduced even by small amounts.

To maintain intracranial pressure at levels below 25 mm of mecury makes good sense if one considers the following points: Normal intracranial pressure is in the range of 5 to 10 mm of mercury. For the pressure to be elevated into seriously abnormal ranges of 15 to 20 mm of mercury, a sizeable increase in intracranial volume is required, as demonstrated by the pressure-volume curve. Actually the first portion of the pressure-volume curve is not flat, but is concave upward.[315] By the time pressures of 20 mm of mercury are recorded in man, much of the buffering capacity has probably been taken up, and if there is no focal mass lesion, this high pressure implies a rather extensive diffuse brain injury with new added intracranial volume. By the time pressures reach levels of 25 or 30 mm of mercury, the amount of new intracranial volume (edema fluid, clotted blood, cerebrospinal fluid, intravascular blood) is no doubt quite large, and in the acutely damaged brain, the elevated pressures are associated with extensive abnormalities.[241] In summary, elevations of intracranial pressure to levels above 20 mm of mercury are probably associated with extensive (but not necessarily irreversible) brain damage, and from a functional standpoint the extensively injured brain has a poor tolerance for pressure levels of 25 to 30 mm of mercury and higher.[28,91]

MANAGEMENT OF ELEVATED INTRACRANIAL PRESSURE IN HEAD INJURY. Early diagnosis and removal of operable mass lesions, and intensive medical management with controlled ventilation will reduce the incidence of seriously elevated intracranial pressure in head injury.[26] Still, the problem exists and indeed 30 per cent of patients with diffuse brain injury, and 50 per cent of postoperative patients will have intracranial pressure above 20 mm of mercury sometime during their early hospital course.[97,208,243]

When intracranial pressure begins to increase, the first step is to be sure there is no positional or systemic medical reason (temperature elevation, electrolyte imbalance) for the elevation. If a CT scan or radiographic contrast study has not recently been done, one should be obtained to rule out development of a new mass lesion. If there is no systemic medical reason for rising intracranial pressure and a new mass lesion has been ruled out, specific measures to control or reduce the pressure should be undertaken. The maneuvers that can accomplish this, in order of safety and the order in which their use is recommended, are (1) increased hyperventilation, (2) ventricular drainage against a positive pressure head, and (3) intermittent administration of mannitol. Other techniques that may be considered if these are not adequate include induced barbiturate coma with or without hypothermia, temporary (less than five minutes) induced hypotension, and the administration of extra-large doses of corticosteroids.[24]

Increased hyperventilation will occasionally reduce the intracranial pressure and control it even when the Pa_{CO_2} had already been reduced to 25 to 30 mm of mercury.[104] This can be accomplished rapidly by manually ventilating the patient with an Ambu bag or by slightly increasing both the tidal volume and the rate (i.e., increase the rate by two to four more breaths per minute, and increase the tidal volume by about 2 cc per kilogram). It has been shown, experimentally, that cerebral vessels still remain sensitive to carbon dioxide alterations after days of hypocarbia, and can constrict further in response to new lower levels of Pa_{CO_2}.[179]

If the pressure remains elevated, then ventricular drainage against a pressure head of 10 to 15 mm of mercury will often adequately control the intracranial pressure. It is critical to use this overflow level of 10 to 15 mm of mercury, for if the ventricle is drained to a pressure level below 5 mm of mercury, the ventricles may collapse, occluding the catheter. In this event, the ability both to drain the ventricle and to record the pressure is lost. The overflow system can be set up so as to still permit intermittent monitoring of the intracranial pressure.[358] Increased hyperventilation and ventricular drainage, along with early evacuation of operable masses and good medical care, will often control seriously rising intracranial pressure.

Mannitol is added to the regimen only if increased ventilation and cerebrospinal fluid ventricular drainage fail to control the pressure. This is because a single bolus of mannitol will usually control the pressure for no more than three to four hours, and then repeated boluses of mannitol are required. While this therapy can clearly be effective in controlling intracranial pressure, and can result in excellent long-term neurological outcomes, the prolonged use of mannitol is difficult at best, and is potentially dangerous. Used properly, however, mannitol can be quite effective at this stage, and may obviate the need for other radical and heroic measures. Two principles should be considered when using mannitol. First, mannitol works by increasing serum osmolarity and thereby drawing water out of the brain. The higher the serum osmolarity, the more the brain will be dehydrated. Second, the osmotic agents draw water off that part of the brain that is only minimally damaged or not injured. Edema fluid in damaged brain is probably little reduced in volume, and there is probably no effect on directly contused brain. Thus, the more extensive the brain injury, and the less normal brain that remains, the more mannitol and higher serum osmolarity will be required to remove enough brain water to lower the intracranial pressure.[23]

Long-term intermittent or continuous administration of mannitol should be accompanied by continuous intracranial pressure monitoring, along with frequent checks of serum osmolarity and serum electrolyte determinations every four hours. The patient should not be permitted to become systemically dehydrated (only the brain is to be dehydrated), and the relatively greater brain dehydration can be accomplished because of the blood-brain barrier. Therefore intravenous fluid volume should replace, milliliter for milliliter, the urine output, and the electrolyte concentration in the intravenous fluid should be adjusted according to the serum electrolyte levels. While urine from an osmotic diuresis is very low in electrolytes, both sodium and potassium are still being depleted in small amounts by the diuresis and must be replaced.

Ordinarily, one should begin with a bolus of mannitol at a dose of 1 gm per kilogram given rapidly. Lower dosages have been recommended, but since the goal is to reduce intracranial pressure quickly, this is best done by adequately raising the serum osmolarity rapidly and to a significant degree.[216] A single bolus of 1 gm per kilogram of body weight will usually raise the osmolarity by 8 to 10 mOsm per liter. If this dose is inadequate to reduce the intracranial pressure sufficiently, a second bolus should be given. If 2 gm per kilogram is inadequate, then mannitol alone will usually not suffice, and other measures may be necessary. This is unusual, for the intracranial pressure can almost always be reduced, at least temporarily, if enough mannitol is used.[21]

After the intracranial pressure is initially brought to a satisfactory range with mannitol, it is probably best to use intermittent doses based on levels of pressure. If brain damage is not very extensive, repeated bolus doses may be needed only every six or eight hours. When there is more extensive edema or contusion, mannitol may be needed every three or four hours. In any event, serum osmolarity should not be left above 325 mOsm per liter for longer than several hours, for at these levels serious complications develop.[23] Serum osmolarity can usually be maintained in ranges of 310 to 320 mOsm per liter for up to seven days without serious side effects. But with higher levels of serum osmolarity for longer periods, there is a high incidence of systemic acidosis and renal failure. In either of these situations the mannitol must be stopped, and intracranial pressure usually will soar. Thus, the mannitol should be used only as often as necessary, in an amount only large enough to control intracranial pressure, and the patient should be weaned from it as soon as feasible.

When brief use of mannitol is inadequate, Shapiro and co-workers have reported success in using barbiturate coma, sometimes combined with hypothermia, to control intracranial pressure.[306,307] Marshall,

Smith, and Shapiro have also reported some very good long-term results in their patients, and their work substantiates the usefulness of aggressive control of rising intracranial pressure.[218]

Finally, transient reduction of arterial blood pressure can quickly capture a rising intracranial pressure and, combined with mannitol, may occasionally salvage the situation in which brain swelling is occurring rapidly and in a malignant fashion. Induced hypotension must be used with caution, and when mean arterial pressure is lowered to 60 mm of mercury, it should not be kept down for longer than two to three minutes because of the already impaired cerebral perfusion pressure.

TREATMENT OF BRAIN EDEMA VERSUS VASCULAR BRAIN SWELLING. When the intracranial pressure is elevated, and hydrocephalus and hematomas have been treated and are accounted for, the cause will be either brain edema, vascular dilatation, or a combination of both. At the present time, remedies for elevated intracranial pressure are not usually used to manage the specific abnormality, but rather to bring down the pressure in any way that is feasible. This fact is mentioned here because it could be more expeditious to treat the offending element directly. For example, increased hyperventilation or transient hypotension, or both, could be effective for diffuse cerebral hyperemia, and large doses of steroids or dehydrating agents better for edema. As diagnostic tools and techniques improve, and therapeutic modalities expand, treatment can proceed in a more specific direction. The Philadelphia head injury research group has already begun to use this approach, having demonstrated hyperventilation as effective in controlling intracranial pressure in some patients who show increased cerebral blood flow in association with their elevated intracranial pressure.[104]

Localized Injuries to the Skull and Brain

A spectrum of injuries is described here, the common theme of which is that the injuring force is applied over a relatively small area of the skull, resulting in inward fracturing of the skull and, if the force-to-area ratio is sufficiently high, in laceration of the scalp, tearing of the dura, and penetration of the brain. Thus, such injuries range from closed depressed skull fracture through perforating injuries or stab wounds of the skull to missile injuries of the head, the most extreme of which is a through-and-through injury with both entrance and exit wounds. All these injuries present particular though related problems of diagnosis and management, which are discussed as a continuum in this section.

Depressed Fractures of the Skull

A skull fracture is defined as depressed if the outer table of one or more of the fractured segments lies below the level of the inner table of the surrounding intact skull (Fig. 58–98).[242] Often the depression is not appreciated on the standard series of plain skull x-rays, and if a depressed fracture is suspected from the appearance of double density or a circular fracture, then tangential views should be obtained in the appropriate area so that the true extent of the depression can be gauged.

As with fractures elsewhere in the body, the principal subdivision of depressed frac-

tures is into closed and compound varieties. Estimates of the proportions of closed depressed fractures to compound ones range from 50 per cent to 10 per cent, though closed fractures are in the minority in most reported series.[199,242] This definition hinges on the presence or absence of a scalp laceration in the vicinity of the fracture, but, properly, closed depressed fractures that involve the paranasal sinuses should be regarded as compound also.

Regardless of whether a depressed fracture is closed or compound, the dura mater underlying the fracture may be intact or lacerated and the underlying brain may be intact, contused, or lacerated. This is a consequence of the configuration of the bone fragments and the depth to which they have been impressed at the time of injury. It is important to state that the position of the fragments on x-ray represents the current end point; the fragments may actually have penetrated much more deeply at the point of impact and then ''bounced'' back. This factor has important implications for two commonly held concepts in the management of depressed fracture of the skull,

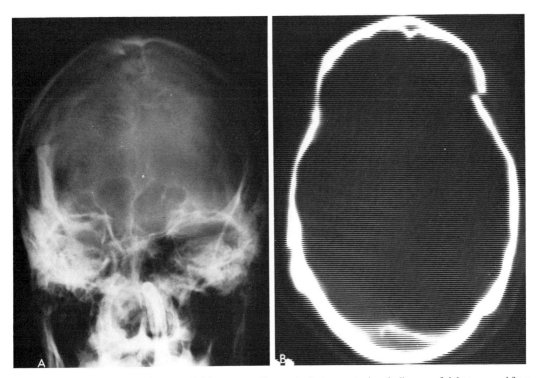

Figure 58–98 Depressed fracture of right temporal bone. *A*. Anteroposterior skull x-ray of right temporal fracture. *B*. CT scan of right temporal fracture. Fracture is depressed more than the thickness of the skull, and elevation should be considered.

namely that the pressure of the indriven bone fragments may be responsible for focal neurological deficits and for the formation of an epileptogenic focus. From this belief it would follow that elevation of bone fragments would be indicated to alleviate neurological deficit and to prevent post-traumatic epilepsy. It follows from the argument concerning the end point of the depression of fragments, however, that if cortical damage has occurred, it is likely to have been produced at the moment of impact and not by later compression. This is borne out by the observation that removal or elevation of depressed fracture fragments does not result in a rapid improvement of neurological deficit, nor does this procedure influence the rate of occurrence of post-traumatic epilepsy.[153]

Since the alteration of neurological deficit and the prevention of post-traumatic epilepsy are indications for operative treatment, the prime indications vary in cases of closed and compound depressed fracture and are therefore discussed separately. The actual operative procedure is, however, so much the same for both that it is described in a single section.

Closed Depressed Fractures of the Skull.

The most common variety of closed depressed skull fracture is the "pond" or "ping-pong ball" type of indentation seen in very young children. This type of fracture in the growing skull is analogous to the "greenstick" fracture in long bones and appears as a dent in the skull. In this variety of fracture, dural tearing is uncommon; but in older patients, closed depressed fractures may be associated with sharp indriven edges of bone that are sufficient to tear dura and lacerate the underlying brain and even a sizeable blood vessel to produce a hematoma.

The first and most common indication for operative treatment is cosmetic. If a forehead fracture is depressed 3 to 4 mm, and certainly if the outer table of the fracture fragment is depressed below the level of the inner table of the skull, a significant deformity may result. In patients with an exceptionally thin scalp, lesser degrees of depression may be unsightly. The location of the fracture, e.g., orbital rim, may be so critical that, with very little displacement, a

major cosmetic defect may be produced. Over 50 per cent of all depressed fractures are frontal, so this is a frequent consideration.[199,248] In the first two or three days after injury, the extent of the bony depression cannot be judged by inspection or palpation because of the scalp swelling. Depressed fractures below the hairline are most likely to be elevated, but large depressions elsewhere may be so disturbing to the patient's body image that elevation may be requested by the patient or family. In such a situation, however, the risks and benefits should be very carefully explained.

Other indications for elevating closed depressed fractures include a radiological appearance of the fracture such that dural tearing is suspected. In such cases there may be a growing fracture, and dural repair may be advised on that account. As stated, the concepts of fracture elevation as a means of alleviating a mass effect, of improving neurological deficit, and of preventing epilepsy are not based on strong evidence. If the fracture is associated with progressive neurological deficit or progressing impairment of consciousness so that an intracranial hematoma is suspected, however, operation is indicated.

In elevating closed depressed skull fractures, there is one technique that is confined to closed fractures in very young children. In such cases, in which the dura is so often intact, it may be permissible to elevate the fracture through a small scalp incision, a burr hole at the edge of the depression, and upward leverage on the depressed area with a periosteal elevator introduced under the fracture site. This, however, is one of those operative techniques that are often easier to describe in print than to apply in practice. The indented fracture may be extremely resistant to reduction, and the dura may be torn so that the instrument is inadvertently thrust onto the pial surface. Thus, the surgeon must always be prepared to convert the procedure to the more conventional exposure and elevation of the fracture as described later.

Compound Depressed Fractures of the Skull

The principal concern with this type of injury is that contaminated material may have been introduced through the wound into the cranial cavity and, if the dura is torn, into the brain at the time of injury. With the passage of time between injury and closure of the wound, bacterial infection of the cranial cavity can occur.[157] The primary emphasis in management of such cases is on establishing the diagnosis as soon as possible so that appropriate operative treatment can be arranged. Several obstacles to the provision of such care may arise. A quarter of patients with depressed skull fracture have never been unconscious, and another quarter have post-traumatic amnesia of less than one hour; thus, unless the fracture is suspected and discovered, the patient may never be admitted to the hospital at all.[153,158] Because of the mobility of the scalp, the laceration may be at some distance from the fracture site and not detected during suture of the skin wound. Because many of these patients are under the influence of alcohol or otherwise uncooperative when first seen, it may be difficult to obtain good quality skull x-rays, so the fracture may be missed. In this way, the stage is set for a delay between injury and repair of the lesion. For these reasons, the infection rate in large reported series of civilian depressed fractures varies between 5 and 10 per cent, a less than optimal figure when compared with the figures achieved under conditions of modern warfare.[38,157]

The other factor that makes early recognition of a depressed skull fracture so important is that associated intracranial hematomas may develop in more than 5 per cent of cases, most of them being intracerebral in location.[38,242] Again, there is the danger that a patient who has never been unconscious will be allowed to leave the hospital with the depressed fracture undiagnosed, only to return when the signs of cerebral compression are manifest.

The overwhelming indication for operative treatment in compound depressed fracture is the prevention of infection by removal of contaminated tissue and foreign material and the exclusion of external infection.[246] Repair of dural laceration and excision of contused necrotic brain and hematoma are other considerations, and restoration of the bony defect is a matter that may be dealt with at the primary operation or as a secondary procedure, according to the circumstances. If these principles are adhered to, the problems of persistent neurological deficit and post-traumatic epilepsy

are thereby reduced, since infection and hematoma complicating depressed fracture are significant factors in increasing the incidence of both adverse sequelae.[157,158,242]

Operative Technique for Depressed Fractures

SCALP INCISIONS. When the scalp is intact over a depressed fracture requiring elevation, the normal indication for operation is cosmetic and the skin incision should also be cosmetically acceptable, i.e., behind the hairline if possible. The elevation of even a simple fracture may become an exercise in frustration if the skin incision is poorly planned. The incision must allow enough exposure of the fractured area to facilitate access to the periphery of the fracture and should be large enough to obtain pericranium for dural grafting or to enlarge the bony defect by craniectomy should dural opening and an intracranial procedure become necessary. The incision should allow for enlargement in the event of unexpected findings. Likewise, draping and skin preparation should take account of potential enlargement of the wound. In the planning stage, it is wise to remember that the fracture is often more fragmented and extensive, particularly at the inner table, than suggested by the x-ray or external inspection.

Two types of scalp incisions are generally useful in *closed* depressed fractures. One is a linear incision or some variant, specifically the curvilinear or S incision, the other a fully developed flap. Linear incisions can be accomplished quickly and with little blood loss. They interfere little with normal blood supply of the scalp and heal easily. They are readily extended should more exposure be required. A theoretical disadvantage is that the suture line will be directly over the area of fracture, but in practice this does not interfere with proper wound healing. A straight incision will often not offer sufficient exposure, and an S curve will be superior. The center of the S should be centered over the fracture.

The second type of incision recommended for closed fractures is the horseshoe flap and its variants. It must be planned with greater care than the linear incision, since it is not readily enlarged; to enlarge this incision usually will require a T arm, which then may interfere with healing.

The flap has the advantage of placing the line of incision at the periphery of the fracture and requires less retraction to maintain

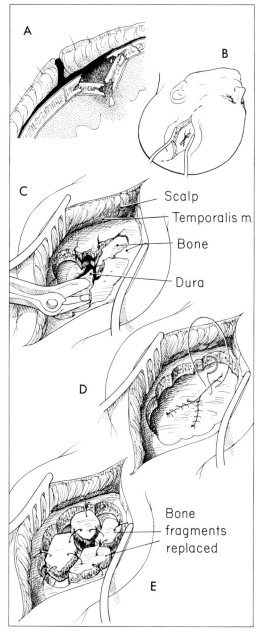

Figure 58–99 Treatment of the compound depressed fracture of the skull. *A*. Type of compound depressed fracture requiring elevation. *B*. Removal of devitalized scalp by splitting incision to create an elipse that includes the margins of the wound. *C*. Removal of impacted bone by burr hole to locate and identify the normal dura, followed by resection of bone fragments. *D*. Watertight closure of the dura following brain debridement. *E*. Replacement and fixation (by silk suture) of bone fragments.

exposure, but it requires somewhat more time to develop and to close than linear incisions.

When a closed depressed fracture complicates blunt mechanical head injury and there is evidence of an operable mass, the fracture should never be approached directly. The basic "trauma flap" presented earlier in this chapter should be used and the fracture dealt with through this incision. This approach will allow proper treatment of both the fracture and the concomitants of blunt head injury.

In *compound* depressed fractures, the wounds are often dirty or contaminated. Indriven skin, hair, or foreign debris can be wedged in between the depressed bone fragments, even when the external appearance of the wound seems relatively clean. Thus, simple irrigation and superficial debridement in the emergency room is inadequate therapy.[59]

Compound fractures may require that contused, lacerated, devitalized scalp be debrided. An S, or curvilinear, incision is usually most applicable here (Fig. 58–99). The incision is split into an ellipse that includes the margins of the wound to be excised. The excision of lacerated, contaminated tissue should extend to the pericranium, and specimens from this block of tissue should be cultured for pathogenic bacteria.

Occasionally, the area of avulsed or devitalized scalp is so large as to preclude closure of the wound. When this occurs, the principles elaborated in the chapter on the management of scalp lacerations are applied, and provisions made for the rotation of flaps and grafting. It is desirable to cover the area of fracture (with or without replaced bone fragments) with a full thickness of scalp.

If the fragments are firmly impacted, a burr hole should be placed at the margin of the fracture to permit identification of normal dura, then rapid separation of the fragments by resection of small amounts of bone becomes possible, as shown in Figure 58–99.

All depressed fractures are comminuted. If the skin incision has been well planned, the area of depression should be well exposed, including a wide margin (2 to 3 cm) of normal calvarium. Pericranium should be preserved, if possible, and placed over the fragments of bone at closure.

Only when the comminuted fragments are completely loose should they be pulled from the wound directly. They should never be levered out in such a way that the hemisphere is compressed or other fragments are pushed deeper into the wound, since the edge of an inner table fragment may be razor sharp.

Preliminary burr holes are mandatory when a fracture overlying a dural venous sinus is to be elevated. These should always be approached with the assumption that the fragments have lacerated the sinus and are tamponading hemorrhage. Burr holes are placed so the area of the sinus can be quickly exposed for control of hemorrhage. The bony exposures may take the form of a free flap cut by craniotomy or craniectomy (working from the periphery toward the center).

The depressed fragments should be left undisturbed until the surgeon has obtained exposure adequate to deal with a lacerated sinus, the scrub nurse has proper instruments ready, and the anesthetist is ready to administer transfusions and alter the angle of the table should massive hemorrhage occur. The technique of dural venous sinus repair is discussed later.

Once dura is visualized, fragment removal becomes easier, and rongeurs or punches may be used to separate impacted fragments quickly and lift them atraumatically from the wound. Bone removal should continue until the surgeon is certain that the dura is intact or the full extent of the dural laceration has been seen. The sharp edges of inner table fragments may produce dural tears at one side of the fracture site. If the fracture extends into a paranasal air sinus, the mucous membrane should be stripped and the ostium plugged with the rolled up membrane and a muscle patch. In compound fractures, complete removal of all foreign material (such as hair, gravel, cartridge wadding, or cloth) and contaminated or devitalized tissue is fundamental.

If, after removal of the bone fragments, the dura is intact but tense, it should be opened and the brain inspected. Nadell and Kline reported that 40 per cent of depressed fractures with intact dura were accompanied by underlying cortical damage requiring debridement.[248] Any hematoma and pulped brain should be removed, and bleeding points should be controlled.

LACERATIONS AND CONTUSIONS OF THE BRAIN. Cerebral laceration is present in 85 per cent of cases in which dural laceration has occurred and, depending on the nature of the wounding instrument, may be much more extensive than the degree of bony disruption.[81,248] The principles described in the section on missile injury are equally applicable here.

DURAL REPAIR. Although some schools of neurosurgical teaching do not insist on complete dural closure at this stage in the repair of a depressed skull fracture, dural closure is strongly recommended. The enormous Korean and Vietnam wartime experience with penetrating cranial metallic fragment and missile wounds attended by a low incidence of postoperative infection, cerebrospinal fluid leakage, or brain herniation attests in part to the value of watertight dural repair in which pericranial or fascial grafts are used where necessary.[135,231] Such closure must follow meticulous debridement and hemostasis, however.

REPLACEMENT OF BONE FRAGMENTS AND CRANIOPLASTY. For many years, after Macewen had demonstrated its feasibility in 1888, it was acceptable practice to replace bone fragments only in cases of closed depressed fracture.[210] Recently, Jennett and Miller, and Braakman reported no increase in postoperative infection after bone fragment replacement, even in cases in which the dura had been torn and up to 24 hours had elapsed after injury.[37,157] In these series there was a slightly higher incidence of postoperative infection in those patients in whom bone was left out, related possibly to the greater contamination of the wound in those cases.

With less than a 5 per cent infection rate even when cases with dural laceration are included, it seems wiser to replace bone fragments at the first operation than to risk the possible complications of a second cranioplasty procedure.[242] If more than 24 hours has elapsed between injury and operation, if the wound is quite dirty, or if there is suspicion of infection already being present, all bone fragments should be left out, and cranioplasty should be performed three or more months later.

Early cranioplasty using acrylic or tantalum at the time of primary operation has not proved successful, carrying a high incidence of wound infection. The infection rate may, however, be the result of using this procedure in situations in which the risk of infection is higher, particularly highly comminuted frontal fractures involving the paranasal air sinuses.[157] In these areas, autologous bone grafts may be preferable.

Anticonvulsant Therapy

The decision to institute prophylactic anticonvulsant therapy should be based on information concerning the risk of post-traumatic epilepsy in the individual patient. Fortunately, this information, based on a study of 1000 patients by Jennett and co-workers, is available for patients with depressed skull fracture.[158] Although the overall incidence of late (persisting) post-traumatic epilepsy was 15 per cent, this ranged from less than 4 per cent in patients with post-traumatic amnesia of less than 24 hours, no early epilepsy, and intact dura to over 60 per cent in patients who had the combination of longer post-traumatic amnesia, early epilepsy, and lacerated dura.[153] Therefore, it is possible to make a decision to prescribe anticonvulsants when calculated risk exceeds a certain level. It would

seem prudent at least to recommend therapy in patients with dural laceration, since this does correspond to a risk of epilepsy of more than 20 per cent, as does the presence of early epilepsy (one or more seizures in the first week) and post-traumatic amnesia of longer than 24 hours.[158]

Perforating (Stab) Wounds of the Skull and Brain

All these wounds are compound, and the dura mater is virtually always torn and the underlying brain lacerated (Fig. 58–100). Because of the localized nature of the injury, most patients remain conscious or have been only briefly unconscious.[79] All the factors mentioned in relation to the operative management of compound depressed skull fracture apply to these patients also. There are, however, some additional considerations in perforating wounds that concern cryptic wound entry sites via the orbit or nose, penetration by radiolucent objects, and the problems produced by the protruding instrument of wounding.

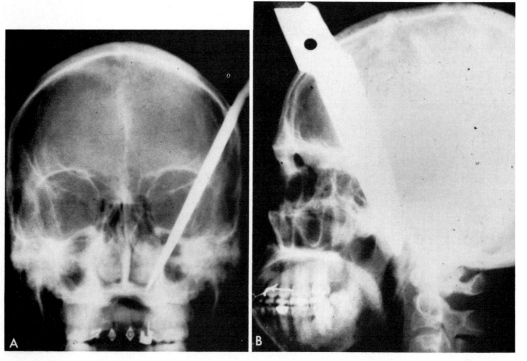

Figure 58–100   Skull x-rays of perforating stab wound of the brain. A scissors blade was driven into the left hemisphere (by hand). The patient had a minimal fifth cranial nerve deficit preoperatively. He made a nearly complete recovery after removal of the blade via craniotomy. *A*. Anteroposterior view. *B*. Lateral view.

All neurosurgeons should be aware of the possibility of penetration of the cranial cavity by sharp objects that enter the eye or the nose.[129] The thin floor of the anterior cranial fossa is easily breached, and subsequent orbital swelling may totally obscure the wound of entry so that the correct diagnosis hinges on a good history and a high index of suspicion. Dujovny and associates pointed out that firm pointed objects may easily penetrate the skull and dura in children because of the thinness of the incompletely ossified skull.[88] Miller and co-workers reviewed 42 cases of intracranial penetration by retained wooden foreign bodies, which revealed a 74 per cent morbidity rate and death in 25 per cent of 28 cases occurring in the postantibiotic era.[240]

The cardinal principle in dealing with skull and brain injuries in which the wounding instrument is still protruding from the skull is that no attempt should be made to pull it out until the surgeon has investigated and is prepared for all the possible consequences, mainly the production of massive hemorrhage. This entails obtaining excellent skull x-rays and performing cerebral angiography if the foreign body looks as though it might involve a major vessel; e.g., carotid artery. In the operating room some ingenuity in preparation and draping may be required. The skin incision and preliminary bone work should be completed prior to withdrawing the penetrating instrument if it is thought likely to have entered a dural venous sinus or major artery. In this way, the bone flap can be turned with the minimum of delay, the dura opened, and the wound track in the brain exposed.[79]

Missile Injuries of the Skull and Brain

Although most of the literature of gunshot wounds of the head derives from the experience of warfare, civilian gunshot wounds are common, the result of domestic or sporting accidents, suicide attempts, and criminal assaults. In conditions of warfare, missile wounds are subdivided into low-velocity injuries due to fragments of grenades, mines, and other explosive debris and high-velocity injuries due to bullets, many of which are of extremely high velocity (2000 feet per second). Civilian missile wounds are usually caused by bullets of varying caliber, fired from a wide assortment of weapons ranging from handguns and shotguns to high-powered rifles fired from close or long range.[136]

Just as in closed blunt head injury and in depressed skull fracture, hypoxemia, hemorrhage, intracranial hypertension, brain shift, and infection may all dramatically influence the outcome from the primary brain injury. There is, however, much more variation in the extent of primary wounding, which depends on the type of weapon and the size, shape, velocity, and trajectory of the missile and the way in which it makes contact with the skull. The brain lesion caused by the missile may be compounded by further brain damage produced by the inward passage of multiple bone fragments (Fig. 58–101). In high-velocity missile wounds, the initial entry wound in the skull may be small, but the skull may shatter from within, beginning along suture lines, as a result of the radial movement of brain tissue during transient cavity formation in the brain created by the tremendous force

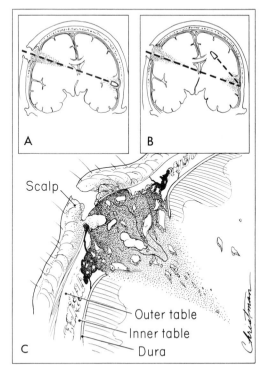

Figure 58–101 Schematic drawing of gunshot missile wound. The brain injury may be complicated by inward passage of bone fragments and intracranial ricochet of the missile. *A*. Initial bullet track. *B*. Ricochet of bullet within brain. *C*. Bone fragments carried into brain.

that has been delivered into the cranial cavity. Such wounds are invariably fatal. With missiles of lower velocity, brain damage may still be extremely severe if the bullet is caused to tumble by its initial contact within the skull, or if it fails to exit and ricochets to another site in the brain. In the past, this process had to be inferred from plain x-rays, but now the track of the bullet in the brain usually is visible on the CT scan, and if an intracranial hematoma is present, this too can be clearly seen.

Bullet wounds are more deadly than those caused by shell fragments. With the development of guns that deliver high-speed missiles, the effect of penetration upon the nervous system became devastating. Guns with muzzle velocity of 2000 or more feet per second kill almost instantly.[135] The higher the velocity, the greater the transmission of energy per unit of time and the larger the transient cavitation, with damage not only along the path of the missile but in areas adjacent to the path as the missile transverses a closed system such as head and skull. With high-velocity wounds, there is added injury and death as a result of sudden sharp increase in intracranial pressure to more than 3000 mm of mercury from the temporary cavity about the missile, which may be 50 or more times as large as the missile. This cavity is formed by the radial motion imparted by the missile, through creation of oscillating positive and negative pressure along the path of the missile. The cavity formation causes compression and stretching of the tissues adjacent to and remote from the missile path. The high intracranial pressure generated by the cavitation in a closed system such as the skull may cause failure of respiratory and cardiac centers in the medulla, resulting in death.[50]

In an experimental model of cerebral missile injury in rhesus monkeys, Crockard and co-workers suggested that the missile produces direct brain stem damage, the extent of which can be related to the wounding energy.[67,68] This group of investigators found that following the initial transient rise and fall of intracranial pressure due to passage of the missile, there was a major increase in intracranial pressure and reduction of arterial pressure and cerebral perfusion pressure, with reduced cerebral blood flow. Death of the animal was most closely related to the combination of these three factors, though cerebral metabolic rates for oxygen and glucose were also reduced. In earlier experiments on monkeys, Gerber and Moody measured intracranial pressure; blood pressure; carotid flow; blood gases; respiratory rate, depth, and volume; and electroencephalograms following missile injury of the head. The most important single parameter that correlated with death was a drop in carotid flow. Since they had seen the same correlation in epidural compression experiments, they hypothesized that reduced cerebral blood flow, as measured by carotid flow, was a common factor in death from craniocerebral missile injuries and epidural compression injuries.[105]

The importance of missile velocity for outcome is pointed out in Hammon's report on a series of military casualties in which gunshot wounds were associated with a 22.73 per cent operative mortality rate, and fragment wounds with a 7.64 per cent mortality rate. Of United States soldiers who did not have an operation, three times as high a percentage died of gunshot wounds (46.56 per cent) as died from fragment wounds (15.1 per cent).[135] Civilian penetrating wounds are generally from lower-velocity missiles than are military wounds and are associated with less tissue damage than occurs during warfare, but nevertheless are associated with a high mortality rate: 40 per cent and 55 per cent in two series.[277,362]

The majority of knowledge concerning the changes in mortality and morbidity rates associated with missile injuries comes from experience with head injuries during wartime. A mortality rate of 73.9 per cent in 898 cases of head wounds was reported in the Crimean War.[228] In the American Civil War, 71.7 per cent in a series of 704 cases of penetrating head wounds were fatal.[230] The development of antiseptic, then aseptic, techniques in surgery was associated with an improved prognosis for patients with penetrating head injuries. During World War I, the mortality rate was reduced from 54.5 per cent to 28.8 per cent, mainly through the efforts of Cushing, who introduced the technique of debridement and closure of open wounds.[71,72] Earlier definitive treatment plus the introduction of chemotherapy and antibiotics contributed to lowering the mortality rate to 14 per cent in World War II and then to 9.6 per cent and 9.4 per cent in the Korean and Vietnam Wars, respectively.[135,151,221,231]

The basic principles of debridement of the scalp wound; removal of hematoma, all pulped brain, and indriven devitalized bone fragments; watertight dural closure; and anatomical galeal and scalp closure without tension have been successfully applied to mass casualties. Employment of rapid evacuation systems and early definitive treatment have been instrumental in lowering mortality rates by reducing infection or the opportunity for large intracranial hematomas to develop. These same principles should be employed in civilian cases of penetrating missile wounds.

Time from Penetrating Injury to Treatment

In order to prevent infection and the development of large intracerebral hematoma, treatment should be undertaken as soon as possible. In World War II and in previous wars, the time to definitive treatment often ranged from 30 hours to eight days, which allowed for deep infection to develop in the missile tract.[15] Soldiers frequently remained in areas of potential contamination for extended periods of time before rescue. During World War II, it became increasingly clear that rapid evacuation for earlier definitive treatment was essential to improve results. Only in the Korean and Vietnam conflicts was rapid evacuation of the wounded regularly achieved so that casualties were operated on usually within two hours of wounding.[52] The evacuation system and method for providing emergency care in Vietnam was an outstanding accomplishment, but as a result, more of those with the most severe head injuries were admitted to the evacuation hospital just in time to die. Also, patients who were in extremely critical condition and who would have died early if not transported so quickly were now being operated upon. Even with these more severe injuries included, the initial in-hospital mortality rate for brain operations was close to 9 per cent, attesting to the improved medical and surgical care that was achieved.[135] In civilian practice, the wounded usually arrive at the hospital promptly and can be operated on within

two hours of wounding, before deep infection occurs. At this stage, deep bone and metal fragments will not have become contaminated and may not need to be removed.[52]

In a study of civilian gunshot wounds, Raimondi and Samuelson showed that a significant worsening of the patient's neurological status and a greater likelihood of death occur with delays in definitive treatment. In their series of 150 consecutive civilian missile wounds to the cranium, progressive respiratory depression was noted to be associated with delay of treatment.[277] Early definitive treatment decreases the chance for intracerebral hematoma and edema to develop and further compress adjacent brain, much as occurs in the area around a contusion in closed head injury. Statistics from the Korean conflict have shown a 10 per cent incidence of intracerebral hematoma in early treatable cases of missile wounds versus a 41 per cent incidence in delayed cases.[20] Thus, the evidence is strong that these hematomas should be located and removed as rapidly as possible. Though most of these hematomas will be located in the missile tract, a few will be distant from the tract or in the ventricles. In these cases, a CT scan is helpful in defining the missile tract and any occult hematomas (Fig. 58–102).

Infection

Routine use of antibiotics has become an integral part of modern treatment of penetrating craniocerebral wounds. In the absence of obvious cerebrospinal fluid fistula, proper operative technique and antibiotics have practically eleminated meningitis as a major factor causing morbidity and death. Brain abscess is the primary infection problem that remains. Brain abscess development is clearly related to the presence of retained devitalized tissue, especially bone fragments, following operation. The reports of military neurosurgeons have shown convincing statistical proof of a relationship between brain abscess and retained devitalized bone fragments. Martin and Campbell found infection to be 10 times as frequent around bone fragments as in their absence in World War II casualties.[220] Hagan reported on 506 consecutive patients evacuated from Vietnam with particular refer-

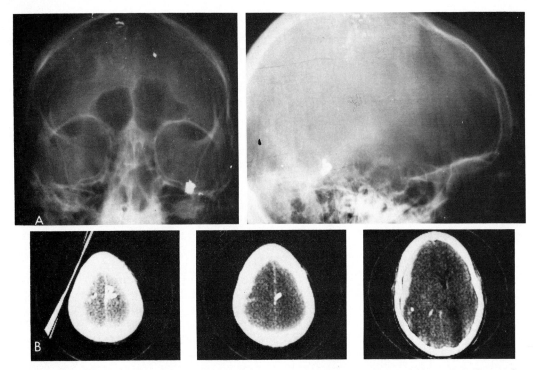

Figure 58–102 *A*. Skull x-rays showing the missile entry wound to the right of midline and the largest fragment resting in the contralateral middle fossa. *B*. The CT scan of the same patient. On the left is shown the entry site of the missile to the right of midline. In the middle scan damage from passage of the missile through midline structures can be seen. On the right the scan shows a contralateral fragment with a subdural hematoma caused by vessel laceration associated with ricochet of the fragment.

ence to early complications.[131] In that series, cultures of the bone fragments from 56.4 per cent of 68 patients who underwent reoperation early (5 to 54 days after injury) for retained bone were positive, even though these patients had been receiving antibiotics preoperatively for an average of two weeks. Hagan pointed out that a retained bone fragment is evidence of incomplete brain debridement. Based on this kind of evidence, the accepted military practice is to re-explore every wound with a retained bone fragment in order to effect its removal, and this policy was vigorously carried out during the Vietnam conflict. The basic principle followed was that all accessible bone fragments be removed at a primary operation, and any accessible bone fragment visible on postoperative x-rays be removed by immediate reoperation.

In civilian practice, the isolated deep or inaccessible bone fragment need not necessarily be removed. In removing it, the patient's neurological condition could be worsened, and since the missile tract becomes contaminated from the surface inward, if the primary operation is performed within two hours of wounding, a deep fragment should not be contaminated. Meirowsky has suggested that in such situations it may be desirable for the patient to accept the possibility of late infection rather than undergo extensive or repeated operation in neurologically hazardous areas of the brain.[232] This concept is further supported by the clinical bacteriological study of Carey and associates, which revealed that only 45 per cent of patients treated within a few hours of being wounded had contaminated indriven bone in cerebral missile tracts. They estimated that up to 75 per cent of all indriven bone chips were sterile.[52] Sukoff and co-workers reported on 70 consecutive cases of penetrating craniocerebral trauma from Vietnam. No complications developed after 12 months of observation in six cases in which retained bone was left in situ. These authors noted that reoperation for retained bone fragment was not without complications and prolonged search was often necessary and often unrewarding. They advocated careful consideration of neurological status, location of the fragments, and their accessibility before undertaking re-exploration.[327]

The experimental work by Pitlyk and coworkers in dogs suggested that an isolated bone fragment peripheral to the main missile tract may be left in place, as such carries little risk, but clusters of retained bone fragments point to potential areas of contamination by skin and hair that justify re-exploration.[271] In clinical practice, clusters of retained bone, as seen in postoperative x-rays, are especially indicative of poor debridement of missile tracts that may well lead to eventual deep infection. These clusters must be removed.

It is commonly held that retained metallic missiles or fragments may have less potential for infection than other debris, since the metal is sterilized when fired and the metal usually tracks deeper, dissociating itself from indriven contaminating material. The metal itself may not always be sterile, however, and it may initiate a granulomatous reaction in the brain.[262] Drew and Fager as well as Maltby have reported late cases of brain abscess developing around a retained metal body.[86,213] They pointed out that an acute abscess is more likely to develop around bone, while a late abscess is most often secondary to retained metal. In Hagan's series of Vietnam War casualties, all the metallic fragments cultured revealed microbial growth.[131] In addition, the metal fragment may be associated with a hematoma, and the fragments may migrate, causing further brain injury.[152,262] Raimondi and Samuelson pointed out that the low-velocity injury of civilian wounds, being less damaging to cerebral tissue, reduced the necessity for total metal fragment removal. They reported no infection in 25 patients with retained metal fragments.[273] Their data would also support the concept of removing only readily accessible metal fragments.

Metals, when embedded in cerebral tissue, can produce various reactions. Most missiles encountered in war have a high ferrous content, whereas most civilian gunshot injuries are produced by predominantly lead missiles. Shotgun wounds generally involve "chilled" or hardened lead shot, whereas most .22-caliber bullets are copper-plated missiles. Lead, if sterile, can be expected to produce only a minimal reaction if retained within the brain, but copper-plated missiles produce a sterile abscess or granuloma and should be removed early after injury.[262,310]

Management of Patients with Craniocerebral Penetrating Wounds

The patient with a penetrating wound of the brain will have brain damage from the missile wound path, the lateral energy forces that have been transmitted to the brain, the intracranial "explosive" forces, and the changes in intracranial pressure. As in closed head injury, multiple pathological processes occur simultaneously. The concepts of primary and secondary brain injury discussed in detail earlier are no less true here. Except for the specifics of surgical care, all the principles of emergency medical care described under closed head injury are to be applied in penetrating wounds. General cardiopulmonary and medical treatment as well as management of intracranial pressure and preanesthetic and anesthetic principles are no different, and urgency and clarity in treatment maneuvers require the same diligence and attention to detail. An important point to remember is that gunshot wounds are often multiple, and the entire body must be thoroughly inspected for entry and exit wounds and appropriate x-rays must be taken. Once the patient's cardiovascular status is stabilized, attention to the specifics of managing missile wounds proceeds.

INDICATIONS FOR OPERATION. Patients with penetrating craniocerebral injuries should receive the same basic neurological examination as those with closed head injuries, and the degree of head injury should be graded in accordance with the same principles. Save for those classified as grade IV, patients should be prepared for immediate operative treatment of the penetrating wound. Patients with no pupillary reflexes, absence of oculocephalic reflexes, and no somatic reflexes of any kind, as often seen in self-inflicted gunshot wounds, should not receive immediate operations, as such patients are at the point of death. Patients with less severe injuries may make a striking clinical recovery, and all should receive urgent operative attention (Fig. 58–103).[177,321]

INITIAL EVALUATION AND DIAGNOSIS. The head should be completely shaved, and

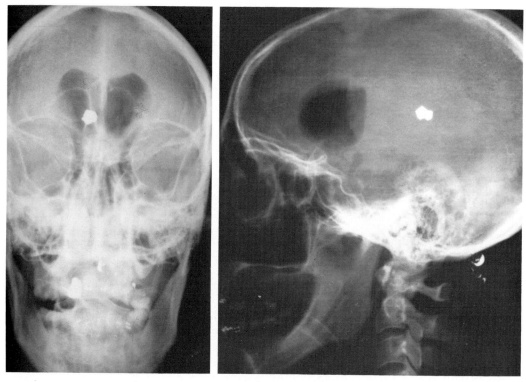

Figure 58–103 Ventriculogram of a patient in deep coma. Acute hydrocephalus appeared within one hour after penetrating missile wound in the suboccipital skull. The patient improved with ventricular drainage prior to debridement.

the entry site and any exit site inspected. If the weapon was fired at close range, the former may show powder burns. The latter will be the larger wound, often with brain visible through the scalp edges. Any scalp bleeding should be controlled by ligature, suture, or coagulation so as not to interfere with subsequent x-rays or CT studies. Clean, sterile dressings should be applied and good quality skull x-rays obtained. Stereo-lateral views are helpful. These x-rays reveal the location and number of bone fragments that should be removed as well as the metal fragment or fragments that should be removed. The number and location of the fragments should be carefully noted to aid in the subsequent debridement. The CT scan has proved especially useful, defining both intracerebral and extracerebral hematomas and bone and metal fragments and often the missile trajectory (Fig. 58–104). Computed tomography rather

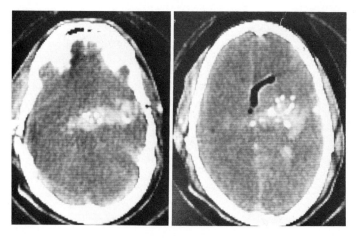

Figure 58–104 CT scan of a patient with a penetrating intracranial missile injury. The trajectory of the missile, showing the tract and indriven bone extending from entry site on right to midline, is defined. Debridement to the midline was necessary to remove the deep bone fragments.

than arteriography is the emergency procedure of choice, as it defines hematoma formation and also the path of any ricocheted bullet, further aiding in performance of the operation. In cases in which the missile track is in the vicinity of a major vessel, however, angiography also should be done if time permits.[136]

PREOPERATIVE TREATMENT. Because of the great hazard of infection in the potentially contaminated wound, antibiotics should be administered promptly in large intravenous doses. Penicillin and chloramphenicol were the most commonly used antibiotics for this problem during the Vietnam conflict.[135] This is still a useful combination in nonallergic patients, but if the drugs are changed, one should keep in mind that broad coverage as well as anti-staphylococcal antibiotic coverage is desirable. The antibiotics should be given during the operation and for five days after it. Corticosteroids are also administered in large doses for the same reasons they are used in closed head injury. There is no evidence that steroid use will increase the likelihood of later intracranial infection. Because epilepsy occurs with 30 per cent of penetrating brain wounds, anticonvulsive therapy is recommended. Mannitol (1 gm per kilogram of body weight) should be administered preoperatively to patients with major missile penetration associated with possible hematomas or brain swelling. This treatment will help reduce dangerously high levels of intracranial pressure, which are often present prior to debridement and hematoma evacuation.

POSITIONING AND DRAPING. Positioning the head is important. There must be no vascular or respiratory obstruction. Observation of the wound or wounds may show progressive brain herniation if intracranial pressure is increased by the induction and maintenance of improper anesthesia or by inadequate ventilation. Access to both the entry site and the exit site, if the latter exists, must be provided. Often the metal fragment to be removed will rest near the opposite inner table or distant from the entry site, and this should be taken into consideration. The necessity for any rotation flaps or plastic procedure should be defined and marked after the sterile preparation. Proper draping should allow for extension of the scalp incisions. Thus, maximum mobility of the head and a wide operative field usually is desirable. Rarely the entry site or the exit wound will be extremely large, and a fascia lata graft may be needed. In this case the thigh area should be prepared for operation as well.

SCALP INCISION. Since the scalp has limited elasticity, a generous curvilinear incision will best distribute tension over a wide area. The entry site should be excised as an ellipse, removing all devitalized and avascular scalp to healthy bleeding scalp edges. Usually, a wide en bloc excision is not necessary. For legal purposes, areas of powder burn that are excised should be sent to the pathological laboratory, and the observed degree of burn should be described in the operation report.

The elliptical opening is enlarged in curvilinear or S-shaped fashion, along the line of any linear fracture, as seen on x-ray. The dermis is usually least damaged; beneath it the fibro-fatty layer may be missing over a larger area, and damage may extend well beyond the torn surface. Such damage to tissue is recognized by infiltration with dark blood and failure to bleed when cut. In such wounds, it may be necessary to sacrifice some intact skin so that the edges of the final wound will be vertical and not beveled inward. The incision direction should allow the craniectomy to be made along the fracture line where the dura may be lacerated. Tripod incisions, though giving concurrent and rapid exposure, may not heal well and should be avoided. Narrow-base scalp flaps with inadequate blood supply must also be avoided, but a semicircular scalp flap is preferred when a craniotomy is to be performed (Fig. 58–105A). The entry site should be centered in the middle of the scalp flap. If temporalis or suboccipital muscle is involved, an especially wide removal of the damaged tissue must be done to prevent further muscle necrosis, which can serve as a nidus for infection. The operation should not proceed until the scalp debridement and opening are completed. All contaminated instruments used on the scalp incision should then be removed from the operative field.

CRANIECTOMY OR CRANIOTOMY. The fractured bone containing the entry site can be removed by circumferential craniectomy with a rongeur after a nearby burr hole opening (Fig. 58–105B). This can be safely done by forming a small craniectomy away from the entry site, then proceeding in a circular fashion over intact dura, staying 2 to 3 cm away from the entry site. The craniec-

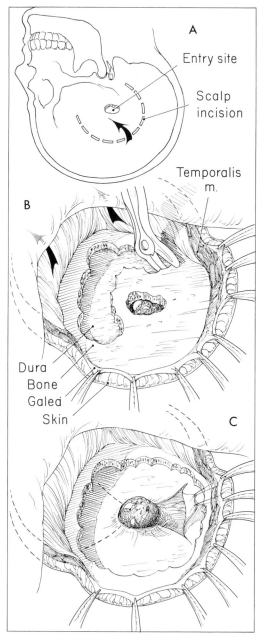

Figure 58–105 Treatment of the penetrating missile wound. *A.* The scalp flap is designed to allow a craniectomy or craniotomy with the entry site in center. Alternatively, an S-shaped incision excising the entry site can be used. *B.* Craniectomy begins away from penetration site, over normal dura, then proceeds toward penetration site. *C.* Minimal dural debridement at penetration site and stellate opening of dura.

tomy should provide for removal of all comminuted bone fragments and be wide enough for adequate exposure and visualization of all damaged dura and contused and necrotic brain. In most civilian wounds, the craniectomy will be about 5 by 5 cm in size. This excised bone is usually discarded. Craniotomy is an alternative to craniectomy, but because of potential bone contamination, is not performed in war casualties. For the civilian patient, craniotomy may be used to avoid a later cranioplasty procedure if the wound is treated early and proper antibiotics are given. Two to four burr holes can be placed 2 to 3 cm from the entry site, and a craniotomy can be performed. Once the bone is removed, the missile entry site in the bone should be drilled or rongeured back to clean bone.

When the bone removal has been completed, the dural defect will expose a conglomerate of pulped brain, blood clot, and bone fragments occupying the hole in the dura, often forming a firm plug. The dura mater should be minimally debrided at the entry site, opened in stellate fashion, beginning at the penetration site, and then retracted by stay sutures (Fig. 58–105*C*).

BRAIN DEBRIDEMENT. This portion is the most vital aspect of the operation. The cortex is inspected, and limits of cortical damage are noted. The pulped brain will usually be tense and herniating slightly. Any hematoma and pent-up debris at or near the cortical surface can be easily removed by gentle suction. Brain resection is begun in a circumferential fashion by using bipolar coagulation and cutting the arachnoid and surface vessels just beyond any obvious devitalized tissue. The removal of brain tissue to the depth of the missile tract and outward to intact surrounding white matter usually insures removal of the indriven bone fragments, pulped brain, and hematoma. The removal of necrotic brain should proceed with a small sucker, No. 8 French suction tip (1.75 mm inside diameter), so as to save, count, and culture the bone chips and compare the number obtained with the number seen on x-ray. The excision should proceed to a depth that allows removal of all bone fragments and ultimately reaches normal brain, but deep midline structures should not be invaded or removed in a blind search for bone fragments (Fig. 58–106*A* and *B*).

If the missile has traversed deep midline structures, one must be careful to debride only within the missile tract. Careful and gentle debridement can be performed here with little if any additional damage to the brain as long as the suction tip does not leave the necrotic tract. When the missile has entered a ventricle, the ventricle should be entered, and debris and hematoma should be removed. Metal fragments that are easily accessible should be removed at the primary operation, but a separate craniotomy may need to be done, as one should not follow a missile tract deep across the brain hoping to grasp or retrieve a piece of metal. Operating loupes giving magnification are helpful, and proper lighting is a necessity for inspecting the tract for bone fragments. Many military neurosurgeons advocate finger palpation of the incision for bone fragments, though small fragments may be missed by this maneuver and it is not recommended.[135] The walls of an adequately debrided missile tract do not collapse. If the debrided missile tract collapses or brain continues to herniate or present as the so-called "closing missile tract," either more pulped brain needs debridement or there is a space-occupying mass, usually a hematoma, distal to the area of debridement. When debridement is adequate, the brain will be pulsating and relaxed away from the dura, and the bleeding will easily cease along the lines of the cortical resection.

DURAL CLOSURE. The dural closure should be watertight. Data accumulated during World War II and the Korean War, when series of patients were treated with and without dural closure, strongly suggested that primary watertight closure of the dura is of the utmost importance if the centripetal infection is to be prevented. Furthermore, careful dural closure aids in preventing cerebrospinal fluid fistulae, which may lead to breakdown of wounds and secondary meningitis. Late cranioplasty is facilitated by good dural closure, as it allows a satisfactory plane of cleavage. Also, by re-establishing a normal anatomical relationship, it may be possible to reduce cortical meningeal scar formation and, potentially, reduce the likelihood of posttraumatic epilepsy.[351]

The graft required for the entry site is usually small, and a quarter-sized piece of

temporal fascia, pericranium, occipital fascia, or galea will often suffice (Fig. 58–106C). For the exit site, a large piece of fascia lata may be necessary. A true watertight closure can be obtained by meticulous placement of the sutures and by testing the graft by injecting saline just prior to place-

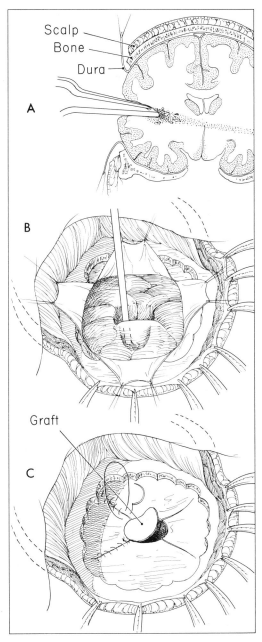

Figure 58–106 *A* and *B*. Brain debridement, beginning at the boundary of normal and damaged brain, proceeding inward, and removing all necrotic brain, devitalized bone, and debris. *C*. The watertight dural closure with a graft.

ment of the last one or two sutures. Artificial dural substitutes should not be used, and cranioplasty should be delayed for a secondary operation until 6 to 12 months have elapsed in order to reduce the risk of infection. The scalp should be closed in an anatomical two-layer fashion.

THE EXIT WOUND AND THE CONTRALATERAL MISSILE FRAGMENT. The exit wound should be managed in a fashion similar to the management of the entrance wound, though often the dural and scalp closure requirements are more complex because of the "blow-out" nature of the exit injury. There will usually be fewer bone fragments for removal at the exit site, as they are carried outward and may often be embedded extradurally in the scalp. Principles of brain debridement remain the same. While the exit site may be grossly larger then the entry site, the lacerated tissue is often healthier than at the entry site, because the energy forces transmitted by the missile are less on the distal side.

An intracranially embedded metal fragment or bullet that is contralateral to the entry site presents a special problem. If it is easily accessible, if it is large, or if it is copper or copper-coated, one should remove the metal fragment at the primary operation. Small pieces of metal deep in the brain and sealed off from the more superficial debris of the entry site need not be removed. Large intact bullets tend to migrate and

should be removed (Fig. 58–107). Late abscess or early or late hematoma formation about the metal will, of course, necessitate its removal.

Special Penetrating Craniocerebral Missile Wounds

There are four types of wounds whose management involves special considerations; tangential missile wounds, air sinus or orbital-facial wounds, intraventricular wounds, and vascular sinus wounds with intracranial penetration.

Tangential Head Wounds

The tangential head wound is caused by a missile grazing the head. It deserves special attention because the forces generated at the point of impact cause more brain damage than the course of the missile per se, which has not entered the brain.[3,71,81,146] In tangential head wounds, the missile, which may be of either moderate or high velocity, strikes the skull at an angle too acute for penetration. The missile ricochets off the skull and may or may not remain in the scalp. The forces generated by the impact may injure not only the scalp but also the skull, dura, and the underlying brain. High-velocity missiles cause much greater damage than do moderate-velocity fragments. Some of the most extensive scalp injuries

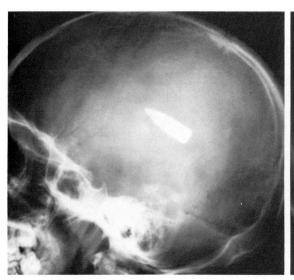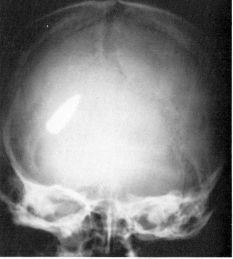

Figure 58–107 Skull x-ray of patient with a spent large bullet in the brain. This large missile should be removed.

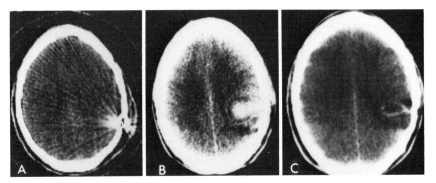

Figure 58–108 CT scan of a patient with a tangential missile wound. *A*. The scan immediately following the injury. It shows a small right parietal depressed fracture with a metal fragment in the scalp. *B*. Computed tomography one month after the injury and bone debridement without durotomy. At this time the patient had papilledema. The scan shows an intracerebral hematoma. *C*. The CT scan two months after injury showing resolution of the contusion. The papilledema also resolved.

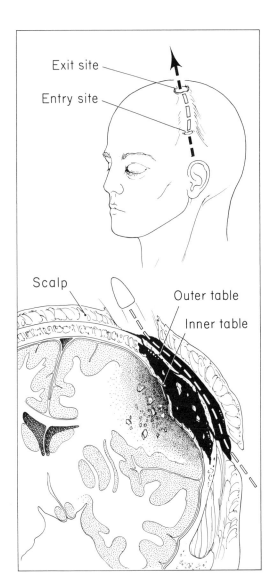

Figure 58–109 The tangential missile wound. Damage to bone and brain may be far greater than suggested from superficial inspection.

are due to this type of wound, and rotated scalp flaps may be required for reapproximation.

Several factors may contribute to the brain injury: brain contusion from the shock of the missile impact, penetration of bone for variable distances into the brain, intra- or extra-axial intracranial hemorrhage, and finally the possibility of secondary pressure effects from expanding blood clots or brain swelling (Fig. 58–108).

A linear fracture may occur at the site of impact, but more often there is a comminuted depressed fracture at the impact site. The outer skull may spring back into normal position while the inner table remains fragmented and depressed. The external wound can appear deceptively benign while there may actually be bone fragments deep in the brain (Fig. 58–109).

The treatment consists of thorough de-

bridement of scalp and brain wound as in other head injuries. A craniectomy or craniotomy will be necessary, and the dura should be opened and the brain inspected even though there is no evidence of dural lacerations. When the brain has been contused and pulped, one should resect nonfunctioning necrotic brain, leaving clean edges. A simple brain laceration with little contusion need not be removed. Watertight dural closure with grafting is also essential here.

Orbital-Facial-Cranial Penetrating Wounds

Penetrating craniocerebral wounds secondary to missiles or foreign bodies entering through the face, maxillary sinus, orbital area, or frontal sinus should be regarded as a greater potential source of in-

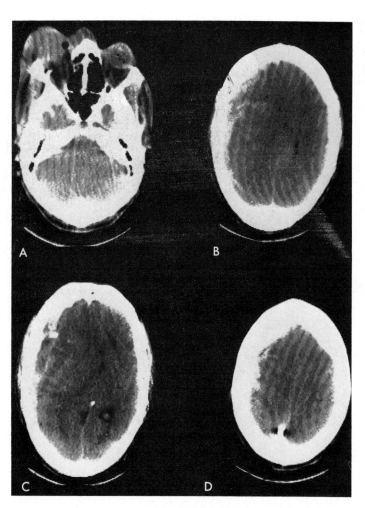

Figure 58–110 CT scan of a patient with an orbital facial penetrating wound. *A.* Computed tomography shows the entry site of the missile at the left proptotic eye. *B.* A left subdural hematoma. *C.* The scan shows the subdural hematoma plus one metal fragment. *D.* The second metal fragment is seen near the inner table of the occipital skull.

fection than those entering the cranial vault directly.[221,298,314] These injuries carry a high incidence of associated subdural and intracerebral hematoma formation (Fig. 58–110).[20,233]

If bone fragments are not visible on x-ray, there is a tendency to do nothing but observe the patient, but this can be disastrous. Antibiotics and expectant care are inadequate treatment, and infection is likely to occur without proper therapy. A hidden cerebrospinal fluid leak and meningitis may develop. Computed tomography greatly aids in defining the location, course, and associated hematoma of a penetrating orbital-facial-cranial wound, as shown in Figure 58–110. The tract of the missile can be plotted, and craniotomy and exploration of the appropriate fossa floor should be done. The pulped brain and bone fragments should be removed, and the dura should be closed. If this is not done, necrotic contaminated brain will be a potential source of infection (Fig. 58–111). If the frontal sinus is penetrated, the posterior wall of bone should be removed and the dura closed. The entire sinus should be entered, and the mucosa should be packed into the ostium. No foreign body should be placed in the ostia of the sinus. Later, when cranioplasty is to be done, autologous bone is favored over methylmethacrylate. Late infection may be lessened, as autologous bone will develop its own blood supply and will not act as a foreign body that can be contaminated by a sinus infection. Orbital-facial wounds occasionally cause a false traumatic aneurysm on one of the major intracranial arteries, and arteriography should be considered before operation.[269]

Intraventricular Foreign Bodies

Intraventricular foreign bodies may cause ventricular obstruction, infection, and mechanical or chemical irritation.[46] Recurrent meningitis and eventual development of hydrocephalus prior to removal of the bullet have been documented.[102] Sherman described the removal of a brass plug from a brain stem in which the breakdown product, copper chloride, had rapidly produced cystic changes.[309] Sudden complete obstruction of the ventricular system can occur.[189] Fortunately, freely moving intraventricular foreign bodies are rare; their removal has sometimes required elaborate methods.

Centrifuge treatment for an intraventricular metallic foreign body has been described by Markham and co-workers. The bullet fragment was immobilized in the ependyma by use of centrifugation in a 5 degrees of freedom of motion simulator at 4 to 6 G's, where it then remained in a fixed position.[214] Stereotaxic procedures have

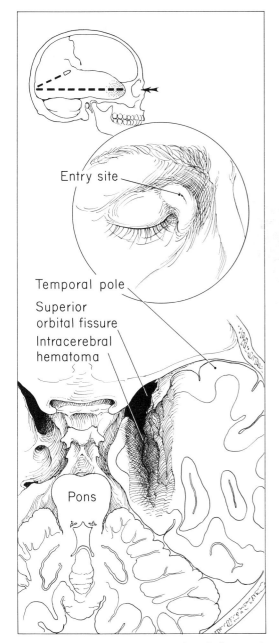

Figure 58–111 Orbital penetrating missile wound. The pulped brain and bone fragments that have penetrated, if accessible, should be removed.

Entry site

Temporal pole

Superior orbital fissure

Intracerebral hematoma

Pons

been used successfully to remove intracranial bullets in brain tissue or the ventricle.[326]

A direct operative approach may be necessary. When the freely movable object is in the lateral ventricle it should be positioned, if possible, in the frontal horn and then removed by a small transcortical incision. Fourth ventricle missiles can be removed via a posterior fossa craniectomy. In the rare case of a fragment in the third ventricle, removal can be accomplished by a transcallosal approach.

Postoperative Rhinorrhea, Otorrhea, and Wound Fistula

Persistent spinal fluid drainage after operation usually means that a dural opening was not recognized at the time of the operation or a completely watertight closure was not obtained. Though daily spinal tap or constant lumbar subarachnoid drainage for three to five days may sometimes heal the fistula, the cerebrospinal fluid leak is less likely to resolve without operative repair than in closed head injury. A postoperative spinal fluid fistula that persists for more than two weeks should be repaired.

In penetrating injuries the path of the missile is usually known from the initial x-rays and operation, so extensive roentgenograms may not need to be done. The dural defect will be near the site of penetration. If the site of the fistula is uncertain before reoperation, a radioactive tracer substance injected into the cerebrospinal fluid by lumbar puncture may confirm the nature and site of the fistula.[80] Special studies including fractional pneumoencephalography with tomograms of the base of the skull and isotope cisternography may be required to define the fistula and should be performed if there is any doubt about its location. Closure with a dural graft is advised, and antibiotic coverage should be continued for 10 days after operation.[150,151,232]

Dural Venous Sinus Injury

Venous sinus injuries may create a great technical challenge, but more often judgment concerning the choice of proper management is the critical factor. The decision revolves around re-establishment of venous drainage from the brain and the control of hemorrhage. Operative management may take the form of ligation of the sinus or reconstruction.

The question of when it is necessary to restore the venous drainage provided by a sinus is critically important, for ligation of an open sinus is relatively easy and quickly accomplished. There is a widely held dictum that the anterior third of the superior sagittal sinus can be safely ligated because of good collateral venous drainage, that ligation of the central third is likely to produce complications related to venous stasis and intracranial hypertension, and that obstructions of the posterior third will invariably lead to severe sequelae.[3,172] This view is supported by Kapp and Gielchinsky's report of a series of 78 Vietnam missile casualties. They ligated the anterior 50 per cent of the superior sagittal sinus in 27 patients with only a single death (4 per cent). This information may extend somewhat the freedom and extent (anterior 50 per cent of the sinus) with which ligation may be employed; it also demonstrates the importance of the posterior half of the sinus, since injuries of that portion were associated with a 24 per cent mortality rate.[165] It may be concluded that injuries to the posterior half of the sagittal sinus should not be permanently ligated but rather should be repaired, re-establishing venous drainage.

Principles concerning the transverse sinuses are more difficult to define, since their contribution to the venous drainage of the supra- and infratentorial spaces is variable. If the superior sagittal sinus drains unilaterally into the right transverse sinus, then ligation here would be disastrous. If, however, the superior sagittal sinus drains bilaterally or through the uninvolved sinus, then ligation may be safe. Preoperative angiography can be helpful.

A depressed fracture that is closed, has no mass effect, and does not require repair for cosmetic reasons, should not be elevated if overlying a venous sinus. If intracranial hypertension without shift is present, occlusion of the sinus may be responsible. This should be confirmed by angiography or venography. The elevation of intracranial pressure produced by unilateral obstruction of the transverse sinus usually subsides in 10 to 14 days, but during that time optic nerve damage may develop as a consequence of the papilledema.

Operative treatment should not begin until the entire operating team is ready to deal with *massive* hemorrhage. Large intravenous cannulae should be placed in multiple sites, and blood and fluids should be *ready* to infuse—if infusion has not already been started. It should be possible to tilt the operating table up and down so that the height of the head in relation to the heart may be altered. In this way, the venous pressure may be lowered to decrease hemorrhage and raised to mitigate air embolism. No obstruction to cerebral venous drainage should be present, which includes cervical intravenous catheter dressings, tracheostomy straps, and even extremes of flexion and rotation of the head upon the shoulders. The depressed fragments should be approached by way of a peripheral craniectomy begun from burr holes placed at the periphery of the wound. The depressed fragments that have potentially lacerated the sinus may then be removed when exposure has been established.

Direct suturing is frequently all that is required, and it can readily be accomplished in most cases. Oversewing with muscle stamps, Gelfoam pad, or Oxycel pack is easily done when the injuries are small. A patch graft is appropriate for wounds with avulsed sections of sinus wall. The patch may be a rotated leaf of dura, pericranium, or fascia; however, the use of the endothelial surface of a vein is preferable, since it is less thrombogenic than other tissue. Care is required to orient the valves with the direction of flow; this is preferable to their removal, which can cause endothelial damage.[287]

At times the sinus is destroyed over too great a distance for conventional repair, and only an interposed graft will restore patency.[312] Many substances, including Dacron prostheses and arteries, have been used, but the best appears to be autogenous saphenous vein. Donaghy and co-workers described a technique using vein-lined siliconized tubing that could be inserted into either end of the completely transected sinus with great speed, though it would seem preferable to use no foreign material if possible.[83] The Kapp-Gielchinsky shunt allows the bridging of avulsed segments of sinus, which can then be repaired at relative leisure (Fig. 58–112).[166,167] This shunt is available in various sizes, has inflatable

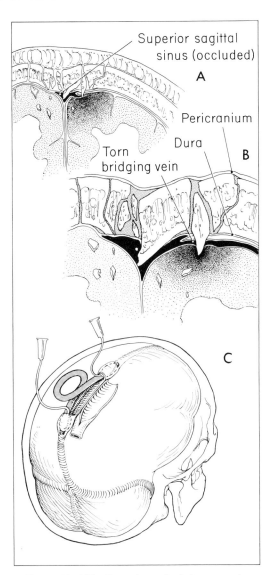

Figure 58–112   Posterior sagittal sinus wounds require treatment designed to preserve the patency of the sinus. The Kapp-Gielchinsky shunt pictured in *C* provides a temporary conduit while microvascular sutures can be placed for grafting of the sinus. An autologous saphenous vein graft is shown in this illustration.

balloons at both ends, and is a good conduit for blood while an autogenous saphenous vein graft is being prepared and sewn into place. Any clots that develop in the sinus should be irrigated out or aspirated before the final sutures are placed.

Traumatic Intracranial Aneurysms

Traumatic intracranial aneurysms are rare, but the result of hemorrhage from them can be devastating. They are usually seen after penetrating injuries or depressed fractures that involve the base of the skull, but on very rare occasions they occur in blunt trauma in which there is only a linear fracture or even no fracture at all.[337] These lesions are often false aneurysms in that part of the wall is made up of the original hematoma, but they may also be true aneurysms that result from an only partial disruption of the arterial wall. When angiography came into wide use in head injury, these lesions were often noted before hemorrhage occurred. Now that computed tomography is replacing angiography as the main diagnostic procedure in severe head injury, it is anticipated that most of the lesions will be discovered because of intracranial hemorrhage or progressive enlargement with cranial nerve compression.

Once discovered, treatment to obliterate the aneurysm should take place as soon as possible, taking into account the patient's overall condition. Those patients who have already bled have a strong propensity to rebleed. Traumatic cerebral aneurysms of peripheral cerebral arteries show an unpredictable course. In a series reported by Asari and co-workers, late catastrophic rupture occurred in 27 of the 60 patients.[14]

The true aneurysms may have a neck that can be clipped and are thus manageable as berry aneurysms. False aneurysms often present a difficult challenge and usually require excision or ligature of the parent vessel to trap the aneurysm. Basal intracranial false aneurysms sometimes can only be satisfactorily managed with reinforcement. Now that intracranial micro-operative arterial bypass procedures are feasible, there may occasionally be an indication for their application here, to be followed later by ligation of the parent vessel.

Other Vascular Complications of Head Injury

Trauma is known to cause a number of vascular complications in and about the head. Some of these are well known, such as occlusion of the extracranial vertebral and carotid arteries. Yet others, such as unilateral or even bilateral middle cerebral artery occlusion, may not be so obvious and may be recorded only as infarction on the CT scan. By 1975, at least 21 cases of middle cerebral artery occlusion attributed

to nonpenetrating head injuries had been described in the literature. Many of the patients had suffered relatively minor head injuries, often without loss of consciousness. Spasm, emboli from the cervical portion of the internal carotid artery, dissecting aneurysm, and thrombus formation all have been suggested as causes for middle carotid artery occlusion.[147]

Cerebral angiography is an important study in the immediate or late follow-up periods in patients with head trauma who are not progressing satisfactorily, who worsen, or who have epistaxis. With rapid widespread employment of computed tomography, certain vascular lesions may be overlooked unless angiography is performed.

CHRONIC SUBDURAL HEMATOMAS

Chronic subdural hematoma presents a problem quite apart from that of acute trauma to the brain. With the chronic subdural hematoma, development of the clinical syndrome is remote in time from the original trauma. The effects of the lesion on the brain relate primarily to brain shift, although focal cortical compression, elevated intracranial pressure, and cerebral vascular insufficiency with brain ischemia occasionally also contribute to the pathogenesis of the symptoms. While the vast majority of chronic subdural hematomas are caused by trauma, they are seen only uncommonly following *severe* brain injury. That is so presumably because chronic subdural hematomas tend to develop in adults with brain atrophy.[274] Younger adults with resilient brains are far less prone to this complication, and younger adults constitute the majority of patients with severe brain injury. For these reasons, discussion of the pathogenesis, diagnosis, and treatment of chronic subdural hematomas is presented separately from that of acute brain trauma.

The etiology and pathogenesis of chronic subdural hematomas has been a subject of great interest since 1863, when Virchow proposed that chronic inflammation of the dura followed by capillary proliferation with an increased tendency to bleeding was responsible for these lesions.[349] Trotter, in 1914, was the first to propose trauma as a cause for chronic subdural hematomas and said that the source of blood in the subdural space was the rupture of veins that drained into the superior sagittal sinus. A study of his four cases showed no inflammatory changes.[342] Putnam and Cushing reviewed the literature in 1925 and gave support to the theory that mild or unnoticed head trauma was the cause of these lesions.[275]

In the last 50 years the treatment of chronic subdural hematomas has changed little, but new theories of pathogenesis have been proposed. Gardner, in 1932, suggested the osmotic theory, which held that chronic subdural hematomas grew by drawing fluid through the semipermeable hematoma wall by the osmotic pressure exerted by hemoglobin proteins in the subdural fluid.[103] This idea was supported by Zollinger and Gross, who further stated that a progressive breakdown of the hemoglobin molecule was responsible for a gradual increase in the osmotic pressure, which was responsible for the growth and late symptoms of chronic subdural hematomas.[365] Munro and Merritt found a progressive dilution of subdural protein concentration and thought that this was consistent with the osmotic theory.[247] Weir disproved this theory in 1971 when, using freezing point determination methods, he showed no differences in subdural fluid, blood, and cerebrospinal fluid osmolalities in 23 patients. Labadie and Glover pointed out that this is an oncotic and not osmotic property of the fluid, which can account for the progressive enlargement of the subdural cavity despite an equivalent osmolality.[185]

The effusion-rebleeding concept was first put forward by Gitlin in 1955, who found increased albumin to gamma globulin ratios and albumin to total protein ratios in subdural hematoma fluid as compared with serum samples. This was used to support the idea that pathologically permeable capillary walls produced an effusion that was responsible for lesion growth.[111] Rabe and associates confirmed these findings with [131]iodine-labeled albumin, which was injected intravenously into an infant and was found in the subdural cavity.[276] Labadie and Glover, in their more recent work, have shown that subdural hematoma fluid accelerates the intrinsic clotting and fibrinolytic systems, and that blood and plasma repeatedly enter the subdural cavity.[186,187]

They have also noted that since some chronic subdural hematomas spontaneously regress, the balance between production and reabsorption of fluid must play a role.[185] The most recent reports of Ito and co-workers in 1976 and 1978 further defined the role of fibrinolytic enzymes in this disorder. [51]Chromium-labeled red blood cells given prior to subdural hematoma aspiration showed mean daily hemorrhage into the cavity equal to 10.2 per cent of its volume. Tissue activator was found to be in the outer membrane and not in the inner membrane. High levels of fibrinogen degradation products were found in the hematoma fluid. Plasmin content was highest in the dura and lacking in the inner membrane. Fibrinogen degradation products themselves inhibit hemostasis, and it is postulated that this could account for continued hemorrhage and growth of the hematoma.[144,145] After years of failure, an animal model has been found in which chronic subdural hematoma acts in the same way as in man and which tends to support the "effusion-rebleeding theory."[12,115,353]

In summary, it is well accepted that the most common cause of chronic subdural hematomas is mild trauma and that it requires from 14 to 21 days to develop to the stage at which it is liquified and can be drained via burr holes.[255,256] This lesion is usually seen in older patients or children under 2 years. This discussion of treatment is concerned only with adults.

Clinical Presentation

Almost all cases are associated with a minor head injury, which may or may not be remembered by the patient or his family. Headache is very common and may be present almost from the time of injury.[237,255,274,342] The headache usually is followed by a latent period during which the patient has very few symptoms. After two or three weeks subtle mental changes may occur, and the patient may become somewhat lethargic with a loss of initiative. Following this stage, at about six weeks after injury, the patient may develop waxing and waning of the level of consciousness. Also a slight paresis with a Babinski's sign is not uncommon at this time. If untreated, these patients may then progressively develop signs and symptoms of tentorial herniation. Alteration of consciousness, confusion, and memory loss are the most frequent signs, and in previous years many patients thought to be psychotic and confined to mental institutions were found to have chronic subdural hematomas on autopsy.[6,224] Seizures are uncommon and are associated with a bad outcome.[224]

The success in achieving a good result lies in early diagnosis and treatment, before herniation states are reached. In order to accomplish this the clinician must consider chronic subdural hematoma in the differential diagnosis of any new mental disturbance or focal neurological deficit in the patient who is 40 years or older, and in all patients with chronic alcoholism.

Diagnosis

As in acute head injury, the CT scan has changed the way in which these patients may best be managed. No longer is angiography necessary to confirm the diagnosis, except in special cases, and no longer are exploratory burr holes on the same and opposite sides necessary, since computed tomography shows both sides of the brain simultaneously as well as demonstrating the lesion. The initial work-up should consist of a skull x-ray series, which, although not diagnostic, will frequently provide useful information. Poppen found 8 skull fractures and 40 shifted pineal glands in his series of 119 chronic subdural hematomas, and McKissock's findings were similar.[224,274] In patients in whom chronic subdural hematoma is suspected, however, CT scanning will give the diagnosis. The hematoma will appear less dense than brain in most cases, with a shift of the ventricular system away from the lesion. Early in their development, however, some chronic subdural hematomas may be isodense with brain, and all that may be seen is a shift of the ventricular system. The greatest diagnostic difficulty arises in the case of bilateral isodense subdural hematomas in which no shift may be seen, but small ventricles and small sulci in an older patient should make one suspicious. In these difficult cases angiography may be necessary.*

---

* See references, 10, 17, 100, 196, 236, 266.

Treatment

Some chronic subdural hematomas will resolve spontaneously, as implied by the existence of calcified "hematomas."[224] Medical treatment has been advocated for certain patients with chronic subdural hematomas. Bender and Christoff have been the main proponents of medical therapy for chronic subdural hematoma, recommending bed rest, mannitol, and steroids. In their series, angiography was used to make the diagnosis and to follow the size of the lesions. Ninety-seven patients were treated this way, seventy-five successfully and twenty-two unsuccessfully. The latter 22 eventually required operative treatment. No patients who were in coma were treated medically.[31] Suzuki and Takau reported 22 of 23 cases successfully managed by treatment with mannitol in doses of 100 to 200 gm per day.[330] Both these groups reported prolonged hospitalizations for these patients.

Despite these reports, with modern operative and anesthetic techniques along with the improved accuracy of diagnosis provided by computed tomography, it would appear that operative treatment will most quickly, effectively, and safely remove the offending mass. It is not possible to compare operative results with nonoperative results, since the sickest patients, who would be expected to do worse, have usually been treated only with operation. The operative mortality rate in McKissock's group's large series, published in 1960, was approximately 6 per cent, and Poppen's operative mortality rate was similar.[224,274] These rates are consistently lower than those reported in the first half of the century, which ranged from 15 to 50 per cent.[58,103,275,342] Presumably earlier diagnosis and treatment have been responsible for the reduction in the number of deaths.

Burr Hole and Twist Drill Drainage

Early in this century it was thought that craniotomy and subtemporal decompression were the best methods of dealing with chronic subdural hematomas. It soon became apparent that these lesions were not infrequently bilateral and that exploratory trephination was needed on the side opposite the suspected lesion in all cases.[58,245,275,342] Coleman advocated bilateral burr holes in the upper temporal region, with craniotomy reserved for solid clots.[58] Of McKissock and co-workers' series of chronic subdural hematomas, 184 were treated with burr hole evacuation alone. Craniotomy was done only if the patient worsened or the lesion did not resolve after repeated tapping.[224] In 1955 Robinson also came out strongly in favor of burr holes as opposed to turning a flap.[290]

Most current writers on the subject prefer to place two or three burr holes on the side of the lesion and to irrigate through small red rubber catheters to wash out the subdural space.[155,169,303] A frontal burr hole placed 3.5 cm from the midline on the coronal suture and a parietal burr hole placed 2 cm above and behind the ear will usually suffice.

Ideally the burr hole locations should be individualized for each patient, depending on the results of the CT scan or angiogram. For chronic subdural hematoma, a frontal and a parietal burr hole will usually be appropriate. Less often the major location of liquid hematoma is in the low temporal or low frontal region. Small red rubber catheters are left in the subdural space for 24 hours. The catheters are brought out through separate incisions and *connected to drainage bags, providing a closed sterile drainage system.* Postoperative drainage might help obliterate the enlarged subdural space and reduce the likelihood of hematoma recurrence. There is, however, no clear evidence that the universal use of postoperative subdural space drainage is beneficial.

Simple twist drill drainage via a ventricular needle can be successful in treating well-liquified hematoma cavities.[252] Repeated drainage may be necessary, however. Recently Tabaddor and Shulman reported the use of twist drill craniostomy and closed-system drainage in 22 patients. Results in patients so treated were superior to the overall results in their patient population when burr holes and drainage or craniotomy was employed.[335]

Failure of the brain to re-expand is often a bad prognostic sign.[58,188,342] Some authors have advocated intrathecal or intraventricular injections of normal saline to re-expand the brain.[188,290] This technique has fallen out of favor, and now most authors prefer general hydration and maintaining the patient in a head-down position, with intraventricular or intrathecal saline being reserved as a procedure of last resort.[155] Postoperatively, patients should be nursed flat or in a slightly head-down position for 24 hours and kept well hydrated with intravenous fluids. Common postoperative neurological complications include failure to improve, recurrent deterioration (which may be secondary to cerebral edema), postoperative hematoma, cerebral ischemia, and failure of the brain to re-expand. Serial computed tomography is very useful in following and sorting out these problems. Metal clips should not be placed on the dura and cortex because they will create artifacts on the CT scan, which is a better means of following these patients than serial skull x-rays of the clips.[264] It is to be hoped that generous hydration will prevent systemic and intracranial hypotension, reduce the risk of cerebral infarction, and encourage brain re-expansion.

Craniotomy for Chronic Subdural Hematoma

While most chronic liquid subdural hematomas are satisfactorily managed by burr hole or twist drill and drainage, some are best dealt with via craniotomy. Craniotomy is recommended under three circumstances: (1) when sizable solid clots return with the irrigation, (2) when the outer membrane is quite thick and the hematoma cavity contains multiple loculations, and (3) when recurrent intractable hematoma formation with a slack brain is still present despite several attempts at burr hole drainage.[275] In all these situations craniotomy almost always reveals a sizable subdural mass lesion that could not be adequately drained through burr holes. For these difficult cases, craniotomy is probably underutilized, and it would seem prudent to proceed with a formal flap when there is doubt about the adequacy of burr hole drainage.[21,222]

Acknowledgment. This work was supported in part by NIH Grant No. 1 P50 NS 12587.

REFERENCES

1. Ad Hoc Committee to Study Head Injury Nomenclature: A glossary of head injury including some definitions of injuries of the cervical spine. Clin. Neurosurg., *12*:388–394, 1966.

2. Adams, J. H.: The neuropathology of head injuries. *In* Vinken, P. J., and Bruyn, G. W., eds.: *Handbook of Clinical Neurology,* Vol. 23. Amsterdam, Oxford, Elsevier–North Holland Publishing Co., 1975, pp. 35–65.

3. Adeloye, A., and Odeku, E. L.: A syndrome characteristic of tangential bullet wounds of the vertex of the skull. J. Neurosurg., *34*:155–158, 1971.

4. Alcala, H., Gado, M., and Torack, R. M.: The effect of size, histologic elements, and water content on the visualization of cerebral infarcts. Arch. Neurol. (Chicago), *35*:1–7, 1978.

5. Alexander, E., Jr.: Medical management of closed head injuries. Clin. Neurosurg., *19*:240–250,1972.

6. Allen, A. M., Moore, M., and Daly, B. B.: Subdural hemorrhage in patients with mental disease. New Eng. J. Med., *223*:324–329, 1940.

7. Allison, T.: Recovery functions of somatosensory evoked responses in man. Electroenceph. Clin. Neurophysiol., *14*:331–343, 1962.

8. Allison, T., Matsumiya, Y., Goff, G. D., and Goff, W. R.: The scalp topography of human visual evoked potentials. Electroenceph. Clin. Neurophysiol., *42*:185–197, 1977.

9. Ambrose, J.: Computerized transverse axial scanning (tomography). Part 2. Clinical approach. Brit. J. Radiol., *46*:1023–1046, 1973.

10. Ambrose, J.: Computerized x-ray scanning of brain. J. Neurosurg., *40*:679–695, 1974.

11. Amendola, M. A., and Ostrum, R. J.: Diagnosis of isodense subdural hematomas by computed tomography. Amer. J. Roentgen., *129*:693–697, 1977.

12. Apfelbaum, R. I., Guthkelch, A. N., and Schulman, K.: Experimental production of subdural hematomas. J. Neurosurg., *40*:336–345, 1974.

13. Armington, J. C.: The Electroretinogram. New York, Academic Press, 1974.

14. Asari, S., Nakamura, S., Yamada, O., et al.: Traumatic aneurysm of peripheral cerebral arteries. Report of two cases. J. Neurosurg., *46*:795–803, 1977.

15. Ascroft, P. B., and Pulvertaft, R. J. V.: Bacteriology of head wounds. Brit. J. Surg. War Surg. suppl. 1:183–186, 1947.

16. Astrup, J., Symon, L., Branston, N. M., and Lassen, N. A.: Cortical evoked potential and extracellular K$^+$ and H$^+$ at critical levels of brain ischemia. Stroke, *8*:52–57, 1977.

17. Baker, H. L., Campbell, J. K., Houser, O. W., et al.: Computer assisted tomography of the head. Mayo Clin. Proc., *49*:17–27, 1974.

18. Baker, R., Gresty, M., and Berthoz, A.: Neuronal activity in the prepositus hypoglossi nucleus correlated with vertical and horizontal movement in the cat. Brain Res., *101*:366–371, 1976.

19. Baratham, G., and Dennyson, W. G.: Delayed traumatic intracerebral hemorrhage. J. Neurol. Neurosurg. Psychiat., *35*:698–706, 1972.

20. Barnett, J. C., and Meirowsky, A. M.: Intracranial hematomas associated with penetrating wounds of the brain. J. Neurosurg., *12*:34–38, 1955.

21. Becker, D. P.: Personal observation.

22. Becker, D. P.: Discussion of Levin, A.: The use of a fiber optic intracranial pressure monitor in clinical practice. Neurosurgery, *1*:266–271, 1977.

23. Becker, D. P., and Vries, J. K.: The alleviation of increased intracranial pressure by the chronic administration of osmotic agents. *In* Brock, M., and Dietz, H., eds.: Intracranial Pressure. Berlin, Springer-Verlag, 1973, pp. 309–315.

24. Becker, D. P., Miller, J. D., Sweet, R. C., et al.: Head injury management 1977. *In* Popp, A J., Bourke, R. S., Nelson, L. R., and Kimelberg, H. K., eds.: Neural Trauma. Seminars in Neurological Surgery. New York, Raven Press, 1979. pp. 313–328.

25. Becker, D. P., Miller, J. D., Ward, J. D., et al.: The outcome from severe head injury with early diagnosis and intensive management. J. Neurosurg., *47*:491–502, 1977.

26. Becker, D. P., Miller, J. D., Young, H. F., et al.: The critical importance of ICP monitoring in head injury. *In* Beks, J. W. F., Bosch, D. A., and Brock, M., eds.: Intracranial Pressure III. Berlin, Springer-Verlag, 1976, pp. 97–100.

27. Becker, D. P., Sullivan, H. G., Adams, W. E., et al.: Controlled hyperventilation in severe mechanical brain injury. *In* McLaurin, R. L., ed.: Head Injuries; Second Chicago Symposium on Neural Trauma. New York, Grune & Stratton Inc., 1976, pp. 157–159.

28. Becker, D. P., Vries, J. K., Sakalas, R., et al.: Early prognosis in head injury based on motor posturing, oculocephalic reflexes, and intracranial pressure. *In* McLaurin, R. L., ed.: Head Injuries. Second Symposium on Neural Trauma. New York, Grune & Stratton Inc., 1976, pp. 27–30.

29. Becker, D. P., Vries, J. K., Young, H. F., et al.: Controlled cerebral perfusion pressure and ventilation in mechanical brain injury: Prevention of progressive brain swelling. *In* Lundberg, N., Ponten, U., and Brock, M., eds.: Intracranial Pressure II. Berlin, Springer-Verlag, 1975, pp. 480–484.

30. Becker, D. P., Young, H. F., Vries, J. K., et al.: Monitoring in patients with brain tumors. Clin. Neurosurg., *22*:364–388, 1975.

31. Bender, M. B., and Christoff, N.: Non-surgical treatment of subdural hematomas. Arch. Neurol. (Chicago), *31*:73–79, 1974.

32. Benson, D. F., and Geschwind, N.: Shrinking retrograde amnesia. J. Neurol. Neurosurg. Psychiat., *30*:539–544, 1967.

33. Benson, D. F., and Geschwind, N.: The aphasiac and related disturbances. *In* Baber, A. B., and Baber, L. H., ed.: Clinical Neurology. New York, Harper & Row, Inc., 1977.

34. Bergeron, T. R., and Rumbaugh, C. L.: Non space occupying sequelae of head trauma. Radiol. Clin. N. Amer. *12*:315–331, 1974.

35. Bergstrom, M., Ericson, K., Levander, B., et al.: Computed tomography of cranial subdural and epidural hematomas: Variation of attenuation related to time and clinical events such as rebleeding. J. Comput. Assist. Tomog., *1*:449–455, 1977.

36. Bickford, R. G., and Klass, D. W.: Acute and chronic EEG findings after head injury. *In*

Caveness, W. F., and Walker, A. E., eds.: Head Injury Conference Proceedings. Philadelphia, J. B. Lippincott Co., 1966, pp. 63–88.

37. Braakman, R.: Survey and follow-up of 225 consecutive skull fractures. J. Neurol. Neurosurg. Psychiat., *34*:106, 1971.

38. Braakman, R.: Depressed skull fracture. Data, treatment and follow-up of 225 consecutive cases. J. Neurol. Neurosurg. Psychiat., *35*: 395–402, 1972.

39. Bricolo, A., Turazzi, S., Alexandre, A., and Rigguto, N.: Decerebrate rigidity in acute head trauma. J. Neurosurg., *47*:680–698, 1977.

40. Brierley, J. B., Graham, D. I., Adams, J. H., and Simpson, J. A.: Neocortical death after cardiac arrest: A clinical, neurophysiological and neuropathological report of two cases. Lancet, *2*:560–565, 1971.

41. Brooks, D. N.: Recognition memory and head injury. J. Neurol. Neurosurg. Psychiat., *37*:794–801, 1974.

42. Brooks, R. A., and DiChiro, G.: Principles of computer assisted tomography (CAT) in radiographic and radioisotopic imaging. Phys. Med. Biol., *21*:689–732, 1976.

43. Browder, J.: A résumé of the principal diagnostic features of subdural hematoma. Bull. N.Y. Acad. Med., *19*:168–176, 1943.

44. Browder, J., and Turney, M. F.: Intracerebral hemorrhage of traumatic origin—its surgical treatment. New York J. Med., *42*:2230–2235, 1942.

45. Brown, H. A., and Naffziger, H. C.: Scalp, cranium and brain. *In* Cole, W. H., ed.: Operative Technique in Specialty Surgery. New York, Appleton-Century-Crofts, Inc., 1949, pp. 413–459.

46. Brown, L., Jr.: Unusual pneumoencephalogram following fragment wound of the brain. J. Neurosurg., *32*:100–102, 1970.

47. Bruce, D. A., Shut, L., Buena, L. A., et al.: Outcome following severe head injuries in children. J. Neurosurg., *48*:679–688, 1978.

48. Bucy, P. C., and Oberhill, H. R.: Subdural hematoma in adults. Arizona Med., *25*:186–189, 1968.

49. Bushnell, L. S.: Acute respiratory failure in the surgical patient: Physiology and management. *In* Skillman, J. J., ed.: Intensive Care. Boston, Little, Brown & Co., 1975, pp. 203–227,

50. Butler, E. G., Puckett, W. O., Harvey, N. E., et al.: Experiments on head wounding by high velocity missiles. J. Neurosurg., *11*:358–363, 1945.

51. Cairns, H., and Holbourn, H.: Head injuries in motorcyclists with special reference to crash helmets. Brit. Med. J., *1*:591–598, 1943.

52. Carey, M. E., Young, H., Mathis, J. L., et al.: A bacteriological study of craniocerebral missile wounds from Vietnam. J. Neurosurg., *34*:145–154, 1971.

53. Caveness, W. F.: Incidence of craniocerebral trauma in the United States in 1976 with trend from 1970–1975. Advances Neurol. *22*: 1–3, 1979.

54. Chambers, J. W.: Acute subdural hematoma. J. Neurosurg., *8*:263–268, 1951.

55. Chatrian, G. E., White, L. E., Jr., and Shaw, Ch.-M.: EEG pattern resembling wakefulness in unresponsive decerebrate state following traumatic brainstem infarct. Electroenceph. Clin. Neurophysiol., *16*:285–289, 1964.

56. Clark, K., Nash, T. M., and Hutchinson, G. C.: The failure of circumferential craniotomy in acute traumatic cerebral swelling. J. Neurosurg., *29*:367–371, 1968.

57. Cody, D. T. R.: Cortical evoked responses in neuro-otologic diagnosis. Arch. Otolaryng. (Chicago), *97*:96–103, 1973.

58. Coleman, C. C.: Chronic subdural hematoma. Amer. J. Surg., *28*:341–363, 1935.

59. Coleman, C.: Treatment of compound fractures of the skull. Ann. Surg., *115*:506–513, 1942.

60. Cooper, P. R., Rovit, R. L., and Ransohoff, J.: Hemicraniectomy in the treatment of acute subdural hematoma: A re-appraisal. Surg. Neurol., *5*:25–28, 1976.

61. Cottrell, J. E., Patel, K., Turndorf, H., et al.: Intracranial pressure changes induced by sodium nitroprusside in patients with intracranial mass lesions. J. Neurosurg., *48*:329–331, 1978.

62. Courjon, J. A.: Post-traumatic epilepsy in electroclinical practice. *In* Walker, A. E., Caveness, W. F., and Critchley, M. T., eds.: The Late Effects of Head Injury. Springfield, Ill., 1969, pp. 215–227.

63. Cracco, R. Q., and Cracco, J. B.: Somatosensory evoked potential in man: Far field potentials. Electroenceph. Clin. Neurophysiol., *41*:5:460–466, 1976.

64. Creutzfeldt, O. D., Watanabe, S., and Lux, H. D.: Relations between EEG phenomena and potentials of single cortical cells. I. Evoked responses after thalamic and epicortical stimulation. Electroenceph. Clin. Neurophysiol., *20*: 1–18, 1966.

65. Creutzfeldt, O. D., Watanabe, S., and Lux, H. D.: Relations between EEG phenomena and potentials of single cortical cells. II. Spontaneous and convulsoid activity. Electroenceph. Clin. Neurophysiol., *20*:19–37, 1966.

66. Crockard, H. A., Coppel, D. L., and Morrow, W. F. K.: Evaluation of hyperventilation in treatment of head injuries. Brit. Med. J., *4*: 634–640, 1973.

67. Crockard, H. A., Brown, F. D., Calica, A. B., et al.: Physiological consequences of experimental cerebral missile injury and use of data analysis to predict survival. J. Neurosurg., *46*:784–795, 1977.

68. Crockard, H. A., Brown, F. D., Johns, L. M., et al.: An experimental cerebral missile injury model in primates. J. Neurosurg., *46*:776–782, 1977.

69. Cullen, K. K., Jr., Ellis, M. S., Berlin, C. I., and Lousteau, R. J.: Human acoustic nerve action potential recordings from the tympanic membrane without anesthesia. Acta Otolaryng., *74*:15–22, 1972.

70. Cushing, H.: Surgery of the head. *In* Keen, W. W., ed.: Surgery—Its Principles and Practice. Vol. 3. Philadelphia and London, W. B. Saunders Co., 1908, pp. 17–276.

71. Cushing, H.: A study of a series of wounds involving the brain and its enveloping structures. Brit. J. Surg., *5*:558–684, 1918.

72. Cushing, H.: Notes on penetrating wounds of the brain. Brit. Med. J., *1*:22–226, 1918.

73. Dandy, W. E.: The brain. *In* Lewis, D., ed.: Practice of Surgery. Vol. 12. Hagerstown, Md., W. F. Prior Co., Inc., 1932, pp. 265–323.

74. Davis, K. R., Ackerman, R. H., Kistler, J. B., et al.: Computed tomography of cerebral infarction: Hemorrhagic, contrast enhancement and time of appearance. Comput. Tomog. *1*:71–86, 1977.

75. Davis, K. R., Taveras, J. M., Roberson, G. H., et al.: Computed tomography in head trauma. Seminars Roentgen. *12*:53–62, 1977.

76. Davis, L. E.: The Principles of Neurological Surgery. Philadelphia, Lea & Febiger, 1946.

77. Dawson, R. E., Webster, J. E., and Gurdjian, E. S.: Serial electroencephalography in acute head injuries. J. Neurosurg., *8*:613–630, 1951.

78. DeVet, A. C.: Traumatic intracerebral hematoma. *In* Vinken, P. J., and Bruyn, G. W., eds.: Handbook of Clinical Neurology. Vol. 24. Amsterdam, Elsevier–North Holland Publishing Co., 1976, pp. 351–368.

79. DeVilliers, J. C.: Stab wounds of the brain and skull. *In* Vinken, P. J., and Bruyn, G. W., eds.: Handbook of Clinical Neurology. Vol. 23. Amsterdam, Elsevier–North Holland Publishing Co., 1975, pp. 477–503.

80. DiChiro, G., Ommaya, A. K., Ashburn, W. L., et al.: Isotope cisternography in the diagnosis and follow-up of cerebrospinal fluid rhinorrhea. J. Neurosurg., *28*:522–529, 1968.

81. Dodge, P. R., and Meirowsky, A. M.: Tangential wounds of the scalp. J. Neurosurg., *9*:472–483, 1952.

82. Dolinskas, C. A., Bilaniuk, L. T., Zimmerman, R. A., et al.: Computed tomography of intracerebral hematomas. 1. Transmission CT observations on hematoma resolution. Amer. J. Roentgen., *129*:681–688, 1977.

83. Donaghy, R. M., Wallman, L. J., Flanagan, M. J., et al.: Sagittal sinus repair. J. Neurosurg., *38*:244–248, 1973.

84. Donchin, E., and Lindsley, D. B., eds.: Diagnostic uses of the average evoked potentials. NASA, SP-101, Washington, 1969, pp. 311–332.

85. Dow, R. S., Ulett, G., and Raaf, J.: Electroencephalographic studies immediately following head injury. Amer. J. Psychiat., *101*:174183, 1943.

86. Drew, J. H., and Fager, C. A.: Delayed brain abscess in relation to retained intracranial foreign bodies. J. Neurosurg., *11*:386–393, 1954.

87. Dublin, A. B., French, B. N., and Rennick, J. M.: Computed tomography in head trauma. Radiology, *122*:365–369, 1977.

88. Dujovny, M., Osgood, C. P., Maroon, J. C., et al.: Penetrating intracranial foreign bodies in children. J. Trauma, *15*:981–986, 1975.

89. Elul, R.: Brain waves: Intracellular recording and statistical analysis help clarify their physiological significance. Data Acquisition and Processing in Biology and Medicine, *5*:93–115, 1966.

90. Enevoldsen, E. M., and Jennsen, F. T.: Autoregulation and CO_2 responses of cerebral blood flow in patients with acute severe head injury. J. Neurosurg., *48*:689–703, 1978.

91. Enevoldsen, E. M., Cold, G., Jensen, F. T., et al.: Dynamic changes in regional CBF, intraventricular pressure, CSF pH and lactate levels during the acute phase of head injury. J. Neurosurg., *44*:191–215, 1976.

92. Faupel, G., Reulen, H. J., Muller, D., et al.: Double-blind study on the effects of steroids on severe closed head injury. *In* Pappius, H. M., and Feindel, W., eds.: Dynamics of Brain Edema, Berlin/Heidelberg/New York, Springer-Verlag, 1976, pp. 337–343.

93. Feinsod, M., and Auerbach, E.: Electrophysiological examinations of the visual system in the acute phase after head injury. Eur. Neurol., *9*:56–64, 1973.

94. Feiring, E. H., and Brock, S.: General considerations of the brain and spinal cord and their coverings. *In* Feiring, E. H., ed.: Brock's Injuries of the Brain and Spinal Cord and Their Coverings. New York, 5th Ed. Springer Publishing Co., 1974, pp. 1–41.

95. Fell, D. A., Fitzgerald, S., Moiel, R. H., et al.: Acute subdural hematomas. Review of 144 cases. J. Neurosurg., *42*:37–42, 1975.

96. Fisher, C. M.: The neurological examination of the comatose patient. Acta Neurol. Scand., *45*:36:1–56, 1969.

97. Fleischer, A. S., Payne, N. S., and Tindall, G. T.: Continuous monitoring of intracranial pressure in severe closed head injury without mass lesions. Surg. Neurol., *6*:31–34, 1976.

98. Fogelholm, R., Heiskanen, O., and Waltimo, O.: Chronic subdural hematoma in adults. J. Neurosurg., *42*:43–46, 1975.

99. Foltz, E. L., and Schmidt, R. P.: The role of the reticular formation in the coma of head injury. J. Neurosurg., *13*:145–154, 1956.

100. French, B. N., and Dublin, A. B.: The value of computerized tomography in the management of 1000 consecutive head injuries. Surg. Neurol., *7*:171–183, 1977.

101. Frost, E. A. M.: Effects of positive end-expiratory pressure on intracranial pressure and compliance in brain-injured patients. J Neurosurg., *47*:195–200, 1977.

102. Furlow, L. T., Bender, M. D., and Teuber, L.: Movable foreign body within the cerebral ventricle. A case report. J. Neurosurg., *4*:380–386, 1947.

103. Gardner, W. J.: Traumatic subdural hematoma with particular reference to the latent interval. Arch. Neurol. Psychiat., *27*:847–855, 1932.

104. Gennerelli, T., Obrist, W., Langfitt, T., et al.: Vascular and metabolic reactivity to changes in pCO_2 reactivity in head injured patients. *In* Popp, A. J., Bourke, R. S., Nelson, L. R., and Kimelberg, H. K., eds.: Neural Trauma. Seminars in Neurological Surgery. New York, Raven Press, 1979, pp. 1–8.

105. Gerber, A. M., and Moody, R. A.: Craniocerebral missile injuries in the monkey: An experimental physiological model. J. Neurosurg., *36*:43–49, 1972.

106. Geschwind, N.: Disconnection syndromes in animals and man. Brain, *88*:585–644, 1965.

107. Geschwind, N.: Current concepts in aphasia. New Eng. J. Med., *284*:654–656, 1971.

108. Gibbs, J. R.: Middle-meningeal hemorrhage. Lancet, *2*:727–731, 1960.

109. Giblin, D. R.: Somatosensory evoked potentials in healthy subjects and in patients with lesions of the nervous system. Ann. N.Y. Acad. Sci., *112*:93–142, 1964.

110. Gissane, W.: The nature and causation of road injuries. Lancet, *2*:695–698, 1963.

111. Gitlin, D.: Pathogenesis of subdural collections of fluid. Pediatrics, *16*:345–351, 1955.

112. Gobiet, W., Bock, W. J., Liesegang, J., et al.: Treatment of acute cerebral edema with high dose of dexamethasone. *In* Beks, J. W. F., Bosch, D. A., and Brock, M., eds.: Intracranial Pressure III. Berlin, Springer-Verlag, 1976, pp. 232–235.

113. Goff, W. R., Matsumiya, Y., Allison, T., and Goff, G. D.: Cross-modality comparisons of average evoked potentials. *In* Donchin, E., and Lindsley, D. B., eds.: Average evoked potentials: methods, results and evaluations. NASA, SP-191, Washington, 1969, pp. 94–141.

114. Goff, W. R., Matsumiya, Y., Allison, T., and Goff, G. D.: The scalp topography of human somatosensory and auditory evoked potentials. Electroenceph. Clin. Neurophysiol., *43*:57–76, 1977.

115. Goodell, C., and Mealey, J.: Pathogenesis of chronic subdural hematoma, Arch. Neurol. (Chicago), *8*:429–437, 1963.

116. Goodkin, R., and Szhiser, J.: Sequential angiographic studies demonstrating delayed development of an acute epidural hematoma. J. Neurosurg., *48*:479–482, 1978.

117. Gordon, E.: Controlled respiration in the management of patients with traumatic brain injuries. Acta Anesth. Scand., *15*:193–208, 1971.

118. Gordon, E., and Ponten, U.: The non-operative treatment of severe head injuries. *In* Vinken, P. J., and Bruyn, G. W., eds.: Handbook of Clinical Neurology. Vol. 24. Amsterdam, Elsevier–North Holland Publishing Co., 1976, pp. 599–626.

119. Graham, D. I., and Adams, H.: The pathology of blunt head injuries. *In* Critchley, M., O'Leary, J. L., and Jennett, B., eds.: The Scientific Foundations of Neurology. Philadelphia, F. A. Davis Co., 1972, pp. 478–491.

120. Greenberg, R. P., and Becker, D. P.: Clinical applications of evoked potential data in severe head injury patients. Surg. Forum., *26*:484–486, 1975.

121. Greenberg, R. P., Mayer, D. J., and Becker, D. P.: The prognostic value of evoked potentials in human mechanical head injury. *In* McLaurin, R. L., ed.: Head Injuries. Second Chicago Symposium on Neural Trauma. New York, Grune & Stratton, Inc., 1976, pp. 81–88.

122. Greenberg, R. P., Becker, D. P., Miller, J. D., et al.: Evaluation of brain function in severe human head trauma with multimodality evoked potentials. Part 2: Localization of brain dysfunction and correlation with post-traumatic neurological conditions. J. Neurosurg., *47*:163–177, 1977.

123. Greenberg, R. P., Mayer, D. J., Becker, D. P., et al.: Evaluation of brain function in severe human head trauma with multimodality evoked potentials. Part 1: Evoked brain injury potentials, methods, analysis. J. Neurosurg., *47*:150–162, 1977.

124. Griffith, R. L., and Becker, D. P.: Physiological monitoring of the head injury patient. Advances Neurol., *22*:51–72, 1979.

125. Grossman, R. G., Turner, J. W., Miller, J. D., et al.: The relation between cortical electrical activity, cerebral perfusion pressure, and CBF during increased ICP. *In* Langfitt, T. W., ed.: Cerebral Circulation and Metabolism. New York, Springer-Verlag, 1975, pp. 232–234.

126. Gurdjian, E. S.: Impact Head Injury. Mechanistic, Clinical and Preventive Correlations. Springfield, Ill., Charles C Thomas, 1975.

127. Gurdjian, E. S., and Thomas, L. M.: Surgical management of the patient with head injury. Clin. Neurosurg., *12*:56–74, 1964.

128. Gurdjian, E. S., and Thomas, L. M.: Traumatic intracranial hemorrhage. *In* Feiring, E. H., ed.: Brock's Injuries of the Brain and Spinal Cord and Their Coverings. 5th Ed., New York, Springer Publishing Co., 1974, pp. 203–282.

129. Guthkelch, A. N.: Apparently trivial wounds of the eyelids with intracranial damage. Brit. Med. J., *2*:842–844, 1960.

130. Gutterman, P., and Shenkin, H. A.: Prognostic features in recovery from traumatic decerebration. J. Neurosurg., *32*:330–335, 1970.

131. Hagan, R. E.: Early complications following penetrating wounds of the brain. J. Neurosurg., *34*:132–141, 1971.

132. Halliday, A. M.: Changes in the form of cerebral evoked responses in man associated with various lesions of the nervous system. Electroenceph. Clin. Neurophysiol., suppl., *25*:178–192, 1967.

133. Halliday, A. M., and Wakefield, G. S.: Cerebral evoked potentials in patients with dissociated sensory loss. J. Neurol. Neurosurg. Psychiat., *26*:211–219, 1963.

134. Hamburger, E.: Vehicular suicidal ideation. Milit. Med., *134*:441–444, 1969.

135. Hammon, W. M.: Analysis of 2,187 consecutive penetrating wounds of the brain from Vietnam. J. Neurosurg., *34*:127–131, 1971.

136. Hammon, W. M.: Missile wounds. *In* Vinken, P. J., and Bruyn, G. W., eds.: Handbook of Clinical Neurology. Vol. 23. Amsterdam, Elsevier–North Holland Publishing Co., 1975. pp. 505–526.

137. Hancock, D. O.: Angiography in acute head injuries. Lancet, *2*:745–747, 1961.

138. Heiskanen, O., and Vapalahti, M.: Temporal lobe contusion and hematoma. Acta Neurochir. (Wein), *27*:29–35, 1972.

139. Holbourn, A. H. S.: Mechanisms of brain injuries. Lancet, *2*:438–441, 1943.

140. Hooper, R.: Observations on extradural hemorrhage. Brit. J. Surg., *47*:71–87, 1959.

141. Hooper, R.: Indications for surgical treatment. *In* Vinken, P. J., and Bruyn, G. W., eds.: Handbook of Clinical Neurology. Vol. 24. Amsterdam, Elsevier–North Holland Publishing Co., 1976, pp. 637–667.

142. Hounsfield, G. N.: Computerized transverse axial scanning (tomography): Part I. Description of system. Brit. J. Radiol., *16*:1016–1022, 1973.

143. Hutcher, N., Silverberg, S. G., and Lee, H. M.:

The effect of vitamin A on the steroid induced gastric ulcers. Surg. Forum., *22*:322–326, 1971.

144. Ito, H., Komai, T., and Yamamoto, S.: Fibrinolytic enzyme in the lining walls of chronic subdural hematoma. J. Neurosurg., *48*:197–200, 1978.

145. Ito, H., Yamamoto, S., Komai, T., and Mizukoshi, H.: The role of hyperfibrinolysis in the etiology of chronic subdural hematoma. J. Neurosurg., *45*:26–31, 1976.

146. Jacobs, G. B.: Tangential wounds of the head. J. Neurosurg., *2*:391–401, 1945.

147. Jacques, S., Sheldon, C. H., Rogers, D. T., et al.: Post-traumatic bilateral middle cerebral artery occlusion. Case Report. J. Neurosurg., *42*:217–221, 1975.

148. Jamieson, K. G., and Yelland, J. D. N.: Extradural hematoma: Report of 167 cases. J. Neurosurg., *29*:13–23, 1968.

149. Jamieson, K. G., and Yelland, J. D. N.: Surgically treated traumatic subdural hematomas. J. Neurosurg., *37*:137–149, 1972.

150. Jamieson, K. G., and Yelland, J. D.: Surgical repair of anterior fossa because of rhinorrhea, aerocele, or meningitis. J. Neurosurg., *39*:328–331, 1975.

151. Jefferson, A., and Reilly, G.: Fractures of the floor of the anterior cranial fossa. The selection of patients for dural repair. Brit. J. Surg., *59*:585–592, 1972.

152. Jefferson, G.: Removal of a rifle bullet from the right lobe of the cerebellum, illustrating the spontaneous movement of a bullet in the brain. Brit. J. Surg., *5*:422–424, 1917.

153. Jennett, B.: Epilepsy After Non-Missile Head Injury. 2nd Ed. London, William Heinemann Ltd., 1975, p. 179.

154. Jennett, B.: Resource allocation for the severely brain damaged. Arch. Neurol. (Chicago), *33*:595–597, 1976.

155. Jennett, B.: An Introduction to Neurosurgery. 3rd Ed. Chicago, Year Book Medical Publishers, 1977, pp. 252–256.

156. Jennett, B.: The clinical problem posed by head injuries. Scot. Med. J., *23*:91, 1978.

157. Jennett, B., and Miller, J. D.: Infection after depressed fracture of the skull. Implications for management of non-missile injuries. J. Neurosurg., *36*:333–339, 1972.

158. Jennett, B., Miller, J. D., and Braakman, R.: Epilepsy after non-missile depressed skull fracture. J. Neurosurg., *41*:208–216, 1974.

159. Jennett, B., Teasdale, G., and Braakman, R., et al: Predicting outcome in individual patients after head injury. Lancet, *1*:1031–1034, 1976.

160. Jewett, D. L.: Volume-conducted potentials in response to auditory stimuli as detected by averaging in the cat. Electroenceph. Clin. Neurophysiol., *28*:609–618, 1970.

161. Jewett, D. L., and Williston, J. S.: Auditory-evoked far fields averaged from the scalp of humans. Brain, *94*:681–696, 1971.

162. Jewett, D. L., Romano, M. A., and Williston, J. S.: Human auditory evoked potentials: Possible brainstem components detected on the scalp. Science, *167*:1517–1518, 1970.

163. Johnston, I. H., and Jennett, B.: The place of continuous intracranial pressure monitoring in neurosurgical practice. Acta Neurochir. (Wein), *29*:53–63, 1973.

164. Johnston, I. H., Johnston, J. A., and Jennett, B.: Intracranial pressure changes following head injury. Lancet, *2*:433–436, 1970.

165. Kapp, J. P., and Gielchinsky, I.: Management of combat wounds of the dural venous sinuses. Surgery, *71*:913–917, 1972.

166. Kapp, J. P., Gielchinsky, I., and Deardourff, S. L.: Operative techniques for management of lesions involving the dural venous sinuses. Surg. Neurol., *7*:339–342, 1977.

167. Kapp, J. P., Gielchinsky, I., Petty, C., and McClure, C.: An internal shunt for use in the reconstruction of dural venous sinuses. J. Neurosurg., *35*:351–354, 1971.

168. Kaufmann, G. E., and Clark, K.: Emergency frontal twist drill ventriculostomy. J. Neurosurg., *33*:226–227, 1970.

169. Kempe, L. G.: Operative Neurosurgery. Vol. 1. New York, Springer-Verlag, 1968, pp. 156–159.

170. Kennedy, F., and Wortis, S. B.: Modern treatment of increased intracranial pressure. J.A.M.A., *96*:1248–1286, 1931.

171. Kerr, F. L., and Hollowell, O. W.: Location of pupillomotor and accommodation fibers in the oculomotor nerve: Experimental observations on paralytic mydriasis. J. Neurol. Neurosurg. Psychiat., *27*:473–481, 1964.

172. Kinal, M. E.: Traumatic thrombosis of dural venous sinuses in closed head injuries. J. Neurosurg., *27*:142–145, 1967.

173. Kishore, P. R. S., Dahlie, J. G., Bartlett, J. E., et al.: Computerized tomography: Management of acute head trauma. J. Kansas Med. Soc., *78*:105–108, 1977.

174. Kishore, P. R. S., Lipper, H. M., Miller, J. D., et al.: Posttraumatic hydrocephalus in patients with severe head injury. Neuroradiology, *16*:261–265, 1978.

175. Kiloh, L. G., McComas, A. J., and Osselton, J. W.: Clinical Electroencephalography. London, Butterworth & Co. Ltd., 1972.

176. Kjellberg, R. N., and Prieto, A., Jr.: Bifrontal decompressive craniotomy for massive cerebral edema. J. Neurosurg., *34*:488–493, 1971.

177. Kline, D. G., and LeBlanc, H. I.: Survival following gunshot wound of the pons: Neuroanatomic considerations. J. Neurosurg., *35*:342–347, 1971.

178. Kobrine, A. I., Timmons, E., Rajjoub, J. K., et al.: Demonstration of massive traumatic brain swelling within 20 minutes after injury. J. Neurosurg., *46*:256–258, 1977.

179. Kontos, H.: Personal communication, 1979.

180. Koo, A. H., and LaRoque, R. L.: Evaluation of head trauma by computed tomography. Radiology, *123*:345–350, 1977.

181. Kooi, K. A.: Fundamentals of Electroencephalography. New York, Harper & Row, 1971.

182. Kooi, K. A., and Bagchi, B. K.: Visual evoked responses in man: Normative data. Ann. N.Y. Acad. Sci., *112*:254–269, 1964.

183. Kramer, S. P., and Horsley, V.: Philosophical Transactions of the Royal Society, *188*:223, 1897.

184. Kurze, T., and Pitts, F.: Management of closed head injuries. Surg. Clin. N. Amer., *486*:1271–1278, 1968.

185. Labadie, E. L., and Glover, D.: Chronic subdural hematoma: Concepts of pathogenesis, a review. Canad. J. Neurol. Sci., *1*:222–225, 1974.

186. Labadie, E. L., and Glover, D.: Local alterations of hemostatic-fibrinolytic mechanisms in reforming subdural hematomas. Neurology (Minneap.), *25*:669–675, 1975.

187. Labadie, E. L., and Glover, D.: Pathogenesis of subdural hematomas. J. Neurosurg., *45*:382–392, 1976.

188. Lalonde, A. A., and Gardner, W. J.: Chronic subdural hematoma, expansion of compressed cerebral hemisphere and relief of hypotension by spinal injection of physiologic saline solution. New Eng. J. Med., *239*:493–496, 1948.

189. Lang, E. K.: Acute hydrocephalus secondary to occlusion of the aqueduct by a bullet. J. Louisiana Med. Soc., *121*:167–168, 1969.

190. Langfitt, T. W.: Measuring the outcome from head injuries. J. Neurosurg., *48*:673–678, 1978.

191. Lanksch, W., Oettinger, W., Baethmann, A., et al.: CT findings in brain edema compared with direct chemical analysis of tissue samples. *In* Pappius, H. M., and Feindel, W., eds.: Dynamics of Brain Edema. New York, Springer-Verlag, 1976, pp. 283–287.

192. Larsen, G. N., Glenn, W., Kishore, P. R. S., et al.: Computer processing of CT images: Advances and Prospects. Neurosurgery, *1*:78–79, 1977.

193. Larson, S. J., Sances, A., Jr., and Christenson, P. C.: Evoked somatosensory potentials in man. Arch. Neurol. (Chicago), *15*:88–93, 1966.

194. Larson, S. J., Sances, A., Jr., Ackmann, J. J., and Reigel, D. H.: Noninvasive evaluation of head trauma patients. Surgery, *74*:34–40, 1973.

195. Lazorthes, G., and Campan, L.: Hypothermia in the treatment of craniocerebral traumatism. J. Neurosurg., *15*:162–167, 1958.

196. Levander, B., Stattin, S., and Svendsen, P.: Computer tomography of traumatic intra- and extracerebral lesions. Acta Radiol. suppl., *356*:107–118, 1975.

197. Levin, A.: The use of a fiberoptic intracranial pressure monitor in clinical practice. Neurosurgery, *1*:266–271, 1977.

198. Levine, J. E., and Becker, D. P.: Reversal of incipient brain death from head-injury apnea at the scene of accidents. New Eng. J. Med., *301*:109, 1979.

199. Lewin, W.: Cerebrospinal fluid rhinorrhea in non-missile injuries. Clin. Neurosurg., *12*:237–252, 1966.

200. Lewin, W.: Changing attitudes to the management of severe head injuries. Brit. Med. J., *2*:1234–1239, 1976.

201. Lewin, W.: The Management of Head Injuries. London, Bailliere, Tindall, & Cassell, 1966.

202. Lewin, W., and Kennedy, W. F. C.: Motorcyclist, crash helmets and head injuries. Brit. Med. J., *1*:1253–1259, 1956.

203. Liberson, W. T.: Study of evoked potentials in aphasics. Amer. J. Phys. Med., *45*:135–142, 1966.

204. Loeb, C., and Poggio, G.: Electroencephalograms in a case with pontomesencephalic haemorrhage. Electroenceph. Clin. Neurophysiol., *5*:295–296, 1953.

205. Long, D. M., and Maxwell, R. E.: Steroids in the treatment of head injury. *In* Vinken, P. J., and Bruyn, G. W., eds.: Handbook of Clinical Neurology. Vol. 24. Amsterdam, Elsevier–North Holland Publishing Co., 1976, pp. 627–635.

206. Long, D. M., Hartman, J. F., and French, L. A.: The response of experimental cerebral edema to glucosteroid administration. J. Neurosurg., *25*:843–854, 1966.

207. Lundberg, N.: Continuous recording and control of ventricular fluid pressure in neurosurgical practice. Acta Psychiat. Neurol. Scand., *36*:149:1–193, 1960.

208. Lundberg, N., Troupp, H., and Lorin, H.: Continuous recording of the ventricular fluid pressure in patients with severe acute traumatic brain injury. A preliminary report. J. Neurosurg., *22*:581–590, 1965.

209. Lynn, C. W.: Repeal and modification of mandatory motorcycle helmet legislation. Virginia Highway and Transportation Research Council. Highway Safety Division of Virginia, 1978.

210. Macewen, W.: Address on the surgery of brain and spinal cord. Lancet, *2*:254–264, 1988.

211. Maciver, I. N., Frew, I. J. C., and Matheson, J. G.: The role of respiratory insufficiency in the mortality of severe head injury. Lancet, *1*:390–393, 1958.

212. Maciver, I. N., Lassman, L. P., Thomson, C. W., et al.: Treatment of severe head injuries. Lancet, *13*:544–550, 1958.

213. Maltby, R. E.: Penetrating craniocerebral injuries: Evaluation of the late results in a group of 200 penetrating cranial war wounds. J. Neurosurg., *3*:239–249, 1946.

214. Markham, J. W., Stein, S., Pelligra, R., et al.: Use of centrifuge in the treatment of an intraventricular metallic foreign body. Technical note. J. Neurosurg., *34*:800–804, 1971.

215. Marr, W. G., and Marr, E. G.: Some observations on Purtscher's disease: Traumatic retinal angiography. Amer. J. Ophthal., *54*:693–705, 1962.

216. Marsh, M. L., Marshall, L. F., and Shapiro, H. M.: Neurosurgical intensive care. Anesthesiology, *47*:2:149–163, 1977.

217. Marshall, C., and Walker, A. E.: The value of electroencephalography in the prognostication and prognosis of post-traumatic epilepsy. Epilepsia, *2*:138–143, 1961.

218. Marshall, L. F., Smith, R. W., and Shapiro, H. M.: The outcome with aggressive treatment of severe head injury. Part I. The significance of intracranial pressure monitoring. J. Neurosurg., *50*:26–30, 1979.

219. Marshall, L. F., Bruce, S. A., Bueno, L., et al.: Vertebrobasilar spasm: A significant cause of neurological deficit in head injury. J. Neurosurg., *48*:560–564, 1978.

220. Martin, J., and Campbell, E. H.: Early complications following penetrating wounds of the skull. J. Neurosurg., *3*:58–73, 1946.

221. Matson, D. D.: The Treatment of Acute Cranio-

cerebral Injuries Due to Missiles. Springfield, Ill., Charles C Thomas, 1948.

222. Mayfield, F.: Personal communication, 1967.

223. McCullough, E. C., Baker, H. L., and Houser, O. W., et al.: An evaluation of the quantitative and radiation features of a scanning x-ray transverse axial tomograph: The EMI scanner. Radiology, *111*:709–715, 1974.

224. McKissock, W., Richardson, A., and Bloom, W. H.: Subdural hematoma. A review of 389 cases. Lancet, *1*:1365–1369, 1960.

225. McKissock, W., Taylor, J. C., Bloom, W. H., et al.: Extradural haematoma. Observations on 125 cases. Lancet, *2*:167–172, 1960.

226. McLaurin, R. L., and King, L. R.: Recognition and treatment of metabolic disorders after head injuries. Clin. Neurosurg., *19*:281–300, 1972.

227. McLaurin, R. L., and Tutor, F. T.: Acute subdural hematoma. Review of ninety cases. J. Neurosurg., *18*:61–67, 1961.

228. McLeod, G. H. B.: Notes on the surgery of the war in the Crimea, with remarks on the treatment of gunshot wounds. Philadelphia, J. B. Lippincott Co., 1862.

229. McNealy, D. E., and Plum, F.: Brainstem dysfunction with supratentorial mass lesions. Arch. Neurol. (Chicago), *7*:10–32, 1962.

230. Medical and Surgical History of the War of Rebellion (1861-1865). Vol. 1, Part 2. Washington, D.C., U.S. Government Printing Office, 1970–1978.

231. Meirowski, A. M.: Penetrating wounds of the brain. *In* Coates, J. B., ed.: Neurological Surgery of Trauma. Washington, D.C., Office of the Surgeon General, Dept. of the Army, 1965, p. 103.

232. Meirowski, A. M.: The retention of bone fragments in brain wounds. Milit. Med., *133*:887–890, 1968.

233. Meirowsky, A. M., and Harsh, G. R.: The surgical management of cerebritis complicating penetrating wounds of the brain. J. Neurosurg., *10*:373–379, 1953.

234. Meldrum, B. S., and Brierley, J. B.: Brain damage in the Rhesus monkey resulting from profound arterial hypotension. II. Changes in the spontaneous and evoked electrical activity of the neocortex. Brain Res., *13*:101–118, 1969.

235. Memon, M. Y., and Paine, K. W. E.: Direct injury of the oculomotor nerve in craniocerebral trauma. J. Neurosurg., *35*:461–464, 1971.

236. Merino-de-Villasante, J., and Taveras, J. M.: Computerized tomography (CT) in acute head trauma. Amer. J. Roentgen., *126*:765–778, 1976.

237. Merritt, H. H.: A Textbook of Neurology. 5th Ed. Philadelphia, Lea & Febiger, 1973, pp. 325–334.

238. Messina, A. V., and Chernick, N. L.: Computed tomography: The "resolving" intracerebral hemorrhage. Radiology, *118*:609–613, 1976.

239. Meyer-Mickeleit, R. W.: Das Elektrencephalogramm nach gedeckten Kopfverletzungen. Deutsch. Med. Wschr., *78*:480–484, 1953.

240. Miller, C. F., Brodkey, J. S., and Colombi, B. J.: The danger of intracranial wood. Surg. Neurol., *7*:95–103, 1977.

241. Miller, J. D.: Pressure and volume in the craniospinal axis. Clin. Neurosurg., *22*:76–105, 1975.

242. Miller, J. D., and Jennett, W. B.: Complications of depressed skull fractures. Lancet, *2*:991–995, 1968.

243. Miller, J. D., Becker, D. P., Ward, J. D., et al.: Significance of intracranial hypertension in severe head injury. J. Neurosurg., *47*:503–516, 1977.

244. Miller, J. D., Sweet, R. C., Narayan, R., et al.: Early insults to the injured brain. J.A.M.A. *240*:439–442, 1978.

245. Munro, D.: Cerebral subdural hematomas. A study of three hundred and ten verified cases. New Eng. J. Med., *227*:87–95, 1942.

246. Munro, D.: Compound fractures of the skull. The results of surgical therapy in two hundred and eighteen cases. New Eng. J. Med., *228*:737–745, 1943.

247. Munro, O., and Merritt, H. H.: Surgical pathology of subdural hematoma. (Based on 105 cases). Arch. Neurol. Psychiat., *35*:64–78, 1936.

248. Nadell, J., and Kline, D. G.: Primary reconstruction of depressed frontal skull fractures including those involving the sinus, orbit, and cribriform plate. J. Neurosurg., *41*:200–207, 1974.

249. Nathanson, M., Bergman, P. S., and Anderson, P. J.: Significance of oculocephalic and caloric responses in the conscious patient. Neurology (Minneap.), *7*:829–832, 1952.

250. National Safety Council: Accident Facts. Chicago, National Safety Council, 1970.

251. National Safety Council: Accident Facts. Chicago, National Safety Council, 1976.

252. Negron, R. A., Tirado, G., and Zapater, C.: Simple bedside technique for evacuating chronic subdural hematomas. Technical note. J. Neurosurg., *42*:609–611, 1975.

253. New, P. F., and Aronow, S.: Attenuation measurements of whole blood and blood fractions in computed tomography. Radiology, *121*:635–640, 1976.

254. Norton, G. A., Kishore, P. R. S., and Lin, J.: Contrast enhancement in cerebral infarctions on CT. Amer. J. Roentgen., *131*:881–885, 1978.

255. Northfield, D. W. C.: The Surgery of the Central Nervous System. Oxford, Blackwell Scientific Publications, 1973, pp. 782–784.

256. Odom, G. L.: Craniocerebral injuries. *In* Sabiston D.C., ed.: Textbook of Surgery. Philadelphia, W. B. Saunders Co., 1977, pp. 1483–1487.

257. Ommaya, A. K., and Gennarelli, T.: Cerebral concussion and traumatic unconsciousness. Correlation of experimental and clinical observations on blunt head injuries. Brain, *97*:633–654, 1974.

258. Ommaya, A. K., and Gennarelli, T. A.: Experimental head injury. *In* Vinken, P. J., and Bruyn, G. W., eds.: Handbook of Clinical Neurology. Vol. 23. Amsterdam, Elsevier–North Holland Publishing Co., 1975, pp. 67–90.

259. Ommaya, A. K., and Gennarelli, T. A.: A physiopathologic basis for noninvasive diagnosis and prognosis of head injury severity. *In* McLaurin, R. L., ed.: Head Injuries. New York, Grune & Stratton Inc., 1976, pp. 49–75.

260. Ommaya, A. K., Murray, G., Ambrose, J., et al.: Computerized axial tomography: Estimation of

spatial and density resolution capability. Brit. J. Radiol., *49*:604–611, 1976.

261. Osborn, A. G.: Diagnosis of descending transtentorial herniation by cranial computed tomography. Radiology, *123*:93–96, 1977.

262. Ott, K., Tarlov, E., Crowell, R., and Papadakis, N.: Retained intracranial metallic foreign bodies. J. Neurosurg., *44*:80–83, 1976.

263. Pagni, C. A.: The prognosis of head injured patients in a state of coma with decerebrated posture. J. Neurosurg. Sci., *17*:289–295, 1973.

264. Parkinson, D., and Chockinov, H.: Subdural Hematomas—some observations on their postoperative course. J. Neurosurg., *17*:901–904, 1960.

265. Patterson, J., and Hardy, E.: Personal communication, 1977.

266. Paxton, R., and Ambrose, J.: The EMI scanner. A brief review of the first 650 patients. Brit. J. Radiol., *47*:530–565, 1974.

267. Pazzaglia, P., Frank, F., et al.: Clinical course and prognosis of acute post-traumatic coma. J. Neurol. Neurosurg. Psychiat., *38*:149–154, 1975.

268. Penry, K.: Personal communication, 1978.

269. Petty, J. M.: Epistaxis from aneurysm of the internal carotid artery due to a gunshot wound. Case report. J. Neurosurg., *30*:741–743, 1966.

270. Picton, T. W., Hillyard, S. A., Krausz, H. I., and Galambos, R.: Human auditory evoked potentials. I. Evaluation of components. Electroenceph. Clin. Neurophysiol., *36*:179–190, 1974.

271. Pitlyk, P. J., Tolchin, S., and Steward, W.: The experimental significance of retained intracranial bone fragments. J. Neurosurg., *33*:19–24, 1970.

272. Plum, F., and Posner, J. B.: The Diagnosis of Stupor and Coma. 2nd Ed. Philadelphia, F. A. Davis Co., 1972.

273. Poole, E. W.: Some aspects of electroencephalographic disturbances following head injury. J. Clin. Path., *23*: suppl. (Roy. Coll. Path.) 4: 187–201, 1970.

274. Poppen, J. L.: Chronic subdural hematomas. Geriatrics, *10*:49–51, 1955.

275. Putnam, T., and Cushing, H.: Chronic subdural hematoma. Arch. Surg. (Chicago), *2*:329–393, 1925.

276. Rabe, E. F., Flynn, R. E., and Dodge, P. R.: A study of subdural effusions in an infant with particular reference to their mechanisms of persistence. Neurology (Minneap.), *12*:79–92, 1962.

277. Raimondi, A. I., and Samuelson, G. H.: Craniocerebral gunshot wounds in civilian practice. J. Neurosurg., *17*:483–485, 1970.

278. Rand, B. O., Ward, A. A., and White, L. E., Jr.: The use of the twist drill to evaluate head trauma. J. Neurosurg., *25*:410–415, 1966.

279. Ransohoff, J., Benjamin, M. V., Gage, E. L., Jr., et al.: Hemicraniectomy in the management of acute subdural hematoma. J. Neurosurg., *34*:70–76, 1971.

280. Ransohoff, J., and Fleischer, A.: Head injuries. J.A.M.A., *234*:8:861–864, 1975.

281. Rapport, R. L., and Penry, J. K.: Pharmacologic prophylaxis of post-traumatic epilepsy. Epilepsia, *13*:295–304, 1972.

282. Rapport, R. L., and Penry, J. K.: A survey of attitudes toward the pharmacological prophy-

laxis of post-traumatic epilepsy. J. Neurosurg., *38*:159–166, 1973.

283. Reeves, A. G., and Posner, J. B.: The ciliospinal reflex in man. Neurology (Minneap.), *19*:1145–1152, 1969.

284. Reilly, P. L., Graham, D. I., Adams, J. H., et al.: Patients with head injury who talk and die. Lancet, *2*:375–377, 1975.

285. Richards, T., and Hoff, J.: Factors affecting survival from acute subdural hematoma. Surgery, *75*:253–258, 1974.

286. Ringkjøb, R.: Care at the road-side—prevention of the second accident. *In* Head Injuries. Proceedings of an International Symposium. Edinburgh and London, Churchill Livingstone, 1971, pp. 32–36.

287. Rish, B. L.: The repair of venous sinus wounds by autogenous venorrhaphy. J. Neurosurg., *35*:392–395, 1971.

288. Roberson, F. C., Kishore, P. R. S., Miller, J. D., et al.: The value of serial computerized tomography in the management of head injury. Surg. Neurol., *12*:161–167, 1979.

289. Robinson, D. A.: Oculomotor control signals in basic mechanisms of ocular motility and their clinical implications. Oxford, Pergamon Press, 1975.

290. Robinson, R. G.: The treatment of subacute and chronic subdural hematomas. Brit. Med. J., *1*:21–22, 1955.

291. Rodin, E. A.: Contribution of the EEG to prognosis after head injury. Dis. Nerv. Syst., *28*:595–601, 1967.

292. Rodin, E., Whelan, J., Taylor, R., Tomita, T., Grisell, J., Thomas, L. M., and Gurdjian, E. S.: The electroencephalogram in acute head injuries. J. Neurosurg., *23*:329–337, 1965.

293. Rose, J., Valtonen, S., and Jennett, B.: Avoidable factors contributing to death after head injury. Brit. Med. J., *2*:615–618, 1977.

294. Rosner, M. J., and Becker, D. P.: ICP monitoring: Complications and associated factors. Clin. Neurosurg., *23*:494–519, 1976.

295. Rossanda, M.: Prolonged hyperventilation in treatment of unconscious patients with severe brain injuries. Scand. J. Clin. Lab. Invest., *22*:suppl. 102:13:E, 1968.

296. Rossanda, M., Selenati, A., Villa, C., et al.: Role of automatic ventilation in treatment of severe head injuries. J. Neurol. Sci., *17*:265–270, 1973.

297. Rowbotham, G. R.: Acute Injuries of the Head. Baltimore, William & Wilkins Co., 1945 and 1966.

298. Rowe, S. N., and Turner, O. A.: Observations on infection in penetrating wounds of the head. J. Neurosurg., *2*:391–401, 1945.

299. Russell, W. R., and Nathan, P. W.: Traumatic amnesia. Brain, *69*:280–300, 1946.

300. Russell, W. R., and Smith, A.: Post-traumatic amnesia in closed head injury. Arch. Neurol. (Chicago), *5*:16–29, 1961.

301. Saunders, B. B., and VanderArk, G. D.: Transverse fracture of the clivus. J. Neurosurg., *39*:271–304, 1963.

302. Schnieder, R. C.: Craniocerebral trauma. *In* Kahn, E. A., Crosby, E. C., Schnieder, R. C., and Taren, J. A., eds.: Correlative Neurosurgery. Springfield, Ill., Charles C Thomas, 1969, pp. 533–596.

303. Schnieder, R. C.: *In* Kahn, E. A., ed.: Neurosurgery. Springfield, Ill., Charles C Thomas, 1969, p. 569.

304. Scotti, G., Terbrugge, K., Melancon, D., et al.: Evaluation of the age of subdural hematomas by computerized tomography. J. Neurosurg., *47*:311–315, 1977.

305. Selhorst, J. B., Hoyt, W. F., Feinsod, M., and Hosobuchi, Y.: Midbrain corectopia. Arch. Neurol. (Chicago), *33*:193–195, 1976.

306. Shapiro, H. M., Wyte, S. R., and Loeser, J.: Barbiturate-augmented hypothermia for reduction of persistent intracranial hypertension. J. Neurosurg., *40*:90–100, 1974.

307. Shapiro, H. M., Galindo, A., Wyte, S. R., et al.: Rapid intraoperative reduction of intracranial hypertension with thiopentone. Brit. J. Anaesth., *45*:1957–2062, 1973.

308. Sharpe, J. A., Rosenberg, M. A., Hoyt, W. F., and Paroff, R. B.: Paralytic pontine exotropia. Neurology (Minneap.), *24*:1076–1081, 1974.

309. Sherman, J. J.: Brass foreign body in the brainstem: A case report. J. Neurosurg., *17*:483–485, 1960.

310. Sights, W. P., and Bye, R. I.: The fate of retained intracerebral shotgun pellets. An experimental study. J. Neurosurg., *33*:646–653, 1970.

311. Simon, R. P.: Delayed forced down gaze during oculovestibular testing in sedative drug-induced coma. Neurology (Minneap.), *27*:346, 1977.

312. Sindou, M., Mayoyer, J., Fischer, G., Pialat, J., and Fourcase, C.: Experimental bypass for sagittal sinus repair: Preliminary report. J. Neurosurg., *44*:325–330, 1976.

313. Skillman, J. J.: Respiratory insufficiency. *In* Skillman, J. J., ed.: Intensive Care. Boston, Little, Brown & Co. 1975, pp. 513–528.

314. Small, J. M., and Turner, E. A.: A surgical experience of 1,200 cases of penetrating brain wounds in battle NW Europe, 1944–1945. Brit. J. Surg., War Surg. suppl. 1:62–74, 1971.

315. Spence, R. W., Celestin, L. R., and McCormick, D. A.: The effect on gastric acid output of three months' treatment with cimetidine. *In* Burland, W. L., and Simkens, M. A., eds.: Cimetidine; Proceedings of the Second International Symposium on Histamine H$_2$-Receptor Antagonists. Amsterdam, Oxford, Excerpta Medica Foundation, 1977, pp. 101–109.

316. Stanley, J. A., and Baise, G. R.: The swinging flashlight test to detect minimal optic neuropathy. Arch. Ophthal. (Chicago), *80*:769–771, 1968.

317. Starr, A.: Auditory brainstem responses in brain death. Brain, *99*:543–554, 1976.

318. Starr, A., and Achor, L. J.: Auditory brainstem responses in neurological disease. Arch. Neurol. (Chicago), *32*:761–768, 1975.

319. Starr, A., and Hamilton, A. E.: Correlation between confirmed sites of neurological lesions and abnormalities of far field auditory brainstem responses. Electroenceph. Clin. Neurophysiol., *41*:595–608, 1976.

320. Staub, R. L., and Black, F. W.: The Mental Status Examination in Neurology. Philadelphia, F. A. Davis Co., 1977.

321. Sternbergh, W. C. A., Watts, C., and Clark, K.: Bullet within the fourth ventricle. Case report. J. Neurosurg., *34*:805–807, 1971.

322. Stockard, J. J., Bickford, R. G., and Aung, M. H.: The electroencephalogram in traumatic brain injury. *In* Vinken, P. J., Bruyn, G. W., and Braaken, R., eds.: Handbook of Clinical Neurology. Vol. 15. New York, Elsevier, 1975, pp. 317–367.

323. Stohr, P. E., and Goldring, S.: Origin of somatosensory evoked scalp responses in man. J. Neurosurg., *31*:117–127, 1969.

324. Stritch, S. J.: Diffuse degeneration of the cerebral white matter in severe dementia following head injury. J. Neurol. Neurosurg. Psychiat., *19*:163–185, 1956.

325. Stritch, S. J., and Oxon, D. M.: Shearing of nerve fibers as a cause of brain damage due to head injury. Lancet, *2*:443–448, 1961.

326. Sugita, K., Doi, T., Sato, O., et al.: Successful removal of intracranial air-gun bullet with stereotaxic apparatus. Case report. J. Neurosurg., *30*:177–181, 1969.

327. Sukoff, M. H., Helmer, F. A., and Plaut, M. R.: Retained intracranial fragments following missile injuries. Bull. Los Angeles Neurol. Soc., *36*:64–71, 1971.

328. Sullivan, H. G., Miller, J. D., Becker, D. P., et al.: The physiological basis of intracranial pressure change with progressive epidural brain compression. An experimental evaluation in cats. J. Neurosurg., *47*:532–550, 1977.

329. Sunderland, S., and Bradley, K. C.: Disturbances of oculomotor function accompanying extradural hemorrhage. J. Neurol. Neurosurg. Psychiat., *16*:35–46, 1953.

330. Suzuki, J., and Takau, A.: Non-surgical treatment of chronic subdural hematoma. J. Neurosurg., *33*:549–553, 1970.

331. Svendsen, P.: Computer tomography of traumatic extracerebral lesions. Brit. J. Radio., *49*:1004–1012, 1976.

332. Sweet, R. C., Miller, J. D., Lipper, M. H., et al.: Significance of bilateral abnormalities on the CT scan in patients with severe head injury. Neurosurgery, *3*:16–21, 1978.

333. Symonds, C.: Concussion and its sequelae. Lancet, *1*:1–5, 1962.

334. Szentagothai, J.: The elementary vestibulo-ocular reflex arc. J. Neurophysiol., *13*:395–407, 1950.

335. Tabaddor, K., and Shulman, K.: Definitive treatment of chronic subdural hematoma by twist drill craniotomy and closed drainage system. J. Neurosurg., *46*:220–226, 1977.

336. Taylor, J., and Ballance, C. A.: A case of large blood cyst in the arachnoid space simulating brain tumor: Operation; recovery. Lancet, *29*:597–599, 1903.

337. Teal, J. S., Bergeron, R. T., Rumbaugh, C. L., et al.: Aneurysms of the petrous or cavernous portions of the internal carotid artery associated with nonpenetrating head trauma. J. Neurosurg., *38*:568–574, 1973.

338. Teasdale, G., and Jennett, B.: Assessment of coma and impaired consciousness. Lancet, *2*:81–84, 1974.

339. Teasdale, G., and Jennett, B.: Assessment and prognosis of coma after head injury. Acta Neurochir. (Wien), *34*:45–55, 1976.

340. Tindall, G. T., Patton, J. M., Durian, J. J., et al.: Monitoring of patients with head injuries. Clin. Neurosurg., *22*:332–363, 1975.

341. Troland, C. E.: Head injuries and infections. *In* Horsley, G. W., and Bigger, I. A., eds.: Operative Surgery, 6th Ed. St. Louis, C. V. Mosby Co. 1953, pp. 1446–1467.

342. Trotter, W.: Chronic subdural hemorrhage of traumatic origin and its relation to pachymeningitis hemorrhagica interna. Brit. J. Surg., 2:271–291, 1914–1915.

343. Tso, M. O. M., and Hayreh, S. S.: Optic disc edema in raised intracranial pressure. Part III. Arch. Ophthal. (Chicago), 95:1448–1457, 1977.

344. Tso, M. O. M., and Hayreh, S. S.: Optic disc edema in raised intracranial pressure. Part IV. Arch. Ophthal. (Chicago), 95:1458–1462, 1977.

345. U.S. Department of Health, Education, and Welfare: Facts of Life and Death. Publication number (HRS) 74-1222. National Center for Health Statistics. Rockville, Md., 1974.

346. U.S. Department of Transportation: News release, 1977.

347. Vaughan, H. C., Jr., and Katzman, R.: Evoked response in visual disorders. Ann. N.Y. Acad. Sci., 112:305–319, 1964.

348. Victor, M.: The amnestic syndrome and its anatomical basis. Canad. Med. J., 100:1115–1125, 1969.

349. Virchow, R.: Diekrankhaften Gasohwelste, Berlin 1, 140, 1863. Cited by Putnam and Cushing, 1925 (ref. 275).

350. Walker, A. E., and Jablon, S.: A follow-up study of head wounds in World War II. VA Medical Monograph 5. Washington, D.C., U.S. Government Printing Office, 1961.

351. Wallace, P. B., and Meirowsky, A. M.: The repair of dural defects by graft. Ann. Surg., 151:174–180, 1960.

352. Walsh, F. B., and Hoyt, W. F.: Clinical Neuro-Ophthalmology. Vol. 3. Baltimore, Williams & Wilkins Co., 1969.

353. Watanabe, S., Shimada, H., and Ishil, S.: Production of the clinical form of chronic subdural hematoma in experimental animals. J. Neurosurg., 37:552–561, 1972.

354. Watts, C., and Clark, K.: Effects of an anti-cholinergic drug on gastric acid secretion in the comatose patient. Surg. Gynec. Obstet., 130:61–63, 1970.

355. Weir, B.: The osmolality of subdural hematoma fluid. J. Neurosurg., 34:528–533, 1971.

356. Whaley, N.: Acute subdural hematoma amenable to surgical treatment. Lancet, 1:213–214, 1948.

357. White, R.: Programmed management of severe head injuries revisited. J. Trauma, 15:779–784, 1975.

358. Wilkins, R. H., and Odom, G. L.: Intracranial arterial spasm associated with craniocerebral trauma. J. Neurosurg., 32:626–633, 1970.

359. Wilkus, R. J., Harvey, F., Ojemann, L. M., and Lettich, E.: Electroencephalogram and sensory evoked potentials. Arch. Neurol. (Chicago), 24:538–544, 1971.

360. Williams, D.: The electroencephalogram in acute head injuries. J. Neurol. Psychiat., 4:107–130, 1941.

361. Wing, S. D., Norman, D., Pollock, J. A., et al.: Contrast enhancement of cerebral infarcts in computed tomography. Radiology, 121:89–92, 1976.

362. Yashon, D., Jane, J. A., Martonffy, D., and White, R. J.: Management of civilian craniocerebral bullet injuries. Amer. Surg., 38:346–351, 1972.

363. Yock, D. H., and Marshall, W. H.: Recent ischemic brain infarcts at computed tomography: Appearances pre- and post-contrast infusion. Radiology, 117:599–608, 1975.

364. Youmans, J. R.: Causes of shock with head injury. J. Trauma, 4:204–209, 1964.

365. Zollinger, R., and Gross, R. E.: Traumatic subdural hematoma. An explanation of the late onset of pressure symptoms. J.A.M.A., 103:245–249, 1934.

59

DIAGNOSIS AND TREATMENT OF HEAD INJURY IN CHILDREN

Children are not little adults; infants are not little children! This adage is particularly emphasized in pediatric craniocerebral trauma, in which major age-related differences exist in the type of head injury; in the clinical pathological reaction of the immature or rapidly growing brain, skull, and dura to injury; and in the long-term prognosis. Probably few children reach adulthood without sustaining some degree of craniocerebral trauma. Injuries are the major cause of childhood death after 1 year of age; they are second only to respiratory infection as reasons for hospital admission.[31] Craniocerebral trauma is the major feature in 30 per cent of accidents. The mortality rate for childhood head injury is about 1.5 per cent. Multiple facets of morbidity remain under active investigation, and many of them still defy attempts at meaningful functional neurological classification.[156]

This chapter focuses on features of craniocerebral trauma that are unique to children or differ significantly from those of the same entity in the adult. One must make a conscious attempt to consider relative developmental maturity of the patient's brain and its coverings in parallel with more obvious aspects of the lesion. For example, endocrine and metabolic responses vary with the temporal development of the relevant organ systems at the time of injury. Psychosocial developmental progress of a child may be seriously disrupted by even apparently minor head injury, and the residua

of trauma may secondarily alter subsequent evolution of behavior, the effects ranging from the ill-defined "minimal brain dysfunction" to severe hyperactivity or learning disorder or frank antisocial behavior.

Included in the broad category of childhood head trauma is the vast complex of pre- and perinatal lesions that present indirectly to the pediatric neurosurgeon. While etiological mechanisms may differ from postnatal injury, one can hardly dispute, for example, that passage through the birth canal is a traumatic event for the infant skull and cerebrum.[117]

A number of nonclinical problems accompany the care of children with head injury, not the least of which are moral and ethical, involving "informed consent" for the child, interpreted by the parent or physician.[41,201] In the child with severe brain injury, the decision to continue therapy, the raison d'être of the physician, itself becomes controversial; the many uncertainties of prognosis and vagaries of newer methods of treatment all too often lead to a respirator stalemate.

EPIDEMIOLOGY

Approximately 10 per cent of all fatal head injuries occur before the tenth year.[50] Granted that the number of children affected by the morbidity of craniocerebral trauma is considerable, certain factors have emerged to subdivide the data.[32,94,194] It has

R. L. McLAURIN AND J. E. McLENNAN

been emphasized that injuries are not "accidents"; a definite epidemiology exists, which allows countermeasures to be set up.[39,75]

Boys are most often involved in head injury at all ages, although sex differences are minor under 5 years of age. In a series of 5800 emergency ward visits during one year by children with craniocerebral injury, Harwood-Nash and co-workers report that 2200 received some form of neurosurgical consultation and 760 were admitted to the hospital.[77,78] Skull fractures accompany 26 per cent of all pediatric head injuries, and the majority of these children are admitted to the hospital for this injury. Skull fracture accompanies about 60 per cent of fatal head trauma in children under 10 years, while in persons over 10 years the rate is about 75 per cent.[50]

The type of trauma to the skull may determine the nature of the bony damage, whether a penetrating wound, a local depressed fracture from a blunt blow, or a fall with coup and contrecoup brain injury. The developmental maturity of the brain is a major determinant of the tissue reaction; the maturity of the skull frequently dictates its response to injury—for example, the thin and pliable infant skull may spontaneously re-expand following focal depression. Open sutures in general protect the brain, particularly from the ravages of increased intracranial pressure; traumatically split sutures, however, have the same significance as a fracture of the parietes.

The peak incidence of childhood head injury occurs under 1 year of age; over 50 per cent of these cases are due to "birth trauma." Despite their mixed etiology, this group of injuries is a major category to be considered by the neurosurgeon. A smaller second peak incidence is found between 3 and 4 years.[77,82] Most children under the

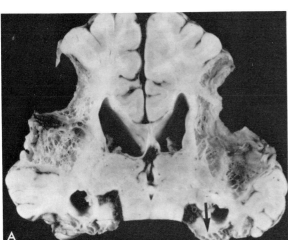 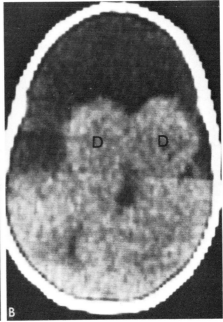

Figure 59–1 Examples of early developmental loss of cerebral tissue. The resulting clinical deficit depends on the area of tissue lost and the age at the time of insult. *A*. Coronal section of the brain from an 11-year-old girl. At 18 months the child fell from a chair and struck the left side of the head. She was not unconscious but became apneic and required resuscitation. Two weeks later she was admitted to the hospital with seizures and progressive obtundation. There was no skull fracture or intracranial hematoma. Metabolic and degenerative diseases were ruled out. The child slowly regained consciousness but remained severely spastic and mentally deficient until her death. The brain weighed 950 gm at autopsy and showed striking symmetrical cystic degeneration of the territory of both middle cerebral arteries. The inferior-medial temporal regions (*arrow*) were also involved. The middle cerebral arteries were most likely occluded by cerebral swelling in their horizontal segments, which led to total infarction of the dependent cerebral tissue. The inferior-medial temporal regions were no doubt compressed at the tentorial hiatus. *B*. Computed tomographic brain scan of an infant demonstrating the entity of "hydranencephaly" resulting from in utero occlusion (or maldevelopment) of major carotid circulation bilaterally. The vertebrobasilar system appears to have developed normally, and diencephalic structures (D) are preserved.

age of 3 are injured in the home environment; during the first year the accident is generally attributed to carelessness of the child's guardian, whether this be dropping the child, allowing a sibling to injure him, or a sin of omission such as failure to protect him from open stairways. The majority of "battered child" instances occur in the first year; the difficulties of discovering the true mechanism of injury are legion. The toddler is at particular risk because eagerness is not tempered with the caution of a few years' experience.

Injury due to the automobile or other moving vehicles increases markedly between ages 4 and 8 years and then falls off, presumably as the child learns of these dangers. In one series, 12 per cent of injuries occurred in school between ages 5 and 13 years.[32] After the age of 13 years the data are not particularly significant epidemiologically. Serious head injury due to participation in sports does not primarily involve children, because the momentum involved is small despite the inexperience of the young athlete.[17,70] A recent exception to this might be the skateboard accident, which has been responsible for many thousand injuries and the cause of at least 10 reported deaths in 1978 alone; the combination of hard surface, high speed, and unstable base make this "vehicle" potentially lethal. In general, cerebral injury in children leads to less permant neurological and behavioral deficit than in adults.[32] The applicability of this widely accepted tenet tails off rapidly, however, with increasing age (particularly after 2 years), and it must be tempered by the limitation of current neurological evaluation and follow-up (Fig. 59–1).

MAJOR DETERMINANTS OF PEDIATRIC BRAIN INJURY

Substrate of Craniocerebral Injury

Figure 59–2 shows the overall mass of the human brain from conception through 2 years of age. This curve was derived from fresh brain weights at autopsy in a total of 415 cases in which there was no cerebral abnormality. The outstanding features of this growth function are (1) rapid exponential gain in brain mass reaching a maximum

acceleration at about 20 weeks and a maximum velocity at about 38 weeks of gestation, just before term; (2) continuation of near-maximum growth rate through term delivery and for several postnatal months; and (3) deceleration of growth beginning at about 1 year to a plateau that provides the 2-year-old child with a brain that has 90 per cent of adult mass.[152] The brain is the only human organ with this preadolescent growth spurt in temporal association with a relatively small body and otherwise small organ systems. The immediate ontogenetic consequence of this growth pattern, perhaps a vital one for evolution of a dominant species, is that the human child is able to benefit comparatively early in life from the experience of previous generations and may master the intellectual tools at a point when he has a number of years remaining to add his own input to the advancement of mankind. Animals with relatively long periods of learning compared with total life span could not develop this potential even if the anatomical complexity of the brain permitted. There is increasing evidence that normal development of the brain, principally the vast arborization of neuronal dendrites and dendritic spines, requires significant contribution from the environment, that is, from more "mature" humans.

Pertinent to cerebral injury, the components that collectively contribute to brain mass may be listed as: (1) neural (somatic) cellular elements, neurons and glia; (2) myelin; accompanied by (3) a vast elaboration of dendrites and axons; and (4) vascular supporting structures (cf. Fig. 59–2). The distribution of water between extra- and intracellular compartments is relatively stable after birth, although its volume decreases as myelin increases. All the neurons are probably present early in the third trimester and are essentially irreplaceable if lost to trauma; the complexity of dendritic interconnections expands tremendously during the first year of life in response to endogenous (genetic) programming and environmental stimulus.

The critical myelinization schedule has been observed by gross and microscopic examination of the developing human telencephalon, diencephalon, and brain stem.[57,59,226] This precise chronological ordering of myelinization accompanying ongoing dendritic synaptic formation, likely, in part, accounts for the so-called "devel-

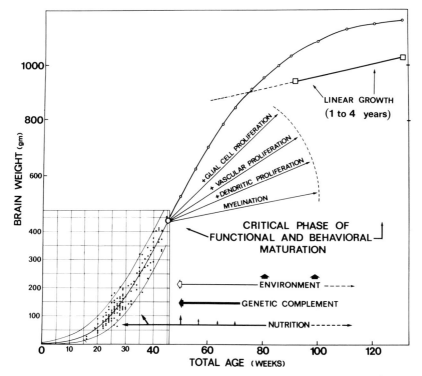

Figure 59–2 Brain growth from conception through two postnatal years. Gain in mass of the human brain is shown from conception through term gestation, 40 weeks (solid line with 95 per cent confidence interval) and from term through 120 weeks total age (O———O). The postnatal portion of the curve is an extrapolation of the double exponential function generated by the prenatal data points. Four major components of mass are noted. Data from the literature of the last 50 years suggest that brain growth is nearly linear from 1 to 4 years after birth (□———□). After the initial exponential growth phase, mass accretion slows markedly by 2 years, when over 80 per cent of the adult brain weight has been reached. This rapid growth phase is permissive of critical functional maturation. Environment, genetic factors, and nutrition have major, temporally variable influence over human brain development and maturation. Outcome of cerebral trauma in this growth period must contend with disruption of these complex developmental interactions. (Data, collected during the Collaborative Perinatal Project of the National Institutes of Health, and curve for prenatal human brain growth from McLennan, J. E., and Gilles, F. H.: A growth model for the total weight of the prenatal human brain. Trans. Amer. Neurol. Ass., *101*:271–272, 1976.

opmental milestones" of the human infant. Even focal trauma may destroy a critical ongoing system development. It is apparent that proper *function* of cerebral, spinal, and peripheral white matter requires myelin (originating from Schwann cells peripherally and oligodendroglia centrally) to effect the only known mechanism for interaction of the neuronal mass with the environment. Considerably less apparent, however, is a dependence of axonal and dendritic growth and differentiation on these wrapping membranes.

Major difficulties occur in defining and following alteration in the various post-traumatic states of cerebral malfunction in children. Prior to injury there is often little evidence regarding the potential intellectual and behavioral development of a young child; the post-traumatic status is therefore ambiguous. Hemiplegia is easily attributed to trauma in a previously "normal" child; hyperactivity or learning disorder is not. The best control for a given child might be a sibling, but this criterion is far from foolproof, and in fact, sibling (or birth order)–precipitated states of behavioral aberration are frequently invoked. Currently a number of studies provide evidence that many facets of neurological and behavioral morbidity from earlier cerebral trauma exist in children who have been found "normal" on follow-up. Experiments on lower animals purporting, for example, to show no permanent effect from simple concussion or even repeated concussion are not relevant to the vastly more complex human situation.[174] The estimation of morbidity can be only as subtle as the current methods of its discovery. Sophisticated tests, such as those for central auditory dysfunction, may well pinpoint the anatomical and functional substrate of post-traumatic morbidity that has been overlooked in the physician's natural tendency toward enthusiasm for "complete" recovery.[105,207] It is apparent that a number of uncomplicated concussions are not totally reversible.

Thus, in what follows, explanations of pathophysiology must be taken at face value. Post-traumatic changes in the cerebrum are largely structural (described from neuropathological studies) or perhaps electrical (derived from electroencephalograms, evoked potentials); these studies do not presume to give much information about functional mechanisms. The ability to unravel complex central circuitry, in fact, presents a problem because of the indeterminacy of the wiring diagram.[178] Understanding of single neuronal responses, biochemical and electrical properties of synapses, and perhaps two or three neuron "circuits" is currently possible and does point to limited principles of function.

Age and Brain Maturity

Mechanisms of cerebral injury and response to injury are different in the child under about 5 months of age.[126] Stress to the head sufficient to cause damage to cerebral tissue results in "tears" in the white matter rather than the contusion and hemorrhage most often found beyond this age. Presumably this response is due to the different elastic properties of the immature brain, the compliance of the infant skull, and the smoothness of the intracranial fossae. The tears, underlying intact dura, result in cavities in the white matter, often containing blood at first and later eventuating in smooth-walled, glial scar–lined excavations or slits with faint brown staining of the walls. These cavities only rarely involve the cortical band; accompanying classic wedge-shaped contusion foci in the same brain are unusual. In many of these cases the apparent contusions are probably the result of ischemia rather than trauma.[51] Although 5 to 6 months after term delivery is a rough dividing point between resulting tears and resulting contusions, obviously myelination is a steadily acquisitional process that varies from child to child; myelin is a major factor in brain compliance.

Courville found in an autopsy study that there is a significant age dependency of lesion distribution.[30] Contrecoup injury occurs in only 10 per cent of children under 3 years, increases to 25 per cent between 3 and 4 years, to 70 per cent in older children, and reaches 85 per cent in the adult. Relevant here is the pliability of the infant skull and the compressibility of the brain; both features allow focal absorption of energy rather than causing acceleration of the cerebrum or, at least, a "fluid wave" across the intracranial cavity to induce a lesion opposite the point of the accelerating force. Because of this age distribution of contrecoup injury, cerebral contusion is relatively rare in young children.

The type of brain injury, as well as its frequency, is also a function of the victim's age. Significant intracerebral hematomas are rare in newborns, as are acute epidural or subdural hematomas; if these lesions occur there are usually contributory circumstances such as traumatic breech delivery.[2,51] The maturity of the brain largely dictates the frequency of intraventricular hemorrhage emanating from the subependymal germinal matrix. Eighty per cent of premature infants studied at postmortem between 28 and 32 weeks of gestation have some degree of matrix hemorrhage; by 35 weeks the matrix has largely involuted, and similar lesions at term must be exceedingly rare. This hemorrhage may be more a physiological mechanism than a traumatic one; in particular, the bleed, or at least the intraventricular rupture, occurs several hours after delivery while the premature infant is safely tucked away in his incubator.[43,60,76,219] Hyaline membranes frequently coexist; the evidence causally linking hyaline membranes and intraventricular hemorrhage is scanty and largely inseparable from the common independent variable of prematurity.[122] One possible separation is that transvaginal delivery predisposes to intracerebral hemorrhage from any site while protecting against hyaline membranes and respiratory distress syndrome; the converse holds for caesarian delivery, but the effect on hemorrhage protection is small.

Figure 59–3 presents a patient who was delivered at term, weighing 8 lb, but nonetheless had a massive intraventricular hemorrhage shortly thereafter that apparently came from the region of the germinal matrix. The age and birth weight of this child

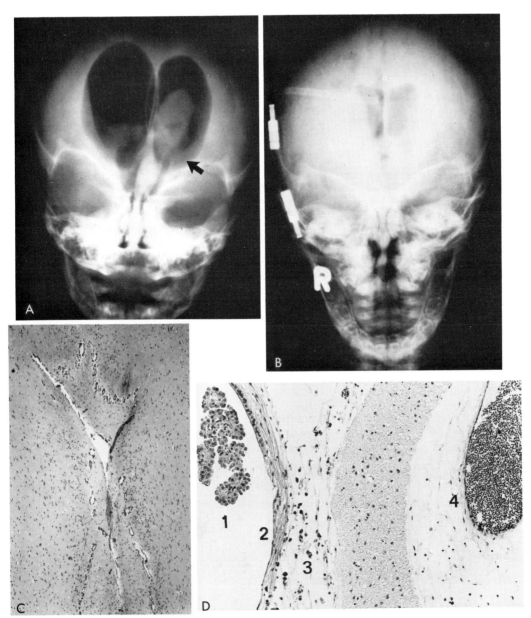

Figure 59–3 Intraventricular hemorrhage. *A*. Ventriculogram made on second day after birth shows acutely enlarged ventricles and a pedunculated mass in the left ventricle extending into the foramen of Monro. The apparent stalk of this clot extends to the region of the former subependymal germinal matrix in the lateral wall of the frontal horn. *B*. Ventriculogram one week after placement of a ventriculoperitoneal cerebrospinal fluid shunt. The ventricles have returned to nearly normal size. *C*. Histological section at 1 year of age demonstrates obstruction of the aqueduct with recanalization, numerous buried ependymal "rosettes," and subependymal residual hemosiderin. *D*. Histological section through lateral wall of the left ventricle demonstrates: (1) normal choroid plexus in ventricular cavity, (2) remote disruption of the ependymal lining of ventricle, (3) cystic gliosis and hemosiderin deep to the ependyma in the region of the former germinal matrix, and (4) normal segment of terminal (striothalamic) vein. All these findings support remote hemorrhage from the germinal matrix. (Histological material kindly provided by the division of Neuropathology, Stanford University School of Medicine and The Santa Clara Valley Medical Center.)

make it exceedingly unlikely that the hemorrhage could have emanated from the subependymal germinal matrix region despite the rather strong histological proof. (Management of intraventricular hematoma in the newborn is considered in a later section.) Intraventricular hemorrhage in a term baby is much more likely to come from the choroid plexus (Fig. 59–4). In the case shown in Figure 59–3 one cannot be dogmatic about the source of the hemorrhage, since evidence supports both plexus and matrix origin. Term babies or preterm babies with large heads may incur posterior fossa subdural hematomas; these are probably due to excessive molding of the occipital region resulting in tears of the underside of the tentorium.[58] Tentorial and falx hematomas are relatively common in newborns dying from other than cerebral causes. Posterior fossa subdural hematoma presents generally as progressive hydrocephalus after the first week of life, but may cause acute brain stem compression as well.

The stage of cerebral development, therefore, determines to a large degree the nature and consequences of pediatric head injury and "birth trauma." Parallel and interdependent development of the skull, sinuses, face, dura, and brain modify these processes.[13] The plasticity of the newborn skull allows amazing overlapping of the parietes during normal transvaginal delivery, generally without consequence for the severely molded cerebrum.[16] This same plasticity of bone and open sutures tempers both the acute nature of the head injury in infants and the later results of intracranial pressure and progressive ischemia. Modulation of these frequently fatal secondary effects of cerebral trauma is a major factor permissive of functional recovery in infants.

Mechanism of Injury

Many studies have been done on the nature of acceleration, deceleration, and torsional force vectors and their consequences for intracranial contents.[172,190] These hold, in general, for the young brain as well as the adult. One of the most attractive physical models for the mechanism of intracranial trauma without skull fracture is the "cavitation" hypothesis for an acutely accelerated fluid-filled spherical shell. The negative pressure that develops at the point opposite the application of the force vector may be a reasonable explanation for contrecoup contusion, and perhaps for superficial and deeper hematomas.[112,190] Most injuries

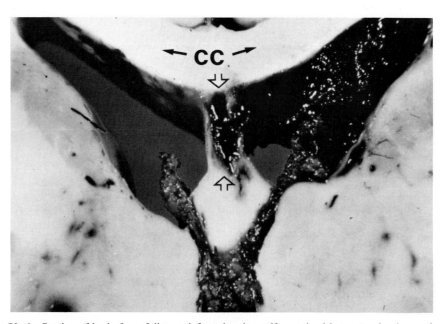

Figure 59–4 Section of brain from full-term infant showing self-contained but extensive hemorrhage in the choroid plexus of the left lateral ventricle, involving the cavum septum pellucidum (*arrows*) and extending into the left foramen of Monro. The germinal matrix region is normal. CC, corpus callosum.

in the perinatal period, particularly parturitional ones, result from low-momentum deforming forces that lead to tears of structures such as the falx, tentorium, sinuses, or bridging veins. This same slow deformation, or "static loading," makes contrecoup lesions rare and allows a number of "surface" injuries, often without consequence for the underlying cerebrum.[172] A "greenstick fracture" of the neonatal skull from forceps application or cephalopelvic disproportion during transvaginal passage is significantly different from a depressed fracture made with a hammer applied to a 5-year-old child's skull.

INITIAL EVALUATION AND INSTITUTION OF THERAPY

Consciousness: Grading and Time Course

Despite many elaborate grading systems that purport to be useful for following clinical course or projecting outcome, a simple scheme that acknowledges level of consciousness and functional (other than mental) deficit serves very well (cf. section on outcome). The so-called Glasgow coma scale described by Jennett and co-workers follows the status of three parameters: eye opening, verbal response, and best motor response. These categories serve for all ages and overlap in predictive value so that parallel confirmatory information may be obtained from each. The quantitative response for each category runs from normal, that is, spontaneous or appropriate to command, through response only to noxious stimulus or stereotyped "reflex," to no response.[96-98]

In the evaluation of infants and young children following head injury, one must use a monitor appropriate for the maturity of the nervous system. For example, the verbal criterion would be of minimal value in an infant, whereas eye and motor status retain their usefulness. It is, therefore, helpful to have information about the child's premorbid status regarding speech, coordination, and behavior.

Level of consciousness following head injury is the single most important predictive parameter, given knowledge of the ictus and postictal progression. Evolution or disappearance of specific neurological signs and symptoms improves reliability of serial evaluations but it almost never overrides the evaluation of consciousness.

The *time course* of progressive change is critical to the proper interpretation of clinical significance (Fig. 59–5). For example, one might note, referring to Figure 59–5: (1) instant coma from cerebral concussion with rapid recovery; (2) "minor" head injury, followed by major motor convulsion and instant coma within one hour after the initial event; (3) brief unconsciousness with recovery, a one-hour period of relatively normal behavior followed by rapid deterioration to coma with localizing signs; or (4) stupor with progressive agitation, interpreted as increasing consciousness but, in fact, heralding herniation from expanding hematoma or cerebral edema.

Management of Mild Injury

Ideally a head injury victim should be managed by a single knowledgeable physician until the clinical course is evident (usually the first few hours). Children and infants are often first examined by a pediatrician, who must decide the significance of the situation. Retaining the child in the office for observation is generally not practicable; the child must either be sent home with appropriate instructions for the parents, or referred to hospital for further evaluation and possible treatment. The ideal criteria on which to base this choice are not likely to be forthcoming, since a balance must be struck between maximum safety for the child and the practicalities of economy and hospital availability. There is no reliable method to discover the occasional child who will develop an intracranial hematoma, other than careful observation.

If the neurosurgeon does not know the referring physician or is unable to communicate satisfactorily by telephone, it is wise to evaluate the child personally. This has the added advantage of an additional time interval for an evolving process to become apparent; appropriate personnel and facilities are usually available for further therapeutic and diagnostic maneuvers.

Parents should be given specific (usually written) criteria, in lay terms, explained by the physician, if a child is discharged from

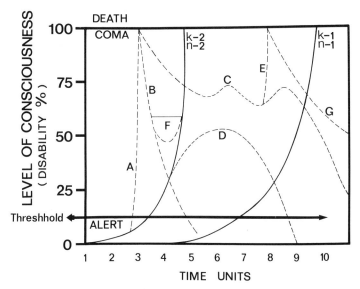

Figure 59–5 Theoretical patterns of alteration of consciousness with time after cerebral injury (A–G). The abscissa represents arbitrary time units, which may vary with the specific patient or type of injury. The ordinate, or "disability" axis, measures the continuum of consciousness from alert (roughly 0–10 per cent disability) through coma and death (100 per cent disability). A, Instant coma of cerebral concussion; B, usual post-concussion course of rapid recovery; C, slower recovery from cerebral contusion with period of fluctuating consciousness; D, plateau and reversal of a process otherwise leading to death (this may be a pharmacological remission or a manifestation of the natural history of the process); E, secondary coma of post-traumatic convulsion (the recovery phase is altered over the preictyl course); F, "lucid interval" during expansion of an epidural hematoma; G, Postconvulsive recovery phase (symptoms are those of the combined primary and secondary cerebral insults). k–2, n–2 and k–1, n–1 are two functions from a family of curves modified from McLennan, J. E.: Letter to the editor. New Eng. J. Med., 269:1323, 1963.

the office or emergency ward following head injury. It should be established that the parents understand the situation, are reliable, live a reasonable distance from the hospital, and have available transportation and telephone. The child who is sent home should, in general, be evaluated again by a physician the following day.

Management of Severe Injury

The child with a head injury should be evaluated with dispatch upon arrival at the emergency ward. In no case should he be required to remain in the waiting area until it has been ascertained by a competent physician or knowledgeable triage nurse that the injury is minor. This decision must be based not only on the appearance of the patient but on the history of the accident. Any trauma to the head involving moderate momentum, e.g., a moving automobile or fall of several feet, has the potential to produce rapid deterioration in a child who is initially alert and ambulatory. It is emphasized that

children with head injury, in comparison with adults, often exhibit marked lability of neurological status; they may appear stable just prior to rapid failure of consciousness. It is the duty of the initial evaluating physician to think expectantly in this situation, to provide adequate monitoring and follow-up, and to be certain that the lines of communication are open.

The lability of children with head injuries should not be attributed to "fear" or other "emotional factors" but rather considered as an integral portion of the response to head injury in terms of general behavior as well as specific neurological factors. Progressive agitation or appearance of "strange behavior" in an initially stable child must be considered a harbinger of impending neurological deterioration. The other aspect of the lability picture shows many children with ultimately minor head injuries who are crying, agitated, disoriented, persistently vomiting, and intermittently lethargic. It is usually prudent to hospitalize all children suffering unconsciousness and those with trauma involving moderate momentum, regardless of possible "normal examination" and normal skull films. An exception might be a case in which several hours have elapsed since the accident when the child is first evaluated.

Patients with severe head injury usually arrive at the hospital comatose and with various manifest neurological signs. There is often trauma to multiple systems. The basic steps of immediate diagnosis and therapy are given here in the pediatric setting; if possible several maneuvers should be undertaken simultaneously.

Nonneurological Evaluation

Respiratory System

Respiratory evaluation, including endotracheal suctioning or intubation and oxygenation to maintain oxygen tension above 100 mm of mercury with appropriate tidal volume for the child's weight, is critical if the patient is cyanotic or apneic. Although 10 cc per kilogram is an average formula for initial respirator tidal volume setting for any child, it is not reliable because of varying chest compliance and respirator compression; observation of chest excursion and auscultation should be used to adjust the inspiratory volume, and arterial blood gases should be checked after 15 to 30 minutes. Hypoxia frequently worsens neurological status acutely; the level of consciousness may improve dramatically with respiratory support. This step may be temporarily bypassed if the patient is hyperventilating and has a clear airway. Frequently, however, hyperventilation is a sign of "air hunger," which may be determined from arterial blood gases, from which the cause of the respiratory change may be deduced (see discussion of treatment of contusion). Auscultation of the chest assures there is no hemopneumothorax; external chest wounds are sealed and chest tubes inserted as indicated.

Cardiovascular System

Cardiovascular evaluation includes cardiac resuscitation for arrest or ventricular arrhythmia, determination and support of systemic blood pressure, and assessment of acute blood loss. Shock may be the result of concomitant abdominal injury or long-bone fracture with internal hemorrhage. It is wise to establish a large-gauge intravenous line at this point; one must be cautious of excess fluid load administered to children with head injury. If blood pressure remains normal, the fluid maintenance rate should be about half the normal daily amount of 1500 ml per square meter per day of 5 per cent dextrose in one fourth–normal saline in divided doses.

Abdomen

Remove the clothing from the entire body, even if the head is the only apparently injured structure. It is not unusual for critical hemorrhage to occur from ruptured liver, spleen, or great vessel while attention is focused on a dilated pupil. Small children may lose a significant amount of their circulating blood volume from internal hemorrhage. A Foley catheter is inserted in the bladder to allow gross evaluation for hematuria and provide a measurement of urine output in response to blood pressure support and osmotic agents.

Neurological Evaluation

Cerebral herniation, as evidenced by decerebrate posturing and dilation of one or both pupils, should be treated immediately if reversal has not already been achieved with earlier measures, including passive hyperventilation. Generally this involves use of intravenous osmotic agents, along with initiation of a plan for further diagnosis and treatment of a possible mass lesion. Mannitol (1 gm per kilogram) given as an intravenous bolus is recommended for reversal of acute herniation.

The remainder of the neurological evaluation should be methodical to the extent permitted by the child's condition. The scalp should be examined for subgaleal hematoma, laceration, and sign of depressed fracture. The latter is often hidden beneath the accompanying hematoma; conversely, a scalp hematoma may have a central fluctuance simulating a depressed fracture. Ecchymosis over the mastoid region (Battle's sign) and periorbital discoloration (raccoon sign) indicate basilar fracture of the temporal and frontal bones respectively (Fig. 59–6). Direct trauma to the orbit should be assessed; this may produce the ecchymosis without fracture and may also cause pupillary and extraocular movement abnormalities that might otherwise be attributed to intracranial causes.

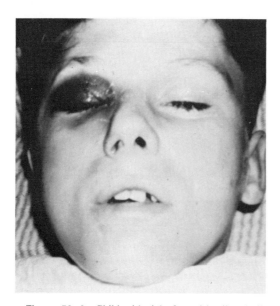

Figure 59–6 Child with right frontal basilar skull fracture, periorbital and eyelid ecchymosis and swelling, the so-called "raccoon" sign.

The tympanic membranes and external auditory canals are examined for disruption and bleeding. Blood loculated in the middle ear or coming through a tear in the ear drum is a good indication of basilar fracture of the temporal bone, often missed on the skull radiograph. Hemorrhage alone may come from the ear lesion; if cerebrospinal fluid is also leaking from the auditory canal, a basilar fracture and dural disruption are present. Cerebrospinal fluid rhinorrhea should be searched for, particularly in frontal bone trauma. It may be present but unnoticed in admixture with hemorrhage and other traumatic exudate from the nostril, or may drip posteriorly into the nasopharynx and not be apparent until the patient is placed in lateral or head-down position.

Evaluation should be made for cervical spine injury prior to excessive manipulation of the head, if indicated by the nature of the trauma or initial examination. Anteroposterior and lateral radiographs of the cervical spine are made without moving the patient if possible. Subarachnoid blood, an invariable occurrence with even moderate head trauma, will not produce neck soreness or stiffness for a few hours, and the patient must be reasonably awake to appreciate it. Immediate soreness indicates cervical strain or fracture. The expected motor and sensory correlates of spinal cord trauma are evaluated in the early phases; paralysis

may be falsely attributed to the comatose state until more detailed neurological examination is made.

The level of consciousness overrides all other neurological signs in importance. This must be assessed early and followed by specific criteria at frequent intervals until a definite trend is discovered. The Glasgow coma scale is a suggested check list to follow and is sensitive to progressive deterioration.[96–98] If possible, a single knowledgeable physician should make repeated evaluations to standardize the stimuli and evaluation of patient response. If deterioration is apparent, action must be taken to prepare for rapid diagnosis and therapy of intracranial mass lesions.

In infancy, anterior and posterior fontanelle tension and open or widened sutures give evidence of either chronic or shorterterm increased intracranial pressure. Widened sutures following trauma usually indicate traumatic diastasis but may also occur with acute increase in intracranial pressure due to cerebral edema, which may develop within an hour of injury, or to a mass lesion. The significance of widened sutures in an infant hinges on the history and the remainder of the neurological examination.

Neurological ocular examination includes evaluation of the fundi, the pupils, and the extraocular muscle function. Size, symmetry, and reactivity of the pupils to light are assessed. Midposition pupils and pinpoint pupils respectively indicate probable midbrain and pontine compromise; light reactivity is generally reduced in these lesions, although cutaneous stimulation of the neck may continue to show the normal ciliospinal reflex, that is, ipsilateral pupillary dilatation. The "swinging flashlight" test should be made to note the presence of the Marcus Gunn phenomenon, an indication of prechiasmal optic nerve imbalance. This test demonstrates a relative suppression in the afferent limb of the pupillary light response on the side of the worst injury. Increasing imbalance during the 24 hours after trauma may be an indication of progressive optic nerve compression. Accentuated hippus, or wide swings in pupillary size, is common and of little diagnostic significance. It is important to know if initially dilated pupils have reverted to normal with hyperventilation or mannitol administration prior to the surgeon's evaluation. A unilaterally dilated, unreactive pupil is a firm sign of medial temporal lobe herniation into the tentorial notch unless it can be attributed to direct orbital or third cranial nerve damage. Drugs affecting pupillary size and reactivity should be avoided following head injury.

Although fundoscopic examination is generally not very helpful in evaluation of acute cranial trauma, it should be made as a baseline for progressive changes. In the older child, papilledema may begin to develop within a few hours of the onset of increased intracranial pressure, and absence of venous pulsations will be an earlier sign. Subhyaloid retinal hemorrhage indicates acute pressure increase, which is not necessarily continuing at the time of examination; it is frequently the result of rupture of an intracranial artery but may occasionally be present with rapid increase in intracranial pressure without intracranial hemorrhage or even in the presence of chronic subdural hematoma of infancy.

Extraocular muscle spontaneous position and excursion should be noted; the oculocephalic maneuver is usually necessary to determine the full range of movement in a patient with severely depressed consciousness. In frontal hemisphere contusion or extracerebral mass lesion, the eyes may be tonically deviated to the side of the lesion. If convulsion occurs, the eyes will deviate away from the origin of the electrical activity. Neutral eye position in response to oculocephalic testing in a comatose patient indicates brain stem damage, generally intra-axial contusion or hemorrhage, and skew deviation represents an asymmetrical or less than complete compromise of the extraocular movement nuclei and their interconnections. Vertical eye movements are of less significance in the immediate examination; they may be elicited by flexing and extending the neck or by forced eyelid opening (Bell's phenomenon).

The fifth and seventh cranial nerves may be partially evaluated. In a comatose patient the corneal reflex and noxious stimuli to the face and oral or nasal mucosa monitor the fifth nerve. The facial nerve is likewise testable unless the patient is in deep coma; supraorbital pressure elicits facial grimacing and wrinkling of the forehead. The two sides are compared, and note is made of a central or peripheral pattern, that is, supranuclear or infranuclear injury. The latter generally occurs in the peripheral course of the facial nerve in the temporal bone or over the angle of the jaw; it is frequently found in temporal bone fractures. Management is discussed in the section on basilar skull fracture. Function of the lower cranial nerves is difficult to test unless the child is awake, although palatal motor asymmetry may be looked for.

Voluntary motor function of the extremities is observed, as is response to noxious stimulus. A stimulus should be given to each limb to note ability to withdraw, and the general pattern of limb movement to a central stimulus, over the nasion or chest, is noted. The patterns of response range from normal, with attempt to remove the stimulus, to decorticate, decerebrate, or flaccid paralysis. In an infant, spontaneous movements should be observed. Distribution of muscle tone is tested by passive manipulation of each extremity. Deep tendon response is tested and quantitated, and plantar response is noted. Severe brain injury may depress deep tendon reflexes completely. If one finds flaccid paraplegia accompanying absence of reflexes, spinal cord injury should be suspected.

The respiratory pattern is observed throughout the examination if breathing is not being controlled by respirator. In general, one may attribute a Cheyne-Stokes pattern to bihemispheral insult, and hyperventilation (in the absence of air hunger), ataxic, or apneustic breathing to various levels of brain stem damage.[179,180] The classic response to acutely raised intracranial pressure is increasing systemic blood pressure and bradycardia; it has been emphasized, however, that these tend to be late and unreliable signs in a child. Persistent hypotension and rapid pulse are of more significance in suggesting ongoing blood loss or initial hypovolemia from accompanying systemic injury. Wide swings in temperature are common in children with severe brain injury. With persistent convulsions or decerebration, the fever must frequently be controlled by external and internal cooling maneuvers. Ongoing fever above 105° F adds certain additional cerebral damage.[83]

When the cerebral injury is determined to be pre-eminent, a CT scan is the diagnostic study of choice. There is seldom a reason to forgo it in dealing with more than moderate cerebral trauma. If the child is agitated, a short-acting sedative such as intravenous diazepam (Valium) in 0.5- to 2-mg aliquots, usually with respiratory control, will be necessary to avoid radiographic artifact that reduces the usefulness of the study. Reasonable alternative procedures include limited cerebral angiography or exploratory burr holes to deal with possible acute extracerebral clots. Echoencephalography may show the midline of the brain, but will generally not indicate the cause of a "shift."

SPECIFIC ENTITIES

Cephalhematoma

This lesion is rather common in the newborn, generally occurring without cerebral damage during transvaginal delivery, although skull fracture may be present.[107] Forceps delivery of the fetal head may add an additional source of trauma. In very large hematomas, significant blood loss may occur, leading to shock; vitamin K deficiency may be implicated.[191] The identical lesion may result from postnatal head injury.

A cephalhematoma should not be aspirated unless (rarely) there is impending compromise of the scalp circulation. The majority of these clots are subgaleal and dissect over wide areas of the scalp; if the hemorrhage is subperiosteal, it tends to stop at suture lines where the cranium is tightly adherent. Subgaleal blood and fluid collections frequently dissect into the areolar connective tissue planes about the orbit; this is noted commonly in frontal trauma or craniotomy. The parent should be warned that this process may make the child look "worse" 12 to 24 hours after the inciting event. In the case of chronic recurrent fluid pockets, aspiration may be done to encourage tissue adhesion; this is always done through the scalp even though fluid involves facial soft tissues. Failure to resorb a fluid collection following trauma or craniotomy suggests continuing cerebrospinal fluid liquorrhea and should be investigated further. On occasion, a subperiosteal cephalhematoma may calcify and require removal.

Skull Injury

Significant brain trauma frequently occurs without disruption of the skull. Con-

versely, skull fracture does not a priori indicate cerebral involvement, although the two lesions are statistically related in any large series of cases.[77,82] If skull fracture or traumatic suture disruption is present, generally a significant force has contacted the head, and the patient should be watched carefully for development of confirmatory signs and symptoms. It is not apparent that all children with head injury should have skull x-rays made; the yield of positive information is slight when routine screening films are done without clinical correlation. If the examining physician plans to alter his disposition of a child, depending on the presence or absence of fracture, he will look at a great many negative x-rays. On the other hand, it is clear that major intracranial hemorrhage can occur in a patient who is initially neurologically normal and has no skull fracture.[54] It is critical to individualize the disposition of a patient with head injury on the basis of the history and the potential for delayed clinical deterioration. It is reasonable to admit to hospital a child who is neurologically normal with a fracture traversing the stem of the middle meningeal artery or a venous sinus. In a study of 4465 children with head injury, Harwood-Nash and associates found 1187 (26 per cent) with skull fracture. Clinical analysis of these cases showed that "the presence of a fracture should not alter the decision for future medical care except with depressed or compounded fracture."[78] Among this entire series, 27 per cent of the fractures were depressed. Of the children with fractures, 3 per cent had associated subdural hematoma and 1 per cent had epidural clot; however, the incidence of these entities in children with head injury without fractures was 6 per cent and 1 per cent respectively. Skull fracture was associated with a significantly higher incidence of brain damage of any type (8 per cent versus 2 per cent without fracture). It has been mentioned that, with the possible exception of a fracture running into a sinus or the middle ear, there is little purpose in obtaining skull films on an urgent basis.[216]

Linear Fracture

The majority of skull fractures fall into the linear group. That is, they follow the normal contour of the skull. These fractures may be single, multiple, or branched, and frequently run into a diastatic suture, which has a similar significance. The vast majority of linear fractures, even if initially diastatic, will heal readily, particularly in younger children. Radiographic diagnosis is essential; the only clinical sign may be a subgaleal hematoma. A number of confusing vascular grooves may be noted on the x-ray. Clues to a true fracture may be double parallel tracks produced by the inner and outer tables of the skull or a sharply branching pattern, in contrast to a vascular marking. Rarely a "growing fracture" will result within a few weeks to months of injury. Very extensive or nearly circumferential fractures of the "blow-out" type may occur in infants (Fig. 59–7). It has been stated that multiple stellate fractures of the occipital bone in a child strongly suggest the "battered child" syndrome; certain didactic rules about the nature and location of skull fractures are helpful.[55] Linear fractures crossing venous sinuses or branches of the middle meningeal artery indicate need for at least 24 hours' observation in hospital. Diastatic fractures, if associated with cerebral contusion, dural laceration, or massive hematoma, should be explored, and the dura should be repaired to avoid future complication.[214]

Enlarging Skull Fracture

Descriptions of cystic lesions of the scalp following skull fracture in infancy and childhood are found in the literature back to the early nineteenth century; historical review is given by Lende and Erickson, who note that Dyke first applied the name "leptomeningeal cyst," which has now been discarded in favor of "enlarging skull fracture of childhood."[120,121] Although the vast majority of diastatic fractures in children heal without incident, occasionally at follow-up weeks or months later a swelling is noted in the scalp over the fracture site. The skull x-ray may show progressive erosion and scalloping of the fracture margin, even with minimal external evidence (Fig. 59–8). The child may present with seizures, most likely from the underlying regional cerebral contusion.

Necessary and sufficient criteria for development of this complication include: (1) diastatic skull fracture, usually in a child less than 1 year old; (2) a diastatic dural defect underlying the fracture; and usually (3) contusion of the underlying brain. The local cerebral injury is often severe and results in necrosis and atrophy, allowing porencephalic dilatation of the nearest ventricular structure, i.e., frontal or temporal horn, as shown in Figure 59–8C, along a vector directed at the fluid accumulation in the surface cyst. It should be incidentally mentioned that similar cystic ventricular outpouchings have been not infrequently documented following simple ventricular needle puncture for aspiration; this should not be considered a totally benign procedure.

The loculated cyst fluid is generally not in communication with the ventricular system

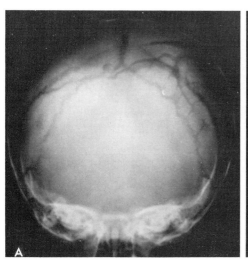 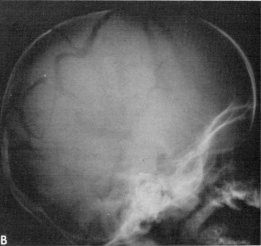

Figure 59–7 Anteroposterior, *A*, and lateral, *B*, skull films demonstrate multiple, stellate, nearly circumferential, "linear" fractures of the "blow-out" variety often found in infants.

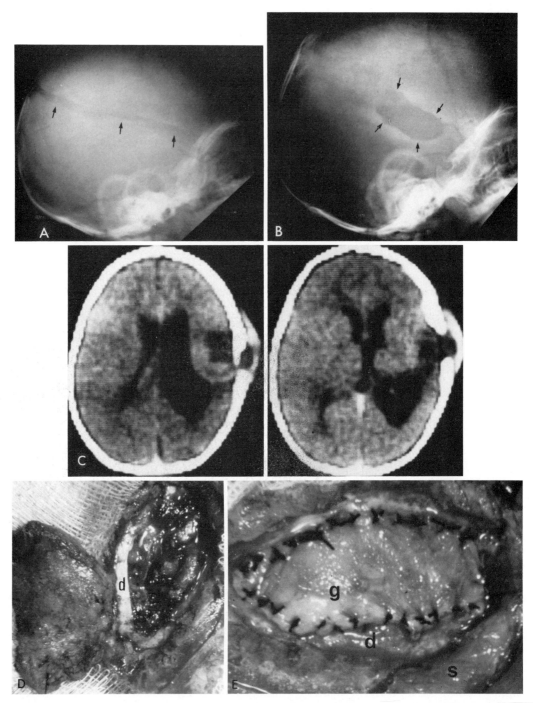

Figure 59–8 Six-month-old child with an enlarging skull fracture. *A*. Lateral roentgenogram showing the original linear diastatic fracture incurred at 2 months of age. *B*. Lateral skull film at follow-up two months after injury demonstrates healing of the posterior portion of the fracture with progressive bony erosion anteriorly. *C*. CT scan shows moderate diffuse ventricular enlargement; the right temporal horn and atrium of the lateral ventricle herniate into a region of cystic degeneration in the bony erosion. *D*. Intraoperative view during repair of enlarging fracture. The eroded bony margin has been removed around the entire periphery of the defect until 1 cm of normal dura (d) is visible. The central dura is missing. The exposed cerebral tissue shows degeneration. *E*. Completed repair using a graft (g) of the resected scar tissue. s, Skull.

or subarachnoid space, although after operative resection of compromised tissue this may occur. Erosion of bone continues because of cerebrospinal fluid pulsations and hydrostatic pressure, as in the experimental model for massive ventricular dilatation following hemicraniectomy and dural release.[86] A leptomeningeal cyst per se is not requisite.[120] At operation the dural defect is found to extend beyond the bony margins, which must then be cut back to allow tight dural patching. Early repair avoids extension of the cerebral damage through continued focal pressure and cystic expansion leading to scarring and atrophy. Occasionally one of these lesions remains stable and is discovered only years later.[211] Recommendation has been made to explore in infancy all diastatic fractures that are associated with marked regional swelling and evidence of underlying cerebral contusion.[214] Cerebral herniation through the bony defect is well known.[212] Attempts to stratify growing fractures into subtypes serve little purpose.[64]

There is general agreement that repair be done as soon as the progressive bone erosion is recognized. The essence of the procedure is definition of the residual dural margins and achievement of watertight dural closure, invariably requiring a graft. Tissue for this graft may be obtained in the operative site by harvesting a sheet of scar tissue covering the cyst or using regional fascia or periosteum; if this is unsatisfactory, fascia lata should be taken from the patient's thigh. It is wise to avoid synthetic materials because of their liability to infection in a region of compromised blood supply. Debridement of the usual extensive, underlying cerebral lesion should be minimal, since one cannot improve tissue function except by arresting progressive damage by repair of the incompetent dura. The surface cyst and adhesions immediately attached to this structure may be removed. The bony defect should be repaired by acrylic cranioplasty to avoid recurrence of the cyst. Anticonvulsants are used in long-term postoperative management.

The thicker adult skull apparently prevents cyst formation under similar circumstances of injury. Recently a variant of the enlarging fracture has been described in occipital fractures; here the cyst expands within the tables of the occipital bone, forming an intraosseous lesion that becomes a compressive mass in the posterior fossa without deforming the external contour of the skull (Fig. 59–9).[42,84]

Basilar Fracture

This entity, generally a linear fracture, extends into the base of the skull; the usual location is the petrous temporal bone, the orbital surface of the frontal bone, or the basiocciput, roughly in this order of frequency. These fractures are often difficult to diagnose by x-ray, and clinical inference is needed to identify, for example, cerebrospinal fluid otorrhea or rhinorrhea, hemotympanum with "Battle's sign" (blood in the mastoid area with surface discoloration), "raccoon sign" (periorbital ecchymoses, as shown in Figure 59–6), or injury to cranial nerves that exit the skull through basal foramina. A vertical fracture may be identified running into the petrous bone and then disappearing. In the horizontal portion of the petrous bone fractures tend to involve the facial canal either longitudinally or transversely and also to lacerate the tympanic membrane and dura overlying the petrous apex. Thus the clinical significance of basilar fractures, other than the accompanying primary brain injury (usually contusion), is that cerebrospinal fluid often leaks to the outside world, and cranial nerves may be involved.

A skull x-ray should be obtained in the "cross-table" lateral, brow-up projection in suspected basilar skull involvement; an air-fluid level in the sphenoid sinus is evidence of fracture.[135] Pneumocephalus seen on the initial skull x-ray is a clue to external communication of a fracture through either a bony sinus, the sella turcica or planum sphenoidale, or a compounded surface wound; since the air is generally subdural, a dural tear is indicated even without frank cerebrospinal fluid leak.

Cranial Nerve Injury

If facial nerve palsy is not initially present with this injury, indicating contusion or transection of the nerve, it should be anticipated in the next 24 hours or so. In this instance, facial nerve malfunction is almost always due to swelling in a tight bony canal; generally good recovery is the rule, and corticosteroids may be administered to facilitate this.

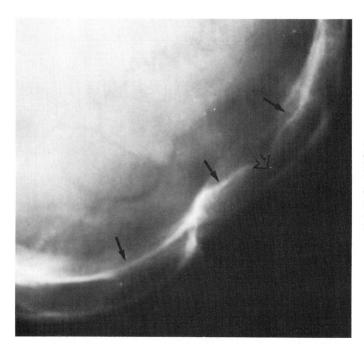

Figure 59–9 Several months after a fracture of the occipital bone this child was found to have a cystic mass behind the cerebellum that is a "growing fracture" expanding in the diploë. Open arrow shows intraosseous nature of this lesion, which is distinct from those found supratentorially.

Return of function in partial facial nerve palsy should be monitored by daily testing of electrical latencies; persistent values exceeding 4.0 msec difference between the two sides may indicate need for nerve decompression.[181] If the eyelid on the injured side fails to close, the cornea should be protected.

Tympanic membrane disruption is common with temporal bone fracture and, with the frequently associated middle ear ossicle disruption and hematoma, can produce a 30-db hearing loss. Adequate examination usually requires extraction of clotted blood from the canal and middle ear and follow-up audiometric testing. In an otherwise severly injured child, these audiological problems are secondary.

Fracture of the anterior fossa and related bony sinuses may injure the olfactory or optic nerves by involvement of the cribriform plate or optic canal. Because this damage is frequently irreversible, careful initial examination should be made for olfaction and afferent pupillary defect (Marcus Gunn pupil). This latter observation is the most reliable test for subtle optic nerve asymmetry; its presence should draw attention to a lesion that may require an attempt at operative or medical reversal. The basis of this test is a depressed direct pupillary reaction to light with preservation of the consensual reaction. Initial unilateral blindness with a nonreactive pupil augurs a very poor prognosis for return of functional vision.

The third, fourth, and sixth cranial nerves may also (less frequently) be injured in fractures involving the sphenoid bone; these lead to expected abnormalities of extraocular and levator muscle function and pupillary size and light reaction. Extraocular muscles may be involved locally in the orbit by entrapment in orbital wall fractures or by massive intraorbital swelling or hematoma; the differential diagnosis between this state and primary nerve injury is made by the ophthalmologist using direct traction on the muscle in question. Generally injuries to cranial nerves three, four, and six may recover over several months, and early operation is not indicated.

Cerebrospinal Fluid Liquorrhea

Cerebrospinal fluid otorrhea is generally mixed with blood initially and should be differentiated from blood alone, which results from a similar injury without dural laceration, or serous drainage alone without cerebrospinal fluid. A drop of blood–cerebrospinal fluid admixture placed on filter paper will leave a central blood stain surrounded by a ring of clear fluid. The cerebrospinal fluid contains a moderate quantity of glucose, whereas serous drainage from the middle ear does not. Bleeding from the ear or hemotympanum following acute head injury is assumed to be caused by basilar skull fracture; definitive radiographic proof may often be obtained by basal views of the skull or tomograms through the petrous bone. This, however, is not indicated in the acute phase; instruments should not be used on the ear, and the drainage should be allowed to flow freely or to collect on a sponge taped over the external canal. Usually otorrhea stops within 48 hours, and antibiotics need not be given if this is the case. The early phases of head injury care are performed as if the basilar fracture were not present.

Cerebrospinal fluid need not necessarily leak externally; it may loculate in the middle ear, exit through the eustachian tube, or drip posteriorly into the nasopharynx from a frontal fracture and not be noted by the patient. It may appear in such occult anatomical sites as the subconjunctival areas (Fig. 59–10).[152] Recurrent meningitis in an infant or child without history of trauma demands thorough search for occult fistulae or congenital tracts involving the temporal bone or trigeminal cistern.[26,103,104] Radionuclide evaluation of the cerebrospinal fluid pathways in the post-traumatic patient with liquorrhea has been helpful in defining delayed and altered cerebrospinal fluid absorption patterns and in localizing the dural and external leak. The dural tear often does not correspond to the external leak, as cerebrospinal fluid may track internally over a long distance.[52,88] The majority of leaks will close spontaneously, particularly those of the temporal bone.[118] Conservative therapy is advisable for at least three weeks before considering work-up for operation. After 48 hours of persistent cerebrospinal fluid leak, antibiotic coverage is probably indicated, particularly in rhinorrhea, which tends to be more persistent than otorrhea. The child should be instructed not to sniff or blow his nose, as this creates positive pressure that drives bacteria (and often air) into the intradural space.

Cerebrospinal fluid rhinorrhea may be delayed for days or weeks owing to initial plugging of the potential dural laceration by swollen tissue or entrapment in the fracture. Delayed meningitis after skull fracture should be a clue to this occurrence.

Operative correction of cerebrospinal fluid liquorrhea should be undertaken after two weeks of persistent drainage. The exploration should be made extradurally, if possible, as one may then easily appreciate the relationship between the fracture and the dural rent. If a dural patch is needed for repair, temporalis fascia or other autogenous tissue is preferred. Synthetic dura and tissue adhesives have, however, had recent success for repair of meninges and bone; synthetic biological products as sealants and dural grafts have some theoretical advantages.[119,204,221] The patient should be nursed with head up 30 to 45 degrees in both the pre- and postoperative periods. Serial lumbar punctures or constant lumbar drainage may aid in reducing cerebrospinal fluid pressure and thus the hydrostatic force at the leak site; one must be persistent, however, to keep up with the cerebrospinal fluid production rate of 0.3 ml per minute.[45]

Controversy exists regarding antibiotic utilization in children with basilar fractures to avoid entrance of bacteria into the subdural and subarachnoid spaces. It is proba-

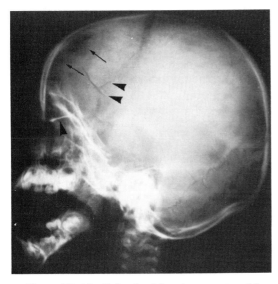

Figure 59–10 Following injury by an automobile tire to the face and frontal skull of an 18-month-old infant, cerebrospinal fluid leaked transiently from the nostrils and persisted as loculations in the subconjunctival sacs, with massive expansion of the eyelids. This film demonstrates a stellate linear fracture (*double arrowhead*) running into a diastatic coronal suture, an internal depression of the left orbital roof (*single arrowhead*), and frontal pneumocephaly (*arrows*). (From McLennan, J. E., Mickle, J. P., and Treves, S.: Radionuclide cisternographic evaluation and follow-up of posttraumatic subconjunctival CSF loculation. J. Neurosurg., *44*:496–499, 1976. Reprinted by permission.)

bly common practice to administer prophylactic antibiotics to these patients even without cerebrospinal fluid liquorrhea. The incidence of meningitis in retrospective series of patients with basilar fracture varies from about 6 to 25 per cent; infection, most often by pneumococci, is more common with frontal than with temporal fracture, since cerebrospinal fluid leak is usually more persistent in the former location.[123] Chemoprophylaxis is contraindicated according to two reports, one of which is a prospective study in which treated patients were at severalfold higher risk of infection than controls; there is a suggestion that more resistant organisms may be involved in treated patients.[91,134]

Depressed Fracture

This entity involves bone driven in below the normal contour of the inner table of the skull. Depressions of the frontal sinus may involve only the outer table. Simple depression of only the outer table has no significance other than possible cosmetic undesirability. Skull depressions usually result from a blow by a blunt object and are accompanied by underlying coup cerebral contusions.

Clinical examination of the traumatized area discloses regional swelling; palpation of a depression is not reliable other than through a compounded scalp wound. If routine skull radiographs fail to quantitate a depression, tangential views, often with the aid of fluoroscopy, will demonstrate the depth of the lesion. Decision to elevate a depressed fracture operatively in an older child is rationally based on: (1) the depth of depression, measured on a tangential view through the lesion; (2) location of the fracture and correlation with underlying neurological deficit or poor cosmetic appearance; and (3) other reason for exploration, such as a compounded wound, active hemorrhage, or a related foreign body.

The last point is widely accepted; the first two points remain open to discussion, and adequate evidence for evaluation may be lacking. Bony depressions may involve internal structures as well as the skull tables, for example, the orbital roof, floor, or lateral margins (cf. Fig. 59–10).

Depressed "ping-pong" fractures of the neonatal skull will occasionally spring back spontaneously within a few weeks. These lesions are "greenstick" in nature, usually have no overriding edges, are not associated with laceration of the scalp or dura, and usually do not involve cerebral damage. They may occasionally be corrected by digital pressure or by suction; operative elevation is accomplished through a suture or small bony trephine opening, popping the depressed area outward.[185] As with a ping-pong ball, the area may again become depressed spontaneously, and care should be taken to avoid pressure over the fracture for several days. The authors usually elevate neonatal fractures that are depressed more than 5 mm and do not operate on those of 3 mm or less.[132]

It is often stated that depressed fractures, particularly over the motor or sensory cortex, are epileptogenic or may produce ongoing focal cerebral damage as the brain pulsates against the bony depression.[141] Although no adequate series in which operation has not been performed exists, this is often given as reason for elevation of even apparently minor lesions. In certain circumstances, location dictates that no operation be done; this applies particularly to fractures overlying the torcular Herophili or the sagittal, transverse, or lateral sinuses. In the absence of significant hematoma, exploration in these areas may cause severe venous hemorrhage, resulting in further compromise of the sinus in the attempt to control blood loss. The presence of dural laceration must be considered in an operative plan (if not apparent from cerebrospinal fluid leak or brain tissue extrusion) but is not necessarily a demand for operative repair. For example, basilar fracture with otorrhea implies dural laceration, but the vast majority of these leaks will seal spontaneously if managed conservatively, and rather extensive operative exposure is usually required to visualize the involved region.[118]

The operative approach to depressed fractures should, if possible, incorporate any overlying scalp laceration in the incision. Exposure is carried to normal outer skull table around the entire depressed area, and entry to the epidural space is gained through either a traumatic opening or a burr hole placed at the edge of the depression. If dural laceration is present, bone must be removed over its entire length and closure accomplished. Depressed fragments of bone may often be pried up to normal position in younger children; in older individuals the fragments must generally be freed by rongeur. If the resultant bony defect is large and the operative field uncontaminated, a cranioplasty may be made at the original procedure. It is usual to wait weeks to months for cranioplasty, particularly if there is any underlying neurological lesion. Emergency repair is indicated in compound depressed fractures, particularly if cerebrospinal fluid leak is present; if the overlying scalp is intact, repair may be delayed. Even minor depression of the frontal bones and supraorbital ridges is of cosmetic significance and should, in general, be elevated. Trauma to the frontal sinuses almost always involves laceration of sinus mucosa; the sinus should be stripped of mucosa and sealed with a plug of muscle. Alternatively the posterior wall of the sinus may be removed to avoid a loculated space that may later give rise to a mucocele or other chronic lesion.

Complications of depressed fractures were documented in 26 per cent of a series of 400 patients, half of whom were less than 16 years of age.[159] Infection occurred in 9 per cent, intracranial hematoma in 7 per cent, and involvement of the dural venous sinuses in 11 per cent. In the cases with any one of these complications there were significant increases in mortality rate, neurological deficit, and late post-traumatic epilepsy. Pulmonary embolism of cerebral tissue is also described as a rare complication during birth injury and in children with severe head trauma.[224] There is experimental support for not removing isolated sterile or "dirty" bone fragments from the cerebrum; in association with hair and skin fragments, however, abscess is the rule if the wound is not debrided.[177] Bone fragments may be safely preserved, washed, and replaced in hopes of avoiding future cranioplasty.[114] Occasionally focal synostosis of a suture follows fracture involving that structure in a child. It is notable that there is little evidence that operative repair of depressed fracture prevents complications.[159]

Venous Sinus Thrombosis

A potentially disastrous complication of depressed skull fracture is venous sinus thrombosis. Depressed fracture at the vertex may occlude the superior sagittal sinus following delivery and also in the older child (Fig. 59–11). The occipital bones may be depressed relative to the parietal bones and cause sinus or torcular compression in newborns lying for long periods on the occiput. Contrast visualization of the involved conduit is the only reliable diagnostic technique. Although one may argue for operative exploration to relieve obstruction, particularly in the posterior two thirds of the sagittal sinus, acute "venous ischemia" has probably already occurred. The late effects are generally related to benign intracranial hypertension, which is self-limiting.[108] Delayed progressive venous thrombosis is, however, well known.[101]

Direct trauma over a venous sinus may cause occlusion, but more commonly the lesion results from a secondary problem such as sepsis, brain swelling, venous sludging and hypercoagulability, or dehydration. Diagnosis of the lesion as a "pure" entity is difficult; it is frequently overlooked as a complication of cerebral trauma because of other ready explanations for symptoms such as convulsions or focal neurological deficit. There is no specific treatment other than correction of the contributory factors. There is controversy about the use of anticoagulants; in the case of coexisting cerebral contusion, anticoagulants other than, perhaps, "mini heparin" would appear contraindicated.[56]

The possibility of delayed hemorrhage from a torn venous sinus is probably minimal because of the effective tamponade of this low-pressure system. The majority of disasters occur at the time of exploration, perhaps with an attempt to remove a spicule of bone penetrating the sinus, or avulsion of cortical veins at their entry into the sinus. A case can easily be made for nonintervention.

Meningeal Hemorrhage

Epidural Hematoma

Traumatic epidural hematomas are rare in infants and young children because sharp-edged fractures are unusual, the branches of the middle meningeal artery do not yet form grooves in the inner table of the skull, and the dura is tightly adherent at the suture lines. In a series of 42 infants with severe head trauma at birth, there were 15 depressed fractures, 24 acute or

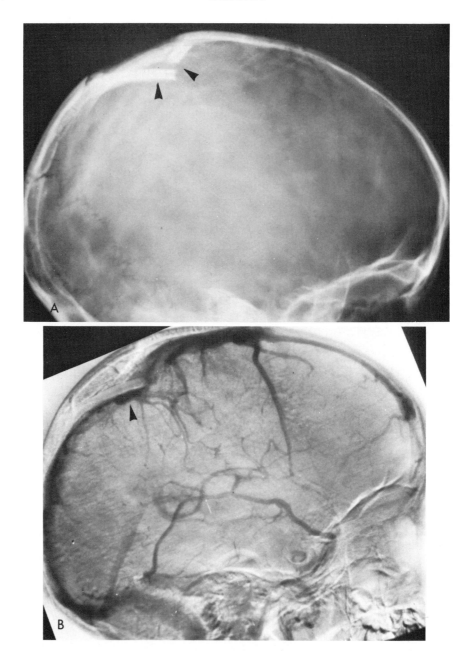

Figure 59–11   Depressed vertex skull fracture in a 3-year-old child, incurred when he was struck by a falling object. *A*. Lateral skull film shows depressed bone fragments. *B*. Lateral venogram demonstrates subtotal occlusion of the sagittal sinus in its posterior segment. (Reprinted by permission from Figure 5, page 359 in Chapter 12 in Pediatric Neurology and Neurosurgery by Richard A. Thompson and John R. Green, Eds. Copyright 1978, Spectrum Publications, Inc., New York.)

subacute subdural hematomas, 13 chronic subdural hematomas, and no epidural clots of significant size.[167] Exceptions include a series of 104 pediatric epidural hematomas, 17 of which were found in newborns; these authors note that the hematoma was widespread in 45 of their patients, and that only the coronal suture acted as a barrier to extension.[28] Only 1 per cent of children of all ages with head injury had epidural hematoma as the dominant intracranial lesion in the large series of Harwood-Nash.[77,78,82] Nonetheless, Matson collected a large series of traumatic epidural hematomas in children, about half of whom were under 2 years of age.[141] The classic epidural hematoma is found in the temporal region underlying a transverse fracture that crosses a branch of the middle meningeal artery; these lesions, however, may occur at any site. Four per cent of all epidural clots occur in the posterior fossa, and there is a prevalence of children in this group.[7] A fracture need not be present; if there is a fracture, which is radiographically defined in only about 50 per cent of temporal epidural hematomas, it is nearly certain that the clot will underlie it. This rule may be used for burr hole placement in emergency situations. It is not unusual to find a fracture at operation that was not appreciated on the skull film. In a series of 46 patients with no skull fracture but with epidural clots, 91 per cent were under age 30 years, and 30 patients were less than 20 years old.[54] It thus appears that absence of fracture is relatively common in children and young adults.

The hemorrhage, in the majority of cases, stems from the middle meningeal artery or its branches; venous epidural clots occur at the cranial apex from tears in the superior sagittal sinus and in the posterior fossa from the occipital sinus around the foramen magnum (Fig. 59–12). Epidural hemorrhage is a true neurosurgical emergency because of the rapidly expanding mass under arterial pressure and the usual temporal clot location, which provides a directly medial vector to impact the uncus on the midbrain. Subacute and chronic epidural hemorrhage that has escaped clinical progression and recognition is much less common.

Although epidural hematomas may accompany head injury of any severity, they are the major acute complication that may follow rather minor cranial trauma, even without skull fracture or loss of consciousness.

The classic "lucid interval" is the period following head trauma when the patient is relatively normal prior to deterioration of consciousness (cf. Fig. 59–5). There need not even be initial concussion. The lucid interval is terminated by a rapid progression of signs and symptoms such as headache, lethargy, vomiting, seizures, hemiparesis, dilation of the ipsilateral pupil, decerebrate posturing, and ultimately respiratory depression and death. This time course is illustrated by curve F of Figure 59–5. The lucid interval appears during recovery (curve B) from concussion (curve A) and then reverses to proceed rapidly to coma and death (k-2, n-2).

Obviously the neurological picture is a function of the stage of progression of brain compression and transmitted shift into the midline region. One must ferret out the clues early on, such as swelling of the temporal or occipital muscles, and unexplained

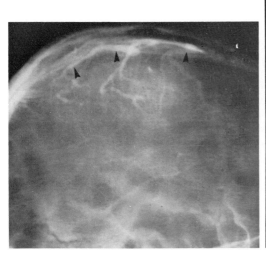 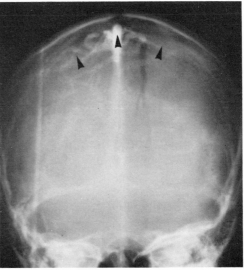

Figure 59–12   Ten-year-old child who demonstrated signs of intracranial hypertension five days after injury. Anteroposterior and lateral venograms show depression of the sagittal sinus away from the inner table of the skull by a subacute epidural hematoma (*arrowheads*). (Reprinted by permission from Figure 3, page 355 in Chapter 12 in Pediatric Neurology and Neurosurgery by Richard A. Thompson and John R. Green, Eds. Copyright 1978, Spectrum Publications, Inc., New York.)

change in the child's behavior, particularly the onset of hyperirritability in a previously lucid patient. At this point the diagnosis must be made rapidly, either by computed tomography (vastly superior for posterior fossa lesions), angiography, or exploratory burr holes. The computed tomographic scan will classically show a well-localized, biconvex, high-density lesion immediately subjacent to the inner table of the skull with appropriate mass effect and anatomical shift (Fig. 59–13). It is relatively unusual to have the clinical signs of progression dispersed in time so that they follow in orderly fashion. Change in vital signs is a late occurrence and must not be awaited before planning therapy.

Perhaps all diagnostic studies but the immediately available CT scan are contraindicated if clinical decline is apparent; mannitol should be administered, the patient intubated and hyperventilated, and burr holes and craniotomy performed with dispatch. If the patient is stable, skull films will often show a linear fracture, which may have a depressed segment and cross a groove of a meningeal vessel. Absence of demonstrated fracture should in no way change one's clinical caution, however. With suspected traumatic mass lesion, lumbar puncture is contraindicated. Ventricular puncture will be helpful only in cases of acute posterior fossa cerebrospinal fluid ob-struction, will provide only transient improvement, and may, in fact, encourage upward herniation through the tentorial hiatus. In confusing cases, cerebral angiography may be definitive in showing inward displacement of dural vessels and sinuses (see Fig. 59–12).

Location of the clot in the posterior fossa may vastly confuse the progression of clinical signs, and decline in consciousness due to brain stem compression and ventricular obstruction will often not be accompanied by pupillary asymmetry or hemiparesis. In this circumstance, lateral ventricular aspiration will show clear fluid under increased pressure, and will likely achieve temporary clinical improvement, allowing time for more definitive intervention.[7]

For an epidural hematoma to form, the anatomical potential space between the skull and dura must open to receive it. Experimentally a steady force of 90 gm applied to the epidural space of dogs will separate the dura inward. If the force is pulsatile, the usual situation with an arterial tear, the necessary force may be reduced to 35 to 70 gm. In this model, it appears that the clot reaches maximum size early in the course; the length of the lucid interval is then determined by the "reaction time" of the brain to the overlying force.[46] This work, however, did not include trauma as the cause of the clot and might not apply to

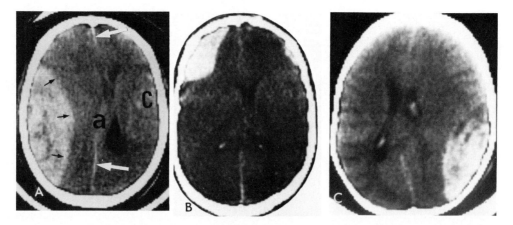

Figure 59–13 Acute and subacute epidural hematomas defined by CT scan. *A*. Left frontoparietal clot showing classic biconvex high-density lesion (*small arrows*). There are compression of the left ventricular system, bowing of the median fissure (marked by subarachnoid blood, *larger arrows*), acute loculation and dilatation of the opposite ventricular atrium (a), and contrecoup cerebral contusion (c). *B*. Left frontal epidural hematoma. Only moderate posterior and rightward shift of left lateral ventricle is seen. Blood in interhemispheric fissure shows little displacement of the midline. *C*. Acute epidural hematoma of the right temporoparietal region with major shift of midline to left.

the human situation that accompanies a concussion or contusion. Often there is no classic lucid interval; the epidural deterioration takes off from a fluctuating recovery course such as curve C of Figure 59–5. Perhaps equally plausible as an explanation for secondary deterioration is the well-known biphasic spasm of arteries following traumatic rupture, wherein the initial spasm may stop arterial hemorrhage within a few minutes but the clot re-expands an hour or so later when the spasm resolves.[155]

The treatment of epidural hematoma should always be operative in acute and subacute cases (within the first 48 to 72 hours). If the patient begins to deteriorate while being observed, or is initially in extremis, intubation, hyperventilation, and intravenous osmotic diuretics should be employed. Although these measures may provide temporary improvement to allow a diagnostic study, they must be followed by craniotomy.

If facilities for diagnostic study are not immediately available, a diagnostic burr hole should be made over the center of the fracture; if there is no fracture, the side ipsilateral to a dilated pupil and contralateral to a hemiparesis should be chosen first. When clot is discovered, it is partially decompressed through the burr hole, and a craniotomy is quickly fashioned. In the temporal region or the posterior fossa, craniectomy is extended from the burr hole. The bony opening should be planned to achieve control of the proximal middle meningeal artery. The authors usually do not open the dura unless insufficient clot is found to explain the clinical course or the dura is tightly re-expanded after clot evacuation. The dura should be sutured to the pericranium at the periphery of the bone flap or craniectomy to obliterate the potential epidural space. Hemicraniectomy has been tried to offset the ravages of severe cerebral edema.[164]

In recounting the classical clinical course of epidural hematoma, it is important to realize that an apparent "lucid interval" may occur with various other cerebral injuries. Reilly and co-workers found 66 of 151 patients with ultimately fatal head injury who were alert enough to talk at some point after injury; 44 of these patients had a significant intracranial clot, and 41 of these clots were other than epidural.[189] These statistics attest to two points: (1) patients with

epidural hematoma have an excellent prognosis if operated on early in the course, and do not fall into this group of ultimately fatal cases, and (2) the cerebral contusion and edema accompanying subdural and intraparenchymal clots greatly increases the mortality rate despite operative intervention. There were 22 patients in this series who died of contusion and brain swelling without frank hematoma, although they were initially alert. Obviously a "lucid interval" may occur with various cerebral injuries other than epidural hematoma. In a larger series of 424 patients with severe, not necessarily fatal, head injury, 32 per cent talked at some point before decline and 13 per cent were initially considered normal.[98] Deterioration occurred within 6 hours of injury in 45 per cent, but 27 per cent of the patients did not fail until after 24 hours.

Outcome in pediatric epidural hematoma depends on the neurological state at the moment of decompression, on the time course of decline, and on accompanying unrelated cerebral injury such as contusion. Death in pediatric acute epidural hemorrhage that has been properly diagnosed and treated is limited to the 5 to 10 per cent of patients whose extremely rapid downhill course thwarts intensive intervention. In some series of unselected cases, however, the mortality rate has been as high as 20 per cent, with an additional 20 per cent showing significant residual neurological deficit.[28]

Subdural Hematoma

Subdural hematoma is a collection of blood between the dura and the pia-arachnoid. Technically, this space is separate from the subarachnoid space, although in trauma there is often disruption of the leptomeninges. Blood may enter the subdural space from a "bridging" vein connecting the cortical surface to a venous sinus in the dura, from a cortical arterial tear, or from a rent in the inner side of a dural sinus. Acute subdural hematoma is almost always arterial in origin or stems from a major sinus rent. The clinical syndrome accompanying a subdural hematoma is determined principally by the source and time course of clot accumulation, by accompanying trauma to the underlying brain, and by potential for expansion of the dura and skull to minimize the effect of increasing intracranial pressure.

Acute Subdural Hematoma

The hallmark of this lesion is rapid clinical deterioration due to an expanding clot of arterial origin overlying cerebral contusion and edema. The patient with an acute subdural hematoma is almost always severely injured. Acute subdural clot as a result of birth injury is quite rare. Usually there is recognized difficulty with parturition, such as breech presentation.[2,150] The skull may not be fractured. The newborn child becomes acutely distressed within 12 hours of delivery, often with dilation of the ipsilateral pupil and respiratory difficulty. It is generally possible to remove enough blood by repeated transcoronal needle aspiration to avoid craniotomy. Seizures may be difficult to control. Any neonate in acute neurological distress should have diagnostic bilateral subdural needle aspiration; if blood is discovered, therapy is immediately initiated by removing enough blood to lower the intracranial pressure.

In the older child, particularly if the cranial sutures are closing, acute traumatic subdural hematoma is an emergency. It is invariably accompanied by cerebral contusion, providing an additional force leading to cerebral edema, increased intracranial pressure, and shift of midline structures. This pressure continues to evolve over several hours after injury. The midline shift accompanying acute subdural hematoma may appear excessive for the thickness of the surface clot because of the edema of cerebral contusion in the same hemisphere. The midline displacement may often be minimal, however, because the subdural hematomas are bilateral.

Diagnosis of acute subdural hematoma is most efficiently and accurately made by computed tomographic scan; a high-density rim of blood is noted overlying the hemisphere, often with collapse of the lateral ventricle on the same side. There may be edema or contusion visible under the clot, and occasionally accompanying intracerebral hematoma. Skull films frequently show a fracture, but this is not requisite. Clinically there are generally contralateral hemiparesis and ipsilateral dilated pupil in a comatose or severely obtunded patient. Emergency use of hyperventilation and osmotic diuretic agents will usually provide sufficient stabilization to allow proper studies to be obtained. A limited cerebral arteriogram, particularly viewed in the anterior-posterior vector, will show an avascular space over the hemisphere and a medial shift of regional vessels. Diagnostic burr holes may occasionally be necessary if contrast studies are not available.

If an acute subdural hematoma is discovered, a craniotomy is fashioned to cover a large portion of the affected area; it is seldom possible to remove enough of a severe clot through burr holes, nor do they allow control of a source of active hemorrhage. If contrast studies have not clearly defined the lesion, the entire head should be shaved, and one or two burr holes should be placed on the side opposite a removed hematoma to insure that clot is not present bilaterally. At craniotomy, the cortex will frequently show regional contusion; usually a ruptured cortical artery will be found after the clot is removed. Massive cerebral swelling will often be in evidence at the time of closure, perhaps requiring a dural graft of regional fascia and removal of the bone flap.[21] Acute subdural hematoma of only a few millimeters' thickness need not be removed unless a decompressive craniotomy is required.

Rapid expansion of the occasional acute subdural clot of venous origin (e.g., dural sinus tear) is difficult to understand; the resulting intracranial pressure is often many times the cerebral venous pressure. The cycle of brain swelling from underlying tissue compromise, severe anatomical shifts, and ultimate ischemia undoubtedly makes this syndrome evolve rapidly.[111] The cerebral contusion makes the acute subdural hematoma a much more lethal lesion than an epidural clot treated with equivalent haste.[150] Drastic measures such as hemicraniectomy have been used to attempt modification of this lethal course.[29]

Chronic Subdural Hematoma

This entity is found most commonly in infancy, with peak incidence at about 3 to 6 months of age. The usual patient with subdural hematoma is noted to have excessive expansion of the head circumference and a tense anterior fontanelle in the first several weeks to months of life, eventually accompanied by distended scalp veins, "setting-sun" eyes, vomiting, lethargy, and increasing cephalofacial disproportion.[141] Many of these infants are discovered only after moderate progression of the symptoms, when failure to thrive and delay of motor and mental milestones cause concern. Only about half of these infants have a documented history of head trauma.[195] Significant subdural hematoma may exist with relatively normal head circumference, particularly if there is cerebral atrophy (Fig. 59–14).

Frequently the clinical presentation is subtle and rather protracted, e.g., a 1-year-old child with a full anterior fontanelle but without significantly increasing head growth and with only moderate feeding problems and slow weight gain. Chronic anemia is frequent owing to repeated subclinical episodes of blood loss into the subdural cavity, often additive to the physiological drop in hematocrit seen within a few months of birth. Only a third of infants with chronic subdural hematoma exhibit macrocrania sufficient to be suspect to the pediatrician; in any case, this feature is subtle compared with that found in obstructive hydrocephalus. The "cracked-pot" sound on skull percussion is common to both entities. Funduscopic examination may show subhyaloid hemorrhages as a clue to the presence of the hematoma. A convulsion may be the initial clinical symptom and will occur during evolution in about half the pa-

tients; this is a result of direct cortical irritation from the blood products rather than an effect of pressure. Chronic seizures after successful therapy are rare. Transillumination of the infant's cranium may be helpful, but contrast studies are necessary for firm diagnosis. Skull fractures are usually absent in chronic subdural hematoma; the initiating traumatic episode is generally minor and often unnoticed. Despite marked degrees of skull molding during transvaginal delivery, this is almost never the cause of the hematoma.

Computed tomography will demonstrate a range of densities in the subdural compartment depending on the chronicity of the hematoma and the presence of repeated bleeding into the space.[199] High-density acute subdural hematoma begins to approach normal brain density from one to two weeks after the original hemorrhage; in this isodense phase, the presence of a subdural mass may be inferred from the regional mass effect (Figs. 59–15 and 59–16). Beyond about two weeks, the density slowly approaches that of cerebrospinal fluid (Figs. 59–14 and 59–17). If there is repeated hemorrhage into a chronically enlarged subdural space, the density may vary with serial scanning; fresh blood (red cells) will often gravimetrically layer under-

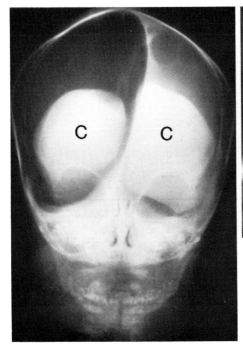

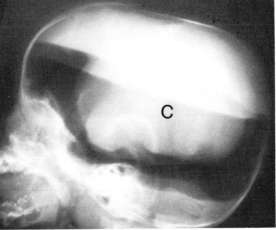

Figure 59–14 Massive congenital subdural hematoma with atrophic brain. This child had only mild macrocrania. Anteroposterior and lateral roentgenograms following exchange of 150 cc of air for an equivalent volume of yellowish fluid show the severely atrophic cerebral hemispheres (c).

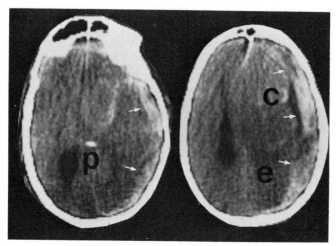

Figure 59–15 Two adjacent slices of a CT scan showing an acute right-sided subdural hematoma covering most of the hemisphere. This lesion appears as a crescentic area of high density (*arrows*), accompanied by swelling and contusion of the underlying cerebrum. There is often displacement of the midline (note blood in the interhemispheric fissure) in excess of that expected from the extra-axial mass alone. Note the scattered, anterior, high-density (white) hemorrhagic contusion (c) and the posterior lower-density edema (e) of the right hemisphere; the right lateral ventricle is absent owing to cerebral swelling, and the left atrium and posterior horn are loculated with early dilatation. The pineal gland (p) is displaced to the left.

neath the more watery phase in the usual occiput-down scanning position. Radioisotope brain scan may clearly show chronic subdural hematoma. With isotope imaging, the frequent confusion with scalp hematoma or swelling and skull fracture makes this study less helpful in acute cases. Cerebral angiography is difficult in small infants and is an occasional cause of femoral artery occlusion; it is, therefore, not a reasonable initial diagnostic study for chronic subdural hematoma and should be reserved for situations in which other studies are equivocal. The most direct diagnostic maneuver is the transcoronal subdural tap; if the tap is positive, therapy is immediately initiated by removing fluid.

It is rather common to find bilateral chronic fluid collections, since the subdural space is continuous over the hemispheres; membranes may form, however, limiting the lesion to one hemicranium.

Recent neomembranes are composed of a thin layer of loose connective tissue with a meshwork of actively proliferating fibroblasts and many distended thin-walled sinusoidal capillary vessels.[51] Acute and chronic inflammatory infiltrates and small foci of hemorrhage or hemosiderin indicate repetitive bleeding; this evidence is cited in favor of membrane stripping to remove the source of the recurrent hemorrhage. Collagen fibers are laid down as the membrane ages; the outer membrane is generally thicker and opaque as compared with the inner (epipial) membrane, which remains translucent except in very chronic lesions. It is common for multiple loculations of hematoma to be found, each enveloped in separate membranes of varying ages. In this situation, craniotomy may be necessary for effective removal of blood products and membranes, but the vast majority of infant subdural hematomas never become inaccessible to transcoronal aspiration.

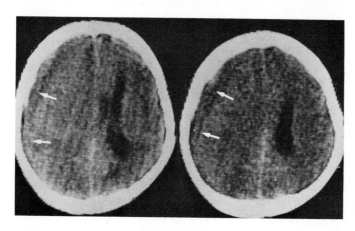

Figure 59–16 CT scans from a patient with an "isodense" subdural hematoma. Compression of the left ventricular system and mild bowing of the midline to the right are present. There is a faint crescentic outline (*arrows*) over the left hemisphere.

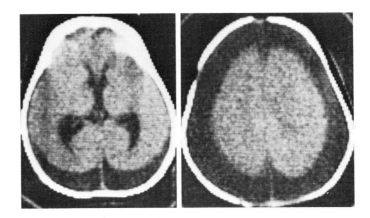

Figure 59–17 CT scans from an infant with chronic bilateral subdural hygroma and macrocrania. The ventricular system is only mildly dilated. Cerebral tissue is surrounded by low-density fluid that is the residuum of earlier subdural hemorrhage. The hygroma is most extensive over the top of the brain and communicates across the midline.

Both the neomembrane formation and the transudation of fluid through existing membranes may be retarded experimentally and clinically by corticosteroids.[12,62] Isotopically labeled protein recovered from subdural fluid comes from circulating blood within 12 hours; additional high-molecular-weight products derive from red blood cell destruction.[183] The mechanism of persistent reaccumulation of subdural fluid collections is controversial; it apparently involves both osmotic and inflammatory factors, to some degree, but the principal factor is most likely recurrent small hemorrhages from the vascular neomembrane, formation of which is repeatedly stimulated by each additional aliquot of fresh blood.[61,115,183]

The obvious goal of therapy in subdural hematoma is to reduce the intracranial pressure. In the subacute or chronic situation, this is generally realized by repeating transcoronal subdural aspiration until the fluid collection remains under low pressure and reduced in volume. Samples of each tap should be retained to provide qualitative serial assessment of fluid color, protein content, and hematocrit. In the absence of repeated hemorrhage, the fluid should clear progressively as the volume aspirated decreases.

There need be little variation in the basic aspiration technique described by Matson.[141] Fluid flow may be aided by moving the infant's head to bring the pool to the tip of the needle; this maneuver should be done by an assistant who is holding the child's head. Additional fluid may be recovered by transiently increasing intracranial pressure by manual compression of the jugular veins. Large-gauge, short-bevel needles may be forced through the coronal su-

ture up to age 7 or 8 years, but this is difficult after about 3 years. Twist drill cranial entry is preferred in older children. If fluid volume is unexpectedly reduced or flow is poor, loculations may be present. It is occasionally necessary to make an exploratory subdural tap through the lamb-doid suture, provided these sutures lie normally above the transverse sinuses. The tap should be 2 to 4 cm off midline (in the pupillary line anteriorly). If this procedure is also unproductive and retention of fluid is suspected, a radiological procedure will define the situation. It is important to realize that fluid will stop flowing when the pressures across the dura equalize; this does not imply that the subdural space has been emptied or that the brain has re-expanded to obliterate the space, although these are the ultimate goals of repeated aspiration over a period of days.

Controversy remains over the tapping schedule and curative therapy of the chronic subdural hematoma of infancy.[144,150,151] It has been taught that persistent reaccumulation of subdural blood should be treated by wide craniotomy and "stripping" of the thickened "outer subdural membrane" that forms in two to four weeks after initial hemorrhage.[92,141]

Craniotomy for membrane removal is anatomically extensive, frequently bilateral, and in a small child has significant operative morbidity. This operation allegedly removes both the source of repeated hemorrhage and a "constricting" factor to future brain growth. There is no adequate evidence that the neomembranes prevent normal growth of the cerebrum or that their removal allows "expansion" of compressed hemispheres. In the absence of cerebral re-expansion, the potential subdural space remains a hazard for future hemorrhage. It is reasonable to continue even prolonged treatment by aspiration to avoid a less than satisfactory craniotomy that creates an immediate potential space and has little current rationale; if the head circumference is stable and the brain growing normally, persistent subdural collections are of little proved liability. The vast majority of chronic subdural fluid collections may be satisfactorily resolved within two weeks of daily aspirations. There is unequivocal documentation that residual fluid may be spontaneously absorbed from the subdural space; thus if the child's condition is clinically stable, taps are discontinued, and the lesion is followed by CT scan.[12,145]

Chronic fluid reaccumulation in the subdural space is greatly enhanced by persistent cephalocranial disproportion, usually a combination of macrocrania and cerebral atrophy.[86,144,183] If repeated tapping does not control the intracranial pressure, various internal shunts of the subdural space or closed temporary external drainage may be utilized.[37,210] Reduction cranioplasty has occasionally been done at the time of membrane stripping.[141] Chronic untreated subdural hematomas may become extensively calcified and are associated with seizures and mental retardation as a consequence of the original brain trauma; operative therapy of this chronic lesion does not appear to alter the clinical course.[148]

Successful treatment of massive hydrocephalus with resultant cerebral mantle collapse and tension on bridging veins is a well-known cause for secondary subdural hematoma, and it may also result in overriding of the frontal and parietal bones and secondary synostosis.[37,87] The concomitant therapy of hydrocephalus and infant subdural hematoma (before or after shunting) may be accomplished by internal subdural shunts aided by an "on-off switch" in the ventricular shunt to force temporary expansion of the ventricles to obliterate the subdural space. Ventricular infusion has been used to advantage in the same way.[206] Generally one should treat the subdural hematoma first and then deal with the dilated ventricles, which represent an "ex vacuo" form of atrophy. Fortunately, coexistence of these pathological conditions is uncommon, because the prognosis is poor. There is chronic parenchymal compromise from stretching of white matter and compression of cortex at the same time, leading to severe loss of cerebral tissue and psychomotor retardation. It is noteworthy that nonabsorptive hydrocephalus is seldom a complication of chronic subdural hematoma of infancy. The compressed subarachnoid space appears to be functionally maintained by at least a thin layer of circulating cerebrospinal fluid.

Posterior Fossa Subdural Hematoma

Infratentorial subdural hematoma in the newborn, usually resulting from a rent in the tentorium, is documented by only nine cases in the literature.[15,58] It is likely that this entity is often missed both clinically and at postmortem examination. The clinical presentation includes change in the baby's cry, vomiting, poor suck and feeding, generalized hypotonia, and progressive hydrocephalus in the first week of life, and, if untreated, may eventuate in neurological disaster from brain stem compression, occlusion of the cerebral aqueduct, and even upward herniation of the cerebellum through the tentorial hiatus.[51,58] Third nerve paresis is absent, and respiratory embarrassment is an early sign. The treatment is operative evacuation of the clot.

Subdural Hygroma

Post-traumatic subdural collections of xanthochromic watery fluid may be found within days of injury or within weeks or months of trauma. In the former situation it likely results from loculation of slightly blood-tinged cerebrospinal fluid.[61] In the chronic situation, it is assumed to be a residuum of an earlier subdural clot that has undergone hydropic change (cf. Figs. 59–15, 59–16, and 59–17).[51,199] These collections may accumulate days or weeks after trauma, when the initial CT scan showed no extracranial mass; this delay in appearance further confuses the issue of etiology. The neomembranes surrounding a chronic hygroma cavity were likely initiated at the time of original hemorrhage and have become invested with collagen and are relatively avascular. Removal of a delayed post-traumatic subdural hygroma does not usually lead to clinical improvement, and most collections resorb with time.[49]

Prognosis

The overriding fact appears to be that the main prognostic criterion in outcome of subdural hematoma is not the method of treatment but rather the antecedent (ictyl) event with associated cerebral compression, contusion, and anatomical shifts.[184] The irreversible lesion caused by this ictus is probably not increased by the presence of chronic subdural fluid collections, although these continue to cause symptoms until removed. By this doctrine, chronic seizures and mental status and developmental abnormality and atrophy all result from initial trauma and not from chronic pressure.

Psychomotor development will be normal following all modalities of appropriate therapy in about three fourths of all patients with chronic subdural hematomas.[145,151,202,227] The children with poor outcome from either acute or chronic subdural hematoma remain those with significant brain contusion at the time of initial trauma. In children with subdural hematoma who do well otherwise, residual seizure disorder is uncommon.

Intracerebral Hematoma

Large intraparenchymal hematomas of the newborn are rare, although a number of case reports in the older literature indicate they may occur with gross mechanical trauma.[51] Many of these lesions are no doubt missed, as evidenced by recorded "uneventful" births of babies who died soon thereafter with pulmonary emboli of macerated cerebral tissue.[224] Infants and newborns are occasionally found to harbor intraparenchymal clots at postmortem examination (death from other causes); many of these apparent clots prove, in fact, to be hemorrhagic contusion foci when examined microscopically.[51] Since they occur frequently without history of head trauma, other mechanisms such as asphyxia and hypotension are likely responsible.

Beginning with the use of computed tomography, it has been possible to study the true incidence of traumatic intracerebral clots and contusions. These lesions were often formerly overlooked entirely, unless responsible for major neurological deficit, and described as an "avascular mass" on cerebral angiography. The incidence of frank hematoma is likely to be much higher than suspected; Figure 59–18 presents two patients who had isolated intraparenchymal hematomas that could only be defined by CT scan—in both cases the clinical correlation was useful but could not differentiate between hematoma and contusion. Hematomas usually occur in the contrecoup location, either as components of a regional contusion or as single or multiple isolated lesions. They may less frequently directly underlie the skull trauma, separated from the surface by a small strip of normal tissue, as shown in Figure 59–18A, or be deep within the diencephalon or brain stem like the isolated lesions seen in Figure 59–18B. Coexisting traumatic subdural hematomas are not unusual.[38,147]

The majority of traumatic intraparenchymal clots are located in the temporal and frontal lobes, the commonest position for contrecoup lesions. Since contrecoup lesions of any sort are unusual in younger children, the relative rarity of intracerebral hematomas in this age group is reasonable on this basis alone. Isolated deep clots of the basal ganglia, thalamus, and brain stem frequently evoke argument as to origin from trauma or, for example, from deep arteriovenous malformation. Since trauma is often a temporally related factor in "spontaneous" hemorrhage from an arteriovenous malformation or aneurysm, and occult arteriovenous malformations may obliterate themselves by bleeding, this situation is not easily unravelled.[155] As is frequently necessary, the patient shown in Figure 59–18B was studied by cerebral angiography, which was entirely normal.

Historically the notion of "Spät-Apoplexie" is important. Realistically, the appearance days after injury of a frank hematoma in a contusion focus is probably unusual, although with initial and follow-up CT scans, it is possible to document.[22,127] The majority of these patients no doubt show delayed deterioration from regional edema and related secondary processes; when studied by CT scan, the original clot is discovered. The recent series of severe pediatric brain injuries reported by Bruce and associates is remarkable for the total absence of intracranial hematomas.[23]

The CT scan is crucial for diagnosis and decision for operative evacuation of intraparenchymal clots. Location and size of the clot and the attendant anatomical shift dic-

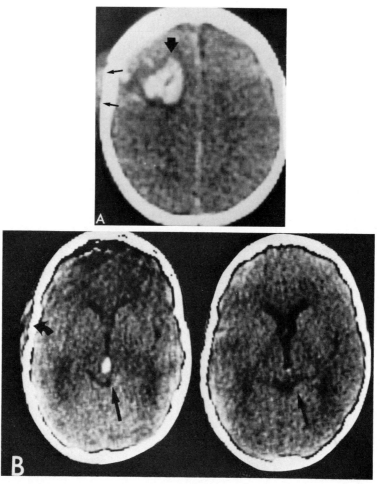

Figure 59-18 Examples of children with intracerebral traumatic hematomas. *A*. Left frontal coup hematoma clearly separated from the surface of the hemisphere (*large arrow*). Also present are overlying hemorrhagic contusion, extracranial swelling, and hemorrhage at the site of skull fracture (*small arrow*). *B*. Traumatic midbrain hematoma of 1.0 cc volume (seen only on one CT slice) in a 16-year-old girl. The arrow indicates asymmetry of the pericollicular cistern from mass effect and regional swelling. The curved arrow shows minimal surface injury.

tate the advisability of intervention. Deeper clots accompanying subdural hematomas and regional contusion may be rationally managed only with CT assistance—formerly, operative exploration leading to discovery of a surface hematoma of significant size satisfied the surgeon, so no further lesion was suspected. Removal should be considered if a clot is accessible and causing regional shift, particularly if correlated with clinical deficit; frequently subsequent functional improvement is rapidly apparent. If the lesion is largely contusion—and the child can be managed conservatively—this is the wisest course of action. Removal of clots, which largely separate white matter tracts, allows rapid recovery of regional function by release of local pres-

sure and displacement, but the rate of recovery for a given contusion focus is slower and impossible to predict accurately. There are a number of reports of improved consciousness following delayed removal of traumatic hematomas.[147] If an operation is avoided, the clot may be followed to resolution by serial CT scans; follow-up postmortem data suggest, however, that isodense residual cavities persist for long periods.[157] This may well be related to the marked increased incidence of late-occurring epilepsy in patients who had acute subdural and intraparenchymal hematomas, even those apparently involving only white matter.[95] It is possible to remove deep clots by suction with minimal brain disruption, much as an abscess cavity is aspirated.[9]

Brain Injury

Concussion

The term "concussion" is a statement of a clinical event; it conveys no mechanistic knowledge. There are two aspects to nervous system injury, a physiological one and an anatomical one; with increased research, the line between these is becoming less distinct. The most common brain injury, cerebral concussion, has recently been re-evaluated. This entity is classically described as a totally reversible, transient, cerebral malfunction manifested by loss of consciousness and postural tone followed by a variable "postconcussion syndrome" of neurological signs, symptoms, and behavioral changes.[149] There is amnesia for the ictus extending retrograde for variable periods, possibly equated quantitatively with severity of the blow to the head. The benignancy of this event has, however, been overestimated; significant residual abnormality exists in many concussed patients, most often involving behavioral and intellectual spheres.[53] The cumulative effect of cerebral concussion, for example, as seen in professional boxers, who also "accumulate" contusions, acknowledges that permanent structural and functional changes occur in the cerebrum, at least in susceptibility to repeated insult.[70] A number of "postconcussive" cerebral syndrones have been described in children and include transient blindness, hemiparesis, somnolence, irritability and vomiting, and migraine attacks.[68,73,156,176] Children who are learning to talk will often be rendered mute for several days following concussion, although otherwise alert; verbal auditory agnosia has been described in children with cerebral birth abnormality and later cerebral trauma.[187]

In clinical parlance, one may grade the severity of cerebral concussion in children. Since it may be difficult to document transient unconsciousness in a young child who, for example, cannot be questioned regarding post-traumatic amnesia, the parent's (or observer's) description might include a "stunned" or quiet (flaccid) child who recovered movement rapidly and then manifested vomiting, drowsiness, pallor, and glassy eyes. A more definitive picture in an older child might include "traumatic automatism," that is, ambulatory confusion and amnesia following head injury

without documented atonic unconsciousness. Delayed vomiting and difficulty rousing from sleep, with waxing and waning confusion, may follow without necessarily signaling a mass lesion. Full-blown concussion in a child involves loss of postural tone, obviously impaired consciousness, and almost routinely, recurrent vomiting, often requiring intravenous fluid administration to avoid significant dehydration. Prolonged vomiting following pediatric concussion does not of itself indicate impending complication; in fact, it has been noted that vomiting will often decrease as a child becomes increasingly lethargic from increased intracranial pressure.[216]

In uncomplicated cerebral concussion the neuropathological examination (death from another cause) is normal by standard criteria; this leads to the idea of completely reversible functional abnormality. Recent techniques have shown subtle disruption of white matter fibers and tracts as a substrate for clinical correlation of residual deficits.[208] It is still common practice for a physician to assure a parent that the child's apparently uncomplicated concussion will have no residuum and certainly no permanent or functionally progressive aftermath. Animal models of concussion add to the belief in complete reversibility, although this appears to be a graded phenomenon dependent on the force applied to the skull and the site of the blow.[170,174] It is readily apparent, however, that the human concussion is considerably more complex in terms of measurable residua than is that in the rat or even the monkey.

Minimal concussive force may be applied experimentally without producing pathological changes in the parenchyma; with small additional force, hemorrhages appear concomitantly in the brain stem and other areas of the brain.[170] These results do not apply to the human condition, since experimental models may be tightly controlled as to total force, vector, and site of application. The pathophysiology of concussion is far from settled; possible mechanisms vary from immediate excitation, akin to coma from a grand mal seizure, to immediate metabolic and electrical depression.[172,174] There is evidence that the brain stem "shock" may induce secondary, slower changes in the supramesencephalic parenchyma, probably of vasogenic (ischemic) nature and likely mediated through the reticular formation.[74,170] It is also likely that the ubiquitous subarachnoid hemorrhage and torsional stress on the cerebral surface cause secondary vascular spasm, edema, and ischemia that may lead to diffuse lesions following brain stem "concussion." Within minutes of experimental injury, reduced cerebral blood flow and energy metabolism occur; but the state of these parameters immediately after injury is difficult to document, since measurements take a finite time to perform.[168,169] A mechanism different from the increased cerebral blood flow or the compartmentalization abnormality following direct trauma to the brain of children may be involved.[23,102]

Contusion

Cerebral Contusion

Beyond the subtleties of neuropathological change in cerebral concussion, the major categories of severe injury within the brain are laceration, contusion, and hemorrhage. These are primary lesions of direct (and perhaps penetrating) cerebral injury; they often coexist in the same brain, and may all be either minor or fatal as individual entities. The clinical significance of these lesions, beyond the focal tissue injury, is related to ischemia and cerebral edema with resultant anatomical shift of critical vascular and brain stem structures, and to obstruction of cerebrospinal fluid pathways; it is these secondary processes that produce neurological deterioration over the initial postinjury status. The effect of anatomical shifts is manifest clinically by herniation of swollen and displaced cerebral tissue through or under relatively fixed anatomical structures: (1) beneath the falx, (2) through the tentorium, and (3) through the foramen magnum. In each, critical blood supply to regional and distal structures is lost, thus extending the effect beyond the compressed tissue itself. The midbrain may be compromised at the tentorium, and the medulla at the foramen magnum.

Contusion of cerebral tissue is classically diagnosed when the patient's post-traumatic status does not reverse according to a concussive time course, as shown in Figure 59–5, and there is no evidence of a progressive clot. Focal neurological signs may be present, or the mental status may remain altered.

Cerebral contusion is invariably accompanied by at least initial loss of consciousness. Unless there is massive telencephalic disruption, unconsciousness of more than a minute or so (cf. Concussion) probably indicates a significant lesion of the brain stem reticular activating system. Recovery from coma often assumes the time course of curve C in Figure 59–5 and may cycle clinically between diffuse response to painful stimulus and purposeful avoidance or verbalization. During this initial "recovery" phase, the child's neurological examination will "localize" to indicate the specific telencephalic region of the contusion foci, for example, aphasia, right hemiparesis, and unilateral up-going toe indicate a left frontotemporal lesion. These findings immediately allow differentiation from the entity of cerebral concussion. During the period of recovery of consciousness, a convulsion is not uncommon (see tracing E, Fig. 59–5).

Mental confusion may persist for hours, days, or weeks, even in a state of alertness; if this cannot be correlated with specific findings of the neurological examination, it is generally attributed to diffuse frontal lobe and perhaps limbic system malfunction. With massive bifrontal contusion, the patient may remain comatose and exhibit a Cheyne-Stokes respiratory pattern.

Temporal Lobe Contusion

This syndrome deserves separate mention because it may be successfully treated by resection of the irreversibly damaged tissue if it progresses to become life-threatening. After initial recovery of consciousness, the child may become more lethargic by 24 to 48 hours, with focal signs appearing that depend upon the side of involvement. As massive focal edema develops in the temporal pole, medial forces cause impingement of the parahippocampal gyrus on the midbrain, with resultant hemiparesis, third nerve dysfunction (pupil dilatation and loss of light reflex), decerebration, and coma. Early clinical recognition of this deterioration, accompanied by appropriate contrast study (arteriography or computed tomography), will allow initiation of vigorous medical therapy to control the edema or ultimately, perhaps, craniotomy and resection of the contused temporal pole tissue.[142,146]

Brain Stem Contusion

In the entity commonly called "brain stem contusion," it is apparent that diffuse cerebral malfunction usually occurs rather than focal brain stem alteration; duration of coma may be more dependent on the former than on the latter.[66,67] Cerebral evoked potentials and clinical analysis indicate that decortication and decerebration are probably controlled above the midbrain.[19,66] Oculomotor abnormality correlates best with primary brain stem dysfunction or secondary stem compression from transtentorial herniation. The predictive value of decerebrate posturing must be evaluated.[19]

Clinically, certain neurological findings indicate brain stem involvement; if these are severe, the more focal findings of accompanying telencephalic contusion foci will be masked by the functionally lower-level lesion.

Pupillary changes (usually bilateral), impairment or absence of extraocular muscle movements, bilateral up-going great toes (Babinski reflex), and decerebrate posturing, point to primary brain stem contusion. These signs, developing later in the clinical course, naturally indicate secondary (extra-axial) brain stem compression from transtentorial (lateral or superior) herniation.

Pathology

Contusion and hemorrhage frequently follow a coup-contrecoup distribution according to the site of the blow to the skull and the interaction of cerebral structures along the force (momentum) vector projected to the opposite side of the cranium. The geometric analysis may become complex,[112,190] for example, with torsional forces or in instances in which the skull never contacts an external object. These mechanisms, beyond the scope of this discussion, are of practical value in the design of safety features for the automobile (e.g., infant seats), protective sports equipment, and so forth. In terms of the care of the patient with head injury, it is largely irrelevant just how the injury occurred.

Infants traumatized before 5 months of age demonstrate lacerations of the white matter; beyond about 5 months the lesion is a contusion similar to the adult entity, often wedge-shaped with the apex innermost, and consisting of multiple petechial and initially perivascular hemorrhages.[126] These hemorrhages increase in size for several hours after injury but seldom become frank hematomas. Microglial activation occurs with the hemorrhagic stimulus, and the "clean up" process begins in about 36 hours. The morphology and mechanism of contusion varies with the nature of injury.[126] In recovered patients, the residual lesion is a cavity extending to the surface and often opening into the subarachnoid space. A focal contusion reaches maximal size due to swelling in five to seven days after trauma and then resolves over two or three months. In minimal form, lesions are found on gyral crests next to intact sulcal cortex; in larger foci the atrophy or residual (acquired) porencephaly extends deep into the white matter.[128,129] Contusion underlying acute subdural hematoma is generally severe; the two components of this injury combine to form a particularly lethal lesion, often leading to massive cerebral edema despite removal of the surface clot.

Secondary pathological changes from increased intracranial pressure and ischemia may rapidly mask the primary lesions; it is apparent that "pure" brain stem lesions are rather rare. Diffuse damage to cerebral white matter probably occurs at the moment of impact in patients who suffer immediate and irreversible coma.[3,162] These lesions no doubt account for the numerous neurological residua in survivors, particularly those residua of intellectual and behavioral nature. The common lesions of the corpus callosum may, for example, produce a post-traumatic disconnection syndrome.[3,193] Many of these primary lesions escape recognition, even by CT scan, and remain for the pathologist to define.[48]

Brains from patients who "die instantly" will not show the secondary processes of cerebral edema, shifts of anatomical structures, or clot; most will show microscopic perivascular hemorrhages, and all show acute vasodilatation and subarachnoid hemorrhage.[125,170] Experimentally, the hemorrhages are essentially always in the brain stem, wherever else they may be.[170] If careful search is made, disrupted axons may be demonstrated; these are perhaps the brain stem "mechanism" for "instant death."[3,162,208]

X-Ray Diagnosis

Prior to the advent of the computer-assisted tomographic scanner, angiographic discovery of an avascular mass lesion that was not on the surface of the brain suggested either deep hemorrhage or contusion. The option for craniotomy depended mainly on clinical evidence of progression of the mass effect, but this did not reliably separate the two conditions. Focal neurological deficit in an otherwise alert patient also suggested regional contusion. The CT scanner has been invaluable in demonstrating the nature and location of cerebral contusion and in defining the spectrum of abnormalities found in pediatric brain injury.[40,44,161,228] The lesions may be quite extensive as single foci or may be multifocal (Fig. 59–19). Conversely, there may be only scanty abnormality visible in a deeply comatose patient. The latter situation, with or without correlative localizing neurological signs, is probably best explained by at least coinvolvement of the brain stem, which is not visualized by computed tomography with any regularity; recent reports have indicated diffuse but subtle changes in the initial CT scan of patients with bilateral supratentorial contusion.[209] Anatomical shifts are determined by the size of a focal lesion, by regional swelling, or by a balance of coup and contrecoup components. The ventricles tend to be compressed unless loculated by shifting structures; the intracranial pressure is generally elevated.

Although computed tomography is the study of choice following any head injury, cerebral angiography will reliably indicate, as an avascular mass lesion, most contusion foci sufficient to cause deterioration in neurological status.[186] Small contusions will not necessarily be demonstrated. Isotope brain scan may show the lesion, particularly if a few days have passed since the trauma; it is not a satisfactory immediate study because of overlying abnormalities due to scalp and skull trauma.

Vital Signs After Contusion

Neurogenic hyperventilation is found in only a small number of patients with brain stem injury, although respiratory irregularity is common.[179,180] Rapid regular respiration, with occasional apnea, correlates with injury to the midbrain and upper pons; ataxic or irregular respiratory patterns usually accompany lower lesions. Proper evaluation of rapid respiratory drive requires arterial blood gas determinations to rule out peripheral causes of "air hunger." Hyperthermia is rather common following cerebral contusion in younger children. Rapid respiration, persistent tonic posturing of the extremities, rigid lordotic spine, and repeated convulsions all contribute to an occasionally severe problem in temperature control. Temperature above 104° F. requires vigorous therapy. The mechanism of poor temperature control is no doubt hypothalamic injury, often additive to the hyperthermic stimulus of blood found almost invariably in the subarachnoid space.

The classic arterial blood pressure response to intracranial hypertension of cerebral contusion is systemic hypertension accompanied by bradycardia, the so-called "Cushing reflex." The opposite effects are found in peripheral hemorrhage, and interaction between these coexisting disorders may be reflected by only moderate vital sign changes despite severe injury. It is emphasized that vital sign changes are not a necessary accompaniment of impending

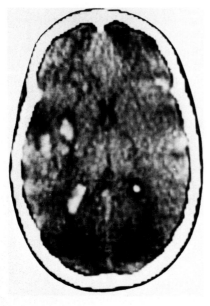

Figure 59–19 CT scan of a 16-year-old involved in a high-speed road accident. Diffuse cerebral contusion is present with numerous small hemorrhages in both hemispheres. There is little alteration of midline position because cerebral swelling is balanced; the ventricular system is still visible on this study made only an hour after injury.

neurological deterioration in children with head injury; if they occur at all, they tend to be late in the early course.

Nonoperative Management

INTRACRANIAL PRESSURE. The principal modalities of therapy directed toward control of the inevitable increased intracranial pressure include respiratory control (hyperventilation) and control of circulating free water through minimal intravenous fluid administration and liberal use of osmotic diuretics. Steroids and barbiturates also affect intracranial pressure. Ventricular drainage is quantitatively inefficient, since the problem is not excessive cerebrospinal fluid production; difficulty keeping the conduit patent in the face of cerebral edema and compressed ventricles also make it impractical.

The absolute level of intracranial pressure above which cerebral damage is progressive is unknown. In normal man, the intracranial pressure may be raised to well over 1000 mm of water by subarachnoid saline infusion without producing more than a headache. In cerebral contusion, the brain edema is of the "vasogenic" type as opposed to intracellular "cytotoxic" edema. It should be noted at the outset that therapy to reduce cerebral edema may simply be lowering intracranial pressure without removing extracellular water from the brain; it has been noted that osmotic agents are not a rational treatment for edema due to leaky blood-brain barrier, whereas steroids are, since they act to decrease membrane permeability. Thus the authors suspect that osmotic agents actually effect water removal through action on residual normal tissue, and that there may be a similar explanation for the enigma that steroids have minimal effect on badly traumatized cerebrum.[217] Massive doses of steroids have been found effective by some workers.[63]

Constant monitoring of intracranial pressure is ideal, with close observation of the respiratory pattern if the child's breathing is not controlled by respirator. An arterial catheter is extremely helpful in the first few days to monitor blood pressure and provide an immediate source of specimens for frequent arterial blood gas analysis. Alarms should be set to indicate respiratory and cardiovascular irregularities. A controlled constant volume infusion device assures that fluid overload does not occur and that precise doses of potent drugs such as the cardiac and vascular tonic and lytic agents are administered.

The major methods of intracranial pressure monitoring utilize epidural or subdural (and subarachnoid) implants; epidural pressure transducers are advantageous in avoiding the requisite dural opening for a subdural cannula, which transmits the surface fluid pressure through a hollow tubing to an external transducer.[93,100] Both methods are useful for prolonged constant monitoring, frequently needed for as long as several weeks.

Continuous pressure monitoring allows rational timing of osmotic or other therapy to avoid peak cycles of intracranial pressure. Generally a pressure above about 350 mm of water should be treated in a child with head injury. The monitor allows notation of clinical setbacks that may not be apparent in the severely injured patient.

Although urea was one of the first osmotic agents found useful for traumatic edema, currently mannitol and glycerol are most widely used. Mannitol intravenously is particularly suitable for immediate therapy in the emergency room; it is administered as a bolus or rapid drip to a total dose of 0.5 to 1.5 gm per kilogram and may be repeated every two or three hours as needed. Urine output should be monitored by indwelling bladder catheter. A rebound effect on intracranial pressure should be anticipated, necessitating repeated administration of mannitol or a definitive operative procedure (clot removal or decompression and resection of a contusion).

Glycerol may be used intravenously as a 10 per cent solution, which carries a significant free fluid load, or orally (per nasogastric tube in comatose patients) as a 50 per cent solution in 5 per cent dextrose in water. The dosage should be 0.5 gm per kilogram every three to four hours initially but may be adjusted depending on the results. This drug is metabolized by the liver and contributes to patient caloric intake during long-term usage. Oral administration is subject to the frequent vagaries of gastric and intestinal absorption, particularly in the first few days after injury; it may also be contraindicated by coexisting abdominal trauma.

If the patient's serum osmolarity reaches

350 mOsm per liter, use of the osmotic agent should be reduced or discontinued. Figure 59–20 shows a direct readout of intracranial pressure recorded by an epidural fiberoptic transducer; a statistical summary of pressure is shown for 20 consecutive treatment periods using oral glycerol.

Respiratory control is of considerable aid in reducing intracranial pressure in the short term. Tracheal intubation and hyperventilation should be accomplished to maintain the serum carbon dioxide tension between 30 and 35 mm of mercury, with even lower levels occasionally required. Intracranial pressure response to this maneuver is apparent within 30 seconds, and will provide sufficient time for diagnostic studies and operative therapy, if indicated, to be achieved. Its use in more protracted management is widespread, although experimental evidence abounds to suggest that the effect on intracranial vascular volume disappears. Even in this case, stepwise reduction in Pco_2 will achieve incremental salutory results.

In addition to the universally used osmotic agents, barbiturates, diphenylhydantoin (Dilantin), and the curarelike compounds have particular indications. Recent work suggests experimentally that barbiturates may reduce the oxygen requirement of the brain.[137,139,143,158,200] The rationale for their use after head injury with significant ongoing pressure or other forms of cerebral "suppression" such as contusion is that one protects the brain from *future* insult by pretreatment. Doses of intravenous pentobarbitol (Nembutal) in the range of 3 to 6 mg per kilogram may achieve rapid reduction of raised intracranial pressure that has been resistant to other therapy. Although this intentional induction of "barbiturate coma" is a newer therapeutic modality, existing studies indicate that one should achieve a serum level of around 3 to 5 mg per 100 ml for maximum protection; clinically this has corresponded to electroencephalographic slow theta rhythm, a useful monitor, since the neurological examination is uninformative.[138] Strict respiratory and arterial blood gas monitoring with controlled ventilation is essential. There would appear to be a dual and probably related purpose to barbiturate use in head injury: reduction of cerebral metabolism and reduction of intracranial pressure. Further

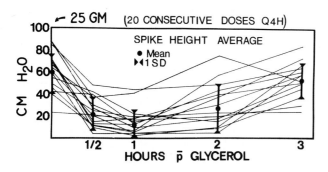

A

Figure 59–20 Intracranial pressure tracings monitored by an epidural fiberoptic transducer. *A*. Intracranial pressure values before and at one half, one, two, and three hours after 20 consecutive doses of 25 gm (0.5 gm per kilogram) of glycerol given by nasogastric tube as a 50 per cent solution. The mean intracranial pressure and standard deviation of the 20 readings are shown. Glycerol was effective for about three hours after each dose in this patient with diffuse cerebral contusion. *B*. Intracranial pressure tracing from a 12-year-old girl with intraventricular hemorrhage and moderate, stable ventricular dilatation. Twenty-five grams of glycerol was given by nasogastric tube roughly every two hours to control her pressure (*arrows*). The left-hand portion of the tracing shows the intracranial pressure when she was given only 12.5 gm of glycerol at three-hour intervals. The patient's level of consciousness was depressed at the peak pressures.

B HOURS

work is needed to discover the place of this treatment in the spectrum of other modalities. Classically, systemic hypothermia has been used to provide a similar reduction in metabolism.

In certain patients who exhibit tonic decerebration, uncontrolled cerebral hyperventilation, or persistent convulsions, systemic paralysis with a curarelike compound is temporarily beneficial. The intravenous dosage varies depending on the compound used; control is best achieved with an agent that requires readministration every two hours or so. This generally has a beneficial effect on raised intracranial pressure as well. All children with major cerebral injury should be given frequent doses of antacid medication to protect the stomach from "stress ulceration" and hemorrhage.[1]

METABOLIC EFFECTS. Maintenance fluid administration is about 1000 ml per square meter per 24 hours (one half to two thirds of normal maintenance requirement); the amount of sodium and potassium given is related to the serum electrolyte profile. Electrolyte levels, blood urea nitrogen, glucose and osmolality of the serum, and arterial blood gas values are obtained at frequent intervals, at least every 12 hours in the acute injury phase. In patients with head injury and systemic trauma, care must be taken to avoid excess fluid load.

Acid-base balance in a traumatized child requires knowledge of carbon dioxide tension, pH, and serum bicarbonate content. Excessive breathing is common after head injury and leads to respiratory alkalosis with serum pH above 7.45. This may be spontaneously a result of hypoxia, cerebrospinal fluid acidosis, or central neurogenic hyperventilation. Hypoxia should be treated appropriately with pulmonary toilet and additions to the inhaled oxygen concentration. The most common cause of respiratory alkalosis is induced ventilator hyperventilation employed in an effort to lower the Pco_2 for its beneficial effect on cerebral blood flow and intracranial pressure. pH in excess of 7.55 may contribute to convulsions.

Respiratory acidosis is uncommon in absence of pulmonary trauma or infection; if discovered, a cause such as post-traumatic pulmonary insufficiency, "neurogenic" pulmonary edema, or pneumonia should be investigated.[65,163]

Metabolic alkalosis is a result of hydrogen ion loss, usually from excessive nasogastric suction in the early days after head injury or from prolonged ileus or abdominal injury. Hypokalemia and hyperaldosteronism both accentuate renal hydrogen ion loss. Potassium chloride should be administered to offset this tendency. A mixed respiratory and metabolic alkalosis appears to be most common following head injury in the absence of systemic shock or poor respiratory gas exchange. Persistent metabolic acidosis is unusual and usually due to shock with excess lactic acid production or to acute renal failure; both of these complications are immediately life-threatening and should be dealt with vigorously.

Serum osmolality is regulated predominantly by input and excretion of salt and water. Neural cellular function is probably affected by hyperosmolality in excess of 320 mOsm per liter, although in cases of severe intracranial hypertension with requisite osmotic diuretic usage, one may accept levels up to 340 to 350 mOsm per liter as the lesser of two evils. Since inadequate water intake is obviated by intravenous administration, the most common source of hypertonicity, in the absence of osmotic diuretic use, is excess urine output, the syndrome of inadequate antidiuretic hormone release or diabetes insipidus due to hypothalamic injury or pituitary disruption. If water replacement needs become excessive, aqueous pitressin may be cautiously administered. Extreme care must be taken to avoid acute reversal and water retention, particularly in a small child. Urine flow and osmolality should be monitored hourly and replacement adjusted accordingly during acute diabetes insipidus.

Equally common is the reverse problem of inappropriate secretion of antidiuretic hormone, which is *normally* seen in the first two days after head injury, usually partially offset by transient "cerebral salt retention," triggered by a decrease in circulatory blood volume. If the antidiuretic hormone secretion persists, it leads to often severe hypotonicity. Inappropriate antidiuretic hormone secretion exists even in cerebrally injured neonates and premature infants, although it has been little appreciated in the literature.[165] Diagnosis of this syndrome requires serum hypotonicity in spite of urinary hypernatremia and normal adrenal and renal function. Major therapy is through restriction of fluid intake to one fourth to one third of normal maintenance fluid, and occasionally use of hypertonic (three times normal) salt solutions in resistant cases. Recently the tetracycline Declomycin has found application in this problem through its interference with renal tubular water retention; it essentially produces nephrogenic diabetes insipidus.[27,47] Prolonged positive-pressure ventilation may contribute to the persistence of inappropriate antidiuretic hormone secretion.[205]

Glucose metabolism is frequently upset by cerebral injury, while hypoglycemia is common in neonates and may add to neurological depression of cerebral trauma.[69] More common is the problem of hyperglycemia in children of all ages. The common use of steroids in this clinical setting increases glucose intolerance. Excess glucose adds to the osmotic load, causes dehydration through concomitant renal water loss, and is most hazardous in the setting of hyperglycemic nonketotic coma, which may produce a number of confusing neurological signs additive to those of the primary injury and has been correlated with massive cerebral edema.[133,173,182] These problems may be severe in a latent or overtly diabetic child. Since the usual manifestations of all the endocrinopathies are masked by traumatic coma, discovery requires anticipatory metabolic monitoring.

Post-traumatic anterior pituitary deficiency usually assumes importance in the later acute or early chronic stages; corticosteroid lack, may, however, become critical early in the course. This is particularly the case for the child who has been receiving long-term premorbid steroid treatment. Anterior pituitary pan-deficiency following concussion and even skull fracture has been reported in a number of children; the pathology of this lesion is well known, and in fatal head injury, 50 per cent of patients show ischemic or hemorrhagic changes of the gland and hypothalamus.[34,35,99,175]

Intermediate and long-term management of children with "closed" or postoperative head injuries is essentially an exercise in maintenance of homeostasis to provide optimal atmosphere for repair of cerebral damage. The child is ideally treated in an intensive care facility until there are independence of respiratory support, no significant ongoing neurological fluctuation, and self-regulation of intracerebral pressure. Even without complications, this may take several weeks. Children with severe neurological compromise are eventually managed in an "extended care facility"; physical therapy is an early adjunct to recovery to avoid joint contracture, and rehabilitation is begun as soon as the patient is physically and mentally able to benefit from it.

SEIZURES. Experimental work has shown that pretreatment with diphenylhydantoin (Dilantin) following head injury may prevent development of subsequent chronic seizure foci.[131,188] Since this drug has been commonly given prophylactically in cerebral trauma, it has proved to be perhaps the basis of a dual salutory effect.[188] Phenobarbital is frequently the drug of choice for posttraumatic seizure control in smaller children. Again this may be a wise choice because of its effect on cerebral metabolism and intracranial pressure. Barbiturates tend to suppress the level of consciousness and may confuse the neurological status, although, as discussed earlier, they have specific therapeutic indications. Cortical contusion and the presence of fresh blood in the immediate epicortical space may cause repetitive or continuous convulsions requiring deep sedation or even systemic paralysis to control. A new antiseizure drug, sodium valproate, should be mentioned, as it has already had major effect in controlling difficult pediatric seizures of the "absence" variety; it is also finding broader use, particularly in so-called mixed seizure varieties, which include many chronic "post-traumatic" cases.

Operative Management

Operative therapy may be indicated if focal contusion causes a pronounced progression of signs and symptoms, and if the tissue can be safely sacrificed. The common contusion involving the anterior temporal lobe and adjacent orbital frontal cortex may be "decompressed" by limited resection of the pulped tissue of the anterior temporal region. This lesion is associated with a recognized clinical syndrome and responds well to internal decompression.[146] With current intracranial pressure monitoring systems and vigorous therapy for increased pressure, resection may often be avoided. The decision to resect an area of contusion must be based on the belief that there is no possible recovery of the regional tissue. Although patients with focal cortical injuries or resections often appear "normal," specific mental status testing may demonstrate significant deficiencies.[160] To save a life this may be justified, but, particularly in children, it must be well considered.

In uncontrolled post-traumatic intracranial hypertension, a decision must be made as to the place of bony operative decompression without resection of tissue. Generally, performance of a wide unilateral, bilateral, or bifrontal cranial decompression is decided on if the child's basic cerebral lesion is thought to be reversible, that is, the parenchyma is suffering principally from pressure-related ischemia without irrecoverable neural loss. Reported results of decompressive procedures for trauma are disappointing; many of these patients, however, have been severely compromised before operative intervention.[29,109,222] Large dural grafts are made, and in the bifrontal procedure, the anterior falx is severed to allow the brain to move upward freely; this necessitates occlusion of the anterior portion of the sagittal sinus, which may add additional venous drainage problems to the traumatically swollen brain. If craniotomy is done for clot resection, and severe swelling is anticipated, it is reasonable to not replace the bone flap and perhaps to enlarge the dural cover by grafting.

Cerebral Wounds From Foreign Body Penetration

Although children are occasionally accidental victims of cerebral gunshot wounds in peacetime, more frequently calvarial penetration results from low-momentum pointed objects such as a stick or nail. Because of the small amount of energy involved, the penetration tends to occur through a thin part of the skull such as the medial or superior orbital wall. A rather common injury stems from a child running with a stick protruding from the mouth, falling forward, and driving the point through the soft palate or tonsilar fossa into the base of the brain. These wounds are difficult to evaluate because of the hidden entrance site. The tip of the foreign body may break off within the skull. A particularly insidious occurrence is the reported insertion of sewing needles through the anterior fontanelles of unwanted children and infants.[6]

The principal cause of death from penetrating injury to the brain is a rapidly forming hematoma due to direct laceration of an artery or venous sinus. Much more common is the secondary complication of infection, which may evolve several weeks after an apparently minor injury as judged by the external wound. Often there will be a missed foreign body, such as a pencil point; this is one of several sources of cerebral abscess in childhood.[89,154]

Therapy for the acute wound is directed to control of hemorrhage, which, if not initially present, may occur when the foreign body is removed, perhaps releasing a tamponaded sinus or vessel—this is a danger if the penetrating object is removed without proper operative exposure. Thorough debridement of the regional injury, closure of the obligate dural laceration, and administration of appropriate antibiotics are general guidelines for management. If the penetrating object is totally removed, and if the patient's condition is stable, computed tomography may show the extent of the injury, and the patient may be managed with antibiotics alone (Fig. 59–21).

PRENATAL AND PERINATAL INJURY

In Utero Injury

The liability to mechanical head injury begins in the womb, reaching significance as the fetal head enlarges in the third trimester; numerous undocumented events earlier in pregnancy may traumatize the fetus, of course, but the magnitude of this problem is totally speculative. The mechanism of fetal head injury is occasionally an external blunt or penetrating force to the maternal abdomen; more usually it is compression of the cranium against the pelvic bones or the sacral promontory.[4,5,55,82] Depressed skull fractures predominate before parturition. The responsible forces are obvious from study of the normal fetal cephalic rotation, engagement, and labor, and the resultant remarkable molding of the fetal skull.[8,16]

In suspected fetal cerebral damage prior to term, an attempt should be made to estimate the gestational age to assess feasibility of early delivery and evaluation and treatment of the injury.[197] Once the child is de-

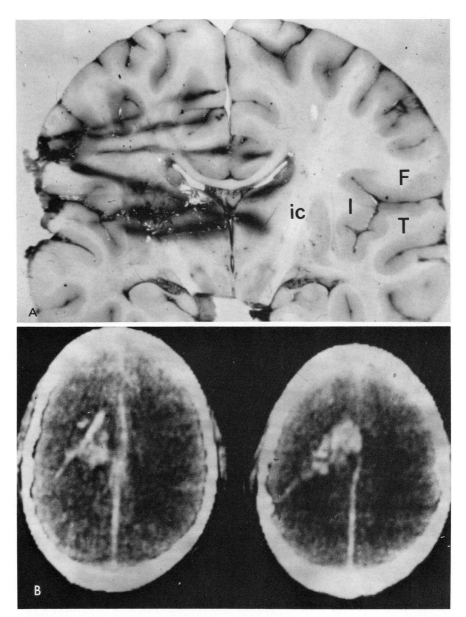

Figure 59–21   Examples of penetrating injury to the brain. *A*. Coronal section of brain through the thalamus showing multiple hemorrhagic tracks in the right hemisphere made by a thin pointed object. Several tracks have penetrated across the midline. ic, Internal capsule; I, insula; F, frontal lobe; T, temporal lobe. *B*. CT scan from a 19-year-old man who was aphasic and hemiparetic from a penetrating wound to the left hemisphere made by a screwdriver. There is a hematoma at the medial end of the track, and bulge of the midline locally to the right. Entry site was above the left ear.

livered, the treatment is identical to that for any other infant of the same age. Trauma to the fetal head in utero may be more common than suspected.

Posterior Fossa Hematoma

Posterior fossa subdural hematoma usually presents as obstructive hydrocephalus at a few weeks of age, although it may cause more acute brain stem compression, block of the cerebral aqueduct, and respiratory arrest.[58] Acute epidural hematomas and intraparenchymal clots in newborns of any gestational age are rare.[51]

Low-birth-weight infants are at risk for cerebellar hemorrhage; if massive, this syndrome presents as progressive apnea necessitating ventilatory support and falling hematocrit leading to death in 12 to 36 hours.[140] Often the diagnosis is missed because there is no bulging of the anterior fontanelle. With early diagnosis these infants may recover completely, aided by the fact that early loss of cerebellar tissue leaves almost no motor or coordination deficit.

Intra-axial or extra-axial hematoma of the posterior fossa large enough to cause brain stem symptoms or cerebrospinal fluid obstruction is an absolute indication for craniectomy and clot evacuation. Smaller lesions should probably also be removed because of the danger of sudden expansion and the uncertainties of their cause.

Nontraumatic Neurological Entities

Neonatal Intracranial Hemorrhage

The subependymal germinal matrix tissue lies over the head of the caudate nucleus in the wall of the lateral ventricle; it reaches maximum mass at about 26 weeks of gestation and then disappears over the next 10 weeks as cells leave to populate other regions of the developing brain. The region is prone to infarction and hemorrhage, often with ventricular rupture in premature infants delivered between 28 and 33 weeks of gestation. It is not a recognized entity at term gestation.

Considerable fetal morbidity stems from the spectrum of matrix infarction and hemorrhage, although definition of the problem or even identification of nonfatal cases is difficult.[198,218] Even without obvious rupture of clot into the lateral ventricle, periventricular damage disrupts normal cerebral development (Fig. 59–22).

If the event of intraventricular rupture is clinically apparent, the infant may become apneic, opisthotonic in status epilepticus, or limp, and show rapid increase in head size and a tight anterior fontanelle. More often, the neurosurgeon will be asked to see a premature infant a week or so after delivery when increasing head circumference accompanies failure to thrive that is out of proportion to the other problems of prematurity. Even without specific history, this clinical picture in an infant born between 28 and 35 weeks almost certainly represents intraventricular hemorrhage from the germinal matrix.

If the infant is seen in the acute phase, CT scan will usually give a definitive diagnosis; in any case, ventricular aspiration will document the problem, and the pressure may be checked and reduced if necessary.[113] The subdural space should be tapped on the way to the ventricle, as the two lesions may coexist. Occasionally a clot may obstruct only one foramen of Monro or predominantly dilate one ventricle during acute rupture, as shown in Figure 59–22; both ventricles should be tapped. The infant is monitored for apnea and given diphenylhydantoin. Generally the intracranial pressure is limited by open sutures, and continuous drainage need not be provided unless rapid head growth supervenes. A 5- to 10-ml air "bubble" may be introduced by transcoronal needle into the lateral ventricle in the nursery; anterior-posterior and cross-table lateral (brow-up and brow-down) skull x-rays will define the ventricular size and perhaps show a mass. If the head circumference continues to enlarge too rapidly, repeated ventricular aspirations will control the internal hydrocephalus and aid in removing high-protein fluid. Ventricular shunting is required in persistent obstruction or malabsorption of cerebrospinal fluid; this is ideally performed when the ventricular fluid has cleared sufficiently to avoid obstruction of the shunt valve mechanism, or drainage may be valveless.

If a premature infant with a chronically large head is given a ventricular tap a few weeks after delivery, brownish thin fluid is obtained as a residuum of the hemorrhage.

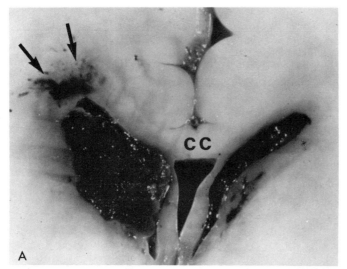

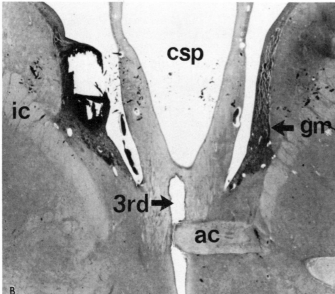

Figure 59–22 Coronal sections of neonatal brains, through the basal ganglia, demonstrating subependymal germinal matrix hemorrhage and intraventricular rupture. Both cases show a normally present cavum septum pellucidum. *A.* The site of hemorrhage is the right germinal matrix (*arrows*); the hematoma ruptured into the ventricular system, causing asymmetrical acute ventricular dilatation. CC, corpus callosum. *B.* Normal germinal tissue (gm) is present lateral to the left ventricle; the right germinal matrix contains a clot that did not rupture into the ventricle until the postmortem examination. The right ventricle is, however, focally dilated by the bulging clot. csp, Cavum septum pellucidum; ac, anterior commissure; 3rd, third ventricle; ic, internal capsule.

Obstruction to cerebrospinal fluid generally occurs at the cerebral aqueduct, shown in Figure 59–3C, the fourth ventricular exit, or the basilar cisterns (Fig. 59–23).

Intraventricular hemorrhage in a newborn of more than 36 weeks' gestation generally comes from the choroid plexus (cf. Fig. 59–4). Babies with larger heads (i.e., term or post-term) are at greater risk for tears of the falx and tentorium leading to subdural blood collections. Breech delivery or otherwise traumatic extraction greatly increases the risk, and acute subdural hematoma after delivery is found almost exclusively in this group.[2] Immediate sub-dural taps may be lifesaving in this situation.

Asphyxia Neonatorum

The notion of "cerebral palsy" is inextricably entwined with both traumatic and asphyxic mechanisms of brain injury. The role of perinatal asphyxia, overall, in death and morbidity from pediatric brain injury is a major one; neurosurgeons must be conversant with the protean manifestations of asphyxia neonatorum to make a reasonable judgment of etiology and therapy in cerebral trauma. Clinical findings frequently

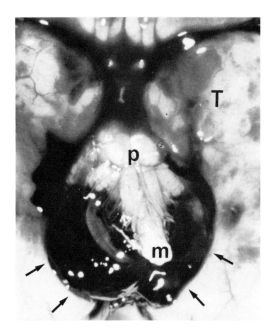

Figure 59–23 Base view, posterior portion of neonatal brain demonstrates acute hematoma loculated about the fourth ventricular outlet foramina; the clot creates a mass between the brain stem and the cerebellum (*arrows*). This infant suffered massive intraventricular hemorrhage from the germinal matrix that filled the ventricular system and created this "subarachnoid" loculation. T, medial temporal lobe; P, pons; m, medulla oblongata.

mimic or coexist with those of mechanical perinatal trauma. In addition, asphyxia invariably complicates the management of a traumatic lesion.

Dramatic physiological changes take place during parturition; oxygen deficit during this transition is frequently associated with functional loss of neural tissue, with complex rules for reversibility. Multiple risk factors are associated with asphyxia neonatorum; the interacting variables of cerebral blood flow and cardiac output, glucose, pH, hypercarbia, and the like are all critical to the type of lesion and to the apparent resistance to insult of the neonatal cerebrum. The type of brain damage incurred depends heavily on the gestational or postnatal age of the infant.[18,166,213,223] Although neurological sequelae in children surviving prolonged mechanical ventilation in the neonatal period include mental, visual, auditory, and major motor deficits, the current opinion is that in the majority of cases, the outcome justifies a concerted effort to resuscitate even very severely asphyxiated neonates.[136,215] Sublethal as-

phyxia from obstetrical complications has been shown compatible with normal intelligence and fine motor development at four years' follow-up.[171]

Porencephaly: "Cerebral Palsy"

Collectively, the infants and children who suffer from fixed lesions of cerebral scarring (gliosis) or missing tissue (cystic residua) constitute the most common neurological "birth trauma" group. The ill-defined entity "porencephaly," in its various manifestations, is often associated with obstruction of the cerebrospinal fluid pathways and thus eventually falls into the neurosurgeon's province.[51,130,144]

A porencephalic cyst is an asymmetrical fluid-filled space formerly occupied by cerebral white matter; often it connects with the ventricular system, and in minimal form may appear as a focal ventricular dilatation or diverticulum. Although many of these lesions are attributed to "birth trauma," they most likely result from in utero or perinatal infarction. The cystic residua of severe cerebral contusion in older children may be difficult to differentiate from the congential lesion (Fig. 59–24). In cases of "porencephaly" in which new clinical deficits evolve, cystic tumors must be considered; although a number of cases of "progressive" cerebral palsy are recorded, usually this progression is a mechanical problem of hydrodynamics and osmotic forces rather than a subtle neoplasia.

Although the porencephalic cysts and accompanying gliosis may commonly be associated with diplegic or hemiplegic spasticity and dysarthria, the specific loss of function depends on the original region of cerebral compromise. Retardation is common with large or multiple lesions. Adequate control of secondary hydrocephalus has been achieved by fenestration of cysts into the ventricular system or subarachnoid space; frequently mechanical internal shunts are required to maintain stable intracranial hydrodynamics.

THE BATTERED CHILD

This topic is of major importance to the pediatric neurosurgeon and may involve virtually any of the entities thus far described. The most severe consequences of

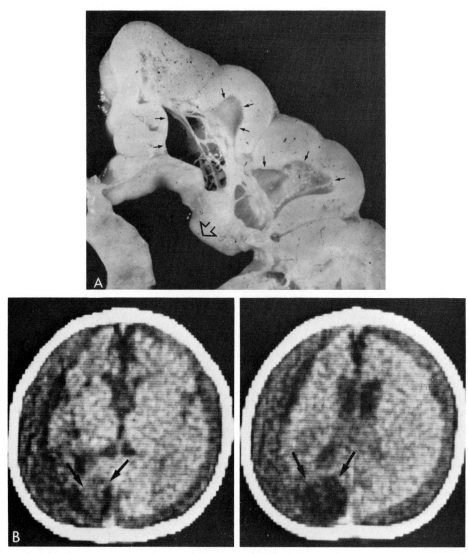

Figure 59–24   Congenital and post-traumatic porencephaly. *A*. Congenital multicystic brain with dilatation of the ventricular system (*open arrow*) due to loss of tissue. Note sharp demarcation between remaining cortical band and destroyed subjacent white matter (*small arrows*). This condition is often attributed to "birth trauma." *B*. CT scans of 7-month-old infant with enlarging head circumference; the patient suffered cerebral contusion and bilateral subdural hematomata at 3 months of age. Multicystic left hemisphere is noted with residual subdural hygroma fluid bilaterally. The posterior left hemisphere shows a large post-traumatic porencephalic cyst (*arrows*).

the "battered child" syndrome, and nearly all the fatalities, involve cerebral injury. It has become a watchword for modern pediatric emergency coverage that this cause must be considered when any child has unexplained subdural hematoma or head injury. Evidence for multiple injuries of varying causes and ages is the hallmark of the classic presentation. One third of all cases occur in children under 6 months of age, and another third before 3 years; there is a severalfold increased incidence among pre-

mature or ill newborns, hyperkinetic or destructive children, stepchildren, and "unwanted" or illegitimate babies.[11,106,110] Social and economic antecedents have been intensively investigated.[90,203]

The explanation for injury offered by the parent is often totally lacking or contains bizarre or contradictory elements. A young sibling is a frequent scapegoat, even though he may be obviously incapable of inflicting the injury. Delay in seeking medical assistance is usual, unless the child is seriously injured. In this situation the nervous system is usually involved. Neurological presentation may vary from intractable seizures or coma to a jittery baby or isolated increased intracranial tension (full anterior fontanelle). In any of these situations, bilateral chronic or acute subdural hematomas may be present without external evidence of injury; 50 per cent of these cases result from violent shaking of the child.[25] This same mechanism is implicated in spinal cord trauma leading to a floppy or frankly paralyzed child.[72] It is recognized as well that hypokinetic, hypotonic infants may result from extreme maternal nutritional and emotional neglect, with the ultimate correlate of retardation.[24] This rather common but often undiscovered situation falls within the broader definition of "Trauma X," that is, "an unhealthy environment for the child" of whatever etiology. Treatment for any of the resulting neurological entities is outlined in the appropriate section of this chapter.

OUTCOME OF CRANIOCEREBRAL INJURY

This discussion is directed primarily at the long-term results following cerebral contusion; other entities may have specific differences in outcome as outlined in the appropriate section. A major effort has been given to prognostic prescience based on clinical findings in the few days after trauma involving cerebral contusion. Adequate qualitative prediction, other than the outcome of survival, is perhaps, currently an insoluble problem. It requires nonexistent understanding of brain function and reaction to traumatic disruption. In children the arrest and setback of developmental processes vastly complicates the situation; this, no doubt, is in part the source of discordant ideas on the recovery potential following trauma to the young brain.[14,85,196] It is known that infants under 2 years of age have a better potential for regaining function after irrevocable loss of specific portions of the telencephalon.[36,81] Beyond this age the potential falls off rapidly, and the issue of tissue recovery becomes pre-eminent.

In an adult, personality and intellectual achievement have generally been established premorbidly. There is no consistent reference for a 2 year old child with brain injury who was compromised at 18 months of age; nor is there a reasonable predictor for future attainment. Thus studies of outcome after head injury are limited to correlations between the frequency of certain early clinical signs and ultimate mental status relative to age, i.e., comatose, severely handicapped, able to perform at "previous level," and so forth. Additionally one may define, at the moment of follow-up testing, residual behavioral and intellectual deficits within the limits of new psychobehavioral technology. Predictions for future improvement in any temporally defined parameter can only be based on progress to date, time interval since injury, and what little is known of the present deficit as a likely compromising influence on acquisition of new knowledge. The nervous system probably cannot continue to improve for years; manifest long-term improvement in a traumatized child is likely a mixture of normally recovered "learning" processes and the so-called "plasticity" of certain totipotential neural components.[33,79,225]

The task of prognostication following pediatric head injury is nearly impossible, in part because of the unpredictability of reaction in the developing brain. There are, nonetheless, some studies appearing that examine specific points of recovery potential, or attempt with computer aid to provide a summary of meaningful cross correlations between a morass of signs and symptoms and outcome. In general, these studies answer the question "Will the child live?" but only superficially the qualification "Will he have brain damage?"[20,124,160]

There is apparent agreement that childhood brain trauma of an "intermediate" severity has a favorable outlook; this lesion involves closed head injury with localized contusion and impairment of consciousness that is neither "extreme nor prolonged."[156] It is also apparent that within the rather pliable limits of this definition, "favorable" means that the child recovers from a hemiparesis, perhaps from transient aphasia, and again becomes a normally functioning person. There is no meaningful measure, in this case, with which to examine whether the injury leads to a specific loss of ultimate achievement.

There is also good agreement on "guarded" prognosis in children who remain in protracted periods of depressed consciousness or persistent neurological dysfunction. It is this group, should they improve at all, that has multiple behavioral and intellectual deficits compounding physical handicaps; both brain stem injury and "diffuse" injury are included in this heterogenous category without specific mechanistic correlation other than coma.[71] The intelligence quotient may be followed serially for several years; although it generally increases a bit, the result is invariably a "retarded" child.

Evaluation of school performance, recognized to be a critical marker of mental and behavioral adjustment, showed, for example, only 17 of 37 children with severe head injury doing "fairly normally" after four years. The children were all under the age of 16 years at the time of injury and sustained contusion as the major cerebral injury without an additional ischemic component. All those who were comatose for two weeks were unable to attend regular school; even brief coma is capable of producing this outcome.[80] Depending on the specific focus of outcome examined, this evaluation is typically carried out by workers who have no involvement in the initial (therapeutic) aspects of the cases. It is recognized that neither a child's mother nor his physician can be relied upon as an accurate judge of his mental status.[53]

Review of the neurological literature discloses little improvement in the outcome of head injury over the past 50 years, despite therapeutic advances of "major" consequence.[79,116] Reports of two recent series of patients, however, appear to indicate that cerebral trauma is not necessarily a definitive event, at least for pediatric populations. One hundred and sixty patients reported by Becker and co-workers, heavily weighted to the pediatric age group, and 53 patients with a mean age of 7.2 years reported by Bruce and associates show surprisingly low morbidity and mortality rates following severe head injury treated with early, intensive, multidisciplinary therapy.[10,23] Immediate computer-assisted diagnosis of operative lesions and monitoring of intracranial pressure and respiratory and metabolic parameters, and use of metabolic depressants are the mainstay of this effective regimen. This approach avoids the recognized factors contributing to death after head injury—such as delay in treatment of mass lesions, poorly controlled epilepsy, meningitis, hypoxia, and hypotension—and focuses heavily on the major unavoidable secondary process of cerebral edema.[192] A modified Glasgow coma scale, with addition of brain stem reflexes, has proved valuable in the initial phase of a multi-institutional study, and serves well for younger patients.[116] These studies are beginning to confirm the older opinion, garnered from postmortem studies, that children indeed suffer different traumatic cerebral lesions than do adults. Computed tomographic brain scans show fewer hemorrhagic contusion foci and intracranial hematomas than expected in severe head injury; these scans allow visualization of lesions that would formerly not have been found and provide the assurance that operative lesions have not been missed.

An important qualification to the dictum that children do well after head injury is discussed by Bruce and co-workers.[23] If children indeed suffer different types of lesions, specifically lacking in contusion, laceration, and clots, their initial neurological status is probably not comparable to adult injury in potential for recovery; that is, an initially bad coma scale rating may be due to reversible causes.

An unexpected dividend from the recent studies is that heroic effort at salvage of children with severe head injury does not necessarily result in increased numbers of severely compromised survivors; it appears that, as with certain childhood encephalopathies, the major lesion of increased intracranial pressure, although probably not edema in the adult sense with reduced parenchymal density on CT scan, may be controlled with some regularity to allow good recovery of temporarily malfunctioning neural elements.

REFERENCES

1. Abramson, D. J.: Curling's ulcer in childhood; Review of the literature and report of five cases. Surgery, 55:321–336, 1964.
2. Abroms, I. F., McLennan, J. E., and Mandell, F.: Acute neonatal subdural hematoma following breech delivery. Amer. J. Dis. Child., 131:192–194, 1977.
3. Adams, J. H., Mitchell, D. E., Graham, D. I., et al.: Diffuse brain damage of immediate impact type. Brain, 100:489–502, 1977.
4. Alexander, E., Jr., and Davis, C. H., Jr.: Intrauterine fracture of the infant's skull. J. Neurosurg., 30:446–454, 1969.
5. Alexander, E., Jr., and Kushner, J.: Intrauterine head injuries. In Vinken, P. J., and Bruyn, G.

W., eds.: Handbook of Clinical Neurology. Vol. 23. Amsterdam, Elsevier–North Holland Publishing Co., 1975, pp 471–476.

6. Ameli, N. O., and Alimohammadi, A.: Attempted infanticide by insertion of sewing needles through fontanelles: Report of two cases. J. Neurosurg., 33:721–723, 1970.

7. Arkins, T. J., McLennan, J. E., and Winston, K. R.: Acute posterior fossa epidural hematomas in children. Amer. J. Dis. Child., 131:690–692, 1977.

8. Axton, J. H. M., and Levy, L. F.: Congenital moulding depressions of the skull. Brit. Med. J., 1:1644–1647, 1965.

9. Backlund, E. O., and vonHolst, H.: Controlled subtotal evacuation of intracerebral haematomas by stereotactic technique. Surg. Neurol., 9:99–101, 1978.

10. Becker, D. P., Miller, J. D., Ward, J. D., Greenberg, R. P., Young, H. F., and Sakalas, R.: The outcome from severe head injury with early diagnosis and intensive management. J. Neurosurg., 47:491–502, 1977.

11. Bell, W. E., and McCormick, W. F.: Increased Intracranial Pressure in Children. Philadelphia, W. B. Saunders, Co., 1972.

12. Bender, M. B., and Christoff, N.: Nonsurgical treatment of subdural hematomas. Arch. Neurol. (Chicago), 31:73–79, 1974.

13. Bergsma, D., ed.: Morphogenesis and Malformation of Face and Brain. Birth Defects: Original Article Series, Vol. 11, No. 7. New York, Alan R. Liss, Inc., 1975.

14. Black, P., Jeffries, J. J., Blumer, D., Wellner, A., and Walker, A. E.: The posttraumatic syndrome in children. In Walker, A. E., Caveness, W., and Critchley, M., eds.: Late Effects of Head Injury. Springfield, Ill., Charles C Thomas, 1969, pp. 142–149.

15. Blank, N. K., Strand R., Gilles, F. H., and Palakshappa, A.: Posterior fossa subdural hematomas in neonates. Arch. Neurol. (Chicago), 35:108–111, 1978.

16. Borell, U., and Fernström, I.: The mechanism of labour. Radiol. Clin. N. Amer., 5:73–85, 1967.

17. Brain damage in sport. (editorial) Lancet, 1:401–402, 1976.

18. Brann, A. W., and Dykes, F. D.: The effects of intrauterine asphyxia on the full term neonate. Clin. Perinatol., 4:149–161, 1977.

19. Bricolo, A., Turazzi, S., Alexandre, A., et al.: Decerebrate rigidity in acute head injury. J. Neurosurg., 47:680–698, 1977.

20. Brink, J. D., Garrett, A. L., Hale, W., WooSam, J., and Nickel, V. L.: Recovery of motor and intellectual function in children sustaining severe head injuries. Develop. Med. Child Neurol., 12:565–571, 1970.

21. Britt, R. H., and Hamilton, R. D.: Large decompressive craniotomy in the treatment of acute subdural hematoma. Neurosurgery, 2:195–200, 1978.

22. Brown, F. D., Mullan, S., and Duda, E. E.: Delayed traumatic intracerebral hematomas. J. Neurosurg., 48:1019–1022, 1978.

23. Bruce, D. A., Schut, L., Bruno, L. A., Wood, J. H., and Sutton, L. N.: Outcome following severe head injuries in children. J. Neurosurg., 48:679–688, 1978.

24. Buda, F. B., Rothney, W. B., and Rabe, E. F.: Hypotonia and the maternal-child relationship. Amer. J. Dis. Child., 124:906–907, 1972.

25. Caffey, J.: On the practice and theory of shaking infants. Amer. J. Dis. Child., 124:161–169, 1972.

26. Carter, B. L., Wolpert, S. M., and Karmody, C. S.: Recurrent meningitis associated with anomaly of the inner ear. Neuroradiology, 9: 55–61, 1975.

27. Cherrill, D. A., Stote, R. M., Birge, J. R., and Singer, I.: Demeclocycline treatment in the syndrome of inappropriate antidiuretic hormone secretion. Ann. Intern. Med., 83:654–656, 1975.

28. Choux, M., Grisoli, F., and Peragut, J. C.: Extradural hematomas in children. Child's Brain, 1:337–347, 1975.

29. Cooper, P. R., Rovit, R. L., and Ransohoff, J.: Hemicraniectomy in the treatment of acute subdural hematoma; A re-appraisal. Surg. Neurol., 5:25–28, 1976.

30. Courville, C. B.: Contrecoup injuries of the brain in infancy. Arch. Surg. (Chicago), 90:157–165, 1965.

31. Craft, A. W.: Head injury in children. In Vinken, P. J., and Bruyn, G. W., eds.:Handbook of Clinical Neurology. Vol. 23. Amsterdam, Elsevier–North Holland Publishing Co., 1975, pp. 445–458.

32. Craft, A. W., Shaw, D. A., and Cartlidge, N. E. F.: Head injuries in children. Brit. Med. J., 4:200–203, 1972.

33. Cragg, B. G.: Plasticity of synapses. Brit. Med. Bull., 30:141–144, 1974.

34. Crompton, M. R.: Hypothalmic lesions following closed head injury. Brain, 94:165–172, 1971.

35. Crompton, M. R.: Hypothalamic and pituitary lesions. In Vinken, P. J., and Bruyn, G. W., eds.: Handbook of Clinical Neurology. Vol. 23. Amsterdam, Elsevier–North Holland Publishing Co., 1975, pp. 465–469.

36. Damasio, A. R., Lima, A., and Damasio, H.: Nervous function after right hemisherectomy. Neurology (Minneap.), 25:89–93, 1975.

37. Davidoff, L. M., and Feiring, E. H.: Subdural hematoma occurring in surgically treated hydrocephalic children, with a note on a method of handling persistent accumulations. J. Neurosurg., 10:557–563, 1953.

38. De Vet, A. C.: Traumatic intracerebral hematoma. In Vinken, P. J., and Bruyn, G. W., eds.: Handbook of Clinical Neurology. Vol. 24. Amsterdam, Elsevier–North Holland Publishing Co., 1976, pp. 351–368.

39. Dodge, T. C.: An injury is no accident. New Eng. J. Med., 298:509–510, 1978.

40. Dolinskas, C. A., Zimmerman, R. A., and Bilaniuk, L. T.: A sign of subarachnoid bleeding on cranial computed tomograms of pediatric head trauma patients. Radiology, 126:409–411, 1978.

41. Duff, R. S., and Campbell, A. G. M.: Moral and ethical dilemmas in the special care nursery. New Eng. J. Med., 289:890–894, 1973.

42. Dunsker, S. B., and McCreary, H. S.: Leptomeningeal cyst of the posterior fossa. J. Neurosurg., 34:687–691, 1971.

43. Emerson, P., Fujimura, M., Howat, P., et al.: Timing of intraventricular haemorrhage. Arch. Dis. Child., 52:183–187, 1977.

44. Epstein, F., Naidich, T. P., Chase, N. E., Kricheff, I. I., Lin, J. P., and Ransohoff, J.: Role of computerized axial tomography in diagnosis and treatment of common neurosurgical problems of infancy and childhood. Child's Brain, 2:111–131, 1976.

45. Findler, G., Sahar, A., and Beller, A. J.: Continuous lumbar drainage of cerebrospinal fluid in neurosurgical patients. Surg. Neurol., 8:455–457, 1977.

46. Ford, L. E., and McLaurin, R. L.: Mechanisms of extradural hematomas. J. Neurosurg., 20:760–769, 1963.

47. Forrest, J. N., Cox, M., Hong, C., Morrison, G., Bia, M., and Singer, I.: Superiority of demeclocycline over lithium in the treatment of chronic syndrome of inappropriate secretion of antidiuretic hormone. New Eng. J. Med., 298:173–177, 1978.

48. French, B. N., and Dublin, A. B.: The value of computerized tomography in the management of 1000 consecutive head injuries. Surg. Neurol., 7:171–183, 1977.

49. French, B. N., Cobb, C. A., III, Corkill, G., and Youmans, J. R.: Delayed evolution of posttraumatic subdural hygroma. Surg. Neurol., 9:145–148, 1978.

50. Freytag, E.: Autopsy findings in head injury from blunt forces. Arch. Path. (Chicago), 75:402–413, 1973.

51. Friede, R. L.: Developmental Neuropathology. New York, Springer-Verlag, 1975.

52. Front, D., Beks, J. F., Georganas, C. L., et al.: Abnormal patterns of cerebrospinal fluid flow and absorption after head injuries: Diagnosis by isotope cisternography. Neuroradiology, 4:6–13, 1972.

53. Fuld, P. A., and Fisher, P.: Recovery of intellectual ability after closed head injury. Develop. Med. Child Neurol., 19:495–502, 1977.

54. Galbraith, S. L.: Age-distribution of extradural hemorrhage without skull fracture. Lancet, 1:1217–1218, 1973.

55. Genieser, N. B., and Becker, M. H.: Head trauma in children. Radiol. Clin. N. Amer., 12:333–342, 1974.

56. Gettelfinger, D. M., and Kokmen, E.: Superior sagittal sinus thrombosis. Arch. Neurol. (Chicago), 34:2–6, 1977.

57. Gilles, F. H.: Myelination in the neonatal brain. Hum. Path., 7:244–248, 1976.

58. Gilles, F. H., and Shillito, J., Jr.: Infantile Hydrocephalus: Retrocerebellar subdural hematoma. J. Pediat., 76:529–537, 1970.

59. Gilles, F. H., Dooling, E., and Fulchiero, A.: Sequence of myelination in the human fetus. Trans. Amer. Neurol. Ass., 101:244–246, 1976.

60. Gilles, F. H., Price, R. A., Kevy, S. V., et al.: Fibrinolytic activity in the ganglionic eminence of the premature human brain. Biol. Neonate., 18:426–432, 1971.

61. Gitlin, D.: Pathogenesis of subdural collections of fluid. Pediatrics, 16:345–352, 1955.

62. Glover, D., and Labadie, E. L.: Physiopathogenesis of subdural hematomas. Part II, Inhibition of growth of experimental hematomas with dexamethasone. J. Neurosurg., 45:393–397, 1976.

63. Gobiet, W., Bock, W. J., Liesgang, J., et al.: Treatment of acute cerebral edema with high dose of dexamethasone. In Beks, J. W. F., Bosch, D. A., and Brock, M., eds.: Intracranial Pressure III. Berlin, Springer-Verlag, 1976, pp. 232–235.

64. Goldstein, F. P., Rosenthal, S. A. E., Garancis, J. C., et al.: Varieties of growing skull fracture in childhood. J. Neurosurg., 33:25–28, 1970.

65. Graf, C. J., and Rossi, N. P.: Pulmonary edema and the central nervous system: a clinico-pathological study. Surg. Neurol., 4:319–325, 1975.

66. Greenberg, R. P., Becker, D. P., Miller, J. D., et al.: Evaluation of brain function in severe human head trauma with multimodality evoked potentials. Part 2: Localization of brain dysfunction and correlation with posttraumatic neurological conditions. J. Neurosurg., 47:163–177, 1977.

67. Greenberg, R. P., Mayer, D. J., Becker, D. P., et al.: Evaluation of brain function in severe human head trauma with multimodality evoked potentials. Part 1: Evoked brain-injury potentials, methods, and analysis. J. Neurosurg., 47:150–162, 1977.

68. Griffith, J. F., and Dodge, P. R.: Transient blindness following head injury in children. New Eng. J. Med., 278:648–651, 1968.

69. Griffiths, A. D.: Association of hypoglycemia with symptoms in the newborn. Arch. Dis. Child., 43:688–694, 1968.

70. Gronwall, D., and Wrightson, P.: Cumulative effect of concussion. Lancet, 2:995–997, 1975.

71. Gruszkiewicz, J., Doron, Y., and Peyser, E.: Recovery from severe craniocerebral injury with brain stem lesions in childhood. Surg. Neurol., 1:197–201, 1973.

72. Guthkelch, A. N.: Infantile subdural hematoma and its relationship to whiplash injuries. Brit. Med. J., 2:430–431, 1971.

73. Haas, D. C., Pineda, G. S., and Lourie, H.: Juvenile head trauma syndromes and their relationship to migraine. Arch. Neurol. (Chicago), 32:727–730, 1975.

74. Haas, W. K.: Cerebral blood flow and metabolism after experimental brain stem trauma. In McLaurin, R. L., ed.: Head Injuries: Second Chicago Symposium on Neural Trauma. New York, Grune & Stratton, Inc., 1976, Chapter 28.

75. Haddon, W., Jr.: Energy damage and the ten countermeasure strategies. J. Trauma, 13:321–331, 1973.

76. Hambleton, G., and Wigglesworth, J. S.: Origin of intraventricular hemorrhage in the preterm infant. Arch. Dis. Child., 51:651–659, 1976.

77. Harwood-Nash, D. C.: Craniocerebral trauma in children. Curr. Probl. Radiol., 3:1–42, 1973.

78. Harwood-Nash, D. C., Hendrick, E. B., and Hudson, A. R.: The significance of skull fracture in children. Radiology, 101:151–155, 1971.

79. Head Injuries—from accident department to necropsy room. Lancet, 1:589–591, 1978.

80. Heiskanen, O., and Kaste, M.: Late prognosis of severe brain injury in children. Develop. Med. Child Neurol., 16:11–14, 1974.

81. Hendrick, E. B., Hoffman, H. J., and Hudson, A. R.: Hemispherectomy in children. Clin. Neurosurg., 16:315–327, 1969.

82. Hendrick, E. B., Harwood-Nash, D. C., and Hudson, A. R.: Head injuries in children: A statistical survey of 4,465 consecutive cases at the Hospital for Sick Children, Toronto, Canada. Clin. Neurosurg., *11*:46–65, 1965.

83. Henschel, E. O., ed.: Malignant Hyperthermia. Current Concepts. New York, Appleton-Century-Crofts, 1977.

84. Hillman, R. S. L., Kieffer, S. A., Ortiz, H., et al.: Intraosseous leptomeningeal cysts of the posterior cranial fossa. Radiology, *116*:655–659, 1975.

85. Hjern, B., and Nylander, I.: Late prognosis of severe head injuries in childhood. Arch. Dis. Child., *37*:113–116, 1962.

86. Hochwald, G. M., Epstein, F., Malhan, C., et al.: The role of the skull and dura in experimental feline hydrocephalus. Develop. Med. Child Neurol., *14*:suppl. 27:65–69, 1972.

87. Hoffman, H. J., and Tucker, W. S.: Cephalocranial disproportion: A complication of the treatment of hydrocephalus in children. Child's Brain, *2*:167–176, 1976.

88. Holman, B. L., and Davis, D. O.: Radioisotope assessment of cerebrospinal fluid pathways. Prog. Nuc. Med., *1*:359–375, 1972.

89. Horner, F. A., Berry, R. G., and Frantz, M.: Broken pencil points as a cause of brain abscess. New Eng. J. Med., *271*:242–248, 1964.

90. Hunter, R. S., Kilstrom, N., Kraybill, E. N., and Loda, F.: Antecedents of child abuse and neglect in premature infants: A prospective study in a newborn intensive care unit. Pediatrics, *61*:629–635, 1978.

91. Ignelzi, R. J., and VanderArk, G. D.: Analysis of the treatment of basilar skull fractures with and without antibiotics. J. Neurosurg., *43*:721–726, 1975.

92. Ingraham, F. K., and Matson, D. D.: Subdural hematoma in infancy. J. Pediat., *24*:1–37, 1944.

93. James, H. E., Bruno, L., and Schut, L.: Intracranial subarachnoid pressure monitoring in children. Surg. Neurol., *3*:313–315, 1975.

94. Jamieson, D. L., and Kaye, H. H.: Accidental head injury in childhood. Arch. Dis. Child., *49*:376–381, 1974.

95. Jennett, B.: Epilepsy and acute traumatic intracranial haematoma. J. Neurol. Neurosurg. Psychiat., *38*:378–381, 1975.

96. Jennett, B.: Assessment of the severity of head injury. J. Neurol. Neurosurg. Psychiat., *39*:647–655, 1976.

97. Jennett, B., and Teasdale, G.: Predicting outcome in individual patients after severe head injury. Lancet, *1*:1031–1034, 1976.

98. Jennett, B., Teasdale, G., Galbraith, S., et al.: Severe head injuries in three countries. J. Neurol. Neurosurg. Psychiat., *40*:291–298, 1977.

99. Joele, L. J., and Endtz, L. J.: Traumatic disorders of pituitary-hypothalmic function. Appl. Neurophysiol., *38*:110–114, 1975.

100. Johnston, I. H.: Intracranial pressure changes after head injury. *In* Vinken, P. J., and Bruyn, G. W., eds.: Handbook of Clinical Neurology. Vol. 23. Amsterdam, Elsevier—North Holland Publishing Co., 1975, pp. 199–222.

101. Kalbag, R. M., and Woolf, A. L.: Cerebral Venous Thrombosis. London, Oxford University Press, 1967.

102. Kasoff, S. S., Zingesser, L. H., and Shulman, K.: Compartmental abnormalities of regional cerebral blood flow in children with head trauma. J. Neurosurg., *36*:463–470, 1972.

103. Kaufman, B., and Bellon, E. M.: The trigeminal nerve cistern. Radiology, *108*:597–602, 1973.

104. Kaufman, B., Jordan, V. M., and Pratt, L. L.: Positive contrast demonstration of a cerebrospinal fluid fistula through the fundus of the internal auditory meatus. Acta Radiol., *9*:83–90, 1969.

105. Keith, R. W., ed.: Central Auditory Dysfunction, New York, Grune & Stratton, Inc., 1977.

106. Kempe, C. H., and Helfer, R. E.: Helping the Battered Child and His Family. Philadelphia, J. B. Lippincott Co., 1972.

107. Kendall, N., and Woloshin, H.: Cephalhematoma associated with fracture of the skull. J. Pediat., *41*:125–132, 1952.

108. Kinal, M. E.: Traumatic thrombosis of dural sinuses in closed head injuries. J. Neurosurg. *27*:142–145, 1967.

109. Kjellberg, R. N., and Prieto, A., Jr.: Bifrontal decompressive craniotomy for massive cerebral edema. J. Neurosurg., *34*:488–493, 1971.

110. Klein, M., and Stern, L.: Low birth weight and the battered child syndrome. Amer. J. Dis. Child., *122*:15–18, 1971.

111. Kobrine, A. I., Timmins, E., Rajjoub, R. K., et al.: Demonstration of massive traumatic brain swelling within 20 minutes after injury. Case report. J. Neurosurg., *46*:256–258, 1977.

112. Kopecky, J. A., and Ripperger, E. A.: Closed brain injuries: An engineering analysis. J. Biomech., *2*:29–34, 1969.

113. Krishnamoorthy, K. S., Fernandez, R. A., Momose, K. J., et al.: Evaluation of neonatal intracranial hemorrhage by computerized tomography. Pediatrics, *59*:165–172, 1977.

114. Kriss, F. C., Taren, J. A., and Kahn, E. A.: Primary repair of compound skull fractures by replacement of bone fragments. J. Neurosurg., *30*:698–702, 1969.

115. Labadie, E. L., and Glover, D.: Physiopathogenesis of subdural hematomas. Part I, Histological and biochemical comparisons of subcutaneous hematoma in rats with subdural hematoma in man. J. Neurosurg., *45*:382–392, 1976.

116. Langfitt, T. W.: Measuring the outcome from head injuries. J. Neurosurg., *48*:673–678, 1978.

117. LeBoyer, F.: Birth Without Violence. New York, Alfred A. Knopf, 1975.

118. Leech, P. J., and Paterson, A.: Conservative and operative management for cerebrospinal-fluid leakage after closed head injury. Lancet, *1*:1013–1015, 1973.

119. Lehman, R. A., Hayes, G. J., and Martins, A. N.: The use of adhesive and lyophilized dura in the treatment of cerebrospinal rhinorrhea. J. Neurosurg., *26*:92–95, 1967.

120. Lende, R. A.: Enlarging skull fractures of childhood. Neuroradiology, *7*:119–124, 1974.

121. Lende, R. A., and Erickson, T. C.: Growing skull fractures of childhood. J. Neurosurg., *18*:479–489, 1961.

122. Leviton, A., Gilles, F. H., and Strassfeld, R.: Caesarian section and the risk of neonatal in-

tracranial hemorrhage. Trans. Amer. Neurol. Ass., *101*:121–124, 1976.

123. Lewin, W.: Cerebrospinal fluid rhinorrhea in nonmissile head injuries. Clin. Neurosurg., *12*:237–252, 1966.

124. Lewin, W.: Severe head injuries. Proc. Roy. Soc. Med., *60*:1208–1212, 1967.

125. Lewis, A. J.: Mechanisms of Neurological Disease. Boston, Little, Brown & Co., 1976.

126. Lindenberg, R.: Morphology of brain lesions from blunt trauma in early infancy. Arch. Path. (Chicago), *87*:298–305, 1969.

127. Lindenberg, R.: Trauma of meninges and brain. *In* Minckler, J., ed.: Pathology of the Nervous System, Vol. 2. New York, McGraw-Hill Book Co., 1971, pp. 1705–1765.

128. Lindenberg, R., and Freytag, E.: Morphology of cortical contusions. Arch. Path. (Chicago), *63*:23–42, 1957.

129. Lindenberg, R., and Freytag, E.: The mechanism of cerebral contusion. Arch. Path. (Chicago), *69*:440–469, 1960.

130. Little, W. J.: On the influence of abnormal parturition, difficult labor, premature birth and asphyxia neonatorum on the mental and physical conditions of the child, especially in relation to deformities. Trans. Obstet. Soc. London, *3*:293–344, 1862.

131. Lockard, J. S., DuCharme, L. L., Congdon, W. C., et al.: Prophylaxis with diphenylhydantoin and phenobarbital in alumina-gel monkey model: Four-month followup period: Seizure, EEG, blood and behavioral data. Epilepsia, *17*:49–57, 1976.

132. Loeser, J. D., Kilburn, H. L., and Jolley, T.: Management of depressed skull fracture in the newborn. J. Neurosurg., *44*:62–64, 1976.

133. Maccario, M.: Neurological dysfunction associated with nonketotic hyperglycemia. Arch. Neurol. (Chicago), *19*:525–534, 1968.

134. MacGee, E. E., Cauthen, J. C., and Brackett, C. E.: Meningitis following acute traumatic cerebrospinal fluid rhinorrhea. J. Neurosurg., *33*:312–316, 1970.

135. Marc, J. A., and Schecter, M. M.: The significance of fluid-gas displacement in the sphenoid sinus in post-traumatic CSF rhinorrhea. Radiology, *108*:603–606, 1973.

136. Marriage, K. J., and Davies, P. A.: Neurological sequelae in children surviving mechanical ventilation in the neonatal period. Arch. Dis. Child., *52*:176–182, 1977.

137. Marsh, M. L., Marshall, L. F., and Shapiro, H. M.: Neurosurgical intensive care. Anesthesiology, *47*:149–163, 1977.

138. Marshall, L. F., and Shapiro, H. M.: Barbiturate control of intracranial hypertension in head injury and other conditions: Iatrogenic coma. Acta Neurol. Scand. *56*:suppl. 64:156–157, 1977.

139. Marshall, L. F., Bruce, D. A., Bruno, L., and Schut, L.: Role of intracranial pressure monitoring and barbiturate therapy in malignant intracranial hypertension. J. Neurosurg., *47*:481–484, 1977.

140. Martin, R., Roessmann, U., and Fanaroff, A.: Massive intracerebellar hemorrhage in low-birth-weight infants. J. Pediat., *89*:290–293, 1976.

141. Matson, D. D.: Neurosurgery of Infancy and Childhood. Springfield, Ill., Charles C Thomas, 1969.

142. Maurice-Williams, R. S.: Temporal lobe swelling: A common treatable complication of head injury. Brit. J. Surg., *63*:169–172, 1976.

143. McGraw, C. P.: Experimental cerebral infarction, effects of pentobarbital in mongolian gerbils. Arch. Neurol. (Chicago), *34*:334–336, 1977.

144. McLaurin, R. L.: Repeated aspiration as the preferred treatment of subdural hematomas in infants. *In* Morley, T. P., ed.: Current Controversies in Neurosurgery. Philadelphia, W. B. Saunders Co., 1976, pp. 561–565.

145. McLaurin, R. L.: Management of chronic subdural hematomas in infancy. In O'Brien, M. S., ed.: Pediatric Neurological Surgery. New York, Raven Press, 1978, pp. 135–146.

146. McLaurin, R. L., and Helmer, F.: The syndrome of temporal-lobe contusion. J. Neurosurg., *23*:296–304, 1965.

147. McLaurin, R. L., and McBride, B. H.: Traumatic intracerebral hematoma, review of 16 surgically treated cases. Ann. Surg., *143*:294–305, 1956.

148. McLaurin, R. L., and McLaurin, K. S.: Calcified subdural hematomas in childhood. J. Neurosurg., *24*:648–655, 1966.

149. McLaurin, R. L., and Titchener, J. L.: Post-Traumatic Syndrome. *In* Youmans, J. R., ed.: Neurological Surgery. Philadelphia, W. B. Saunders Co., 1973, pp. 1023–1035.

150. McLaurin, R. L., and Tutor, F. T.: Acute subdural hematoma. A review of ninety cases. J. Neurosurg., *18*:61–67, 1961.

151. McLaurin, R. L., Isaacs, E., and Lewis, H. P.: Results of nonoperative treatment in 15 cases of infantile subdural hematoma. J. Neurosurg., *34*:753–759, 1971.

152. McLennan, J. E., and Gilles, F. H.: A growth model for the total weight of the prenatal human brain. Trans. Amer. Neurol. Ass., *101*:271–272, 1976.

153. McLennan, J. E., Mickle, J. P., and Treves, S.: Radionuclide cisternographic evaluation and follow-up of posttraumatic subconjunctival CSF loculation. J. Neurosurg., *44*:496–499, 1976.

154. McLennan, J. E., Fischer, E. G., Suzuki, Y., and Treves, S.: Cerebral abscess in children. Amer. J. Dis. Child., in press.

155. McLennan, J. E., Rosenbaum, A. E., Hedley-Whyte, E. T., et al.: Angiographic visualization of fatal hemorrhage from a cerebral arteriovenous malformation. J. Neurosurg., *41*:622–626, 1974.

156. Mealey, J., Jr.: Pediatric Head Injuries. Springfield, Ill., Charles C Thomas, 1968.

157. Messina, A. V., and Chernik, N. L.: Computed tomography: The "resolving" intracerebral hemorrhage. Radiology, *118*:609–613, 1975.

158. Michenfelder, J. D., and Sundt, T. M.: Anesthesia, cerebral metabolism and cerebral ischemia. *In* McLaurin, R. L., ed.: Head Injuries, Proceedings of the Second Chicago Symposium on Neural Trauma. New York, Grune & Stratton, Inc., 1976, pp. 175–180.

159. Miller, J. D., and Jennett, W. B.: Complications

of depressed skull fracture. Lancet, 2:991–995, 1968.

160. Milner, B.: Residual intellectual and memory deficits after head injury. In Walker, A. E., et al., eds.: The Late Effects of Head Injury. Springfield, Ill., Charles C Thomas, 1969, pp. 84–97.

161. Milstein, J. M., Rennick, J., and Goetzman, B. W.: Computerized axial tomography of the brain in neonates and young infants. Surg. Neurol., 8:59–62, 1977.

162. Mitchell, D. E., and Adams, J. H.: Primary focal impact damage to the brainstem in blunt head injuries—Does it exist? Lancet, 1:215–218, 1973.

163. Moore, F. D., Lyons, J. H., Pierce, E. C., et al.: Post-Traumatic Pulmonary Insufficiency. Philadelphia, W. B. Saunders Co., 1969.

164. Morantz, R. A., Abad, R. M., George, A. E., and Rovitt, R. L.: Hemicraniectomy for acute extracerebral hematoma: An analysis of clinical and radiographic findings. J. Neurosurg., 39:622–628, 1973.

165. Moylan, F. B. M., Herrin, J. T., Krishnamoorthy, K., Todres, I. D., and Shannon, D. C.: Inappropriate antidiuretic hormone secretion in premature infants with cerebral injury. Amer. J. Dis. Child., 132:399–402, 1978.

166. Myers, R. E.: Two patterns of perinatal brain damage and their conditions of occurrence. Amer. J. Obstet. Gynec., 112:246–276, 1972.

167. Natelson, S. E., and Sayers, M. P.: The fate of children sustaining severe head trauma during birth. Pediatrics, 51:169–174, 1973.

168. Nilsson, B., and Nordström, C. H.: Experimental head injury in the rat. Part 3: Cerebral blood flow and oxygen consumption after concussive impact acceleration. J. Neurosurg., 47:262–273, 1977.

169. Nilsson, B., and Ponten, U.: Experimental head injury in the rat. Part 2: Regional brain energy metabolism in concussive trauma. J. Neurosurg., 47:252–261, 1977.

170. Nilsson, B., Ponten, U., and Voigt, G.: Experimental head injury in the rat. Part 1: Mechanics, pathophysiology, and morphology in an impact acceleration trauma model. J. Neurosurg., 47:241–251, 1977.

171. Niswander, K. R., Gordon, M., and Drage, J. S.: The effect of intrauterine hypoxia on the child surviving to 4 years. Amer. J. Obstet. Gynec., 121:892–899, 1975.

172. Ommaya, A. K., and Gennarelli, T. A.: Cerebral concussion and traumatic unconsciousness: Correlation of experimental and clinical observations on blunt head injuries. Brain, 97:633–654, 1974.

173. Park, B. E., Hester, R. W., and Netsky, M. G.: Closed head injury complicated by nonketotic hyperglycemic hyperosmolar coma. Surg. Neurol., 4:330–332, 1975.

174. Parkinson, D.: Concussion. Mayo Clin. Proc., 52:492–496, 1977.

175. Paxson, C. L., and Brown, D. R.: Post-traumatic anterior hypopituitarism. Pediatrics, 57:893–896, 1976.

176. Pickles, W.: Acute focal edema of the brain in children with head injuries. New Eng. J. Med., 240:92–95, 1949.

177. Pitlyk, P. J., Tolchin, S., and Stewart, W.: The experimental significance of retained intracranial bone fragments. J. Neurosurg., 33:19–24, 1970.

178. Platt, J. R.: Man and the indeterminacies. Perspect. Biol. Med., 10:67–80, 1967.

179. Plum, F., and Posner, J. B.: The Diagnosis of Stupor and Coma. 2nd Ed. Philadelphia, F. A. Davis Co., 1972.

180. Plum, F., and Swanson, A. G.: Central neurogenic hyperventilation in man. Arch. Neurol. (Chicago), 81:535–549, 1959.

181. Potter, J. M., and Braakman, R.: Injury to the facial nerve. In Vinken, P. J., and Bruyn, G. W., eds.: Handbook of Clinical Neurology. Vol. 24. New York, Elsevier–North Holland Publishing Co., Inc., 1976.

182. Prockop, L. D.: Hyperglycemia, polyol accumulation, and increased intracranial pressure. Arch. Neurol. (Chicago), 25:126–140, 1971.

183. Rabe, E. F., Flynn, R. E., and Dodge, P. R.: A study of subdural effusions in an infant. Neurology (Minneap.), 12:79–92, 1962.

184. Rabe, E. F., Flynn, R. E., and Dodge, P. R.: Subdural collections of fluid in infants and children. Neurology (Minneap.), 18:559–570, 1968.

185. Ragnor, R., and Parsa, M.: Non-surgical elevation of depressed skull fracture in an infant. J. Pediat., 72:262–264, 1968.

186. Raimondi, A. J.: Pediatric Neuroradiology. Philadelphia, W. B. Saunders, Co., 1972, Chapter 2.

187. Rapin, I., Mattis, S., Rowan, A. J., et al.: Verbal auditory agnosia in children. Develop. Med. Child Neurol., 19:192–207, 1977.

188. Rapport, R. L., and Penry, J. K.: A survey of attitudes toward the pharmacological prophylaxis of posttraumatic epilepsy. J. Neurosurg., 38:159–166, 1973.

189. Reilly, P. L., Graham, D. I., Adams, J. H., et al.: Patients with head injury who talk and die. Lancet, 2:375–377, 1975.

190. Ripperger, E. A.: The mechanics of brain injuries. In Vinken, P. J., and Bruyn, G. W., eds.: Handbook of Clinical Neurology. Vol. 23. Amsterdam, Elsevier–North Holland Publishing Co., 1975, pp. 91–107.

191. Robinson, R. J., and Rossiter, M. A.: Massive subaponeurotic haemorrhage in babies of African origin. Arch. Dis. Child., 43:684–687, 1968.

192. Rose, J., Valtonen, S., and Jennett, B.: Avoidable factors contributing to death after head injury. Brit. Med. J., 2:615–618, 1977.

193. Rubens, A. B., Geschwind, N., Mahowald, M. W., et al.: Posttraumatic cerebral hemispheric disconnection syndrome. Arch. Neurol. (Chicago), 34:750–755, 1977.

194. Rune, V.: Acute head injuries in children. Acta Paediat. Scand., suppl. 209, 1970.

195. Russell, P. A.: Subdural haematoma in infancy. Brit. Med. J., 2:446–448, 1965.

196. Russell, W. R.: Brain, Memory, Learning: A Neurologist's View. Oxford, Clarendon Press, 1959.

197. Schreiber, M. H., and Morettin, L. B.: Antepartem prediction of fetal maturity. Radiol. Clin. N. Amer., 5:21–28, 1967.

198. Schwartz, P.: Birth Injuries of the Newborn. New York, Hafner Publishing Co., 1961.

199. Scotti, G., Terbrugge, K., Melancon, D., et al.: Evaluation of the age of subdural hematomas by computerized tomography. J. Neurosurg., *47*:311–315, 1977.

200. Shapiro, H. M., Lafferty, J., Keykhar, M. M., Behar, M. G., and Van Horn, K.: Barbiturates and intracranial hypertension. *In* McLaurin, R. L., ed.: Head Injuries, Proceedings of the Second Chicago Symposium on Neural Trauma. New York, Grune & Stratton, Inc., 1976, pp. 181–184.

201. Shaw, A.: Dilemmas of "informed consent" in children. New Eng. J. Med., *289*:885–890, 1973.

202. Shulman, K., and Ransohoff, J.: Subdural hematoma in children: The fate of children with retained membranes. J. Neurosurg., *18*:175–181, 1961.

203. Sills, J. A., Thomas, L. J., and Rosenbloom, L.: Non-accidental injury: A two-year study in central Liverpool. Develop. Med. Child Neurol., *19*:26–33.1977.

204. Silverberg, G. D., Harbury, C. B., and Rubenstein, E.: A physiological sealant for cerebrospinal fluid leaks. J. Neurosurg., *46*:215–219, 1977.

205. Sladen, A., Laver, M. B., and Pontoppidan, H.: Pulmonary complications and water retention in prolonged mechanical ventilation. New Eng. J. Med., *279*:448–453, 1968.

206. Smyth, H. S., and Livingston, K. E.: Ventricular infusion in the operative management of subdural hematoma. *In* Morley, T. P., ed.: Current Controversies in Neurosurgery. Philadelphia, W. B. Saunders Co., 1976, pp. 566–571.

207. Stockard, J. J., and Rossiter, V. S.: Clinical and pathologic correlates of brain stem auditory response abnormalities. Neurology (Minneap.), *27*:316–325, 1977.

208. Strich, S. J.: Shearing of nerve fibers as a cause of brain damage due to head injuries. Lancet, *2*:443–448, 1961.

209. Sweet, R. C., Miller, J. D., Lipper, M., Kishore, P. R. S., and Becker, D. P.: Significance of bilateral abnormalities on the C.T. scan in patients with severe head injury. Neurosurgery, *3*:16–21, 1978.

210. Tabaddor, K., and Shulman, K.: Definitive treatment of chronic subdural hematoma by twist-drill craniostomy and closed-system drainage. J. Neurosurg., *46*:220–226, 1977.

211. Taveras, J. M., and Ransohoff, J.: Leptomeningeal cysts of the brain following trauma with erosion of the skull. J. Neurosurg., *10*:233–241, 1953.

212. Tenner, M. S., and Stein, B. M.: Cerebral herniation in the growing fracture of the skull. Radiology, *94*:351–355, 1970.

213. Terplan, K. L.: Histopathologic brain changes in 1152 cases of the perinatal and early infancy period. Biol. Neonat., *11*:348–357, 1967.

214. Thompson, J. B., Mason, T. H., Haines, G. L., et al.: Surgical management of diastatic linear skull fractures in infants. J. Neurosurg., *39*:493–497, 1973.

215. Thomson, A. J., Searle, M., and Russell, G.: Quality of survival after severe birth asphyxia. Arch. Dis. Child., *52*:620–626, 1977.

216. Till, K.: Paediatric Neurosurgery. Oxford, Blackwell Scientific Publications, 1975.

217. Tornheim, P. A., and McLaurin, R. L.: Effect of dexamethasone on cerebral edema from cranial impact in the cat. J. Neurosurg., *48*:220–227, 1978.

218. Towbin, A.: Mental retardation due to germinal matrix infarction. Science, *164*:156–161, 1969.

219. Tsiantos, A., Victorin, L., Relier, J. P., et al.: Intracranial hemorrhage in the prematurely born infant. J. Pediat., *85*:854–859, 1974.

220. Valdes-Dapena, M. A., and Arey, J. B.: Pulmonary emboli of cerebral origin in the newborn. Arch. Path. (Chicago), *84*:643–646, 1967.

221. VanderArk, G. D., Pitkethly, D. T., Ducker, T. B., et al.: Repair of cerebrospinal fluid fistulas using a tissue adhesive. J. Neurosurg., *33*:151–155, 1970.

222. Venes, J. L., and Collins, W. F.: Bifrontal decompressive craniectomy in the management of head trauma. J. Neurosurg., *42*:429–433, 1975.

223. Volpe, J. J.: Perinatal hypoxic-ischemic brain injury. Clin. Perinatol., *4*:383–397, 1977.

224. Wacks, M. R., and Bird, H. A.: Massive gross pulmonary embolism of cerebral tissue following severe head trauma. J. Trauma, *10*:344–348, 1970.

225. Witelson, S. F.: Early hemisphere specialization and interhemisphere plasticity: An empirical and theoretical review. *In* Segalowitz, S. J., and Gruber, F. A., eds.: Language Development and Neurological Theory. New York, Academic Press, 1977, Chapter 16, pp. 213–287.

226. Yakovlev, P. I., and Lecours, A. R.: The myelogenetic cycles of regional maturation of the brain. *In* Minkowski, A., ed.: Regional Development of the Brain in Early Life. Oxford, Blackwell Scientific Publications, 1967.

227. Yashon, D., Jane, J. A., White, R. J., and Sugar, O.: Traumatic subdural hematoma of infancy: long-term follow-up in 92 patients. Arch. Neurol. (Chicago), *18*:370–377, 1968.

228. Zimmerman, R. A., Bilaniuk, L. T., Bruce, D., Dolinskas, C., Obrist, W., and Kuhl, D.: Computed tomography of pediatric head trauma: Acute general cerebral swelling. Radiology, *126*:403–408, 1978.

60

PROGNOSIS AFTER HEAD INJURY

Head injuries occur frequently. At least seven million a year occur in the United States. Unfortunately, a large proportion of them have an unsatisfactory outcome. If account is taken of the nuances of neurological and intellectual dysfunction, of socioeconomic and sexual maladjustment, and of behavioral and emotional disturbances, then it becomes clear that head injuries exact a dreadful toll on society.

For many years, neurosurgeons with experience in the management of patients with head injuries have recognized certain clinical factors as important because of their influence on outcome. These clinical factors have been viewed largely in terms of their usefulness in predicting death versus survival. However, the identification of those patients who will require extensive supportive care for long periods following injury and the assessment of what benefits such care is likely to offer are of no less importance. Thus, prediction of outcome must be more detailed than a simple indication of who will live and who will die after injury.

Since the more important clinical prognostic factors were first recognized, many changes and improvements have evolved in the management of head injury. Examples are the development of neurosurgical intensive care units with 24-hour monitoring of the patient's neurological state, early intubation, tracheostomy, and intermittent positive-pressure ventilation that can be continued safely for days or even weeks. Intracranial pressure monitoring has come into widespread use only in the last 10 years, and even more recently the rapid, safe, and informative technique of CT scan-ning has made an enormous impact on head injury management. Among other therapeutic advances is the use of hyperosmolar agents, barbiturates, chlorpromazine, and steroids in both normal and very high levels of dosage. These agents are being applied against a background of improved understanding of the pathophysiology of primary and secondary brain damage following head injury. Finally, in the overall management of the injured patient, the development of improved emergency treatment services, rapid transport, shock teams, and multidisciplinary trauma groups have all made contributions to improving outcome.

DESCRIPTION OF OUTCOME

The number of outcome categories selected to provide a clear description of the extent of disability must be large enough to define the post-traumatic patient population accurately and still have sufficiently large numbers in each group to permit accurate statistical analysis. This latter factor assumes immense importance when comparative studies of therapy within a given center or between centers are envisaged.

Firm predictions of outcome become less feasible when outcome categories are established that make fine distinctions between levels of intellectual, behavioral, and socioeconomic disability. Currently, prognosis in head injury falls far short of such subtle predictions. This in no way diminishes the importance or desirability of such information; the present limit of knowledge on the subject must, however,

D. P. BECKER, J. D. MILLER, AND R. P. GREENBERG

be recognized. Toward that end, the first part of this chapter provides an evaluation of those factors that have a known and often a quantifiable influence on outcome when this is defined in broad categories without regard for finer differences in neurological dysfunction. The emphasis is largely on identifying in patients those combinations of factors that are associated with a high risk of death or severe disability from head injury. In the second section, factors are discussed that influence outcome in a more subtle way, affecting the quality of survival rather than influencing life or death. The emphasis here is on defining the patterns of recovery and disability present in those patients who in broad categorical terms would be said to have made good recovery or have moderate disabilities.

DEFINITION OF OUTCOME

After surveying many of the problems associated with assignment of outcome categories, Jennett and Bond concluded that at the present time five categories represented the most practical solution.[57] Such a division was most compatible with many of the best-documented studies of outcome from head injury that had already been reported. The Glasgow outcome scale, proposed by these authors, therefore contains five exclusive categories: death, persistent vegetative state, severe disability, moderate disability, and good recovery.

Within the category "death" efforts should be made to distinguish those patients who die as a result of primary or secondary brain damage, usually associated with uncontrollable intracranial hypertension, from those who die because of either secondary systemic complications or other causes that occur after the patients have recovered consciousness. Secondary problems that may occur during prolonged coma include pneumonia, pulmonary embolism, and renal failure. Knowledge of the relative numbers of patients who die in these different circumstances influences the strategy that is adopted to manage patients with head injury.

The term "persistent vegetative state" was coined by Jennett and Plum as the best description of a state that has been variously labeled "apallic syndrome," "akinetic mutism," "vigil coma," or "pro-

longed coma."[58] The essential component of the syndrome is absence of adaptation to the environment and of any speech or evidence of mental function in a patient who is apparently awake at times with spontaneous eye opening.

"Severe disability" applies to patients who are dependent on the help of others for activities of daily living. The actual disability, however, may be predominantly either mental or physical.

"Moderate disability" implies that such patients are independent insofar as activities of daily living are concerned but are unable, because of their physical or mental disability, or both, to return to their former occupational level.

The term "good recovery" indicates that patients have been able to return to their former occupational level though not necessarily to their former occupation. Such patients may have minor deficits in neurological or mental function. It should be emphasized that the scale does not include a category for patients who are said to have "recovered completely" or made an "excellent recovery" from injury. Clearly, the two upper categories in the Glasgow coma scale include many problems of emotional, intellectual, sexual, and social disability. A few moments' thought about the problems of discriminating objectively between levels of such subtle disabilities will, however, convince most clinicians of the value of this simple five-point outcome scale.

DEFINITION OF INPUT DATA

If descriptive clinical and laboratory data about patients with head injury are to be related to outcome, then it is clear that the input data must be clearly defined in terms that are universally understood and acceptable, especially when collaborative or comparative studies are proposed. There is little value in comparing outcome in two series of patients if the clinical status of the patients cannot be compared, either because the information is not available, or because the descriptions are not in universally understandable terms. Factors that may influence the outcome from a head injury are protean. More important input variables are shown in Tables 60–1 and 60–2. The nature of such data determines that they can be broadly divided into two main

TABLE 60–1 DATA ON PATIENTS WITH HEAD INJURY THAT CAN BE EXPRESSED IN NUMERICAL (CONTINUOUS) OR DISCRETE (CATEGORICAL) FORM.*

CONTINUOUS DATA	CATEGORICAL DATA
Age	Age groups
Times	Time bands (e.g., coma 1 to 3 days)
Blood pressure	Blood pressure groups
Intracranial pressure	Intracranial pressure groups, groups, course, waves
Blood gases	Blood gas groups, responses
Respiratory rate, volumes	Respiratory patterns
Pupil size (mm)	Pupil size, light response
Cerebral blood flow	Cerebral blood flow level, response to stimuli
Cerebral oxygen metabolism ($CMRO_2$)	$CMRO_2$ groups
Brain shift (mm)	Brain shift groups
Evoked potential latency, amplitude	Evoked potential classes of abnormality

* Continuous data may not be normally distributed.

groups. Continuous data, which are recorded in numerical form (age, arterial blood gas concentrations, blood pressure, and the like), are easy to define and to compare in different groups of patients, provided the circumstances in which the measurements are made are known. Categorical data consist of two forms of nonnumerical information. One group of data can be assigned to fixed points on a defined ranking scale (examples would be the oculocephalic and the oculovestibular responses). The Glasgow coma scale is the clearest example of this system. The other type of data can only be grouped into mutu-

TABLE 60–2 DATA ON PATIENTS WITH HEAD INJURY THAT CAN BE EXPRESSED ONLY IN CATEGORICAL FORM*

RANKABLE CATEGORICAL DATA

Eye opening
Motor response
(to standard stimuli) } = Glasgow coma scale
Verbal response
Oculocephalic response (head turning)
Oculovestibular response (ice water)
Limb strength

NONRANKABLE DATA

Sex
Cause of injury
Other injuries
X-ray and CT findings

* The first group of data can be ranked in order of severity. The second group can be arranged only in exclusive classes.

ally exclusive categories (for example, sex or cause of injury).

Many different forms and complexities of single-element coma scales have been devised, but most, like the bed of Procrustes, deform the subject in order to fit the scale. Overgaard and his colleagues used a multi-element scale, but the most useful coma scale is the one from Glasgow that was devised by Teasdale and Jennett.[99,143] This scale, which ranks separately eye opening, best motor response, and verbal response to standardized stimuli, is described in Chapter 58. There are four points on the eye opening scale, six on the motor scale, and five on the verbal scale.[144] The points on these scales can be allotted with over 80 per cent concurrence by different observers.[147,148] Although it is possible to add the numbers on the three scales, this rather defeats the purpose of a three-element system, which, as it stands, conveys a considerable amount of information about the level of responsiveness of the patient.[59]

Both the oculocephalic response to head turning and the oculovestibular responses to ice water irrigation of the ear can be ranked into four definable levels. For the oculocephalic response, these are suppression of eye movements (normal response in the conscious subject), intact response (bilateral conjugate righting), impaired response (dysconjugate), and absence of response. For the oculovestibular response, the four levels are nystagmus (normal response in the conscious but also the lethargic subject), tonic conjugate deviation to the irrigated side, dysconjugate response, and no response.[108] Although these scales appear strictly comparable, they are not. The oculovestibular test uses a much more powerful stimulus. Eye movement reflexes cannot be declared absent unless the oculovestibular test is used. Teasdale and Smith have carried out an extensive comparison of the two tests in patients with severe injury. They found comparable grades of response in only 63 per cent of 160 patients, and where the grading differed the oculovestibular test usually gave a higher level of response. Thus, on 15 tests in which the oculocephalic response was absent, dysconjugate or tonic conjugate responses were obtained on oculovestibular testing.[145]

The reaction of the pupil to light can reliably be assigned as present or absent. Many observers interpolate a category of sluggish reaction to light, but there may be considerable variation between observers in assignment of this category of response.

In assessing the strength of the limbs as contrasted with the level of response, the most commonly used ranking scale is that proposed by the Medical Research Council of Great Britain, which uses six levels of strength ranging from normal power to no response and describes the levels in objectively discernible terms.[112] All of the foregoing information can easily be recorded and displayed on one progress chart.[146]

With this terminology, defining the patient's condition in terms of the Glasgow coma scale (pupil response to light, eye movement reflexes, and motor power) together with a clear definition of the time after injury at which assessment is made, head injury populations that appear closely comparable can be developed in different centers.[62,63] Thus, by defining terms applicable to individual patients and defining entry criteria for individual patients into any given study, it is possible to define the total population of head injuries studied.

In the following discussion, reference is made to a series of 160 patients with closed head injuries whom the authors have followed to death or recovery.[5] At the time of admission or later in their hospital course, these patients failed to obey commands and gave no verbal response to painful stimulation. Motor responses ranged from failure to obey commands to no motor response at all. Patients in whom the depressed level of consciousness was later recognized to be due to alcohol, drug overdosage, or early epilepsy were excluded from the series. Patients with gunshot wounds of the head and those whose state on arrival at the hospital already fulfilled the clinical criteria of brain death were excluded. The management protocol for the patients admitted to the series was uniform. It was based on the concept of achieving the earliest possible diagnosis, evacuating all intracranial mass lesions related to the injury, and preventing or detecting and treating secondary cerebral insults such as hypoxia or intracranial hypertension. All patients were artificially ventilated and had continuous monitoring of intracranial pressure.[87] All patients were managed in a neurosurgical intensive care unit, and any cardiopulmonary dysfunction, fluid electrolyte imbalance, or increase in body temperature was vigorously

investigated and treated. The outcome of surviving patients was assessed at three months and one year from the time of injury.

OVERALL OUTCOME FROM SERIOUS INJURY

In many reported series there has been variation in the criteria used to describe a serious head injury. Most authors consider failure to obey commands and absence of verbal response to stimulation, including painful stimulation, as criteria for inclusion in this group. Jennett and colleagues also require failure to open the eyes in response to pain, and stipulate that this state must have been present for at least six hours following injury. Patients who were initially less obtunded but then deteriorated are included if the comatose state is of at least six hours' duration.[62,63] Other reported series have included all patients who died without regaining consciousness or who remained in coma for 12 to 24 hours.[16,50,102]

Mortality rates from several series are summarized in Table 60–3. They range from 35 to 50 per cent. Corresponding rates of survival with good recovery or only moderate disability range between 60 and 35 per cent. There is also a large variation (5 to 25 per cent) in the numbers of patients considered severely disabled. This difference may in part reflect variations in criteria for assignment to the category. In series in which the same terminology is used to define the category, variation is much less (5 to 10 percent of patients severely disabled). There is least variation in the smallest category, partly because it is so easily recognized. This is the permanent vegetative state, and all reported series show 1 to 3 per cent of patients in this category.*

These figures are for all head injuries. When specific subgroups are followed the outcome figures are quite different. Lower mortality rates are found in series restricted to children.[14,51] In patients with acute subdural hematoma or extensor rigidity, much higher mortality rates are found. These subgroups are considered in more detail later.

---

* See references 5, 16, 50, 62, 63, 99, 100, 102, 120.

TABLE 60-3 OUTCOMES ASSESSED ON GLASGOW COMA SCALE FROM RECENT REPORTS ON PATIENTS WITH SEVERE HEAD INJURY*

AUTHORS	YEAR	NUMBER OF PATIENTS	OUTCOME (PER CENT)		
			Good Recovery/ Moderate Disability	Severe Disability/ Vegetative	Dead
Carlsson et al.†	1968[a]	496	53	12	35
Overgaard et al.‡	1973	139	31	28	41
Pagni§	1973	1091	—	—	52
Rossanda et al.‖	1973	223	—	—	52
Pazzaglia et al.¶	1975[b]	282	40	11	49
Jennett et al.**	1977[c]	700	38	11	51
Becker et al.††	1977	148	57	11	32

[a] Patients with intracranial hematoma excluded: coma for 12 hours.
[b] Coma for 24 hours.
[c] Coma for 6 hours.

* Patients were comatose on admission unless otherwise specified.

† Factors affecting the clinical course of patients with severe head trauma. Part 1: Influence of biological factors. Part 2: Significance of post-traumatic coma. J. Neurosurg., 29:242–251, 1968.

‡ Prognosis after head injury based on early clinical examination. Lancet, 2:631–635, 1973.

§ The prognosis of head injured patients in a state of coma with decerebrated posture. J. Neurosurg. Sci., 17:289–295, 1973.

‖ Role of automatic ventilation in treatment of severe head injuries. J. Neurosurg. Sci., 17:265–270, 1973.

¶ Clinical course and prognosis of acute post-traumatic coma. J. Neurol. Neurosurg. Psychiat., 38:149–154, 1975.

** Severe head injuries in three countries. J. Neurol. Neurosurg. Psychiat., 40:291–298, 1977.

†† The outcome from severe head injury with early diagnosis and intensive management. J. Neurosurg., 47:491–502, 1977.

At the authors' institution the outcomes of a first series of 160 cases and of a subsequent series of 100 similarly defined and managed patients are closely comparable (Table 60–4).[5,86]

Many of the deaths from head injury occur early. If a patient survives the first 48 hours after injury, his chances for long-term recovery are good. The clearest exposition of this point has been of Carlsson and his colleagues, who found the time course of survival of patients to be monoexponential; 96 per cent of those patients who were to die from brain damage and its immediate sequelae had died within 48 hours of injury. The 50 per cent mark was reached at 17.5 hours.[16] This particular series of cases did not include patients with intracranial hematomas, but it is unlikely that the inclusion of such cases would greatly alter these conclusions.

The high early mortality rates can be used to support a fatalistic view that these deaths are due to irreparable brain damage and therefore unavoidable. Many early deaths are, however, due to intracranial mass lesions with fulminating intracranial hypertension and brain shift, which can be alleviated in some cases. As a result, it is in this early phase that the surgeon ought to be active and aggressive in his treatment.

CLINICAL FACTORS THAT INFLUENCE OUTCOME

Factors Existing Prior to Injury

Age

It is commonly asserted that age is the most important single factor determining

TABLE 60-4 OUTCOMES IN TWO CONSECUTIVE SERIES OF PATIENTS WITH SEVERE HEAD INJURY*

SERIES OF PATIENTS	MEAN AGE (YEARS)	MASS LESIONS PRESENT (PER CENT)	OUTCOME (PER CENT)				
			Good Recovery	Moderate Disability	Severe Disability	Vegetative	Dead
First 160	27	39	36	24	8	2	30
Next 115	30	40	33	23	6	2	36

* Patients were treated at the Medical College of Virginia. The same management protocol was used.

outcome from serious head injury.* In support of this, examples are cited of "miraculous" recoveries in young patients, and statements are made that patients over 60 years old who remain comatose for more than 24 hours seldom recover. Although it is true that in most large series of head injuries a significant positive correlation exists between increasing age and an increasing mortality rate, this mathematical correlation should not be interpreted as proof of a direct causal relationship. Carlsson and his colleagues pointed out that the age-related mortality rate of head injury in their series of 496 patients was almost exclusively due to death from medical causes to which the elderly are more susceptible.[16] This has been confirmed in the authors' own study (Table 60–5).[5]

Two other factors contribute to an association between age and morbidity from head injury. Older patients are more likely than younger patients to have pre-existing brain damage due to prior trauma or cerebrovascular disease, which will make a good recovery from a head injury less likely. Intracranial hematomas complicating head injury are more frequently encountered in older patients in head injury series in which the entry criterion is failure to obey commands following injury. As is

---

* See references 14, 35, 49, 50, 56, 62, 63, 99, 100, 102, 115, 120.

TABLE 60–5 MORTALITY RATE FROM SEVERE HEAD INJURY RELATED TO AGE IN A SERIES OF 160 PATIENTS*

AGE GROUP (YEARS)	NUMBER OF PATIENTS	MORTALITY RATE (PER CENT)		
		Total Deaths	Systemic Cause	Cerebral Cause
0–20	67	22	9	13
21–40	64	33	19	14
41–60	22	36	23	13
61–80	7	57	43	14
Total	160	30	16	14

* When deaths are divided into those from systemic medical cause and elevated intracranial pressure, the relationship between mortality rate and age is restricted to deaths from medical causes. (Data from Becker, D. P., Miller, J. D., Ward, J. D., Greenberg, R. P., Young, H. F., and Sakalas, R.: The outcome from severe head injury with early diagnosis and intensive management. J. Neurosurg., 47:491–502, 1977; and Miller, J. D., Becker, D. P., Ward, J. D., Sullivan, H. G., Adams, W. E., and Rosner, M.J.: Significance of intracranial hypertension in severe head injury. J. Neurosurg., 47:503–516, 1977.)

shown later, the presence of intracranial hematomas exerts a profound influence on outcome from injury.

Pre-Existing Brain Damage

Many neurosurgeons have had the distressing experience of following a patient through the recovery phase from a serious head injury to resumption of his former level of activity, only to see the same patient devastated by a second head injury that seemed initially to be much milder than the first. This is a dramatic example of the concept of cumulative brain damage after injury. Another example is the punch-drunk syndrome of boxers.[114] Pre-existing brain damage need not be traumatic, however; hydrocephalic patients who have been restored to full function by cerebrospinal fluid shunting or patients who have recovered well from stroke may be totally disabled by an apparently minor head injury.

Nature of the Injury

The Force Involved

The force causing the injury has a considerable influence on the outcome. Unfortunately, accurate information on it seldom is obtained. In the authors' experience, relatively few patients who are injured in high-speed automobile accidents and have been unconscious from the time of injury and remain so on admission to hospital are discovered to have intracranial hematomas. Unconsciousness in these patients is due to diffuse brain injury caused by the considerable forces involved in impact. In contrast, a much higher proportion of those patients who have become unconscious following a blow to the head or a fall from a low height, in which much less injuring force is involved, are found to have intracranial hematomas. In these patients persisting unconsciousness when the patient reaches hospital or deterioration into coma after a lucid interval is due to secondary brain compression and distortion rather than to the primary brain injury.

Observation of only the conscious level on admission to hospital of comatose patients fails to make the crucial differentiation between the patients whose unconsciousness is due to diffuse brain injury and those who have become unconscious because of brain compression from a mass lesion. Knowledge of the forces involved in the initial injury is clearly of major importance in making this differentiation. Sequential examination is also vital. It is most important to recognize that the way in which entry criteria for a series of patients with head injury are defined influences the outcome. For patients with diffuse brain injury it matters little whether the comatose state is defined on admission, after 6 hours, or after 24 hours. On the other hand, for the patient with an intracranial hematoma, these differences in timing are literally life or death matters, since a comatose patient with an acute subdural hematoma may be salvageable after 1 to 6 hours of coma due to brain compression but not after 6 to 24 hours of unrelieved brain compression.

Intracranial Mass Lesions

The importance of entry criteria and of age has been stressed in evaluating outcome from head injury and in comparing results from one series with another. Of equal importance, however, is the proportion of patients in a series who are suffering from an intracranial mass lesion as a complication of head injury. Not only is the number of patients with mass lesions important in assessing outcome but also the type of mass lesion, i.e., epidural, subdural, or intracerebral hematoma. The definition of a significant unilateral mass lesion is that it produces 5 mm or more of midline shift. Intracranial hematoma is by far the most significant "avoidable factor" leading to the death of patients following head injury.[118]

The outcome of patients with mass lesions is significantly worse in several respects than in patients with diffuse brain injury.[5] For example, in the authors' series of 160 patients, 62 had intracranial mass lesions that were treated by operative decompression. The average brain shift was 9 mm. In these 62 patients a significantly greater incidence of abnormal motor response (abnormal flexor, extensor, or nil as best response) was found, i.e., 56 per cent as compared with a 49 per cent incidence in the remaining 98 patients, who were categorized as suffering from "diffuse brain injury." Of course, many patients with mass lesions also have diffuse brain damage. Similarly, there was a significantly higher percentage of patients with impaired reflex eye movements and bilateral absence of pupillary light response in the mass lesion group. This finding is important, since these two signs are reliable indices of brain stem dysfunction.

As would be expected from their neurological findings, the group of patients with mass lesions fared worse, having a 40 per cent mortality rate compared with a 23 per cent mortality rate in the diffuse injury group. Correspondingly the rate of good recovery in the mass lesion group was only 29 per cent compared with 40 per cent in the patients with diffuse brain injury (see Table 60–4). This difference has also been stressed by Pazzaglia and by Gutterman.[48,102]

To this point, all mass lesions have been lumped together even though there may be pronounced differences between the subgroups; e.g., patients with epidural hematomas fare better than those with acute subdural hematoma. Furthermore, patients with predominantly intracerebral mass lesions, whether primarily hematoma or contusion, have the worst outcome (Table 60–6).

TABLE 60–6 OUTCOME IN 107 COMATOSE PATIENTS WHO REQUIRED OPERATIVE DECOMPRESSION OF ACUTE EXPANDING INTRACRANIAL MASS LESION*

LOCATION OF MASS LESION	NUMBER OF CASES	OUTCOME (PER CENT)		
		Good Recovery/ Moderate Disability	Severe Disability/ Vegetative	Dead
Epidural	17	76	6	18
Subdural	52	42	12	46
Intracerebral	38	21	21	58

* This group of 107 patients treated at the Medical College of Virginia is 39 per cent of all comatose patients with head injury who were seen during a five-year period.

Epidural Hematoma

Although generally considered the most benign of the intracranial hematomas complicating injury, epidural hematoma nevertheless produces awesome mortality and morbidity rates in many reported series. Overall mortality rates range from 10 to 55 per cent but are relatively meaningless since death is the result of the interplay of many factors such as intradural brain damage and duration of coma due to brain compression.[39,52,55] Thus, among patients in coma at the time of operative decompression there are three times as many deaths as among those who are drowsy but able to converse. If a patient in coma has never had a lucid interval, the risk of death is twice as great as in the patient who has had a lucid interval. If cerebrospinal fluid is bloody, the mortality rate is twice as high as in those patients who have clear cerebrospinal fluid.[39] If patients have bilateral dilated pupils or bilateral decerebrate rigidity at the time of operation, then very few of them make a good recovery following operation, whether these signs are the result of intradural brain damage or secondary to severe brain compression.

A more useful concept is the "ideal mortality rate" from head injury complicated by epidural hemorrhage. Since a certain number of patients will have severe intradural damage associated with the epidural hematoma, this ideal figure can never be zero. Given a management protocol such that all patients have access to definitive diagnostic measures within a few hours of injury, the mortality rate should be under 20 per cent; probably 5 to 10 per cent is the most realistic range.[52,55]

Acute Subdural Hematoma

The mortality rate from acute subdural hematoma has remained high over the past 40 years, ranging in different reported series from 50 to 95 per cent.* Clearly the factor of associated brain damage weighs heavily in these deaths. Other factors of importance that increase their number are bilateral lesions, severe visible disruption of brain, the use of burr holes rather than craniotomy for evacuation of hematoma, and advanced age. Below 60 years of age, the

outcome does not seem to be influenced by the age factor. In a series with an overall mortality rate of 70 per cent, decerebrate rigidity had no particular influence on that rate, while in the series with a lower mortality rate overall, this sign significantly increased the rate.

It is difficult to suggest an "ideal mortality rate" for patients with acute subdural hematoma, since this group shades into the next group to be considered, patients with intracerebral lesions. With optimum deployment of present-day methods, however, it should be possible to hold the number of deaths to below 50 per cent.

Intracerebral Mass Lesion

This group of patients continues to present the greatest challenge to the neurosurgeon involved in the management of head injury. Large external decompressions are favored by some and have been abandoned by others.[20,22,70,111,156] Internal decompression by frontal or temporal lobectomy has generally been used, but the incidence of postoperative intracranial hypertension remains high at 71 per cent. This group has the highest mortality rate at 58 per cent and the lowest rate for good and moderately disabling recoveries at 21 per cent compared with death of 46 per cent and good recoveries of 40 per cent of all of the authors' patients with mass lesions (see Table 60–6).

Chronic Subdural Hematoma

Since initial brain damage is minimal, the mortality rate and morbidity of chronic subdural hematoma are entirely related to the rapidity with which the diagnosis is made. If brain compression and shift progress to the point at which signs of brain stem dysfunction emerge, the chances of a good recovery recede rapidly. Since chronic subdural hematoma commonly afflicts the elderly, many of whom may have had previous head injury or cerebrovascular disease, prolonged disability is common. In subdural effusion of infancy it may be close to impossible to gauge the quality of outcome. Children with this lesion commonly appear rather passive and often have sunny personalities, so they are popular with nursing staff. This very engaging appearance, however, may in itself indicate severe brain dysfunction.

---

* See references 22, 35, 49, 56, 111, 113, 140.

Blunt Versus Penetrating Injury

Differentiation between blunt and penetrating injury is important to the outcome of head injury for two reasons. First, the presence of a penetrating injury implies that the force applied to the skull has been more locally distributed, and the associated brain damage in these cases is likely to be severe but localized in the area of penetration. Many such patients do not lose consciousness or lose it only briefly. In blunt injury in which the force is applied to the skull as a whole, brain damage is likely to be diffuse. As a result, coma and polar damage leading to frontal or temporal swelling may occur. Penetrating injuries may introduce infection, which can adversely affect outcome in a patient whose brain injury and initial neurological status would have suggested a good outcome.

Early Insults to the Injured Brain

Between injury and the patient's arrival at the hospital primary brain damage that the patient may have suffered can be compounded by secondary insults. These are important to document, as they may greatly influence outcome and increase the severity of the original injury.

Respiratory Problems

In experimental studies of head injury, a brief period of apnea is a common sequel to impact. It seems likely that this also occurs in patients.[137] Clearly, spontaneous respiration is resumed in most cases. Aspiration of emesis or blood also can occur at this early stage when gag reflexes are depressed. Concomitant facial or chest injuries are other common contributors to respiratory problems that are encountered following head injury.

Shock

Although reduced blood pressure is commonly attributable to internal or external hemorrhage from concomitant injuries, another possible cause of systemic hypotension that may contribute adversely to outcome is seen in the patient who loses consciousness while caught in an upright position, for example, the patient trapped in the front seat of a crushed automobile.

Documentation of such circumstances by rescue squad personnel or police may shed light on an unexpectedly poor outcome from head injury.

Early Seizures

Epilepsy soon after injury is often viewed as a warning that an intracranial hematoma is present, but the hypoxia, cerebral vasodilatation, and intracranial hypertension that accompany seizures may produce significant secondary brain damage and profoundly affect outcome. The occurrence of seizures after injury may have considerable diagnostic import. The presence of early seizures has clear prognostic value in that their occurrence has been associated with an increase in the incidence of late (and continuing) post-traumatic epilepsy.[65,66]

Clinical Factors Observed in Hospital

Systemic Factors

Hypoxemia

The adverse influence of hypoxemia on outcome from head injury has been well documented.[53,110,119] In one population of patients with severe head injury the incidence of hypoxemia (defined as arterial Po_2 less than of mercury 65 mm on spontaneous air breathing) was 30 per cent.[86] If this figure is added to the number of patients who have an abnormally high alveolar to arterial oxygen gradient, then the incidence of impaired oxygenation rises to over 85 per cent in unconscious patients with head injury.[37]

Arterial Hypotension and Anemia

Arterial hypotension, (systolic blood pressure less than 95 mm of mercury) in 13 per cent of cases, and anemia (hematocrit less than 30 per cent) in 12 per cent of patients have been found on admission.[86] Although these two systemic insults occur almost exclusively in patients with multiple injuries, 57 per cent of those with head injuries have multiple injuries. Therefore arterial hypotension and anemia constitute a significant problem in the total population of patients with head injury.

The effect of all three of these disorders is to reduce oxygen delivery to the brain, particularly when normal mechanisms that protect against such insults have been deranged by the effects of trauma. It is important, therefore, to assess whether the presence of such insults is associated with a poorer outcome. One must first consider separately those patients who have intracranial mass lesions and those with diffuse brain injury in whom operative decompression is not required. In the former group, neurological dysfunction is worse and outcome is significantly poorer than in diffuse injury. Although the outcome in patients with mass lesions was worse when systemic insults were present on admission, the difference in outcome between those with and those without insults was not statistically different. In the group with diffuse brain injury, on the other hand, patients who also had hypoxia and hypotension or anemia or both on admission fared significantly worse (Table 60-7).[86]

Neurological Signs

Glasgow Coma Scale

While the Glasgow coma scale was not intended for use as a prognostic indicator, nevertheless the level of responsiveness and the duration for which a patient may remain at a given point on the scale correlate

TABLE 60-7 INFLUENCE OF EARLY SYSTEMIC INSULTS (HYPOTENSION, HYPOXIA, AND ANEMIA) ON OUTCOME IN HEAD INJURY WITH INTRACRANIAL MASS LESIONS AND WITH DIFFUSE BRAIN INJURY

		OUTCOME (PER CENT)	
PATIENT GROUP	NO. OF PATIENTS	Good Recovery/ Moderate Disability	Severe Disability/ Vegetative/ Dead
Mass lesions			
No insult	24	50	50
Systemic insult	16	25	75
Diffuse Injury			
No insult	28	87	13
Systemic insult	32	64	36
			(P < 0.05)

* Forty patients had intracranial mass lesions; sixty patients had diffuse brain injury. In the latter group the presence of systemic insults on admission is significantly related to a poorer outcome. (From Miller, J. D., Sweet, R. C., Narayan, R., and Becker, D. P.: Early insults to the injured brain. J.A.M.A., *240*: 439–442, 1978. Reprinted by permission.)

TABLE 60-8 RELATIONSHIP BETWEEN BEST RANKING ON GLASGOW COMA SCALE AND OUTCOME*

	OUTCOME (PER CENT)	
RESPONSIVENESS ON GLASGOW COMA SCALE AT 24 HOURS	Good Recovery/ Moderate Disability	Vegetative/ Dead
11–15	91	6
8–10	59	27
5–7	28	54
3–4	13	80

* Best ranking on Glasgow coma scale equals the sum of eye opening, motor response, and verbal response figures at 24 hours from injury. The outcome was assessed at six months from injury. (Data from Jennett, B., Teasdale, G., Braakman, R., Minderhoud, J., and Knill-Jones, R: Predicting outcome in individual patients after severe head injury. Lancet, *1*:1031–1034, 1976.)

closely with outcome (Table 60-8).[59,62,63] The best motor response obtained is the single most important prognostic element. Among the six levels of response on the motor scale, a significant prognostic dividing point can be found between normal and abnormal flexion—that is, between semipurposeful withdrawal without localization and a decorticate response in which there is an element of wrist flexion and pronation often accompanied by tucking of the thumb under the fingers. In some ways this natural cutoff point can be problematic because it is precisely the area on the motor scale at which there is difficulty in making a clear distinction between two adjacent responses. In the original description of the Glasgow coma scale the distinction was not made at all, all of these responses, both normal and abnormal, being classed as flexor.[43] In a later amendment flexor responses were subdivided into normal and abnormal flexion.[144]

In the authors' series of cases, the patients were initially subdivided into two groups, those with mass lesions and those with diffuse injury. Abnormal motor responses (abnormal flexion, extension, or nil) were then noted to carry a significant adverse prognosis for outcome only in the patients with diffuse brain injury. In patients with mass lesions who had been evaluated prior to operative decompression, the presence of abnormal motor responses did not correlate statistically with an adverse outcome (Table 60-9).[5]

Failure to open the eyes on command or on painful stimulation carries an adverse

TABLE 60–9   INFLUENCE OF ABNORMAL MOTOR RESPONSE, IMPAIRMENT OR ABSENCE OF OCULOCEPHALIC RESPONSE, AND BILATERAL ABSENCE OF PUPILLARY LIGHT RESPONSE ON OUTCOME*

| | OUTCOME | | | | | | | |
| | Mass Lesion | | | | Diffuse Injury | | | |
RESPONSE	No. of Patients	Good Recovery/ Moderate Disability	Severely Disabled/ Vegetative	Dead	No. of Patients	Good Recovery/ Moderate Disability	Severely Disabled/ Vegetative	Dead
Best motor response								
Localize/flexion	30	60%	10%	30%	61	92%	2%	6%
Abnormal flexion/ extension	32	41%	9%	50%	37†	24%	24%	52%
Oculocephalic response								
Intact	28	75%	7%	18%	69	84%	4%	12%
Impaired/absent	34†	29%	12%	59%	29†	24%	24%	52%
Pupil light response								
Present	39	67%	8%	25%	81	75%	9%	16%
Bilaterally absent	23†	22%	13%	65%	11†	0%	18%	82%
† P < 0.05								

* There were 62 patients with intracranial mass lesions and 98 patients with diffuse brain injury. Daggers indicate a significantly poorer outcome for that group of patients. Note that abnormal motor responses (prior to operative decompression) do not significantly affect outcome in patients with mass lesions. (Data from Becker, D. P., Miller, J. D., Ward, J. D., Greenberg, R. P., Young, H. F., and Sakalas, R.: The outcome from severe head injury with early diagnosis and intensive management. J. Neurosurg., 47:491–502, 1977.)

significance in the first 72 hours after injury. Eye opening at a later stage after injury does not necessarily imply a good prognosis, however, since patients who remain in a vegetative state commonly open their eyes spontaneously, and many even appear to follow sounds and moving objects with their eyes.

The return of a verbal response is a usual signal for the end of coma, and is accompanied by ability to obey commands. It should be appreciated, however, that emergence from coma by these criteria does not correspond with the end of the period of post-traumatic amnesia. Patients who remain unconscious for several days will often speak for a period of several more days but remember nothing afterward.

Signs of Brain Stem Dysfunction

In all series of head injuries, the presence of fixed pupils (not necessarily dilated) and impairment or absence of oculocephalic and oculovestibular responses is an ominous sign no matter whether recorded early or late after injury. Supporting the statistical correlation of such signs with high morbidity and mortality rates, there is sound clinicopathological evidence showing brain stem damage in patients who during life showed this type of neurological dysfunction. Furthermore, in neurophysiological studies these abnormal signs correlate closely with abnormalities of brain stem evoked potentials (see Table 60–9).[45,46]

Similar statements can be made about the adverse significance of absence of the corneomandibular and ciliospinal reflexes, although these are less frequently reported. The ciliospinal reflex, although not named as such, was used over a hundred years ago by Macewen as a means of differentiating between alcoholic and traumatic coma.[77]

Duration of Coma and Post-Traumatic Amnesia

These factors represent respectively the objective and subjective determinations of duration of disordered consciousness following injury. End of coma may best be signaled by the attainment of a certain level on the Glasgow coma scale, but this point may be difficult to judge in individual cases. For example, resumption of speech may be impossible because of a tracheostomy or aphasia due to focal brain damage. Spontaneous eye opening occurs in the permanent vegetative state, and the fact that a patient is obeying commands, albeit briskly, does not convey full emergence from coma.

Thus, this determination, intended to be objective, may become very subjective as far as the observer is concerned.

The concept of post-traumatic amnesia, the time between injury and return of continuous memory, was developed as a yardstick of the severity of brain damage by Russell and Nathan in 1946, and its value has since been attested to by others.[31,125,126,157] Contrary to what might be expected, the patient is often quite clear as to exactly when he "came around" and began to remember. Post-traumatic amnesia always lasts longer than the observed coma, and the difference between the two durations may be more than a week in some cases in prolonged post-traumatic confusion. As a rough guide, the post-traumatic amnesia may be expected to last approximately three times as long as the duration of the coma. Thus, two days of coma is likely to be associated with six days of amnesia. Relatively broad categories of duration of post-traumatic amnesia are sufficient to discern differences in degree of injury and in outcome. Thus, an amnesia of less than one hour signifies a minor brain dysfunction and occurs mainly in patients who are thought never to have been unconscious. An amnesia lasting between one hour and one day signifies mild dysfunction and is most commonly seen in a patient who has been stunned for a few minutes. An amnesia lasting between one day and one week indicates a significant degree of diffuse brain damage at the time of injury, and an amnesia lasting longer than a week indicates severe brain dysfunction after injury. Anomalous situations will arise in certain cases because the patient cannot communicate or because there is a prolonged period of post-traumatic confusion following a relatively short duration of coma. This problem is seen most commonly in the elderly patient. Carlsson and his colleagues noted that whereas duration of coma was not influenced by age, the duration of amnesia did appear to increase with age, other factors being equal.[16] This suggests that the duration of the amnesia is influenced by the type of brain that has been injured as well as by the severity of injury.

The duration of amnesia after the injury probably is the best simple yardstick for determining the severity of diffuse head injury and the total toll of brain dysfunction.[31] The prognostic significance of post-traumatic amnesia is discussed further in the section on the quality of recovery.

SIGNIFICANCE OF DIAGNOSTIC STUDIES FOR OUTCOME

Diagnostic studies performed in patients with head injury and the information provided by such studies that is relevant to outcome are summarized in Table 60–10.

Plain X-Rays of Head and Neck

These x-rays may demonstrate the presence of intracranial air or gas and foreign bodies, which imply potential intracranial infection and therefore an unexpectedly adverse prognosis. The discovery of a fracture-dislocation of the cervical spine is quite significant when limb motor responses are absent in a patient with a severe head injury. If, in this case, the absence of motor function reflects spinal cord damage, then clearly an estimate of level of consciousness by limb motor response on the coma scale would be inappropriate and misleading. As a result, it is important to test the face as well as the limbs for responses to painful stimuli.

CT Scan, Angiogram, Ventriculogram

The most important contribution of these studies for prognosis is the identification of an intracranial mass lesion. As mentioned earlier, the significance of abnormal motor responses for outcome is different in patients with mass lesions and those without them, and, as will be seen, the significance of early intracranial hypertension for outcome is also dependent on whether or not a mass lesion has been shown to exist. If this fact is added to the finding that the most common cause of death in patients who become unconscious following a lucid interval is intracranial hematoma, it can be seen that confirmation or exclusion of an intracranial mass lesion is the most important contribution of these radiographic studies, both for management and for determination of outcome.

One advantage that computed tomography offers over other types of diagnostic

TABLE 60–10　DIAGNOSTIC STUDIES PERFORMED IN HEAD INJURY THAT ARE RELEVANT TO OUTCOME

DIAGNOSTIC STUDY	INFORMATION PROVIDED FOR OUTCOME
Plain skull x-rays	Fracture, foreign body, air (risk of infection)
CT scan	Mass lesion—location and type
	Intracerebral lesions—unilateral or bilateral
Angiogram	Mass lesion, vascular lesion, circulation time
Ventriculogram	Mass lesion, intracranial pressure
Intracranial pressure measurement	Level of pressure, waves, trend, response to therapy, compliance (risk of mass lesion)
Respiratory evaluation	Rate, volume, pattern, response to stimuli
Cerebral circulation studies	Transit time, mean flow, regional changes, response to stimuli and therapy, sequential changes
Cerebral oxygen metabolism study ($CMRO_2$)	Mean value for brain, response to therapy
Electroencephalogram	Diffuse vs. focal hemisphere dysfunction
Evoked potential studies	Location, hemisphere vs. brain stem dysfunction, sequential changes, response to therapy
Cerebrospinal fluid studies	pH and gases, lactate and pyruvate levels, neurotransmitter levels

studies is that it can often differentiate between epidural, subdural, and intracerebral lesions, information that has important implications for outcome. In addition to the value of detecting and possibly identifying the type of intracranial mass lesions, each of these neuroradiological studies has some additional and separate contribution to make in relation to outcome.

Computed tomography permits a survey of the entire brain. It also permits some differentiation between edema and infarction shown as low-density abnormalities and between hemorrhage and contusion seen as increased-density abnormalities. Diffuse isodense brain swelling is signaled by the disappearance of the convolutional marking of the sylvian fissure and compression or disappearance of the ventricles in the absence of marked density change in the cerebral hemispheres themselves. This diffuse swelling does not carry an implication for poor outcome, whereas bilateral lesions of increased density, whether seen soon after injury or after the evacuation of an intracranial mass lesion, are associated with a significant increase in the mortality rate and a decrease in the number of patients who make a good recovery (Fig. 60–1).[139] In parallel with these implications for outcome, the presence of bilateral increased-density abnormalities correlates with a high incidence of decorticate or decerebrate posturing together with a greater incidence of severe intracranial hypertension. Most of the additional deaths among these patients are due to uncontrollable intracranial hypertension (Table 60–11).

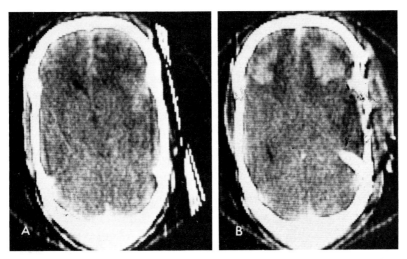

Figure 60–1　CT scans on successive days from a patient with right frontal contusion and right-to-left midline shift. *A.* Scan on admission. *B.* Scan 24 hours later showing bilateral dense frontal lesions.

**TABLE 60–11   RELATIONSHIP BETWEEN FINDINGS ON INITIAL
CT SCAN AND OUTCOME***

CT SCAN FINDINGS	NO. OF PATIENTS	OUTCOME (PER CENT)		
		Good Recovery/ Moderate Disability	*Severe Disability/ Vegetative*	*Dead*
Normal	26	81	11	8
Bilateral isodense swelling	29	72	3	24
Unilateral dense lesion	62	66	11	23
Bilateral dense lesions	23	28	4	70
Total	140	63	9	28

* There were 140 comatose patients with head injury. The outcome was evaluated three months from injury. (From Sweet, R. C., Miller, J. D., Lipper, M., Kishore, P. R. S., and Becker, D. P.: Significance of bilateral abnormalities on the CT scan in patients with severe head injury. Neurosurgery, 3:16–21, 1978. Reprinted by permission.)

Cerebral arteriography provides important information concerning the speed of the cerebral circulation.[47] The most extreme example of this is found in circulatory arrest, which can be taken as a confirmation of brain death if it is shown after injection into both carotid arteries. Slowing of the circulation time, particularly with reflux of contrast into the basilar artery from a carotid injection, carries a very bad prognosis. In the study of Scialfa and Cristi no patient with a cerebral circulation time of 7 seconds or more survived, and patients with circulation time of between 5.5 and 6.5 seconds were all deeply comatose and had a correspondingly poor level of recovery.[129]

Appearance of severe spasm in major cerebral arteries shows correlation with the occurrence of ischemic brain damage in fatal cases, and with low values of cerebral blood flow, which in turn are suggestive of a bad outcome from injury.[80]

In addition, the cerebral arteriogram may show other lesions that have a bearing on outcome, such as aneurysms, in which the cause of coma may be related to spontaneous subarachnoid hemorrhage rather than to head injury.

The ventriculogram provides the most limited information radiologically, but does have the great advantage of permitting measurement of intraventricular pressure at the time of ventricular puncture. Early measurement of pressure is of some value in prognosis, as is discussed in the following section.[87]

Intracranial Pressure

In patients with severe head injury, intractable intracranial hypertension is the mode of death in about half of the patients who die.[87] In such cases, the intracranial pressure rises inexorably to the level of the blood pressure; this event is followed by abolition of all motor response, dilatation of the pupils, and loss of electroencephalographic activity. The onset of apnea and confirmation of the disappearance of all brain stem reflex activity in such patients constitutes brain death.

Severe elevation of intracranial pressure to sustained levels in excess of 40 mm of mercury has been associated in many published series with a very poor outcome and a large number of fatalities.[68,87,153–155] In the presence of a normal blood pressure this level of intracranial pressure would produce a perfusion pressure at the lower limits of tolerance of normal autoregulation. At this level of intracranial pressure, the frequency of abnormal evoked potentials in patients with head injury is significantly increased.[43] This evoked potential finding can be linked with studies that show that under controlled experimental conditions abnormal cortical evoked potentials emerge at that level of cerebral perfusion pressure at which cerebral blood flow begins to decrease, whether this cortical perfusion pressure is attained by reduction of blood pressure or elevation of intracranial pressure.[149]

The significance of lesser degrees of intracranial hypertension, between 20 and 40 mm of mercury, to outcome from head injury is less well established, and no close correlation between the occurrence of such levels of pressure and mortality and morbidity rates has been observed in published series of patients with head injuries in whom intracranial pressure has been monitored continuously. In some series these intermediate levels of intracranial hypertension have been associated with the lowest mortality rates.[67,68] This surprising finding emerges because in the "low-pressure group" (0 to 20 mm of mercury) a larger number of patients died without regaining consciousness—a confusing observation that arises if deaths are enumerated in a single category without regard to cause. The fatalities in the low-pressure group are nearly all due to extracranial causes in patients who remain unconscious for prolonged periods. Most of these patients show extensive diffuse brain damage but little evidence of the neuropathological sequelae of intracranial hypertension.[1]

All authorities agree that an intracranial pressure level of 10 mm of mercury or less is normal and that a sustained pressure in excess of 20 mm of mercury mean is abnormal, but there is dispute as to the significance of intermediate levels of intracranial pressure.

For intracranial pressure to be unequivocally normal, an upper level of 10 mm of mercury is needed, while for it to be unequivocally elevated, a lower limit on intracranial pressure of 20 mm of mercury is necessary. In the authors' series of 160 patients, intracranial pressure monitoring was begun very soon after injury and continued in the intensive care unit, both in patients without mass lesions and in the 40 per cent of patients who had had mass lesions evacuated. Correlations were made of the eventual outcome and the intracranial pressure levels occurring both earlier and later in the course after the head injury (Fig. 60–2).[87] In assessing the significance of early measurements of intracranial pressure, it was found that virtually all the patients with intracranial mass lesions had some degree of intracranial hypertension early in their course. Initial intracranial pressure levels in excess of 40 mm of mercury could be positively correlated with a poorer outcome. Intermediate levels of intracranial hypertension had no particular significance for outcome. In patients with diffuse brain injury, in whom no mass lesion was present, two thirds of the group had initial intracranial pressure levels in excess of 10 mm of mercury. Morbidity and mortality rates increased in these patients in parallel with the initial intracranial pressure. Thus, in this subgroup it did appear that early measurements of intracranial pressure gave

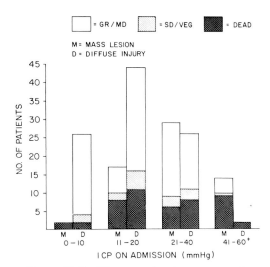

Figure 60–2 Histogram showing outcome of patients with different intracranial pressure (ICP) levels on admission to hospital. Comparison is made between patients with mass lesions (prior to their evacuation) and patients with diffuse brain injuries in whom intracranial pressure bore a close relationship to outcome. GR/MD, good recovery/moderate disability; SD/VEG, severe disability/vegetative.

information concerning eventual outcome, and any pressure level above 10 mm of mercury was of adverse significance.

To assess the behavior of intracranial pressure in the intensive care unit after endotracheal intubation, with artificial ventilation, and after intracranial masses had been removed, patients were divided into three broad categories: those in whom the intracranial pressure remained below 20 mm of mercury or was restored to this level by the management regimen; those in whom intracranial pressure rose over 20 mm of mercury in a sustained manner but could be reduced below that level by appropriate treatment with hyperventilation, cerebrospinal fluid drainage, or osmotherapy; and the final group of patients in whom intracranial pressure remained high or rose over 20 mm of mercury and could not be controlled by therapy. In this last group of patients, intracranial pressure rose to the level of arterial blood pressure, and death was due to fulminating intracranial hypertension (Fig. 60–3).

Comparisons were made between the pressure patterns in patients who had had intracranial mass lesions removed and patients with diffuse brain injury who had never had an intracranial mass lesion. There was no difference between these two

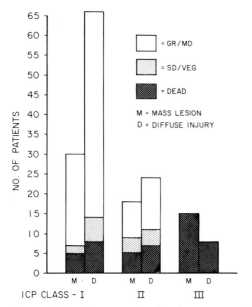

Figure 60–3 Histogram showing the outcome of patients with different classes of intracranial pressure (ICP) response to management regimen. Class I patients are those in whom intracranial pressure remained below 20 mm of mercury after evacuation of mass lesions and institution of artificial ventilation. Class II patients are those in whom intracranial pressure rose over 20 mm of mercury mean but could be controlled by further hyperventilation, cerebrospinal fluid drainage, and intravenous mannitol. Class III patients are those with uncontrollable intracranial hypertension, all of whom died. There is no difference in outcome between those patients who had mass lesions removed and those with diffuse injury in each intracranial pressure class, but a greater proportion of patients with mass lesions fall into classes II and III. GR/MD, good recovery/moderate disability; SD/VEG, severe disability/vegetative.

groups of patients. Patients who had had mass lesions evacuated behaved now like patients with "diffuse brain injury." Persistent or secondary elevation of intracranial pressure was associated with a poorer outcome, even if the rise in pressure could be controlled by medical therapy. This finding could be interpreted to mean that elevations in intracranial pressure cause brain damage and that, even if they are subsequently controlled, the patient fares poorly. An alternative and more likely interpretation of the data is that secondary or persistent elevation of intracranial pressure is another manifestation of the extent and severity of brain damage, whether primary or secondary, and for this reason it signals a poorer outcome even if it is possible to control the phenomenon of intracranial hypertension.

Respiration and Outcome

Apnea is a crucial and, in many cases, final point in the process of brain herniation with raised intracranial pressure. Prior to cessation of respiration, however, severely ill patients with neurological disorders may exhibit a variety of abnormalities of respiratory pattern such as Cheyne-Stokes, apneustic, or ataxic respiration.[103,105] The adverse effects of respiratory obstruction and the contribution of early intubation and tracheostomy was one of the major advances in the care of serious head injury 20 years ago.[30,78,79] In addition, other studies have demonstrated that certain combinations of increased ventilation and low arterial carbon dioxide tension show correlation with a poor outcome from head trauma.[53,119,155] Aspects of respiration that influence outcome are: the pattern of breathing, posthyperventilation apnea, the ventilatory response to carbon dioxide, blood gas concentrations and pH, and cerebrospinal fluid gas concentrations and pH.

Pattern of Breathing

Although abnormal patterns of respiration have long been recognized, it was only relatively recently that Plum and Posner popularized the idea that the pattern of respiration could be used as a sign to localize areas of brain damage.[103–105] Thus, Cheyne-Stokes respiration was held to be associated with bilateral deep hemispheral lesions, apneustic breathing with lesions of the lower pons, and ataxic breathing with lesions of the medulla.[13] Since this proposal the most extensive study of respiratory patterns in patients with acute brain damage has been carried out by North and Jennett in 227 patients, 90 of whom had suffered severe head injury.[93] The respiratory pattern was recorded by transthoracic impedence pneumography, and the patterns were classified into three categories according to objective criteria. Periodic breathing consisted of a regularly occurring variation in tidal volume with more than 50 per cent variation; tachypnea consisted of a respiratory rate of more than 25 breaths per minute; irregular breathing was an erratic variation in frequency and in tidal volume with more than 50 per cent variation between the smallest and largest breaths. Abnormal respiratory patterns were observed in 60 per cent of patients, and more than one abnormal pattern was observed in more than 20 per cent of patients during even a relatively brief period of several hours of respiratory monitoring.

Respiratory pattern abnormalities were most common in patients at the lower levels of consciousness who responded only to pain, but there was no association between any particular respiratory pattern and conscious level. Abnormal respiration was equally common in each of the three main diagnostic groups, head injury, brain tumor, and intracranial hemorrhage. Tachypnea was slightly more frequent in the patients with head injuries as compared with the other patients. It occurred in almost a quarter of those with head injury.

The correlation of abnormal respiratory patterns with the site of brain damage was rather disappointing. The only constant factor to emerge was that all 12 patients with proved medullary lesions had abnormal breathing patterns. Patients with combined cerebellar and medullary lesions also had a high incidence of abnormal breathing, as did patients with pontine lesions, but in patients with lesions confined to the cerebellum there was no significant association with abnormal breathing. Irregular breathing was the form that was most significantly associated with medullary and pontine lesions. No significant association was found between periodic respiration and any particular site of brain damage as determined by clinical examination, multiple diagnostic investigations, or autopsy.

There was a correlation between abnormal respiratory patterns and outcome in that a significantly higher percentage of those with any type of abnormality died as compared with those patients who had a normal respiratory pattern during the monitoring period. The type of abnormal respiration that correlated most significantly with poor outcome was tachypnea, and of those patients with tachypnea most deaths occurred in those whose arterial carbon dioxide tension was less than 30 mm of mercury on spontaneous ventilation. Low arterial PCO_2 alone was not significantly associated with poor outcome.

Posthyperventilation Apnea

Plum and his colleagues found posthyperventilation apnea lasting more than 12 seconds was confined to patients with bilateral damage in the cerebral hemispheres.[106] Others, however, have reported that this phenomenon may occur in the normal person.[36] Jennett and her colleagues compared a group of 50 normal volunteer subjects with 50 patients suffering from brain damage, of whom more than a third had a severe head injury.[64] Respiration was monitored by impedance pneumography, and end-tidal carbon dioxide concentration was monitored continuously. In the test the subject was asked to take five deep breaths, and the successive apneic period, if present, was measured in seconds. In healthy subjects apnea of more than five seconds' duration was seen in only four instances out of 172 tests. When the same test was applied to the 50 patients with brain damage there was an extremely high incidence of posthyperventilation apnea lasting more than five seconds. No correlation, however, was found between differing sites and severity of brain damage and the duration or frequency with which posthyperventilation apnea was encountered. It was concluded that any brain damage and lethargy in combination was sufficient to produce this sign and that it was not of value in localizing damage or in predicting outcome.

Ventilatory Response to Carbon Dioxide

It has been proposed that in patients with brain injury an increased sensitivity to carbon dioxde is encountered. The minute volume is believed to increase much more steeply with increasing arterial carbon dioxide content (PCO_2) than would otherwise occur, and this may indicate areas or degrees of brain damage that are crucial to the patient's recovery.[104] This proposal was tested by North and Jennett in a larger number of patients with brain damage, and the only abnormality that was encountered was a decrease in the sensitivity of the ventilatory response in patients with severe damage.[94] The decrease in carbon dioxide response was not a parameter of severity of injury and did not relate well to the patient's recovery.

Arterial Blood Gases and Gas Exchange

As stated earlier, many studies attest to the poor outcome that accompanies marked derangements of arterial blood gases and acid-base balance in patients with severe head injury.* In particular, any degree of hypoxemia correlates with an increase in mortality rate in virtually all series of reported cases. Extremely low arterial carbon dioxide levels, if accompanied by tachypnea, have been correlated with an increased number of patients ending in the severely disabled and vegetative groups. Increased values for alveolar-arterial oxygen tension gradients have been reported in large numbers of patients with head injury, but this abnormality is so common that the correlation with outcome has not been a close one.[9,53,119] Increased levels of arterial carbon dioxide have correlated with a high mortality rate, but this is an unusual respiratory abnormality in these patients unless there is associated chest injury.

Cerebrospinal Fluid Measurements

In patients with severe head injury there may be considerable cerebral tissue acidosis that may be at least in part responsible for spontaneous hyperventilation. This in turn will produce cerebrospinal fluid lactacidosis at a time when there is a systemic respiratory alkalosis. For this reason it may be more crucial for patient outcome from head injury to assess cerebrospinal fluid gases and acid-base status.[38,133] Gordon and Rossanda performed extensive measurements of the P_{CO_2}, P_{O_2}, and pH levels of fluid obtained either from lumbar or cisternal puncture, or from the lateral ventricle in patients with head injury.[40,41] Increases in the normally small difference in carbon dioxide content between cerebral venous blood and cerebrospinal fluid were attributed to reduced cerebral blood flow and indicated a poor outcome. Since low cerebrospinal fluid pH occurring when arterial pH is on the alkaline side because of the hypocapnia has been attributed to cerebral ischemia and an increase in cerebrospinal fluid lactate, Crockard and co-workers proposed that the level of cerebrospinal fluid lactate obtained from the lumbar spinal fluid might be an index to the outcome from severe head injury. Of 38 patients studied, all patients with a cerebrospinal fluid lactate level of over 55 mg per 100 ml (6.1 mEq per

liter) died.[24,25] This close correlation between cerebrospinal fluid lactate and outcome has not, however, been confirmed by others.[33] Lactate leakage from red blood cells in the cerebrospinal fluid clearly is a major problem with such studies. Crockard points out that early measurements are essential. To some extent cerebrospinal fluid lactate may also be an index of traumatic subarachnoid hemorrhage.

Measurements of Cerebral Circulation and Metabolism

Mean Cerebral Blood Flow and Oxygen Consumption

In general, the greater the severity of a patient's injury, the lower is the mean cerebral flow value for the entire hemisphere and the lower is the level of cerebral oxygen consumption (CMR_{O_2}). When cerebral blood flow falls below 25 ml per 100 gm per minute and when oxygen consumption falls below 1 ml of oxygen per 100 gm per minute, then a fatal or poor outcome is to be expected provided that the effects of depressant agents such as barbiturates can be ruled out.

Occasionally patients in deep coma following a head injury may be found to have global increases in cerebral blood flow above the normal range but with a low rate of oxygen metabolism. This finding is also of adverse significance with a strong chance of a fatal or vegetative outcome or severe disability. It is much more common, however, to find hyperemia limited to regions of the brain.*

Regional Cerebral Blood Flow

Since it became possible to measure cerebral blood flow in multiple areas several studies of regional cerebral blood flow have been made in patients with head injury. Both abnormally low levels and abnormally high levels have been found in areas that correspond to those areas that suffer the worst visible damage, namely frontal and temporal lobes.[15,33,98] The [133]xenon technique of measuring cerebral blood flow with external detectors mea-

---

sures mainly cortical blood flow. The value for the flow should therefore correspond with externally visible pathological changes, and in many cases this has been confirmed. What is less clear, however, is the significance of these flow alterations for outcome. More evidence is awaited to show that the measurement of a given level of flow over the motor strip correlates closely with hemiplegia that is either temporary or persistent and can be confidently predicted to be so.

Responsiveness of the Cerebral Circulation

The observation of the effect of alterations in blood pressure and arterial carbon dioxide tension has enabled workers to examine the capacity of the cerebral circulation to respond to physiological stress on a regional basis. Complementing observations of regional abnormalities in flow, further abnormalities have been uncovered in many cases to show that even when resting blood flow is not altered there is a reduced capacity to respond to vasoactive stimuli in certain areas. Once again, these areas correspond rather closely with the areas of the brain that are most frequently damaged on the surface.[15,32,98] The significance of such changes in cerebral vascular responsiveness in terms of final outcome and for the persistence of focal neurological signs remains to be firmly established.

Sequential Measurements of Cerebral Blood Flow

The adoption of the atraumatic technique of measuring cerebral blood flow following an intravenous injection or inhalation of [133]xenon has permitted two major extensions of blood flow measurement, namely the capacity to measure the flow in both hemispheres at the same time and to measure flow sequentially two or three times over a period of a week. In these studies it has been shown that a better correlation with eventual outcome can be obtained by observing whether cerebral blood flow that has started at an elevated or reduced level becomes normal over the next two or three days. Such studies are at an early stage and are rather limited, since few centers have the capacity to make these measurements, but already the results appear promising.[95]

Measurements of Cerebral Vascular Transit Time

Because of the complexity of making measurements of total and regional cerebral blood flow, several workers have turned to simpler techniques that provide more limited information. The simplest example of this is measurement of the transit time of the contrast material during cerebral angiography.[47] Broadly speaking, the only significant finding to outcome in patients with severe head injury is the observation of severe slowing of the cerebral circulation.

An intravenous isotope technique was developed by Oldendorf and Kitano in which the mode transit time of the isotope was calculated by differentiating the cranial curve of radioactivity detected following intravenous injection of a nondiffusible tracer.[96] Differentiation of head curve produces a value that represents the time in seconds between the most rapid increase of activity coming into the head and the most rapid decrease of activity leaving the head. This then is the mode transit time and is different from the mean transit time, which would be a true parameter of cerebral blood flow. Essentially, such transit time measurements are measurements of velocity only and not of volume flow. Rowan and his colleagues assessed such transit time measurements in humans and experimental animals and concluded that long transit times do correlate fairly closely with reduced cerebral blood flow.[122] As blood flow increases, however, the decrease in the transit time is not a linear function of increasing flow, since the relationship between volume and velocity flow is a curve of the form $Y = X^2$.

In practical terms the problem with such transit time measurements lies in the wide variability of normal measurements. Although it may be possible to discern a significant difference between the mean values for transit time between a group of normal volunteers and a group of patients with severe head injury, the standard deviation for the normal group is so wide that it is difficult to decide whether or not a moderately increased transient time is within the normal range.[101,121] It has been claimed that sequential measurements in the same patient with the patient acting as his own control provide more reliable information concerning changes in the cerebral circulation.

Little information is available from normal volunteers as to the variability of these measurements over time, however. Until such information becomes available, measurements of cerebral transit time by means of nondiffusible indicators in patients with severe head injury must be regarded as limited in value.

Electroencephalography and Evoked Potentials

The Electroencephalogram

Electroencephalographic data have not proved to be particularly useful in helping predict the outcome after a head injury with regard to survival, degree of recovery, or even persistence of focal neurological deficit. It is common practice in some clinical units to obtain a single electroencephalogram in the early period following head injury. One record adds little prognostic information and fails to detect late changes that may occur after the single study has been done. If serial studies are not obtained, intracranial hemorrhage, for example, accumulating some days following the initial one will not be recognized and will, thus, bias assessments of the electroencephalogram's prognostic value. But, even taking into account both data skewed owing to secondary insults and data from carefully done serial studies in head injury, the electroencephalogram remains of limited value in head injury prognosis.

Electroencephalogram Parallels Clinical Severity

In head injury the degree of electrical abnormality uncovered by serial electroencephalographic studies commonly parallels the severity of the patient's clinical course.[6,26,107] Thus, severe depression of amplitudes and generalized slowing of frequencies below 4 Hz indicate, in most cases, a worse prognosis than normal- to high-amplitude records with frequencies above 4 Hz (Fig. 60–4A).[69,160] Significant exceptions exist that make attempts to correlate wave amplitude and frequency with post-traumatic clinical condition unsatisfactory.

Studies by Dow and co-workers on electroencephalograms recorded immediately following mild head injury indicated that abnormalities related to central nervous system trauma may disappear within 30 minutes of injury.[30] A normal electroencephalogram, therefore, may fail to alert the physician to the occurrence of the brain trauma and the possibility of post-traumatic sequelae. Dow also observed that records taken immediately following mild head injury were less reliable than clinical judgement in predicting time loss from work. Individuals who have sustained mild head injuries may have abnormal records in spite of being asymptomatic.[6,107] The abnormalities may have predated the mild trauma, or the electroencephalogram may suggest a greater degree of brain dysfunction than is, in fact, present.[134] The opposite result, a "normal" electroencephalogram in the face of rather severe clinical symptoms, is also possible. So-called "alpha coma," which occurs with pontomesencephalic tegmental injury, is characterized by a "normal" record while the patient's condition and prognosis are grave.[19,76,159]

Electroencephalographic Changes Lag Behind Clinical Changes

It has been noted by many investigators that changes in post-traumatic electroencephalograms often lag behind clinical improvement or deterioration of the patient, and it is difficult to determine the patient's progress from the electroencephalographic data.[6,26,107,117] Conversely, generalized slowing, even into the delta range, may persist days after a patient has made a significant clinical recovery.[116] Especially noteworthy in traumatized children is the presence of high-amplitude delta frequencies both during the early period following head injury while the patients are comatose and days after they have regained consciousness.[21]

Dissociation of Electroencephalographic and Clinical Findings

Rodin studied the electroencephalograms in acute fatal head injuries and observed no significant difference between the data from patients who died of their injury within 48 hours and the data from those who survived the 48-hour period other than a tendency to have records with lower amplitudes in the fatal cases.[117] General suppression of am-

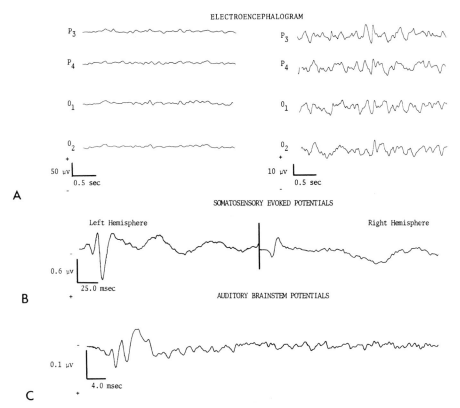

Figure 60–4 Electroencephalogram and evoked potential studies obtained from a 54-year-old man less than 24 hours after head trauma. The patient had a right subdural hematoma that was removed. He did not move the left upper extremity to nociceptive stimulation, and the right upper extremity assumed the decrerebrate position. Death occurred two weeks later. *A*. Suppression of all frequencies (*left*) was seen on the electroencephalogram. The electrical activity (4 to 6 Hz range), apparent at higher amplification (*right*), did not reveal focal or lateralized abnormality. *B*. Somatosensory evoked potentials (right and left median nerve stimulation) recorded over the right parietal lobe demonstrated severe abnormality with loss of electrical activity after 20 msec from time of stimulation. The potential recorded over the left parietal lobe was less abnormal, and electrical activity could be seen as long as 250 msec after stimulation. These data agreed with the clinically apparent left hemiparesis. *C*. Auditory brain stem potentials were abnormal, indicating probable brain stem dysfunction as well as more rostral cerebral dysfunction.

plitude was noted by Dawson to have a fatal prognosis if it appeared within 30 hours of injury (see Fig. 60–4*A*).[26] Widespread suppression of the electroencephalogram secondary to acute barbiturate ingestion should be carefully ruled out before interpreting low amplitude or isoelectric records.[6,69,73]

In nearly half of patients with severe brain damage following head trauma the electroencephalogram can appear normal within the first six months after injury.[83,158] If it becomes normal before the clinical condition has improved, this may indicate a poor prognosis for recovery, as the patient's overall clinical condition may have peaked.[105] It would appear that the electroencephalogram is most likely to return to normal within the first three months following injury, and after six months it stabilizes and exhibits little further change even years later (Fig. 60–5).[116,134,158]

Focal Neurological Deficits and the Electroencephalogram

Predicting the persisting focal neurological deficits by use of electroencephalographic data has proved difficult both with data collected early and with data collected in the later post-traumatic stage. Patients with lateralized lesions such as cerebral contusion who manifest permanent hemiplegia often have diffusely rather than focally abnormal records in the early period following head trauma and normal records six months later despite a residual neurological deficit. Walker and Jablon found

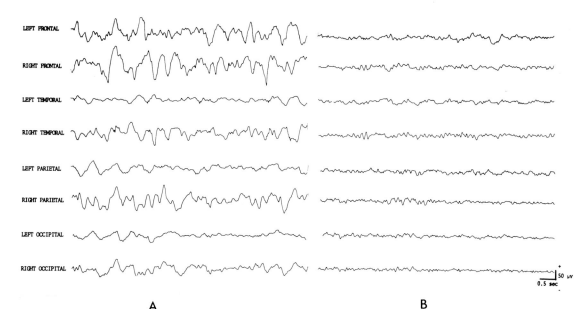

Figure 60–5   The patient had a severe contusion of the left hemisphere as well as a left acute subdural hematoma that was operatively removed. *A.* The electroencephalogram four days following trauma indicated left temporal, parietal, and occipital suppression of amplitudes. A dense right hemiparesis was present at the time of this study. *B.* Approximately two and a half months later the electroencephalogram no longer manifested lateralized or focal suppression, yet the right hemiparesis persisted.

that 50 per cent of patients with hemiplegia or hemiparesis caused by head trauma had normal electroencephalograms in follow-up studies. They also noted that only 43 per cent of soldiers with penetrating head injuries had abnormal records in the same follow-up period.[158] Meyer-Mickeleit, on the other hand, stated that in cases of cerebral contusion accompanied by focal neurological signs, diffuse electroencephalographic abnormalities disappeared in six months while focal alterations persisted for two years (25 per cent) or more (five years in 15 per cent of cases).[85]

Significance of Electroencephalographic Suppression

Suppression of electroencephalographic wave amplitude is widely regarded as an indication of a surface hematoma. Illustrated in Figure 60–5 are the records of a patient who at the time of operation was noted to have severe contusion of the left hemisphere as well as an acute subdural hematoma. The patient's electroencephalogram four days following evacuation of the hematoma still indicated suppression of amplitude in the left temporal (T_3), parietal (P_3), and occipital (O_1) regions. He was hemi-

paretic on the right side at this time. Eighty-one days after the injury, his record no longer manifested lateralized suppression, yet his hemiparesis was unchanged. Focal suppression of electroencephalographic amplitude has been described by Dawson and co-workers as occurring without frequency slowing in 75 per cent of cases. The remaining 25 per cent of cases had both suppression and frequency slowing. Focal suppression appeared early in Dawson's series, in the majority of cases within the first 48 hours, and cleared in adults before or by the time of clinical recovery. In children he observed the persistence of focal slowing as long as four months after clinical recovery.[26]

Significance of Focal Delta Activity

Localized cortical lesions can also be manifested by slowing of electroencephalographic frequencies accompanied by normal to high wave amplitudes. Williams reported that while abnormal focal discharges could be found to correlate with clinical symptoms, it was also quite common to observe abnormal focal electroencephalographic patterns without corresponding clinical findings and focal clinical symptoms with normal electroencephalograms.[160] Both Dawson's group and Rodin and associates reported delta foci in head injury that shifted location within and across hemispheres.[26,117] They concluded that there was no general rule for the behavior of delta foci and that they were of little clinical importance in head injury.

Post-Traumatic Epilepsy and the Electroencephalogram

There is a degree of correlation between the extent and severity of brain damage and the nature, persistence, and degree of electroencephalographic abnormality at varying times after head injury. For example, duration of post-traumatic amnesia, presence of dural tearing, depressed skull fractures, intracerebral hematoma, and missile injury (as contrasted with blunt injury) are associated with a higher percentage of electroencephalographic abnormalities.[158,160] These factors are also associated with an increased incidence of post-traumatic seizures. Thus, the likelihood exists of spurious correlations between electroencephalographic abnormalities (particularly focal changes) and the occurrence of post-traumatic epilepsy.[60,83] Even allowing for this possibility, a poor association exists between electroencephalographic patterns and clinical observations in patients who develop post-traumatic epilepsy. Whether the electroencephalogram is recorded in the initial six months following trauma or more than five years later, it can be normal in half the patients who develop epilepsy.[23,83] Furthermore, the presence of an abnormal electroencephalogram does not increase the chances of developing epilepsy.[83] Factors that might bear on this disparity between electroencephalographic patterns and epilepsy include the failure to attempt activation with hyperventilation or drugs, the location of the seizure focus on basal cerebral cortex (i.e., subtemporal), and the as yet unknown suppressing mechanism that inhibits an epileptogenic focus in the brain from initiating a clinically detectable seizure.[6,83,85,116,134]

Though a change in the pattern after head injury from slow wave to focal spike activity was associated in some cases with development of post-traumatic epilepsy, Courjon found that 25 per cent of 100 patients who developed epilepsy had normal records at the time.[23] In a study of 772 patients, Jennett found no difference in the incidence of diffuse or focal electroencephalographic abnormalities between those patients who did and those who did not develop post-traumatic epilepsy. Many patients with persisting abnormalities (especially after depressed skull fracture) never developed epilepsy, and even some who developed local spike activity did not have seizures. Conversely, some of those patients who developed post-traumatic epilepsy had normal records that became abnormal only after the post-traumatic seizures had become established. Jennett has concluded that the electroencephalogram as routinely used did not contribute materially to the prediction of post-traumatic epilepsy in individual patients.[60]

Multimodality Evoked Potentials

Evoked potential data can be correlated with the patient's prognosis perhaps more closely than it can with the diagnosis.[42,44] By utilizing a functional grading system, as described in Chapter 58, to analyze abnormal evoked potential data, encouraging results have been obtained associating the data recorded in the first few days following head injury with the patient's neurological condition at different times following injury.[45] Whether used to evaluate single neural pathways or areas of brain traversed by many neural systems, Greenberg and associates noted severe evoked potential abnormalities (grade III or IV) correlated well with residual or permanent neuronal dysfunction, while mild evoked potential abnormalities (grade I or II) bespoke eventual functional recovery.[45,46] It is possible, in certain instances, to predict in the first few days following trauma while the patient may still be in coma the chance of functional recovery of specific areas of compromised brain.[45]

Focal Neurological Deficits and Evoked Potentials

Severe depression or absence of an evoked potential of any modality (visual, auditory, or somatosensory) recorded early after head injury indicates permanent dysfunction of the specific neural system tested.[45] Moreover, correlations of evoked potential data with intraoperative and autopsy findings demonstrate that severely abnormal evoked potentials are usually obtained only in the most profoundly injured brains (Fig. 60–6).[45,132,159] Mild to moderate evoked potential abnormalities predict functional recovery, assuming the absence of secondary insults (Fig. 60–7B).[45] The capacity for early evoked potential studies to forecast persisting focal deficits has been shown by the authors to apply to visual (persisting blindness), to auditory (persisting deafness), and to somotosensory (persisting hemiplegia) evoked potentials.

The capacity of evoked potential data to forecast functional recovery of a neural system, even when the data are recorded in the first week following trauma and functional recovery takes place months later, may be related to the number of compromised neurons, their location, or the re-

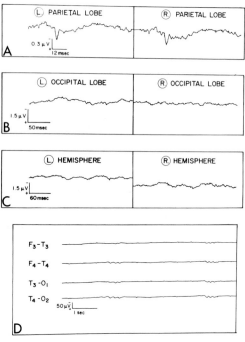

Figure 60–6 Tonsillar herniation and brain death. This multimodality evoked potential study was obtained on day 1 postinjury from an areflexic, flaccid patient who also had an isoelectric electroencephalogram. Somatosensory response, *A*; visual response, *B*; and auditory response, *C*, were all severely abnormal (grade IV), indicating little probability of functional recovery. *D*. The potentials detected in the electroencephalogram represent respirator artifact. The patient subsequently died. (From Greenberg, R. P., et al.: Evaluation of brain function in severe human head trauma with multimodality evoked potentials. J. Neurosurg., 47: 150–177, 1977. Reprinted by permission.)

versibility of cellular dysfunction. It would appear that evoked potential waveforms become profoundly altered only when the neuronal substrate has been irreversibly damaged. Milder evoked potential abnormalities result perhaps from neurons with reversible dysfunction or from areas of injury that are small and whose function can be assumed by surrounding undamaged cells.[4,84] The somatosensory evoked potential data in Figure 60–7A were recorded from a patient whose left hemisphere, especially the parietal and frontal lobes, was severely contused, as confirmed by intraoperative diagnosis. The somatosensory evoked potential recorded from scalp overlying the left parietal lobe had not regained its normal appearance almost four months after the head injury. The patient's right hemiplegia persisted and was unchanged 18 months later. Even with the patient comatose, it was possible on the fourth day after the head injury, when the first evoked potential study was done, to predict that there would be a permanent neurological motor deficit.

Coma and Multimodality Evoked Potentials

The duration of coma following head trauma has been more closely related to multimodality evoked potentials such as visual, somatosensory, and auditory ones than to one modality alone. With multimodality evoked potentials, more extensive areas of brain can be sampled than with the single one.[46] At least 80 per cent of patients with head injury who were comatose and from whom mildly abnormal visual, somatosensory, and auditory evoked potentials of grade I or II were obtained within the first week after injury (mean day 3) became responsive within 30 days of their injury. Those patients whose multimodality evoked potential study was mildly abnormal and who did not regain consciousness within 30 days usually were over 55 years old. According to the multimodality evoked potential data, the duration of coma following head injury was dependent on bilateral cerebral hemispheric dysfunction rather than brain stem dysfunction (Table 60–12).[45]

The oft-repeated assertion that patients who have prolonged coma following head injury yet do not have an intracranial mass

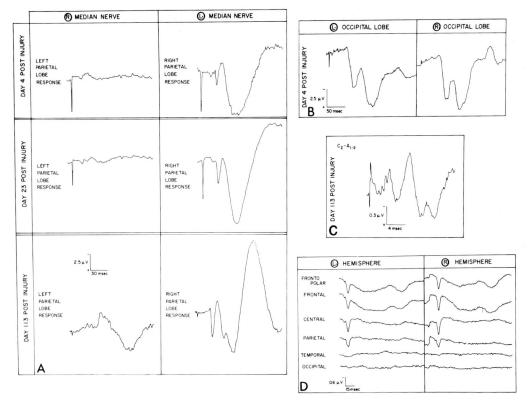

Figure 60–7 Left parietal lobe lesion. Postoperative multimodality evoked potential study from a patient who had had a generous left frontal lobectomy and in whom a severe left parietal lobe contusion was diagnosed intraoperatively. *A*. Serial somatosensory evoked potential study recorded from scalp overlying left parietal lobe on days 4, 23, and 113 postinjury. There was little recovery of normal somatosensory evoked potential waveform from the left parietal lobe, and the patient's dense right hemiparesis did not resolve. The right parietal lobe response was mildly abnormal on day 4 and recovered by day 113. The patient never demonstrated left hemiparesis. *B*. This moderately abnormal visual evoked potential correctly predicted full functional visual recovery even though it was obtained only 4 days after trauma while the patient was still comatose. *C*. The patient's auditory far-field potentials and middle latency auditory near-field potentials were normal. *D*. A topographical study following right median nerve stimulation shows absence of a somatosensory evoked response anywhere on the scalp. (From Greenberg, R. P., et al.: Evaluation of brain function in severe human head trauma with multimodality evoked potentials. *J. Neurosurg.*, *47*: 150–177, 1977. Reprinted by permission.)

lesion are suffering from primary brain stem damage has been challenged by Strich, by Oppenheimer, and more recently by Mitchell and Adams.[1,90,97,135,136] The latter authors were unable to identify isolated brain stem damage at autopsy in 18 patients in whom histological evidence of increased intracranial pressure was absent. They suggest, moreover, that ". . . the principal reason for the difficulty in defining primary localized brain stem damage due to blunt head injury is that it does not exist as a pathological entity." The so-called clinical syndrome of primary brain stem damage ". . . may equally easily result from a lesion above the brain stem. . . ."[90] The evoked potential data discussed in this section show a high degree of correlation

between prolonged coma and hemispheric dysfunction rather than brain stem dysfunction, and may well be an in vivo physiological confirmation of this aspect of the pathology of head injury.

Evoked Potentials and Final Outcome

Multimodality evoked potentials recorded early (mean day 3) and later (mean day 14) in the hospital course of patients with head injury have been correlated with the patients' final outcome.[44–46] Outcome categories were divided into two groups: good recovery and moderate disability in one group, and severe disability, vegetative survival, and death in the other group.[57] In

TABLE 60–12 CORRELATION OF MULTIMODALITY EVOKED POTENTIALS WITH DURATION OF COMA*

DURATION OF COMA (DAYS)	Visual $I–II^a$	Visual $III–IV$	Somatosensory $I–II$	Somatosensory $III–IV$	Auditory $I–II$	Auditory $III–IV$	Brain Stem $I–II$	Brain Stem $III–IV$	NUMBER OF PATIENTS
1–7	9	3	11	1	10	2	10	2	12
8–30	13	4	15	2	14	3	13	4	17
30	5	9	4	10	6	8	9	5	14
Totals	27	16	30	13	30	13	32	11	43
	$(P < .05)^b$		$(P < .005)$		$(P < .05)$		$(P > .25)$		

[a] Injury potential grade determined by best response.
[b] Based on X^2 test of association.

* Data were obtained in 43 patients with severe head injury. Mean study was performed on day 3. All patients were unresponsive when study was done. Patients who subsequently died were not included. (From Greenberg, R. P., Becker, D. P., Miller, J. D., and Mayer, D. J.: Evaluation of brain function in severe human head trauma with multimodality evoked potentials: Part II. Localization of brain dysfunction and correlation with post-traumatic neurological conditions. J. Neurosurg., 47:163–177, 1977. Reprinted by permission.)

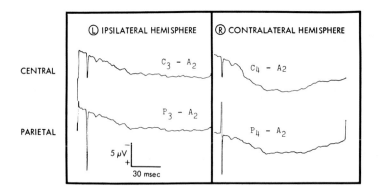

Figure 60–8 Representative somatosensory evoked potential obtained on left median nerve stimulation three days after head injury. The severely abnormal waveform (grade IV) correctly predicted the patient's poor final outcome.

TABLE 60–13 CORRELATION OF MULTIMODALITY EVOKED POTENTIALS AND OUTCOME*

STUDY AND OUTCOME CATEGORY	Visual $I–II^a$	Visual $III–IV$	Somatosensory $I–II$	Somatosensory $III–IV$	Auditory $I–II$	Auditory $III–IV$	Brain Stem $I–II$	Brain Stem $III–IV$	NUMBER OF PATIENTS
Initial (mean day 3)									
Good recovery or moderate disability	21	13	28	6	24	10	27	7	34
Severe disability, vegetative, or dead	8	9	3	14	9	8	11	6	17
Totals	29	22	31	20	33	18	38	13	51
	$(P > .10)^b$		$(P < .01)$		$(P > .10)$		$(P > .10)$		
Serial (mean day 14)									
Good recovery or moderate disability	22	9	28	3	22	9	27	4	31
Severe disability, vegetative, or dead	8	6	1	13	6	8	6	8	14
Totals	30	15	29	16	28	17	33	12	45
	$(P > .10)^b$		$(P < .001)$		$(P > .10)$		$(P < .05)$		

[a] Injury potential grade determined by best response.
[b] Based on Fisher's exact test for 2 × 2 table.

* Relationship between outcome and multimodality evoked potentials was studied early and later following severe head injury. (From Greenberg, R. P., Becker, D. P., Miller, J. D., and Mayer, D. J.: Evaluation of brain function in severe human head trauma with multimodality evoked potentials: Part II. Location of brain dysfunction and correlation with post-traumatic neurological conditions. J. Neurosurg., 47:163–177. Reprinted by permission.)

the early period studied, only the somatosensory evoked potential could be clearly associated with the patients' final outcome three months or more after the trauma (Fig. 60-8 and Table 60–13). By the second time period, abnormal auditory far-field (brain stem) as well as somatosensory evoked potentials were significantly related to a poor outcome (Fig. 60–9 and Table 60–13).

If somatosensory evoked potentials performed in the first week following trauma were only mildly abnormal (grade I or II), 90 percent of patients could be expected to have a good recovery or to be only moderately disabled, assuming no secondary insult occurred after the first week. Therefore, graded somatosensory evoked potentials appear to be promising prognostic tools for evaluating outcome within a few days of head injury.

THE QUALITY OF SURVIVAL FROM HEAD INJURY

Just as a glass may be viewed as half full by the optimist and half empty by the pessimist, the same series of patients with head injury may be viewed in entirely different ways by different people. Miller and Stern commented on the surprisingly good recovery made by a group of patients who had sustained severe head injuries.[89] Fahy and his colleagues, discussing another but similar series of patients, emphasized the frequency of permanent neurological sequelae.[34]

The more rigorously patients are scrutinized and tested following head injury, the more frequent and subtle the deficits that are disclosed. Documentation of such deficits must always be coupled with an assessment of how disabling they will be to the individual patient. Mild dysphasia or minor hemiparesis may have vastly different consequences for the unskilled manual worker than for the university lecturer, the skilled manual worker, or the musician.

Merely to categorize or classify the deficits that may follow head injury is difficult. It is important to attempt the classification, however, as programs of rehabilitation are without meaning unless it is clear what the deficits are, what is being treated, and whether there is improvement.[7,27,91] One group of deficits may be classed as neuro-

physical problems, which include neurological deficits and nonneurological handicaps. Dysphasia is a neurological deficit but introduces other difficulties related to the next category of problems, which can be classified as mental. The mental changes include alterations in cognitive function and memory, and frankly abnormal mental symptoms that may shade into psychoses. The third category of post-traumatic problems are social in nature. These social problems may be personality disorders that can be attributed to mental changes and manifested as changes in work performance, leisure pursuits, family cohesion, sexual behavior, abuse of alcohol, and decreased sociability.[8]

The nature of post-traumatic problems depends on many factors other than the type and location of the brain damage incurred in the trauma and its sequelae. The preinjury status of the brain, the personality of the patient and the family, and the employment and home milieu are important also. The location, severity, and extent of brain injury is the most important factor. In this regard an important point must be made before proceeding further. Many of the outstanding contributions to the literature on psychological disturbances following head injury have been based on study of focal brain lesions—missile wounds, depressed skull fractures. Such injuries have the obvious attraction for the psychologist that the area of brain damage is known and can be correlated with tests of function thought to be specific for that part of the brain.[92,130,150,151] Caution should be exercised before extrapolating results of testing in these patients to patients who have suffered blunt head injury with loss of consciousness and diffuse brain damage. Clearly this subject is a difficult one, and the discussion that follows only highlights important factors that contribute to disability in the patient who has survived a head injury.

Neurological Deficits

Dysphasia

Whether predominantly motor, sensory, or mixed, dysphasia is a serious handicap for the patient who may have made an otherwise good recovery from his head injury. Apart from the obvious difficulty in com-

AUDITORY BRAINSTEM POTENTIALS

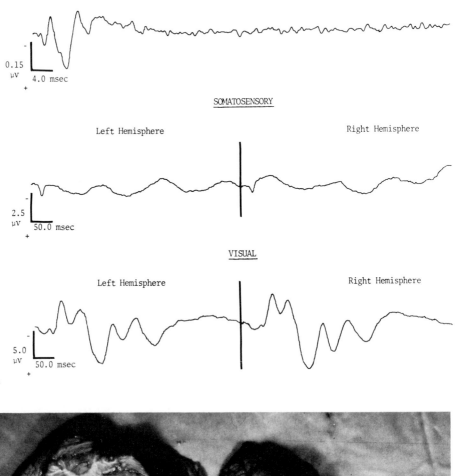

0.15
μV
−
4.0 msec
+

SOMATOSENSORY

Left Hemisphere   Right Hemisphere

2.5
μV
−
50.0 msec
+

VISUAL

Left Hemisphere   Right Hemisphere

5.0
μV
−
50.0 msec
+

A

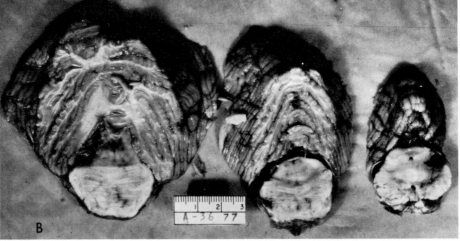

B

Figure 60–9 *A*. Multimodality evoked potential study recorded two weeks following head injury in the patient whose early somatosensory evoked potential study was shown in Figure 60–8. At two weeks, abnormal somatosensory potentials persisted. Auditory brain stem potentials were highly abnormal also, but the visual response was normal, indicating that the abnormal somatosensory evoked potential was due to severe brain stem dysfunction. *B*. The patient died three weeks after injury. Postmortem examination revealed extensive brain stem hemorrhages, especially in the inferior collicular tegmental area.

munication, it is a frequent source of frustration and may provoke antisocial behavior. The problem is a common one, particularly with severe blunt head injuries. Levin and his colleagues noted dysphasia in 50 per cent of patients who were unconscious on admission to the neurosurgical unit. All the patients who had dysphasia had been in coma for more than 24 hours.[74] Thus, the frequency of dysphasia was significantly related to duration of coma. It was also related to the presence of signs of brain stem dysfunction such as abnormal eye movements.

This last finding is interesting because it suggests that brain stem dysfunction may have a relationship with dysphasia, which in the past has been thought to be a cerebral hemisphere deficit. If, however, one considers that any patient with a blunt head injury who has signs of brain stem dysfunction will also have widespread hemisphere damage including frontal and temporal lobe involvement, then the correlation becomes clearer. A final word of caution in assessing aphasia is the observation by the Sarnos that there may not be a good correlation between test performance and the ability of the patient to function in everyday life.[127,128]

Anosmia

This neurological deficit is commonly ignored by the examining physician and, surprisingly, is something of which few patients spontaneously complain. The impact of anosmia on the quality of life is considerable, however, for not only is the sense of smell absent but the subtleties of taste sensation are absent also. A most eloquent description of the problem of anosmia is to be found in the small book on head injury management by John Potter.[109]

Anosmia occurs in 5 to 10 per cent of patients with head injuries and is thought to be due to the avulsion of olfactory filaments following frontal or occipital impact injury. Sumner found that most cases of post-traumatic anosmia followed blunt head injuries. If post-traumatic amnesia was longer than 24 hours, the incidence rose to 30 per cent.[138] When the patient has bilateral periorbital hematoma indicative of an anterior cranial fossa fracture, the incidence of anosmia is even higher. Anosmia is permanent in more than half the patients in whom it is found.

Visual Problems

Following head injury, visual problems may be extremely troublesome. These may take the form of blindness or abnormal visual patterns due to optic nerve damage, which progresses to atrophy. The optic nerve is most often damaged in the optic canal as an extension of bony injury. Therefore, its occurrence is not an index of the severity of brain damage. It is important to detect this deficit early in order to warn the patient and family of the likelihood of impaired vision, since useful recovery of vision occurs in so few cases. Visual field deficits after temporal lobe injury are common and may not be appreciated by the patient. Thus, patients who have recovered from head injuries and resumed driving their automobiles may be involved in a series of unexplained minor accidents before the true nature of the problem is revealed by testing the visual fields. Eye movement disorders due to brain stem or peripheral cranial nerve lesions may cause considerable problems, particularly during the recovery phase before true fusion of the images or suppression of one image is obtained.

Facial Weakness

Whether due to upper motor neuron lesions associated with temporal lobe injury or to facial nerve damage caused by petrous fractures, weakness of facial muscles usually recovers, especially if the facial palsy is of delayed onset. These deficits in any case present mainly a cosmetic and body image problem for the patient.

Deafness

Conductive deafness is usually due to damage to the tympanic membrane or bleeding in the auditory canal. This has a much better prospect for recovery than nerve deafness in which restoration of hearing virtually never occurs. Dizziness and vertigo due to associated labyrinthine damage may occur when the injury has disrupted the inner ear and its connections, but these symptoms usually subside after some weeks or months. Milder degrees of injury may be responsible for some of the symptoms of the post-concussional syndrome. Thus 30 per cent of patients who complain of dizziness following head injury have been shown by electronystagmographic recording to have a peripheral labyrinthine dysfunction.[17]

Dysarthria

Dysarthria may be a prominent feature during the recovery phase from serious head injury, particularly in young people who have during the acute phase after injury exhibited intense decerebrate spasms and other forms of abnormal motor posturing. Not infrequently these same patients will exhibit spontaneous *abnormal movements* of an athetoid nature even progressing in rare cases to ballistic types of movement disorder. As a rule such abnormalities are temporary, although they may last several weeks or even months. By contrast, frank signs of cerebellar dysfunction are rare following head injury. Presumably, this is accounted for by the relatively protected nature of the cerebellum and the nature of the movement disorders, which are more suggestive of basal ganglia dysfunction.

Hemiplegia

By far the best-understood neurological deficit following head injury, hemiplegia is probably the single deficit best compensated for by the patient and his family. Patients with hemisensory deficits fare less well in this regard. Minor degrees of dysfunction in the form of apraxia or weakness of the hand that appears only on fatigue are very common after head injury and may not be remarked upon by the patient or the examining physician. Finger tapping tests are aimed at eliciting such minor degrees of dysfunction.

Recovery from Deficits

In assessing the final outcome from head injury, a frequent problem is deciding when objective recovery has ceased. It is commonly stated that improvement may proceed for two or three years following an injury. Such studies as are available, however, would suggest that patients with severe head injuries have achieved virtually all objectively discernible neurological improvement by the end of the first year. In terms of the five broad categories of outcome, more than 90 per cent of recovery has occurred by six months.[7,65] It is possible, however, particularly for the less

severely injured, for patients to continue making functional improvement for longer periods of time as they learn to compensate for their physical disabilities.[28,71] Therefore, it is of the greatest importance for the doctor, the patient, and the family to be aware of the neurological deficits that have followed the injury so that a realistic approach can enable the patient to cope with them.

Post-Traumatic Epilepsy

This neurological complication of head injury presents a special problem, since many of the victims are considered to have made a good recovery from injury at the time of appearance of post-traumatic seizures. The significance of the seizures may not be appreciated, and information concerning their occurrence may never be known by the doctor who initially treated the patient for his head injury. Thus their true incidence may be underestimated.

The most extensive study of post-traumatic epilepsy in blunt head injuries has been made by Jennett and Lewin.[65,66] These investigators made a plea, for which they presented a very convincing case, that epileptic seizures occurring in the first week after injury should be regarded as a separate and different entity from seizures that start later. Most of the later seizures occur three months or more from the time of injury. The reasons for considering the two forms of seizures as separate are that risk factors for each are different and that the nature of the seizures is different. Temporal lobe attacks are rare in the first week after injury and common as manifestations of late post-traumatic epilepsy. The significance of early epilepsy is that it increases the risk of developing late post-traumatic epilepsy, which tends to persist. Other factors that increase the risk of late epilepsy are summarized in Table 60–14. In brief, these factors are missile wounds of the head with dural penetration; intracranial hematomas, whether epidural, subdural, or intracerebral; infection; and depressed skull fractures associated with dural tearing and prolonged post-traumatic amnesia.[18,61]

The significance of post-traumatic epilepsy in adversely affecting the outcome from head injury should not be underestimated. Hypoxia, cerebrovasodilatation,

TABLE 60–14 FACTORS THAT RAISE RISK OF EPILEPSY IN FOUR YEARS FOLLOWING HEAD INJURY TO MORE THAN 25 PER CENT

PRIMARY FACTORS (Only 1 Required)	SECONDARY FACTORS (Combination of Any 2 Required)
Penetrating missile injury	Depressed skull fracture
Intracranial hematoma	Dural penetration
Early epilepsy (in first week)	
	Intracranial infection
	Focal neurological signs
	Post-traumatic amnesia longer than 24 hours

and raised intracranial pressure that occur as a result of the seizure may be devastating in patients who have already suffered a critical amount of brain damage.

The Postconcussional Syndrome

The postconcussional syndrome may be defined as a symptom complex that follows minor head injury and consists of headache, dizziness, and nervous instability. In the 40 or so years that the syndrome has been recognized controversy has persisted concerning the relative contributions to the syndrome of genuine organic disturbances, of preinjury psychological abnormalities, of the effects of litigation, and of frank malingering. Because of the recognized association between mild injuries and prolonged complaints, Miller in particular opted strongly for a nonorganic basis for the syndrome.[88] Others have claimed that there is sound pathophysiological evidence to support an organic basis for the syndrome, consisting of the known cellular alterations seen in the concussed brain, abnormalities of the blood-brain barrier and cerebral circulation time, and a high incidence of positional nystagmus.[141] Cartlidge followed up 372 survivors of head injury and was able to identify two groups of patients in terms of their complaints of post-traumatic headache and dizziness, which were present in approximately 25 and 20 per cent of patients respectively at long-term follow-up.[17] Broadly speaking, it was found that one group of patients who were already complaining of headache and dizziness at the time of discharge from hospital improved progressively, the majority returning to normal by two years from injury. These pa-

tients showed a high incidence of positional nystagmus. The second group of patients developed their symptoms only after discharge from hospital. They had a much lower incidence of nystagmus, and a much higher proportion of these patients made legal claims for compensation and had symptoms of depression. In this second group there was a much greater tendency for the symptoms to persist for indefinite periods of time. It was proposed that in the former group organic factors played a predominant causative role in the postconcussional syndrome and in the latter, psychological factors were pre-eminent.

Psychological Deficits and Mental Symptoms

Prolonged Confusion and Post-Traumatic Amnesia

During recovery, patients with head injury will pass through a phase of disorientation for person, place, or time and may remain in this confused state for a rather prolonged period in some cases. Upon further recovery they have no recollection of the events that occurred during their period of post-traumatic confusion. The time span between injury and the recovery of continuous memory is defined as the period of post-traumatic amnesia. This was discussed earlier. When patients are in a confused state it can be confidently asserted that they are still within their period of post-traumatic amnesia. It is important that this judgment be made because the duration of post-traumatic amnesia is at present one of the most important correlates with the extent and severity of psychological as well as physical deficits following injury. There are obvious difficulties in making psychological measurements within the period of post-traumatic confusion.[81] There is a close association between the duration of post-traumatic amnesia and many aspects of the sequelae of head injuries, such as the incidence of post-traumatic epilepsy and psychological sequelae, and the length of time before the patient returns to work.

Intellectual Deficit

Although it is commonly stated that some patients suffer marked intellectual impairment as a result of severe or even moderate head injuries, this statement requires closer analysis.[123,124,152] Subsequent testing of such patients will often reveal that some aspects of previous intellectual capacity remain unimpaired, for example, the size of the vocabulary. Factors that lead to impairment of intellectual function following injury relate to disorders of recent memory and disorders of attention or concentration.[11,12,72,82,161] Many patients suffer from problems related to communication with others. Examples are minor degrees of dysphasia, dyslexia, dysgraphia, or disorders or pattern recognition. Thus the patient may not be able to comprehend fully the tests that are given to him. There is, however, a significant correlation between post-traumatic amnesia and poor performance on the Wechsler Memory Scale and the Performance IQ on the Wechsler Adult Intelligence Scale.[11,12,82]

Serial testing of patients following severe head injury reveals that after they emerge from post-traumatic amnesia, the maximum improvement as measured by psychological tests occurs during the first six months following injury.[82] Some recovery does persist beyond six months, but it is much less by comparison. Patients with lesser degrees of initial damage may show recovery over a prolonged period.[28] As yet, there is no convincing evidence that early intensive rehabilitation of these patients will speed this intellectual recovery or advance it beyond its current stage.[7,8]

Disorders of Behavior

The other main group of nonneurological disorders following injury is usually classified as change in personality and behavior. The components of these sequelae are usually impaired emotional control leading to bursts of anger or weeping with depression and inability to persist in any constructive behavior. This type of alteration in the patient's personality is the most difficult for the relatives and close friends of the injured person to accept. As with many of the so-called minor sequelae of head injury, this pattern of disorder may not at first be mentioned by the family, and the patient may suffer from lack of insight so that he is only partially aware of the extent of the problem. The physician should always ask the family about these disorders. In many cases, a simple question will trigger a flood of complaints. This change in the patient's personality is often the principal disappointment that the family may experience after witnessing what initially appeared to be a good recovery from injury. Sometimes the outbursts of anger are sufficiently abrupt to raise suspicions of a form of temporal lobe epilepsy, but this seldom turns out to be the case.

Psychiatric Disorders and Disorders of Social Function

There is an indeterminate point beyond which abnormalities of behavior following head injury can be regarded as evidence of a psychiatric disorder. This change is a particularly common problem in children. Shaffer and his colleagues noted a 62 per cent rate of psychiatric disorder in 98 children who had had a depressed fracture of the skull. Psychiatric disorders were, however, closely related to a variety of psychosocial factors such as broken marriages and parental psychiatric disturbances.[130] In adults, emotional disturbances are also common after injury, though frankly psychotic disturbances are much rarer.[2,29] As in the study of childhood psychiatric disturbances, there is a strong relationship between psychiatric disorders following head injury and preinjury and environmental factors.[75] When such disturbances occur they are much harder for the patient's family and medical advisors to cope with than physical handicaps, and this may account for the greater degree of social disablement that such problems can bring.[7,34,75,130]

In determining the degree and nature of recovery a patient makes from head injury, a further group of disorders must be considered in addition to the neurological and psychological deficits. These disorders may be grouped together under the category of social impairment, although there is no clear separation between them and the previously listed mental sequelae.

Difficulties with emotional control, insight, and ability to persevere with tasks as well as other factors may combine to make a patient ineffective at his work and unable to hold his previous job or to pursue worthwhile leisure activities. The patient may become estranged from his own family and friends and sit for hours in front of the television set, unwilling or unable to initiate any form of spontaneous activity. If he is more active, the pattern of behavior disturbance may predispose to alcohol abuse or even to criminal conduct.

Finally, a common problem in the patient who recovers from a severe head injury is sexual incompetence. This may be coupled with general lack of interest in most activities but can also be due to specific impotence.

It is in this area that expert and sympathetic counseling both for patients and for their families is required early in the recovery phase. This is important if domestic antagonism is not to arise at a time when the patient must lean most heavily for support on those nearest and dearest to him.

Factors Influencing the Quality of Survival

In addition to the type and severity of deficits suffered by the patient, several other important factors interact to determine the final quality of survival or recovery from injury for that particular patient. These factors may be grouped under those relating to the brain injury itself, preinjury factors relevant to the patient, his home circumstances, the nature of his occupation, and whether or not legal claims are under consideration.

Many of the factors relating to brain injury have already been covered in detail, but of particular importance is the differentiation between blunt injury producing diffuse brain damage and penetrating injury that may produce severe but focal neurological deficits. There is still a general lack of understanding of the widespread neural devastation that can follow a blunt injury to the head with no skull fracture but with immediate and prolonged coma. The appearance of brain tissue extending from a penetrating wound of the skull always seems to command more respect. The presence of complicating factors such as infection or hypoxemia, which produce diffuse brain damage in addition to the traumatic lesion, is also clearly important, but the duration of coma and of post-traumatic amnesia are probably the factors of greatest importance for the ultimate outcome of the patient.

Of the factors that relate to the status of the patient prior to his injury the most important are his age, the presence of any pre-existing brain damage or disease, and the general level of his intelligence. It may be noted at this point that in many cases this can be accurately assessed from school or service records. The preinjury personality of the patient and his degree of self-confidence and self-assertion are also important.

Home circumstances may exert a powerful influence on the recovery process from injury once the patient leaves the hospital. The presence of an understanding family who adopt a positive and realistic attitude toward recovery from the injury and who are able to understand the difficulties that the patient faces as he tries to readjust to his previous environment constitutes a strong positive influence. On the most basic level, the economic position of the family is clearly important in terms of the facilities that they may be able to provide for him. Physical recovery may also be influenced by the geographic area where the patient lives and the quality of social services and support that the community can provide.

The preinjury occupation that the patient followed is important in the determination of how easy it is for him to return to his former occupational level. This will be related both to the skills that are required for the work, whether these were predominantly intellectual or manual, and also to the attitude that the patient adopts toward work and the readiness with which colleagues will smooth the way to a return to full activity.

Finally, the matter of pending litigation is of great importance. Most physicians have had the experience of a patient who continues with indefinite complaints for as long as it takes for his legal claim to be settled and then effects a rapid recovery. To be fair, this attitude is virtually imposed upon the patient by his legal advisors for the satisfactory pursuance of his claims. Clearly it is not in the patient's interest to declare spontaneously that the symptoms and signs have completely cleared.

From the foregoing it is apparent that a multiplicity of factors interact to determine the quality of recovery or survival that a patient makes following an injury, be it trivial or severe. The more finely one attempts to analyze the various patterns of recovery, the more one must sacrifice quantitative prognosis as related to the input data gathered at the time of injury. On the other hand, it is important that such efforts continue to be made because the very process of such inquiry continues to shed new light on the mechanisms underlying brain damage and forces a review of the concepts of what constitutes reversible and irreversible damage to the brain and the brain's capacity for recovery and adaptation.

Acknowledgment. This work was supported in part by NIH Grant No. 1 P50 NS 12587.

REFERENCES

1. Adams, J. H., Mitchell, D. E., Graham, D. I., and Doyle, D.: Diffuse brain damage of immediate impact type. Its relationship to "primary brain stem damage" in head injury. Brain, *100*:489–502, 1977.
2. Aita, J. A., and Reitan, R. M.: Psychotic reactions in the late recovery period following brain injury. Amer. J. Psychiat., *105*:161–169, 1948.
3. Andrew, J.: Tracheostomy and management of the unconscious patient. Brit. Med. J., *2*:328–332, 1956.
4. Astrup, J., Symon, L., Branston, N. M., and Lassen, N. A.: Cortical evoked potentials and extracellular K + and H + at critical levels of brain ischemia. Stroke, *8*:52–57, 1977.
5. Becker, D. P., Miller, J. D., Ward, J. D., Greenberg, R. P., Young, H. F., and Sakalas, R.: The outcome from severe head injury with early diagnosis and intensive management. J. Neurosurg., *47*: 491–502, 1977.
6. Bickford, R. G., Klass, D. W.: Acute and chronic EEG findings after head injury. *In* Caveness, W. F., and Walker, A. E., eds.: Head Injury Conference Proceedings. Philadelphia, J. B. Lippincott Co., 1966, pp. 63–88.
7. Bond, M. R.: Assessment of the psychosocial outcome after severe head injury. *In* Outcome of Severe Damage to the Central Nervous System. Ciba Foundation Symposium 34 (new series). Amsterdam, Elsevier Publishing Co., 1975, pp. 141–153.
8. Bond, M. R., and Brooks, D. N.: Understanding the process of recovery as a basis for the investigation of rehabilitation for the brain injured. Scand. J. Rehab. Med., *8*:127–133, 1976.
9. Brackett, C. E.: Respiratory complications of head injury. *In* Head Injuries; Proceedings of an International Symposium. Edinburgh and London, Churchill Livingstone, 1971, pp. 255–265.
10. Brodersen, P., and Jorgensen, E.: Cerebral blood flow and oxygen uptake and cerebrospinal fluid biochemistry in severe coma. J. Neurol. Neurosurg. Psychiat., *37*:384–391, 1974.
11. Brooks, D. N.: Recognition, memory and head injury. J. Neurol. Neurosurg. Psychiat., *37*:794–801, 1974.
12. Brooks, D. N.: Wechsler Memory Scale performance and its relationship to brain damage

13. Brown, W. H., and Plum, F.: The neurologic basis of Cheyne-Stokes respiration. Amer. J. Med., 849–860, 1961.
15. Bruce, D. A., Langfitt, T. W., Miller, J. D., Shutz, H., Vapalahti, M. P., Stanek, A., and Goldberg, H. I.: Regional cerebral blood flow, intracranial pressure and brain metabolism in comatose patients. J. Neurosurg., *38*:131–144, 1973.
14. Bruce, D. A., Schut, L., Bruno, L. A., Wood, J. H., and Sutton, L. N.: Outcome following severe head injuries in children. J. Neurosurg., *48*:679–688, 1978.
16. Carlsson C. A., von Essen, C., and Löfgren, J.: Factors affecting the clinical course of patients with severe head trauma. Part 1: Infuence of biological factors. Part 2: Significance of post-traumatic coma. J. Neurosurg., *29*:242–251, 1968.
17. Cartlidge, N. E. F.: Post-concussional syndrome. Scot. Med. J., *23*:103, 1978.
18. Caveness, W. F.: Onset and cessation of fits following craniocerebral trauma. J. Neurosurg., *20*:570–583, 1963.
19. Chatrian, G., White, L. E., and Shaw, C. M.: EEG pattern resembling wakefulness in unresponsive decerebrate state following traumatic brain stem infarct. Electroenceph. Clin. Neurophysiol., *16*:285–289, 1964.
20. Clark, K., Nash, T. M., and Hutchison, G. C.: The failure of circumferential craniotomy in acute traumatic cerebral swelling. J. Neurosurg., *29*:367–371, 1968.
21. Cook, A. W., Browder, E. J., and Lyons, H. A.: Alterations in acid-base equilibrium in craniocerebral trauma. J. Neurosurg., *18*:366–370, 1961.
22. Cooper, P. R., Rovit, R. L., and Ransohoff, J.: Hemicraniectomy in the treatment of acute subdural hematomas: A re-appraisal. Surg. Neurol., *5*:25–29, 1976.
23. Courjon, J. A.: Post-traumatic epilepsy in electroclinical practice. *In* Walker, A. E., Caveness, W. F., and Critchley, M.: eds.: The Late Effects of Head Injury. Springfield, Ill., Charles C Thomas, 1969, pp. 215–227.
24. Crockard, H. A., and Taylor, A. R.: Serial CSF lactate/pyruvate values as a guide to prognosis in head injury coma. Europ. Neurol., *8*:151–157, 1972.
25. Crockard, H. A., Coppel, D. L., and Morrow, W. F. K.: Evaluation of hyperventilation in treatment of head injuries. Brit. Med. J., *4*:634–640, 1973.
26. Dawson, R. E., Webster, J. E., and Gurdjian, E. S.: Serial electroencephalography in acute head injuries. J. Neurosurg., *8*:613–630, 1951.
27. Denny-Brown, D.: Disability arising from closed head injury. J.A.M.A., *127*:429–436, 1945.
28. Dikmen, S., and Reitan, R. M.: Psychological deficits and recovery of functions after head injury. Trans. Amer. Neurol. Ass., *101*:72–77, 1976.
29. Dikmen, S., and Reitan, R. M.: Emotional sequelae of head injury. Ann. Neurol., *2*:492–494, 1977.
30. Dow, R. S., Ulett, G., and Raaf, J.: Electroen-

cephalographic studies immediately following head injury. Amer. J. Psychiat., *101*:174–183, 1943.

31. Editorial: The best yardstick we have. Lancet, 2:1445–1446, 1961.

32. Enevoldsen, E. M., and Jensen, F. T.: Autoregulation and CO_2 responses of cerebral blood flow in patients with acute severe head injury. J. Neurosurg., *48*:689–703, 1978.

33. Enevoldsen, E. M., Cold, G., Jensen, F. T., and Malmros, R.: Dynamic changes in regional CBF, intraventricular pressure, CSF pH and lactate levels during the acute phase of head injury. J. Neurosurg., *44*:191–214, 1976.

34. Fahy, T. J., Irving, M. A., and Millac, P.: Severe head injuries: A six year follow up. Lancet, 2:476–479, 1967.

35. Fell, D. A., Fitzgerald, S., Moiel, R. H., and Caram, P.: Acute subdural hematomas: Review of 144 cases. J. Neurosurg., *42*:37–42, 1975.

36. Fink, B. R.: Influence of cerebral activity in wakefulness on regulation of breathing. J. Appl. Physiol., *16*:15–20, 1961.

37. Froman, C.: Alterations of respiratory functions in patients with severe head injuries. Brit. J. Anaesth., *40*:354–360, 1968.

38. Frowein, R. A., and Karimi-Nejad, A.: Sauerstoffversorgung des Hirngewebes nach schweren Hirnschädigungen. Acta neurochir. (Wien), *19*:1–31, 1968.

39. Gallagher, J. P., and Browder, E. J.: Extradural hematoma: Experience with 167 patients. J. Neurosurg., *29*:1–12, 1968.

40. Gordon, E.: Some correlations between the clinical outcome and the acid-base status of blood and cerebrospinal fluid in patients with traumatic brain injury. Acta Anaesth. Scand., *15*:209–288, 1971.

41. Gordon, E., and Rossanda, M.: The importance of the cerebrospinal fluid acid-base status in the treatment of unconscious patients with brain lesions. Acta Anaesth. Scand., *12*:57–73, 1968.

42. Greenberg, R. P., and Becker, D. P.: Clinical applications of evoked potential data in severe head injury patients. Surg. Forum, *26*:484–486, 1975.

43. Greenberg, R. P., Mayer, D. J., and Becker, D. P.: Correlation in man of intracranial pressure and neuroelectric activity determined by multimodality evoked potentials. *In* Beks, J. W. F., Bosch, D. A., and Brock, M., eds.: Intracranial Pressure III. Berlin, Springer-Verlag, 1976, pp. 58–62.

44. Greenberg, R. P., Mayer, D. J., and Becker, D. P.: The prognostic value of evoked potentials in human mechanical brain injury. *In* McLaurin, R. L., ed.: Head Injuries: Second Chicago Symposium on Neural Trauma. New York, Grune & Stratton, Inc., 1976, pp. 81–88.

45. Greenberg, R. P., Becker, D. P., Miller, J. D., and Mayer, D. J.: Evaluation of brain function in severe human head trauma with multimodality evoked potentials: Part II. Localization of brain dysfunction and correlation with posttraumatic neurological conditions. J. Neurosurg., *47*:163–177, 1977.

46. Greenberg, R. P., Mayer, D. J., Becker, D. P.,

and Miller, J. D.: Evaluation of brain function in severe human head trauma with multimodality evoked potentials. Part I: Evoked brain injury potentials, methods, analysis. J. Neurosurg., *47*:150–162, 1977.

47. Greitz, T.: Radiologic study of brain circulation by rapid serial angiography of the carotid artery. Acta Radiol., suppl. 140:1–128, 1956.

48. Gutterman, P., and Shenkin, H. A.: Prognostic features in recovery from traumatic decerebration. J. Neurosurg., *32*:330–335, 1970.

49. Harris, P.: Acute traumatic subdural hematomas: Results of neurosurgical care. *In* Head Injuries —Proceedings of an International Symposium. Edinburgh, Churchill-Livingstone, 1971, pp. 321–326.

50. Heiskanen, O., and Sipponen, P.: Prognosis of severe brain injury. Acta Neurol. Scand., *46*:343–348, 1970.

51. Heiss, W. D., Gerstenbrand, F., Prozenz, P., and Krenn, J.: The prognostic value of CBF measurements in patients with the apallic syndrome. J. Neurol. Sci., *16*:373–382, 1972.

52. Hooper, R.: Observations on extradural hemorrhage. Brit. J. Surg., *47*:71–87, 1959.

53. Huang, C. T., Cook, A. W., and Lyons, H. A.: Severe craniocerebral trauma and respiratory abnormalities. Arch. Neurol. (Chicago), 9: 113–122, 1963.

54. Ingvar, D. H.: Cerebral blood flow and metabolism in complete apallic syndromes, in states of severe dementia and in akinetic mutism. Acta Neurol. Scand., *49*:233–244, 1973.

55. Jamieson, K. G., and Yelland, J. D. N.: Extradural hematoma: Report of 167 cases. J. Neurosurg., *29*:13–23, 1968.

56. Jamieson, K. G., and Yelland, J. D. N.: Surgically treated traumatic subdural hematomas. J. Neurosurg., *37*:137–149, 1972.

57. Jennett, B., and Bond, M. R.: Assessment of outcome after severe brain damage. Lancet, *1*:480–484, 1975.

58. Jennett, B., and Plum, F.: Persistent vegetative state after brain damage. Lancet, *1*:734–737, 1972.

59. Jennett, B., and Teasdale, G.: Aspects of coma after severe head injury. Lancet, *1*:878–881, 1977.

60. Jennett, B., and Van der Sande, J.: EEG prediction of post-traumatic epilepsy. Epilepsia, *16*:251–256, 1975.

61. Jennett, B., Miller, J. D., and Braakman, R.: Epilepsy after non-missile depressed skull fracture. J. Neurosurg., *41*:208–216, 1974.

62. Jennett, B., Teasdale, G., Braakman, R., Minderhoud, J., and Knill-Jones, R.: Predicting outcome in individual patients after severe head injury. Lancet, *1*:1031–1034, 1976.

63. Jennett, B., Teasdale, G., Galbraith, S., Pickard, J., Grant, H., Braakman, R., Avezaat, C., Mass, A., Minderhoud, J., Vecht, C. J., Heiden, J., Small, R., Caton, W., and Kurze, T.: Severe head injuries in three countries. J. Neurol. Neurosurg. Psychiat., *40*:291–298, 1977.

64. Jennett, S., Ashbridge, K., and North, J. B.: Post-hyperventilation apnoea in patients with brain damage. J. Neurol. Neurosurg. Psychiat., *37*:288–296, 1974.

65. Jennett, W. B.: Epilepsy After Blunt Head Injuries. 2nd Ed. London, William Heinemann Ltd., 1975.

66. Jennett, W. B., and Lewin, W. S.: Traumatic epilepsy after closed head injuries. J. Neurol. Neurosurg. Psychiat., 23:295–301, 1960.

67. Johnston, I. H., and Jennett, B.: The place of continuous intracranial pressure monitoring in neurosurgical practice. Acta Neurochir., 29:53–63, 1973.

68. Johnston, I. H., Johnston, J. A., and Jennett, W. B.: Intracranial pressures following head injury. Lancet, 2:433–436, 1970.

69. Kiloh, L. G., McComas, A. J., and Osselton, J. W.: Clinical Electroencephalography. London, Butterworth & Co. Ltd., 1972.

70. Kjellberg, R. N., and Prieto, A.: Bifrontal decompressive craniotomy for massive cerebral edema. J. Neurosurg., 34:488–493, 1971.

71. Klonoff, H., Low, M. D., and Clark, C.: Head injuries in children: A prospective five year follow-up. J. Neurol. Neurosurg. Psychiat., 40:1211–1219, 1977.

72. Klove, H., and Cleveland, C. S.: The relationship of neuropsychological impairment to other indices of severity of head injury. Scand. J. Rehab. Med., 4:55–60, 1972.

73. Kooi, K. A.: Fundamentals of Electroencephalography. New York, Harper & Row, 1971.

74. Levin, H. S., Grossman, R. G., and Kelly, P. J.: Aphasic disorder in patients with head injury. J. Neurol. Neurosurg. Psychiat., 39:1062–1070, 1976.

75. Lishman, A.: The psychiatric sequelae of head injury: A review. Psychol. Med., 3:304–318, 1972.

76. Loeb, C., and Poggio, G.: Electroencephalograms in a case with pontomesencephalic hemorrhage. Electroenceph. Clin. Neurophysiol., 5:295–296, 1953.

77. Macewen, W.: The diagnosis of alcoholic coma. Glasgow Med. J., 11:1–14, 1879.

78. MacIver, I. N., Frew, I. J. C., and Matheson, J. G.: The role of respiratory insufficiency in the mortality of severe head injuries. Lancet, 1:390–393, 1958.

79. MacIver, I. N., Lassman, L., Thomson, C. W., and McLeod, I.: Treatment of severe head injuries. Lancet, 2:544–550, 1958.

80. Macpherson, P., and Graham, D. I.: Arterial spasm and slowing of the cerebral circulation in the ischemia of head injury. J. Neurol. Neurosurg. Psychiat., 37:1069–1072, 1974.

81. Mandleberg, I. A.: Cognitive recovery after severe head injury. 2. Wechsler Adult Intelligence Scale during post-traumatic amnesia. J. Neurol. Neurosurg. Psychiat., 38:1127–1132, 1975.

82. Mandleberg, I. A., and Brooks, D. N.: Cognitive recovery after severe head injury. 1. Serial testing on the Wechsler Adult Intelligence Scale. J. Neurol. Neurosurg. Psychiat., 38:1121–1126, 1975.

83. Marshall, C., and Walker, A. E.: The value of electroencephalography in the prognostication and prognosis of post-traumatic epilepsy. Epilepsia, 2:138–143, 1961.

84. Meldrum, B. S., Brierley, J. B.: Brain damage in the Rhesus monkey resulting from profound arterial hypotension. II. Changes in the spontaneous and evoked activity of the neocortex. Brain Res., 13:101–118, 1969.

85. Meyer-Mickeleit, R. W.: Das Elektroencephalogramm nach gedeckten Kopfverletzungen. Deutsch. Med. Wschr., 78:480–484, 1953.

86. Miller, J. D., Sweet, R. C., Narayan, R., and Becker, D. P.: Early insults to the injured brain. J.A.M.A., 240:439–442, 1978.

87. Miller, J. D., Becker, D. P., Ward, J. D., Sullivan, H. G., Adams, W. E., and Rosner, M. J.: Significance of intracranial hypertension in severe head injury. J. neurosurg., 47:503–516, 1977.

88. Miller, H.: Accident neurosis. Brit. Med. J., 1:919–925; 992–998, 1961.

89. Miller, H., and Stern, G.: The long-term prognosis of severe head injury. Lancet, 1:225–229, 1965.

90. Mitchell, D. E., and Adams, J. H.: Primary focal impact damage to the brainstem in blunt head injuries. Does it exist? Lancet, 2:215–218, 1973.

91. Najenson, T., Groswasser, Z., Stern, M., Schechter, I., Davis, D., Bourghans, N., and Mendleson, L.: Prognostic factors in rehabilitation after severe head injury. Scand. J. Rehab. Med., 7:101–105, 1975.

92. Newcombe, F.: Missile Wounds of the Brain. A Study of Psychological Deficits. London, Oxford University Press, 1969.

93. North, J. B., and Jennett, S.: Abnormal breathing patterns associated with acute brain damage. Arch. Neurol. (Chicago), 31:338–344, 1974.

94. North, J. B., and Jennett, S.: Response of ventilation and of intracranial pressure during rebreathing of carbon dioxide in patients with acute brain damage. Brain, 99:169–182, 1976.

95. Obrist, W. D., Langfitt, T. W., terWeeme, C. A., O'Connor, M. J., Gennarelli, T. A., Zimmerman, R. A., and Kuhl, D. E.: Non-invasive, long-term, serial studies of rCBF in acute head injuries. Acta Neurol. Scand., 56:suppl. 64:178–179, 1977.

96. Oldendorf, W. H., and Kitano, M.: Radioisotope measurement of brain blood turnover time as a clinical index of brain circulation. J. Nucl. Med., 8:570–587, 1967.

97. Oppenheimer, D. R.: Microscopic lesions in the brain following head injury. J. Neurol. Neurosurg. Psychiat., 31:299–306, 1968.

98. Overgaard, J., and Tweed, W. A.: Cerebral circulation after head injury. Part I. Cerebral blood flow and its regulation after closed head injury with emphasis on clinical correlations. J. Neurosurg., 41:531–541, 1974.

99. Overgaard, J., Christensen, S., Hvid Jansen, O., Haase, J., Land, A. M., Pederson, K. K., and Tweed, W. A.: Prognosis after head injury based on early clinical examination. Lancet, 2:631–635, 1973.

100. Pagni, C. A.: The prognosis of head injured patients in a state of coma with decerebrated posture. J. Neurosurg. Sci., 17:289–295, 1973.

101. Papo, I., Caruselli, G., Occhipinti, C., and Di Pietrantoni, F.: Prognostic value of cerebral transit time (radiocirculography) in head injury. J. Neurosurg. Sci., 17:208–211, 1973.

102. Pazzaglia, P., Frank, G., Frank, F., and Gaist, G.: Clinical course and prognosis of acute post-traumatic coma. J. Neurol. Neurosurg. Psychiat., *38*:149–154, 1975.

103. Plum, F.: Neural mechanisms of abnormal respiration in humans. Arch. Neurol. (Chicago), *3*:484–487, 1960.

104. Plum, F., and Brown, H. W.: The effect of respiration of central nervous system disease. Ann. N.Y. Acad. Sci., *109*:915–931, 1963.

105. Plum, F., and Posner, J. B.: The Diagnosis of Stupor and Coma. Philadelphia, F. A. Davis Co., 1966.

106. Plum, F., Brown, H. W., and Snoep, E.: Neurologic significance of post-hyperventilation apnea. J.A.M.A., *181*:1050–1055, 1962.

107. Poole, E. W.: Some aspects of electroencephalographic disturbances following head injury. J. Clin. Path. (suppl. Roy. Coll. Path.), *23*:4:187–201, 1970.

108. Poulsen, J., and Zilstorff, K.: Prognostic value of the caloric-vestibular test in the unconscious patient with cranial trauma. Acta Neurol. Scand., *48*:282, 1972.

109. Potter, J. M.: The practical management of head injuries. London, Lloyd-Luke Ltd., 1963, pp. 1–84.

110. Price, D. J. E., and Murray, A.: The influence of hypoxia and hypotension on recovery from head injury. Injury, *3*:218–224, 1972.

111. Ransohoff, J., Vallo, B., Gage, E. J., and Epstein, F.: Hemicraniectomy in the management of acute subdural hematomas. J. Neurosurg., *34*:70–76, 1971.

112. Riddoch, G.: Aids to the Investigation of Peripheral Nerve Injuries. Medical Research Council War Memorandum 7. His Majesty's Stationery Office, 1942.

113. Richards, T., and Hoff, J., Factors affecting survival for acute subdural hematoma. Surgery, *75*:253–258, 1974.

114. Roberts, A. H.: Brain damage in boxers; a study of the prevalence of traumatic encephalopathy among professional boxers. London, Pitman Publishing Ltd., 1969.

115. Robertson, R. C. L., and Pollard, C.: Decerebrate state in children and adolescents. J. neurosurg., *12*:13–17, 1955.

116. Rodin, E. A.: Contribution of the EEG to prognosis after head injury. Dis. Nerv. Syst., *28*:595–601, 1967.

117. Rodin, E., Whelan, J., Taylor, R., Tomita, T., Grisell, J., Thomas, L. M., and Gurdjian, E. S.: The electroencephalogram in acute head injuries. J. Neurosurg., *23*:329–337, 1965.

118. Rose, J., Valtonen, S., and Jennett, B.: Avoidable factors contributing to death after head injury. Brit. Med. J., *2*:615–618, 1977.

119. Rossanda, M., Bozza-Marrubini, M., and Beduschi, A.: Clinical results of respirator treatment in unconscious patients with brain lesions. *In* Brock, M., Fieschi, C., Ingvar, D. H., Lassen, N. D., and Schürmann, K., eds.: Cerebral Blood Flow. Berlin, Springer-Verlag, 1969, pp. 260–262.

120. Rossanda, M., Selenati, A., Villa, C., and Beduschi, A.: Role of automatic ventilation in treatment of severe head injuries. J. Neurosurg. Sci., *17*:265–270, 1973.

121. Rowan, J. O., Cross, J. N., Tedeschi, G. M., and Jennett, W. B.: Limitations of circulation time in the diagnosis of intracranial disease. J. Neurol. Neurosurg. Psychiat., *33*:739–744, 1970.

122. Rowan, J. O., Harper, A. M., Miller, J. D., Tedeschi, G. M., and Jennett, W. B.: Relationship between volume flow and velocity in the cerebral circulation. J. Neurol. Neurosurg. Psychiat., *33*:733–738, 1970.

123. Ruesch, J.: Intellectual impairment in head injuries. Amer. J. Psychiat., *100*:480–496, 1944.

124. Ruesch, J., and Moore, B. E.: Measurement of intellectual function in the acute stage of head injury. Arch. Neurol. Psychiat., *50*:165–170, 1943.

125. Russell, W. R., and Nathan, P. W.: Traumatic amnesia. Brain, *69*:280–300, 1946.

126. Russell, W. R., and Smith, A.: Post-traumatic amnesia in closed head injury. Arch. Neurol. (Chicago), *5*:4–17, 1961.

127. Sarno, M. T., and Levita, E.: Natural course of recovery in severe aphasia. Arch. Phys. Med. Rehab., *52*:175–186, 1971.

128. Sarno, J. E., Sarno, M. T., and Levita, E.: Evaluating language improvement after completed stroke. Arch. Phys. Med. Rehab., *52*:73–78, 1971.

129. Scialfa, G., and Cristi, G. F.: Prognostic value of cerebral angiography in non-surgical cases of traumatic coma. J. Neurosurg. Sci., *17*:202–204, 1973.

130. Shaffer, D., Chadwick, O., and Rutter, M.: Psychiatric outcome of localized head injury in children. *In* Outcome of Severe Damage to the Central Nervous System. Ciba Foundation Symposium 34(New series). Amsterdam, Elsevier Publishing Co., 1975, pp. 191–213.

131. Shalit, M. N., Beller, A. J., Feinsod, M., Drapkin, A. J., and Cotev, S.: The blood flow and oxygen consumption of the dying brain. Neurology (Minneap.), *20*:740–748, 1970.

132. Starr, A., and Hamilton, A. E.: Correlation between confirmed sites of neurological lesions and abnormalities of farfield auditory brain stem responses. Electroenceph. Clin. Neurophysiol., *41*:595–608, 1976.

133. Steinbereithner, K., and Wagner, O.: Untersuchungen über das Verhalten des Säurebasenhaushaltes und der Atemgase in Liquor und arteriellen Blut bei schweren Schädeltraumen mit besonderer Berücksichtigung des Hyperventilationssyndroms. Klin. Wochenschr., *45*:126–133, 1967.

134. Stockard, J. J., Bickford, R. G., and Aung, M. H.: The electroencephalogram in traumatic brain injury. *In* Vinken, P. J., and Bruyn, G., eds.: Handbook of Clinical Neurology. Vol. 23. Amsterdam, Elsevier–North Holland Publishing Co., 1975, pp. 317–367.

135. Strich, S. J.: Diffuse degeneration of the cerebral white matter in severe dementia following head injury. J. Neurol. Neurosurg. Psychiat., *19*:163–185, 1956.

136. Strich, S. J.: Shearing of nerve fibres as a cause of brain damage due to head injury. A pathological study of 20 cases. Lancet, *2*:443–448, 1961.

137. Sullivan, H. G., Martinez, J., Becker, D. P.,

Miller, J. D., Griffith, R., and Wist, A. O.: Fluid-percussion model of mechanical brain injury in the cat. J. Neurosurg., *45*:520–534, 1976.

138. Sumner, D.: Post-traumatic anosmia. Brain, *87*:107–120, 1964.

139. Sweet, R. C., Miller, J. D., Lipper, M., Kishore, P. R. S., and Becker, D. P.: Significance of bilateral abnormalities on the CT scan in patients with severe head injury. Neurosurgery, *3*:16–21, 1978.

140. Tallala, A., and Morin, M. A.: Acute traumatic subdural hematoma: A review of one hundred consecutive cases. J. Trauma, *11*:771–777, 1971.

141. Taylor, A. R.: Post concussional sequelae. Brit. Med. J., *2*:67–71, 1967.

142. Taylor, A. R., and Bell, T. K.: Slowing of cerebral circulation after concussional head injury. Lancet, *2*:178–180, 1966.

143. Teasdale, G., and Jennett, B.: Assessment of coma and impaired consciousness. A practical scale. Lancet, *2*:81–84, 1974.

144. Teasdale, G., and Jennett, B.: Assessment prognosis of coma after head injury. Acta Neurochir. (Wien), *34*:45–55, 1976.

145. Teasdale, G., and Smith, J.: Eye movements and brain stem dysfunction after head injury. J. Neurol. Neurosurg. Psychiat., *38*:822–829, 1975.

146. Teasdale, G., Galbraith, S., and Clarke, K.: Acute impairment of brain function. 2. Observation record chart. Nurs. Times, June 19, 1975.

147. Teasdale, G., Knill-Jones, R., and Jennett, B.: Assessing and recording "conscious level." J. Neurol. Neurosurg. Psychiat., *37*:1286, 1974.

148. Teasdale, G., Knill-Jones, R., and Van der Sande, J.: Observer variability in assessing impaired consciousness and coma. J. Neurol. Neurosurg. Psychiat., *41*:603–610, 1978.

149. Teasdale, G., Rowan, J. O., Turner, J., Grossman, R., and Miller, J. D.: Cerebral perfusion failure and cortical electrical activity. Acta Neurol. Scand., *56*:suppl. 64:430–431, 1977.

150. Teuber, H. L.: Disorders of memory following penetrating missile wounds of the brain. Neurology (Minneap.), *18*:287–288, 1968.

151. Teuber, H. L.: Recovery of function after lesions of the central nervous system. Neurosci. Res. Program Bull., *12*:197–209, 1974.

152. Tooth, C.: On the use of mental tests for the measurement of disability after head injury. J. Neurol. Neurosurg. Psychiat., *10*:1–11, 1947.

153. Troupp, H.: Intraventricular pressure in patients with severe brain injuries. J. Trauma, *5*:373–378, 1965.

154. Troupp, H.: Intraventricular pressure in patients with severe brain injuries II. J. Trauma, *7*:875–883, 1967.

155. Vapalahti, M., and Troupp, H.: Prognosis for patients with severe brain injuries. Brit. Med. J., *3*:404–407, 1971.

156. Venes, J. L., and Collins, W. F.: Bifrontal decompressive craniectomy in the management of head trauma. J. Neurosurg., *42*:429–433, 1975.

157. Von Wowern, F.: Post-traumatic amnesia and confusion as an index of severity in head injury. Acta Neurol. Scand., *42*:373–378, 1966.

158. Walker, A. E., and Jablon, S.: A follow up of head injured men of World War II. J. Neurosurg., *16*:600–610, 1959.

159. Wilkins, R. J., Harvey, F., Ojemann, L. M., and Lettich, E.: Electroencephalogram and sensory evoked potentials. Arch. Neurol. (Chicago), *24*:538–544, 1971.

160. Williams, D.: The electroencephalogram in acute head injuries. J. Neurol. Psychiat., *4*:107–130, 1941.

161. Williams, M., and Zangwill, O. L.: Memory defects after head injury. J. Neurol. Neurosurg. Psychiat., *15*:54–58, 1952.

61

POST-TRAUMATIC SYNDROME

A discussion of the post-traumatic syndrome is difficult because of the problem in defining it. A syndrome includes a set of symptoms or signs that lead to a specific disease diagnosis, the elements of which can usually be attributed to certain pathophysiological mechanisms. By definition the post-traumatic syndrome should include all the consequences of head injury, regardless of the severity and nature of the injury. By usage, however, it includes a rather specific group of symptoms that frequently follow minor craniocerebral trauma but that may have ill-defined and variable pathophysiological bases. It is also known as the "post-concussion syndrome" or the "minor contusion syndrome." The usual components of the syndrome are headache, dizziness, and nervous instability.

In addition to this triad of symptoms the syndrome is also characterized by a tendency to become worse instead of improving as expected after injury, treatment, and convalescence; lack of correlation between the occurrence of the syndrome and the severity of injury, length of coma, duration of amnesia, or other indices of the extent of craniocerebral trauma; resistance to treatment, a lengthy course, and multiple visits to an expanding list of medical specialists; and an overlapping complexity of psychic and neurological symptoms interacting with disturbances of behavior and neural function.

A further difficulty in describing the syndrome arises from the lack of agreement on whether the symptoms are psychogenic in origin or due to organic damage. Cogent arguments can be offered on each side of the question, and it seems likely that, in the individual patient, either or both factors may be operative. The practical question, however, is whether the syndrome is either preventable or reversible. To answer this question, inquiry into its pathophysiology is essential. The fact that the syndrome consists of a group of nonspecific symptoms that may be of diverse etiologies permits it to occur rather consistently despite the variable pathophysiological mechanisms.

Traditional disputes on whether the syndrome arises principally from mental and emotional reactions to head trauma or from disordered neurophysiological mechanisms and brain damage may be avoided if the discussion of it is based on an orderly conceptual framework.[2,7,10] Clearly there are some structural and functional changes in the neural system responsible at times for major aspects of the clinical picture. In some cases the major manifestations develop from the impairing effect of chronic anxiety that has been generated during the initial trauma, the emergency treatment, and the hospital stay. This anxiety seeks discharge or containment through neurotic or occasionally psychotic symptoms, but mainly through personality change. In other cases the elements of the syndrome are psychophysiological in origin, usually expressed through changes in neural function such as autonomic disturbances, tinnitus, weakness, and changes in sensation in varying patterns. Finally, the search continues for as yet unknown mechanisms to explain more completely the mystifying and obstinate symptoms of the condition. In summary, the syndrome can be viewed as representing the effect of complex causal chains powered by neurophysiological, psychophysiological, psychiatric, and probably some unknown factors.

Based on the foregoing conceptual framework, the discussion will necessarily divide the considerations of pathogenesis, diagnosis, and management into those of

---

R. L. McLAURIN AND J. L. TITCHENER

organic cause and those of psychic origin. Prior to this discussion, however, a description of the syndrome is presented.

DESCRIPTION OF SYNDROME

Somatic Complaints

Headache

Headache constitutes the most consistent component of the syndrome, although its character is extremely variable. Jacobsen reported that in a series of 297 patients with head injury the incidence of headache in the post-traumatic period was 78 per cent.[5] The headache may be generalized or localized, and localization, when present, is usually to the area of the head that received the initial impact. At times it simply involves the entire side of the head that the patient associates with the injury. The discomfort is described variously as consisting of a bandlike tightness, a sensation of expanding pressure within the cranium, or a throbbing, aching, or sharp pain. It may be continuous or intermittent, with some relation to physical exertion and posture. Most commonly it is aggravated by emotional and physical stress.

The relationship between the period of amnesia associated with head injury and the occurrence of a post-traumatic syndrome, particularly headache, has been explored by a number of authors.[*] The period of unconsciousness has also been investigated; the duration of unconsciousness is, however, usually much more difficult to define, as the period of amnesia frequently extends well beyond general reappearance of environmental contact and orientation. Attempts have also been made, notably by Russell, to equate retrograde amnesia with post-traumatic headache.[7] Jacobsen concluded by statistical analysis that there was no difference in the incidence of headaches in patients with and those without amnesia following injury.[5] Moreover, in further analysis of his data in which the cases were subdivided according to the duration of amnesia, no prognostic relationship could be defined. The obvious implication of these findings is that post-traumatic headache is not due to intracranial injury.

Dizziness or Giddiness

Subjective disorders or equilibrium constitute the second most common component of the post-traumatic syndrome, occurring in approximately 50 per cent of patients with head injuries. The complaint is usually not one of true spontaneous vertigo, and when this occurs there is invariably found evidence of brain stem or vestibulocochlear damage. The symptoms are, more often, a sensation of giddiness, faintness, or unsteadiness related to sudden movements of the head. The feeling may be described as one of movement of the environment in relation to the patient or a sense of movement within the subject. Another form of this symptom is described as a loss of balance accompanied by transient visual deficit and a dazed sensation; this usually occurs on rising from a stooped or recumbent posture. The individual episodes of dysequilibrium are usually brief, lasting only a few seconds, and the relationship to movement of the head or the entire body is fairly consistent.

Jacobsen, attempting to correlate the incidence of vertigo with the severity of the head injury, found that there existed an increasing incidence of the symptom with injuries resulting in longer periods of unconsciousness.[5] This relationship has been cited to support the organic basis of the symptom.

Psychogenic Complaints

The somatic complaints and the communication of the patient about them are an integral part of the psychiatric aspects of the syndrome. These painful problems acquire an intense meaning in the life of the patient and appear to vary with arousal of underlying emotional conflict in his life situation. This correlation of waxing and waning complaints with the inner conflictual life of the patient requires an empathic study of the person and his relations with others and should not be discarded as a factor because the patient resists the idea that there are external and emotional stresses in his past and present experience. This acceptance of the superficial picture and the word of the pa-

---

* See references 3–6, 8, 9, 12–14.

tient is the major mistake of those who fail to understand psychogenetic factors in the causation of such complex syndromes.

Second, anxiety over the headache and dizziness, and depression over the disabling condition may be manifested by quiet fearful resignation or by agitation, irritability, or querulousness with family and physician as often as by the more familiar symptoms of withdrawal moodiness and open despair.

The personality changes are the most difficult to describe briefly. The patient's physical symptoms become the center of his life; he notices and is interested in very little else about himself or, most poignantly, about his personal interactions or loss of meaningful relations with others. *He literally becomes a headache and a dizziness,* assuming the role of the sick, head-injured person, though he may once have been an active, interesting, participating individual with flexibility in social roles, enthusiasms in vocation, enjoyment of marriage and sexuality, and a pleasure in social relations. More specific and narrowed changes in personality include paranoid and counterphobic acting-out traits that replace previous ways of adapting.

In the paranoid post-traumatic personality the symptoms are still the center of the person's way of life but with an added element—a constant undercurrent of communication and expression of feeling that the injury, the pains, and the neural problems have been somehow "done to" the person. A vague, or sometimes specified, external agency is held responsible, and usually physicians play essential roles in this belief system. They are viewed with resentful contempt for their inadequacies, dishonesties, indifference, and incompetence in the care of the patient. The mode and tone of the complaining is the tip-off to the underlying paranoid trend in the personality change.

Counterphobic acting-out traits refer to behavior in which the individual overcomes or endures his traumatically engendered anxiety by variations on the theme of the behavior that led to his trauma. The easiest example would be a man whose injury occurred in an auto accident after he had been drinking. He would fight his phobias by acting as though he were unafraid, by drinking heavily, and by driving fast. He would explain that alcohol was used to dull the pain

of his headache, hiding the true unconscious motive, which is to master the anxiety by approaching a reliving of the trauma. Considering this mechanism, it is not surprising that individuals who have suffered head trauma are liable to have further accidents.

PATHOGENESIS

Headache

Numerous mechanisms have been implicated in the pathogenesis of post-traumatic headache. Certain of these are of historical interest only as they have been progressively exonerated by extensive observation and analysis. In general, the mechanisms that have been suspected may be divided into those that involve organic effects of the injury and those that are primarily psychogenic. The present authors believe that in most instances there are combinations of these mechanisms in operation.

The organic mechanisms to be considered may be conveniently subdivided into those involving intracranial structures, those involving extracranial structures, and those originating from associated neck injury.

Headache occurring during the first few days and weeks after injury is more likely to be based on intracranial damage than that which persists for months or years. In the early stages after injury, subarachnoid or epidural hemorrhage may be responsible for discomfort, and the character of the headache may or may not indicate the generalized or localized nature of the process. The pain from a localized hematoma results from traction and displacement of pain-sensitive structures, particularly at the base of the brain. The pain from subarachnoid blood, on the contrary, is probably secondary to a sterile inflammatory reaction of the meninges.

Headache due to accumulation of blood or fluid in the subdural space may persist for several weeks or months, but rarely longer than six months. Blood within the subdural compartment may cause progressively greater displacement of the subjacent brain (whether actual enlargement of the hematoma occurs is still debated) or it may be slowly absorbed. Subdural hygroma, presumably due to tearing of the arachnoid membrane, likewise may be responsible for pain caused by displacement of structures for a period of weeks or a few months.

Intracranial hypotension has been implicated as a cause of post-traumatic headache, but this would necessarily depend on the occurrence of a cerebrospinal fluid leak, which in most instances repairs itself within a few days. Again, the mechanism of this headache is traction by the unsupported brain on pain-sensitive structures, and it is dependent on the postural attitude. The converse of this situation is the intracranial hypertension that may result from defective absorption secondary to subarachnoid blood. Although this is a rare long-term complication of head injury, it must be considered in the clinical evaluation, as it may persist for months and years beyond the traumatic event.

Penfield and Norcross proposed that chronic post-traumatic headache might be related to adhesions between the arachnoid and the dura.[8] They noted that normally there is a small amount of fluid in this space, allowing movement between the brain with its leptomeninges and the dura, and that trauma caused adhesions between these layers. The sensitive area affected by the adhesion was felt to be a meningeal artery or a dural sinus. Therapy was directed toward lysis of the adhesions by collapse of the brain away from the dura, achieved by insufflation of air into the subdural space and removal of cerebrospinal fluid. This pathogenetic mechanism and its therapy, however, have been subsequently abandoned.

More recently, Taylor and Bell demonstrated slowing of the intracranial circulation persisting for many months after head injury.[14] This intriguing observation was made by using a bolus of radioactive iodine; a significant relationship between the severity of postconcussional symptoms and the slowing of cerebral circulation was demonstrated. Although the importance and the mechanism of this phenomenon are unknown, it is tempting to attribute postconcussion symptoms to an ischemic state.

The extracranial causes for head pain, exclusive of those related to neck structures, in the post-traumatic period include muscle contraction, changes in vascular tone, and the presence of painful nerve endings adjacent to a scar.

Numerous studies have been undertaken to determine the relationship between muscle contraction in the neck and scalp and head pain occurring after trauma. That excessive muscle contraction does occur can be readily demonstrated electromyographically. The question is then raised whether the discomfort is actually a result of relative or absolute muscle ischemia or whether the pain is due to some other factor that secondarily produces muscle spasm. In either event, the pathway for referral of pain from muscular contraction is presumed to include the cervical posterior roots, which make contact through collateral fibers with the descending trigeminal nucleus.

The relationship between vascular changes and headache are clearly recognized outside the field of head injury. That such vasomotor tone changes may occur as a result of trauma has not been firmly established, but the character of post-traumatic headache frequently is similar to that seen in cluster headaches. There is no evidence, however, that migraine is either precipitated or aggravated by trauma. It has been postulated, without convincing evidence, that basal skull injuries may lead to vasomotor changes because of injury to the greater superficial petrosal nerve and the afferent branches of the sphenopalatine ganglion.

Scar formation in the scalp may, as in other superficial areas, be accompanied by painful nerve endings and neuroma formation. This mechanism of headaches is easily diagnosed by the discrete tenderness and the clear-cut response to local injection of an anesthetic agent.

That cervical spine injuries may be associated with head trauma is well recognized. This has led to the implication of cervical structures as a cause for headache. The relationship of muscle contraction to head pain has already been noted. Other supporting structures include nuchal ligaments and muscle tendons as well as bones and intervertebral discs. Each of these structures has a nerve supply that may, by means of collateral fibers, cause referral of discomfort to the upper cervical or trigeminal nerve distribution. Probably more post-traumatic discomfort is attributed to these structures than is deserved, but the theoretical mechanism still enjoys a certain immunity to critical evaluation clinically.

Dizziness

There is increasing evidence to indicate that disturbances of equilibrium have an organic basis, although there remains considerable disagreement as to the location of the responsible pathological change. The possible areas of damage include the inner ear, the eighth cranial nerve, and the brain stem.

Longitudinal fractures of the temporal bone are the most commonly recognized fractures and are usually due to an impact in the temporal or parietal areas. The fracture is parallel to the long axis of the petrous bone and there is usually only minor injury to the auditory or vestibular mechanisms. Transverse fractures, however, are at right angles to the long axis of the petrous bone, usually result from blows to the frontal or occipital areas, and are much more likely to cause damage to the inner and middle ear. The exact location of the disorder responsible for vestibular dysfunction following head injury is often difficult to determine, but if a transverse fracture extends into the labyrinth it can be reasonably assumed that damage to the end-organ is responsible to some degree.

Symonds drew attention to the evidence favoring the organicity of the symptoms and sequelae of concussion.[9] Experimental concussion required acceleration of deceleration of the brain and brain stem within the cranium. Pathological observations demonstrated loss of neurons after concussion as well as widespread diffuse degeneration of cerebral white matter. In addition the existence of retrograde and post-traumatic amnesia was considered consistent only with organic damage. Thus, Symonds suggests that the basis of postconcussion dizziness may be brain stem injury. Jacobsen has noted, however, that if brain stem damage were the cause of vertigo it would be logical to expect that there would be a common association with other evidences of brain stem dysfunction such as cranial nerve involvement and disturbances of long-fiber tracts passing through the pons and medulla.[4] Such associated findings are rare.

Taylor more recently has reviewed post-concussion sequelae and concluded that physical and biochemical abnormalities have been neglected in reaching the assumption about the neurotic basis of symptoms.[13] He noted that vertical nystagmus has been recorded in more than half the patients with post-traumatic symptoms. Moreover, there are specific changes in rhythm and amplitude of electronystagmographic recordings. These changes are different from those found in damage to the labyrinth but are like those seen in vertebrobasilar insufficiency. Thus, the brain stem has been seriously implicated as the source of subjective dysequilibrium.

Favoring the concept of damage to the inner ear as a basis for dysequilibrium is an abundance of experimental data and some postmortem observations on humans. Schuknect demonstrated hemorrhages in the cochlea and damage to the organ of Corti in experimental head injury.[8] Human material has demonstrated transverse fractures of the petrous bone with damage to the labyrinth.

Probably the strongest evidence favoring injury to the vestibular labyrinth is derived from a type of postconcussion dysequilibrium known as benign paroxysmal positional vertigo. This seems to be due to utricular trauma resulting from blows to the occipital and temporal regions. Patients with this type of positional vertigo have demonstrated disorganization of the sensory epithelium of the utricular macula, degenerative changes beneath the epithelium, and absence of the otolithic membrane.

Psychogenic Symptoms

In an attempt to define the psychopathogenesis of this component of the syndrome, the crucial emotional issue of head injury is described and this is followed by a conceptual model of the etiology and course of the post-traumatic syndrome.

In the perception of the person with a head injury and in the image of himself he has experienced a major threat to centers known by him to provide the essence of himself as a unique animal, man, and as a unique human individual. There is no other physical injury with quite the same effect and degree of threat to human and individual uniqueness. This quality of the head injury experience needs to be remembered for full appreciation of the defensive stance of the post-traumatic patient. Another crucial meaning of the experience is threatened loss of the integrity, organization, and continuity of thinking and feeling.

From the psychogenetic point of view the syndrome is increasingly dominated by responses to the *experience* of damage to and paralysis of that part of self that gives life continuity and meaning, the head, the brain, and the mind. The very fact that a prominent feature of the syndrome includes forms of giving up some of the richness, the drive, and the zest for life, and submitting to emotional constriction and degrees of cognitive paralysis serves to prove this point. The principle of conservation has been allowed to operate in the system. The individual constricts feeling, withholds ambition, and sacrifices hope in order to avoid losing all. Patterns of action and behavior that formerly expanded into social, vocational, sexual, and relational aspects of functioning—in brief, the joys of living—are surrendered; there is a falling back to a lower level of complexity of thinking and feeling to avoid obliteration of the flow and regulation of thought and feeling.

Another way of stating the basic change is that anxiety released by a massively threatening situation, injury to the head, rather than structural damage to the central nervous system, is the cause of impairment, and the impairment caused by anxiety tends to resemble in many ways the impairment sometimes caused by brain damage.

The clinical picture presented by a patient after head injury is so dreadfully complex and so often discouragingly fixed when seen 12 months or more after release from hospital that most specialists in the medical field seize desperately upon a number of different therapies or become attracted to a great range of various theories about its cause or become secretly angry at the patient and think puritanical thoughts about what the wishes for compensation will do to some people.

For a synthesis and clarification of the many ambiguous factors at work before and after the trauma that tend to produce the syndrome, a model is constructed that may bring conceptual order to the problem. The model for the syndrome shall be a telescopic device of a series of lenses, each lens progressively transforming the original image of the person and his head trauma and finally producing the clinical picture at the other end (Fig. 61–1). Each lens in this device transforms the image provided to it by the preceding lens. Following is a list of the lenses with a word or two about each to be amplified by discussion of the contribution of each toward the final clinical picture.*

Telescopic Model of Post-Traumatic Syndrome

1. Trauma, coma, stupor, amnesia, acute distress.
2. Traumatic neurosis, with disorganization of "executive functions" such as judgment, thinking, memory, and orientation.
3. Somaticized traumatic neurosis. A somatic component blends with psychic disturbance.
4. Somaticized traumatic neurosis becomes part of or an element in pre-existing *psycho*neurosis.
5. Personality constriction—withdrawal of object-interests toward a defensive posture on many fronts, thus affecting broad areas of living. Personality change.
6. Trauma as a screen.
7. Interaction with family.
8. Social interaction.
9. Secondary gain, compensation problems, litigation, struggle, rage, and humiliation.

In a more or less progressive fashion, with allowances for different sequences and varying emphases, the course of the patient after head injury passes through such a psy-

---

* Some will note the plagiarism from Freud (Standard Edition V, *The Interpretation of Dreams*, pp. 540–542), who used the same model in an entirely different way and for a different concept.

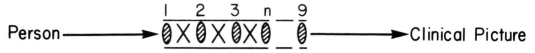

Figure 61–1   Telescopic model of post-traumatic syndrome.

chological telescopic device, being modified by each lens, toward the production of a full-blown clinical picture of a post-traumatic syndrome.

The elements of this compound system may be examined to see how each makes its contribution to the final picture.

Physical Impact, Coma, Stupor, Shock, Amnesia, and Other Disturbances of Consciousness

In each case it is possible to discover the amount of helplessness and the specific details of helplessness experienced by the victim just before and for a period after the head injury. We recover these details from accident reports, from the patient himself, and from witnesses. It is possible, imaginatively, to reconstruct the emotional experience of the victim whose car sped out of control or who fell or who was struck by an assailant. Some of the physiodynamics of the accident can be analyzed for details of the victim's active or passive participation in the accident, and for degrees of responsibility of the self or others in the traumatic event. Did the victim have a period of "contemplation" of the accident; i.e., did he see it begin to happen and move inexorably toward his injury? Could he have taken action to avert the final result? Were there others injured? Or killed? What was the relationship of others involved? Was there conscious intent to damage by anyone, the victim or others? Does the victim's account differ from those of others with regard to responsibility or intent?

A different, less drastic helplessness is felt during emergency treatment. This state consists of disturbances in awareness and sensation, in confusion and the paralysis of thought, in the immobilization or the need for tubes and resuscitative apparatus. This enforced infancy, often in an environment of disorienting over- and understimulation in a recovery room, has its effect on every victim of head injury. The recovery room has been described in many studies as a prime instance of biological technology leaping far ahead of the understanding of human needs. To take just one aspect of the frightening sights and sounds of a recovery room: Not many physicians or nurses who work or visit in these places realize that man, who is biologically and psychologically conditioned to a circadian cycle, has no way of knowing day from night if he is a patient in such a place and has not yet regained the initiative to ask.

Traumatic Neurosis

Now the problem moves from a biological stage of helplessness to its psychological counterpart, from the actual flooding of the psychic apparatus with the terror of the moment and from the reality-enforced state of infancy and immobilization to the recurring *memory* of the overwhelming of adaptive resources. This stage is at the interface between the biological factors and the more clearly psychological ones.

Some studies have shown that any severe physical injury including head injury is regularly accompanied by some degree and some form of traumatic neurosis, meaning that an overwhelming of the adaptive capacity of the mind leads to disorganization of ego functions, the controlling, regulating, expressive, and communicative aspects of behavior. The response at such a point of disorganization of mental functions calls for strong attempts, both realistic and wildly distorted, to *master* the excessive excitation provided by the traumatic experience of the accident and bodily injury. "Realistic" attempts at mastery include trying to remember details, investigating and inquiring about what happened, thinking through and sorting out responsibilities and causal sequences. At another level of mental functioning there are attempts at mastery of the excitation through repetitive dreams, distorted reconstructions of the event, denying personal participation or responsibility, and many other irrational and unconsciously operating mechanisms.

The traumatic neurosis consists of a flooding of the psychic apparatus with levels of excitation beyond its capacity to respond. There is insufficient containment of the arousing stimuli and therefore a relative loss of equilibrium and disorganization of central adaptive functions. The feeling is that of helplessness. In the process of recovery from this state there is an attempt to master the traumatic event in memory by reliving it in dreams and, in the waking state, by an excessive guarding and intense vigilance against the slightest risk of repeating the chance of further stimuli overwhelming the adapative apparatus.

The Traumatic Neurosis Somaticizes

The next lens in the hypothetical telescopic device is a psychopathological process that begins early and stays late in those cases in which the post-traumatic syndrome becomes severe and chronic. The massive excitation from the terrifying experience and the threat to the head, paralysis of thought and feeling, loss of memory, and destruction of mechanisms of control over the self system evokes, in addition to the state of helplessness, large quantities of emotion that have the quality and intensity of basic and primitive drives. Such aggressive energies can be only partly discharged in expressions of anger toward those in the environment because there is reflexive fear of the power of these destructive feelings and fear of retaliation from those who are targets of the feeling. Libidinous drives having the intensity and qualities of infantile states are stirred in the form of self-concern and needs to be taken care of. If those in the environment are unable to respond effectively, or if the patient's adaptive, channeling resources are at a low level, these impulses are turned on the self to become highly charged concerns for the body and body parts, in this case the nervous system and its functions. It is as though these primitive energies had nowhere else to go but to the self—*the somatic self*, the body. The rage during recovery from the helpless state, also having nowhere else to go, is turned to the body or body parts and is known through pain, a strange sensation in some part of the system, a disturbance in function, or it finds partial, indirect discharge in the form of a permanent reproach toward significant persons and toward the world, especially doctors who can do nothing to change the symptoms. Thus the patient is intensely involved in the somatic function and more and more accusatory of the physician when efforts fail to obtain relief. These aggressive and libidinous impulses turned toward the somatic self and the body are the representation of the helplessness of the terrifying experience and reflection in the patient of the dehumanizing threat to the systems of control, expression, thinking, and feeling.

The Somaticized Traumatic Neurosis Becomes Part of or a Modification of Latent or Pre-Existing Psychoneurosis

As the storm of the immediate trauma dies down and neurotic reactions to trauma have begun to show, being partly expressed through complaints or disturbances in nervous function, whatever problems in overall social and emotional adjustment or symptomatic psychic disorder or sexual or other difficulties that exist, instead of being crowded aside by these new problems, blend with them to form a new pattern of psychoneurosis. For example, an individual whose way of life is moderately depressive because of conflicts that engender guilt over unresolved hostility is likely, after head trauma that has caused the problems we have described, to have an intensified conflict between unconscious hostility and guilt and therefore a potential for a newly aggravated neurotic illness along the lines that had been established before the injury.

A stiffening of the personal adaptation is the consequence of the increased defensiveness of a personality that has a prolonged traumatic neurosis, and this is added to the pre-existing psychoneurotic system with an increase of psychic symptom formation. To the framework of a latent or active psychoneurosis are added the rigidifying and constricting effects of a somaticizing traumatic neurosis.

Personality Constriction

In the circumstances so far outlined there develops a demand for yet another process of change. The need for a greater degree of defensiveness means a pulling back of interests and a decided change in relations with the outside world. These changes are summed up as personality, or ego, constriction, meaning that in the state of crisis the person unwittingly takes a turn toward greater conservatism and much less willingness to risk being hurt (in the emotional and social senses of being hurt as well as the physical). Simultaneously, he is more interested in protecting the self against every sort of change. There is less hope, less interest in others, a stiffening of character that resists novel experiences and tends to avoid the experience of overstimulation by reducing the perception of feelings in the self. A narrower range of experience, feeling, ambition, and relationships with others is accepted at the cost of flexibility and pleasure seeking. This constriction and fearing to venture is the most imposing obstacle to acceptance of help because psychotherapy means a new relationship, and such an exploration of thought and feeling is strongly resisted by faintly hostile complaining and insistence that the source of all personal problems is truly damage to the body, specifically the head and the nervous system. Ego constriction tends to focus all thinking about the self upon totally somatic and nonpsychological causation of individual problems.

The Trauma Becomes a Screen

The traumatic event becomes a screen for the victim's view of his own life; all problems, suspected shortcomings, and conflicts are viewed as truly arising from the traumatic event and the physical disabilities it caused. This phenomenon should *not* be confused with conscious self-justifying or unconscious secondary gain. When the trauma becomes a screen for a life problem the individual begins to think of himself as though nothing good or bad happened before the trauma; everything in his character is explained by what happened to him in his accident. If he felt inadequate before the accident for reasons he could not understand he now sees the idea of inadequacy as a feeling forced upon him by the accident and the limitation it caused. Now he feels a failure at work or thinks he is a dependent person because of what has happened rather than as the result of long-standing inner difficulties. Occasionally this screening effect can bring about an actual recovery from psychological problems because a new light is thrown upon them. Some experience the ordeal and survival as an impetus to make a new life and to forget old inhibitions and rationalization. However, such unconsciously motivated acting and thinking as though everything in life started with the physical injury usually forces the patient toward less acceptance of personal responsibility for problems and less availability for therapy and recovery.

Family Interaction

The model and its diagram fall short in conceptualizing the influence of the family interaction system and a head injury patient's changing participation in it during the course of the acute illness and development of the syndrome. The model fails at this point in the telescopic sequence because there are no strong reasons for placing the family interaction lens at this point in the device; the actual influence of this factor is exerted along the whole course and is hardly ever actually concentrated at one point. The family interaction is placed at this particular position in the sequence because at a time when the impairing effects of anxiety have become chronic and the somaticizing blend of traumatic neurosis and psychoneurosis is crystalizing and taking shape, the interaction system also begins to change—the family awakens bitterly to the fact that there has been a change in role and role functions within it. A neurotic problem has been recognized at some level of awareness in the total family system, with consequent changes in feeling and communication in all parts of the system that involve many facets of function of family life.

But let us go back to consider the problems of the interaction of the family system and the individual system throughout the course of the development of our difficult syndrome.

In most sizable studies of series of individuals who have suffered injuries requiring hospitalization, states of severe psychological conflict have been in evidence prior to the physical trauma in a high percentage of the patients. Serious accidents tend to occur in the context of inner emotional conflict or external crises in the individual's life or in the context of a combination of both crisis and conflict situations. It is not always a hidden suicidal drive that is responsible; it may be that the violence of the external event, the accident, matches the violence of the inner turmoil.

That such conflictive states intensely involve individuals who are brought to the emergency services after serious accidents has been often demonstrated, and it is probably true of head injury patients also. It is not only the individual, however, but the family with which he is interacting that is involved either in the crisis or in sharing the emotional conflict. The traumatic event may be as much a symptom of family conflict (an intense quarrel, an increase in doubt or mistrust or suspicion, an increase

of feelings of indifference and meaningless-
ness) as it is an outbreak of individual turmoil.

Though the injury itself occurs at least
partly as a result of family conflict or family
crisis, it is unlikely that a head injury with
hospitalization and continuing threat to
family stability will improve the already impaired family interaction system. Sometimes the shock effect will do so, but in a
larger proportion of cases family adaptation
will be more difficult. A variety of responses of the family as a system will occur
throughout the remainder of the course of
development of our syndrome.

For example, attitudes of doubt or disappointment in the psychological strength of
the injured individual may predispose to an
infantilization of the patient and continuing
subtle restrictions that prevent progressive
rehabilitation. Tendencies to project feelings that are unacceptable to himself to
others in the family system may lead to hidden accusations flowing both ways regarding the responsibility or blame for the mis-
fortune. As these feelings build up and are
unexpressed overtly and verbally, they lead
to disabling distortion of feeling and behavior such as the patient's unconscious need
to remain sick to prove he is truly the injured one and the true victim.

A patient affected by all the changing
forces suggested in this model would have
little chance of recovery. It is used only as a
conceptual device; most patients will be
only partially affected by most of these con-
verging psychogenic factors. This conceptual device, the system of lenses, only helps
to show a sequential arrangement of the
varieties of experience these patients undergo and how a synergism from one stage
to another leads to a final clinical picture
that is very resistant to treatment. The con-
verging pathogenic processes are difficult if
not impossible to undo.

DIAGNOSIS

Headache

Generally speaking, the diagnostic evaluation of postconcussion headache is evaluation for operatively correctible lesions.
When no such lesion is found the headache
is attributed, by exclusion, to the postconcussion state, and speculation then begins

whether it is organic or functional, and if
organic, which of the unproved pathogenetic mechanisms may be responsible.

The character of the headache, as described previously, is helpful in diagnosis,
and the duration of symptoms may also be
useful in excluding certain lesions such as
post-traumatic hematomas. The neurological examination is used to detect evidence
of intracranial hypertension or focal neurological deficit and may also detect evidence
of muscle spasm, particularly in the suboccipital area, which may be responsible for
the headache.

X-rays of the skull are important in determining the existence of a fracture, displacement of a calcified pineal gland or choroid
plexus, or rarely the presence of air within
the cranial vault indicating cerebrospinal
fluid leakage. Even more rarely, a calcified
hematoma may be visualized.

Electroencephalography and isotope
scanning may be employed to detect focal
or generalized dysrhythmia or areas of increased permeability of the blood-brain
barrier. Computed tomography or contrast
studies may be necessary to rule out an expanding lesion, and air encephalography is
essential if normal-pressure hydrocephalus
is being sought. At present, studies of cerebral circulation have no practical application in the management of the postconcussion syndrome.

It may be repeated that the diagnosis of
post-traumatic headache is usually made
purely by the history, as positive findings of
organic damage are usually lacking. Because of the absence of definite signs, the
headache is easily attributable to a psychogenic basis.

Dizziness

In addition to the history and routine
neurological evaluation, certain special observations and tests should be directed toward vestibular evaluation. Audiological
testing is done to determine whether damage to the temporal bone has produced conductive or sensorineural hearing loss. The
latter is much more commonly seen and
occurs more frequently in head injury accompanied by skull fracture. By the use of
certain methods of testing, such as delayed
auditory feedback, nonorganic or functional hearing loss can be detected; this is

of considerable importance in medicolegal evaluation of the syndrome.

Vestibular function is specifically studied by nystagmus identification. Nystagmus should be sought first with the patient's head erect and his eyes open. The incidence of this type of nystagmus after head injury is approximately 10 per cent. It can be increased by posturing. This nystagmus, however, has been noted to decay after a period of 6 to 12 months following the injury.

Examination for nystagmus with the eyes closed is performed by electronystagmography. This nystagmus may be "spontaneous," i.e., unrelated to posture, or positional. It is found in approximately 60 per cent of persons with head injuries. Decay of this type of nystagmus is less constant with the passage of time after injury. It is noteworthy, however, that spontaneous and positional nystagmus are also frequently seen in normal subjects.

Caloric testing can be used also with electronystagmographic recording. Dysrhythmia in postcaloric nystagmus is considered by some to be characteristic of head injury and is thought to be caused by a central lesion of the vestibular centers in the medulla. Thus, as Taylor has suggested, it is a concrete sign of the postconcussion state and implicates the brain stem.[10]

A specific type of post-traumatic vestibular disturbance has become known as benign paroxysmal positional vertigo and is thought to be due to utricular injury. It is provoked when the patient is recumbent with the affected ear downward. There is a delay of several seconds before onset of vertigo, which spontaneously stops after about 10 to 15 seconds. The accompanying nystagmus is rotatory.

These diagnostic procedures are valuable when one is attempting to delineate the cause of subjective dysequilibrium and also to determine if there is organic damage. While they are valuable diagnostically, they do not assist significantly in planning therapeutic management.

Psychogenic Symptoms

The best treatment is preventative. Therefore the need for it must be noticed and its application accomplished while the patient is in close contact with the physician, that is, during the hospital treatment of the acute injury or during convalescence and return for postdischarge follow-up.

The following indicators of concern may be looked for: (1) signs of traumatic neurosis—easy startle reaction, traumatic dreams, irritability, shakiness, and restlessness; (2) doubts of the self and physical capacities exaggerating whatever residuals remain, doubts of the family that the injury victim can possibly resume his former roles at work and in the family, questions and worries about sexual capacity; (3) any indications of melancholy when hopefulness and mood should be improving along with neurological recovery—accounts from the family of withdrawal and hopelessness may help in noticing this problem; (4) signs of personality change and constriction as described earlier; and (5) an emphasis or an alteration in tone of complaints about headache or other residuals of the injury.

If these indicators are apparent there is evidence that the course of recovery from the head injury is not routine and that inquiry is needed, perhaps a psychological examination by an expert.

TREATMENT

Headache

The principal means of treating headache on a symptomatic basis is by use of analgesics. The antipyretic analgesics can be used safely, but it is imperative that narcotic and morphine-like analgesics be totally avoided. Regardless of the role of psychogenic factors in the cause of the headaches, the patient can easily fall into a state of addiction if such drugs are prescribed.

Other drugs that may have occasional usefulness include tranquilizers and central-acting skeletal muscle relaxants. These may be useful if psychogenic factors are prominent and if muscle spasm is a part of the headache. While ergot preparations are extremely valuable in the treatment of vascular headaches, they have little or no role in the management of postconcussion headache.

Dizziness

The principal therapeutic agent useful in the treatment of vertigo and dizziness has been dimenhydrinate (Dramamine). This can be used in sizable doses, either orally or intramuscularly. It may also be supplemented by meclizine hydrochloride (Bonamine), cyclizine (Marezine), or meclizine and nicotinic acid (Antivert).

Psychogenic Symptoms

Reflecting once again on the psychological processes discussed earlier, we observe that the post-traumatic syndrome appears in large part, but not in a pejorative or condemning sense, to be iatrogenic. It is iatrogenic in the sense that much of it arises from interaction with doctors, hospitals, treatments, medical systems, and concepts of the self provided by surgical and medical diagnoses and treatments. It is not that the diagnosis and treatment are bad, but rather that during the course of the diagnosis and treatment processes there are multiple implants of anxiety and psychic conflict that burgeon into the problems seen in the deeply rooted and resistant post-traumatic syndrome.

Experience with related or similar conditions suggests that patients with the theoretically premonitory signs of later development of the post-traumatic syndrome can best be treated, in the neurosurgical situation itself, by recognizing their depressive or anxiety symptoms and probably by delaying hospital discharge until the surgical or medical staff and *the patient himself* can be assured that everything is in order in the central nervous system. We guess that many individuals who are strong potential candidates for the syndrome have simply been discharged too early! The psychological defense of denial will work to cover up even neurological deficits and even more to conceal anxiety, depression, or beginning somatization. Sensitivity to and recognition of them will do much to prevent the advance of these psychiatric problems, and if not, a more formal psychological treatment can intervene.

In treating the deeply rooted syndrome, as the patient passes from one specialist to another, the physician must not become angry and particularly should not develop puritanical rages about compensation. In most instances the problem consists not of laziness or greed but of deep-seated conflicts having to do with a sequence of inca-

pacity, humiliation, rage, and despair of doing any better with the world. It is better for the physician to have a scientific attitude and to avoid the compensation neurosis concept in diagnosis. A scientific attitude toward the problem of chronic pain entails recognition of the function of the reiterated expression of pain. These communications serve to discharge feelings that arise from unconscious conflicts and that can find no other means of expression.

The neurosurgeon may help his patient best by being willing to continue the relationship and by being sensitive to the psychological problems underlying the symptoms. He can avoid confrontations over the "real" cause of the problem and use medications judiciously if he attends to the thoughts and feelings associated with his prescriptions. Rehabilitation through job retraining and physical medicine is a useful adjunct. Referral for supportive psychotherapy, with the comment that the trauma has surely had emotional effects, will be most helpful if the neurosurgeon is willing to continue his relationship and can respond skillfully to the hostility that may arise. It is difficult to predict the correct responses for all patients. An example would be, if shame about the referral is causing anger, to emphasize the courage it takes to face problems and the truth about the self.

Generally, the psychological treatment of the syndrome requires a slowly progressive, gradual lessening of the severity of the problem and associated disabilities through acceptance of the patient and his difficult situation. To accomplish this, the physician must hold in check the pressures of therapeutic ambition.

REFERENCES

1. Barber, H. O.: Head injury: Audiological and vestibular findings. Ann. Otol., 78:239–252, 1969.
2. Cartlidge, N. E. F.: Post-concussional syndrome. Scot. Med. J., 23:103, 1978.
3. Caveness, W. F.: Posttraumatic sequelae. In Caveness, W. F., and Walker, A. E., eds.: Head Injury Conference Proceedings. Philadelphia, J. B. Lippincott Co., 1966.
4. Friedman, A. P.: The so-called posttraumatic headache. In Walker, A. E., Caveness, W. F., and Critchley, M., eds.: The Late Effects of Head Injury. Springfield Ill., Charles C Thomas, 1969.
5. Jacobsen, S. A.: The Posttraumatic Syndrome Following Head Injury. Springfield, Ill., Charles C Thomas, 1963.

6. Jacobsen, S. A.: Mechanisms of the sequelae of minor craniocervical trauma. *In* Walker, A. E., Caveness, W. F., and Critchley, M., eds.: The Late Effects of Head Injury. Springfield, Ill., Charles C Thomas, 1969.

7. Jennett, B.: Late effects of head injuries. In Scientific Foundations of Neurology. Critchley, E., ed. Philadelphia, F. A. Davis Co., 1972, pp. 441–451.

8. Penfield, W., and Norcross, N. C.: Subdural traction and posttraumatic headache study of pathology and therapeusis. Arch. Neurol. Psychiat., *36*:75–95, 1936.

9. Russell, W. R., and Smith, A.: Posttraumatic amnesia in closed head injury. Arch. Neurol., *5*: 4–17, 1971.

10. Rutherford, W. H., Merrett, J. D., and McDonald, J. R.: Sequelae of concussion caused by minor head injuries. Lancet, *1*:1–4, 1977.

11. Schuknect, H. F., Neff, W. D., and Perlman, H. B.: An experimental study of auditory damage following blows to the head. Ann. Otol., 60: 273–290, 1951.

12. Symonds, C.: Concussion and its sequelae. Lancet. *1*:1–5, 1962.

13. Taylor, A. R.: Postconcussional sequelae. Brit. Med. J., *3*:67–71, 1967.

14. Taylor, A. R., and Bell, T. K.: Slowing of cerebral circulation after concussional head injury. Lancet, *2*:178–180, 1966.

62

POST-TRAUMATIC
EPILEPSY

Even apparently trivial head injuries can be implicated as the basis for the genesis of single or chronically recurring seizures. Clearly, however, not all patients who sustain even severe head injuries develop seizures. Therefore, so that such patients can be given prognostic information, conditions that are likely to lead to seizures should be defined. In addition, if patients who are susceptible to seizures can be identified prior to the onset of the seizures, there is the hope that therapeutic measures can be applied to prevent the development of this chronic, and often difficult to treat, disorder.

The overall incidence of seizures following nonpenetrating head injuries is generally quoted at approximately 5 per cent and following injuries associated with penetrating wounds, at 20 to 60 per cent. The clinical value of these estimates is severely limited, however, by the great variability within these groups of patients. Attempts have therefore been made to define more precisely the likelihood of individual patients to develop seizures.

PROGNOSTIC VALUE OF FACTORS THAT INCREASE RISK OF POST-TRAUMATIC SEIZURES

Focal and Diffuse Brain Injury

Lacerations of the brain associated with depressed skull fractures appear to have the most serious consequences, as reflected by one estimate that as many as 90 per cent

of such patients may develop seizures.[21] This figure is higher than is generally reported, and more commonly reported figures are closer to 60 per cent for the patients who have the most severe of the penetrating injuries.[4,12,17]

The presence of intracranial hemorrhage with or without a penetrating wound also increases the risk of seizures. Seizures commonly follow intracerebral and subdural hemorrhages (40 per cent) while epidural hemorrhages are followed by seizures less frequently (10 per cent).[14,15]

A persistent focal neurological deficit such as hemiplegia testifies to both the severity and the location of the damage. In this case, the location of the injury as manifest by lateralized weakness is important, since lesions near the central sulcus are more likely to cause seizures than are wounds near the frontal or occipital poles,[19,27,28] For example, in one series 65 per cent of patients with wounds in the parietal region developed seizures, while only 39 per cent of patients with frontopolar lesions and 38 per cent of patients with occipital lesions were similarly afflicted.[27]

Evidence of diffuse brain dysfunction is an important predictor of the evolution of seizures. In this regard, the presence of post-traumatic amnesia of more than 24 hours' duration increases the likelihood of chronic seizures, especially in those patients with depressed fractures.[12] Why amnesia should have a greater significance in patients with open head injuries than in those with closed injuries is not clear.

The factors just enumerated are more or less indicators of the so-called "severity" of the lesion. "Severity" in this context remains undefined, however. Specifically, it is unclear whether the spatial extent of the damage has the same significance as the intensity or density of the pathophysiological changes. At present, available diagnostic techniques provide information regarding primarily the anatomical extent of the lesion. The intensity of pathophysiological abnormalities within the spatial limits of the lesion may only be surmised in most cases. Previous reports have not attempted to differentiate these two factors because of the inherent difficulties in making such distinctions.

Some studies have raised the interesting speculation that the relatively well-localized cortical lesion or cicatrix generally considered to be the fundamental cause of post-traumatic seizures may represent only a part of the pathophysiological condition induced by the injury.[25-27] It is argued that chronic seizure disorders will develop only if cortical scar formation is associated with more widespread or "centrally" located changes in neuronal activation and inhibition. These unresolved problems may be part of the reason that the occurrence of post-traumatic epilepsy cannot be predicted with any degree of accuracy in a particular case.

Pathophysiological Changes Associated With Injury

The various pathophysiological changes that may accompany head trauma include acute and chronic changes in cerebral circulation, mechanical effects of gliosis and the meningocerebral cicatrix, alterations in the blood-brain barrier and glial-neuronal relationships, as well as alterations of complex interneuronal relationships such as disruption of inhibitory systems.[11] It is also possible that some pathophysiological changes may be better predictors than others of the occurrence of seizures.

For example, Westrum and co-workers, after examining chronic experimental epileptogenic lesions and comparing them with human biopsy specimens, suggested that the neurons within epileptogenic foci may have fewer synaptic endings on their dendrites than those in normal tissue. They regarded this as evidence of partial deafferentation leading possibly to postsynaptic hypersensitivity.

Since it is very difficult to characterize directly and precisely the status of these potentially significant pathophysiological mechanisms following head injury, the clinically determined risk factors outlined earlier have been used to estimate the epileptogenic nature of the cerebral damage.

Interval Between Injury and Seizures

Seizures Occurring Soon After Injury

Jennett has provided evidence that the chance of recurrent or chronic seizures increases significantly if the patient's first seizure occurs within the first week after head injury. In a series of 1000 patients, late epilepsy occurred in 3 per cent of patients who had no seizures in the first week, but in 25 per cent of patients who did have a seizure in the first week. Further analysis revealed that while early epilepsy was associated with a greater incidence of late seizures, irrespective of the character of the injury, the effect was most striking following closed head injuries without intracranial hematomas (compare with opposite relationship of these two groups of patients with regard to post-traumatic amnesia.).[13-15]

Seizures during the first week represent a different entity from seizures after the first week.[14] This opinion is supported by the observation that the seizures during the first week are frequently of focal motor type (41 per cent), while similar seizures occurring later represent only 3.2 per cent of the total. In contradistinction, after the first week, partial complex seizures represent a significant percentage (22 per cent); this type is only rarely seen during the first week. Finally, while a seizure during the first week increases their likelihood, later more chronic seizures actually occur in less than one third of such patients. In contrast, 86 per cent of patients having their first seizure between one week and three months after the injury develop recurrent seizures.

Seizures immediately following head trauma (within the first hour), however, are distinct from those occurring between 1 and 24 hours after the injury. These occur only rarely and have no prognostic implications for later seizures.

The correlation of early seizures with late and generally more chronic seizures raises interesting questions in addition to being empirically valuable. It would be interesting to know what factors responsible for the development of late post-traumatic seizures are manifest in the occurrence of the early seizures. It is possible that early seizures are a reflection of the intensity and spatial extent of the damage caused by the trauma. This is unlikely, however, because seizures within the first week following apparently trivial head trauma carry the same implications as early seizures following severe brain damage.[12] An alternative view is that these early seizures may reflect congenital or constitutional factors in the patient's response to injury. On the other hand, although it is reasonable to assume that such factors exist, their presence remains to be demonstrated.[15] Evaluation of such constitutional factors is confounded, however, by the multifactorial basis for an individual's susceptibility to seizures.[16]

Chronic Seizure Disorders

In most instances post-traumatic epilepsy becomes most disabling when it is chronic in nature and is manifest as recurrent seizures. Earlier reports do not clearly differentiate between a chronic seizure disorder requiring continuing medications and one or more seizures that may occur after a head injury and then abate, never to recur. Part of the reason for such ambiguity is the difficulty of defining "recurrent seizures." There is no agreement as to how many seizures over what period of time should be considered as chronic or recurrent.

As already indicated, seizures occurring within the first week have been analyzed to determine their significance with regard to later, more chronically recurring seizures. Viewed from another perspective, however, approximately 50 per cent of patients having one or more seizures following a head injury stop having seizures. The criterion for cessation of seizures is a two-year seizure-free period.[2,4] The remission of the seizures is not related to the effects of anticonvulsant therapy and is thought to be a manifestation of the natural history of the disorder. The single most important criterion for determining whether seizures will cease is the frequency of the attacks. Those patients who have more than 10 seizures per year are likely to have persistent seizures. In addition, patients with fewer than 10 seizures per year are more likely to continue having seizures if the disorder has been present for five years or more.[3]

Patients who have sustained head injuries continue to be likely to develop a chronic seizure disorder for many years after the injury. In one series of 265 patients undergoing operations for intractable seizures, 24 per cent had had their first seizure within 6 months of the injury, 43 per cent within 12 months, 58 per cent within two years, 66 per cent within three years, and 78 per cent within five years.[23] In 8 per cent of the patients the first seizure occurred 10 years or more after the injury, the longest interval being 27 years.[12]

Age-Dependent Considerations

The age of the patient at the time of injury may alter the outlook for the future.[15] Early seizures occur more frequently in children under 5 years of age (9 per cent) as compared with patients 5 years of age or older (4 per cent), but there is no statistical difference in the incidence of late seizures (less than 5 years of age 19 per cent, more than 5 years old 26 per cent). Late seizures following early seizures occur more frequently, however, in patients 16 years of age or older (33 per cent) than in patients below the age of 16 (17 per cent), a statistically significant difference. It would appear, therefore, that children under the age of 5, and especially under the age of 1 year, develop early seizures more frequently than older persons, but may be less likely to develop a late chronic seizure disorder.[9]

Relative Influence of Individual Risk Factors

The relative importance of each of the risk factors has recently been outlined in a report offering a consise mathematical method of predicting post-traumatic epilepsy.[7] Each risk factor was given a value that was to be substituted into equations estimating the probability of post-traumatic seizures for a time between one week and five years after the injury. These risk factors are listed here to provide a concise description of their relative weight. The weight of each factor is represented by a number scaled to fit the equations and cannot be used directly to predict probability of seizures. For example, a depressed skull fracture is twice as important as a linear skull fracture and half as important as a dural tear.

0.05	Unconsciousness or amnesia for one hour or more
	Linear skull fracture
0.10	Persisting electroencephalographic abnormality
	Prefrontal or occipital damage
	Depressed skull fracture
	Infection (central nervous system)
0.15	Seizures in first week
	Temporal lobe damage
0.20	Hemiplegia, aphasia
	Intracranial hemorrhage
	Dural tear or missile wound
0.25	Central or parietal damage

According to the authors, when these factors are used in their formulae, which account for age and interval of time since the injury, they provide results that fit published data and predict with 95 per cent confidence the chance of post-traumatic epilepsy in single cases. Whether or not predictions based upon these formulae prove to be dependable remains to be determined.

The Electroencephalogram

The electroencephalogram offers little assistance defining the risk of chronic seizures. In fact, unequivocal epileptiform abnormalities (diffuse spike and wave complexes) are commonly found in children after injury and are not associated with the occurrence of later seizures.[5] When similar abnormalities are seen in adults the implication is that the trauma happened to a patient with pre-existing epilepsy.

In one study, repeated electroencephalograms were obtained on 80 patients who had sustained head trauma.[6] The first tracing was obtained during the first few hours following the injury. During the first few days abnormal patterns were the rule and provided no insight with regard to prognosis. Focal as well as diffuse abnormalities were seen. These abnormalities tended to disappear, and 40 per cent of the patients who eventually developed seizures had normal electroencephalograms prior to the first seizure.

Fifty per cent of the patients recovered clinically and their electroencephalograms became normal within 3 to 15 years. The abnormalities disappeared gradually, first becoming intermittent before disappearing entirely. In 25 per cent of the cases the electrical abnormalities persisted but the clinical manifestations disappeared. The electroencephalogram did provide prognostic information, however, after the first seizure. Under these conditions, the presence of focal electrographic abnormalities was associated with a recurrent seizure disorder in later years.

PROPHYLACTIC ANTICONVULSANT THERAPY

Within the past 10 years there has been increasing interest in the use of prophylactic anticonvulsant therapy for patients sustaining head trauma. The underlying assumption is that patients who sustain a head injury may develop a sequence of pathophysiological changes that will eventually lead to one or more seizures. It is further argued that some form of therapy shortly after the injury will interrupt the sequence of events in such a way as to decrease the likelihood of seizures in general and, most importantly, the development of a chronic seizure disorder. Only three partially controlled investigations may offer some support for this hypothesis.

In the first study, 100 World War II veterans were divided randomly into two groups. One group received 200 mg of diphenylhydantoin daily, while the other group served as controls. After four years, seizures had occurred in 38 per cent of the untreated groups, but only 4 per cent of the treated group had been similarly afflicted. These same patients were followed for an additional three years, and by that time 51 per cent of the untreated group and 6 per cent of the treated group had had seizures.[1] All types of seizures were included, and a patient with a single seizure was not differentiated from a patient with chronic recurrent seizures.

A subsequent study evaluated drug prophylaxis in 73 adults. The patients were randomly divided into a treated group (diphenylhydantoin 200 mg, phenobarbital 30 mg, daily) and an untreated group. None of the patients in the treated group had seizures, and the medication was discontinued after two years. No seizures were documented in these patients for another 32 months after the medications were discontinued. In contradistinction, 20.8 per cent of the patients not treated with prophylactic anticonvulsants developed seizures. Furthermore, even these patients became entirely seizure-free upon the introduction of anticonvulsants after their first seizure.

It is difficult to accept these data as being representative of all patients with head injuries. For example, in the earlier series, over 50 per cent of untreated patients developed seizures.[1] This is at considerable variance with other published figures and represents an expected frequency of occurrence that would be consistent only for the most severely injured patients.[4] Therefore, it is not easy to make the assumption that the treated and control groups are comparable. The later study offers figures that appear more representative.[20] In this case, however, there is some question about the criteria used to define genuine epileptic seizures as opposed to seizure-like phenomena, and the response to medications after the onset of seizures is considerably better than might ordinarily be expected.[22]

None of these reports provide information regarding serum levels of anticonvulsant agents. It is likely, however, that no more than a few of the patients achieved levels that could be considered therapeutic, considering the dosages used. This provides a basis for an entirely new notion: that anticonvulsants in subtherapeutic levels could conceivably have a prophylactic effect upon a developing post-traumatic seizure disorder.

In fact, not only is this concept innovative, it is the fundamental assumption underlying all reports supporting the use of prophylactic anticonvulsant medications. To date, there is no published evidence in support of this notion based upon documentation of serum anticonvulsant levels.

In order to test this hypothesis directly, a prospective, double-blind study was begun in 1970 and completed recently. The object of the study was to determine whether epileptogenic lesions could be prevented from developing after head injury if daily doses of 60 mg of phenobarbital and 200 mg of di-

phenylhydantoin were given prophylactically for 18 months. At the end of a 36-month period as well as in a three to six year follow-up of 103 patients there was no significant difference in seizure occurrence between the treated and untreated groups.[18] It appears, therefore, that prophylactic subtherapeutic doses of anticonvulsants (as determined by serum levels) are ineffective in reducing the probability of seizures in patients who have sustained head injuries.

Prophylactic anticonvulsant medications were also used in Vietnam between 1967 and 1970. A retrospective study to evaluate the occurrence of early seizures used the Registry of Head and Spinal Cord Injuries and reports of field surgeons to provide information on 1614 patients.[24] Of this group, 70 per cent (1136) received anticonvulsant therapy, while 29 per cent (465) received no prophylactic therapy. In 1 per cent (13) of the cases the presence or absence of a prophylactic regimen was unknown. Anticonvulsant therapy was begun within six hours of injury in about half the cases. Diphenylhydantoin was most commonly used in doses of 300 to 400 mg per day. Phenobarbital was used alone or in combination with diphenylhydantoin in 4 per cent and 3 per cent of the cases respectively. The usual route of administration was intramuscular initially and subsequently changed to oral. In 83 per cent of the cases the dura had been penetrated and the cortex damaged; linear depressed skull fractures accounted for 17 per cent. The incidence of early seizures in the treated group was 1.6 per cent (18 of 1136) and 3.7 per cent (17 of 465) in the untreated group. The difference of 2.1 per cent is not statistically significant.

In this series the effect of anticonvulsants on seizures occurring only within the first week was reviewed, and under the conditions of the study it is difficult to evaluate the effectiveness of the anticonvulsants. Since therapeutic levels of diphenylhydantoin or phenobarbital may not be reached for two weeks when the drugs are administered by the oral route, it is unlikely that any of these patients achieved therapeutically significant levels. In addition, the intramuscular route for administration of diphenylhydantoin is unreliable and is considered by many to be inappropriate under any circumstances.[31] Since it is possible to achieve therapeutic levels of diphenylhydantoin in a matter of hours, this no longer needs to be a problem in future studies.[29]

Therefore, evidence that is now available regarding the use of prophylactic anticonvulsant medication applies only to subtherapeutic levels of the drugs and the results of the existing studies are inconclusive at best. No studies that evaluate the effect of prophylactic anticonvulsants when used in dosages sufficient to produce therapeutic drug levels have been published.

Potential Difficulties Associated With Prophylactic Anticonvulsant Medications

Anticonvulsant drugs have potentially serious side effects. The risk admittedly is small, but nevertheless it is present. In addition, under certain circumstances they may be contraindicated in this population of patients. For example, Haque and associates have shown that the metabolic clearance rate of dexamethasone is increased by an average of 140 per cent after the administration of diphenylhydantoin.[8] Therefore, under conditions in which dexamethasone is being used to control brain edema, anticonvulsant therapy with diphenylhydantoin may be contraindicated.

The use of prophylactic anticonvulsants poses the additional problem of knowing when to discontinue the medication. Assuming that a patient who has never had seizures is started on anticonvulsants, what criteria can be used to determine when medications should be withdrawn?

The electroencephalogram offers a potential measure of the vulnerability of a patient to seizures. As indicated earlier, however, even a normal electroencephalogram, some time after the injury, provides no assurance that the patient will remain seizure-free. In addition, most physicians are hesitant to discontinue anticonvulsant medication in the face of an abnormal electroencephalogram, even in patients who have never had a seizure. The implication is that unequivocal epileptiform abnormalities on a record even in seizure-free patients suggest the presence of a potentially epileptogenic abnormality. This point of view is supported by Zivin and Ajmone Marsan, who found that 14.1 per cent of patients with unequivocal epileptiform complexes

on their electroencephalograms and no history of previous clinical seizures eventually develop seizures.[32] It is unknown whether these statistics can be applied to patients with a history of head trauma who are receiving anticonvulsant medications.

In summary, the benefit of prophylactic anticonvulsants to patients sustaining head trauma remains an unproved hope. Anticonvulsant therapy in such patients is not without risk, and the effect of the drugs upon coincident therapeutic measures needs to be considered. Finally, no criteria have been established for discontinuance of such medications.

If prophylactic anticonvulsants are to be employed in patients who have sustained head trauma before conclusive data regarding their efficacy have been obtained, the following guidelines are recommended:

1. The potential deleterious effects of anticonvulsant medications upon coincident therapeutic regimens should be considered.

2. Anticonvulsant levels should be monitored on a regular basis and therapeutic levels attained.

3. Appropriate routes of administration should be employed to maintain relatively constant blood levels of the drugs.

4. Periodic electroencephalographic evaluation, while of unproved benefit, may provide some indication of when to discontinue the medications.

5. Under ideal circumstances patients should be followed for five years.

REFERENCES

1. Birkmayer, W.: Die Behandlung der traumatischen Epilepsie. Wien. Klin. Wschr., 63:606–609, 1951.
2. Caveness, W. F.: Onset and cessation of fits following craniocerebral trauma. J. Neurosurg., 20:570–583, 1963.
3. Caveness, W. F.: Etiologic and provocative factors: Trauma. In Vinken, P. J., and Bruyn, G. W., eds.: Handbook of Clinical Neurology. Vol. 15. Amsterdam, North-Holland Publishing Co., 1974, pp. 274–294.
4. Caveness, W. F.: Epilepsy, a product of trauma in our time. Epilepsia, 17:207–215, 1976.
5. Courjon, J. A.: Posttraumatic epilepsy in electroclinical practice. In Walker, A. E., Caveness, W., and Critchley, M., eds.: The Late Effects of Head Injury. Springfield, Ill., Charles C Thomas, 1969, pp. 215–227.
6. Courjon, J.: A longitudinal electroclinical study of 80 cases of post-traumatic epilepsy observed from the time of the original trauma. Epilepsia, 11:29–36, 1970.

7. Feeney, M., and Walker, A. E.: Mathematical prediction of human post-traumatic epilepsy. Society for Neuroscience Abstracts III, 1977, p. 140.

8. Haque, N., Thrasher, K., Werk, E. E., Knowles, H. C., and Sholiton, L. J.: Studies on dexamethasone metabolism in man: Effect of diphenylhydantoin. J. Clin. Endocr., 34:44–50, 1972.

9. Hendrick, E. B., Harwood-Hash, D. C. F., and Hudson, A. R.: Head injuries in children. A survey of 4465 consecutive cases at the Hospital for Sick Children, Toronto, Canada. Clin. Neurosurg., 11:46–65, 1963.

10. Hoff, H., and Hoff, H.: Fortschritte in der Behandlung der Epilepsie. Mschr. Psychiat. Neurol., 114:105–118, 1947.

11. Jasper, H. H.: Physiopathological mechanisms of post-traumatic epilepsy. Epilepsia, 11:73–80, 1970.

12. Jennett, W. B.: Predicting epilepsy after blunt head injury. Brit. Med. J., 1:1215–1216, 1965.

13. Jennett, W. B.: Early traumatic epilepsy. Definition and identity. Lancet, 1:1023–1025, 1969.

14. Jennett, W. B.: Epilepsy after blunt (non missile) head injuries. In Walker, A. E., Caveness, W. F., and Critchley, M., eds.: The Late Effects of Head Injury. Springfield, Ill., Charles C Thomas, 1969, pp. 201–214.

15. Jennett, W. B.: Early traumatic epilepsy. Incidence and significance after nonmissile injuries. Arch. Neurol., 30:384–398, 1974.

16. Metrakos, J. D.: Genetics of epilepsy. The Lennox Lecture. American Epilepsy Society. 1975.

17. Ommaya, A. K.: Head injury in the adult. In Conn, H. F., ed.: Current Therapy. Philadelphia, W. B. Saunders Co., 1972, pp. 692–697.

18. Penry, J. K., White, B. G., and Brackett, C. E.: A controlled prospective study of the pharmacologic prophylaxis of post traumatic epilepsy. Neurology (Minneap.) 29:600–601, 1979.

19. Phillips, G.: Traumatic epilepsy after closed head injury. J. Neurol. Neurosurg. Psychiat., 17:1–10, 1954.

20. Popek, K., and Musil, F.: Klinický pokus o prevenci posttraumatické epilepsie po těžkých zraněnick mozku u dospělých. Čas. Lék. Čes., 108:133–147, 1969.

21. Ransohoff, J., Doyle, A., and Fleischer, A.: Head trauma—management of acute injury. In Conn, H. F., ed.: Current Therapy. Philadelphia, W. B. Saunders Co., 1977, pp. 767–770.

22. Rapport, R. L., and Penry, J. K.: Pharmacologic prophylaxis of post-traumatic epilepsy. Epilepsia, 13:295–304, 1972.

23. Rasmussen, T.: Surgical therapy of post-traumatic epilepsy. In Walker, A. E., Caveness, W. F., and Critchley, M., eds.: The Late Effects of Head Injury. Springfield, Ill., Charles C Thomas, 1969, pp. 277–305.

24. Rish, B. L., and Caveness, W. F.: Relation of prophylactic medication to the occurrence of early seizures following craniocerebral trauma. J. Neurosurg., 38:155–158, 1973.

25. Russell, W. R.: Disability caused by brain wounds; review of 1,166 cases. J. Neurol. Neurosurg. Psychiat., 14:35–39, 1951.

26. Russell, W. R.: The development of grand mal after missile wounds of the brain. Johns Hopkins Med. J., 122:250–253, 1968.

27. Russell, W. R., and Whitty, C. W. M.: Studies in traumatic epilepsy: Factors influencing the incidence of epilepsy after brain wounds. J. Neurol. Neurosurg. Psychiat., 15:93–98, 1952.

28. Walker, A. E., and Erculei, F.: Head Injured Men Fifteen Years Later. Springfield, Ill., Charles C Thomas, 1969.

29. Wallis, W., Kutt, H., and McDowell, F.: Intravenous diphenylhydantoin in treatment of acute repetitive seizures. Neurology (Minneap.), 18:513–525, 1968.

30. Westrum, L. E., White, L. E., and Ward, A. A.: Morphology of the experimental epileptic focus. J. Neurosurg., 21:1033–1046, 1964.

31. Wilensky, A. J., and Lowden, J. A.: Inadequate serum levels after intramuscular administration of diphenylhydantoin. Neurology (Minneap.) 23:318–324, 1973.

32. Zivin, L., and Ajmone-Marsan, C.: Incidence and prognostic significance of "epileptiform" activity in the EEG of non-epileptic subjects. Brain, 91:751–778, 1968.

63

PSYCHOLOGICAL TESTING AFTER CRANIOCEREBRAL INJURY

Neuropsychological studies of craniocerebral trauma have been concerned principally with identifying the nature of psychological deficits and the recovery process. These two areas (initial deficit and recovery potential) are obviously intertwined, and within them, a number of more specific questions have been investigated. For example, are there some types of initial deficits from which recovery occurs promptly, but others that represent, over time, persisting disabilities? To what extent can identification of the initial disability, coupled with an understanding of recovery potential, foster and promote the development and application of rehabilitation and training programs? Is it possible to develop a testing procedure that will permit accurate prediction for the individual patient of his recovery potential and eventual outcome? Plum has commented, "The capacity to predict accurately the outcome of serious neurological disease within the first few days of illness would possess many advantages."[15] Jennett has given a somewhat more detailed list of major questions concerning recovery from craniocerebral trauma. "What is the nature of the persisting disability? Can more scientifically based rehabilitation, including physical, mental, and social components, either accelerate the rate of recovery or reduce the ultimate degree of disability? Can the ultimate outcome be predicted in the acute stage; and can the amount of further improvement be estimated in the later stages of recovery?"[10] Jennett goes on to note that in his studies two factors appear to be most important: the patient's age and the duration of coma. These factors, however, would seem to be related to the severity of damage or degree of impairment, and the degree of impairment is quite variable among persons of any given age or for any duration of coma. Thus, it might be more productive to measure the degree of impairment directly as a basis for predicting outcome, as was done by Dikmen and Reitan and which is reported later in this chapter.

NEUROPSYCHOLOGICAL DEFICITS

There has been extensive research on late psychological effects of head injuries, particularly those sustained in war.[13,20–22] Systematic psychological studies of the recovery process, using extensive objective measures for evaluation, have been relatively lacking. Reports in the literature, as well as clinical observations, however, clearly indicate that recovery does occur. The criteria used to define recovery often are subjective, vague, or quite general in nature.[4,5,18] In some instances the recovery process has been studied only in specific areas of performance or with narrowly selected patient populations.[2,9] Few reports have dealt specifically with prediction of the capability of resuming pre-injury activities such as employment and self-care.[8,22] A

R. M. REITAN

number of more recent studies have, however, attempted to relate results obtained on the first clinical examination, very shortly after the injury, to general outcome criteria. Variables such as age, severity of the head injury, and pre-injury mental status have been identified in general terms as being related to eventual capability for occupational employment.

Dikmen and Reitan investigated a group of patients with cerebral concussion, cerebral contusion, and post-traumatic epilepsy as compared with control subjects, using an extensive battery of neuropsychological tests.[7] The battery consisted of 25 variables derived from the Wechsler-Bellevue Scale, Halstead's Neuropsychological Test Battery, and the Trail Making Test. The group with evidence of cerebral contusion (hemiplegia or hemiparesis, aphasia, homonymous visual field losses, or hemianesthesia) showed significant neuropsychological impairment, performing more poorly than either of the other groups on all 25 variables. The group with cerebral concussion (loss of consciousness, amnesia, confusion, irritability, headaches, nervousness, easy fatigability, and difficulty concentrating) showed some degree of impairment, but their test scores more closely resembled those of the controls than those of the group with cerebral contusion. When post-traumatic epilepsy was used as a criterion, the subjects, even though they had no signs of cerebral contusion, tended to perform less well than the group with concussion alone and, in fact, resembled the group of patients with both post-traumatic epilepsy and signs of cerebral contusion more closely than they did the controls. Thus, clinical signs of cerebral contusion seem to represent a significant variable with respect to the degree of neuropsychological deficit sustained by persons with head injuries, and the same seems to be true of post-traumatic epilepsy. In general, these results indicate that when cerebral tissue damage has been sustained, significant neuropsychological deficits are likely to be present. Of course, such deficits, even though often difficult to recognize in casual or even clinical examination of the patient (as contrasted with neuropsychological examination), may be of great significance with respect to the eventual ability of the patient to resume pre-injury activities and responsibilities.

PREDICTION OF POTENTIAL FOR RECOVERY

Jennett and his colleagues have made major progress in predicting outcome in individual patients following severe head injury, using clinical findings in the first few days following the injury. Teasdale and Jennett have devised a simple scale for assessing depth and duration of impaired consciousness and coma. The scale is based on three aspects of behavior: motor responsiveness, verbal performance, and eye opening.[19] These authors thought that the tests must be simple in order to achieve general acceptance and use in a wide range of hospitals staffed by persons without special training. Although the authors claim good agreement among judges, the evaluations are based essentially on subjective observations. Jennett and co-workers have shown that such sources of information can provide a relatively good basis for predicting outcome six months after severe head injury.[12] The predictive variables, evaluated on clinical examination during the first few days after the injury, include eye movements, pupillary response, motor responses, rankings from the coma scale just described, and age of the patient. While the criteria may seem to be based on information from rather simple sources, Jennett and his colleagues note that these values may yield up to 300 points of information for each subject, considering the fact that the examinations are repeated over several days. Thus, an extensive set of data is available for each subject. These data were used to predict outcome classified in the following categories: death, persistent vegetative state, severe disability, moderate disability, and good recovery. The time of six months after the injury was selected because Jennett and his co-workers believe that most of the recovery has occurred in the first six months.[3] The types of predictions made from the data were classified as those that could be made confidently and those in which confidence was less. Confident predictions could be made in 44 per cent of the cases in which examinations were made in the first 24 hours following severe head injury and in 52 to 61 per cent when data gathered over three days were available. When confident predictions were made, 96 to 98 per cent were correct as judged by the actual six-months outcome in 200 cases.

Overgaard and associates studied 201 patients who had sustained head injuries in road traffic accidents. They evaluated level of consciousness, motor patterns, and neuro-ophthalmological signs, and also considered the patient's age and blood pressure, and the presence of major complicating intracranial or extracranial injuries. They estimated adequacy of recovery in terms of the extent to which the patient was able to resume pre-injury activities. They found that the basic clinical signs, together with age and post-traumatic blood pressure, were related to functional recovery two to three years after the injury.[14] Bond, reporting on psychosocial outcome after severe head injury, used a neurophysical scale, a mental scale, and a social scale in 58 patients.[3] These scales have the advantage of being relatively simple to understand, but they are rather rough measures because they involve subjective ratings under only a limited number of categories. Bond found that duration of post-traumatic amnesia was significantly related to results obtained on these scales. In addition, he evaluated cognitive recovery by using the Wechsler Adult Intelligence Scale. This scale, however, was developed to measure intelligence in normal subjects rather than those with brain injury. While the Wechsler Scale is affected by brain injury, studies have shown that it is not as sensitive as tests developed specifically to measure neuropsychological deficits in patients with brain injury.[16] Thus, the validity of the results reported by Bond may be limited by the insensitivity of the tests used. Bond concluded that daily living was affected primarily by impairment of intellect and personality and, to a lesser extent, by physical incapacity. He found, however, that outcome was only rarely related to development of symptoms of mental illness.

Dikmen and Reitan have reported results of an extensive longitudinal study, conducted over an 18-month period, of 34 subjects with head injury.[6,7] Not all their subjects had sustained serious or severe head injuries and they probably were considerably less damaged than those reported by Jennett and his colleagues. Criteria for their inclusion in this study, however, were an altered state of consciousness (or objective evidence of brain damage when consciousness was not lost) plus a sufficiently serious head injury to require hospitalization. Each subject was given an extensive battery of neuropsychological tests within about 30 days after the injury, and the same battery was repeated at 12 and 18 months following the first testing. The measures covered areas of general intelligence, concept formation, problem-solving ability, memory, attention, and motor and emotional functions. This test battery required cooperation and a degree of alertness from each subject and, obviously, could not be administered until the subject had regained consciousness and was reasonably alert and able to cooperate. Thus, the conditions under which this study by Dikmen and Reitan was performed were basically different from those reported by many other investigators. The neuropsychological test battery had been specifically designed and previously tested for its adequacy in representing the full range of abilities included in normal and impaired brain functions, and it was not administered until the patient was ready for discharge from the hospital. In addition, the follow-up period extended for 18 months rather than only six months. While Jennett and his co-workers believe that most of the recovery occurs during the first six months (as is very probably true), more sensitive measures often show a significant degree of deficit that may extend for a considerably longer time. The longer-term follow-up is particularly important in patients who continue to have adjustment problems. The results of Dikmen and Reitan's study revealed that subjects with head injuries showed neuropsychological deficits, as compared with control subjects, across a broad range of measures, but, on repeated measurements at 12 and 18 months, showed significant improvement. The improvement from the first examination to the 12-month examination was appreciably greater than the improvement from 12 to 18 months. Improvement occurred on nearly every measure of intellectual and cognitive ability, but did not show up as consistently on measures of emotional status.[6,7]

Dikmen and Reitan divided the group of 34 subjects into those with more serious initial deficits and those with milder deficits for comparison of recovery potential. The group with greater initial deficits demonstrated a greater absolute degree of recovery on the various tests, although even at 18 months following the injury they continued to show greater residual deficits than the group with milder damage. Since no special retraining or rehabilitation procedures were applied to any of the subjects (the improvement represented natural biological processes and environmental factors) it is interesting to note that these influences were "kinder" to those with more severe initial impairment even though the more severely injured never reached the level of those with initially milder impairment.[6,7]

Dikmen and Reitan also did a detailed evaluation of the clinical findings for each subject. Even in individual cases the area of greatest recovery represented the functions that initially showed the greatest deficit. Thus, it appeared that the weakest or most impaired areas of ability showed the greatest degree of recovery over the 18-month period. The clinical evaluation of each subject also revealed an unexpected result. Eight of the thirty-four subjects, who had shown improvement at the 12-month examination, demonstrated definite deterioration at the time of the 18-month examination. This deterioration tended to occur in the areas of initial impairment. No corresponding positive signs were present on clinical neurological examination or were elicited on electroencephalography in these eight subjects. Computed tomography was not available. The neuropsychological impairment was definite, however, even though unexplained, and should be further investigated.

The final aspect of the study by Dikmen and Reitan concerned prediction of neuropsychological status to be expected at 18 months following the injury. On the basis of neuropsychological variables obtained during the first examination (within about one month following the head injury), an attempt was made to predict outcome. The 34 subjects were divided into groups; those who had essentially normal results or showed only mild impairment, and those who were definitely impaired at 18 months following the injury. The initial neuropsychological data had classified 31 of the 34 patients (91 per cent) in their correct group. The three "errors" were instances in which patients were, at the end, more impaired than had been predicted on the basis of the

initial neuropsychological data. Obviously, these findings must be replicated in order to determine the clinical usefulness of the results and the extent to which they will hold up. It does appear, however, that detailed neuropsychological evaluation may elicit findings that are closely related to the long-term outcome in patients with head injuries.

ILLUSTRATIVE CASE HISTORIES

A Question of Brain Damage

In many instances of brain injury the diagnosis is well established because clear evidence of brain damage has been observed. In other instances, especially those involving closed head injuries, it is more difficult to determine whether any significant damage to the brain has been sustained.

In the case of the 19-year old man described here, neurological findings were minimal.

The subject had been in an auto accident six months before the current examination. He had sustained a head injury and, though not unconscious, was in a confused state for about one week. Because of a serious fracture of the femur he had been hospitalized for four months at that time. Since the head injury, he had experienced frequent headaches, he tired easily, and he complained of difficulty in concentrating. The subject had completed one year in college and at present was in his second year. He had been a good student in high school and in his first year in college. After the first semester of the second year, he had transferred to another school because his performance had dropped off; his parents felt that the standards of the school he had been attending might be somewhat stringent. Nevertheless, he continued to have academic difficulties even in the college to which he had transferred. Because of this the parents were concerned about the possibility that the patient might have sustained brain damage in the accident. Upon physical examination, neurological findings were essentially normal. Electroencephalographic tracings were obtained and the results indicated the presence of a dysrhythmia, grade I, involving both temporal areas. No further positive results were obtained, and the question of possible brain damage in association with the head injury sustained six months earlier was not definitely resolved. The patient was referred for neuropsychological evaluation because the neurological surgeon who had examined him was aware that neuropsychological deficits might well be present, even though results of the neurological examination were essentially negative.

The Wechsler-Bellevue Scale and Halstead-Reitan Battery were administered to the subject. The Wechsler-Bellevue Scale yielded a full-scale IQ of 105, with a verbal IQ of 112 and a performance IQ of 95. In spite of these relatively adequate IQ values, the patient obtained a Halstead Impairment Index of 0.8, which is well into the range characteristic of cerebral damage. The Halstead Impairment Index is a summary value based on the tests in the Halstead Neuropsychological Test Battery. Inspection of the results for the individual tests in this battery failed to indicate any striking or severe areas of deficit. In most respects this patient performed reasonably well, although he consistently obtained scores that were just within the limits characteristic of brain damage as contrasted with normal brain function.

The major indications of cerebral damage, however, were not derived from the level of performance shown by this subject but instead from comparisons of the functional efficiency of the two sides of the body. Tests of lateral dominance indicated that the patient was strongly right-handed, right-footed, and right-eyed, but, nevertheless, he performed poorly with his right hand as compared with his left hand. For example, finger tapping speed was somewhat slower with the right hand than with the left hand (highly unusual for persons with normal brain function). The patient also performed poorly with his right hand as compared with his left hand on the Tactual Performance Test and, when using both hands on the same task, did more poorly than when using his left hand alone. This provided rather definite evidence that the right hand tended to impair efficiency of performance in a complex psychomotor task when a bimanual effort was being made. While these results, indicating deficit on the right side, seem to implicate the left cerebral hemisphere, other findings suggested some bilateral cerebral damage. The subject had difficulties relating to tactile form recognition in both hands.

The overall set of test results indicated some impairment in level of performance on those tests that are especially sensitive to the organic integrity of the cerebral hemispheres and implicated both cerebral hemispheres, although the left cerebral hemisphere seemed to be principally involved. Independent interpretation of these results, without reference to the history of the subject or other findings, suggested that brain injury might be responsible for some impairment of academic aptitude and proficiency, since the left cerebral hemisphere subserves language functions and the symbolic aspects of verbal communication. Thus, the neuropsychological test results not only recapitulated the history of this patient with respect to traumatic involvement of the brain but also provided a basis for understanding the difficulty he was having in his college work.

Resolution of problems of this type may be particularly helpful inasmuch as they provide an understanding of the patient's complaints and, in many instances, forestall the tendency to jump to the conclusion that emotional or affective factors are responsible for the patient's difficulties. In this case, it was apparent that the patient needed some special tutoring in order to make better progress in college and that a direct and straightforward approach in academic instruction in all probability was most appropriate to his academic difficulties. Although the results on this patient indicate that neuropsychological examination may contribute directly to knowledge of the organic status of the brain, it should be noted that the principal expectation from neuropsychological testing should relate to description of abilities of the subject and that conclusions regarding the organic condition of the brain represent inferences based on behavioral measurements rather than direct evidence.

Psychiatric Complications Associated with Closed Head Injury

This patient, a 15-year-old boy, had sustained a head injury when he collided with a car while riding his bicycle. The automobile hit the back of the bicycle and the patient was thrown into the air. His head hit the windshield of the car with sufficient force to shatter the glass. The patient had a swollen area at the back of his head and was unconscious for 15 to 20 minutes. He was relatively incoherent for an additional period of time after regaining consciousness. Physical examination was performed immediately following this and showed the presence of multiple abrasions and superficial lacerations of the head, face, upper and lower extremities, and abdomen. Skull x-rays, however, showed no fracture. Although the patient had some tenderness and swelling in the right occipital area, the optic discs were flat. The patient went to bed shortly after the physical examination and slept for almost 24 hours. He seemed to be normal upon rising.

Ten months after the accident the parents brought the boy to a neurological surgeon for further examination because they had observed behavioral changes. They reported that the patient seemed moody, was sometimes quite withdrawn and irritable, and had engaged in unusual and erratic behavior. For example, a number of times the patient had arisen after the rest of the family had been asleep for several hours and had wandered about the city. He seemed to be unclear about these activities when questioned and may possibly have had some degree of amnesia for these episodes. Physical neurological examination was essentially normal at this time, and electroencephalographic examination also yielded normal results. The patient was referred for neuropsychological examination not because of the possibility of brain injury per se but instead to determine whether brain damage might have been a contributing factor to the boy's behavioral changes.

Neuropsychological test results indicated that the general intelligence of this subject was in the average range, but low scores on the Picture Arrangement and Block Design subtests of the Wechsler-Bellevue Scale suggested the possibility of some right cerebral dysfunction. More convincing evidence was obtained from Halstead's Neuropsychological Test Battery. Not only did the level of performance indicate mild cerebral damage but a number of comparisons of the functional efficiency of the two sides of the body, as well as the relationships of various test scores, indicated involvement of both cerebral hemispheres. Independent interpretation of the test results suggested that the findings were perfectly compatible with a hypothesis of a closed head injury sustained sometime in the past. It was noted, however, that the basic adaptive abilities of the patient were not severely impaired. Evidence from the Minnesota Multiphasic Personality Inventory indicated that the patient was quite disturbed from an affective point of view and functioned under a great deal of emotional tension. In fact, the indications of emotional disturbance were sufficiently severe to recommend that the patient obtain psychiatric treatment. It appeared, since his basic abilities were intact, that he was potentially able to profit from this type of treatment with respect to solution of his problems.

Prior evidence has suggested that trauma of the brain might, in certain instances, be a factor that tends to precipitate the expression of pre-existing behavioral aberrations.[1] In fact, among those patients who demonstrate psychotic behavior following brain injury, a review of premorbid personality indicates that the psychotic behavior seems only to represent an exaggeration of the earlier tendencies. It would appear from such findings that development of bizarre or deviant behavioral tendencies may be precipitated by injuries of the brain and that neuropsychological examination may contribute to understanding of such patients.

Recovery of Function Following Severe Brain Injury

The patient was a 21-year-old man who was in his third year of college when he sustained a head injury in a football game. Although he was conscious and rational for about one half hour after the injury, he complained of a severe headache. Then he lapsed into a deep coma after experiencing a decerebrate type of seizure. On admission to the hospital, a lumbar puncture revealed blood-tinged cerebrospinal fluid. He was extremely ill for the next week, although various diagnostic procedures did not reveal any specific lesion. Pneumoencephalography, performed one week after admission, showed a shift of the ventricular system from right to left. The patient underwent an operation at which a solid subdural hematoma, approximately 4 to 5 mm in maximal thickness, was removed from over the entire right cerebral hemisphere. The patient showed gradual improvement during the next two and one half weeks although he had weakness of his right limbs and the right side of his face. Language functions and spontaneous speech also were impaired. One month after the injury he was able to be up, and his speech and level of consciousness appeared to be approximately normal. Neurological examination at this time showed the presence of a left lower quadrantic homonymous visual field defect and a slight residual right hemiparesis. He was, however, noted to be quite alert and was able to engage in normal daily activities. Neuropsychological examination was performed the day before the patient's discharge, just less than seven weeks after the injury occurred.

The results indicated that the patient was seriously impaired and had evidence of bilateral cerebral damage. He showed no definite symptoms of aphasia, but certain mild difficulties that he had in dealing with the symbolic aspects of language functions implied the presence of deficits in that area. The Wechsler-Bellevue Scale yielded a verbal IQ of 110, performance IQ of 88, and full-scale IQ of 99. The patient did poorly on the Block Design and Digit Symbol subtests as well as on the Digit Span subtest. Since the patient had been a successful third-year college student prior to the injury, these scores strongly suggested that at present he was considerably impaired.

Even more pronounced evidence of impairment was obtained from Halstead's Neuropsychological Test Battery. The patient obtained an Impairment Index of 1.0, indicating that on all the tests in this battery his scores fell in the range characteristic of persons with cerebral damage as compared with persons having normal brain function. The patient also did poorly on the Trail Making Test and had great difficulty in alternating between numbers and letters in Part B. While he performed reasonably well on certain sections of the Category Test, on other parts he demonstrated great confusion with respect to organizing diverse stimulus material in a meaningful way, formulating hypotheses that were relevant to his observations of the stimulus material, and understanding the essential nature of the problem situations. It was clear that the patient was seriously impaired in analytical reasoning and logical analysis. He also performed very poorly on the Tactual Performance Test and had great difficulty placing the blocks in their proper spaces in the board while blindfolded. It was apparent that this subject had some impairment in ability to deal with spatial configurations and also in adapting to the novel aspects of this type of problem.

Additional results indicated that the patient was impaired in incidental memory, since he did poorly when asked to recapitulate aspects of situations to which his attention had not been immediately directed. Motor and sensory-perceptual tasks also were performed poorly, especially on the right side. Although the patient was definitely right-handed, his finger tapping speed, though somewhat slow in both hands, was clearly impaired in his right hand as compared with the left. He had mild difficulty in tactile finger localization on both hands but was seriously impaired in fingertip number writing perception on his right hand only. These various results clearly implicated both cerebral hemispheres but suggested that the left hemisphere was actually somewhat more seriously damaged than the right, in spite of the fact that the subdural hematoma had been removed from the right cerebral hemisphere.

The patient was examined again three months later. At this time his verbal IQ was 121, performance IQ 122, and full-scale IQ 124. It was apparent that he had made excellent progress in recovering his general intelligence, the greatest improvement occurring in the areas that previously had been identified as showing the major deficits. Even more striking improvement occurred in the patient's ability in logical analysis and analytical reasoning. He performed well within the normal range on this type of task, as contrasted with the severe impairment shown on the initial examination. He improved greatly on the Tactual Performance Test and required just more than one third of the original time for completion of the task. In addition, evidence of incidental alertness and memory was now well within the normal range. The patient continued to have some difficulty on the Trail Making Test

and found it especially difficult to keep both the alphabetical and numerical series in mind at the same time as he alternated between them. Finger tapping speed was still somewhat depressed in both hands but showed clear improvement, especially on the right side. The overall results, while still indicating some mild impairment, were approaching the normal range. On the basis of these findings it was recommended that the patient begin preparing for resumption of his college education the following fall. Even though the test results were essentially within the normal range, past experience has indicated that the intellectual and cognitive abilities of persons who have been impaired are not as capable of withstanding pressure and stress as are those of the person who has sustained no impairment to begin with. Thus, it was recommended that the patient begin studying on his own and possibly auditing classes rather than immediately accepting full responsibility for his academic performance. It was thought that this type of preparation would enable him to resume his regular college program in the fall, approximately six months later.

In order to be sure that improvement was continuing, however, the patient was re-examined shortly before the beginning of the fall semester. The results indicated continued improvement. The few remaining areas of deficit were now within normal limits, and the general picture of recovery appeared to be nearly complete. The subject resumed his academic training and made satisfactory progress. Psychological testing was done annually for the next two years; the improvement achieved by this patient appeared to be secure. The last examination, which was essentially within normal limits for a person of superior general intelligence, was done after the subject had successfully completed college.

It is apparent that difficulties exist in correlating the exact location of the lesion with the psychological deficits in many patients with brain injuries. Nevertheless, assessment of the initial deficits and the rate of recovery can represent important contributions, particularly because of the inaccuracies inherent in gross observational judgments of the potential of individuals for undertaking high-level tasks. It is entirely possible that with the usual clinical assessment this patient might have been encouraged to re-enter college after missing only a single semester. Retrospectively it appears that this would have been a mistake. Even though the patient had made good progress by this time, he showed areas of weakness and probably would have had difficulty resuming his normal academic role. If a patient experiences failure after sustaining a brain injury, it often can seriously impair his confidence and undermine his ability to exploit his full potential after his recovery has become more complete. In many instances in which recommendations are made on the basis of casual observations of the patient's deficits and strengths, the patient is not able to fulfill the responsibilities implicit in the task he has undertaken and consequently experiences failure. Often the next step is to recommend undertaking somewhat less demanding tasks, only to have the patient fail again. After several such experiences of failure, the patient is unable to do tasks or meet demands that should be well within his range of capability. It is, therefore, particularly important that patients with injuries of the brain be permitted to start with relatively simple tasks from which it is possible to derive a sense of mastery and success and to experience the positive reinforcement that is implicit in successful performance, rather than to experience the sense of failure and personal inadequacy that accompanies deficient performance.

Approaches to Rehabilitation and Training

Relatively little formal work has been done to develop methods of retraining higher-level brain functions following deficits resulting from injury. It has been well demonstrated in individual cases, however, that considerable improvement may occur. Sometimes the improvement occurs spontaneously, as in the previous patient, but in other instances deficits remain relatively permanent and a special training program must be instituted.

The following case is a typical example of such a problem.

A 28-year-old-man fell and suffered severe injury of both frontal lobes while climbing a utility pole. A crosspiece of the pole pierced his forehead, causing a compound depressed skull fracture and damage to the frontal lobes. The brain was extremely edematous, and bilateral frontal tissue removal was necessary to relieve the pressure. For two weeks following the operative repair the patient was not responsive. After 17 days he began to talk and was rational in a general sense even though his responses to many situations seemed rather inappropriate. His

physical recovery, however, continued to be routine.

Neuropsychological examination was performed one month after the injury had been sustained and shortly before the patient was ready for discharge from the hospital. The results indicated that he was impaired in a number of ways, but his most outstanding difficulty was impairment on the Category Test. He appeared almost completely unable to comprehend relationships among the stimulus figures, to generate hypotheses concerning their organization, or to understand the essential nature of the problems involved. Although able to describe his observations of the stimulus material in concrete terms, he was entirely unable to analyze relationships or engage in logical reasoning processes. This type of deficit has frequently been attributed specifically to frontal lobe damage and certainly is seen in such instances, but it is also one of the significant aspects of impairment in many patients with brain lesions, regardless of their location. In this instance, it constituted a very significant feature of the deficits shown by the patient.

Approximately six months after the injury the patient was able to return to work, although it was recognized that the type of job he could fill must be a very routine one. He obtained a job with a maintenance crew of a small town and was able to perform simple routine jobs of a concrete nature, such as cutting weeds. When given a specific task that was repetitive in nature and did not require independent decisions or serial judgment, he performed reasonably well. It was apparent that he was motivated to do well and did his best to follow instructions. As his supervisor began to give him more responsibility, however, his difficulties became apparent. Although the supervisor had known the patient before the injury and had considered him to be a competent person, he soon decided that he could not continue to employ him. For example, when the patient was asked to care for a vehicle belonging to the city, he applied paste wax directly on top of accumulated dirt instead of washing the car first. It seemed that he had little ability to recognize the sequential aspects of procedures that involved multiple steps. In a second incident the patient was asked to back up a truck that was being used for collecting trash. He complied, but without wondering if anyone was behind the truck and without giving any advance warning; he almost ran down another worker. In reporting this incident the supervisor concluded that it was not possible to let the patient try to do anything on his own, that the patient did not put "two and two together," and that he did not seem to have the basic common sense of a child. Essentially, it appeared that the patient's difficulties were in line with expectation on the basis of the type of serious impairment shown in neuropsychological examination. It was finally decided to attempt to retrain this patient with special emphasis on developing ability in seeing relationships between events and in using good judgment.

The retraining efforts began with having the patient sort simple material into groups according to principles that he devised himself. In his first efforts the principles obviously did not apply to the groupings that he effected, and only with careful coaching and instruction was he able gradually to begin to understand how various items and objects went together. He had particular difficulty learning to substitute one criterion or principle for another. For example, when he had grouped objects on the basis of a particular criterion, such as color, it was impossible for him to think of the objects according to other possible criteria, such as functional utility. Another training procedure involved repeated administration of forms of the Category Test until gradually he began to understand the principles that were implicit in organization of the stimulus material. During this training the patient did not show particular progress in practical everyday activities. Following one training session, the patient failed to arrive home in his car at the usual time. His wife borrowed a neighbor's car and retraced the route that the patient would have taken. She found him in his car, pulled over to the side of the road, about three blocks from the neuropsychology laboratory. He had been sitting there for about three hours. When asked what the problem was, he said he didn't know; the car had just stopped. He had not been able to postulate the reason, but a quick inspection showed that he was out of gasoline. He was asked why he had not made a telephone call for help from one of the adjacent buildings and responded that he hadn't thought of that. He finally was asked what he *had* been doing and he indicated that he had been observing all license plates of passing cars so that he would be able to recognize one coming from his home town, jump out of his car, stop the vehicle, and ask for help.

After several months of working with the patient, another plan for training was devised. The patient was given several words at the top of a piece of paper and was told to write a story that would incorporate each of the words as essential features in the story. His first attempts consisted merely of writing separate sentences, each of which contained one of the words. There was no apparent relationship between the sentences nor did they tell any meaningful story. This kind of effort, together with careful explanation and illustration of what could be done with the words, was continued with the patient until he gradually began to form some connection between them. Eventually the patient reached a point at which he was rather proficient in this type of task and began to see relationships that might possibly exist between the words. In fact, eventually he showed a considerable degree of flexibility in performance and was able to take the same set of words and generate a new story. It was at this point that the patient's supervisor reported that he had begun to make practical progress in his working situation. In time the patient returned to the point at which he was judged to be a useful and satisfactory employee even though he needed close supervision and was not able to plan and carry out his own activities in an independent fashion. Nevertheless, he had become occupationally productive, whereas previously he had not been able to fill even the most simple type of job.

It appears that there are three major areas of psychological deficit that are associated with cerebral damage. One relates to the use of language for communication, another to organization of spatial and temporal relationships, and a third to logical analysis, concept formation, and reasoning ability. Many patients demonstrate deficits in all these areas simultaneously, but others have their major problems in one area or another. Careful evaluation of the psychological strengths and weaknesses of individual subjects following cerebral damage may provide a sound basis for developing appropriate rehabilitation programs, even though a great deal of developmental work is needed in this area. Prior results indicate that the Halstead-Reitan Neuropsychological Test Battery is especially useful in this regard because of its sensitivity to the many complex aspects of psychological functions represented by the brain.[17]

REFERENCES

1. Aita, J. A., and Reitan, R. M.: Psychotic reactions in the late recovery period following brain injury. Amer. J. Psychiat., *105*:161–169, 1948.
2. Becker, B.: Intellectual changes after closed head injury. J. Clin. Psychol., *31*:307–309, 1975.
3. Bond, M. R.: Assessment of psychosocial outcome after severe head injury. *In* Porter, R., and Fitzsimons, D. W., eds.: Outcome of Severe Damage to the Central Nervous System: CIBA Foundation Symposium 34 (New Series). Amsterdam, Elsevier, 1975, pp. 141–157.
4. Carlsson, C. A., Essen, C. V., and Lofgren, J.: Factors affecting the clinical course of patients with severe head injuries. J. Neurosurg., *29*: 242–251, 1968.
5. Cole, E. M.: Intellectual impairment in head injury. Chapter 19. Ass. Res. Nerv. Ment. Dis. Proc., *24*:473–479, 1945.
6. Dikmen, S., and Reitan, R. M.: Psychological deficits and recovery of functions after head injury. Trans. Amer. Neurol. Ass., *101*:72–77, 1976.

7. Dikmen, S., and Reitan, R. M.: Neuropsychological performance in post-traumatic epilepsy. Epilepsia, *19*:177–183, 1978.

8. Dresser, A. C., Meirowsky, A. M., Weiss, G. H., McNeel, M. L., Simon, A. G., and Caveness, W. F.: Gainful employment following head injury. Arch. Neurol., *29*:111–116, 1973.

9. Gronwall, D. M. A., and Wrightson, P.: Delayed recovery of intellectual function after minor head injury. Lancet, *14*:605–609, 1974.

10. Jennett, B.: Scale, scope and philosophy of the clinical problem. *In* Porter, R., and Fitzsimons, D. W., eds.: Outcome of Severe Damage to the Central Nervous System. CIBA Foundation Symposium 34 (New Series). Amsterdam, Elsevier, 1975, pp. 3–21.

11. Jennett, B., and Bond, M. R.: Assessment of outcome after severe brain damage—a practical scale. Lancet, *1*:480–484, 1975.

12. Jennett, B., Teasdale, G., Braakman, R., Minderhoud, J., and Knill-Jones, R. P.: Predicting outcome in individual patients after severe head injury. Lancet, *1*:1031–1034, 1976.

13. Newcombe, F.: Missile Wounds of the Brain. London, Oxford University Press, 1969, pp. vi, 145.

14. Overgaard, J., Hvid-Hansen, O., Land, A. M., Pedersen, K. K., Christensen, S., Haase, J., Hein, O., and Tweed, W. A.: Prognosis after head injury based on early clinical examination. Lancet, *2*:631–635, 1973.

15. Plum, F.: Opening remarks. *In* Porter, R., and Fitzsimons, D. W., eds.: Outcome of Severe Damage to the Central Nervous System. CIBA Foundation Symposium 34 (New Series). Amsterdam, Elsevier, 1975, pp. 1–2.

16. Reitan, R. M.: The comparative effects of brain damage on the Halstead Impairment Index and the Wechsler-Bellevue Scale. J. Clin. Psychol., *3*:281–285, 1959.

17. Reitan, R. M., and Davison, L. A., eds.: Clinical Neuropsychology: Current Status and Applications. Washington, D.C., V. H. Winston & Sons, 1974.

18. Russell, W. R.: The Traumatic Amnesias. London, Oxford University Press, 1971.

19. Teasdale, G., and Jennett, B.: Assessment of coma and impaired consciousness. A practical scale. Lancet, *2*:81–84, 1974.

20. Teuber, H.-L.: Neglected aspects of the posttraumatic syndrome. *In* Walker, A. E., Caveness, W. F., and Critchley, M., eds.: The Late Effects of Head Injury. Springfield, Ill., Charles C Thomas, 1969, pp. 13–34.

21. Walker, A. E., and Erculei, F.: Head Injured Men. Springfield, Ill., Charles C Thomas, 1969.

22. Walker, A. E., and Jablon, S.: A Follow-up Study of Head Wounds in World War II. V. A. Monograph, Washington, D.C., U.S. Government Printing Office, 1961.

64

POST-TRAUMATIC ARACHNOID CYSTS

A skull fracture occurring in infancy or childhood ordinarily heals without difficulty. Rarely, steady enlargement of a skull fracture following a head injury, particularly in the first year of life, is caused by a post-traumatic arachnoid cyst.

ETIOLOGY AND PATHOLOGY

In 1953, Taveras and Ransohoff proposed that the mechanism for production of expanding fractures was as follows: "Trauma produces a skull fracture and an underlying dural tear. At the same time there is probably sufficient subarachnoid hemorrhage to hinder the local circulation of cerebrospinal fluid. The arachnoid membrane projects out through the dural tear into the fracture site. This trapped arachnoidal hernia, aided by the normal pulsations of the brain, gradually erodes the edges of the bone and at the same time compresses the underlying cortex. There must be some degree of ball valve mechanism at work also, with the cerebrospinal fluid having easier ingress into than egress from the cyst. Arachnoidal adhesions about the margin of the lesion probably also play a part in trapping the fluid locally." The authors felt that the "dural tear is the single most important factor in the pathogenesis of these lesions and that without it the fracture would heal as expected."[13] At operation, the skin and galea are intact. The pericranium is intact or enters the fracture to attach to one dural edge (Fig. 64–1A and B). The inner table of the bone is more eroded than the outer, producing a saucer shape. The dural edges may be markedly recessed, necessitating removal of bone for its identification. The arachnoid cyst is filled with clear fluid and is sealed off from the surrounding subarachnoid space by scar tissue. The brain may be depressed. If the pia is torn, brain may be herniated upward and fill the cyst and fracture (Fig. 64–1C). Brain may be embedded in pericranium. With loss of brain substance, the ventricle may be enlarged and, rarely, may communicate with the cyst. Destruction of underlying brain is variable.

In 1961, Lende and Erickson reviewed the literature and felt there were more factors involved in the production of meningeal cysts than "an unsuspected dural tear," for in his fifth case the "loss of the dura mater was greater in extent than the loss of bone," indicating a deficiency of the dura mater greater than a simple tear occurring at the time of injury.[7]

Few experimental studies related to this problem are recorded. Müller advanced the hypothesis that the endocranial surface is molded by the surface of the arachnoid, which in turn duplicates the contours of the brain because it is held in place by the arachnoid trabeculae. If these trabeculae are severed, local unrestricted pressure of the cerebrospinal fluid is transmitted to the overlying bone, causing elevation of the skull.[8] Darlington showed that experimentally induced irregularity on the surface of the brain imprinted itself on the inner surface of the skull.[1] Keener, studying the effect of dural defects under normal bone, concluded that the primary pathological factor in the production of growing fractures in childhood was the presence of a "persistent dural defect."[6]

In 1967, Goldstein and co-workers noted that experimentally produced expanding

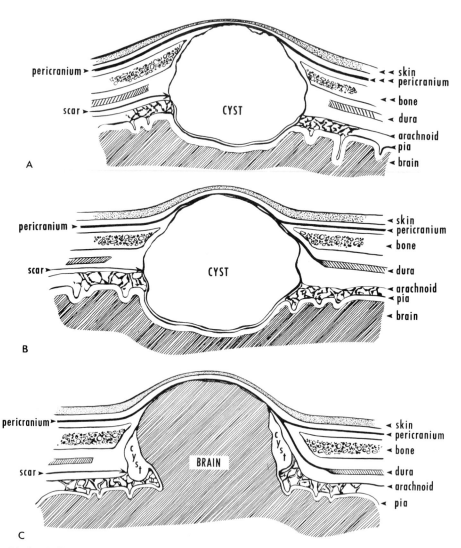

Figure 64–1 *A*. Post-traumatic arachnoid cyst with intact pericranium, erosion of internal table, recession of dura beneath bone edges, partitioning of cyst from subarachnoid space by scar, and depression of underlying brain. *B*. In this variety, pericranium with underlying dura is continuous through the fracture line. *C*. Pial tear with herniation of the brain into the cyst and fracture line.

craniotomy lines did not occur unless there was an open dura and arachnoid.[2] Additional pial, brain, or ventricular damage did not increase the incidence of growing fracture. Therefore, these latter components appeared to be of secondary importance in the production of growing fractures. It was also noted that the formation of a cyst or pouch increased the incidence of enlarging craniotomy lines more than simple opening of the dura and arachnoid. It appeared that it was not the simple pulsation of fluid against the bone, but rather fluid in a cyst or pouch that produced the higher incidence of bone erosion (cf. Fig. 64–1). In a later

study, Rosenthal and associates showed that the traumatic arachnoid cyst did not communicate with the rest of the subarachnoid space.[11]

SYMPTOMS AND CLINICAL COURSE

Commonly, a linear or diastatic parietal skull fracture occurs in a child under the age of three. Nothing unique can be noted about the manner in which the initial cranial trauma occurs. The scalp overlying the fracture is almost never broken at the time

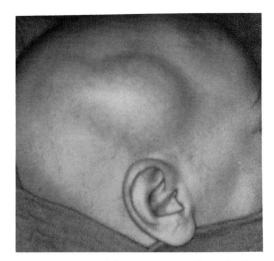

Figure 64–2 Clinical appearance of growing fractures.

of injury. A cephalhydrocele, or collection of cerebrospinal fluid beneath the scalp, commonly follows the head injury (Fig. 64–2). This may occur rapidly or be delayed in onset. Initial differentiation from hematoma may be difficult, and early puncture may yield bloody fluid, but later development of pulsation and aspiration of clear fluid establish its origin. Ordinarily such a collection of cerebrospinal fluid is transient, and the detail of its existence may be missing from the history when the patient presents with a cranial defect months or years later.

A latent period from 2 to 12 years occurs, during which unsuspected enlargement of the fracture line occurs. When the bony defect is large enough for the parents to see or feel a pulsating cranial mass, the child is brought to the hospital, and x-rays reveal a lens-shaped bony defect following the long axis of the fracture line.

A second mode of presentation is due to underlying brain damage secondary to the initial trauma, which results in focal seizures, hemiparesis, or hemiatrophy in association with a pulsating lens-shaped bony defect.

DIAGNOSIS

Distinctive changes in the roentgenograms of the skull occur with an arachnoid cyst of the brain. An initial skull fracture may be seen in the parietal bone, occasionally in the occipital or frontal bone. Instead of healing normally as expected, the fracture line enlarges (Fig. 64–3). The edges of the defect are irregular, wavy, and scalloped in contour. Areas of rarefaction of bone edges may coexist with other areas of increased density of bone, suggesting a process of bone absorption and deposition. The edges may be thinned or thickened, with greater erosion of the inner table than the outer table creating a saucer-like edge.

An arteriogram may be normal or may reveal displacement such as would be seen with a developmental arachnoid cyst, subdural hygroma, or other surface lesion. The vessels involved show stretching and displacement around an avascular mass.

The diagnosis is made from the x-ray findings of a lens-shaped defect of the skull in an infant or child who has a pulsating cra-

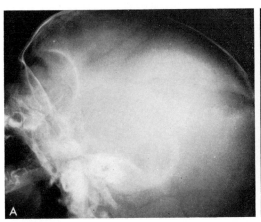
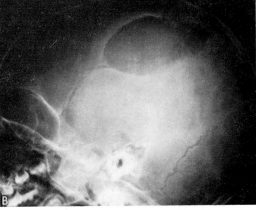

Figure 64–3 *A.* Beginning enlargement of parietal diastatic skull fracture six months postinjury. *B.* Same patient at nine months showing marked enlargement.

nial defect and a history of a previous linear or diastatic skull fracture. A computed tomogram will show the extent of the arachnoid cyst. An associated porencephalic cyst or ventricular dilatation may also be observed.

Rare and Unusual Variations

The foregoing description is of the classic syndrome. Rare and unusual variations have been sporadically reported. Sartawi and co-workers reported an adult with traumatic arachnoid cyst of the occipital bone without demonstrable fracture.[12] Jelsma and Ross reported a 58-year-old woman with arachnoid cyst, presumably traumatic, in the region of the gasserian ganglion, that produced facial pain.[5] Nichols and Manganiello reported a traumatic arachnoid cyst in the cerebellopontine angle that simulated acoustic tumor.[9] Hillman and associates described two instances of intradiploic arachnoid involving the occipital bone following fracture.[3] Intraspinal arachnoid cysts causing progressive compression of the spinal cord following brachial plexus avulsion have been observed in three instances.[12,13]

TREATMENT

Treatment consists of excision of the cyst and repair of the dural and bony defects. It should be noted that the dural defect is larger than the bony defect. Thus the bony edges must be rongeured away until normal dura is found. The dural defect is closed in a watertight fashion with a fascia lata or pericranial graft. The bony defect is repaired with rib graft. Although artificial membranes for the dura and plastic for the skull defect may be used, natural tissues are preferable in growing children. Diagnosis and treatment must be prompt. The lesion is inherently benign and may be completely redeemable, but if it is untreated, the bony and dural defects will continue to enlarge.

REFERENCES

1. Darlington, D.: The convolution pattern of the brain and endocranial cast in the ferret. J. Anat., 91:52–60, 1957.
2. Goldstein, F. P., Sakoda, T., Kepes, J. J., Davidson, K., and Brackett, C. E.: Enlarging skull fractures: An experimental study. J. Neurosurg., 27:541–550, 1967.
3. Hillman, L. R. S., Keiffer, S. A., Ortiz, H., and Clubb, R.: Intraosseous leptomeningeal cysts of the posterior cranial fossa. Radiology, 116:655–659, 1975.
4. Hoffman, E. P., Garner, J. T., Johnson, D., and Shelden, C. H.: Traumatic arachnoid diverticulum associated with paraplegia. J. Neurosurg., 38:81–85, 1973.
5. Jelsma, F., and Ross, P. J.: Traumatic intracranial arachnoid cyst involving the Gasserian ganglion. J. Neurosurg., 26:439–441, 1967.
6. Keener, E. B.: An experimental study of reactions of the dura mater to wounding and loss of substance. J. Neurosurg., 16:424–447, 1959.
7. Lende, R. A., and Erickson, R. C.: Growing skull fractures of childhood. J. Neurosurg., 18:479–489, 1961.
8. Müller, F. W.: Uber die Beziehungen des gehirns zum windungsrelief (G. Schwalbe) an der Aussenseite de Schlafengegend beim menschlichen Schädel. Arch. Anat., pp. 57–118, 1908.
9. Nichols, P. J., and Manganiello, L. O. J.: Traumatic arachnoidal cyst simulating acoustic neurinoma. J. Neurosurg., 10:538–539, 1953.
10. Pye, I. F., and Hickey, M. C.: Traumatic arachnoid diverticula: A report of two cases causing spinal cord compression. Brit. J. Radiol., 48:889–893, 1975.
11. Rosenthal, S. A. E., Grieshop, J., Freeman, L. M., and Goldstein, F. P.: Experimental observations on enlarging skull fractures. J. Neurosurg., 32:431–434, 1970.
12. Sartawi, M., Schwartz, F. T., and Fox, J. L.: An unusual osteolytic lesion of the skull due to a traumatic arachnoid cyst. Neuroradiology, 6:180–181, 1973.
13. Taveras, J., and Ransohoff, J.: Leptomeningeal cysts of brain following trauma with erosion of the skull; Study of seven cases treated by surgery. J. Neurosurg., 10:233–241, 1953.

65

DURAL FISTULAE AND THEIR REPAIR

Dural cerebrospinal fluid fistulae occur when there is a defect in the pia-arachnoid that permits the cerebrospinal fluid to escape from the subarachnoid to the extra-arachnoid space. This condition is most commonly manifested as rhinorrhea or otorrhea, but also is evidenced by spinal fluid leakage through a scalp defect or a pia-arachnoid tear along the spinal subarachnoid pathway.

Galen, in the second century A.D., was the first to observe that the brain contained fluid-filled ventricles. Willis described cerebrospinal fluid rhinorrhea in 1676, and Bidloo described the first case of post-traumatic rhinorrhea in a patient in Holland in 1700.[63,100] The first description of a case of nontraumatic rhinorrhea in the English medical literature has been credited to Miller in 1826.[63] Although Magendie wrote extensively on the anatomy and physiology of cerebrospinal fluid in 1842, it was not until 1899, when St. Clair Thomson wrote a monograph reviewing 21 cases of spontaneous cerebrospinal fluid rhinorrhea, including one of his own, that this clinical entity became well recognized.[72,94]

The principle of closing a dural defect was first proposed by Grant in 1923. He reported the case of a 19-year-old man who was in an automobile collision. A skull film revealed intracranial air and a fracture through the frontal sinus. Grant stated, " . . . we felt that an attempt should be made to find and close the tear in the dura through which the air had entered. It was feared that infection might pass in from the frontal sinus, producing meningitis." Unfortunately, the operative intervention planned by Grant was foiled because the osteoplastic flap was placed too high to permit access to the floor of the frontal fossa. In addition, profuse bleeding from the dura was encountered, presumably from the superior sagittal sinus, in the anteroinferior portion of the incision, which required closure of the incision with tampons in place. Since no intracranial air was found at the second operation to remove the tampons, Grant assumed that the dural rent had been obliterated spontaneously.[31]

The successful operative repair of a cerebrospinal fluid leak was first reported in 1926 by Dandy, who closed a traumatic dural tear over a frontal sinus fracture with a muscle and fascia lata graft.[20] Cushing reported three additional successful repairs later that same year.[19] Since that time, operative intervention has remained the major therapeutic strategy in the treatment of persistent dural fistulae, mandated by the associated high risk of intracranial infection. The seriousness of these infections, particularly meningitis, has not been eliminated by the use of modern antibiotics.

Modern operative treatment of cerebrospinal fluid fistulae remains basically the same as the original approaches devised by Grant and Dandy, but the apparent simplicity of this solution is misleading. Preoperative localization of the fistula is difficult, sometimes impossible, and operative exploration and treatment are not uniformly successful. In short, the management of

R. F. SPETZLER AND C. B. WILSON

dural fistulae remains a formidable challenge to the skill of the modern neurosurgeon.

ETIOLOGY OF DURAL FISTULAE

All dural fistulae have in common a defect in the pia-arachnoid that allows cerebrospinal fluid to leak from the subarachnoid space to the extra-arachnoid space. Their most common manifestation is rhinorrhea or otorrhea, the leakage of spinal fluid through the nose or the ear. More apparent, and for this reason easier to treat, are dural fistulae directly through the skull and scalp. Another common cerebrospinal fluid leak occurs following lumbar puncture; although these iatrogenic leaks are rarely troublesome, a few require operative closure of the dura.

The most common cause of a cerebrospinal fluid leak is trauma. Although trauma may cause a pia-arachnoid perforation anywhere along the cerebrospinal axis, the tear is most often confined to the basal areas of the skull. The floor of the frontal fossa is thin and therefore particularly susceptible to fracture. The cribriform plate is especially vulnerable, since the pia-arachnoid is adherent to the bone, and small arachnoid pouches enter the skull perforations at the exit of the olfactory nerve rootlets.

Nontraumatic fistulae occur much less frequently, and may be caused by hydrocephalus, tumor, infection, and congenital anomalies. Ommaya has classified the causes of rhinorrhea by dividing cerebrospinal fluid fistulae into traumatic and nontraumatic categories (Fig. 65–1).[73] Traumatic fistulae are further subdivided into accidental and iatrogenic, and then into acute and delayed. Nontraumatic fistulae are subdivided into high-pressure and normal-pressure leaks; high-pressure leaks are classified as those caused by tumor and those secondary to hydrocephalus, and normal-pressure leaks as congenital anomalies, "focal atrophy," and osteomyelitic erosion. In this classification system, Ommaya has abandoned previously used terminology, such as "spontaneous," "primary spontaneous," "secondary spontaneous," and "idiopathic" rhinorrhea, since these vague terms bear no relationship to either the pathogenesis or natural history of the disease.[73–75] Unfortunately, despite the advantage Ommaya's classification offers by identifying the cause of the fistula, his system is not entirely satisfactory. The subdivisions often overlap, and it becomes difficult, in many cases, to determine whether a patient has a delayed traumatic fistula or a normal-pressure, nontraumatic leak. Furthermore, hydrocephalus may play a role in fistulae in any of the categories.

An alternate classification of dural fistulae, based on their causes and the cerebrospinal fluid pressure, is summarized in Table 65–1. This classification system has the advantage of simplicity, and provides a basis for rational treatment: the juxtaposition of the cause with the presence or absence of abnormal cerebrospinal fluid

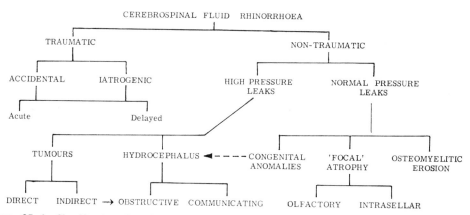

Figure 65–1 Classification of cerebrospinal fluid rhinorrhea. (From Ommaya, A. K., Di Chiro, G., Baldwin, M., and Pennybacker, J. B.: Nontraumatic cerebrospinal fluid rhinorrhoea. J. Neurol. Neurosurg. Psychiat., *31*:214–225, 1968. Reprinted by permission.)

TABLE 65–1 CEREBROSPINAL FLUID FISTULA MANAGEMENT CLASSIFICATION

CAUSE	INTRA-CRANIAL PRESSURE	MANAGEMENT
Traumatic		
Accidental		
Immediate	Normal	Nonoperative for 10 days; if persistent, same as delayed
Delayed	Normal	Direct repair
	High	Shunt for hydrocephalus or removal of cause (e.g., hematoma)
Iatrogenic		
Intracranial opera-	Normal	Direct repair
tion	High	Direct repair and shunt, or shunt alone
Transsphenoidal		
operation		
Immediate	Normal	Conservative for 4 days; if persistent, repacking of sella
Delayed	Normal	Repacking of sella
	High	Shunt
Radiation therapy of		
pituitary tumor	Normal	Transsphenoidal packing
Lumbar puncture	Normal	If leak persists longer than 2 weeks, autologous epidural blood patch; rarely direct repair
Space-occupying lesion	(e.g., tumor, cyst, aneurysm)	
Erosion, focal	Normal	Removal of causative lesion and repair of dural defect
Increased intra-cranial pressure	High	Removal of causative lesion; shunt may be required as a secondary procedure
Empty sella	Normal	Transsphenoidal packing of sella
	High	Transsphenoidal packing of sella and shunt
Hydrocephalus		
Communicating	High	Lumbar-peritoneal shunt
Obstructive	High	Ventriculoperitoneal shunt
Congenital anomalies	Normal	Direct repair
	High	Shunt; infection or pneumocephalus is an indication for direct repair

pressure suggests the appropriate treatment.[89] It cannot be overemphasized that operative treatment directed only at the actual leak, without appropriate management of the abnormal pressure, is likely to fail. Since all patients with dural fistulae may have either aseptic or septic meningitis, communicating hydrocephalus is a possible complication of any spinal fluid leak.

TRAUMATIC FISTULAE

Post-traumatic cerebrospinal fluid fistulae occur in an estimated 2 to 3 per cent of all patients with head injuries and in as many as 6 per cent of patients who have suffered severe head trauma.[9,63,79,82] There appears to be little correlation between the severity of a head injury and the occurrence of a dural fistula; in a series of 1745 patients with head injuries reported by Mincy, 25 of the 54 patients who developed a cerebrospinal fluid leak, or nearly 50 per cent, suffered only a brief or no loss of consciousness and had no neurological deficit.[63] The danger of undiagnosed post-traumatic fistulae is documented by the prominence

of head trauma as the leading cause of meningitis in adults.[6,34,99]

Cerebrospinal fluid fistulae that result from a direct skin-skull-dural defect require routine debridement with closure of all layers. Since these fistulae are usually apparent to the examining physician and present neither a diagnostic nor a therapeutic dilemma, this discussion is limited to the post-traumatic fistulae that lead to otorrhea or rhinorrhea.

Post-traumatic rhinorrhea and otorrhea can be divided into two types: the type that is apparent immediately or soon following trauma, and the type that commences weeks to years following head injury.[30] Immediate post-traumatic rhinorrhea ceases spontaneously within the first week in 85 per cent or more of patients; otorrhea ceases spontaneously in nearly all cases.[7,63,80–82] Of 1250 patients with head injuries reviewed by Brawley and Kelly, 24 per cent had basal skull fractures, and of these, 11.5 per cent developed rhinorrhea or otorrhea immediately.[7] The delayed appearance of a cerebrospinal fluid fistula occurs within three months following injury in 95 per cent of cases, but may be delayed for many years. One such case of long-delayed onset was reported by Kraus, whose patient developed post-traumatic rhinorrhea 22 years following trauma.[50]

Traumatic dural fistulae are not uncommon in childhood; the adult to child ratio is about 10 to 1.[13,32,35,37] Their occurrence below the age of two is decidedly rare, however, probably because the base of the skull is still flexible and the sinuses are not yet fully developed.[13]

Pathophysiology of Traumatic Fistulae

A dural fistula can occur anywhere along a break in the pia-arachnoid. The fragile base of the skull is particularly vulnerable to the formation of a fistula as a result of head trauma. A basal fracture may lacerate the pia-arachnoid and may, in fact, lead to herniation of the dura, the arachnoid, and the brain into the fracture site. Bone fragments may become displaced through the dura. Because the pia-arachnoid adheres closely to the base of the frontal fossa, particularly at the cribriform plate, small tears in the pia-arachnoid can occur when minor head trauma causes a shift of the intracranial contents in relation to the base of the skull. These arachnoid tears can result in an immediate extracranial escape of cerebrospinal fluid, or if they are partially plugged, can produce a ball-valve effect that results in an intermittent or delayed cerebrospinal fluid leak. The majority of delayed post-traumatic leaks probably result from a partial tear that weakens the pia-arachnoid, which then becomes susceptible to delayed perforation when sudden increases of cerebrospinal fluid pressure occur, as with straining and coughing.

A cerebrospinal fluid leak persists if the injured tissue does not heal properly. A persistent leak may occur if there is lack of tissue approximation—for example, in a displaced fracture—or if a continuous or intermittent increase of cerebrospinal fluid pressure resulting from hydrocephalus, coughing, or respiratory or arterial pulsation exceeds the tensile strength of the healing tissue. In a patient with an arachnoid fistula, sneezing or coughing may force air through the fistula, resulting in pneumocephalus.

Location of Post-Traumatic Fistulae

The fragility of the cribriform plate and the juxtaposition of the arachnoid investment to the bone where the first cranial nerve perforates the skull makes this area of the skull the most common site of a dural fistula. So fragile is the cribriform plate that it is the pathway for most high-pressure fluid leaks. Fractures that result in arachnoid tears through the frontal, ethmoid, and sphenoid sinuses are the next most frequent cause of dural fistulae and source of rhinorrhea (Figs. 65–2 and 65–3).[83]

It is important to remember that the lateral extensions of the sphenoid sinus in the middle fossa may make detection of a fistula there difficult.[66] Fractures through the petrous bone into the mastoid air cells may cause otorrhea, arising from either the middle or posterior fossa.[51] Paradoxical rhi-

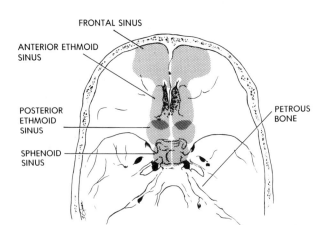

FRONTAL SINUS
ANTERIOR ETHMOID SINUS
POSTERIOR ETHMOID SINUS
SPHENOID SINUS
PETROUS BONE

Figure 65–2 Frequent sites of cerebrospinal fluid leakage. View from above.

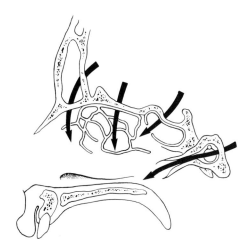

Figure 65–3   Common cerebrospinal fluid leakage pathways.

norrhea may occur as a result of a petrous arachnoid fistula in the middle ear with the tympanic membrane intact; since the cerebrospinal fluid can enter the nasal passage via the eustachian tube, the leak can be manifested as rhinorrhea. A rare cause of rhinorrhea is a cerebrospinal fluid fistula occurring between the sphenoid bone and Rosenmüller's fossa.[41]

Intracranial Infections

Although the rationale for operative repair of dural fistulae has long been based on the risk of meningitis in patients with rhinorrhea and otorrhea, the actual rates of morbidity and death from meningitis associated with cerebrospinal fluid fistulae are not well documented. Before the era of modern antibiotics, it was assumed that any patient with a cerebrospinal fluid leak ultimately would succumb to an intracranial infection. With the use of these antibiotics, morbidity and death from meningitis have decreased significantly. Nevertheless, meningitis has not been eradicated, nor has it been controlled with uniform success.[4,6]

The reported incidence of meningitis in patients with post-traumatic dural fistulae varies from 3 to 50 per cent; the infection rate tends to be higher if the cerebrospinal fluid leak persists longer than seven days.[7,52,63,80] Pneumococcal meningitis, the infection most frequently associated with a dural leak, occurred in as many as 83 per cent of all post-traumatic meningitic epi-

sodes reported in one series. Although the mortality rate for adult patients with pneumococcal meningitis approaches 50 per cent, the mortality rate for patients with pneumococcal meningitis associated with a dural fistula is less than 10 per cent.[14,99] There are a number of case reports of patients having as many as 12 recurrent attacks of meningitis without apparent neurological sequelae.[6,18,99]

Dandy pointed out that recurrent meningitis associated with a dural fistula is relatively benign, and attributed this to the free drainage of cerebrospinal fluid through the fistula.[21] A factor more important than free cerebrospinal fluid drainage may be that patients with recurrent meningitis from a dural fistula usually are young and otherwise healthy, in contrast to adult patients in whom meningitis is not associated with a dural defect.[34] The relatively benign course of post-traumatic meningitis in no way diminishes its seriousness, but it does suggest that not all dural fistulae require immediate operative correction at the time of detection, as some authors have recommended.[12,53–55,64] It appears, however, that the prognosis for children with meningitis secondary to dural fistula is poorer, warranting a more aggressive operative approach in pediatric cases.[13]

Post-traumatic meningitis associated with a dural fistula should be treated aggressively with appropriate antibiotics. Whether or not prophylactic antibodies should be used in treating patients with an asymptomatic dural leak remains a controversial issue.[3,7,33,48,52] There appears, however, to be a real risk of producing drug-resistant meningitis in patients receiving prophylactic antibiotics. In one neurosurgical intensive care ward, the use of prophylactic antibiotics led to an epidemic of *Klebsiella aerogenes* infection that resulted in the deaths of eight patients with *Klebsiella* meningitis. This epidemic was promptly controlled by the drastic measure of withdrawing both prophylactic and therapeutic antibiotics.[78] In one study of comatose patients, it was found that antibiotics failed to provide any prophylactic benefit; on the contrary, the patients who were treated with antibiotics were three times as likely to develop pulmonary infection as those who were not.[76] A prospective and retrospective study of an admittedly small number of patients failed to demonstrate any benefit in the use of prophylactic antibiotics to treat patients with cerebrospinal fluid leaks.[48,58] Many cases of meningitis have been reported to have developed despite the use of prophylactic antibiotics; of particular significance are those in which pneumococcal meningitis developed despite prophylactic antimicrobial therapy with drugs effective against the offending organism.[7,63]

It appears that prudent management of the patient with a cerebrospinal fluid fistula and concurrent active meningitis must include vigorous treatment with appropriate antibiotics, but that the prophylactic use of antibiotics is probably ineffective, possibly hazardous, and should be abandoned.

NONTRAUMATIC DURAL FISTULAE

The first account of a case of nontraumatic cerebrospinal fluid rhinorrhea is credited to Miller, who in 1826 reported the case of a boy who had a progressively enlarging head and recurrent bouts of profuse fluid discharge from his nose. A cribriform dural fistula was verified at necropsy.

Nontraumatic dural cerebrospinal fluid leaks are rare.[68,75] They may be caused by increased intracranial pressure resulting from a mass lesion or an obstructive process occurring along the normal cerebrospinal fluid pathways.[56,67,85] Because of the intimate anatomical relationship between the subarachnoid space and the nasal passages at the lamina cribrosa, increased intracranial pressure can lead to perforation of the pia-arachnoid along one of the olfactory rootlets and result in rhinorrhea.[72] This pathway was demonstrated experimentally by Locke and Naffziger, who injected celloidin under pressure into the subarachnoid space in dogs.[57] The celloidin often escaped into the nose through the fragile cribriform plate along one of the olfactory nerve filaments.

Mass lesions or infectious processes may also cause dural fistulae by direct erosion of the pia-arachnoid and bone.[85] These cases rarely present a diagnostic or therapeutic dilemma, since the dural leak is usually a late manifestation of the primary disorder.

Congenital anomalies, such as "focal atrophy" of the cribriform plate or sella turcica, may present as cases of spontaneous rhinorrhea.[1,70,71] O'Connell described a case in which the anterior half of the olfactory bulb had atrophied.[72] He postulated that the pressure of the cerebrospinal fluid on the exposed lamina cribrosa caused distention of the subarachnoid pouches in the empty neural foramina and eventually led to the establishment of a fistula. It is probably on a similar basis that rhinorrhea occurs in the presence of an empty sella; atrophy of the contents of the sella followed by protrusion of the pia-arachnoid through an incomplete diaphragma sellae, either because of increased intracranial pressure or constant pulsation of the cerebrospinal fluid, eventually results in a cerebrospinal fluid leak.[8,14,26,65]

Cerebrospinal fluid fistulae of nontraumatic spontaneous origin have also been reported in the anteromedial aspect of the middle cranial fossa in the temporal bone.[39,49] Their pathogenesis in this area is similar to that of fistulae elsewhere and has been thought to be secondary to pulsatile cerebrospinal fluid pressure causing thinning of pneumatized areas of the middle fossa. Additional thinning of the bone leads to the development of a small hole or enlargement of normally present pit holes and the subsequent herniation of dura, arachnoid, and brain through these holes. Further progression of this process leads to thinning and fenestration of the dura, resulting in an arachnoid diverticulum, which, when it ruptures, results in a cerebrospinal fluid fistula.[45,46]

A less subtle congenital anomaly, such as a nasal encephalocele, may present either as spontaneous rhinorrhea or as iatrogenic rhinorrhea following ill-advised biopsy of a suspected nasal polyp (Fig. 65–4).[80]

SYMPTOMS AND DIAGNOSIS OF DURAL FISTULAE

A cerebrospinal fluid fistula should be suspected in all patients who have suffered head trauma, and in all adults who have one or more bouts of meningitis without an underlying disease. Clinical signs that suggest the presence of a dural fistula include anosmia, a fluid level behind the tympanic membrane, and more obviously, drainage of serosanguinous fluid from the nose, ear, or wound. The sudden onset of clear-fluid drainage from the nose or a bout of menin-

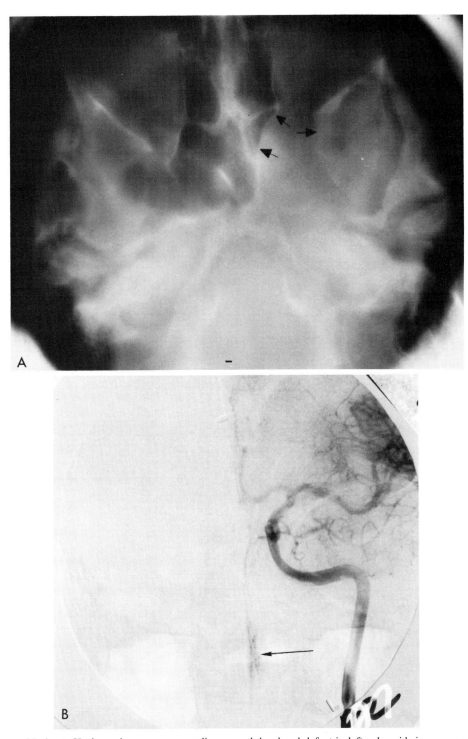

Figure 65–4 *A*. Horizontal tomogram revealing smooth-bordered defect in left sphenoid sinus area outlined with arrows. *B*. Selective angiography reveals abnormal midline vessel extending into the nasopharynx where a blush is present (*arrow*). Patient presented with rhinorrhea of many years' duration and had had four previous episodes of meningitis. ^{99m}Technetium-labeled serum

gitis usually indicates the presence of a delayed or nontraumatic leak.

The voluntary production of cerebrospinal fluid rhinorrhea with head position has been referred to as the reservoir sign.[21] This sign, usually elicited by flexion of the head in the erect position, has been proposed to be specific for a dural fistula into the sphenoid sinuses, whereas a cerebrospinal fluid leak through the frontal sinus has been supposed to be associated with free flow of the fluid. Cerebrospinal fluid in the sphenoid sinus will, on flexion of the head, be discharged through the ostium, which is situated halfway up the anterior wall of the sinus. Although the reservoir sign is in all likelihood not specific, it is well to remember that head positioning, particularly in the morning when the fluid has accumulated in the various sinuses overnight, may lead to a momentary profuse discharge that will establish the diagnosis as well as allow the collection of an ample fluid sample for chemical analysis. Recognition of dural fistulae in children is complicated by the frequency of runny noses in that age group; a high index of suspicion is warranted when treating a child who is at risk of a cerebrospinal fluid leak.

If enough nasal drainage, uncontaminated by blood, can be collected, the diagnosis of a cerebrospinal fluid fistula can be confirmed if the fluid shows a glucose level that is greater than 30 mg per 100 ml; however, the spinal fluid glucose level may be less than 30 mg per 100 ml if the patient has meningitis. Dextrostix and Uristix are not useful for cerebrospinal fluid glucose determinations because they are so sensitive that they frequently show a positive result on normal nasal discharge.[27,36,47]

If the dural fistula is secondary to a mass lesion, an infection, or an obstructive process, a neurological symptom complex that identifies the primary process is usually present. In order to confirm and localize a cerebrospinal fluid fistula, an orderly diagnostic work-up must be performed. One reasonable diagnostic plan is presented in Figure 65–5.

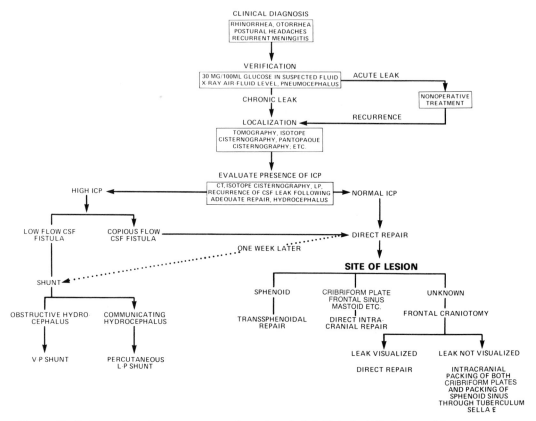

Figure 65–5 Flow chart for management of cerebrospinal fluid leak. ICP, intracranial pressure. (From Spetzler, R. F., and Wilson, C. B.: Management of recurrent CSF rhinorrhea. J. Neurosurg., *49*:393–397, 1978. Reprinted by permission.)

Skull films including erect and supine views should be obtained on all patients suspected of harboring a cerebrospinal fluid leak.[92] They may demonstrate a fracture, pneumocephalus, or an air-fluid level in one of the sinuses (Fig. 65–6). When an injury is the result of trauma, hypercycloidal tomography may reveal a subtle basilar skull fracture or a displaced bone spicule. The results of the clinical evaluation will deter-

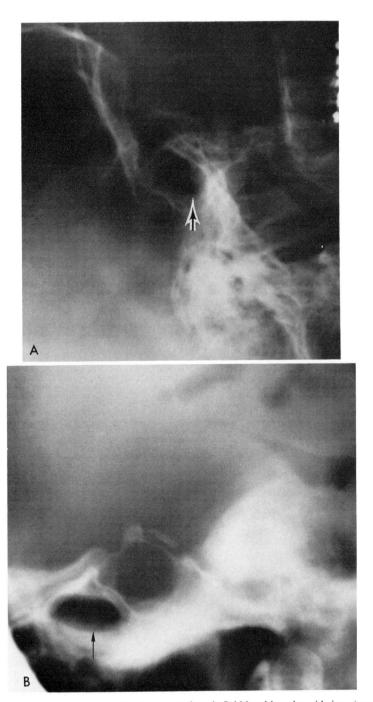

Figure 65–6 *A*. Brow-up lateral skull film demonstrating air-fluid level in sphenoid sinus (*arrow*). *B*. Midline tomogram during pneumoencephalogram demonstrating air-fluid level in sphenoid sinus (*arrow*) with patient in sitting position. Also notice ballooned sella. Patient had pituitary tumor of which the presenting symptom was rhinorrhea.

mine the area that should be studied; for example, anosmia indicates the area of the base of the frontal fossa, while hearing loss indicates the petrous bone.

In the past, various substances have been introduced into the lumbar subarachnoid space to verify a leak, including such dyes as methylene blue, phenolsulfonphthalein, and indigo carmine (Table 65–2). The hazard of methylene blue injected into the subarachnoid space has been well documented, and under no circumstances is its use in the subarachnoid space justified.[25,87,102] Fluorescein has also been injected intrathecally, but on rare occasions its use has resulted in status epilepticus.[59,97]

These techniques are now largely obsolete and have been replaced by radioisotope-labeled serum albumin cisternography, which not only verifies the presence of a cerebrospinal fluid leak, but usually localizes the site of the leak as well.* Although [131]iodine-labeled albumin (RISA) has been used for radioisotope cisternography, [99m]technetium-labeled albumin is a more efficient isotope, despite its shorter half-life, and permits better visualization and localization of fistulae with minimal cerebrospinal fluid flow (Figs. 65–7, 65–8, and 65–9).

In performing cisternographic studies, [99m]technetium-labeled serum albumin is introduced into the subarachnoid space, after which the patient's head is placed in front

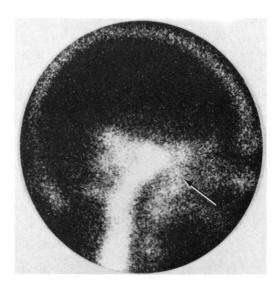

Figure 65–7 Technetium cisternography of a patient with a four-year history of rhinorrhea and two episodes of meningitis. [99m]Technetium-labeled serum albumin (5 mc) was injected into cervical subarachnoid space. At six hours, this cisternogram was obtained. This right lateral view reveals the cervical subarachnoid space, the basilar cisterns, the ambient cistern, the sylvian cistern, and extensive activity in the hypopharynx (*arrow*) through a tract in the sphenoid sinus.

of a gamma camera and the transit of the isotope is recorded. The isotope can be visualized as it leaves the subarachnoid space and accumulates extradurally in areas such as the hypopharynx or nasopharynx, often

---

* See references 2, 5, 22, 23, 38, 40, 62.

TABLE 65–2 DIAGNOSTIC PROCEDURES FOR LOCALIZATION OF CEREBROSPINAL FLUID LEAKS

PROCEDURE	SUBSTANCES
Dyes for subarachnoid injection	Indigo carmine Phenolsulfonpthalein Methylene blue (do not use!)
Photoluminescent substance for subarachnoid injection	Fluorescein
X-rays	Skull films Tomography Pneumoencephalography Subdural pneumography Computed tomography
Isotopes for subarachnoid injection	RISA ^{99m}Tc serum albumin
Elective increase of intracranial pressure	With ^{99m}Tc serum albumin
Intraoperative test	Nasal air insufflation

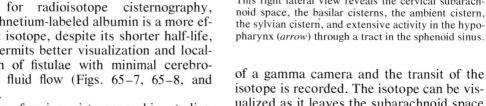

Figure 65–8 Right lateral [131]iodine-labeled albumin cisternogram revealing radioisotope activity in hypopharynx (*arrow*). Notice lack of detail in contrast to technetium study shown in Figures 65–7 and 65–9.

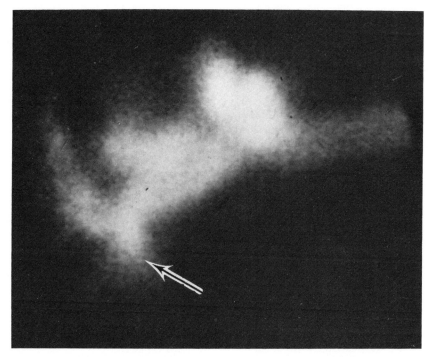

Figure 65–9 Left lateral technetium cisternogram demonstrating cervical subarachnoid space, basilar cistern, ambient cistern, and sylvian cistern. Below the sylvian cistern a small inferior area of radioisotope activity demonstrates the cerebrospinal fluid leakage site, which was through the posterior ethmoid sinus (*arrow*).

leaving a trail that localizes the actual site of the fistula. Head positioning and straining may facilitate active cerebrospinal fluid flow. If the leak is small, packing the nasal passageway with cottonoids will facilitate collection of the cerebrospinal fluid containing the isotope and will obviate its loss through swallowing and a resultant negative study. Abnormal fluid dynamics suggesting hydrocephalus may be demonstrated by ventricular reflux of the isotope.

The radioisotope-labeled serum albumin may be introduced into the subarachnoid space by either the lumbar or the lateral cervical route. The Cl-C2 lateral cervical route is advantageous in that it minimizes the risk of obtaining a suboptimal study as a result of injecting the radioisotope into the extra-arachnoid space—a frequent complication of lumbar injections. Furthermore, cervical injection provides a shorter route to the base of the skull and allows a high isotope concentration to bathe the basal cisterns, resulting in better visualization of the dural fistula.

If the isotope cisternogram is negative, despite good clinical or radiographic evidence of the presence of a dural fistula, a repeat study, including elective elevation of the intracranial pressure, may be performed by using the following technique.[88] After the [99m]technetium-labeled albumin has been injected into the cervical subarachnoid space, normal saline is infused into the lumbar subarachnoid space by means of a spinal needle that is attached to a Harvard pump equipped with a manometer. Saline infusion is continued until the leak is demonstrated or until the intracranial pressure has been raised to 600 mm of water.

Iophendylate (Pantopaque) encephalography may aid in localizing dural fistulae, particularly those of the middle and posterior fossa.[15,43,91] For this study, 6 to 10 ml of Pantopaque is introduced into the subarachnoid space and manipulated to the area of interest in the posterior or middle fossa. Radiographic demonstration of Pantopaque in the extracranial space is diagnostic of a cerebrospinal fluid leak. A negative radioisotope or Pantopaque study in the presence of an active leak is diagnostic of a direct ventricular fistula. Because the Pantopaque or isotope fails to enter the ventricular system, and as no cisternal component to the fistula is present, clear cerebrospinal fluid ventricular drainage may occur in the presence of a negative cisternogram; a ventriculogram would be diagnostic.[88] Pneumoencephalography may also demonstrate the site of a dural fistula on occasion, particularly if the "hanging head" position is employed.[60]

If either the clinical presentation or an abnormal isotope cisternogram suggests the presence of hydrocephalus, computed tomography (CT) is useful in determining ventricular size; however, since cerebrospinal fluid flow through the fistula constitutes external drainage, the ventricular size on the scan may lead one to underestimate the degree of hydrocephalus. Computed tomography is also helpful in detecting an infectious process, whether diffuse or localized, as well as the presence of intracranial air, displaced bone fragments, cerebral edema, or a foreign object (Fig. 65–10).

There are times when a fistula cannot be demonstrated, despite the use of all the available tests to localize a cerebrospinal fluid leak. In these cases, operative ex-

ploration may be the only resort. Since most fistulae are located in the anterior fossa, operative exploration should be directed to this area initially. If no leak can be seen in the anterior fossa, then the surgeon should be prepared to expose the middle fossa as well.

When operative exploration fails to demonstrate the site of the fistula, Ray and Bergland suggest using an intraoperative technique of air insufflation in which the nasal passageway is isolated by inserting balloons anteriorly and posteriorly in the nose.[82] Air is introduced into this sealed-off nasal passage, and bubbles appearing in the operatively exposed, saline-irrigated, frontal fossa demonstrate the elusive arachnoid defect.

If the fistula cannot be detected, the cribriform plates can be covered and the sphenoid sinuses packed bilaterally in an attempt to obliterate any microscopic arachnoid rent.

TREATMENT OF DURAL FISTULAE

Dural fistulae can be managed by either nonoperative or operative procedures. The appropriate treatment depends on the cause, extent, severity, and location of the cerebrospinal fluid leak.

Neurosurgeons may be reluctant to authorize the early reduction of facial fractures in the presence of a cerebrospinal fluid leak, for fear that the manipulation of the craniofacial disjunction will increase the risk of meningitis.[55] Nevertheless, except when the patient's clinical condition contraindicates the procedure, early reduction has definite advantages. Although leakage of cerebrospinal fluid may be increased temporarily, it more often ceases or is reduced following reduction. The early reduction of facial bones also lessens the risk of introducing virulent hospital microbes into the nasopharynx; later reduction may cause a closed dural fistula to reopen. In addition, reduction is accomplished more easily and with better cosmetic results if it is done early following trauma.[24]

Collins reported 19 patients whose facial fractures had been reduced within 48 hours; operative repair of a fistula was necessary in only 2 of these patients.[17] In a large series of Le Fort III fractures, no single intracranial infection complicated early reduction;

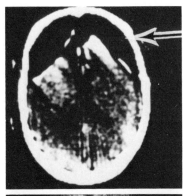
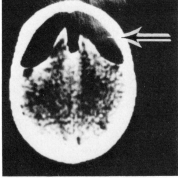

Figure 65–10 Computed tomogram of patient presenting with suspected rhinorrhea, demonstrating subdural air and verifying the presence of a dural perforation.

in fact, even severe cerebrospinal fluid rhinorrhea often ceased following reduction. Although antibiotic coverage during the reduction procedure has been recommended, its value has not been documented.[24] Intranasal packing should be loose to permit posterior nasal drainage.

Obviously, the presence of an intracranial abscess, with or without pneumocephalus, associated with a dural fistula requires prompt operative management.[31,84] If a patient with pneumocephalus is endangered by increased intracranial pressure, the amount of intracranial air can be reduced significantly by having the patient breathe 100 per cent oxygen. As the nitrogen is washed out of the blood stream by pure oxygen, the nitrogen in the intracranial air pocket diffuses into the blood stream, resulting in a prompt reduction in the volume of intracranial gas (Fig. 65–11).

Nonoperative maneuvers are summarized in Table 65–3. Bed rest should be instituted, and the patient should be cautioned to avoid sneezing, coughing, and nose blowing. Stool softeners and laxatives should be ordered to minimize straining. Medication to decrease cerebrospinal fluid production, such as acetazolamide (Diamox) or digoxin, may be prescribed, although their usefulness has not been established. Although cerebrospinal fluid pressure can be decreased by means of dehydration or diuretics or both, drainage techniques are more effective and the simplest is repeated lumbar punctures with removal of cerebrospinal fluid to obtain an intracranial pressure at or slightly above atmospheric pressure. Continuous drainage can be obtained by inserting a catheter into the lumbar subarachnoid space and draining cerebrospinal fluid into a sterile receptacle.[61] An alternative siphoning procedure, particularly applicable if communicating hydrocephalus plays a role in the pathogenesis of the leak, is the percutaneous insertion of a lumboperitoneal shunt.[90] There is a potential risk of introducing organisms through the dural defect by the siphoning techniques, but this has not occurred in the authors' experience. Overshunting should be avoided to prevent pneumocephalus.[77]

Patients with rhinorrhea secondary to obstructive or communicating hydrocephalus seldom require direct operative repair of the cerebrospinal fluid fistula following a shunting procedure. A patient harboring a mass lesion with a cerebrospinal fluid leak from secondary erosion of the pia-arachnoid and skull requires removal of that lesion and, as part of the procedure, repair of the dural defect.

Operative treatment for a patient with a demonstrated leak can be directed intra- or extracranially. The major advantage of the intracranial approach is that it allows direct visualization of the dural perforation and inspection of the cortex adjacent to the defect. In addition, a graft placed intracranially over the dural defect will be tamponaded in place by the overlying brain and the intracranial pressure.[86] The transsphenoidal approach has the advantage of minimizing operative trauma and allowing the repair of dural defects, such as a leak through the tuberculum sellae, that are often difficult to visualize when the intracranial approach is used.[11,96,101] The disadvantages of the extracranial approach are that it is impossible to visualize the extent of associated brain damage and it is difficult, from the outside, to plug the dural defect against the pressure. Optimal management requires that the neurosurgeon consider both approaches in choosing the appropriate procedure for any individual patient; a tuberculum sellae leak is probably treated more effectively by using an extracranial approach, whereas a cribriform plate, middle fossa, posterior fossa, or unidentified leak requires an intracranial approach.

The most common intracranial approach for the repair of a dural fistula requires exposure of the frontal fossa. If the fistula is lateralized, a limited exposure is possible. If the location of a fistula has not been identified preoperatively, a bifrontal bone flap is preferable.

The initial coronal scalp incision should be outlined to the zygomatic arches so that the surgeon can extend the initial craniotomy by rongeuring the temporal bone in the event that the middle fossa must be visualized. The use of an operating microscope is mandatory to achieve optimal illumination, visibility, and magnification. A dental mirror, used judiciously, allows the surgeon to visualize the lateral extent of the sphenoid sinus and much of the middle fossa through a limited exposure. A small but significant number of patients will have two, rarely more, fistulae, and one should inspect the floor of the anterior fossa on both sides by using a dental mirror if necessary.

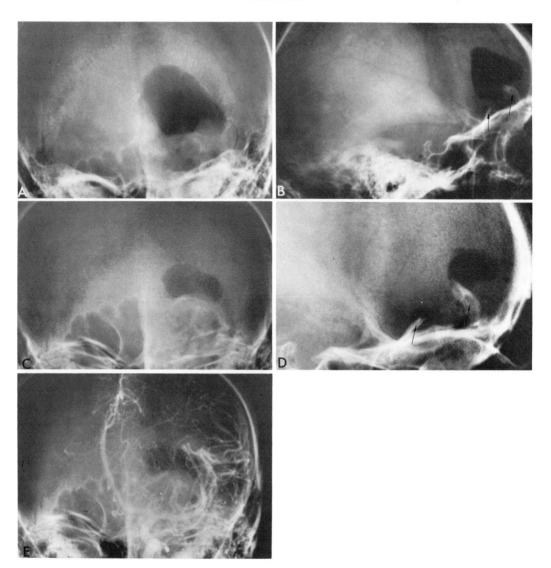

Figure 65–11 *A* and *B*. Lateral and anteroposterior skull films demonstrating pneumocephalus and bone displacement (*arrows*) of left orbital roof. The patient presented with meningitis and rhinorrhea and a history of trauma four days prior to admission. Signs of an intracranial mass effect with decreasing level of consciousness were treated by having the patient breathe 100 per cent oxygen, thereby decreasing the pneumocephalus by a significant amount as the nitrogen from the intracranial air diffused into the vascular system. *C* and *D*. Second set of skull films demonstrates marked decrease in size of pneumocephalus. Only 10 minutes had elapsed between the first set of films and the second. *E*. Anteroposterior angiogram performed at the same time as skull films and *D*. A large left anterior mass effect is evident.

Illustration continued on opposite page

When the dural leak is identified, an underlying bony defect should be suspected. Small bony defects can be repaired with bone wax; larger ones with wire mesh or methylmethacrylate.[93] The dural defect can be closed with many substances, but the use of autologous material avoids reactions associated with the introduction of foreign substances. Fascia lata, temporalis fascia, and pericranium are suitable patch materials;

gelatin sponge has been advocated, but fascia is preferable.[16] Stenting the graft to the dura can be performed with many small sutures placed through the graft and dura, or the graft can be secured by the judicious use of small amounts of tissue adhesive.[69,95] German's technique of freeing a portion of the anterior falx and using it as a flap to hold a muscle patch over an olfactory groove fistula also appears to be effective.[29]

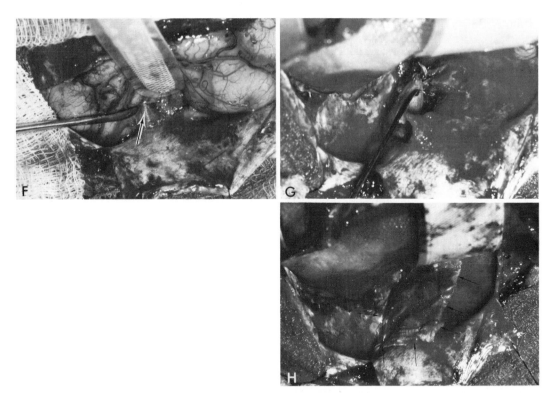

Figure 65-11 (*continued*)   *F.* Operative view of left frontal craniotomy. The floor of the frontal fossa is visualized. The frontal lobe is elevated, exposing a bone spicule penetrating the cortex (*arrow*)—the same bone fragment that was visualized on the skull films. *G.* Further elevation of the frontal lobe demonstrates the free bone fragment (at tip of instrument) and large opening into orbit and ethmoid sinus. *H.* Repair of floor of frontal fossa. Fascia lata patch is tacked to remaining dura with 5–0 stainless steel sutures (*arrows*). The patient made a full recovery.

Should preoperative tests, as well as operative exposure, fail to demonstrate the fistula, packing of both cribriform plates and the sphenoid sinus is indicated; prior to the operation, the patient should be informed about the risk and the expected disability of anosmia. Both cribriform plates are covered with muscle, which is held in place with falx flaps, pericranium, temporalis fascia, or fascia lata. The graft is held in place with either sutures or tissue adhesive. In addition, the periosteum is incised and reflected over the tuberculum sellae, which is resected to expose the sphenoid sinus. The sphenoidal mucosa is either removed or mobilized and pushed downward, and the sphenoid sinus is packed with muscle on either side of the septum. A graft is secured to obliterate the opening over the tuberculum sellae.[83]

A fistula located in the middle or posterior fossa can be approached by the route with which the surgeon feels most comfortable; the techniques for closure of the dural fistula in these locations are the same as those described for fistulae occurring in the frontal fossa. A mastoid subtemporal approach may be used for exposing temporal bone fistulae.[42]

An extracranial approach is particularly suitable for fistulae located in the pituitary fossa, sphenoid sinus, tuberculum sellae, and posterior ethmoid sinus.[98] If the neurosurgeon is familiar only with the transsphenoidal approach, an otolaryngologist

TABLE 65-3 NONOPERATIVE MANAGEMENT OF CEREBROSPINAL FLUID LEAK

Medications for decreasing cerebrospinal fluid
Diamox	250 mg every 6 hours
Digoxin*	0.25 mg per day
Decadron	4 mg every 6 hours

Procedures for decreasing cerebrospinal fluid pressure
  Mannitol
  Lasix
  Dehydration (500 ml per 24 hours)
Cerebrospinal fluid drainage
  Repeated lumbar punctures
  External lumbar drainage
  Percutaneous lumboperitoneal shunt

---

* Efficacy doubtful.

should be consulted when a fistula in another area is to be corrected from an extracranial route.

When the transsphenoidal approach is used, the fistula should be entirely exposed. A graft, preferably with a small amount of tissue adhesive, should be placed over the dural defect, and the edges of the graft should be tucked under the bony edges. The graft is supported by packing the sphenoid sinus with muscle or fat, which is held in place with septal cartilage or a stainless steel strut. If a patient has rhinorrhea following a trans-sphenoidal operation, then a trial of conservative management is in order.

When the dural fistula is to be managed operatively, the presence of a concomitant cerebrospinal fluid absorption defect must be recognized in order to determine whether a shunting procedure is necessary, either as the only treatment or in addition to a direct repair of the cerebrospinal fluid leak. If concomitant communicating hydrocephalus is present, a shunt should not be inserted at the time of an intracranial procedure. At least a week should be allowed to elapse between the craniotomy and the insertion of a shunt in order to avoid a subdural hematoma or hygroma from the decreased intracranial pressure caused by the shunt. A lumboperitoneal shunt, which can be inserted percutaneously, is both simple and effective.[90] As noted earlier, in some instances, particularly in patients with small dural defects associated with hydrocephalus, shunting alone constitutes adequate treatment.

Cerebrospinal fluid leaks occur in the lumbar region also. Although the vast majority of post–spinal puncture headaches clear up spontaneously, a small number of patients will require treatment other than bed rest. A lumbar arachnoid tear can be demonstrated by injecting a radioactive isotope into the cervical subarachnoid space and using a gamma camera to monitor the pooling of the isotope in the lumbar region.[28,44] The initial treatment of a persistent lumbar subarachnoid tear consists of injecting 10 ml of autologous blood, taken from a peripheral vein, into the epidural space in the region of the suspected leak. With the patient at bed rest, this blood patch usually will seal the dural tear. If a cerebrospinal fluid leak persists, operative exploration and closure of the dural tear may become necessary.[10]

PROGNOSIS

The prognosis is excellent for patients with dural fistulae that have been successfully repaired. Unless an underlying disease is present, the patient's life expectancy is normal. Patients who have a continuing cerebrospinal fluid leak are predisposed to repeated episodes of meningitis with its associated morbidity and mortality. Many of these patients may tolerate multiple bouts of meningitis, however, particularly if they receive prompt, aggressive treatment.

CONCLUSION

Dural fistulae remain a difficult and often perplexing problem to the neurosurgeon. Localization of the fistula and recognition of associated complicating factors require an array of diagnostic procedures. Although it may be necessary to perform repeated preoperative tests and, in some cases, operative exploration, persistence on the part of the neurosurgeon will result in the localization and closure of the fistula. Operative closure of dural defects is indicated in any patient with a persistent cerebrospinal fluid leak or recurrent meningitis. Concomitant recognition and treatment of increased intracranial pressure is mandatory; otherwise direct closure of the fistula will fail. If operative closure of the fistula is successful, the prognosis for the patient is excellent.

Acknowledgment: This study was supported by NIH Trauma Fellowship NIGMO-7032.

REFERENCES

1. Adson, A. W., and Uihlein, A.: Repair of defects in ethmoid and frontal sinuses resulting in cerebrospinal rhinorrhea. Arch. Surg., *58*:623–634, 1949.
2. Allen, M. B., Jr., Fammal, T. E., Ihnen, M., and Cowan, M. A.: Fistula detection in cerebrospinal fluid leakage. J. Neurol. Neurosurg. Psychiat., *35*:664–668, 1972.
3. Anderson, W. M., Schwartz, G. A., and Gammon, G. D.: Chronic spontaneous cerebrospinal rhinorrhea. Arch. Intern. Med., *107*: 723–731, 1961.

4. Appelbaum, E.: Meningitis following trauma to the head and face. J.A.M.A., *173*:1818–1822, 1960.

5. Ashburn, W. L., Harbert, J. C., Briner, W. H., and DiChiro, G.: Cerebrospinal fluid rhinorrhea studied with the gamma scintillation camera. J. Nucl. Med., *9*:523–529, 1968.

6. Boe, J., and Huseklepp, H.: Recurrent attacks of bacterial meningitis. Amer. J. Med., *29*:465–475, 1960.

7. Brawley, B., and Kelly, W.: Treatment of skull fractures with and without cerebrospinal fluid fistula. J. Neurosurg., *26*:57–61, 1967.

8. Brisman, R., Hughes, J., and Mount, L.: Cerebrospinal fluid rhinorrhea and the empty sella. J. Neurosurg., *31*:538–543, 1969.

9. Brisman, R., Hughes, J., and Mount, L.: Cerebrospinal fluid rhinorrhea. Arch. Neurol., *22*:245–252, 1970.

10. Brown, B. A., and Jones, W. W.: Prolonged headache following spinal puncture. Response to surgical treatment. J. Neurosurg., *19*:349–350, 1962.

11. Burian, N.: The microsurgical treatment of rhinorrhea. *In* Koos, W., Bock, F., and Spetzler, R., eds.: Clinical Microneurosurgery. Stuttgart, Georg Thieme Publisher, 1976, pp. 67–69.

12. Cairns, H.: Injuries of the frontal and ethmoidal sinuses with special references to cerebrospinal rhinorrhea and aeroceles. J. Laryng., *52*:589–623, 1937.

13. Caldicott, W. J. H., North, J. B., and Simpson, D. A.: Traumatic cerebrospinal fluid fistulas in children. J. Neurosurg., *38*:1–9, 1973.

14. Calkins, R. A., Pribram, H. F. W., and Joynt, R. J.: Intrasellar arachnoid diverticulum. A case report. Neurology (Minneap.), *18*:1037–1040, 1968.

15. Cantu, R. C., Michelsen, J. J., and New, P. F. J.: Demonstration of a ventriculo-mastoid fistula (paradoxical cerebrospinal fluid rhinorrhea) by Pantopaque ventriculography. Neurochirurgia, *10*:35–44, 1967.

16. Cloward, R. B., and Cunningham, E. B.: The use of gelatin sponge in prevention and treatment of cerebrospinal rhinorrhea. J. Neurosurg., *4*:519–525, 1947.

17. Collins, W. F.: Dural fistulae and their repair. *In* Youmans, J. R., ed.: Neurological Surgery. Philadelphia, W. B. Saunders Co., 1973, pp. 981–992.

18. Crossley, R. B., and Spink, W. W.: Recurrent meningitis; meningeal defects found after 12th attack. J.A.M.A., *215*:331, 1971.

19. Cushing, H.: Experience with orbito-ethmoidal osteomata having intracranial complications. Surg. Gynec. Obstet., *44*:721–742, 1927.

20. Dandy, W. E.: Pneumocephalus (intracranial pneumatocele or aerocele). Arch. Surg., *12*:949–982, 1926.

21. Dandy, W. E.: Treatment of rhinorrhea and otorrhea. Arch. Surg., *49*:75–85, 1944.

22. DiChiro, G., Reames, P. M., and Matthews, W. B.: RISA-ventriculography and RISA-cisternography. Neurology (Minneap.), *14*:185–191, 1964.

23. DiChiro, G., Ommaya, A. K., Ashburn, W. L., and Briner, W. H.: Isotope cisternography in the diagnosis and follow up of cerebrospinal fluid rhinorrhea. J. Neurosurg., *28*:522–529, 1968.

24. Dingman, R. O.: Maxillofacial injuries. *In* Youmans, J. R., ed.: Neurological Surgery. Philadelphia, W. B. Saunders Co., 1973, p. 931.

25. Evans, J. P., and Keegan, H. R.: Danger in the use of intrathecal methylene blue. J.A.M.A., *174*:856–859, 1960.

26. Gabriele, O. F.: The empty sella syndrome. Amer. J. Roentgen., *104*:168–170, 1968.

27. Gadeholt, H.: The reaction of glucose-oxidase test paper in normal nasal secretion. Acta Otolaryng., *58*:271–272, 1964.

28. Gass, H., Goldstein, A. S., Ruskin, R., et al.: Chronic postmyelogram headache. Isotopic demonstration of dural leak and surgical cure. Arch. Neurol., *25*:168–170, 1971.

29. German, W. J.: Cerebrospinal rhinorrhea—surgical repair. J. Neurosurg., *1*:50–66, 1944.

30. Gotham, J. E., Meyer, J. S., Gilroy, J., and Bauer, R. B.: Observations on cerebrospinal fluid rhinorrhea and pneumocephalus. Ann. Otol., *74*:214–233, 1965.

31. Grant, F. C.: Intracranial aerocele following fracture of the skull. Report of a case with review of the literature. Surg. Gynec. Obstet., *36*:251–255, 1923.

32. Greenblatt, S. H., and Wilson, D. H.: Persistent cerebrospinal fluid rhinorrhea treated by lumboperitoneal shunt. Technical Note. J. Neurosurg., *38*:524–526, 1973.

33. Hagan, R. E.: Early complications following penetrating wounds of the brain. J. Neurosurg., *34*:132–141, 1971.

34. Hand, W. L., and Sanford, J. P.: Post-traumatic bacterial meningitis. Ann. Intern. Med., *72*:869–874, 1970.

35. Hardwood-Nash, D. C.: Fractures of the petrous and tympanic parts of the temporal bone in children: A tomographic study of 35 cases. Amer. J. Roentgen., *110*:598–607, 1970.

36. Healy, C. E.: Significance of a positive reaction for glucose in rhinorrhea. Clin. Pediat., *8*:239, 1969.

37. Hendrick, E. B., Harwood-Nash, D. C., and Hudson, A. R.: Head injuries in children: A survey of 4,465 consecutive cases at the Hospital for Sick Children, Toronto, Canada. Clin. Neurosurg., *11*:46–65, 1964.

38. Holman, B. L., and Davis, D. O.: Radioisotopic assessment of cerebrospinal fluid pathways. Progr. Nucl. Med., *1*:359–375, 1972.

39. Hooper, A. C.: Sphenoidal defects—a possible cause of cerebrospinal fluid rhinorrhea. J. Neurol. Neurosurg. Psychiat., *34*:739–742, 1971.

40. Jacobson, I., and Maran, A. G.: Localization of cerebrospinal fluid rhinorrhea. Arch. Otolaryng., *93*:79–80, 1971.

41. Jaffe, B., Welch, K., Strand, R., and Treves, S.: Cerebrospinal fluid rhinorrhea via the fossa of Rosenmuller. Laryngoscope, *86*:903–907, 1976.

42. Jones, H. M.: The problem of recurrent meningitis. Proc. R. Soc. Med., *67*:1141–1147, 1974.

43. Jungmann, A., and Peyser, E.: Roentgen visual-

ization of cerebrospinal fluid fistula with contrast medium. Radiology, *80*:92–95, 1963.

44. Kadrie, H., Drieger, A., and McInnis, W.: Persistent dural cerebrospinal fluid leak shown by retrograde radionuclide myelography: Case report. J. Nucl. Med., *17*:797–799, 1976.

45. Kaufman, B., Nielsen, F., Weisr, M., et al.: Acquired spontaneous, nontraumatic normal-pressure cerebrospinal fluid fistulas originating from the middle fossa. Radiology, *122*:379–387, 1977.

46. Kaufman, H. H.: Non-traumatic cerebrospinal fluid rhinorrhea. Arch. Neurol., *21*:59–65, 1969.

47. Kirsch, A. P.: Diagnosis of cerebrospinal fluid rhinorrhea: Lack of specificity of the glucose oxidase test tape. J. Pediat., *71*:718–719, 1967.

48. Klastersky, J., Sadeghi, M., and Brihaye, J.: Antimicorbial prophylaxis in patients with rhinorrhea or otorrhea: A double-blind study. Surg. Neurol., *6*:111–114, 1976.

49. Kramer, S. A., Yanagisawa, E., and Smith, H. W.: Spontaneous cerebrospinal fluid otorrhea simulating serous otitis media. Laryngoscope, *81*:1083–1089, 1971.

50. Kraus, H.: Schadelverletzungen mit Eroffnung der Nebenhohlen. J. Int. Coll. Surg., *38*:372–376, 1962.

51. Lang, E. R., and Bucy, P. C.: Cerebrospinal fluid otorrhea. Arch. Otolaryng., *75*:415–418, 1962.

52. Leech, P. J., and Paterson, A.: Conservative and operative management for cerebrospinal fluid leakage after closed head injury. Lancet, *1*:1013–1015, 1973.

53. Levin, S., Nelson, K. E., Spies, H. W., and Lepper, M. D.: Pneumococcal meningitis: The problem of the unseen cerebrospinal fluid leak. Amer. J. Med., *10*:264, 1972.

54. Lewin, W.: Cerebrospinal fluid rhinorrhea in closed head injuries. Brit. J. Surg., *42*:1–18, 1954.

55. Lewin, W.: Cerebrospinal fluid rhinorrhea in nonmissile head injuries. (Proceedings of the Congress of Neurological Surgeons.) Clin. Neurosurg., *12*:237–252, 1964.

56. Locke, C. E., Jr.: The spontaneous escape of cerebrospinal fluid through the nose: Its occurrence with brain tumor. Arch. Neurol. Psychiat., *15*:309–324, 1926.

57. Locke, C. E., and Naffziger, H. C.: Cerebral subarachnoid system. Arch. Neurol. Psychiat., *12*:411–418, 1924.

58. MacGee, E. E., Cauthen, J. C., and Brackett, C. E.: Meningitis following acute traumatic cerebrospinal fluid fistula. J. Neurosurg., *33*:312–316, 1970.

59. Mahalay, M. S., Jr., and Odom, G. L.: Complication following intrathecal injection of fluoroescein: Case report. J. Neurosurg., *25*:298–299, 1968.

60. Marc, J. A., and Schecter, M. M.: The significance of fluid-gas displacement in the sphenoid sinus in post-traumatic cerebrospinal fluid rhinorrhea. Radiology, *108*:603–606, 1973.

61. McCallum, J., Maroon, J. C., and Janetta, P. J.: Treatment of postoperative cerebrospinal fluid fistulas by subarachnoid drainage. J. Neurosurg., *42*:434–437, 1975.

62. McKusick, K. A., Malmud, L. S., Kordela, P. A., and Wagner, H. N., Jr.: Radionuclide cisternography: Normal values for nasal secretion of intrathecally injected ^{111}In-DTPA. J. Nucl. Med., *14*:933–934, 1973.

63. Mincy, J. E.: Post-traumatic cerebrospinal fluid fistula of the frontal fossa. J. Trauma, *6*:618–622, 1966.

64. Morley, T. P., and Hetherington, R. F.: Traumatic cerebrospinal fluid rhinorrhea and otorrhea, pneumocephalus and meningitis. Surg. Gynec. Obstet., *104*:88–98, 1957.

65. Morley, T. P., and Wortzman, G.: The importance of the lateral extensions of the sphenoidal sinus in post-traumatic cerebrospinal rhinorrhea and meningitis. J. Neurosurg., *22*:326–332, 1965.

66. Mortara, R., and Norrell, H.: Consequences of a deficient sellar diaphragm. J. Neurosurg., *32*:565–573, 1970.

67. Norsa, L.: Cerebrospinal rhinorrhea with pituitary tumors. Neurology (Minneap.), *3*:864–868, 1953.

68. Nussey, A. M.: Spontaneous cerebrospinal fluid rhinorrhea. Brit. J. Med., *1*:1579–1580, 1966.

69. Nystrom, S. H. M.: On the use of biobond in the treatment of cerebrospinal rhinorrhea and frontobasal fistula. Int. Surg., *54*:332–340, 1970.

70. Obrador, S.: Primary non-traumatic spontaneous cerebrospinal fluid rhinorrhea with normal cerebrospinal fluid pressure. Schweiz. Arch. Neurol. Neurochir. Psychiat., *111*:369–376, 1972.

71. Obrador, S., Roda, J. E., and Gomez-Bueno, J.: Cerebrospinal fluid rhinorrhea in empty sella. Acta Neurochir., *26*:285–291, 1972.

72. O'Connell, J. E. A.: Primary spontaneous cerebrospinal fluid rhinorrhea. J. Neurol. Neurosurg. Psychiat., *27*:241–246, 1964.

73. Ommaya, A. K.: Cerebrospinal fluid rhinorrhea. Neurology (Minneap.), *14*:106–113, 1964.

74. Ommaya, A. K.: Spinal fluid fistulae. Clin. Neurosurg., *23*:363–392, 1976.

75. Ommaya, A. K., DiChiro, G., Baldwin, M., and Pennybacker, J. B.: Non-traumatic cerebrospinal fluid rhinorrhea. J. Neurol. Neurosurg. Psychiat., *31*:214–225, 1968.

76. Petersdorf, R. G., Curtin, J. A., Hoeprich, P. D., et al.: A study of antibiotic prophylaxis in unconscious patients. New Eng. J. Med., *257*:1001–1009, 1957.

77. Price, D. J. E., and Sleigh, J. D.: Control of infection due to Klebsiella aerogenes in a neurosurgical unit by withdrawal of all antibiotics. Lancet, *2*:1213–1215, 1970.

78. Raaf, J.: Post-traumatic cerebrospinal fluid leaks. Arch. Surg., *95*:648–651, 1967.

79. Raskin, R.: Cerebrospinal fluid rhinorrhea and otorrhea: Diagnosis and treatment in 35 cases. J. Int. Coll. Surg., *43*:141–154, 1965.

80. Raskind, R., and Doria, A.: Cerebrospinal fluid rhinorrhea and otorrhea of traumatic origin. Int. Surg., *46*:223–226, 1966.

81. Rasmussen, P. S.: Traumatisk Liquorrhea: en Oversigt Og en Analyse at 90 Tilfarlde. Ugeskr. Laeg., *127*:397–403, 1965.

82. Ray, B. S., and Bergland, R. M.: Cerebrospinal

fluid fistula: Clinical aspects, techniques of localization and methods of closure. J. Neurosurg., 30:399–405, 1969.

83. Robinson, R. G.: Cerebrospinal fluid rhinorrhea, meningitis and pneumocephalus due to nonmissile injuries. Aust. N. Z. J. Surg., 39:328–334, 1970.

84. Rovit, R. L., Schechter, M. M., and Nelson, K.: Spontaneous "high pressure cerebrospinal rhinorrhea" due to lesions obstructing flow of cerebrospinal fluid. J. Neurosurg., 30:406–412, 1969.

85. Schneider, R. C., and Thompson, J. M.: Chronic and delayed traumatic cerebrospinal rhinorrhea as a source of recurrent attacks of meningitis. Ann. Surg., 145:517–529, 1957.

86. Schultz, P., and Schwartz, G. H.: Radiculomyelopathy following intrathecal instillation of methylene blue. A hazard reaffirmed. Arch. Neurol., 22:240–244, 1970.

87. Spetzler, R. F., and Wilson, C. B.: Management of recurrent CSF rhinorrhea. Presented at the Sixth Annual Neurosurgery Postgraduate Course, San Francisco, May 20–27, 1976.

88. Spetzler, R. F., and Wilson, C. B.: Management of recurrent CSF rhinorrhea of the middle and posterior fossae. J. Neurosurg., 49:393–397, 1978.

89. Spetzler, R. F., Wilson, C. B., and Schulte, R.: Simplified percutaneous lumboperitoneal shunting. Surg. Neurol., 7:25–29, 1977.

90. Teng, P., and Edalatpour, N.: Cerebrospinal fluid rhinorrhea with demonstration of cranionasal fistula with Pantopaque. Radiology, 81:802–806, 1963.

91. Teng, P., and Papatheodorou, C.: Cerebrospinal fluid rhinorrhea and otorrhea. Arch. Otolaryng., 82:56–61, 1965.

92. Thomas, L. M., Webster, J. E., and Gurdjian, E. S.: A note on the use of methylmethacrylate for sealing the bony portion of a cranio-nasal fistula. J. Neurosurg., 17:355–356, 1960.

93. Thomson, St. C.: The Cerebrospinal Fluid: Its Spontaneous Escape from the Nose. London, Cassell & Co., Ltd., 1899.

94. Vandeark, G. D., Pitkethly, D. T., Ducker, T. B., and Kempe, L. G.: Repair of cerebrospinal fluid fistulas using a tissue adhesive. J.Neurosurg., 33:151–155, 1970.

95. Vrabec, D. P., and Hallberg, O. E.: Cerebrospinal fluid rhinorrhea. Arch. Otolaryng., 80:218–229, 1964.

96. Wallace, J. D., Weintraub, M. I., Mattson, R. H., and Rosnagle, R.: Status epilepticus as a complication of intrathecal fluorescein: A case report. J. Neurosurg., 36:659–670, 1972.

97. Weiss, M. H., Kaufman, B., and Richards, D. E.: Cerebrospinal fluid rhinorrhea from an empty sella: Transsphenoidal obliteration of the fistula. J. Neurosurg., 39:674–676, 1973.

98. Whitecar, J. P., Reddin, J. L., and Spink, W. W.: Recurrent pneumococcal meningitis. New Eng. J. Med., 274:1285–1289, 1966.

99. Willis, T.: Opera omnia; cerebri antomia, nervorumque descriptio et usus. Geneva, 1676.

100. Wilson, C. B., Hankinson, H., and Powell, M. R.: Neurosurgeon's view of the role of diagnostic radioisotopic studies. Symposium on Clinical Uses of Radionuclide: Critical Comparison with Other Techniques. U. S. Atomic Energy Commission Series, 27:73–78, 1972.

101. Wilson, C. B., Rand, R. W., Grollmus, J. M., Heuser, G., Levin, S., Goldfield, E., Schneider, V., Linfoot, J., and Hosobuchi, Y.: Surgical experience with microscopic transsphenoidal approach to pituitary tumors and non-neoplastic parasellar conditions. Calif. Med., 117:1–9, 1972.

102. Wolman, L.: The neuropathological effects resulting from the intrathecal injection of chemical substances. Paraplegia, 4:97–115, 1966.

66

CRANIAL DEFECTS
AND THEIR REPAIR

Skull defects—man-made, accidental, and the result of disease—have been known since antiquity. Various types of repair have been attempted for almost as long. This subject has been reviewed by Grant and Norcross, by Woolf and Walker, and by Reeves.[21,56,74] Although the frequency of this problem increases during wartime, it is part of the everyday practice of most neurosurgeons during peace.

ETIOLOGY OF CRANIAL DEFECTS

Trauma

Trauma is the most important cause of cranial defects in civilian as well as military neurosurgery. The majority of these lesions are made by the neurosurgeon in the course of adequate excision of compound depressed skull fractures and penetrating wounds of the brain. Management of these injuries requires primary repair of the dura and scalp, but not necessarily of the cranium. Contaminated, comminuted fragments of bone, without periosteal attachment, are usually discarded. Closed depressed skull fractures may occasionally be so comminuted that retention of the bone fragments is not practical. Closed linear skull fractures in children can, with underlying dural laceration, become "growing skull fractures" and thus produce cranial defects.

In the military, head injuries resulting in cranial defects are usually from shell or mine fragments, because rifle and machine gun wounds of the head are more often le-thal. In civilian life, the high and apparently increasing incidence of automobile accidents, industrial injuries, and gunshot wounds of the head presages an endless flow of patients who have lost some portion of their cranium. With improved methods of care, both operative and nonoperative, more of them will survive to the time of possible need for cranioplasty.

Infection

Osteomyelitis of neurosurgical significance is most often frontal, a complication of pyogenic frontoethmoiditis. Huge bifrontal defects may result from excision of infected bone. Another source of cranial defect is wound infection or aseptic necrosis of the bone flap following craniotomy. Both these complications require that the wound be excised and, almost always, that the bone flap be discarded.

Neoplasms

Osteomas of the skull, hyperostosing meningiomas, dermoids, and eosinophilic granulomas may leave large defects after their excision. Cranial defects caused by destructive tumors, such as metastatic carcinoma, are usually not significant clinical problems. Rarely, however, after radical excision of a locally invasive malignant tumor, with or without radiotherapy, the prognosis is sufficiently good to warrant repair of the defect.

R. L. TIMMONS

Congenital Defects

Congenital defects of the skull are usually associated with more extensive dysraphic disorders such as cranial meningocele or meningoencephalocele. The cranial defect does not itself constitute the clinical problem until the meningeal hernia has been repaired with retention of nearly normal neurological function. Matson, however, reported congenital skull defects, usually midline, that were not associated with other evidence of craniocerebral dysraphism.[43]

External Decompression

Craniectomy and the removal of bone flaps are now rarely necessary for management of intracranial mass lesions or diffuse brain swelling. A possible exception is lead encephalopathy, and there have recently been renewed attempts to control posttraumatic increased intracranial pressure that has not responded to other measures by removal of large bone flaps.

Regardless of the cause of cranial defect, there are three questions that the neurosurgeon contemplating repair must answer. The first is whether the defect needs to be repaired, because the presence of a cranial defect does not in itself justify cranioplasty. One must define the significance of cranial defects and the indications for their repair. The second question concerns the timing of cranioplasty, and the third concerns the method of cranioplasty. Some degree of controversy and personal preference have been involved in the answers to these questions, especially the one regarding method. As in other fields of neurosurgery, however, different methods may be equally successful in different hands.

CRANIAL DEFECTS AS INDICATIONS FOR CRANIOPLASTY

Most authors have discussed the possible significance of cranial defects under six headings. The first two are accepted generally as definite indications for cranioplasty, while the clinical evidence in support of the other four is controversial.

Cosmetic Significance

The appearance of the skull, especially the fronto-orbital region, is probably secondary in importance only to the appearance of the face. Large cranial defects carry the implication of intellectual or personality disorder, even if the underlying brain is intact. Achieving social acceptance and obtaining or holding a job become difficult. The patient with an unsightly skull defect withdraws from society and accepts total disability, even though this is not justified on the basis of neurological or mental deficit. Defects that underlie temporal or occipital muscle usually are not cosmetic problems, nor are the smaller defects that lie posteriorly, especially if they are covered with hair.

Protection of the Brain

It is difficult to establish the degree of increased susceptibility to brain injury, if any, that is caused by a skull defect of any given size. Brain injury as a consequence of cranial defect is a rare clinical experience. This might be because most cranial defects above a given size are repaired, and when they are not, the patient is so fearful of injury that he avoids all activity that might possibly lead to trauma of any sort. This anxiety or feeling of insecurity caused by a cranial defect may interfere with rehabilitation of the patient as much as a cosmetic problem. Cranioplasty may therefore be justified for imagined as well as real danger of subsequent cerebral injury.

The real dangers apply to the following occupations or groups of patients: (1) military service, which disqualifies an individual with an unrepaired defect over 2 to 3 cm; (2) heavy industry, construction, and mining; and (3) contact sports and racing. These activities or occupations usually require that a helmet be worn over a normal skull, and it must be assumed that an individual with an unrepaired cranial defect larger than the arbitrary 2 to 3 cm would be at increased risk. (4) Children, because their behavior and activity are difficult to control, and (5) patients with seizures, who constitute a significant proportion of those with cranial defects, are included. Helmets or heavy caps are frequently prescribed for these latter two groups prior to cranioplasty.

Local Discomfort

Tenderness or pain may be referred to the cranial defect, but this varies. Some patients have no local symptoms, while others cannot bear palpation of the defect and complain of pulsating pain that is aggravated by exertion, dependency of the head, or exposure to heat or the sun. The size and location of the defect bear no relation to these symptoms. Some patients complain of defects little larger than a burr hole, while others with large bifrontal defects have no local symptoms. Walker and Erculei studied men with cranial defects from World War II after 15 years.[69] Most of them had had a cranioplasty (tantalum), but some had not had the defect repaired. There was no difference between the two groups with regard to local symptoms. The patients who had had a cranioplasty complained of local tenderness and pain in the same proportion as, or greater proportion than, those with residual cranial defects. While there seems to be little doubt that some patients with local complaints are benefited symptomatically by cranioplasty, the basis for symptoms in these patients might be psychological and therefore come under the cosmetic or protective indications for cranioplasty listed earlier. Dural defects and intradural disorders such as increased intracranial pressure, infection, or retained foreign body could produce local symptoms similar to those just described, but the clinical problem here is not the cranial defect.

"Syndrome of the Trephined"

This syndrome has been described by almost everyone writing on the subject of cranial defects and cranioplasty, and it is apparently fixed in the literature. The symptoms are extremely variable and nonspecific. They include local discomfort, generalized headache, dizziness or vertigo, intolerance of vibration and noise, irritability, easy fatigability, loss of incentive and ability to concentrate, anxiety and depression. These are the same symptoms that we now describe under the heading of "postconcussion syndrome" or "post-trau-matic syndrome." The syndrome is not affected by the size or location of the cranial defect, nor by its repair.[22,69] The pathogenesis of this syndrome may be primarily related to social and psychological factors, in which case the patient might be improved by cranioplasty for the reasons discussed under cosmetic and protective indications. On the other hand, the syndrome might also be related to dural or intradural abnormality, in which case cranioplasty should have no bearing upon the clinical course.

Seizures

The relation of a cranial defect to the development of seizures, and conversely, the effect of cranioplasty on either pre-existing seizures or the subsequent development of a convulsive disorder, have been discussed in the literature. Prevention of seizures and improvement of an existing seizure disorder have been listed as reasons for cranioplasty, often with little supporting experimental or clinical evidence. Some reports that describe clinical improvement of a seizure disorder after cranioplasty include only short-term follow-up, while others concern patients who had dural as well as cranial defects. The operative procedure in these instances involved dural repair or excision of a meningocortical cicatrix as well as cranioplasty. Walker and Erculei compared men with head injuries who had unrepaired defects with others who had had cranioplasty, both early and late, and found no difference in clinical course or subsequent development of post-traumatic epilepsy between the two groups.[18,69] Other authors agree that the convulsive disorder is related to intradural disease, i.e., the effect on the brain of the same injury or disease that produced the cranial defect, and not the cranial defect itself. A patient who has lost a bone flap because of postoperative craniotomy infection and refused later repair provides an appropriate clinical illustration. The resulting cranial defect does not produce a convulsive disorder, nor does it adversely affect a pre-existing one.

Cerebral Atrophy

Pneumoencephalography has demonstrated dilatation of the lateral ventricle underlying a cranial defect and shift of the ventricular system toward that side. This has been described as "migration" of the ventricle toward the defect. That these changes indicate atrophy of cerebral tissue underlying the defect is not disputed, but the same question arises that has been discussed under the previous three headings. Does the cerebral atrophy result from or is it affected by the cranial defect itself so that cranioplasty is indicated to prevent further atrophy? Or, is the atrophic process caused by the effect on the brain of the same injury or disease that produced the cranial defect so that repair of the cranium would have no effect on development of cerebral atrophy? Recent clinical opinion supports the latter concept except possibly in children and in adults with huge defects.

Large unrepaired defects in adults remain flat if the dura is intact and there is no intradural abnormality. These patients rarely show progressive neurological deterioration, although a recent report by Tabaddor and LaMorgese describes an exception.[66] Their patient had a very large defect, almost a hemicraniectomy, and they related progressive concavity of the defect to the progressive neurological deficit that occurred two months postoperatively. The pathogenesis of the progressive neurological deficit in this patient is unclear, but it was apparently reversed by cranioplasty. Tabaddor postulated that with defects below a given size, the weight of the stretched scalp is borne by the bone margins, while with huge defects, the unsupported scalp sags against the brain, transmitting atmospheric pressure directly to it. Langfitt has stated that lumbar puncture pressure in the sitting position is higher in patients with cranial defects.[34] The rigid nature of the intact cranium prevents application of atmospheric pressure directly to the system, causing reduction of pressure (below "normal") as fluid is displaced into the manometer. With a cranial defect, the system becomes elastic, the scalp may move inward as fluid is displaced into the manometer, and thus atmospheric pressure is applied directly to the system. Whether one accepts the clinical significance of these hydrodynamic phenomena or not, the intact calvarium certainly supports or suspends the dura away from the brain, thus providing a subarachnoid space through which pass all of the arterial supply to and part of the venous drainage from the cerebral cortex. The obliteration of the subarachnoid space under a cranial defect could theoretically interfere with cortical perfusion. Nevertheless, Tabaddor's patient remains an isolated or at least rare clinical example of this phenomenon.

In contrast with cranial defects in adults, those in children may bulge, even in the absence of known dural or intradural abnormality (Fig. 66–1). The margins of the defect sometimes become everted, as though an intracranial force were pushing them out. Yet, there are no symptoms or signs of increased intracranial pressure. Sequential pneumoencephalography has, in some such instances, shown progressive ventricular dilatation underlying the defect. Probably the difference is simply that between the growing and the nongrowing brain. Brain growth produces cranial enlargement, and in the presence of a large cranial defect, this expansile force might be distributed in an asymmetrical fashion. The resulting tendency of the growing brain to bulge through a cranial defect could produce the hemodynamic alterations known to exist with cerebral hernia.

In summary, cranial defects should be repaired for cosmetic and protective reasons, including the social, economic, and psychological factors that are frequently involved. Local and generalized symptoms that are not related to these factors may be caused by dural or intradural abnormality and would not be relieved by cranioplasty. The same can be said of convulsive disorders and cerebral atrophy, except in children, who probably need an intact cranium for normal cerebral growth, and possibly in adults with very large cranial defects. In these two instances, cranioplasty may prevent the development of local hemodynamic forces that would adversely affect the underlying brain.

TIMING OF CRANIOPLASTY AND PREOPERATIVE MANAGEMENT

There is a natural tendency to hope for spontaneous regeneration of cranium. Growth of bone from the margins of a defect is slight and clinically insignificant. Regeneration of bone is mostly from the outer layer of dura, which is periosteum. This tissue loses its osteogenic potential after 5 or 6 years of age. In younger patients, there is

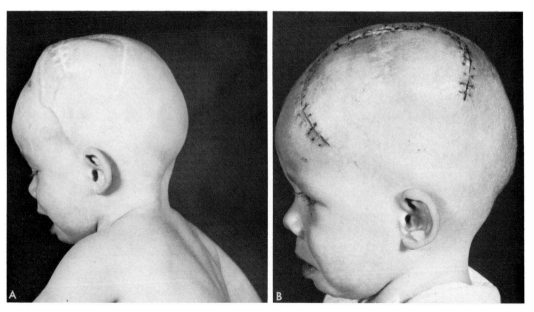

Figure 66–1 *A.* Bulging of brain through left parietal defect in a 20-month-old boy. *B.* Defect repaired with autogenous rib (see Fig. *66–9*).

rapid regeneration of bone as is seen, for example, after craniectomy for craniosyn-ostosis. Osseous regeneration cannot be expected, even in these young patients, if the dura has been replaced by a fascia lata graft. Because the important regeneration is from the dura, the size of the defect should have no bearing on the rapidity or completeness of spontaneous repair.

Patients older than 5 or 6 years show little or no spontaneous regeneration of cra-nium with one notable exception. Huge bi-frontal craniectomies for osteomyelitis in older children and teen-agers have been fol-lowed by rapid complete reformation of the skull (Fig. 66–2). The inflammatory process must have some effect on the osteogenic property of dura. Although one cannot oth-erwise anticipate significant spontaneous regeneration of defects in older children and adults, there is a progressive thickening or decreased elasticity of scalp and dura, so

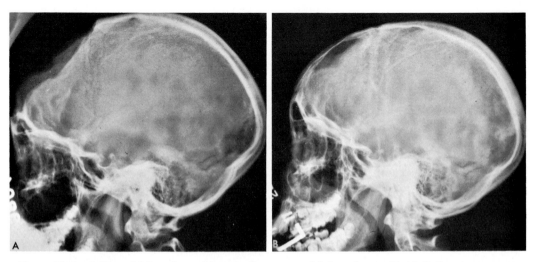

Figure 66–2 *A.* Frontal defect after craniectomy for osteomyelitis in an 8-year-old girl. *B.* Spontaneous regen-eration 10 months later. Although the regenerated bone is not as dense as original cranium, observation and palpa-tion of the defect give the impression of normal skull.

that pulsations decrease in amplitude and may disappear altogether.

Significant spontaneous repair, if it is going to occur, is evident within the first six months. Delay in the performance of cranioplasty is more often related to two other factors: overt or latent infection, and the condition of the scalp.

Regardless of the method of cranioplasty, the material used to fill the defect must be considered a foreign body, temporarily in the case of osteoplastic cranioplasty, permanently in the case of alloplastic cranioplasty. It is therefore unreasonable to expect healing to occur in the presence of overt sepsis. Despite scattered claims of success following cranioplasty performed in this situation, the great majority of neurosurgeons believe that cranioplasty of any sort should not be done until at least 6 to 12 months have elapsed following the last overt sign of wound infection. Furthermore, if unexpected infection is encountered during the course of exposure, the cranioplastic procedure should be terminated, and attention should be directed toward eradication of infection.

Primary repair of a cranial defect is of course perfectly feasible following surgical excision of hyperostosing meningiomas and other tumors of the skull. Some divergence of opinion exists regarding compound wounds that have been made surgically clean by excision. Primary cranioplasty may be successful in such instances and would save the patient a second operative procedure. The argument against primary repair of the cranial defect following excision of compound wounds is twofold: (1) These recently injured patients ought to have the shortest procedure and the shortest anesthesia time consistent with adequate excision and closure. (2) Viable tissue with an intact blood supply will tolerate and control a degree of contamination that will not be controlled in the presence of foreign material or even autogenous bone that lacks a blood supply. Free bone fragments have been successfully replaced following early excision of compound wounds.[31] There has recently been an even greater tendency to replace bone fragments, including areas of potential contamination such as frontal sinus, orbit, and cribriform plate.[49] This would obviate the need for a cranioplastic procedure or make it simpler, i.e., a smaller, less complicated defect. The attempted salvage of the patient's own skull fragments is, however, quite different from risking an iliac or rib graft, and it takes far less time. Primary alloplastic cranioplasty carries an even higher risk of failure in the face of otherwise insignificant contamination, but is utilized by some neurosurgeons. Most prefer to wait three to six months after primary healing of a compound wound before considering repair of the cranial defect.

Successful cranioplasty, regardless of method, requires not only the absence of infection and contamination but also the presence of full-thickness well-vascularized scalp. Split-thickness skin grafts should be replaced by pedicle flaps of scalp or other full-thickness skin. Wide, thin, poorly vascularized scars should be excised and closed before or as part of the cranioplastic procedure.

METHODS OF CRANIOPLASTY

The many techniques for repair of cranial defects resolve themselves into two major groups, alloplastic and osteoplastic. Each group has its neurosurgical adherents, because each method possesses advantages and disadvantages. Several authors have observed that alloplastic methods became popular during both world wars, while enthusiasm for osteoplastic methods recurred during the peace that followed.[30,39,48]

Alloplastic Cranioplasty

Gold was used to fill cranial defects as far back as the sixteenth century.[56] The modern era of cranioplasty began in the late nineteenth and early twentieth centuries when bone grafting methods were developed. Most procedures during this period were osteoplastic, but gold, silver, lead, aluminum, and celluloid underwent considerable trial, especially during World War I. These methods, with sporadic exceptions, proved unsatisfactory, and apparently most surgeons returned to osteoplastic methods during the interval between World Wars I and II. Renewed interest in metallic cranioplasty developed in the early 1940's, stimulated by the great need for repair of cranial defects that occurred during and after World War II.

Tantalum Cranioplasty

The ideal substance for cranioplasty should be strong, light, malleable, and inert. Some of the earliest trials involved Vitallium, an alloy of cobalt, chromium, and molybdenum, but this substance has never received the attention from neurosurgeons that it has from other fields such as orthopedics because it is not malleable and cannot be shaped at the operating table. Ticonium, an alloy similar to Vitallium, with nickel replacing some of the cobalt, seemed to fulfill the foregoing requirements experimentally, but it never received a clinical trial. The widest clinical application, by far, has been given tantalum, a metal that fulfills the requirements perhaps more closely than any metallic substance.[44,54,58,70,73] Perforated sheets of tantalum 0.015 inch (0.38 mm) thick are light, malleable enough to allow some shaping at the operating table, and strong enough to afford adequate protection, although not approximating the strength of the intact skull.[67] In the absence of infection, the surrounding host tissue forms a thin translucent fibrous membrane, which envelops the plate. The metal itself remains essentially inert, so plates removed years after their insertion are reportedly unchanged, indicating the absence of electrolysis or corrosion. As recently reported by McFadden, no metal or metallic alloy is completely inert, completely corrosion resistant.[46] The methods used to cut, shape, and fix the metallic prosthesis, including the use of tools containing other metals or alloys, tend to break down the mechanisms that resist corrosion and may lead to electrolysis.

The techniques of tantalum cranioplasty have been described in detail by Reeves.[56] The plate may be preformed by means of a complicated procedure involving the construction of a die and counterdie. This is preferred for complex fronto-orbital defects. A simpler method is to shape the plates at the operating table by hammering them on convex and concave metal casts that approximate the convexity of the human skull.[43] Available to the neurosurgeon are precut, preformed, perforated tantalum plates in various shapes and sizes, amazingly adaptable to most cranial defects, even fronto-orbital ones (Fig. 66–3). Once formed and fitted, the plate is applied to the calvarium by an onlay or an inlay method. The former is satisfactory for most cosmetic purposes because of the thinness of tantalum plates, while the inlay method may be preferable in the frontal region or under thin scalp. The latter method involves the removal of the outer table of the skull around the margins of the defect to a width of 5 mm and a depth of 2 mm. Fixation can be achieved with tantalum wedges

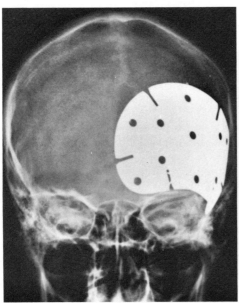
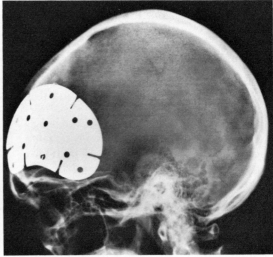

Figure 66–3   Left frontal tantalum cranioplasty with preformed plate.

for an inlaid plate, tantalum wires or screws for either an onlaid or an inlaid plate. Reeves stated that the wedges and screws are mechanically superior to wires. Most neurosurgeons have preferred perforated plates to allow escape of epidural blood and fluid. Some have reported that daily aspirations from the subgaleal space are necessary following tantalum cranioplasty. Subgaleal fluid accumulation has not, however, been frequent, provided there are good fit and fixation, no dural defect, and no infection or contamination. Eventually, the perforations become filled with fibrous tissue, and this provides better fixation of the plate.

Tantalum has several specific disadvantages. It is extremely expensive. Like other metals and metallic alloys, it is an excellent conductor of heat, so some patients have experienced discomfort when exposed to extremes of temperature. Even if well fixed, tantalum can be dented or depressed by an external blow. It is radiopaque, with the result that subsequent contrast studies are difficult to read. Finally, a newer and major disadvantage of tantalum is its interference with subsequent CT scanning (Fig. 66–4).

Other Metallic Prostheses

Most of the metallic cranioplasties done during and following World War II used tantalum, but there have been several subsequent reports concerning other metallic substances. Scott and co-workers reported their extensive experience with stainless steel, which has the same general advantages as tantalum and also is radiolucent and inexpensive.[61] They emphasized the use of a specific type of stainless steel (316), which, according to McFadden, is one of the most inert, most corrosion-resistant of all stainless steels.[46] It is also softer than other types, which may be an advantage in cranioplasty in which malleability is required, but is a disadvantage in the manufacture of vascular clamps and aneurysm clips.

Bates reported experiments with zirconium, which compared favorably with tantalum in regard to inertness and lack of tissue reaction.[5] It is lighter, softer, and more malleable than tantalum; hence, plates must be thicker.

Titanium has been used by Simpson.[63] It is also radiolucent and cheaper than tantalum, and according to McFadden, it is theo-

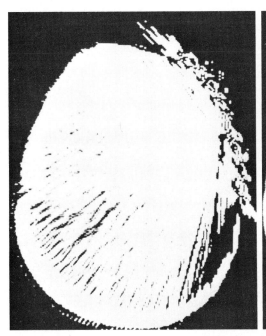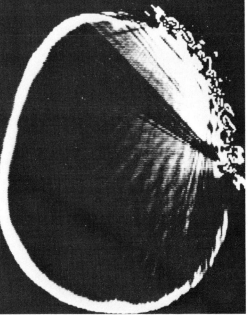

Figure 66–4 Computed tomographic scans following right frontal tantalum cranioplasty.

retically the most inert of all metallic substances studied as far as electrolysis and corrosion are concerned.[46] It is, however, harder and less malleable than tantalum, and should therefore be more difficult to shape.

A metal that was used at the end of the nineteenth and the beginning of this century, aluminum, has been reintroduced by Black and co-workers who claim it is as light, strong, malleable, and corrosion-resistant as tantalum, but cheaper and radiolucent.[7] The perforated plates are made from the Fox eye shield and are thicker (0.025 inch or 0.64 mm) than the standard tantalum plate. Black has more recently reported the successful repair of even fronto-supraorbital defects with aluminum. Some of the defects were so large that two Fox eye shields were welded or tied together. Rounded metal blocks serve as anvils on which to shape the aluminum plate at the operating table, and "sturdy instruments" are required to further shape and cut the plate so as to reconstitute the supraorbital margin. Apparently, silk sutures provide adequate fixation. Of considerable importance, however, is the fact that two of Black's patients had satisfactory CT scans following aluminum cranioplasty.[6]

Theoretically, all metallic plates should be fixed with wires, wedges, or screws of the same metallic substance in order to avoid electrolysis and corrosion.

Acrylic Cranioplasty

The first attempts to repair cranial defects with the acrylic resin methyl methacrylate were also made in the 1940's, after the successful use of this material for dental prostheses.[17,23,64] In lightness, strength, and tissue tolerance, acrylic compares favorably with tantalum. It has the additional advantages of being cheap, radiolucent, and a thermal nonconductor. As used initially in the completely processed form, however, the plastic was rigid and unmalleable, so the early acrylic cranioplasties involved impression techniques just as complex as those for tantalum. The indirect method required the construction of molds or dies that conformed to the cranial defect through the intact scalp. The resulting preformed acrylic plate usually required adjustment by reheating when the defect was exposed. The direct method involved the making of a mold from the cranial defect itself at the time of operative exposure. The mold was then sent to the laboratory where the acrylic plate was made. This required either a delay in the procedure, the patient lying in the operating room, usually under general anesthesia, with a sterile towel over the wound, or else a two-stage procedure. It is not surprising that tantalum, which could be cut, beaten, and shaped at the operating table, was preferred by most World War II surgeons despite the other advantages of acrylic.

Following World War II the one-stage acrylic method appeared, and this has completely changed the picture of alloplastic cranioplasty.[57,65] Previously, the process of polymerization that produced the finished plastic required both heat and pressure, thus necessitating the impression techniques just described and the production of the finished acrylic plate in a laboratory. A process was developed whereby autopolymerization occurred following mixture of the liquid monomer and the powdered polymer in approximately a 1:2 ratio. No pressure was required, and the process produced its own heat. The process of polymerization could now be made to occur in situ so that the plate could be made to conform to the cranial defect before it became rigid. Because of the excellent fit, the good cosmetic result, and the simplicity of the procedure, few neurosurgeons who have trained since World War II have had a great deal of experience with metallic cranioplasty.

Spence emphasized another advantage of acrylic over metallic cranioplasty.[65] The metal plate, especially if onlaid but even if inlaid, left a variable space between it and the dura. The acrylic plate can be made not only to conform to the surface contour of the missing skull but also to fill the entire space of the cranial defect. The obliteration of dead space is laudable in any operative procedure, although there is some residual space between dura and bone flap following any craniotomy. Spence claimed, however, that by completely filling the defect, the acrylic plate "splinted" the brain and prevented its herniation into the defect as Weiford and Gardner alleged for tantalum cranioplasty.[70] There is little evidence, however, that the adult brain requires such "splinting" or tends to herniate into a cranial defect, provided the dura is intact and there is no intradural abnormality producing increased intracranial pressure.

The technique of acrylic cranioplasty is well known to most neurosurgeons. After exposure of the circumference of the defect, irregularities in the cranial margin may be removed to provide a simpler contour for molding the acrylic. The liquid and powder are mixed in a metal container. The liquid is not only sterile as it comes from the manufacturer but also bacteriostatic, so thorough mixing of the two serves to sterilize the resulting plastic. The mixture is at first a thick paste, but with stirring becomes a viscous liquid that can be rolled into a sheet of proper size and thickness to fill the defect. The process of polymerization is exothermic, and if it is allowed to occur in contact with the dura, the latter will be burned. Many surgeons protect the dura with moist cottonoid strips because they are not concerned with a small amount of space between dura and plate. A useful technique is to place the material in a polyethylene bag while it is still a viscous liquid. The bag itself is laid over the defect, and the viscous plastic is molded to exactly fit the contours of the cranial margin as well as the convexity of the missing bone. There may be no margin in certain areas such as the supraorbital ridge and glabella. Here the plastic is shaped to provide what the operator considers to be a satisfactory cosmetic contour, the other side of the cranium being used for comparison if possible. The fingers of the surgeon and his assistants press the soft plastic against the cranial margin around the entire circumference of the defect, thus thinning the plastic wherever it extends over cranium. Irrigation with cold saline helps to dissipate heat, but the plate becomes firm enough to hold its shape before the period of maximal heat production. At this point it is removed from the defect, extracted from the bag, and allowed to become hard and cool. The thin flange of plastic, representing that portion that extended over cranium, may be removed with a rongeur. A carborundum wheel is used to finish the plate, smoothing rough edges or surfaces, thinning it where necessary. Holes are drilled in the plate and the cranium for fixation with wire. Perforations for drainage of epidural fluid are unnecessary. The fit between plate and cranium is not watertight, nor would this serve any particular purpose. The goals are (1)

adequate fit so that cosmetically the plate has the external appearance of the intact skull and (2) solid fixation so that it will not slip or be dislodged by mild trauma. Postoperative fluid collection under the scalp does not seem to be any more frequent than following ordinary craniotomy.

The technique just described is probably the most common method of cranioplasty in use today. It produces satisfactory results according to the criteria listed (Fig. 66–5 and 66–6). There is no interference with subsequent CT scanning, and as a matter of fact, from the radiographic point of view, an acrylic cranioplasty acts like a cranial defect. It has been established that there is no tissue response to acrylic on the part of bone or soft tissue.[13] Long-term follow-up reports are now available.[12,25,52] These are discussed later under advantages and complications of alloplastic cranioplasty.

Some surgeons are still reporting experience with impression techniques, direct or indirect, claiming superior cosmetic results, better fit, and a plate of more uniform thickness.[4,10,42,59,60] The indirect impression technique also saves operative time, since the plate is fabricated preoperatively. Impression techniques are not, however, familiar to most neurosurgeons and require in addition the services of a dental or prosthetics laboratory. When such services are available, including a dentist with training and interest in the problem of cranioplasty, these techniques seem to produce excellent results. Most neurosurgeons, however, are repairing skull defects on their own.

Combined Acrylic and Stainless Steel Mesh Cranioplasty

A method combining acrylic with stainless steel mesh has been described by Galicich and Hovkind.[19] The mesh is cut and molded by hand to fit the defect and then coated with the plastic to a thickness of 1 mm. The resulting plate has the radiolucency of acrylic and the strength of stainless steel. This overcomes one of the drawbacks of acrylic plates, especially in children, namely that thin plates are extremely brittle and easily cracked by ordinary trauma.[27,28]

Follow-up CT scans on one of Galicich's patients show that the stainless steel mesh does reduce the quality somewhat, but un-

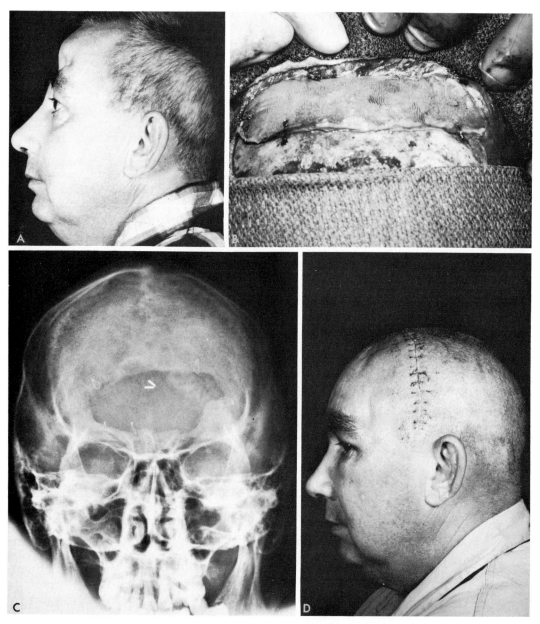

Figure 66–5 *A.* Frontal defect eight months after craniectomy for compound depressed skull fracture. *B.* Acrylic plate wired into defect (patient facing upward). *C.* Postoperative x-ray shows that acrylic is radiolucent. *D.* Postoperative appearance of patient.

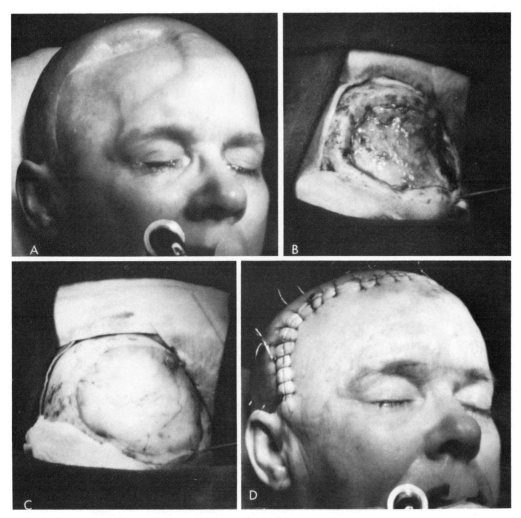

Figure 66–6 *A*. Right frontal defect following loss of bone flap. *B*. Operative exposure of defect. *C*. Acrylic cranioplasty. *D*. Postoperative appearance.

like the CT scan after tantalum cranioplasty, the study is still diagnostically useful (Fig. 66–7).[20] There have been further reports of acrylic–stainless steel mesh cranioplasty, including a prefabrication method.[15,68] Lake and associates have reported experimental work with mesh-reinforced acrylic, using tantalum and aluminum mesh as well as stainless steel.[32] They found a coarse mesh preferable to a fine one because it was stronger yet easier to mold. External trauma to mesh-reinforced plastic produced less fragmentation than it does to acrylic alone or even bone. Aluminum mesh was just as strong as tantalum or stainless steel and had the advantage of radiolucency. CT scans should be unaffected by acrylic–aluminum mesh cranioplasty.

Polyethylene Cranioplasty

Alexander and Dillard reported their experience with another plastic, polyethylene, in 1950.[3] This substance is radiolucent, a thermal nonconductor, inert in tissue, and can be shaped at the operating table because it becomes soft and malleable after immersion in hot water, hard again following immersion in cold water. Despite satisfaction with polyethylene, Alexander did not continue to use it because of the development of the one-stage acrylic technique and the difficulty in obtaining supplies of polyethylene that had been histologically tested.[2] Apparently one of the problems with any plastic prosthetic material is that histological inertness of a

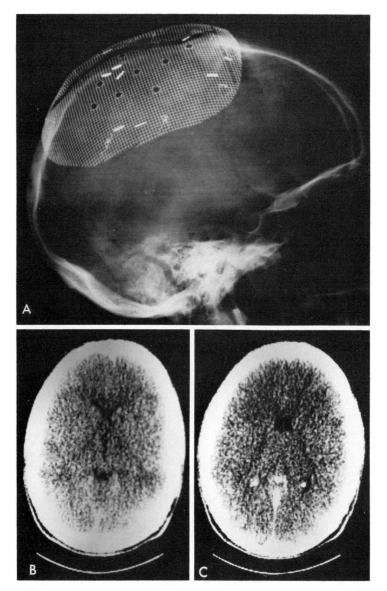

Figure 66–7 *A*. Sixteen-year-old boy with right parietal defect following removal of meningioma. The defect was repaired by acrylic–stainless steel mesh cranioplasty. *B* and *C*. Postoperative CT scans. (Courtesy of Dr. Joseph H. Galicich.)

given batch does not guarantee similar behavior by subsequent batches. Clark has continued to use polyethylene, and he reports that it is not sarcogenic, as intimated by others, and produces no histological reaction in its pure form.[14] Problems with tissue toxicity that had developed in the past resulted from contaminants or additives involved in the manufacturing process. Clark uses a 5-mm polyethylene plate, and he believes that some preoperative molding is necessary. The plate is cut larger than the defect, softened under an infrared lamp, and then molded into the defect through the intact scalp. Further shaping can be done during the operation by additional molding after immersing the plate in very hot water and also by using rongeurs or by whittling the plastic with a scalpel. A significant advantage of polyethylene, according to Clark, is that it does not become as brittle as acrylic.

Recently, prefabrication (i.e., indirect impression) techniques have been reported for using polyethylene.[29,53,59] The listed advantages include absence of infection, flexibility despite tensile strength that assures that the plate cannot be fractured (like acrylic) or dented (like tantalum), radiolucency, and noninterference with CT scanning.

Silastic should be mentioned as yet another substance used in alloplastic cranioplasty.[16,36] This material is inert, easily contoured, and easily fixed with silk or nylon sutures. The softness that makes Silastic easy to handle, however, provides none of the strength or rigidity inherent in normal skull and preferred for any type of skull repair.

Advantages and Complications of Alloplastic Cranioplasty

Neurosurgeons who favor alloplastic cranioplasty list three general advantages over osteoplastic cranioplasty: (1) the availability of the prosthetic material, so that the size of the defect is not a factor, (2) the need for only one operative incision, and (3) the alleged superiority of the cosmetic result since these materials can be either cut, bent, beaten, pressed, or molded, as the case may be, into any shape or contour. The disadvantage of alloplastic cranioplasty is that the material is and remains a foreign body. Even after encapsulation by fibrous tissue, the prosthesis is separate from host tissue, surrounded by potential space, and susceptible to infection or dislodgment, which may occur months or years after initial healing. Sinus tracts between plate and skin, epidural granulomas between plate and dura, and pneumatocele around the plate have been reported.[47,72] These complications occur especially in the fronto-orbital region because of communication between frontonasal duct or residual frontal sinus mucous membrane and the fibrous capsule surrounding the plate. Blatt and Failla have reported successful acrylic cranioplasty even in the fronto-orbital region, provided frontal sinus mucous membrane is completely excised and the nasofrontal duct is occluded.[8] Another common problem has been infection from without such as occurs when a poorly fitted, poorly fixed, or dislodged plate erodes through overlying scalp or skin. Thin poorly vascularized scalp predisposes to this complication. Fracture of an acrylic plate with production of cerebrospinal fluid fistula and erosion of a plate re-

placing the supraorbital margin through the upper eyelid have been reported.[27,41]

Regardless of the cause of loss of skin or scalp over a plate, the prosthesis must be removed.[9,33,71] Despite scattered claims of control of infection and healing of overlying scalp after antibiotic treatment, the general result if the plate is left in situ will be progressive formation of infected granulation tissue around the prosthesis and progressive loss of overlying skin, leaving more and more of the plate exposed (Fig. 66–8). Even if the overlying scalp is intact, dented or depressed tantalum plates and fractured acrylic plates have lost their cosmetic and protective function.

Complications of alloplastic cranioplasty requiring operative intervention have been reported variously as from 6 to 12 per cent in patients followed up to two years.[71] Longer follow-up reports now available indicate complication rates from as low as 2 per cent to a high that is still about 12 per cent.[12,25,52] Infection still constitutes the most common reason for failure, with fracture of an acrylic plate next. One series reported no infection following acrylic cranioplasty, but follow-up was far from complete.[25] Because these complications are more common in the fronto-orbital region than elsewhere, some surgeons who otherwise prefer alloplastic methods believe they should not be used to repair fronto-orbital defects. Alloplastic methods may be even more strongly contraindicated in the fronto-orbital region of growing children because deformities of the orbit are said to result.[41] These factors tend to vitiate the alleged cosmetic superiority of alloplastic cranioplasty.

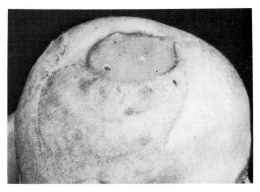

Figure 66–8 Exposure of acrylic plate three years after right parietal cranioplasty. The scalp flap has retracted laterally.

Osteoplastic Cranioplasty

As described earlier, the use of autogenous bone to repair cranial defects began before World War I. Outer table of adjacent skull was popular initially because it was believed that bone should not be separated from its periosteal blood supply. This of course severely limited the size of the defect that could be repaired. It has since been shown repeatedly that fresh autogenous bone may be transplanted and will heal as a free bone flap, which heals in the same way as one left attached to periosteum.[55] The principles of bone transplantation have been outlined by Peer and by Longacre.[37,51] When fresh autogenous bone such as ilium or rib is transplanted to soft tissue such as muscle or fat, it disappears in 8 to 12 months. In contact with living bone such as cranium, it can heal in the same way as a craniotomy bone flap. Peer and Longacre believe that some of the graft osteocytes survive if near the surface of cancellous bone. Survival of the cells is not necessary for survival of the graft, however, because it is invaded by vascular tissue and osteoblasts from surrounding host bone. The invading cells presumably come from the haversian canals and endosteum of the diploë, while the vascular tissue may be derived not only from the diploë but also from underlying dura or overlying scalp. Factors that might be expected to lead to graft failure include: (1) eburnated cranial defect margins or, possibly, heavy waxing of bleeding diploë; (2) dural replacement by fascial graft; (3) thin, poorly vascularized scalp; (4) a graft consisting essentially of cortical bone; and (5) a graft that is poorly fitted or poorly fixed. Conversely, a good contact between cancellous bone graft and bleeding diploë, good fixation, and normal vascularity of both cranium and soft tissue should favor graft survival.

The invading cells and blood vessels construct new bone on the structure of the graft, and this has been described as "creeping substitution." It should be emphasized, however, that the new bone is laid down on a "scaffold" that consists of living bone, not just a source of inorganic salts. For this reason, it cannot be expected that preserved autogenous bone or homologous bone would be as successful as a fresh autogenous bone graft. Craniotomy bone flaps that are replaced after autoclaving

sometimes heal, but in one large series, 40 per cent were lost through infection or reabsorption.[26] The heat of autoclaving or boiling denatures bone protein, and the now-dead autogenous bone flap is little different from boiled homologous or heterogenous bone, as far as the host is concerned. The inflammatory reaction that is produced by the denatured protein hastens absorption. Refrigeration of bone has produced better results.[1,50] Success following replacement of refrigerated bone flaps may be related to the facilities available for aseptic handling and storage under controlled refrigeration. It has been stated that bone may be stored indefinitely at $-23°$ C.[11] There has even been some reported success with refrigerated homologous bone.[1,11] In general, however, except for occasional success with immediate replacement of an autoclaved bone flap and variable success with delayed replacement of a refrigerated flap, preserved (and therefore dead) autogenous, homologous, and heterogenous bone have not gained much acceptance for the repair of cranial defects.

There are three objections to the use of fresh autogenous bone: (1) the possibility that the bone graft will be absorbed, (2) the difficulty in obtaining cosmetic results that compare with preformed tantalum or plastic plates and plastic plates that have been molded in situ, and (3) the difficulty in obtaining enough bone to repair large defects.

Absorption is always a possibility with unfavorable vascular circumstances or with infection (Fig. 66–9). When first inserted, the fresh autogenous bone graft is a foreign body as much as the alloplastic plate because it lacks a blood supply. Infection at this stage leads to sequestration and absorption, so the bone graft, like an infected bone flap following craniotomy, must be removed. As the graft becomes progressively vascularized, it becomes as resistant to infection as normal cranium, while the alloplastic plate is of course just as much a foreign body years later as it was at the time of insertion. In addition, there is always a potential space between an alloplastic plate and its surrounding fibrous tissue envelope, while the living bone graft develops the same relationship to surrounding soft tissue as has normal cranium. The stress and strain factors that produce exuberant callus in long bones are absent in the cranium, so despite solid healing, the graft may never

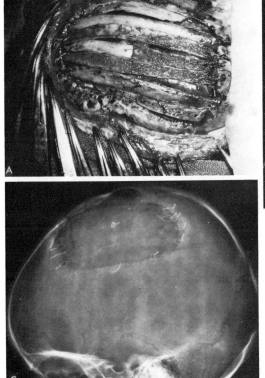

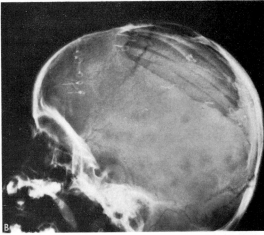

Figure 66–9 *A*. Autogenous split rib cranioplasty (same patient as 66–1). *B*. Early postoperative x-ray. *C*. X-ray two months later, showing resorption of rib. Prior repair of dura with fascia lata graft and waxing of bleeding diploë at time of cranioplasty may have contributed to failure in this case. This defect was subsequently repaired successfully with ilium.

be quite as dense radiographically as surrounding skull. Postoperative films may even show some progressive loss of density despite satisfactory cosmetic appearance and a solid graft by palpation (Fig. 66–10).

The cosmetic problem resolves itself into personal experience and preference of the surgeon. Surgeons skilled in metallic cranioplasty can achieve excellent cosmetic results with tantalum, but for the complicated fronto-orbital defects, this requires preformed plates made according to the com-

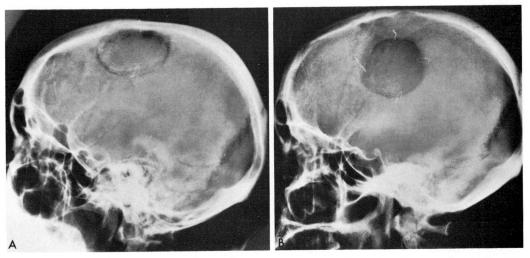

Figure 66–10 *A*. Repair of left frontoparietal defect with autogenous iliac graft. *B*. Four months later the graft has lost density, but the cosmetic result remains satisfactory, and the graft is still solid to palpation.

plex methods described in Reeves's monograph. Acrylic and other types of plastic cranioplasty, by direct or indirect impression techniques, also achieve excellent cosmetic results. A prosthetics laboratory is required, however, as noted earlier. One-stage acrylic cranioplasty is much simpler but has the already described drawbacks (along with tantalum and other alloplastic methods) in the fronto-orbital region where the cosmetic problem is greatest. As described frequently by those who have used it, ilium has a number of curves, which may be adapted to various cranial contours, and rib is equally adaptable (Figs. 66–9, 66–11, 66–12, 66–13. and 66–14).[30,38,39,48] The outer, or occasionally the inner, table of the entire iliac crest is removed subperiosteally with straight and curved chisels. The whole rib is taken from transverse process to costochondral junction and then split. The result in both cases is a graft with cortical bone on one side, cancellous bone on the other. The former provides the strength or rigidity, the latter the scaffold for vascular and osteoblastic ingrowth. It does not matter whether cortical or cancellous bone is outside, next to the scalp, or inside, adjacent to dura. Orientation of the graft is determined by the desired contour. Tibia has also been used but is less satisfactory because it consists mainly of cortical bone. Pure cancellous bone can be molded or shaped, but lacks the rigidity for satisfac-

tory repair of full-thickness cranial defects. It can be used over a more rigid bone graft to build up certain areas such as supraorbital margins or frontal boss, thereby enhancing the cosmetic effect. Cancellous bone and bone chips are also used in a combined method that is described later. Split ilium and rib are not only adequately rigid, but "workable" in that some degree of bending is possible, and they may be easily cut and shaped with saws, chisels, rongeurs, and air drills. An absent glabella or supraorbital margin may be constructed from bone from either source (Fig. 66–12).

Obtaining enough autogenous bone to repair large defects can be a problem. The two iliac crests add up to a great deal of bone, but this would involve a two-stage repair, since both iliac crests should not be taken at one time. One iliac crest, however, and two or more ribs on the same side may be removed at one time with little difficulty. The resulting amount of bone is adequate to fill a large defect (Fig. 66–14). There has been some reluctance to use ilium in young children because of possible involvement of growth centers. It would be necessary to excise bone almost all the way to the acetabulum for this to happen, but in any case, rib may be preferable. As pointed out by Longacre, the thorax contains an almost limitless supply of bone, especially in the young.[38,40] Ribs removed subperiosteally regenerate in several months, and their os-

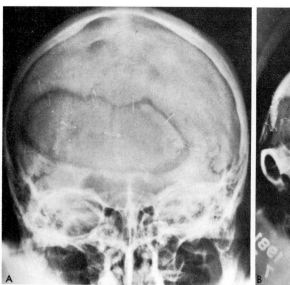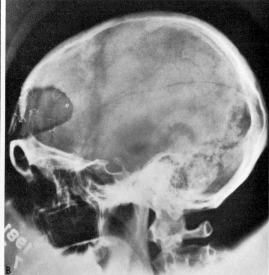

Figure 66–11   Frontal, *A*, and lateral, *B*, views of bifrontal iliac cranioplasty.

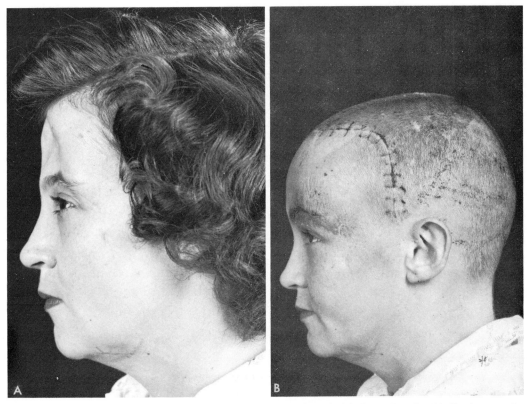

Figure 66–12　*A*. Frontal defect, including supraorbital margin and glabella. *B*. Repair with iliac bone graft.

teogenic potential as graft material exceeds any other bone. Subperiosteal removal of the entire rib is consistent with satisfactory thoracic function provided alternate ribs are removed, two or three at one time.

Osteoplastic methods require more preparation of the cranial defect than do alloplastic methods. Eburnated bone must be excised back to bleeding diploë, and waxing should be held to a minimum. The heat generated by high-speed drills may kill osteocytes and vascular tissue. Contact, cancellous bone to diploë, is probably critical, and fixation is just as important as splinting is with long-bone fractures. In adults, split rib may be inlaid by removing outer table for about 1 cm around the circumference of the defect. The ends of the ribs are fixed to inner table by wire. This is not possible in young children because the skull is not thick enough. The ribs are therefore cut to fit the defect as a full-thickness inlay graft and wired to surrounding cranium. Split ilium is usually so thick that it is likewise inserted as a full-thickness inlay graft, in adults as well as children, without removal of surrounding outer table. Fit and fixation

are more easily achieved than with split rib because the surgeon is dealing with thicker bone and fewer fragments.

Obtaining an autogenous graft requires another incision, and preparation of the recipient site must be more meticulous than for alloplastic cranioplasty. The extra time, effort, and surgical manipulation are well worth it, however, if the result is a solidly healed graft, indistinguishable in appearance and function from normal cranium. It would seem that this type of procedure is especially justified in children and in patients with fronto-orbital defects or large defects. On the other hand, the extra operative manipulation may not be justified in adults with convexity defects of smaller size.

Combined Alloplastic-Osteoplastic Method

As would be obvious to any surgeon, the multiplicity of methods for cranioplasty already described indicates that none of them are ideal, that all have some advantage and

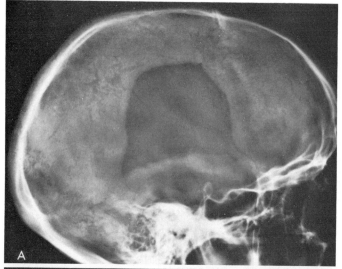

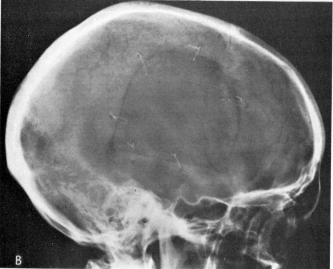

Figure 66–13 *A*. Right temporal post-traumatic defect. *B*. Iliac cranioplasty.

some disadvantage. It is therefore not surprising that neurosurgeons are still looking for new methods or at least new combinations of old methods. As described earlier, vascular ingrowth from host bone (cranial defect margin), dura (endosteum), and probably even scalp is essential for autogenous bone graft survival. Vascular penetration is facilitated if the graft is cancellous bone, bone chips, or bone dust, as described by Shehadi.[62] He used the bone dust from burr holes, mixed with saline to form a paste, spread over the dura and held in place by closure of the scalp. After several weeks, in both experimental and clinical cases, there was new bone that resembled normal skull. The problem with this

technique is that the graft initially has no rigidity or structure. This must limit the repair of large or complicated defects, although Shehadi reports successful repair of a 12-cm defect.

Recent reports describe a method combining autogenous cancellous bone chips with an alloplastic net.[24,35] Polyethylene terephthalate cloth mesh is saturated with polyether urethane to form a "polyurethane terephthalate" net. The latter requires a degree of fabrication. It may be draped over a model of the defect while still wet, and then "cured" with the appropriate contour. Even after cured and rigid, it can be further contoured at the operating table. It is autoclavable and can be cut with scis-

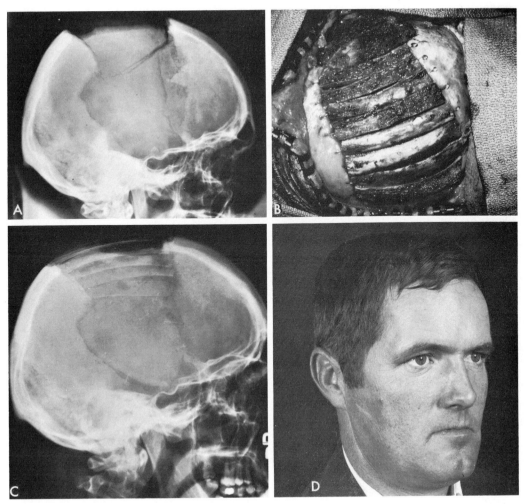

Figure 66-14 *A*. Right temporoparietal and vertex defect, post-traumatic. *B*. Cranioplasty with ilium and two ribs. Ilium fills the right temporal area, while rib fills the right parietal and vertex regions. *C*. Postoperative x-ray. *D*. Postoperative appearance of patient after five months.

sors. The autogenous bone particles, cancellous bone, bone chips, or bone dust from ilium or rib are laid over the dura and molded to fill the defect, the margins of which have been freshened to enhance vascular penetration. The polyurethane terephthalate net, contoured to the shape of missing bone, is placed over the particulate bone and fixed to the margins of the defect with stainless steel wire or Vitallium screws. New bone formation occurs in the form imposed by the alloplastic net. With this method, the advantages of particulate bone grafting (vascular penetration and ease of molding) are realized, and the disadvantage (lack of rigidity or structure) is compensated for by the alloplastic net. The structural advantage of bone grafting and the cosmetic advantage of alloplastic methods are thus combined.

SUMMARY

Decisions concerning the *need* for cranioplasty are rarely difficult. The younger the patient, the larger the defect, the more strategic its location from both cosmetic and protective viewpoints, the easier will be the decision that it should be repaired. Small defects, less than 2 to 3 cm, situated posteriorly, protected by muscle or hair, can be left alone, especially in the older patient. Some elderly patients and some not-so-old ones with cerebral dysfunction will refuse cranioplasty even when recommended by their neurosurgeon.

Decisions concerning the *method* of cranioplasty are more difficult owing to the multiplicity of methods available, each with its own set of advantages and disadvantages. Neurosurgeons have and will develop their own individual approach to this problem, depending upon their individual experience and preference plus the availability of ancillary services such as a dental prosthetics laboratory. Despite variability of individual experience and preference, certain general statements can be made.

1. *Tantalum,* despite the fact that it is well tolerated and produces excellent cosmetic results in experienced hands, has the major drawback of interference with subsequent contrast studies and CT scanning.

2. *Aluminum* may be a reasonable metallic alternative to tantalum, since it seems to be as well tolerated, and just as malleable but does not interfere with radiographic studies.

3. *Acrylic,* well tolerated, cosmetically successful even without much operative experience, and completely radiolucent, seems to be the most adaptable alloplastic method. The major disadvantages of acrylic are encountered in its use in children, whose skulls are still growing and are thin, with the result that brittle plates are easily broken.

4. *Combined acrylic–metallic mesh* methods would appear to resolve the problem of brittleness of the acrylic plate without sacrificing malleability or radiolucency.

5. *Polyethylene* is a possible alternative to acrylic cranioplasty but has received much less trial. The plates are less brittle but more difficult to mold in situ at the operating table.

6. *Osteoplastic* methods, more time consuming and sometimes less satisfactory cosmetically, offer the advantages of permanency, once healed, and adaptability to the growing skull. In very young children with thin skulls, however, fixation and support of ilium and rib are more difficult. Huge defects at any age present the problem of finding enough bone as well as that of adequate fixation and vascular support.

7. *Combined alloplastic and osteoplastic* methods for using particulate bone supported by a plastic net may help to solve these latter problems. Even with further development and refinement of technique, it is unlikely that a single method will ever satisfy all requirements or solve all problems involved in the repair of cranial defects.

REFERENCES

1. Abbott, K. H.: Use of frozen cranial bone flaps for autogenous and homologous grafts. J. Neurosurg., *10*:380–388, 1953.
2. Alexander, E., Jr.: Personal communication, 1969.
3. Alexander, E., Jr., and Dillard, P. H.: The use of pure polyethylene plate for cranioplasty. J. Neurosurg., *7*:492–498, 1950.
4. Asimacopoulos, T. J., Papadakis, N., and Mark, V. H.: A new method of cranioplasty: technical note. J. Neurosurg., *47*:790–792, 1977.
5. Bates, J. I., and Reiners, C. R.: The repair of cranial defects with zirconium. J. Neurosurg., *5*:340–348, 1948.
6. Black, S. P. W.: Reconstruction of the supraorbital ridge using aluminum. Surg. Neurol., *9*: 121–128, 1978.
7. Black, S. P. W., Kam, C. C. M., and Sights, W. P., Jr.: Aluminum cranioplasty. J. Neurosurg., *29*:562–564, 1968.
8. Blatt, I. M., and Failla, A.: Acrylic implants for frontal bone defects. Milit. Med., *137*:22–25, 1972.
9. Bradford, F. K., and Livingston, K. E.: Failure in early secondary repair of skull defects with tantalum. J. Neurosurg., *3*:318–328, 1946.
10. Brown, K. E.: Fabrication of an alloplastic cranioimplant. J. Prosth. Dent., *24*:213–224. 1970.
11. Bush, L. F.: The use of homogenous bone grafts. J. Bone Joint Surg., *29*:620–628, 1947.
12. Cabanela, M. E., Coventry, M. B., MacCarty, C. S., and Miller, W. E.: The fate of patients with methyl methacrylate cranioplasty. J. Bone Joint Surg., *54-A*:278–281, 1972.
13. Charnley, J.: The reaction of bone to self-curing acrylic cement. A long-term histological study in man. J. Bone Joint Surg., *52-B*:340–353, 1970.
14. Clark, G.: Personal communication, 1970.
15. Cooper, P. R., Schechter, B., Jacobs, G. B., Rubin, R. C., and Wille, R. L.: A preformed methyl methacrylate cranioplasty. Surg. Neurol., *8*:219–221, 1977.
16. Courtemanche, A. D., and Thompson, G. B.: Silastic cranioplasty following craniofacial injuries. Plast. Reconstr. Surg., *41*:165–170, 1968.
17. Elkins, C. W., and Cameron, J. E.: Cranioplasty with acrylic plates. J. Neurosurg., *3*:199–205, 1946.
18. Erculei, F., and Walker, A. E.: Post-traumatic epilepsy and early cranioplasty. J. Neurosurg., *20*:1085–1089, 1963.
19. Galicich, J. H., and Hovind, K. H.: Stainless steel mesh–acrylic cranioplasty. J. Neurosurg., *27*:376–378, 1967.
20. Galicich, J. H.: Personal communication, 1978.

21. Grant, F. C., and Norcross, N. C.: Repair of cranial defects by cranioplasty. Ann. Surg., *110*:488–512, 1939.

22. Grantham, E. G., and Landis, H. P.: Cranioplasty and the post-traumatic syndrome. J. Neurosurg., *5*:19–22, 1948.

23. Gurdjian, E. S., Webster, J. E., and Brown, J. C.: Impression technique for reconstruction of large skull defects. Surgery, *14*:876–881, 1943.

24. Habal, M. B., Leake, D. L., and Maniscalco, J. E.: A new method for reconstruction of major defects in the cranial vault. Surg. Neurol., *6*: 137–138, 1976.

25. Hammon, W. M., and Kempe, L. G.: Methyl methacrylate cranioplasty. Thirteen years experience with 417 patients. Acta Neurochir. (Wein), *25*:69–77, 1971.

26. Hancock, D. O.:The fate of replaced bone flaps. J. Neurosurg., *20*:983–984, 1963.

27. Henry, H. M., Guerrero, C., and Moody, R. A.: Cerebrospinal fluid fistula from fractured acrylic cranioplasty plate. J. Neurosurg., *45*:227–228, 1976.

28. Jackson, I. J., and Hoffman, G. T.: Depressed comminuted fracture of a plastic cranioplasty. J. Neurosurg., *13*:116–117, 1956.

29. Karvounis, P. C., Chin, J., and Sabin, H.: The use of prefabricated polyethylene plate for cranioplasty. J. Trauma, *10*:249–254, 1970.

30. Kiehn, C. L., and Grino, A.: Iliac bone grafts replacing tantalum plates for gunshot wounds of the skull. Amer. J. Surg., *75*:395–400, 1953.

31. Kriss, F. C., Taren, J. A., and Kahn, E. A.: Primary repair of compound skull fractures by replacement of bone fragments. J. Neurosurg., *30*:698–702, 1969.

32. Lake, P. A., Morin, M. A., and Pitts, F. W.: Radiolucent prosthesis of mesh-reinforced acrylic: technical note. J. Neurosurg., *32*:597–602, 1970.

33. Lane, S., and Webster, J. E.: A report of the early results in tantalum cranioplasty. J. Neurosurg., *4*:526–529, 1947.

34. Langfitt, T.: Increased intracranial pressure. Clin. Neurosurg., *16*:436–471, 1968.

35. Leake, D. L., and Habal, M. B.: Osteoneogenesis: A new method for facial reconstruction. J. Surg. Res., *18*:331–334, 1975.

36. Lehman, J. H., Jr.: Silastic cranioplasty. Ohio State Med. J., *69*:441–444, 1973.

37. Longacre, J. J.: Transplantation of bone. *In* Converse, J. M., ed.: Reconstructive Plastic Surgery. Philadelphia and London, W. B. Saunders Co., 1964, Vol. 1, pp. 140–160.

38. Longacre, J. J.: Deformities of the forehead, scalp, and cranium. *In* Converse, J. M., ed.: Reconstructive Plastic Surgery. Philadelphia and London, W. B. Saunders Co., 1964. Vol. 2, pp. 575–583.

39. Longacre, J. J., and de Stefano, G. A.: Reconstruction of extensive defects of the skull with split rib grafts. Plast. Reconstr. Surg., *19*:186–200, 1957.

40. Longacre, J. J., and de Stefano, G. A.: Further observations of the behavior of autogenous split-rib grafts in reconstruction of extensive defects. Plast. Reconstr. Surg., *20*:281–296, 1957.

41. Longacre, J. J., Kahl, J. B., and Wood, R. W.: Reconstruction of extensive defects in and about the orbit. Amer. J. Ophthal., *61*:763–768, 1966.

42. Maniscalco, J. E., and Garcia-Bengochea, F.: Cranioplasty: A method of prefabricating alloplastic plates. Surg. Neurol., *2*:339–341, 1974.

43. Matson, D. D.: Neurosurgery of Infancy and Childhood. 2nd Ed. Springfield, Ill., Charles C Thomas, 1969, chaps. 9 and 22.

44. Mayfield, F. H., and Levitch, L. A.: Repair of cranial defects with tantalum. Amer. J. Surg., *67*:319–332, 1945.

45. McClintock, H. G., and Dingman, R. O.: The repair of cranial defects with iliac bone. Surgery, *30*:955–963, 1951.

46. McFadden, J. T.: Metallurgical principles in neurosurgery. J. Neurosurg., *31*:373–385, 1969.

47. Meirowski, A. M., Hazouri, L. A., and Greiner, D. J.: Epidural granulomata in the presence of tantalum plates. J. Neurosurg., *7*:485–491, 1950.

48. Money, R. A.: The repair of cranial defects by bone grafting. Surgery, *19*:627–650, 1946.

49. Nadell, J., and Kline, D. G.: Primary reconstruction of depressed frontal skull fractures including those involving the sinus, orbit, and cribriform plate. J. Neurosurg., *41*:200–207, 1974.

50. Odom, G. L., Woodhall, B., and Wrenn, F. R., Jr.: The use of refrigerated autogenous bone flaps for cranioplasty. J. Neurosurg., *9*:606–610, 1952.

51. Peer, L. A.: Transplantation of Tissue. Baltimore, Williams & Wilkins Co., 1955, Vol. 1, pp. 181–236.

52. Petty, P. G.: Cranioplasty. A follow-up study. Med. J. Aust., *2*:806–808, 1974.

53. Polisar, R. S., and Cook, A. W.: Use of polyethylene in cranial implants. J. Prosth. Dent., *29*: 310–316, 1973.

54. Pudenz, R. H.: The repair of cranial defects with tantalum; an experimental study. J.A.M.A., *121*:478–481, 1943.

55. Ray, B. S., and Parsons, H.: The replacement of free bone plates in routine craniotomies. J. Neurosurg., *4*:299–308, 1947.

56. Reeves, D. L.: Cranioplasty. Springfield, Ill., Charles C Thomas, 1950.

57. Rietz, K.: The one-stage method of cranioplasty with acrylic plastic. J. Neurosurg., *15*:176–182, 1958.

58. Robertson, R. C. L: Repair of cranial defects with tantalum. J. Neurosurg., *1*:227–236, 1944.

59. Sabin, H., and Karvounis, P.: The neurosurgeon-dentist team in cranioplasty. J. Amer. Dent. Ass., *79*:1183–1188, 1969.

60. Schupper, N.: Cranioplasty prosthesis for replacement of cranial bone. J. Prosth. Dent., *19*:594–597, 1968.

61. Scott, M., Wycis, H. T., and Murtagh, F.: Long term evaluation of stainless steel cranioplasty. Surg. Gynec. Obstet., *115*:453–461, 1962.

62. Shehadi, S. I.: Skull reconstruction with bone dust. Brit. J. Plast. Surg., *23*:227–234, 1970.

63. Simpson, D.: Titanium in cranioplasty. J. Neurosurg., *22*:292–293, 1965.

64. Small, J. M., and Graham, M. P.: Acrylic resin for the closure of skull defects. Brit. J. Surg., *33*:106–113, 1945.

65. Spence, W. T.: Form-fitting cranioplasty. J. Neurosurg., *11*:219–225, 1954.

66. Tabaddor, K., and LaMorgese, J.: Complication of a large cranial defect. J. Neurosurg., *44*:506–508, 1976.

67. Turner, O. A.: Tantalum cranioplasty and repeated trauma. J. Neurosurg., *9*:100–103, 1952.

68. Tysvaer, A. T., and Hovind, K. H.: Stainless steel mesh–acrylic cranioplasty. J. Trauma, *17*:3: 231–233, 1977.

69. Walker, A. E., and Erculei, F.: The late results of cranioplasty. Arch. Neurol. (Chicago), *9*:105–110, 1963.

70. Weiford, E. C., and Gardner, W. J.: Tantalum cranioplasty. J. Neurosurg., *6*:13–32, 1949.

71. White, J. C.: Late complications following cranioplasty with alloplastic plates. Ann. Surg., *128*:743–755, 1948.

72. Woodhall, B., and Cramer, F. J.: Extradural pneumatocoele following tantalum cranioplasty, J. Neurosurg., *2*:524–529, 1945.

73. Woodhall, B., and Spurling, R. G.: Tantalum cranioplasty for war wounds of the skull. Ann. Surg., *121*:649–671, 1945.

74. Woolf, J. I., and Walker, A. E.: Cranioplasty: Collective review. Int. Abstr. Surg., *81*:1–23, 1945.

67

FACIAL, AUDITORY, AND VESTIBULAR NERVE INJURIES ASSOCIATED WITH BASILAR SKULL FRACTURES

ANATOMY

The critical anatomical features of the temporal bone that may become involved in fractures of this bone are: (1) the eighth nerve, its main trunk in the auditory meatus and canal and its various vestibular and auditory branches that penetrate the cribriform depths of the canal; (2) the seventh nerve and its closely associated nervus intermedius; (3) the bony and membranous labyrinthine structures of the inner ear, consisting of the cochlea and the vestibular labyrinth; (4) the large venous dural sinuses, including the sigmoid sinus and the superior and inferior petrosal sinuses; (5) the internal carotid artery; (6) the eustachian tube and middle ear, including the middle ear ossicles and mastoid air cells; (7) the external auditory canal and the tympanic membrane; and (8) the dural attachments of the temporal bone in the middle and posterior fossae (Fig. 67–1).

TYPES OF TEMPORAL BONE FRACTURES

Classically, two types of temporal bone fractures have been described, longitudinal and transverse, these terms referring to the direction of the fracture in relation to the long axis of the petrous pyramid (Fig. 67–2).

Longitudinal fractures are clinically more common than transverse fractures. They usually begin in the squamosal portion from a lateral blow to the head and extend downward into the mastoid, or more anteriorly down into the external auditory canal and middle ear. The fracture then extends medially into the anterior portion of the petrous apex, possibly as far medially as the foramen lacerum, or occasionally even to the petrous apex of the opposite side. As the fracture extends downward from the squama into the external canal, it will usually create an obvious bony deformity of the external canal and will also often tear the tympanic membrane. Either of these injuries causes bleeding from the ear. If the dura is torn by the fracture, there may also be leakage of cerebrospinal fluid from the ear.

More severe longitudinal fractures that extend downward into the middle ear may disrupt the ossicular chain, most commonly causing dislocation of the incus, but occasionally, luxation of the stapes. It is also in such severe fractures that the fallopian canal surrounding the facial nerve in its middle ear course may become involved, resulting in facial paresis or paralysis in about 20 per cent of such fractures.

If the fracture extends downward from the squama more posteriorly into the mastoid portion of the temporal bone, the sigmoid venous dural sinus may be torn, which may lead not only to bleeding into the mastoid and middle ear spaces or intracranially but also to bleeding beneath the pericranium over the mastoid. This mastoid

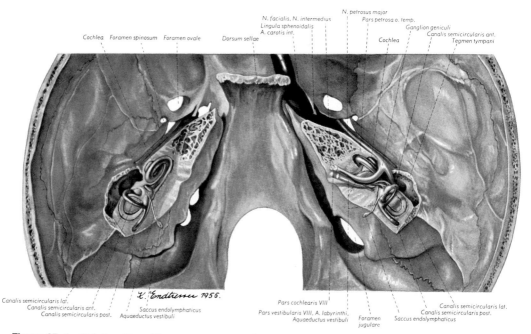

Figure 67–1 Relationships of important structures in the petrous pyramid. The top of the pyramid is chiseled off on both sides. (From Pernkopf, E.: Atlas of Topographical and Applied Human Anatomy, Vol. I. Philadelphia and London, W. B. Saunders Co., 1963. Reprinted by permission.)

swelling and hematoma becomes clinically most apparent after two to three days and is known as Battle's sign.

As a longitudinal fracture extends into the petrous apex, it usually does so along the anterior aspect in the middle cranial fossa, usually avoiding the inner ear labyrinthine structures and the structures in the internal auditory canal. The dura may be torn along this fracture line, and cerebrospinal fluid may leak into the middle ear and escape through the external auditory canal if the tympanic membrane is also torn. If the tympanic membrane remains intact, the cerebrospinal fluid may escape down the eustachean tube into the nasopharynx, where it may be very difficult or impossible to detect. With the head down and forward, however, the fluid from the eustachean tube may run forward out of the nose.

Transverse fractures occur at a right angle to the long axis of the petrous portion of the temporal bone and most commonly result from occipital or occiptomastoid blows to the skull. Transverse fractures are less often encountered as a clinical problem than are longitudinal fractures because of the substantially higher immediate and early mortality rate of the more severe central nervous system injuries associated with basilar skull fractures of the transverse type. The petrous portion may be fractured transversely anywhere along its long axis. More medial fractures traverse the internal auditory canal and the cochlear portion of the labyrinthine capsule anteriorly. The seventh and eighth nerves may be stretched or severed in the internal auditory canal. About 50 per cent of transverse fractures result in facial paralysis. More lateral fractures of the petrous part tend to disrupt both the vestibular and the cochlear components of the labyrinthine capsule. They may shatter the medial wall of the middle ear and dislocate the stapes. The fallopian canal may be disrupted in its horizontal middle ear course and cause injury to the facial nerve in this location. Unlike longitudinal fractures, transverse fractures almost always result in some injury to the labyrinthine capsule. On the other hand, the middle ear, the tympanic membrane, and the external auditory canal are usually not involved in transverse fractures. The transverse fracture, therefore, seldom causes bleeding or leakage of cerebrospinal fluid from the ear. Combinations of transverse and longitudinal fractures may occur and may give a mixed clinical picture of both.

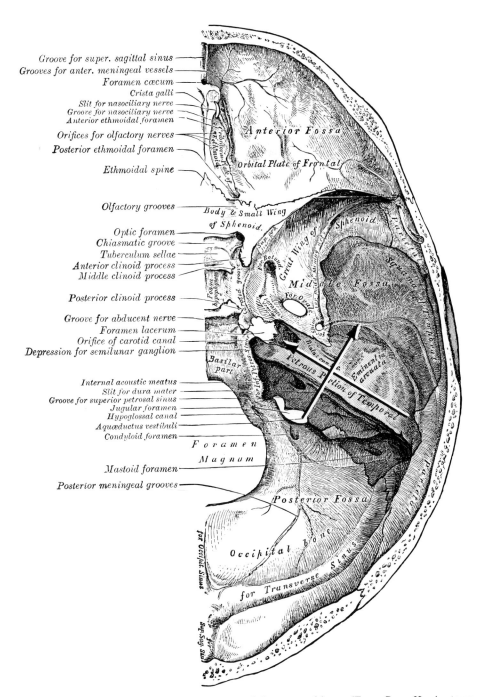

Figure 67–2 Longitudinal and transverse fractures of the temporal bone. (From Gray, H.: Anatomy of the Human Body. 27th Ed. Philadelphia, Lea and Febiger, 1959. Reprinted by permission.)

DIAGNOSIS AND LOCALIZATION OF INJURY

Early neurotological examination is important in any patient with head trauma in whom a basilar skull fracture is suspected and should include evaluation of the presence of blood or cerebrospinal fluid in the external auditory canal; the presence of blood or cerebrospinal fluid in the middle ear behind an intact tympanic membrane; fracture lines in the external auditory canal; ecchymosis over the mastoid area; facial paralysis or paresis; dizziness or vertigo, especially when associated with nystagmus; tinnitus; hearing impairment; and x-ray evidence of temporal bone fracture.

Particular attention should be paid to the following points in the examination of patients with head trauma in whom temporal bone fracture is present or strongly suspected: (1) the ear canal wall; (2) the tympanic membrane; (3) the mastoid process; (4) the eyes for nystagmus or, in the unconscious patient, conjugate deviation; (5) hearing, tested by using live voice and tuning forks; and (6) facial nerve function.

Bleeding and Cerebrospinal Fluid Leakage from Ear

Bleeding from the ear after head trauma is almost always due to a basilar skull fracture, usually of the longitudinal variety. Blood that has run into the ear canal from extrinsic facial or scalp lacerations may be difficult or impossible to distinguish from primary middle ear or ear canal bleeding. The traditional principle of not cleaning such an ear canal to make a specific anatomical diagnosis for fear of introducing an intracranial infection through the fracture and possible dural tear is still probably sound in most cases. When specific localization of such bleeding does seem particularly important for establishing an accurate diagnosis, however, one is justified in carefully cleaning and examining the ear—using strict sterile technique.

Cerebrospinal fluid leakage from the ear may be difficult to ascertain early because of the masking effect of associated bleeding. One can strongly suspect cerebrospinal fluid otorrhea, however, by the clear halo of moisture that it usually creates around the centrally pigmented bloodstain on a clean piece of linen or porous paper. Ultimately, as bleeding subsides and only clear fluid drainage persists, the identity of cerebrospinal fluid can be confirmed by the reaction of its reducing sugars with commercially available testing tapes.

Bleeding may occur into the middle ear from any type of temporal bone fracture, but is most commonly due to longitudinal fractures. The same is true for cerebrospinal fluid in the middle ear from a dural tear. Blood in the middle ear gives the tympanic membrane a characteristic blue or purple appearance. Cerebrospinal fluid in the middle ear may be very difficult to detect and may escape down the eustachian tube and present as rhinorrhea when the patient leans forward with his head down.

Ecchymosis over the mastoid is the classic sign of a basilar skull fracture but is not actually seen very frequently. Known as Battle's sign, it generally appears four to five days following the injury. It results from longitudinal fractures that extend into the mastoid and may be quite extensive if the sigmoid sinus is disrupted.

Facial Paralysis

Facial paralysis is seen in about half the transverse fractures of the temporal bone and in about 20 per cent of the longitudinal fractures. It is important to diagnose the injury accurately and to follow it carefully because in some instances paralysis can be treated surgically and, if it persists untreated, it creates a serious cosmetic and functional deformity. Traumatic facial paralysis can be characterized in the following ways: (1) as paralysis (complete) or paresis (incomplete), (2) immediate or delayed in onset, (3) caused by neurapraxia or axonal degeneration, and (4) by location of the injury either proximal or distal to the geniculate ganglion.

It is important to distinguish between paralysis and paresis, since the prognosis in paresis is usually excellent while that in complete paralysis can be very variable and sometimes poor. The residual motion of paresis may be very subtle and limited to only one part of the face. Complete paralysis can also be overlooked occasionally, as the unparalyzed side of the face transmits a certain degree of its mobility across the midline, giving the illusion of some motion on the paralyzed side. In order to avoid this error, the examiner should always splint the active side of the patient's face with the heel of his hand as he asks the patient to make various voluntary movements of the face.

Immediate versus delayed onset is also a very important distinction to make, since the prognosis in paralysis of delayed onset is considerably better than in paralysis that appears immediately at the time of the fracture. Immediate paralysis almost always results from direct trauma to the nerve by tearing, stretching, or actual sectioning. Delayed paralyses can appear at any time during the first two weeks after fracture has occurred and may be complete or incomplete. Delayed paralyses are usually due to the pressure of hemorrhage or edema or even granulation tissue within the fallopian canal.

Establishing the exact time of onset and the degree of paralysis may be difficult in the unconscious patient. An earnest attempt should be made, however, and all such information should be carefully recorded in serial fashion along with other critical information such as the state of consciousness and vital signs. Recordings should begin with the very first examination in the emergency room and should continue throughout the ensuing days and weeks of hospital observation.

Whether paralysis is simply due to a physiological blockage of impulses along an otherwise intact and viable nerve or whether there is actual axonal degeneration, with or without disruption of the nerve, is an extremely important distinction to make as early as possible. This distinction requires relatively simple electrical testing devices. The results of such tests add crucial objective data to the previous clinical observations of onset and degree of paralysis.

There are a number of different techniques for electrically testing a motor nerve. The two tests most commonly relied upon for diagnosis in facial nerve lesions are the percutaneous nerve excitability test and electromyography of facial muscles.

The percutaneous nerve excitability test is easy to perform and can be interpreted by any physician. It requires an electrical nerve stimulator, which is available in most hospitals. Because of its simplicity, this test can be done daily and at the patient's bed-

side if necessary. It has the advantage of detecting axonal degeneration within 72 hours of the onset of the paralysis, compared with electromyography, which takes 10 to 14 days to show such changes. The test is done by simply placing the electrode on the skin over the area of the main trunk of the facial nerve as it exits from the stylomastoid foramen (Fig. 67–3). A threshold stimulus of known duration is given. A normal response will be observed, such as twitching of the facial muscles on the side stimulated. A nerve that has not undergone degeneration will respond to between 3.0 and 7.0 ma of current. Both the normal and paralyzed sides of the face are tested and the thresholds of electrical excitability of the two sides are compared. If the paralyzed side develops a progressive increase in threshold of between 3 and 5 ma greater than the normal side, or if it has a substantially greater threshold than the normal side from the onset, the assumption of axonal degeneration is made.

Electromyography is a time-honored electrical test for motor nerve degeneration and is valuable for confirmation of the percutaneous nerve excitability test. It can also be used to predict the return of function of a degenerated nerve. From the standpoints of early diagnosis and efficient daily evaluation of a paralyzed nerve, the electromyogram has several disadvantages. Besides the 10- to 14-day latency between

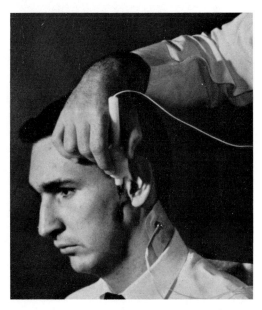

Figure 67–3 Percutaneous nerve excitability test.

onset of paralysis and first appearance of the fibrillation potentials of nerve degeneration, there is also a mild to moderate discomfort from insertion of needle electrodes into the facial muscle groups. Electromyographic equipment lacks simplicity and portability, and usually trained personnel are required to perform the test and to interpret the results. It does, however, have singular prognostic value in predicting return of function in a nerve that is regenerating. Electromyographic evidence of axonal regeneration usually precedes by several weeks or months actual visible recovery of facial motion.

Localization of the facial nerve injury either proximal or distal to the geniculate ganglion is important because the surgical approach differs for different sites of injury. If the nerve is injured in the middle ear or mastoid portions of the fallopian canal distal to the geniculate ganglion, the surgical approach to the nerve is relatively simple, using rather standard mastoid and middle ear operative procedures (Fig. 67–4). If the injury is proximal to the geniculate ganglion in the internal auditory canal or posterior fossa, then the approach is more difficult, requiring an intracranial exposure of the injured nerve.[6] Since the greater petrosal

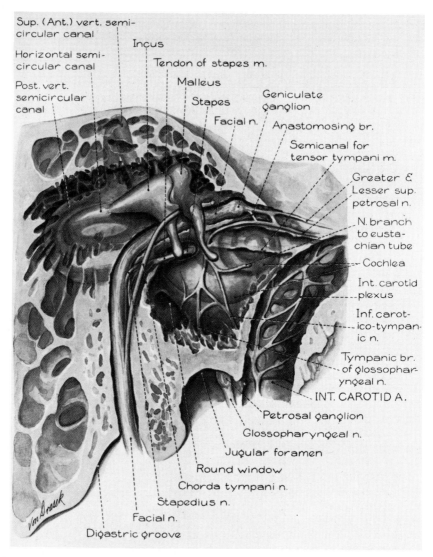

Figure 67–4 Facial nerve in the middle ear and mastoid portions of the temporal bone showing geniculate ganglion and greater petrosal nerve. (From Shambaugh, G. E., Jr.: Surgery of the Ear. Philadelphia and London, W. B. Saunders Co., 1959. Reprinted by permission.)

nerve leaves the facial nerve at the geniculate ganglion to innervate the lacrimal gland, a relatively simple test for tearing, the Schirmer test, can be performed to distinguish between injuries proximal and distal to the ganglion. The Schirmer test is performed by placing a narrow strip of filter paper in the conjunctival sac of each lower eyelid and comparing the wetting of the paper of the two sides over a five-minute period (Fig. 67–5). The normally innervated lacrimal gland should be able to wet at least 2 to 3 cm of this filter strip over a period of five minutes, while a denervated gland may wet no more than a few millimeters. Therefore, injuries to the facial nerve and its nervus intermedius medial to the geniculate ganglion will give a dry eye on the involved side, whereas injuries to the facial nerve in the middle ear and mastoid portions of the fallopian canal lateral to the ganglion will not interfere with lacrimation on the ipsilateral side.

Dizziness and Vertigo

Some variety of dizziness probably occurs in the vast majority of head injuries and certainly in almost all basilar skull fractures. Dizziness is a rather nonspecific term for what may be a variety of peculiar subjective feelings of the patient, usually related to his state of "steadiness." Vertigo, however, is a very specific kind of dizziness in which the patient experiences a definite disorientation in space accompanied by a specific directional motion, either spinning or linear. Vertiginous dizziness is always due to a vestibular disorder, either central or peripheral, and this vestibular dizziness is always associated with nystagmus. It is,

therefore, always important in the early examination of the awake patient with a head injury to note and record the presence or absence of nystagmus and its direction, if present. In transverse fractures of the temporal bone, the vestibular nerve may be torn or stretched in the internal auditory canal, or the vestibular labyrinth itself may be disrupted in more lateral fractures through the otic capsule. In either case, the patient becomes immediately severely vertiginous with nystagmus if he is conscious. This vertigo will subside only slowly over three to four weeks, and thereafter the patient will respond little or not at all to vestibular caloric testing in the involved ear. With such severe injuries to the peripheral vestibular mechanism, there is often an associated severe cochlear injury resulting in sudden sensorineural hearing loss in the involved ear. Longitudinal fractures less frequently result in serious and persistent vestibular injury. Concussion injuries of the otic capsule often cause microhemorrhages into the inner ear, which may give mild transient vertigo with less conspicuous and less persistent nystagmus. Full eventual recovery of response to vestibular caloric testing is the rule rather than the exception in such injuries. The problem of distinguishing central from peripheral vestibular injuries is sometimes difficult, since both may give very similar symptoms and signs and similar responses to caloric testing.

In recent years, electronystagmography (ENG), the technique that electrically measures and records as a permanent tracing the direction, amplitude, and speed of the eye movements in nystagmus, has been developed. With this technique, eye movements can be recorded with the eyes either open or closed, which is often helpful in the differential diagnosis of vestibular and other central nervous system injuries.

Tinnitus and Hearing Impairment

Tinnitus may result from trauma to the auditory nerve, the labyrinth, the blood supply to the ear, or any of the major vessels in or about the ear. Tinnitus due to inner ear or acoustic nerve injury may be quite variable in both intensity and quality as well as duration. It is usually a buzzing or ringing sensation and is usually constant. This contrasts with the tinnitus secondary

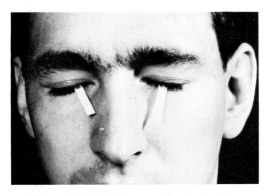

Figure 67–5   Schirmer test for lacrimation.

to injury of the larger vessels around the ear, with or without bleeding into the middle ear, which is usually low pitched and pulsates in synchrony with the heart beat. It may be associated with an audible bruit, particularly in carotid artery injuries. The prognosis for post-traumatic tinnitus is extremely unpredictable. No reliable treatment is known for tinnitus resulting from inner ear or acoustic nerve trauma.

Hearing impairment of some degree almost always follows temporal bone fractures. It may be unilateral if only one side is involved, or it may be bilateral if both temporal bones are injured. Unilateral loss is sometimes subtle and not readily appreciated by either the patient or the examiner, since the patient continues to hear well for ordinary purposes with the intact opposite ear. The hearing loss may be of the conductive type in which sound pressure waves are impeded from reaching the inner ear through the external auditory canal or across the middle ear, as when the external canal or middle ear fills with blood, or the ossicular chain in the middle ear is disrupted. The hearing loss may also be sensorineural as a result of injury to the inner ear structures, the auditory nerve, or even the more central auditory centers and pathways. Following the acute injury, there is usually a mixture of both types of hearing loss.

After full recovery from the acute injury, there is almost always persistence of some degree of sensorineural loss in the involved ear. It is always important in the conscious patient with a suspected temporal bone fracture to include hearing testing as part of the early evaluation. This may be done rather crudely at first with whispered and spoken voice and tuning forks, since even these relatively crude but easily performed tests will give important information regarding the nature of the acute injury to the hearing mechanism. Severe injuries to the inner ear or acoustic nerve, as in transverse fractures, will cause a sensorineural hearing loss, often profound. In such instances, the patient will not even hear a loud spoken voice in the involved ear if the normal ear is adequately masked. Using tuning forks, the Weber test will lateralize to the normal ear, and air conduction will exceed bone conduction on the Rinne test, if the ear still hears at all. On the contrary, in most conductive hearing losses from middle ear or tympanic membrane injuries, as in most longitudinal fractures, the hearing will not be so profoundly affected, and the patient will be able to hear in the whispered voice or softly spoken voice range. The Weber test with tuning forks will lateralize to the injured ear in these cases, and the Rinne test will show bone conduction exceeding air conduction. Mixed types of hearing loss resulting from combinations of inner ear and middle ear injuries will give somewhat more equivocal results on these cruder hearing tests, but these results are still valuable as baseline information and can be better interpreted by later electrical audiometry when the patient's condition warrants. For the hearing tests to be valid for individual ears, one must remember to introduce some sort of masking noise into the ear not being tested. Simply crumpling a piece of paper near the opposite ear may provide adequate masking for low-intensity testing. A louder masking noise, such as is produced by a Baranay noise box, will have to be used for testing in the spoken voice range. More severe sensorineural hearing losses are often accompanied by vertigo and nystagmus, since the cochlear and vestibular labyrinths and nerves are so intimately related, and severe injury to one often results in injury to the other.

Roentgenograms

The clinical value of routine x-ray diagnosis of the skull for demonstrating basilar skull fractures has been variously reported. Longitudinal fractures are particularly difficult to demonstrate except for fracture lines in the squamosal portion of the vault. Transverse fractures are more often visible by x-ray, and this radiographic defect often persists years later, since the enchondral bone of the otic capsule has little capacity for repair. Of the routine x-ray views, the mastoid series is probably better than any other for demonstrating temporal bone fractures, and this includes a Law or Schuller view and Stenver and Towne views. Laminagraphy may reveal localized detail that plain films do not, such as the status of the middle ear and the ossicles or the internal auditory canal. More recently, polytomography has proved to be particularly helpful in revealing in great detail fractures and other injuries of the temporal bone.

TREATMENT OF INJURIES ASSOCIATED WITH TEMPORAL BONE FRACTURES

Facial paralysis that has an immediate onset coinciding with fracture injury of the temporal bone should be treated in almost all instances by operative exploration of the facial nerve as soon as the patient's general condition has stabilized. Paralysis that is delayed in onset or that is only partial should, in most instances, be treated expectantly, since most of these patients will recover spontaneously. This expectant treatment should, however, include day-by-day serial percutaneous electrical testing for all delayed paralysis that is complete. Should electrical evidence of axonal degeneration develop, exploration should be seriously considered. If there is a question whether paralysis was immediate or delayed, it can be followed with electrical testing as though it were delayed, until the degree of injury is better understood. The method of exploration will be dictated by the location of the injury to the facial nerve. Injuries distal to the geniculate ganglion, in which lacrimation is still intact on the involved side, should be explored through a standard mastoid approach. Injuries proximal to the geniculate ganglion, in which lacrimation is usually erased on the ipsilateral side, may be approached through the middle or posterior cranial fossae or by a translabyrinthine approach.[2,6]

If, on exploration of the nerve, its continuity is confirmed and it is merely found to be contused or swollen or to have fractured bone fragments impinging upon it, it should be decompressed by removing the bony fallopian canal from around the involved part and by removing the impinging fragments of bone. If the nerve is actually severed or even deficient in part, a graft may be inserted between its intact proximal and distal ends. Cervical cutaneous nerves are excellent for facial nerve grafting purposes. Results of facial nerve grafting have been very good and are far superior to other substitution procedures for facial paralysis such as fascial slings, eleventh or twelfth to seventh nerve anastamoses, or contralateral facial myotomies.

Most of the conductive hearing losses associated with middle ear injuries of temporal bone fractures are transient and resolve spontaneously as edema, hemorrhage, and serous effusions gradually resorb and subside. Even most traumatic tympanic membrane perforations will heal spontaneously. Those more disruptive injuries in which the middle ear ossicles are dislocated or the tympanic membrane or ear canal is badly disrupted will cause persistent conductive hearing losses and will require eventual otosurgical correction if the hearing is to be improved and the tympanic membrane defect corrected. The vast majority of such injuries, unfortunately, also have an associated inner ear injury that cannot be improved by medical or surgical means and that often limits the degree of hearing recovery even after rather successful middle ear repair.

Tearing and stretching injuries to the auditory and vestibular nerves always result in severe functional deficits in the affected end-organs, which are irreparable by any presently known surgical or medical treatment. The severe vertigo that usually follows severe injuries to the vestibular labyrinth or nerves can sometimes be partially relieved by the use of vestibular suppressant drugs such as meclizine hydrochloride and dimenhydrinate. Most such acute vestibular symptoms subside gradually over three to four weeks. Occasionally, postural vertigo, poor equilibrium in the dark, and tinnitus persist following such injuries, but there is no consistently successful treatment for such conditions.

REFERENCES

1. Boles, R.: Early management of facial nerve trauma. Michigan Med., *68*:39–44, 1969.
2. Dott, N. M.: Facial paralysis: Restitution by extra-petrous nerve graft. Proc. Roy. Soc. Med., *51*:900–902, 1958.
3. Drake, C. G.: Intracranial facial nerve reconstruction. Arch. Otolaryn., *78*:456–460, 1963.
4. Grove, W. E.: Otologic symptoms and complications of craniocerebral injuries. Surg. Gynec. Obstet., *74*:581, 1942.
5. Grove, W. E.: The otoneurology of head injuries including temporal bone fractures. *In* Coates and Schenck, eds.: Otolaryngology. Chapt. 32. Hagerstown, Md., W. F. Prior Co., 1960.

6. House, W.: Surgery of the petrous portion of the VII nerve. Ann. Otol., 72:802, 1963.
7. Maxwell, J. H., and Magielski, J. E.: The management of facial paralysis associated with fractures of the temporal bone. Laryngoscope, 66:599, 1956.
8. McHugh, H. E.: Facial paralysis in birth injury and skull fractures. Arch. Otolaryn., 78:443, 1963.

9. McHugh, H. E.: The surgical treatment of facial paralysis and traumatic conductive deafness in fractures of the temporal bone. Ann. Otol., 68:855, 1959.
10. Richardson, A. T.: Electrodiagnosis of facial palsies. Ann. Otol., 72:569, 1963.

68

MAXILLOFACIAL INJURIES

It is important that the neurological surgeon attending patients with multiple system injuries be familiar with the early management of facial injuries, even though a plastic surgeon may ultimately become responsible for the definitive treatment. An appreciation of the needs of both the patient and the plastic surgeon relative to these injuries will give the neurological surgeon the best perspective in allocating priorities.

A high percentage of the patients coming to the emergency room with multiple system injuries have sustained them in automobile accidents.[4] Of these patients, approximately 54 per cent will have significant facial trauma (Fig. 68–1). Typically, there are injury to the soft tissues and fractures of facial bones.

The early management of facial injuries plays an important role in their final outcome, but the extent of the early treatment is dependent on the nature of the associated injuries. Sometimes there are complications even after the most competent treatment, and these may eventually require complex multistaged reconstructive procedures (cf. Figs. 68–28, 68–29, and 68–30).

TRIAGE

In terms of timing, definitive treatment of most facial injuries ordinarily deserves low priority in the total care of the patient. With the exception of animal bites and accidental tattoo, treatment of soft-tissue trauma can usually be safely delayed up to 24 hours if the wound is given proper preparatory care. Most facial fractures are best treated several days after resorption of edema. Whether the delay is mandatory or elective, neurological, abdominal, thoracic, orthopedic, and urological injuries should be evaluated first.

Emergency Management

The priorities of early management for the patient with extensive facial trauma are the same as for the patient with any other trauma. They are assurance of a clear airway, control of hemorrhage, treatment of shock, and evaluation of associated injuries. After these measures have been completed, the facial injuries can be evaluated, and if appropriate, treatment can be initiated.

The cause of airway problems following facial trauma are varied. Obstruction from dentures, bone fragments, blood, or vomitus should be treated immediately by manual removal or aspiration. Although tracheostomy is often suggested for the patient with extensive facial injury, it is seldom indicated unless there are associated injuries of the head, neck, or chest. Occasionally the mandibular arch of a patient with a bilateral mandibular fracture will collapse, with retrodisplacement of the tongue and subsequent airway obstruction, but the obstruction can usually be relieved by placing the patient in the sitting position, allowing the arch to fall forward.

Hemorrhage from facial trauma usually has diminished by the time the patient arrives in the emergency room. In most instances, persistent bleeding can be controlled by pressure alone. Major vessels may have to be clamped and ligated through the wound. If so, care should be taken to avoid injury to important adjacent structures such as the facial nerve, parotid duct, or lacrimal sac.

As with any other patient sustaining ex-

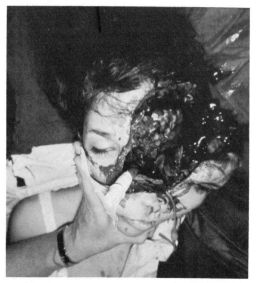

Figure 68–1   Cleaving fracture of skull and face from auto accident. Victim survived eight hours.

tensive trauma, shock must be treated aggressively. Blood loss from the facial injury alone, however, is seldom of sufficient magnitude to cause hypotension. Therefore, it should be anticipated that the shock is more likely to be due to neurological or other associated injuries.

After the patient's vital signs have stabi-lized, other organ systems can be more definitively evaluated. Primary attention is directed toward the facial injuries only after it has been established that no other life-threatening injury needs immediate care. While the relatively low priority of definitive facial injury treatment is stressed, it must also be emphasized that early evaluation cannot be ignored. If the patient's general condition permits, he should be observed and transported in the semi-sitting position to minimize venous ooze and formation of edema in the facial tissues. The patient will be made more comfortable at the same time.

The facial injuries should be evaluated radiographically at the initial x-ray examination for other injuries. A minimum number of facial x-rays are required to supplement the plastic surgeon's clinical evaluation for facial fractures. The Water's view (occipitomental) is the most valuable x-ray for studying the maxilla, the zygoma, and the frontal sinuses (Fig. 68–2) Oblique views of the mandible give the most information about fractures of the lower third of the face. When available, a Panorex view of the mandible may be included for a more sophisticated view of the entire mandible on a single film.

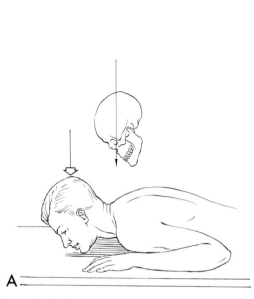
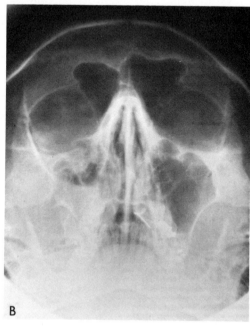

Figure 68–2   Waters x-ray view of facial bones. *A.* Patient must assume prone position. *B.* Depressed fracture of right zygoma. X-ray demonstrates fracture at inferior orbital rim and frontal-zygomatic suture. Right maxillary antrum shows opacity and fluid level.

The taking of proper facial x-rays initially should be stressed. If they are not done early, awkward situations may develop later. The plastic surgeon may be called to the operating room for concurrent treatment of facial injuries while a craniotomy, a laparotomy, or an orthopedic procedure is being performed. In this circumstance, the plastic surgeon will be treating the facial injuries without necessary information that could have been made available. Another problem is presented by the patient who has been set up in balanced traction on the ward; the dilemma then is when to put the patient through the ordeal of a second trip to the x-ray room to obtain the facial films.

The importance of routinely obtaining cervical spine x-rays during the initial x-ray examination for the facial injuries must be emphasized. In a series of 400 patients with facial injuries of varied extent, 4 per cent were found to have cervical spine fractures, many of which were asymptomatic.[4] In patients with extensive multiple system injuries, the incidence would likely be significantly greater (Fig. 68–3).

SOFT-TISSUE INJURIES

After hemostasis, the most important early treatment of soft-tissue injuries is cleansing of the wound. Ideally the wound is treated definitively in the first few hours after injury. When definitive treatment is delayed, however, soft-tissue repair can safely be performed after up to 24 hours if the wounds have been properly cleansed and dressed (Fig. 68–4). The exceptions to this rule are animal bites and retained foreign bodies, which should be treated soon after injury to reduce the likelihood of infection and tissue entrapment of foreign material.

To cleanse the wound, the surrounding skin is washed with soap or an antiseptic preparation (Betadine or pHisoHex). Care should be taken to avoid soaking the wound itself with the solution. The wound is irrigated with saline solution by using a bulb syringe or a jet lavage that incorporates a pulsating water stream. Solutions other than normal saline can be injurious to wounds and do not provide any significant antibacterial effect.

Types of Wounds

Soft-tissue trauma may vary in degree of severity, but usually can be categorized as contusion, abrasion, puncture, laceration, avulsion flap, avulsion defect, or accidental tattoo.

Contusion is usually the result of blunt trauma and is managed by cleansing and a dressing when needed. Contusions may have an underlying hematoma. A hematoma of significant size should be evacuated rather than being allowed to resorb (Fig. 68–5). Evacuation of a hematoma overlying the ear or nasal cartilage is especially important. Spontaneous resolution will often result in resorption of cartilage, subcutaneous scarring, and deformity. An untreated nasal septal hematoma will typically resorb and destroy the septal cartilage, leaving a "saddle nose" deformity. During the early stage (the first 7 to 10 days), a hematoma can be evacuated through a small incision. Where cartilage is not involved, a more conservative approach to treatment is needle aspiration. This operation usually is performed successfully after 10 to 14 days.

Abrasions and puncture wounds are properly treated with cleansing only, provided care is taken to remove any imbedded foreign body. The treatment of accidental tattoo requires scrubbing with a stiff scrub brush (Fig. 68–6). Care must be taken to avoid overzealous scrubbing, which may convert a partial-thickness injury into a full-thickness dermal defect that requires a skin graft.

Simple lacerations should be treated with skin cleansing, wound irrigation with normal saline, and primary closure. If there are beveled or "feathered" wound edges, or if there is obviously devitalized tissue, appropriate debridement should be performed (Fig. 68–7).[3] Most facial wounds, however, should be managed with very conservative debridement. Because of the excellent blood supply of the face, questionably viable facial tissue often will survive. Overly aggressive debridement may result in the loss of vital bits of soft tissue needed for later reconstruction.

Lacerations are closed in layers with a minimal but adequate number of sutures. In the face, buried sutures are a potential nidus of infection, but so also is dead space filled with blood or serum.

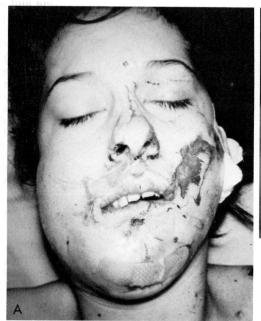

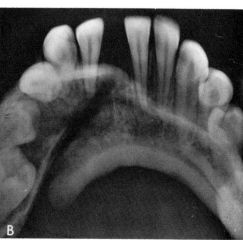

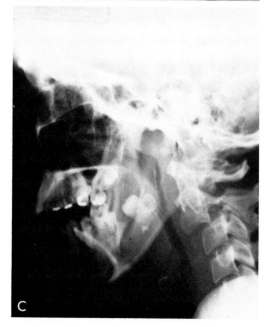

Figure 68–3 *A.* Clinical appearance of front-seat passenger in automobile accident. *B, C,* and *D.* Associated fractures of the mandible (corpus and condyle) and cervical spine (C2). *E.* All three fractures resulted from same force vectors. *F.* Reduction of cervical spine fracture in presence of mandibular fractures. Concomitant fractures complicate patient management. *G.* Postoperative appearance.

Illustration continued on opposite page

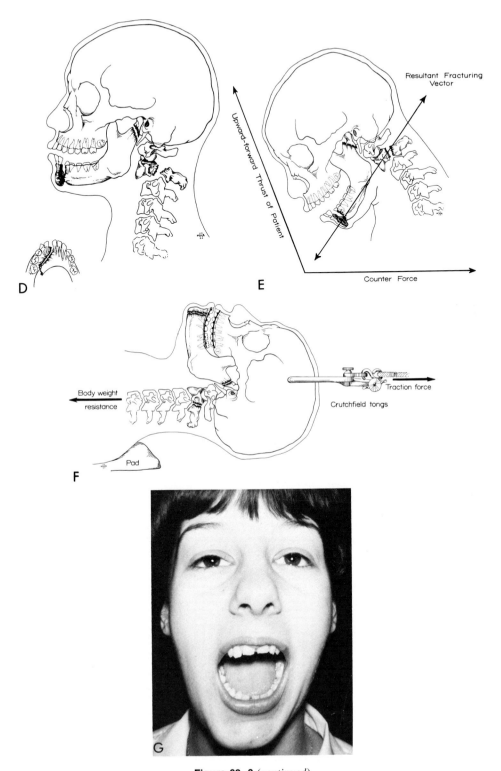

Figure 68–3 (*continued*)

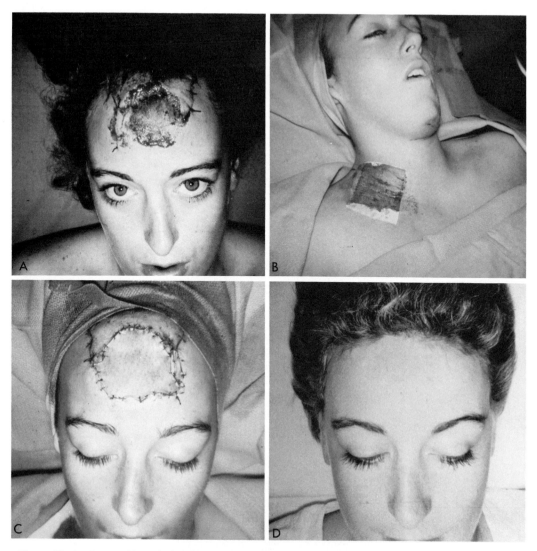

Figure 68–4   Auto accident victim with avulsion of tissue from forehead. *A*. Because of associated closed head injury, wounds were initially only cleaned and dressed. *B* and *C*. Skin graft was subsequently taken from neck under local anesthesia 72 hours following injury. *D*. Final photograph taken one year after grafting.

Soft-Tissue Repair

The cheek is the area of the face most frequently lacerated. Deep structures of concern are the facial nerve, the parotid gland, and the parotid duct.

Nerve Injury

Facial nerve injury should be diagnosed on the basis of physical examination and anatomical landmarks. Under ordinary circumstances, muscle paralysis on the involved side of the face indicates nerve injury. An uncooperative patient, an extensive soft-tissue injury, or extensive edema may make the physical examination inconclusive. A functional as well as cosmetic deformity results from an unrepaired proximal facial nerve laceration.

Most surgeons believe that division of branches of the facial nerve medial to the midpupillary line do not require repair. Branching cross-innervation is likely to reinnervate the appropriate muscle spontaneously. Lateral to the midpupillary line, nerve repair should be attempted in order to guide the advancing axons to the motor end-plate in the muscle.

Section of the temporal branch of the facial nerve causes a more severe functional deficit in the face than section of any other single branch. It causes paralysis of the

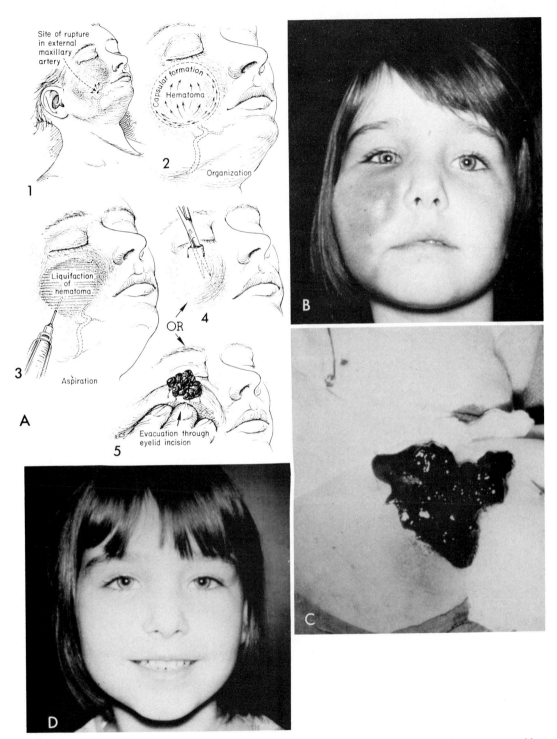

Figure 68–5 *A*. Treatment of hematoma of cheek. *B*. Hematoma of cheek and fracture of zygoma, caused by falling object. *C*. Hematoma was evacuated and fracture was reduced through lower eyelid incision. *D*. Healed eyelid scar is barely visible three months following injury.

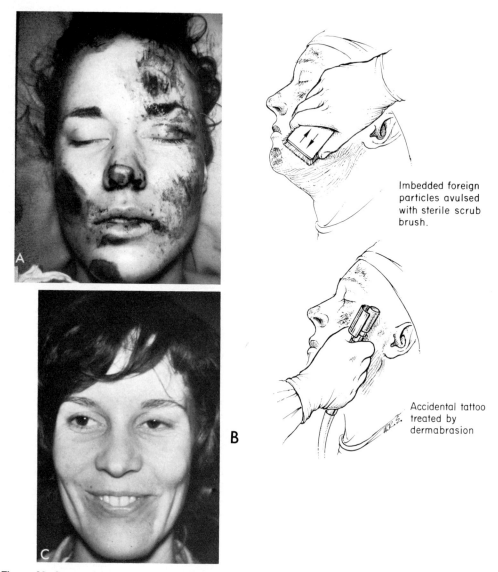

Imbedded foreign
particles avulsed
with sterile scrub
brush.

Accidental tattoo
treated by
dermabrasion

Figure 68-6   *A* and *B*. Accidental tattoo from road dirt must be scrubbed promptly to avoid tissue fixation, or a more formal dermabrasion becomes necessary to remove these small foreign particles. *C*. Final photograph taken three months after treatment with scrub-brush.

eyelid and subsequent exposure of the cornea. This branch courses superiorly at a point halfway between the tragus and the lateral canthus, becoming superficial along its course.

The mandibular branch of the facial nerve also is injured frequently. This branch is always deep to the platysma muscle when posterior to the facial artery. Anterior to the facial artery, it becomes more superficial and, though usually found above the lower border of the mandible, may be found 1 cm below the mandible.

When a proximal laceration of a branch of the facial nerve is suspected, exploration

should be undertaken to identify the nerve ends. The epineurium should be reapproximated with fine suture material. Magnification should be used. Injury of a major nerve trunk is repaired with fascicular sutures and with the aid of an operating microscope.

Parotid Injury

The parotid duct courses along a line from the tragus of the ear to the midportion of the upper lip. It lies deep near the anterior border of the masseter muscle, emptying into the oral cavity adjacent to the first

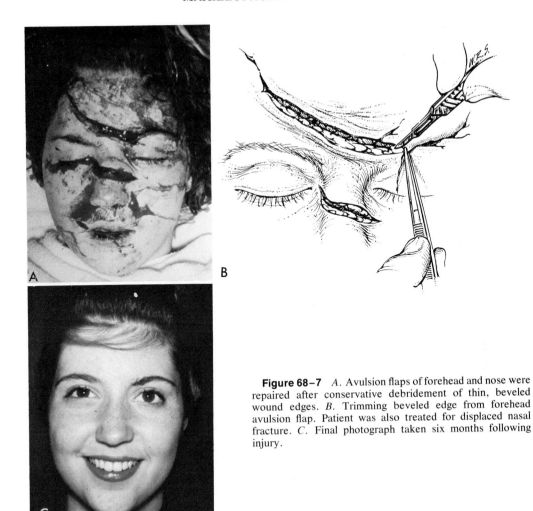

Figure 68–7 *A.* Avulsion flaps of forehead and nose were repaired after conservative debridement of thin, beveled wound edges. *B.* Trimming beveled edge from forehead avulsion flap. Patient was also treated for displaced nasal fracture. *C.* Final photograph taken six months following injury.

maxillary molar tooth (Fig. 68–8). It can be divided by a deep laceration posterior to the anterior border of the masseter muscle. These lacerations also frequently damage the buccal branch of the facial nerve. When there is complete laceration of the parotid duct, end-to-end anastomosis over a small Silastic catheter can be performed (Fig. 68–9). As an alternate procedure to maintain parotid function, the proximal cut end of the duct can be sutured to the oral mucosa.

When clear fluid is seen leaking from a wound in the parotid region, injury to the gland should be suspected. The gland itself need not be sutured. Salivary fistula is a common complication following skin repair of an underlying glandular laceration (Fig. 68–10). The fistula usually closes without further treatment in about three weeks.

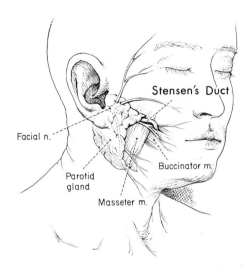

Figure 68–8 Location of Stensen's duct in relation to the parotid gland and facial nerve.

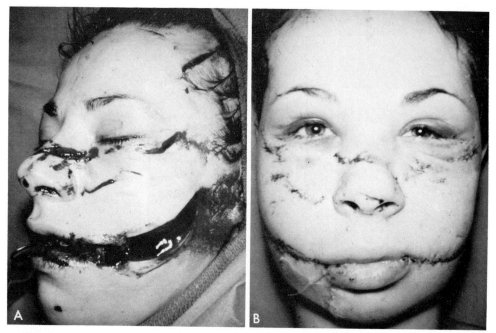

Figure 68–9 *A*. Auto accident victim with complete division of cheek bilaterally. *B*. Stensen's duct was repaired over cannulation with thin Silastic catheter on one side; cut end was sutured into oral mucosa on other side.

Eyelid Injury

Injuries to thin eyelid skin may result in small avulsion flaps that appear questionably viable. These flaps usually survive if replaced anatomically (Fig. 68–11). Divided muscle and tarsal plate should be identified and sutured separately with fine absorbable suture. Simple direct anatomical repair is the best approach. The tarsal plate is adherent to the conjunctiva and can be repaired with the conjunctiva. Lacerations of the thin orbital septum usually do not require separate closure provided the orbicularis oculi muscle is repaired.

Lacerations of the lacrimal apparatus must be recognized and repaired to prevent epiphora and dacryocystitis postoperatively. The divided lacrimal duct may be cannulated with a heavy nylon suture and then reapproximated with fine absorbable sutures. After a week, the nylon stent is removed. Fine, soft polyethylene catheters can also be used for cannulation. When injury to the lacrimal system is severe, primary dacryorhinocystostomy should be considered.

Ear Injury

Lacerations through the full thickness of the ear are best repaired by cutaneous-perichondrial sutures (Fig. 68–12). The cartilage margins may require conservative trimming to facilitate skin closure, but cartilage itself need not be sutured.

As stated earlier, hematoma of the ear from blunt trauma may be potentially disfiguring if left untreated. Aspiration or incision and drainage will evacuate the hematoma in the early stages. If untreated, the hematoma undergoes organization and fibrosis leading to the classic "cauliflower ear."

Nasal Injury

Lacerations through the nostrils are repaired by closure of the mucous membrane with absorbable sutures and the skin with monofilament nylon (Fig. 68–13). Care should be taken to align the nostril border accurately, but ordinarily suturing of the alar or upper lateral cartilages is not necessary. Nasal fracture, of course, should al-

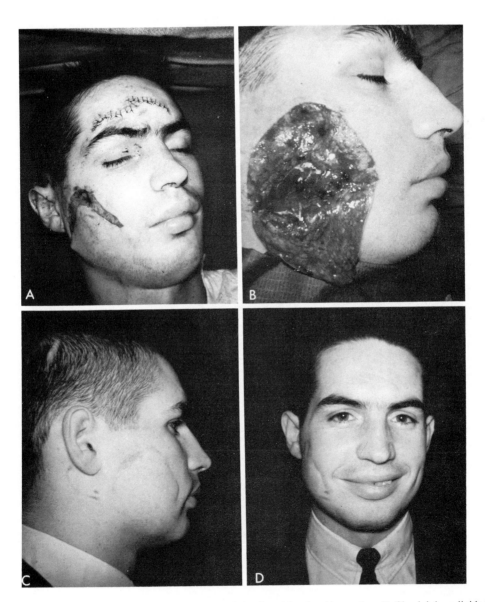

Figure 68–10 *A*. Patient with deep avulsion flap of cheek and forehead laceration. *B*. Cheek injury divided the buccal branch of the facial nerve and lacerated the parotid gland. *C*. Patient developed salivary fistula following repair, but this closed spontaneously in three weeks. *D*. Final photograph taken four months following injury.

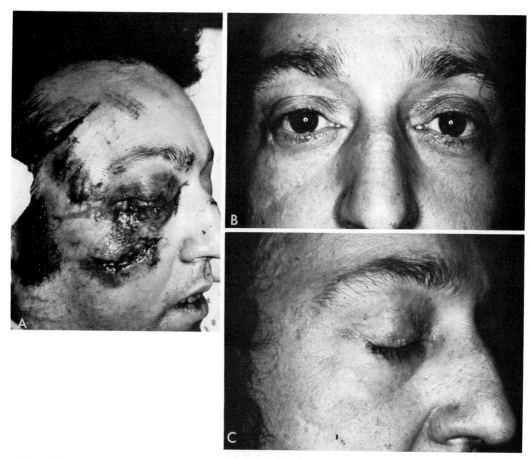

Figure 68–11   *A.* Victim of assault sustained multiple lacerations about the orbit and eyelids. *B.* Tissue was replaced anatomically and repaired with fine sutures. *C.* Final photograph taken three months following injury.

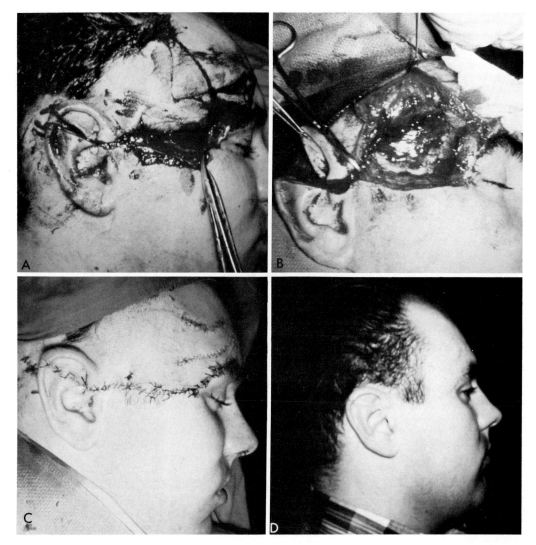

Figure 68–12 *A*. Deep lacerations of forehead, brow, and temporal area, and near-amputation of the superior pole of the ear. *B* and *C*. Repair of ear accomplished under local anesthesia by direct approximation of skin and perichondrium. *D*. Final picture taken six months following injury.

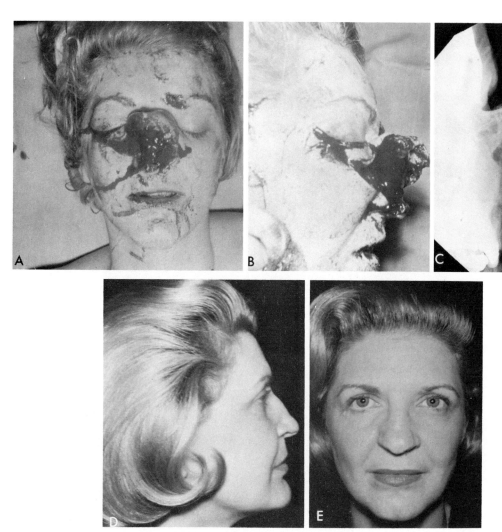

Figure 68–13 *A* and *B*. Avulsion injury of nose, sustained on penetrating automobile windshield. Note complete reversal of nasal-glabellar angle, seen also on lateral x-ray view of nasal bones. *C*. Nasal fractures were reduced and soft tissues repaired by direct anatomical approximation under local anesthesia. *D* and *E*. Final photographs taken one year after injury.

ways be suspected. These fractures often can be diagnosed clinically and treated at the time of soft-tissue repair. Techniques of closed reduction of displaced nasal fractures are discussed later.

FACIAL BONE FRACTURES

Diagnosis

The patient with extensive facial fractures can present an awesome appearance. As previously discussed, forces sufficient to fracture the bony facial structure may also cause disfiguring soft-tissue injury.

Displacement of the bony fragments further distorts the facial contour. The severity of soft-tissue destruction should not distract the examiner from a complete examination of the facial skeleton. The initial x-ray examination may not demonstrate facial fractures. As a result, the diagnosis of bony injuries may depend on the clinical evaluation alone.

Careful observation can disclose depressed frontal sinuses, a deviated nasal complex, a depressed zygoma, enophthalmos, an asymmetrical mandible, or a malaligned dental arch. Poor dental occlusion may be the first clue to mandibular or maxillary fracture. Diplopia may be the only positive finding associated with a fractured orbital floor. Systematic bimanual palpation will help to avoid missing less obvious fractures (Fig. 68–14). Palpation of the bony parts can usually elicit tenderness and sometimes motion and crepitus at the fracture sites.

To simplify and systematize facial bony fracture diagnosis, the facial skeleton can be divided into three zones: upper, middle, and lower. (Fig. 68–15)

Fractures of the Upper Third of the Face

Fractures of the upper third of the face are less common than those of the lower two thirds of the face because of the protection afforded by the nose, which serves as an energy-absorbing projecting part. Fractures of the frontal area usually involve the thinner bones of the frontal sinuses or the supraorbital ridges. Because of the close proximity to the brain, injuries in this area

are more likely to be accompanied by greater morbidity and to be more life-threatening than any other facial fractures (cf. Fig. 68–1).[5]

Positive physical findings usually appear in the ocular region because of extravasation of blood into the orbital area. Periorbital ecchymosis is observed in nearly all cases. Diplopia is inconstant. It is seen with depressed supraorbital fractures, but is not commonly found with glabellar fractures. Nasal fractures and overlying lacerations of the forehead often are found in association with fractures of the upper third of the face.[5]

Treatment of these fractures involves reduction of the bony fragments by either the direct or the indirect approach, and interosseous fixation when required for stabilization (Fig. 68–16).[5] Appropriate debridement of avascular or pulped sinus mucosa, accurate replacement of soft tissue, and systemic antibiotic therapy should accompany the bony reduction. Some surgeons advocate removal of the comminuted bone

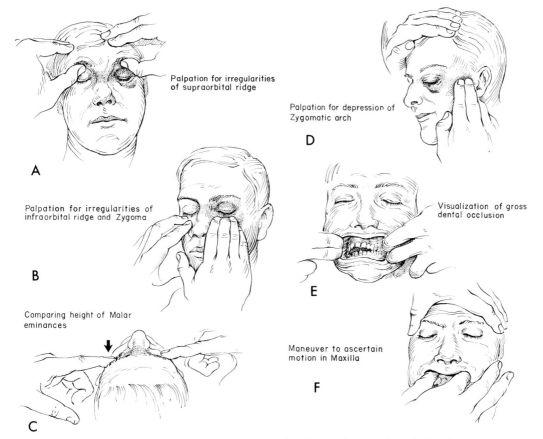

Palpation for irregularities of supraorbital ridge

Palpation for depression of Zygomatic arch

D

Palpation for irregularities of infraorbital ridge and Zygoma

A

B

Visualization of gross dental occlusion

E

Comparing height of Malar eminances

Maneuver to ascertain motion in Maxilla

F

C

Figure 68–14 Systematic bimanual palpation will help avoid missing less obvious fractures.

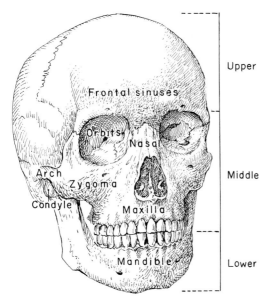

Figure 68–15 The facial skeleton is divided into upper, middle, and lower zones to simplify and systematize facial bone fracture diagnosis.

fragments and extirpation of the sinus, but this bone loss results in gross deformity. These deformities require extensive secondary reconstructive procedures to correct, whereas primary bony reconstruction as just outlined gives excellent functional and aesthetic results without complications (cf. Figs. 68–27, 68–29, and 68–30).[5]

Fractures of the Middle Third of the Face

Fractures in this region of the face often result from injury to unrestrained passengers within an automobile (Fig. 68–17). They range from the nasal fracture, which is the simplest, to the maxillary fracture, which is the most complex of all facial fractures. Because of the prominence of the nasal complex and the thinness of the bones supporting it, nasal fractures are the most common of all facial fractures.[6] Other fractures frequently seen in the middle third of the face involve the maxilla, the zygoma, the zygomatic arch, and the bones making up the orbit.

Nasal Fractures

Clinical findings are the most reliable means of making the diagnosis of a nasal fracture. Positive x-ray visualization is sometimes absent even when the nose shows gross traumatic deformity.[8] A history of a nosebleed following injury, deviation of the nasal pyramid, and crepitus on palpation are the most helpful clinical findings. Sometimes, lateral and occlusal projections of the nasal bones will document these fractures precisely, but often they will not do so even with repeated attempts (Fig. 68–18). The history of a previous fracture or nasal deviation is important, since a healed displaced nasal fracture often cannot be reduced by the usual closed reduction techniques.

Unless the patient can be treated prior to the onset of edema, closed reduction should be delayed five to seven days to allow for its resolution. Reduction can be delayed up to two to three weeks if necessary. The need for reduction can best be determined after the edema has resorbed. Undisplaced nasal fractures require no reduction.

Anesthesia of the nose is accomplished by insertion of intranasal packs soaked in a 5 per cent cocaine solution accompanied by an external block using 1 per cent lidocaine with epinephrine (Fig. 68–19).[8] After the nose has been anesthetized, disimpaction and reduction of the nasal bone fragments are done with three nasal reduction instruments (Fig. 68–20). Reduction of the fracture is followed by immobilization of the fragments with a plaster splint for one week.

Although a severely displaced nasal fracture may be reducible by closed techniques for several months, a minimally displaced fracture will often become fixed by fibrous union within three to four weeks. Efforts to correct the deformity after such healing often requires open reduction and osteotomies.

Maxillary Fractures

The mechanism of injury in maxillary fractures is usually direct impact to the midface as in an automobile or motorcycle accident. In 1901 the French surgeon Le Fort described three common lines of fracture of the maxilla based on weak points of the midface (Fig. 68–21).[2] Clinically, however, maxillary fractures are often a modification or combination of these classic fracture lines. Combinations of such fractures

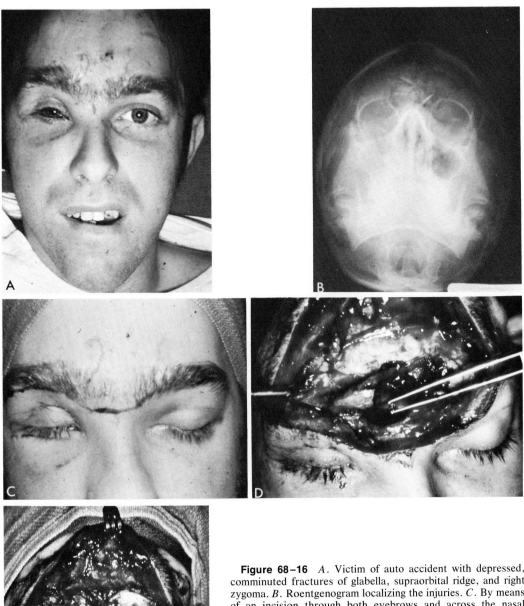

Figure 68–16 *A*. Victim of auto accident with depressed, comminuted fractures of glabella, supraorbital ridge, and right zygoma. *B*. Roentgenogram localizing the injuries. *C*. By means of an incision through both eyebrows and across the nasal bridge, a large forehead flap was raised, and the multiple fractures of the upper third of the face were exposed. Pulped mucous membrane from the frontal sinuses was excised. *D*. Glass foreign bodies were removed from the recesses of the frontal sinuses. After elevation of the posterior wall, the anterior bone fragments were replaced and fixed with key wire sutures. *E*. Right zygoma was reduced and wired.

Illustration continued on following page

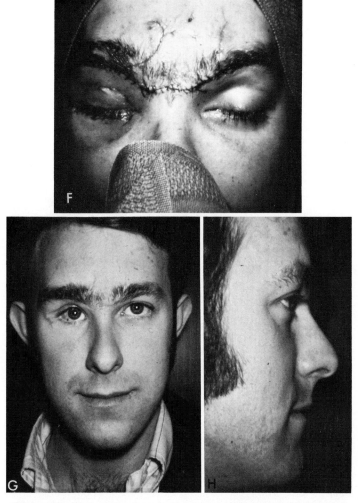

Figure 68–16 (*continued*) *F*. Forehead flap was returned. Convalescence was uncomplicated; no mucocele, pyocele, or wound inflammation occurred. *G* and *H*. Final photographs taken nine months following treatment.

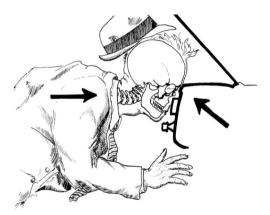

Figure 68–17 Fractures of the middle third of the face commonly result from injury to unrestrained passengers within the automobile. (From Schultz, R. C.: Facial Injuries. 2nd Ed. Chicago, Year Book Medical Publishers, 1977. Reprinted by permission.)

have given rise to the term "panfacial fractures."

Transverse Maxillary Fracture (Le Fort I)

This fracture is often associated with a blow to the upper lip. The detached portion is often a single segment made up of the alveolar process, the palate, and the pterygoid process. Inspection of the dental arches usually demonstrates an open bite with superior displacement of the maxillary incisors. With this fracture, motion of the entire upper dental arch and palate may be detected by grasping the upper teeth. An isolated alveolar ridge fracture also may permit motion of the upper dental arch.

Treatment of a transverse maxillary fracture consists of reduction and immobilization. The reduction and immobilization usually are accomplished best by intermaxillary fixation with arch bars and suspension from the lateral orbital rims. In some cases, however, interosseous wire fixation at the fracture site combined with intermaxillary fixation may be sufficient for stabilization.

Pyramidal Fracture (Le Fort II)

An impact higher on the midface may result in a fracture that passes from the alveolus posteriorly along the nasal processes of the maxillary bone, across the root of the nose, and posteriorly through the lacrimal bones, the floor of the orbit, and the pterygoid process. The isolated maxillary fragment is pyramid-shaped. Unless the blow has impacted the maxilla posteriorly or superiorly, motion can be detected at the medial portion of the orbital floors by grasping the upper teeth and rocking them back and forth. Reduction and immobilization of this fracture can be accomplished with wire suspension from the frontal bone or zygoma (Fig. 68–22). This fracture is quite unstable because of the tendency to become displaced posteriorly. Direct wiring at the infraorbital rim may add to the stability of the repair. Comminution sometimes is found at these points, however, and makes interosseous wiring difficult.

Craniofacial Disjunction (Le Fort III)

Powerful forces delivered to the maxilla may completely separate the facial bone structures from the base of the skull. The only remaining attachment of the face to the skull is soft tissue. This injury is more severe than the pyramidal fractures because the fractures extend transversely across the nasal bridge, both posterior orbital walls, the lateral orbital rims, and the zygomatic arch, separating the face from the cranium. Patients with this facial fracture often have an associated intracranial injury.

Treatment consists of reduction and immobilization of the fracture similar to those used in the Le Fort II fracture with the addition of interosseous wiring at the zygomaticofrontal suture to provide greater immobilization. Cerebrospinal fluid rhinorrhea is not a contraindication to operative reduction of this fracture. In some instances, this reduction will stop the rhinorrhea. The deformity that results from inadequate treatment of a severe maxillary fracture is a flattened, elongated, or depressed midface.

Zygomatic Fractures

The zygoma has two components: the malar eminence and the zygomatic arch. Fractures may occur in either segment sep-

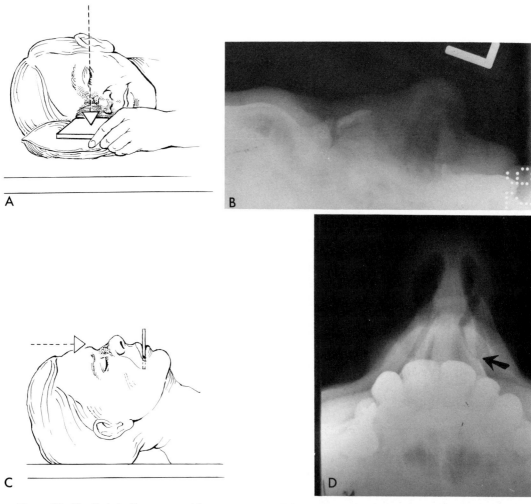

Figure 68–18 To help diagnose nasal fractures, x-rays of the nose are taken in the lateral, *A* and *B*, and occlusal, *C* and *D*, views. (From Schultz, R. C.: Facial Injuries. 2nd Ed. Chicago, Year Book Medical Publishers, 1977. Reprinted by permission.)

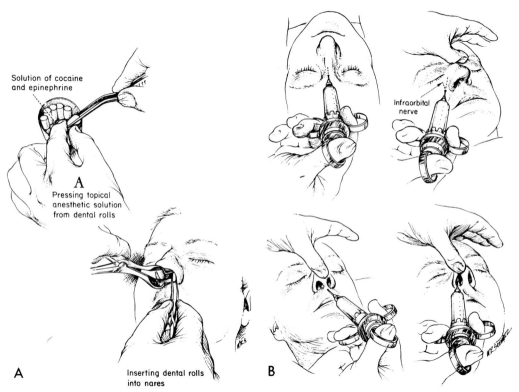

Solution of cocaine and epinephrine

A

Pressing topical anesthetic solution from dental rolls

Infraorbital nerve

A

Inserting dental rolls into nares

B

Figure 68–19 Anesthesia of the nose is provided by cocaine applied on cotton dental rolls, *A*, and by local block by injection of an anesthetic solution, *B*.

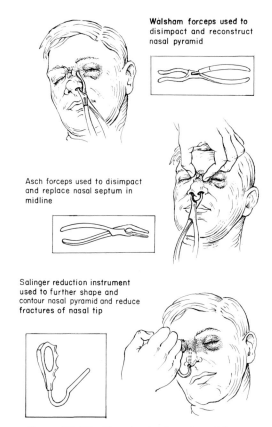

Walsham forceps used to disimpact and reconstruct nasal pyramid

Asch forceps used to disimpact and replace nasal septum in midline

Salinger reduction instrument used to further shape and contour nasal pyramid and reduce fractures of nasal tip

Figure 68–20 Closed reduction of nasal fractures is accomplished with three special instruments.

arately or in both, but an isolated arch fracture is uncommon. The most common fracture of the zygoma involves depression of the malar eminence. This type of fracture consists of three parts—thus the terms "tripod fracture" and "trimalar fracture." The fracture sites are usually found at the zygomaticotemporal and zygomaticofrontal suture lines and the infraorbital foramen. The fractured zygoma may undergo varying degrees of rotation and depression, depending on the mechanism of injury. Treatment usually requires open reduction and internal interosseous fixation at two of the three fracture sites. The inferior and lateral orbital rims are the sites that are fixed (Fig. 68–23). Failure to effect an anatomically stable reduction often results in a flattened and depressed malar eminence after the swelling has resorbed. Some authors have advocated semiclosed reduction in which the force is applied under the arch through an intraoral approach or scalp incision. Without interosseous wiring, however, this

method of reduction can allow recurrence of the displacement and result in late postoperative deformity.

Another technique of reduction of zygomatic fractures is through a Caldwell-Luc incision into the maxillary sinus. The reduction is performed through the sinus. The sinus is then packed to maintain reduction. This technique is somewhat hazardous; blindness has been reported secondary to compression and thrombosis of the ophthalmic vessels or from injury to the optic nerve by bony fragments at the time of manipulation. If packing of the maxillary sinus is necessary to maintain reduction, it should be done with the orbital floor under direct vision.

Orbital Fractures

The bones making up the orbital walls include the zygoma, maxilla, frontal, sphe-

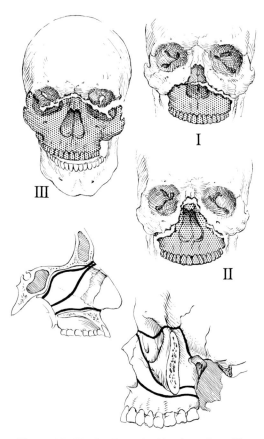

Figure 68–21 Le Fort classification of maxillary fractures: I (transverse), II (pyramidal), and III (craniofacial disjunction).

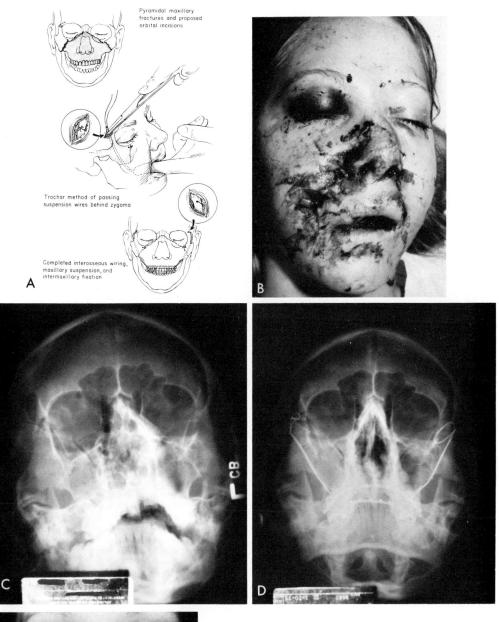

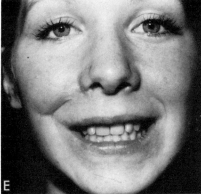

Figure 68–22 *A*. Most displaced maxillary fractures require internal wire suspension from the frontal bones. *B*, *C*, and *D*. This patient sustained a displaced pyramidal maxillary fracture in a motorcycle accident. Burst-type soft-tissue injuries of the right cheek and nose were repaired primarily by anatomical tissue approximation. *E*. Final photograph taken six months following injury.

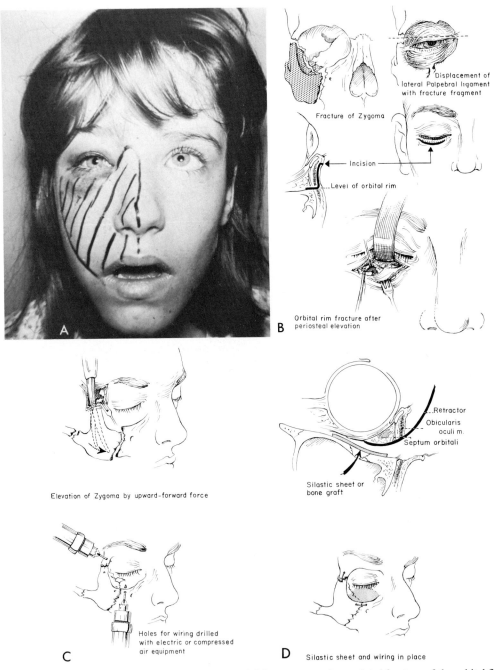

Figure 68–23 *A.* Patient with depressed fracture of right zygoma and associated fracture of the orbital floor, with entrapment of the inferior rectus muscle. (Patient is attempting upward gaze.) Hatched area is anesthetic from injury to the inferior orbital nerve. *B, C,* and *D.* Operative treatment is illustrated. Entrapped inferior rectus was freed to restore normal extraocular movements.

Illustration continued on opposite page

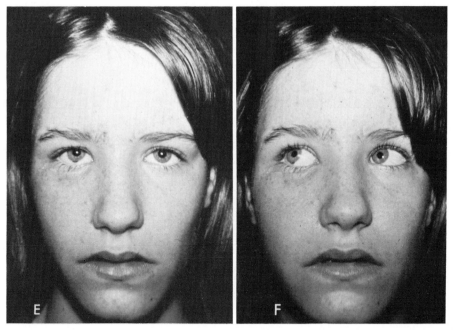

Figure 68–23 (*continued*) *E* and *F*. Final photographs taken three months following injury.

noid, and ethmoid. Any of these bones may be fractured in extensive midface fractures. Commonly, however, an orbital floor fracture, involving the thin maxillary portion, accompanies a depressed zygoma fracture. Rarely, an isolated fracture of the orbital floor leaves the orbital rims intact. The usual injury is a blow to the globe, which transmits the force posteriorly and inferiorly through the weakest point in the orbital walls, the paper-thin orbital floor. Because of the mechanism of injury, this fracture has been named a "blowout" fracture. Clinical findings may include diplopia, enophthalmos, and malfunction of the extraocular muscles. Entrapped periorbital fat and eye muscles may have to be freed from the fracture site. Often the floor is reinforced with a thin Silastic sheet at the time of the reduction, as shown in Figure 68–23.

Some authors advocate waiting for resolution of the swelling and hematoma so that the permanency of the enophthalmos, diplopia, and muscle entrapment can be evaluated more adequately. Experience has shown, however, that the presence of posttraumatic induration and fibrosis often precludes an acceptable functional and aesthetic result when treatment is delayed.

Fractures of the Lower Third of the Face (Mandibular Fractures)

Among facial fractures, those involving the mandible rank third in frequency behind those of the nose and zygoma.[6] Patients with mandibular fracture, in contrast to other facial bone fractures, sometimes experience pain because of muscular distraction of the fragments. The fracture sites frequently are predictable on the basis of the mechanism of injury. Treatment of a fractured mandible is dependent on the location of the fracture, the angle of the fracture line, and the amount of displacement. The directions of muscular pull about the mandible are shown in Figure 68–24. A fracture line angulated anteroinferiorly from above and behind would tend to be impacted into a favorable position because of the action of the masseter and internal pterygoid muscles inserting on the lower border of the mandible at the angle. Conversely, the muscle pull on a fracture line angulated in the opposite direction would draw the fragments farther apart.

A nondisplaced unilateral mandibular fracture can usually be treated by intermaxillary fixation with the teeth held in occlusion by arch bars or Blair-Ivy loops (Figs.

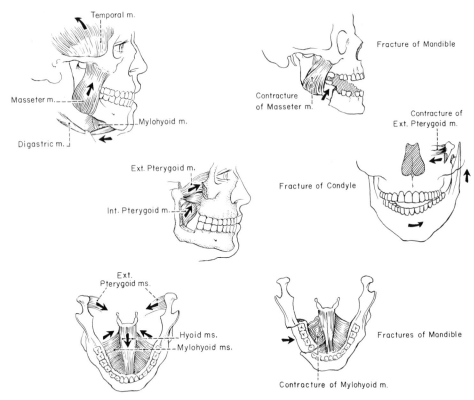

Figure 68–24   Major muscular attachments to mandible and their distracting effects on mandibular fractures.

68–25 and 68–26). A fracture that is unstable because it is markedly displaced, has an unfavorable angle, or is bilateral usually will require open reduction and interosseous fixation, for which either a cutaneous or intraoral incision can be used (Fig. 68–27). Stabilization by means of intraoral splinting, percutaneous Kirschner wires, or external traction devices has been used in various circumstances, but the indications for these methods are limited.

Facial Fractures in Children

In general, the mechanism of injury, the diagnosis, and the management of facial bone fractures in children do not differ greatly from those in the adult; a few differences do exist, however. Because of lack of cooperation on the part of the patient, the diagnosis may rest more heavily on x-ray findings than on clinical examination.

Because of greater resiliency in the facial bones of children, greenstick fractures are more common than completely displaced fractures. Because bony union may occur early in children, fractures should be reduced in the first week after injury.

Subcondylar fractures in children, especially when bilateral, may involve the epiphyseal growth center and cause a growth problem. As with adults, closed treatment is the preferred method of management even in instances of a medially displaced condyle. Intermaxillary fixation is more difficult in children because of the instability of deciduous teeth, instability that occasionally precludes using the teeth to maintain occlusion.

AUTOGENOUS BONE GRAFTS

Despite timely and skillful reduction, postoperative deformities occasionally cannot be avoided. They may result from a severe comminution or displacement that cannot be adequately corrected. Reconstruction of these defects with many different materials has been described; the most physiological and in many ways the most satisfactory reconstruction graft material, however, is autogenous bone.

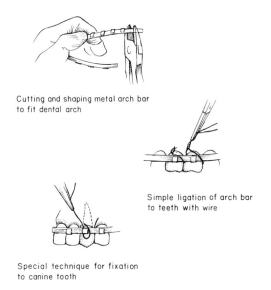

Cutting and shaping metal arch bar to fit dental arch

Simple ligation of arch bar to teeth with wire

Special technique for fixation to canine tooth

Intermaxillary fixation with dental elastics

Figure 68–25 Prefabricated metal arch bars, tailored in length and shape to each patient, are ligated with fine wire to the upper and lower dental arches. They are then used to stabilize mandibular fractures by intermaxillary fixation with additional wire or elastics.

Bone grafts for facial reconstruction usually are taken from rib, iliac crest, or tibia, depending on the specific requirements at the recipient site. All three areas contain cortical bone. Large amounts of cancellous bone can be obtained from the iliac crest and the tibia.

Recipient areas requiring structural support must be grafted with cortical bone. When large defects must be spanned, split rib grafts are usually the most suitable (Fig. 68–28). A smaller defect can easily be filled with an iliac bone graft cut to the shape that is needed.

The disadvantage of cancellous bone is the unpredictable resorption that may take place. The healing that occurs following bone grafting is one of continuing resorption and new bone formation. Successful incorporation of a bone graft is dependent upon a net increase in viable osteocytes in the graft following bony union to the recipi-

ent bone. Adding chips of porous cancellous bone will often increase the volume of a viable bone graft.

Areas of the facial structure most amenable to bone grafting include the nose, mandible, forehead, and orbital rims. In the healing of a severely comminuted nasal fracture there may be insufficient bone available to reshape the pyramid adequately. A saddle nose deformity may result.· After approximately one year of wound maturation, an iliac bone graft can be shaped to correct the problem effectively (Fig. 68–29). Other materials, including cartilage and silicone rubber, have been used for augmenting the nasal dorsum; bone grafts, however, have been found to have a much lower incidence of resorption or extrusion. Iliac bone gives the necessary support and has cancellous bone in sufficient quantity. If an appropriate pocket and bony platform have been created to allow for sufficient bony contact between it and

Text continued on page 2296

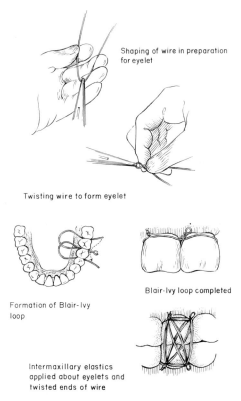

Shaping of wire in preparation for eyelet

Twisting wire to form eyelet

Formation of Blair-Ivy loop

Blair-Ivy loop completed

Intermaxillary elastics applied about eyelets and twisted ends of wire

Figure 68–26 Simple four-point fixation on both sides of the mouth can be fashioned by ligating single lengths of wire about upper and lower molar teeth. Resultant wire eyelets are then joined with either additional wire or elastics to immobilize the mandible by intermaxillary fixation.

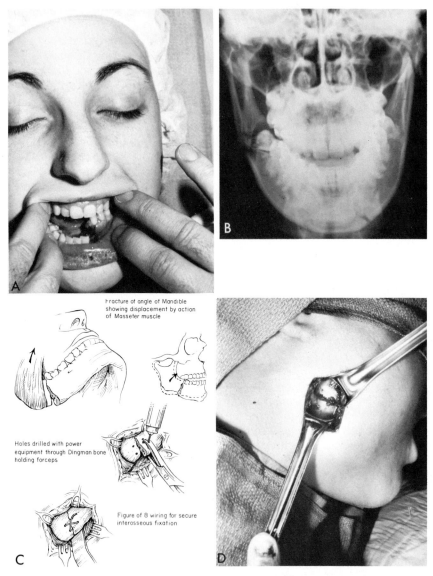

Figure 68–27 *A* and *B*. Patient with displaced fractures of the right mandibular angle and body of the left mandible. *C* and *D*. Fracture of the angle is treated by open reduction.

Illustration continued on opposite page

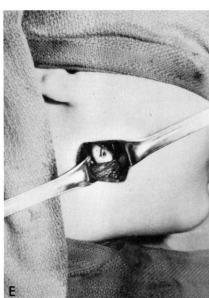

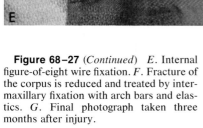

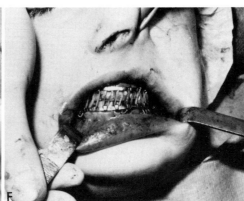

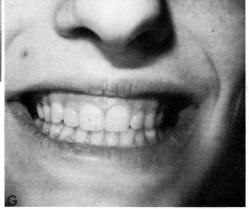

Figure 68–27 (*Continued*) *E*. Internal figure-of-eight wire fixation. *F*. Fracture of the corpus is reduced and treated by intermaxillary fixation with arch bars and elastics. *G*. Final photograph taken three months after injury.

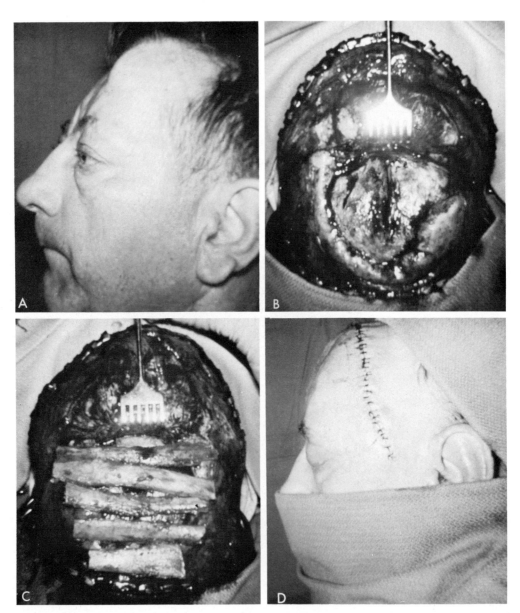

Figure 68–28 *A*. Glabellar and frontal defect in patient treated by another surgical discipline by bone resection for fractures of the upper third of the face. *B*, *C*, and *D*. Defect exposed through a bitemporal forehead flap and reconstructed with split-rib grafts.

Illustration continued on opposite page

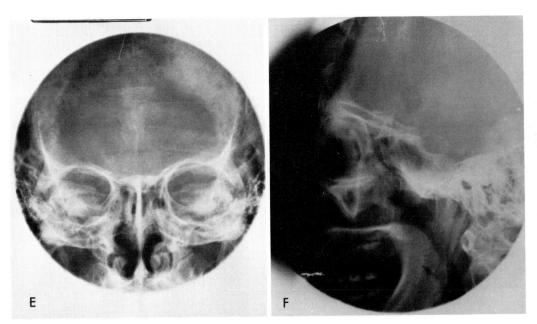

Figure 68–28 (*continued*)   *E* and *F*. X-rays taken two years following reconstruction show viable rib grafts with some coalescence.

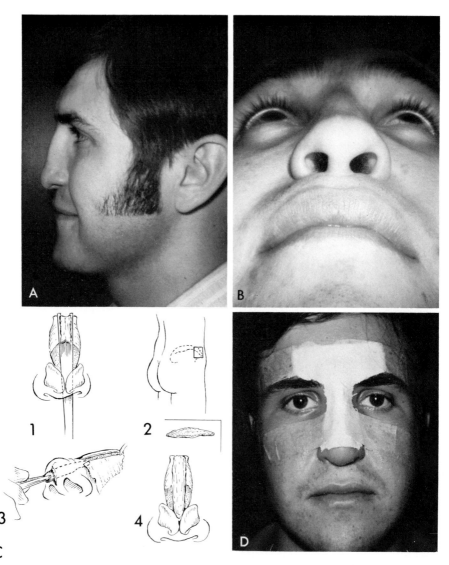

Figure 68–29   *A* and *B*. Saddle nose deformity in an athlete who sustained repeated nasal fractures. *C*. Under local anesthesia the dorsal bony convexity was resected, and the nasal framework was reconstructed with a bone graft taken from the iliac crest. *D*. Nose was protected in a plaster splint.

Illustration continued on opposite page

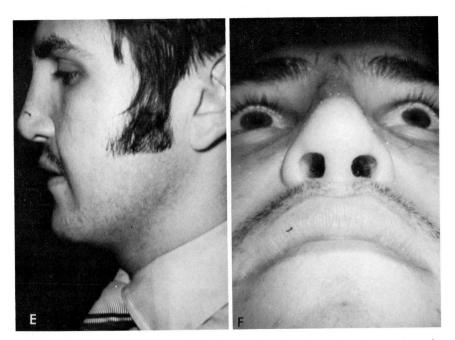

Figure 68–29 (*continued*)   *E* and *F*. Final photographs taken six months after reconstruction.

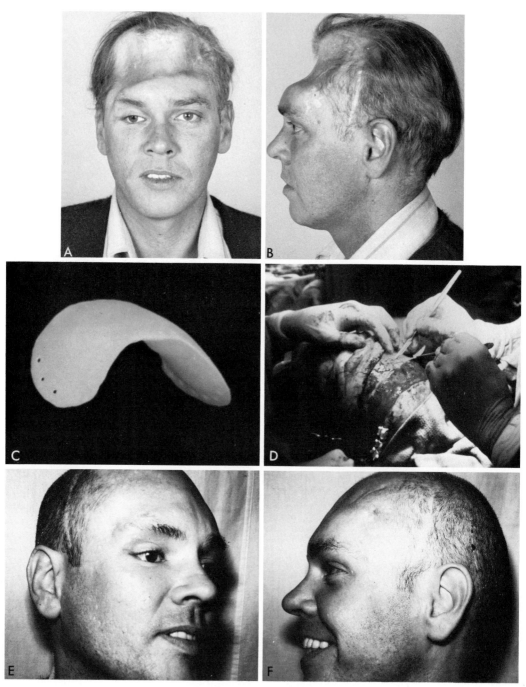

Figure 68–30 *A* and *B*. Patient with frontal bone defect following operative treatment of gunshot wound of the head. Defect is reconstructed with a prefabricated Silastic implant, *C*. Defect is exposed through a bitemporal forehead flap. *D*. Implant required tailoring during the operation to fit precisely before being fixed to adjacent frontal bone with nonabsorbable sutures. Convalescence was entirely uncomplicated. *E* and *F*. Final pictures taken six months following reconstruction.

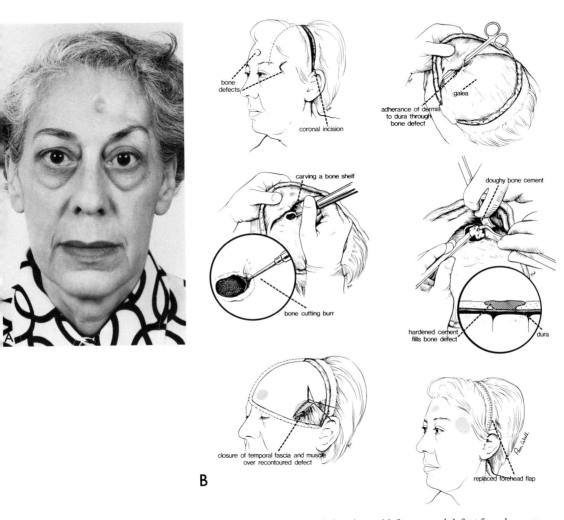

Figure 68–31 *A*. Patient was disfigured by frontal burr hole deformity and left temporal defect from bone resection for cerebral decompression. *B*. Reconstruction of frontal defect with bone cement.

Illustration continued on following page

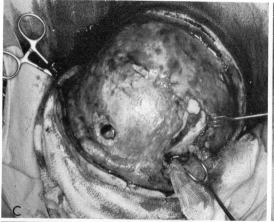
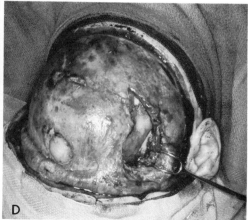

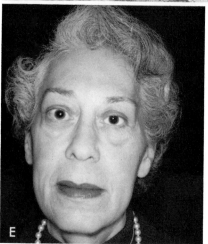

Figure 68–31 (*continued*) *C.* Both defects were exposed through a bitemporal forehead flap. *D.* Undersurface of the dermis was divided carefully from the dura, and bone defects were then reconstructed with moldable bone cement. Convalescence was entirely uneventful. *E.* Final photograph taken 10 months following reconstruction.

the recipient nasal bones, the graft is readily incorporated into the nasal complex.

The superior and inferior orbital rims are vulnerable to violent external forces. Bone grafts may be indicated to restore their contour following unreduced fractures with bone resorption. Rib or iliac bone may be shaped to provide suitable reconstruction in these areas.

ALLOPLASTIC MATERIAL

As new compounds are developed, alloplastic materials are being implanted with increasing frequency. Silicone rubber and methylmethacrylate are currently the most commonly used. Each one has its own advantages.[7]

Silicone rubber must be custom prefabricated to fit the existing defect (Fig. 68–30). It is inert, having essentially no antigenic potential. It is, however, a foreign body and has a higher incidence of extrusion than do autogenous bone or cartilage grafts.

Methylmethacrylate is a cold-curing acrylic that has the advantage of being molded in situ. It is available as a powdered polymer that rapidly hardens into solid form after being mixed with a liquid catalyst (monomer). While still puttylike, the mixture can be placed directly into the exposed defect and molded into the desired shape (Fig. 68–31). Upon hardening, it often becomes firmly attached to the bony crevasses so that final shaping can be accomplished with a power tool. These alloplastic materials are most applicable for reconstruction of the glabellar, supraorbital, and infraorbital areas.[7]

REFERENCES

1. Baker, S. P., and Schultz, R. C.: Recurrent problems in emergency room management of maxillofacial injuries. Clin. Plast. Surg., 2:65, 1975.
2. Le Fort, R.: Experimental Study of Fractures of the Jaw. Rev. Chir. Paris, 479, 1901. Trans. by P. Tessier: Plast. Reconstr. Surg., 50:600, 1972.
3. Schultz, R. C.: Facial injuries from automobile accidents: A study of 400 consecutive cases. Plast. Reconstr. Surg., 40:415, 1967.
4. Schultz, R. C.: One thousand consecutive cases of major facial injury. Rev. Surg., 27:394, 1970.
5. Schultz, R. C.: The changing character and management of soft tissue windshield injuries. J. Trauma, 12:1, 1972.
6. Schultz, R. C.: Frontal sinus and supraorbital fractures from vehicular accidents. Clin. Plast. Surg., 2:93, 1975.
7. Schultz, R. C.: Facial Injuries. 2nd Ed. Chicago, Year Book Medical Publishers, 1977.
8. Schultz, R. C., and De Villers, Y. T.: Nasal fractures. J. Trauma, 15:319, 1975.

69

SCALP INJURIES AND THEIR MANAGEMENT

The scalp is a specialized structure that nourishes and protects the cranium; it is also the most frequently injured part of the body. It is so vulnerable to injury because of its location over the hard, nongiving skull. Indeed, the 1961 automobile crash research project of Cornell University revealed that in the 5959 automobile accidents in the United States, 72 per cent of the people involved had injuries of the head, these wounds varying from simple to complex. In view of the frequency of head injuries, and with the implications associated with scalp injuries, knowledge of proper management is important.

HISTORICAL BACKGROUND

Both minor and major scalp injuries are or have the potential to be a threat to the victim. Historically, untreated wounds of the scalp such as occurred in Biblical times and in scalpings by the American Indian usually resulted in death from blood loss or, later, from local infection and sepsis. With continuing involvement and experience in war, the care of the scalp injury has improved. Using wartime experience, Cushing upgraded the care of scalp injuries by teaching that a scalp wound must be considered a compound injury and it should be *cleansed, explored, debrided,* and *closed*.[2,3,5-7] If these guidelines are utilized, the complications of scalp injuries can be substantially reduced.

ANATOMY OF THE SCALP

The scalp is made up of five layers: the skin, dense connective tissue, the galea aponeurotica, loose connective tissue, and the pericranium (Fig. 69–1).[1,8]

Skin

This structure consists of epidermis and dermis and contains hair, sebaceous glands and sweat glands.

Connective Tissue

This layer lies between the skin and the epicranial muscles and aponeurosis. It contains the nerves and major vessels of the scalp. These vessels anastomose within this connective tissue layer.

When cut, the vessels in this compact layer do not retract and may continue to bleed. Hemostasis is most readily obtained by applying pressure against the bone. Bleeding vessels are difficult to control. One method of checking vigorous scalp bleeding, if pressure is not possible, is to grasp the galea with hemostats and lay it back, thus everting the edges. This maneuver compresses the vessels very effectively. Suturing with a running through-and-through stitch is also an effective hemostatic manuever.

W. M. COCKE, JR.

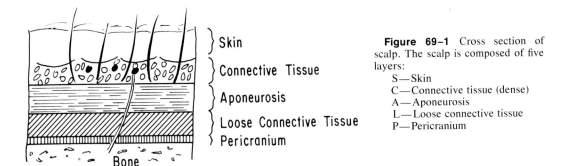

} Skin

} Connective Tissue

} Aponeurosis

} Loose Connective Tissue

} Pericranium

Bone

Figure 69–1 Cross section of scalp. The scalp is composed of five layers:
　　S—Skin
　　C—Connective tissue (dense)
　　A—Aponeurosis
　　L—Loose connective tissue
　　P—Pericranium

Aponeurosis (Galea)

The galea aponeurotica is a flat tendinous structure that extends between the occipitalis and frontalis muscles to its insertion at the superior nuchal line posteriorly and the zygomatic arch, root of the nose, and eyelids anteriorly. When the scalp is cut, this layer spreads and a gaping wound results. The operative handling of this tissue is difficult because the galea is nonelastic. The surgeon does not have the leeway that he does with other tissues such as skin, and this factor must be taken into consideration when designing flaps of the scalp. Failure to suture the galea in compound scalp wounds can lead to the formation of "cerebral fungus," which is actually necrotic, infected brain tissue that protrudes from the wound. Laterally, the temporal muscle is covered with a dense fascia (temporal fascia), which, when wounds in this area are probed, may give the feel of bone and a false impression of a skull fracture.

Loose Connective Tissue

The loose areolar layer can be seen by elevating the scalp. It lies beneath the galea and is an excellent plane for dissection and elevation of skin flaps. There are emissary veins in this layer through which bacteria and septic emboli can pass into the dural sinuses via the suture lines. Blood from intracranial hemorrhage can escape into this layer, as can cerebrospinal fluid.

Pericranium

This layer is similar to periosteum and is loosely attached to the surface of the skull. It blends with the periosteum of the internal portion of the skull and the outer layer of the dura. Bleeding in this layer can strip it up, but the hematoma will not extend past the suture lines. For this reason, bleeding in the pericranium will take the shape of the bone, and this characteristic can be helpful in diagnosis.

The surgeon can reflect the pericranium if necessary without jeopardizing the blood supply to the bone. The skull gets its blood supply from the vessels that enter at the muscle attachments and also from the inner layer of the periosteum.

Nerve Supply

The sensory supply to the scalp arises from the first division of the fifth cranial nerve and the second cervical nerve (Fig. 69–2). The former supplies the anterior portion of the forehead, and the latter supplies the posterior portion. The great auricular nerve supplies the area on the lateral side of the scalp and the region of the ear. The zygomaticotemporal branch of the maxillary division of the fifth cranial nerve supplies sensation to the temporal portion. They can be blocked by local anesthesia when exploration and repair of a scalp wound are indicated.

Blood Supply

An abundance of blood is supplied to the scalp by the occipital, superficial temporal, and postauricular arteries (Fig. 69–3). These vessels are terminal branches of the external carotid artery and form anastomoses with the supraorbital vessels, which arise from the internal carotid system. There are numerous communications, and these communications result in the scalp

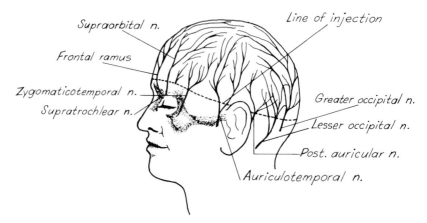

Figure 69–2   Nerve supply to scalp. Dotted line shows appropriate level for injection of local anesthetic to block nerve.

having an extremely rich blood supply. This ample anastomatic system is of practical importance in the planning of skin flaps and in reconstructive procedures following injury to the scalp. Incisions in the scalp can be made with confidence because the collateral circulation assures an adequate blood supply.[4]

The veins follow the arteries and they too provide communication between the scalp and the intracranial cavity. From a practical standpoint, veins draining the pterygoid plexus connect with the veins draining the scalp. If there is infection present, there is the possibility that this infected drainage may reach the dural sinuses, where it can cause meningitis and brain abscess.

Lymphatic Drainage

The scalp itself does not have any lymph nodes, and the lymph drainage of the scalp is to parotid, preauricular, and postauricular nodes anteriorly and laterally, and into the occipital deep jugular and spinal accessory nodes from its posterior aspect.

EVALUATION OF THE INJURED PATIENT

The same rules apply for the evaluation of a scalp injury as for any other injury or disease. An adequate history must be taken. If the patient is unconscious, the his-

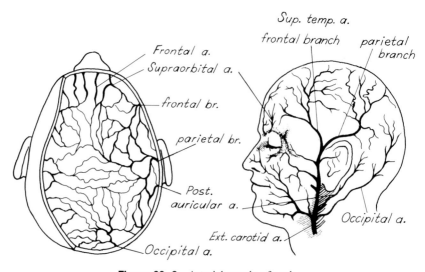

Figure 69–3   Arterial supply of scalp.

tory can be obtained from accompanying relatives or friends. The history should contain the full details of the mechanism of injury so that the physician may be aware of possible associated injuries such as a long bone fracture or a ruptured spleen. The history also should give a detailed account of the patient's medical condition.

After the history has been taken, a thorough examination is undertaken. The examination should consist of "looking before feeling." It is of vital importance to examine the whole patient so as not to overlook an associated injury.

Scalp injuries are usually obvious. They can result from falls, falling objects, vehicular or home or industrial accidents, cutting or avulsion or penetrating wounds, thermal or electrical or radiation burns, and animal and human bites. Blood loss may be rapid. Bleeding can be controlled by compression or by grasping the galea with hemostats and everting the edges. This maneuver compresses the vessels. Clips can be applied, and suturing of the scalp provides definitive hemostasis. Skull fractures and depressions may be detected by palpation.

Special studies should be added to the physical evaluation as needed. Such studies are radiography, computed tomography, and arteriography.

CLASSIFICATION AND MANAGEMENT OF INJURIES

Scalp Injuries

Contusions

Any injury causing contusion of the scalp should alert the surgeon to the possibility of possible intracranial injury. If seroma and hematoma are present, and if there is evidence of impending skin necrosis, evacuation may be indicated.

Lacerations

Scalp lacerations should be thoroughly cleansed, irrigated, and explored. The nonviable tissue is debrided, and the wound is closed (Fig. 69–4). The scalp is most easily closed with large nonabsorbable sutures that penetrate all layers of skin to galea. These sutures may be either interrupted or continuous.[11] They serve also to arrest the blood loss by accurately opposing the cut surfaces to one another and thus compressing the ends of the bleeding vessels. If there is a more complicated injury with tissue loss, it may be necessary to close the wound by either a split skin graft or a skin flap. The typical slicing forehead laceration usually creates a posteriorly based flap,

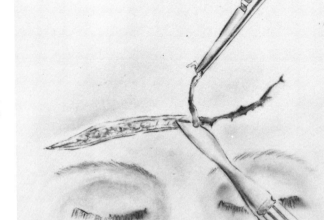

Figure 69–4 Technique of sharpening and debriding the edges of a jagged laceration.

which often heals in a "trap door" deformity caused by accumulating edema fluid (Fig. 69–5*A*). Proper debridement of the skin edges to maintain right angles, followed by postoperative application of pressure dressings, helps to prevent the formation of this chronic edema and trap door scarring (Fig. 69–5*B*). Once the general condition of the patient has been stabilized the wound is infiltrated with a local anesthetic with epinephrine. The irregular and necrotic edges are debrided with a scalpel. The wound is copiously irrigated, and all foreign materials and debris are removed. The wound is then closed in layers with fine absorbable sutures for the galea and through-and-through 4-0 nylon sutures for the soft tissue. A small drain can be placed at the point of dependency, and a pressure dressing is applied. In many avulsion injuries with no tissue loss, the straight line laceration can be broken up by inserting a small V-to-Y type of closure (Fig. 69–6). Closure of a wound of the frontal portion of the scalp will yield a better result if small 6-0 sutures are used and are removed in three to four days, and the wound is supported with adhesive strips. If scarring develops, a secondary revision can be done 6 to 12 months later under more elective conditions, which can improve the scar in many patients.

Soft-Tissue Avulsion

Soft-tissue losses usually are secondary to automobile accidents; many times the injury is not as severe as it looks. By lining up the tissues that are present and viable, one can assess the damage (Fig. 69–7). Soft tissue that appears to be absent may actually not be absent but only displaced (Fig. 69–8). One has simply to restore the tissue to its normal position and hold or suture it in place. If tissue has been lost, it has to be replaced before proper closure can be accomplished (Fig. 69–9). Closure of areas of tissue loss can be accomplished by skin grafts or flaps. An example of this maneuver would be placement of a full-thickness skin graft to replace lost skin. When brain tissue or bare bone is exposed, a skin flap will be needed for safe closure. Such a flap can be designed and trimmed over the defect. A free split graft is then used to cover the flap donor site (Fig. 69–10).

Total Avulsion of the Scalp

Scalp avulsion came into prominence as a problem during World War II, when women who worked in factories had their hair caught in rotating machinery (Figs. 69–11 and 69–12). These injuries may be accompanied by massive blood loss and shock requiring resuscitative measures.

Text continued on page 2308

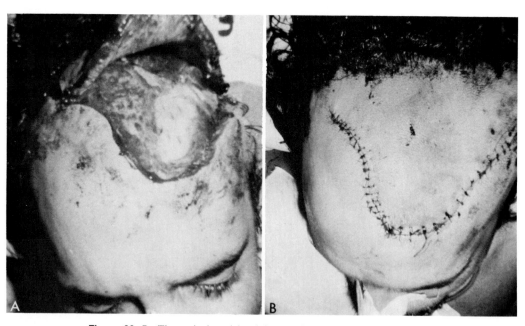

Figure 69–5   The typical avulsion injury to the scalp without tissue loss.

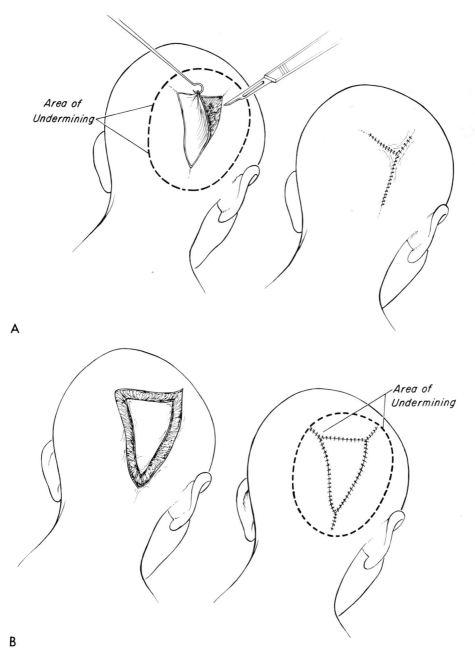

Figure 69–6 *A.* Technique of undermining to gain tissue for closure. *B.* Method of closure of soft-tissue avulsion by undermining edges and closing center with split-thickness skin graft.

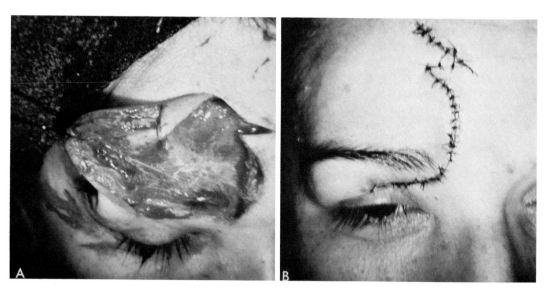

Figure 69–7 *A.* Forehead portion of the scalp that has been avulsed from its attachment. *B.* Use of the Z-plasty to break up a vertical laceration that goes perpendicular to the natural skin creases. A part of the injury is placed horizontally in the natural skin crease, thus camouflaging it.

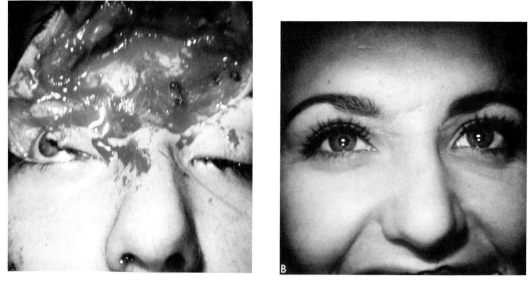

Figure 69–8 *A.* Wound appeared to be an avulsion with partial loss of soft tissue. *B.* Careful reapproximation revealed all tissues to be present.

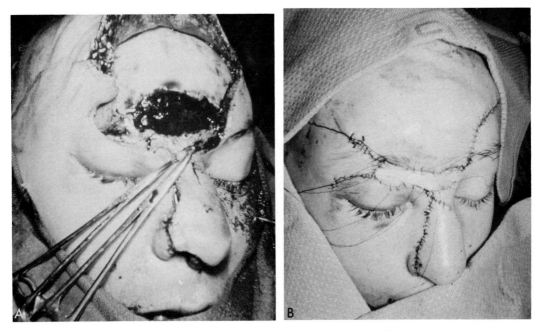

Figure 69–9   *A.* Soft-tissue injury with loss of portion of frontal scalp and soft tissue. *B.* Lost soft tissue was replaced with similar tissue by a full-thickness skin graft from behind the ear.

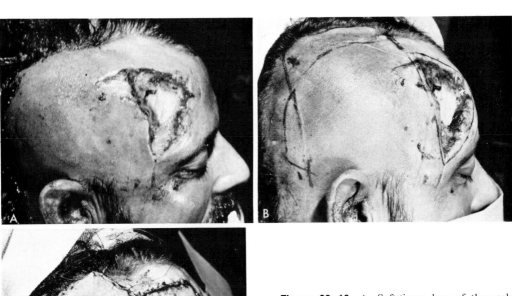

Figure 69–10   *A.* Soft-tissue loss of the scalp. Bare bone has been exposed, and a rotational flap is required for closure. *B.* Outline of rotational flap to cover avulsed area. Note outline of edges of avulsed area to be cleanly incised. *C.* The scalp flap has been rotated forward. Donor area has been covered with a split-thickness graft.

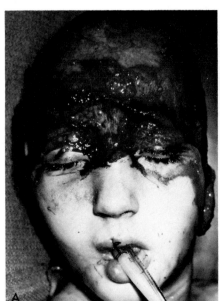

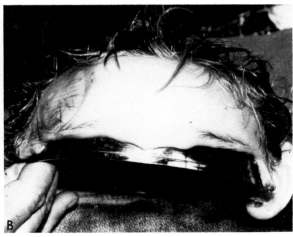

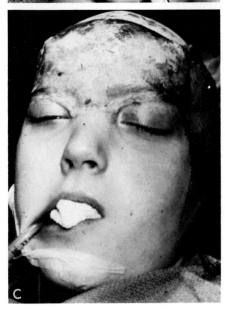

Figure 69–11 *A*. Total avulsion of the scalp by rotary drive of a machine. *B*. Specimen of avulsed scalp, which should be placed in an iced plastic bag for transfer to operative treatment center. *C*. Early results of treatment with split-thickness graft. Avulsed scalp was too traumatized to replace by microvascular technique.

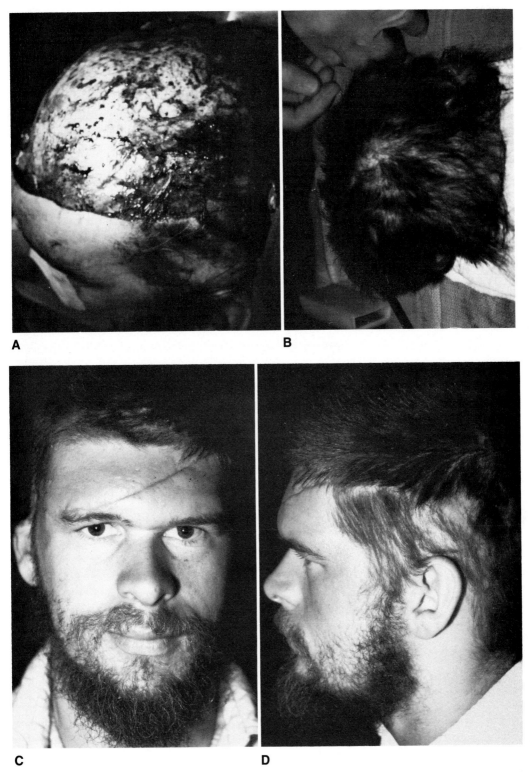

Figure 69–12 *A.* Scalp avulsed, leaving denuded skull. *B.* Avulsed portion of scalp. *C.* Anterior view after replacement of avulsed scalp and micro-operative repair of vascular supply. Note suture line running diagonally across forehead and along right temple area. *D.* Lateral view after replacement of avulsed scalp. (From Buncke, H. J., Rose, E. H., Brownstein, M. J., and Chater, N. L.: Successful replantation of two avulsed scalps by microvascular anastomoses. Plast. Reconstr. Surg., *61*:666–672, 1978. Reprinted by permission.)

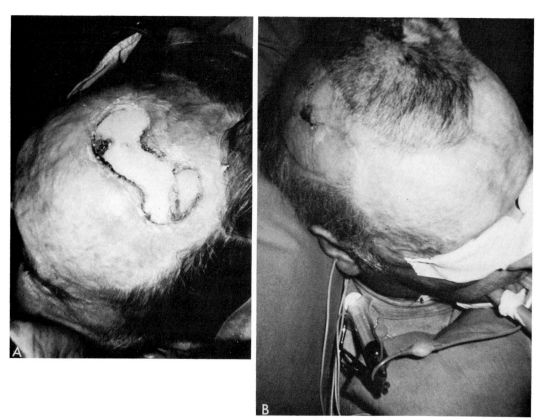

Figure 69–13 *A.* Thermal burn of the scalp that destroyed the full thickness of the tissue in the central portion. Because bare bone was exposed, closure was accomplished by removing the dead cortical bone to allow granulating buds to grow from the marrow space. *B.* Application of a split-thickness skin graft. Because of good tissue at the periphery of this wound, a rotation scalp flap was accomplished to cover the bare bone and also to move hair into the hairless area. A split-thickness skin graft was then used to cover the flap donor area and was applied directly to the temporalis fascia.

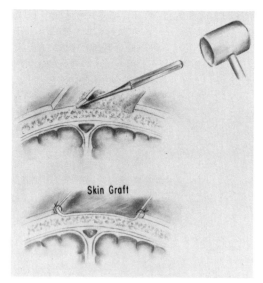

Figure 69–14 Removal of necrotic outer table to expose the viable marrow space between the outer and inner tables. Granulating buds will form from the blood vessels present here, and this tissue will then support a split-thickness skin graft.

The scalp is usually avulsed through the loose areolar tissue that lies between the galea aponeurotica and the pericranium. The avulsed scalp is too thick to "take" as a free graft. With modern microvascular operative techniques, however, scalp tissue such as this, if not too badly damaged, can be replaced, and the small vessels can be anastomosed under microscopic magnification. If the pericranium is intact, it can be grafted; if there is no pericranium present, closure is more difficult. One technique is to drill holes through the outer table or to remove the outer table, enabling granulations to grow. A split skin graft will then take. Transfer of a flap from a distant site on a carrier such as the wrist can be considered to close the defect.

Direct microvascular anastomosis and replantation of the avulsed scalp has been successfully accomplished (see Fig. 69–12).[10] In such cases the patient is at once fully examined for other injuries. Immedi-

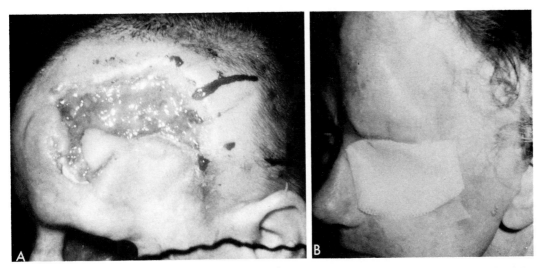

Figure 69–15 *A.* Irradiation necrosis of left side of forehead. *B.* A flap was moved from the right side of the forehead to cover the defect over the left. A skin graft was then placed over the flap donor site.

Figure 69–16 Traditional method of moving blocks of tissue to a distant area. In total avulsion or severe injuries of the scalp, including bony loss, a flap can be moved on the arm from the lower abdomen to the scalp and laid in position. This procedure takes multiple stages and six to eight weeks to accomplish. With newer microvascular surgical techniques a similar block of tissue can be moved from the groin and anastomosed directly to the remaining recipient arteries and veins under magnification.

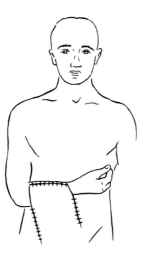
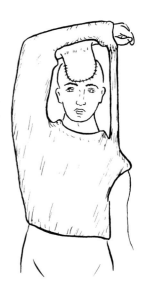

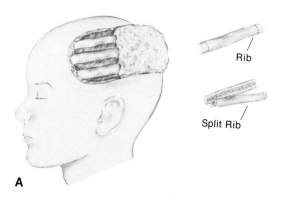

A

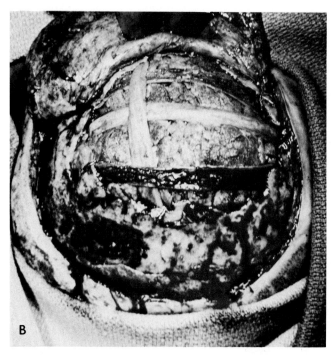

B

Figure 69-17 *A.* Use of split ribs to fill in a defect created following bony loss secondary to trauma or tumor surgery. *B.* Ribs are taken and split longitudinally and laid in position with bone-to-bone continuity, and this is then covered with a local pedicle flap that has been elevated.

ate attention is given to maintaining the airway. Hemorrhage should be controlled with pressure dressings, but bleeding points should not be clamped, as this may damage vessels vital for microvascular anastamoses and subsequent viability of the avulsed scalp. A careful history is taken, which may reveal contraindications to a lengthy operative procedure—such as pulmonary disease, cardiac disease, peripheral vascular disease, neoplasia, or advanced diabetes. The patient is then given suitable analgesia, antibiotics, and antitetanus prophylaxis, but is allowed nothing by mouth.

For transportation to a replantation center the avulsed scalp is cleaned with normal saline, wrapped in damp sterile gauze, and covered with a sterile towel. The specimen is put into a watertight plastic bag, which is then placed in an ice chest filled with crushed ice. It is important not to freeze the part by placing it in dry ice or to pickle it by placing it in formaldehyde.

At the replantation center the avulsed scalp is reconnected to the patient by microvascular anastamoses, which in this region almost always requires a reversed vein graft to provide arterial continuity.

Thermal and Irradiation Injuries

The scalp and forehead are frequently the sites of thermal and electrical burns, and the treatment for these follows the same general rules for burns in other regions of the body. Because of the numerous epithelium-lined hair follicles, regeneration of scalp skin sometimes will occur even when the scalp appears to have suffered a full-thickness burn. When it is clear that the burn actually is full-thickness, early debridement and skin grafting or skin flap closure should be considered (Fig. 69–13). An acceptable alternative is to remove the outer table or penetrate it with drill holes or osteotomes to allow granulations to form, and to follow this procedure with split-thickness skin grafting (Fig. 69–14).

Radiation injuries of the scalp can be quite serious. This problem occurs less frequently than formerly because of the improvements in radiation technique, but it does occur. The treatment is to excise the radionecrotic tissue and repair the defect with a skin flap from adjacent healthy tissue (Fig. 69–15). A split-thickness skin graft can be placed on the flap donor site. A flap

may have to be transferred to the scalp from a distant source. This transference can be done by attaching an abdominal skin flap to the arm and "carrying" it up to the head (Fig. 69–16). The use of the greater omentum as a free flap with direct microvascular anastomoses has been reported.[9]

Skull Defects

Reconstruction of a defect left in the skull following trauma can be done with autogenous bone from the ilium, sternum, or rib, or with one of the alloplastic materials (silicone, acrylic).[12] In these procedures the surgeon has to be both very careful and sure that he has soft-tissue coverage.

In general, the author believes that pa-

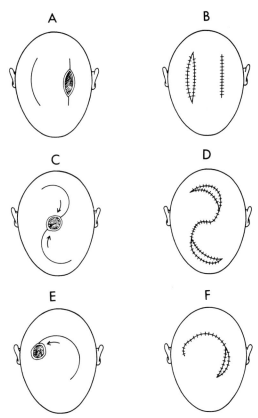

Figure 69–18 Different designs of flaps that can be used to cover defects of the scalp. *A.* Relaxing incision at distant site. *B.* A bipedicle or bucket-handle flap. A skin graft is used to cover the flap donor site. *C* and *D.* Two transposition flaps have been shifted to cover a central defect. Split-thickness grafts are used to cover donor sites. *E* and *F.* Simple rotational-type flap. This type is a layer flap and can be shifted and moved easily.

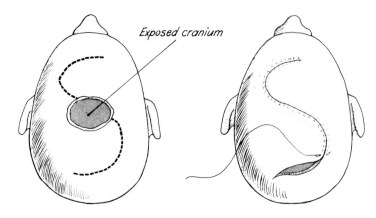

Figure 69–19 Two transposition scalp flaps turned to cover a scalp defect.

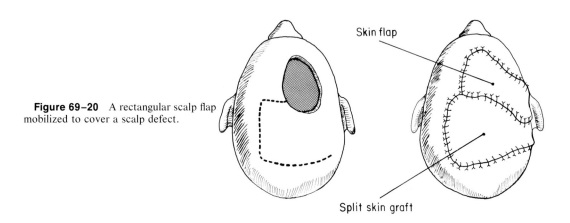

Figure 69–20 A rectangular scalp flap mobilized to cover a scalp defect.

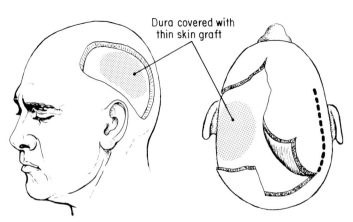

Figure 69–21 A flap based on the frontal scalp blood supply that will be used to cover defect with exposed brain or bone. A large flap is preferable to a small one.

tient's own tissue (autogenous bone graft) is preferable to the alloplastic materials (Fig. 69–17).

There are many options for the design of skin flaps required for closure of scalp defects. In general, the larger the flap, the safer is the blood supply (Fig. 69–18). Because the scalp blood supply is quite abundant, however, most scalp flaps will remain viable and be successful unless there are abnormal circumstances such as scars or irradiation injury (Figs. 69–19, 69–20, and 69–21).

REFERENCES

1. Anson, B. J., and McVay, C. B.: Surgical Anatomy. Philadelphia, W. B. Saunders Co., 1971, pp. 3–51.
2. Cloward, R. G.: Simple suture closure of scalp. Neurosurg., *21*:142, 1964.
3. Coates, J. B., and Meirowsky, A. M.: Neurological Surgery of Trauma. Washington, D.C., U.S. Government Printing Office, 1965, p. 75.
4. Corso, P. S.: Variations of the arterial, venous and capillary circulation of the soft tissues of the head by the methylmethacrylate injection technique and application to the construction flaps and pedicles. Plast. Reconstr. Surg., *27*:160, 1961.
5. Cushing, H. C.: A study of a series of wounds involving the brain and its enveloping structures. Brit. J. Surg., *5*:555, 1918.
6. Dingman, R. O., and Fairbanks, G. R.: Injuries to the scalp. *In* Youmans, J. R., ed.: Neurological Surgery. Philadelphia, W. B. Saunders, Co., 1973, pp. 906–921.
7. Dingman, R. O., and Johnson, H.: Surgery of the scalp. Surg. Clin. Amer., *57*:1011, 1977.
8. DuPlessis, D. J.: A Synopsis of Surgical Anatomy, 11th Ed. Bristol, England, John Wright & Sons, Ltd., 1975.
9. Ikuta, Y.: Autotransplant of omentum to cover large denudation of the scalp. Plast. Reconstr. Surg. *55*:490, 1975.
10. Okada, T., and Tsukada, S.: Past and present treatment of complete scalp avulsion. Chir. Plast. *4*:21, 1977.
11. Otenasek, R. J., and Waslker, A. E.: The use of adhesive tapes for closure of scalp and skin. J. Neurosurg., *20*:812, 1963.
12. Rees, T. D., and Coburn, R. J.: Reconstruction of the scalp, forehead, and calvaria. *In* Grabb, W. C., and Smith, J. W., eds.: Plastic Surgery: A Concise Guide to Clinical Practice. Boston, Little, Brown, & Co., 1973.

70

TRAUMA TO CAROTID ARTERIES

The first report of carotid occlusion due to a nonpenetrating injury was made by Verneil in 1872.[21] It has been estimated that post-traumatic internal carotid artery occlusion follows 0.2 per cent of head injuries.[6] Reports are becoming increasingly frequent, however, giving evidence of the progressive knowledge and awareness of physicians regarding this uncommon condition. Although traumatic occlusion of the carotid artery has been reported many times, its diagnosis before the onset of irreversible brain damage remains a challenge, since many patients have other injuries that may mask the arterial injuries.

Penetrating wounds leading to carotid artery thrombosis are seen most frequently after battle injuries.[8] As expected, a vascular injury is more frequently associated with penetrating wounds than with blunt trauma, although it is not necessary for the artery to be penetrated to produce a thrombosis or partial occlusion. A high-velocity missile may induce thrombosis in the internal carotid artery, although the missile passes some distance from the vessel.[3] Because signs of penetrating wounds of the neck region make the surgeon aware of and concerned with the nearby vessels, injuries from these penetrating-type wounds are not as easily overlooked as similar injuries from blunt trauma to the cervical area.

PATHOLOGICAL PHYSIOLOGY

The most common injury to the carotid artery by blunt trauma is an intimal tear of the arterial wall. One early report placed the frequency of this type of injury at 62 per cent; it may, however, be higher.[22] Other changes associated with injuries of the carotid artery that can promote the development of either thrombosis or partial occlusion include spasm, contusion, intramural hematoma, mural fibrosis, aneurysmal dilatation, and arteriovenous fistula formation.[2,7,22] In older patients with associated atheromatous disease, there may be a fracture of an atheromatous plaque, which usually is at the carotid bifurcation. In younger patients, the arterial injury may occur anywhere along the course of the common carotid or internal carotid artery; it is, however, most common in the internal carotid artery about 1 to 3 cm above the bifurcation. There are rare reports of a similar injury of the vertebral artery in the region of the junction of the atlas and axis where the artery is subject to more strain from bony injury and direct compression.[4,15]

Mechanisms of the intimal tear have been reviewed extensively. There are four basic types of injury that can result in the damage to the vessels.[2,9,20] These are: (1) A direct blow to the anterior cervical region that results in direct trauma to the carotid artery. There is a high incidence of mandibular fractures associated with this type of injury. Also, it is the mechanism of injury in approximately half the patients with atherosclerotic disease who have a fracture of the plaque and resulting stenosis or occlusion. (2) Hyperextension and contralateral rotation of the head from a blow to the side of the head that causes a stretch injury to the carotid artery across the lateral masses of

J. R. YOUMANS AND T. J. MIMS, JR.

the first or second cervical vertebra or the transverse process of the third vertebra. This stretch results in rupture of the intima and media but spares the more elastic adventitial layer. Because of tortuous elongation of the vessel in older patients, this age group usually is spared. (3) Blunt intraoral trauma, which can injure the artery where it lies close to the surface of the tonsillar fossa. (4) Injuries resulting in basilar skull fractures, which may cause thrombosis of the intrapetrous portion of the internal carotid artery and retrograde proximal thrombosis. Other infrequent causes that have been reported include an abnormal styloid process and pharyngeal inflammation resulting in periarterial adhesions and tethering.

In the cervical portion, the principal strength of the artery is in the adventitial elastic tissues. Blunt contusion and stretching of the artery tend to lacerate the intima and media, while the adventitia is preserved.[16] Since there is a natural cleavage plane between the intimal and medial layers, the intimal layer can easily be dissected and elevated. At this stage complete thrombosis is not as common as partial occlusion. The intimal elevation can, however, precede a more drastic arterial dissection, spasm, and other entities.[9] The intimal tear usually is partial, although it can be completely circumferential and still result in only a stenotic lesion.[12] Rupture of the vaso vasorum has also been implicated in the formation of the intimal flap and dissection.[5]

SYMPTOMS AND CLINICAL COURSE

The majority of patients who develop traumatic carotid occlusion present with a history of head injury rather than neck injury. Approximately one third have a history of neck injury, and half have evidence of trauma to the neck on examination. Most of these, however, have only an innocent-appearing bruise or abrasion. Only 6 per cent in one large series were admitted with a diagnosis of carotid artery injury.[22] Vehicle accidents are the most common cause of carotid occlusion due to nonpenetrating injury, but a significant number of cases have resulted from direct or indirect cervical trauma secondary to fighting or brawling.

The penetrating wounds that produce thrombosis of the carotid arteries usually are missile wounds.

Because of the different pathological entities that may cause or be associated with the carotid injury, the symptoms may vary widely. Stenosis or total occlusion may occur, the effects of each being influenced by the intracranial collateral circulation. Cerebral embolization may further complicate the clinical picture. Also, a few patients have transient ischemic attacks.[1,11,18]

Carotid artery injuries should be suspected in patients with blunt trauma to the neck or lower facial region resulting in a hematoma of the anterior triangle of the neck, a Horner syndrome, transient ischemic attacks, jaw fractures or other intraoral damage, shoulder fractures, evidence of chest trauma, basilar skull fractures, and cervical fractures.[9,14] Palpation of a strong carotid pulse or absence of a bruit is not sufficient evidence that injury to the carotid artery has not occurred.

The usual evolution of the signs and symptoms is slower than might be expected with a thrombosis of a major vessel due to acute trauma. The thrombotic occlusion or stenosis is a gradual process and it usually progresses over a period of several hours. Less than 10 per cent of the patients have obvious deficits within the first hour after injury. The usual time of onset of symptoms is 8 to 10 hours following the trauma. A significant number of patients, 17 per cent, do not develop signs for more than 24 hours.[22] Because of this delay in the onset of symptoms, an incorrect diagnosis of intracranial hematoma is often made. In many cases, a clue to the correct diagnosis is the marked hemiparesis combined with alert mental status.[9,15,20] A markedly lowered level of consciousness is an ominous sign, as the majority of patients who have it progress to coma and death.

Nearly all the patients in whom a traumatic occlusion of the carotid artery has been diagnosed have had hemiparesis or hemiplegia. Most also have a unilateral sensory disturbance, and many have visual disturbances. Aphasia is also present when the involved carotid artery supplies the dominant hemisphere. Seizures occur in about 15 per cent of the cases. Severe personality derangements have been noted rarely.[5] Because of the common presentation with cerebral contusion or other intracranial lesions, the symptoms due to the vascular injury are often incorrectly attributed to the concomitant head injury.

Rarely patients may present with vascular disease and a history of cervical injury many months or years prior to the onset of their difficulties.[2] The prolonged time of the course may also give sufficient time for formation of delayed aneurysmal dilatation or formation of an arteriovenous fistula.[18] Traumatic cervical carotid aneurysms are rare, however, because of the strength of the adventitia. Arteriovenous fistula formation occurs three times as commonly as a result of penetrating injuries as it does of blunt injuries.[13] It should be emphasized that the hallmark of blunt traumatic vascular injury is a time delay from the time of injury to the initial presentation of symptoms.

DIAGNOSIS

Modern medical centers rely on computed tomography to evaluate patients with head injuries. If the CT scan does not explain the patient's neurological findings, it should be followed by an arteriogram, which gives the definitive diagnosis of vascular injury (Fig. 70–1). Further, the presence of a head injury with or without neck injury followed by the development of lateralized neurological signs several hours later should arouse the suspicion of a traumatic carotid occlusion.

TREATMENT

In the past, a variety of treatments including anticoagulation, antispasmodic drugs, cervical sympathectomy, and trapping of the involved areas have been tried. The outcome generally was unsatisfactory.[17]

The most important considerations in deciding the treatment are the time elapsed since the onset of symptoms, the type of pathological change, and the degree of the neurological deficit. If a total thrombosis and a marked neurological deficit have been present for many hours, an endarterectomy is not warranted. If the neurological impairment and the carotid narrowing are only minimal, then it may be possible to avoid an operation. If the diagnosis is made within 6 to 12 hours after injury in patients falling

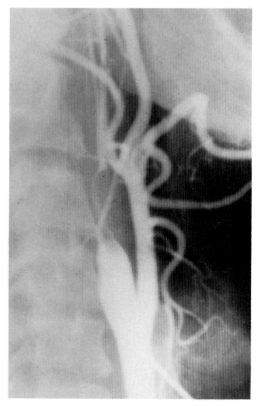

Figure 70–1 Preoperative angiogram showing nearly total occlusion of internal carotid artery. (From Yamada, S., Kindt, G. W., and Youmans, J. R.: Carotid artery occlusion due to nonpenetrating injury. J. Trauma, 7:333–342, 1967. Reprinted by permission.)

between these extremes, then an endarterectomy and removal of intraluminal clots are indicated (Fig. 70–2).

When the patient has cerebral edema from ischemia or infarction, intracranial pressure monitoring is helpful in deciding on other diagnostic and therapeutic measures. The value of extracranial-intracranial anastomosis procedures in the management of traumatic carotid occlusion is not well defined; it does appear to have a role, however.[1] Other methods of treatment such as use of thrombolysin are controversial and probably not worthwhile.[9]

PROGNOSIS

In the past, lack of appreciation of the course of the disease and delay in diagnosis have resulted in the poor outcome of patients with this lesion. Often valuable time has been lost while the patient with head injuries was observed without the possible

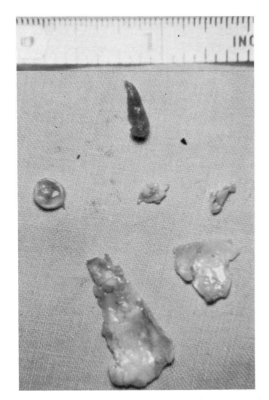

Figure 70-2 Atheroma and thrombus removed during endarterectomy. The thrombus, which partially occluded the internal carotid artery, is located at the top of the picture. (From Yamada, S., Kindt, G. W., and Youmans, J. R.: Carotid artery occlusion due to nonpenetrating injury. J. Trauma, 7:333–342, 1967. Reprinted by permission.)

cervical vascular injury being considered. The mortality rate has been 40 per cent, and the majority of the survivors have had a severe neurological deficit.[22] A high index of suspicion by neurological surgeons and earlier diagnosis should bring higher survival rates of patients with fewer neurological deficits.

REFERENCES

1. Cobb, C. A., and Keller, T.: Microsurgical vascular anastomosis for traumatic middle cerebral artery occlusion. J. Trauma, 18:738–741, 1978.
2. Crissey, M. M., and Bernstein, E. F.: Delayed presentation of carotid intimal tear following blunt craniocervical trauma. Surgery, 75:543–549, 1974.
3. Ecker, A. D.: Spasm of the internal carotid artery. J. Neurosurg., 2:479–84, 1945.
4. Fletcher, R., Woodward, J., Royle, J., and Buxton, B.: Cerebral embolism following blunt extracranial vascular trauma: A report of two cases. Aust, N. Z. J. Surg., 44:269–272, 1974.
5. Friedenberg, M. J., Lake, P., and Landau, S.: Bilateral incomplete traumatic occlusions of internal carotid arteries. Amer. J. Roentgen., 118:546–549, 1973.
6. Gleave, J. R. W.: Thrombosis of the carotid artery in the neck in association with head injury. Third International Congress of Neurological Surgery: Excerpta Medica. International Congress Series 110. Amsterdam, Excerpta Medica, 1966, pp. 200–206.
7. Gurdjian, E. S., Audet, B., Sibayan, R. W., and Thomas, L. M.: Spasm of the extracranial internal carotid artery resulting from blunt trauma demonstrated by angiograph. J. Neurosurg., 35:742–747, 1971.
8. Hughes, J. T., and Brownell, B.: Traumatic thrombosis of the internal carotid artery in the neck. J. Neurol. Neurosurg. Psychiat., 31:307–314, 1968.
9. Kaufman, H. H., Lind, T. A., and Clark, D. S.: Nonpenetrating trauma to the carotid artery with secondary thrombosis and embolism: Treatment by thrombolysin. Acta Neurochir. (Wein), 37:219–244, 1977.
10. Kusunoki, T., Rowed, D. W., Tator, C. H., and Lougheed, W. M.: Thromboendarterectomy for total occlusion of the internal carotid artery: A reappraisal of risks, success rate and potential benefits. Stroke, 9:34–38, 1978.
11. Loar, C. R., Chadduck, W. M., Nugent, G. R.: Traumatic occlusion of the middle cerebral artery. J. Neurosurg., 39:753–756, 1973.
12. McGough, E. C., Helfrich, L. R., and Hughes, R. K.: Traumatic intimal prolapse of the common carotid artery. Amer. J. Surg. 123:724–725, 1972.
13. Robinson, N. A., and Flotte, C. T.: Traumatic aneurysms of the carotid arteries. Amer. Surg., 40:121–124, 1974.
14. Saletta, J. D., Folk, F. A., and Freeark, R. J.: Trauma to the neck region. Surg. Clin. N. Amer., 53:73–85, 1973.
15. Schneider, R. C., Gosch, H. H., Taren, J. A., Ferry, D. J., and Jerva, M. J.: Blood vessel trauma following head and neck injuries. Clin. Neurosurg. 19:312–354, 1972.
16. Shaw, C. M., and Alvord, E. C.: Injury of the basilar artery associated with closed head trauma. J. Neurol. Neurosurg. Psychiat., 35:247–257, 1972.
17. Silvernail, W. I., Croutcher, D. L., Byrd, B. R., and Pope, D. H.: Carotid artery injury produced by blunt neck trauma. Southern Med. J., 68:310–313, 1975.
18. Sullivan, H. G., Vines, F. S., and Becker, D. P.: Sequelae of indirect internal carotid injury. Radiology, 109:91–98, 1973.
19. Thal, E. R., Snyder, W. H., Hays, R. J., and Perry, M. O.: Management of carotid artery injuries. Surgery, 76:955–962, 1974.
20. Towne, J. B., Neis, D. D., and Smith, J. W.: Thrombosis of the internal carotid artery following blunt cervical trauma. Arch. Surg., 104:565–568, 1972.
21. Verneil, M.: Contusions multiples; délire violent; hémiplégie à droite, signes de compression cérébrale. Bull. Acad. Nat. Med. (Paris). 36:45–56, 1872.
22. Yamada, S., Kindt, G. W., and Youmans, J. R.: Carotid artery occlusion due to nonpenetrating injury. J. Trauma, 7:333–342, 1967.

71

INJURIES TO THE CERVICAL SPINE AND SPINAL CORD

The true incidence of injuries to the cervical spine for the United States per year is not clearly known. At Parkland Memorial Hospital in Dallas, about two patients a week are seen with cervical spinal fracture, dislocation, or fracture-dislocation, with and without spinal cord or nerve root injuries. There are approximately 29,000 admissions per year, so cervical injuries account for about 0.2 per cent of the total number of admissions. The vast majority of these injuries, fortunately, are trivial and require only brief or no hospitalization or operative procedures. This figure does not include another large number of patients who sustain purely ligamentous or muscular injuries. These individuals are usually treated as outpatients.

Spinal cord injury in the cervical region occurs at a rate of over 10,000 new cases per year. This figure may be too low, as it represents an annual rate of 50 per million population. Such injury is a disease of the industrial developed nations.[40] Traffic accidents are the leading cause, accounting for 30 to 50 per cent of all injuries.[25,40,60]

In a recent survey of spinal column injuries treated at the Parkland Memorial Hospital, Maravilla, Cooper, and Sklar found that, in 90 patients, 72 per cent of the injuries were due to automobile accidents, 12 per cent to personal assault, and 1 per cent to other causes.[36] In southern California, the second leading cause is water sports.[25,40,60]

Typically, this injury occurs in young adults. The average age of a patient suffering cervical spinal cord injury is in the mid-twenties, and the vast majority are male.[40]

The economics of injury to the cervical spine are staggering. When accompanied by severe neurological deficit, their cost for medical and hospital care alone is in the range of $50,000 per patient. Further, if the deficit is permanent, additional cost continues for many years. Medicine's ability to rehabilitate a quadriplegic patient to a level of independence is limited. The likelihood of returning such an individual to gainful occupation is even less. Detailed discussion of the rehabilitation of patients with spinal injuries is given in Chapter 148.

PREVENTION OF INJURY

Before the mechanics of spinal injury are dealt with, a discussion of prevention is warranted. Rarely do surgeons realize their obligation to the public to instruct in safety. At present and for the foreseeable future, quadriplegia can be treated, at best, poorly. It should, therefore, be prevented when possible. Most diving accidents are preventable, and many injuries suffered in automobile accidents can be reduced in severity by the use of seat belts or shoulder harnesses. Transportation to, and in, the hospital must be carefully done to prevent worsening of the injury. Rogers has reported that 10 per cent of quadriplegic patients become so after the accident.[52] The reasons for this appalling figure are multiple. Failure to recognize that a fracture of the cervical spine is present is the most common. All personnel dealing with accident victims must be instructed to ask about pain and soreness. If any is present, the patient must be moved and transported on a spine board. Sandbags at the sides of the head for immobilization are useless. Movement from ambulance stretcher to emergency room stretcher to x-ray table must be kept to a minimum—and done with the head immobilized. All patients who have been subjected to severe trauma should have x-rays of the neck.

The next most common cause of late onset of neurological deficit is failure to recognize that the fracture is an unstable one. The criteria for stability are discussed later. If there is any question, either because there is insufficient information available or because the surgeon is not sure, skeletal traction should be used until the issue is resolved.

MECHANISM OF INJURY

The cervical spine is particularly susceptible to injury, as it furnishes a bridge between the rigidly supported thorax and the heavy, extremely mobile head. It is therefore subjected to major stress and distortion when there is an impact. The direction of impact and the precise mechanism of injury become of some import because they dictate the type of injury the patient will sustain.

If the spine is injured in flexion, an anterior vertebral body injury is produced. If more force is applied, the posterior element, the facets, may give way, and a dislocation occurs. The spine may be injured in extension, with fracture of the posterior elements. Rotation injuries occur when axial forces produce pure compression fractures of the vertebral body. In the clinical world of the emergency room, it is obvious that many injuries to the spine are caused by combinations of those forces.

When the force is applied along the long axis of the cervical spine, a fracture without very much displacement results. The classic example of this is the bursting fracture of Cl, the Jefferson fracture.[28] This injury occurs when the individual strikes the vertex of the head, driving the occipital condyles against the ring of Cl, and it bursts. Axial forces farther down the cervical spine produce compression fracture of the vertebral body.

If a slight degree of flexion is present when compression occurs, the anterior part of the vertebral body will be compressed. If the force is severe, the disc may be thrust backward into the canal. If no flexion is present, the disc may be driven into the vertebral body, producing a burst fracture of the body (Fig. 71–1).[7]

Alternatively, with compressive forces, the intervertebral discs may herniate through the ligaments.[69] If the disc prolapses into the spinal canal, the patient usually suffers severe neurological injury. Such patients may present with an anterior cervical cord syndrome, showing loss of all spinal cord function save that of the dorsal columns.[56] The patient with anterior cord syndrome is quadriplegic and quadrianesthetic to pinprick and temperature, but retains position sense and touch as well as deep pain sensation. In most compression injuries, there is little ligamentous damage, so usually this type of injury is stable.

Flexion injury is the most common form of injury of the cervical spine. It occurs when the patient's head is bent forward at the time the force is applied. An example is the diving injury in which the head strikes the bottom and is forcibly bent forward. The range of injury in flexion accidents is very wide.[7] There may be total disruption of the entire structure of the cervical spine, i.e., bones, ligaments, muscles, joints, and spinal cord (Figs. 71–2 and 71–3). The facet joints may be dislocated and become locked in flexion injuries, or a simple chip fracture of the anterior aspect of the vertebral body may be all that occurs.

The major ligamentous injury to the cervical spine that occurs with flexion is tearing of the interspinous ligament and the posterior longitudinal ligament. The anterior longitudinal ligament remains intact. In flexion injuries, indications of instability are fractures of both anterior and posterior elements of the vertebral body, persistent widening of the distance between spinous processes, and recurrent dislocation.[72]

Extension injuries occur when the patient falls, or is in an accident, and the head is forced backward vigorously. This is an injury that results in a specific type of neurological deficit: the central cervical cord syndrome.[58] It is often seen in elderly people because of their narrowed cervical canals. This injury is characterized by rupture of the anterior longitudinal ligament at one or more joints. Should the patient have either a congenitally narrow cervical canal

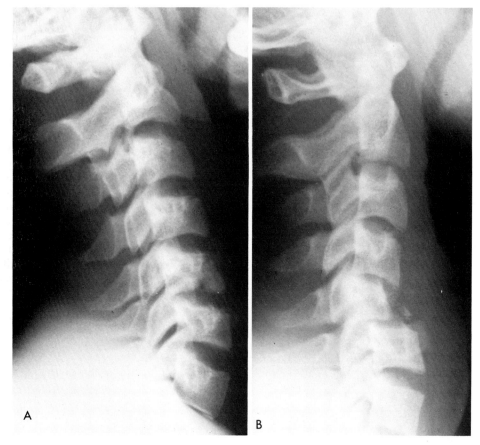

Figure 71-1 *A*. Simple "burst" fracture of C5. The body is split in a coronal plane. C6 has a chip fracture of the anterior part of the body. *B*. Fracture-dislocation of C5–C6 with burst fracture of the body of C6.

or one narrowed by cervical spondylosis, compression of the spinal cord over several segments may occur. The ligamentum flavum is infolded into the narrow canal, producing spinal cord compression over several segments. This compression may be accentuated by the laminar arches in severely narrowed canals. Fracture of the facets may occur at the level of the major ligamentous rupture, and pieces of the facet may impinge on the nerve roots in the foramina.

Compression of the cord by hyperextension produces its greatest effect on the perforating arteries of the spinal cord running to the central gray matter of the cord. The circumferential arteries running around the periphery of the cord are spared. This ischemic lesion produces the neurological picture of quadriparesis, worse in the upper extremities, worse distally in the upper extremities than proximally, and with greater motor loss than sensory loss.

Rotatory injuries occur when the application of force occurs when the head is turned or when the force produces head rotation. A blow to the jaw is a common example. Rotatory injuries produce disruption of the facet joint on the side of rotation (cf. Fig. 71-3).

A type of injury unique to the cervical spine is the acceleration-deceleration injury. The victim is seated in a car that is stopped and is struck from behind. His head oscillates between an extreme extension and an extreme flexion. This type of injury is highly regarded by litigious individuals, yet it does have an anatomical basis. There is damage to the anterior supporting muscles, the longus colli, and the lateral mass of the vertebral body, and to the posterior elements less often.[15]

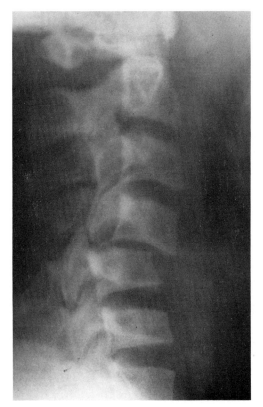

Figure 71-2 Fracture-dislocation of the cervical spine at C4–C5: a flexion injury.

DIAGNOSIS

Early recognition of a cervical spine or cervical cord injury is of paramount importance. For instance, the person who has dived into a swimming pool should not be pulled out of the swimming pool violently but should be supported in the water until professional help arrives. Individuals involved in automobile accidents or falls should be carefully questioned about the presence of paralysis, numbness, paresthesias, or neck pain before they are moved. Ambulance drivers should be thoroughly instructed in recognition of spinal column injuries. All ambulances should be equipped with spinal boards, and a patient who has paralysis, paresthesias, or cervical pain, should be transported on a back board with his head rigidly fixed to it by straps. When admitted to the emergency room, such a patient should not be taken from the back board until a cervical x-ray has been obtained and a neurological baseline established.

Individuals who are unconscious may have cervical spine injuries. In the review of head injuries at Parkland Memorial Hospital, an incidence of 10 per cent of con-

Figure 71-3 Fracture-dislocation of C1–C2, unilateral, due to a rotatory injury. Note the associated fracture of the mandible. The arrow is on the lateral mass C1; the arrow head is pointing to the dislocation.

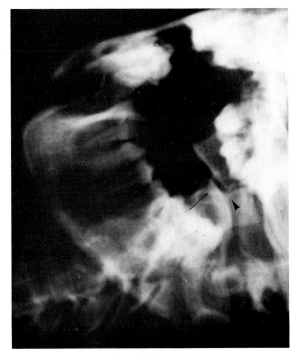

comitant cervical spine fractures was found. All patients who have suffered head injuries should have a single lateral cervical spine film obtained early in their emergency room care.[64] Upon arrival at the emergency room, the patient should be briefly examined and tested for neurological loss. The physician should ask about neck pain, should ask the patient to move the legs and arms. The neck should be gently palpated, and any particular point of pain should be carefully noted. Sensory examination should be performed briefly, testing the upper extremities as well as the lower extremities.

X-ray examination should consist of a single lateral cervical spine film initially. The principal disadvantages of limiting the x-ray examination to a single lateral view are two. First, a fractured odontoid may well be missed, as appreciation of this fracture on the lateral film can be difficult. Second, the physician must be sure that the entire cervical spine is covered by the x-ray. Obviously the lower cervical segments may be missed if the patient is muscular or obese, or has shoulders that ride higher than normal. If the lateral cervical spine film reveals any abnormal or suspicious findings, then more complete films, up to and including polytomography, should be obtained to determine the extent of the injury (Fig. 71–4). Anteroposterior, lateral, and oblique films are helpful. An open-mouth view of the odontoid is part of the routine examination. The surgeon should be careful that the entire cervical spine is x-rayed. In large or heavily muscled individuals, it may be difficult to visualize C6, C7, or the C7–T1 interspace. By pulling the arms down, one may obtain an adequate film. If not, the ''swimmer's'' view is helpful. This is a lateral view, with one arm elevated over the head (Fig. 71–5). The ''pillow'' view should be reserved because it requires rather sharp flexion of the neck; in the presence of dislocation of the spine, spinal cord injury might well occur. This view is obtained by having the patient supine on the x-ray table, flexing the neck with a pillow under the occiput, and angling the beam of the x-ray tube caudad. This throws the laminae and lateral masses in relief, and one may see fractures that are otherwise invisible. With the availability of polytomography, however, its use probably is redundant.

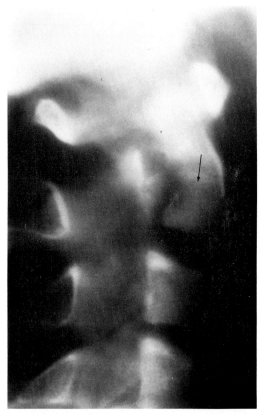

Figure 71–4 The use of polytomography to clarify fractures of the cervical spine. A fracture of the body of C2 is seen (*arrow*).

MANAGEMENT

There are three goals in management of the patient with a cervical spinal injury. The first and foremost one is to do no additional damage to either the bony, ligamentous, or neural components. The second is to treat the neurological injury. The third is to realign the spine to insure stability and freedom from pain. Part of this third aspect is the treatment of any of the ligamentous or muscular injuries that may have occurred.

If there is neither neurological deficit nor x-ray evidence of fracture, and the patient's complaints are of pain localized to the neck, the most likely diagnosis is that of acceleration injury to the cervical spine. This entity produces a variety of symptoms with a paucity of objective findings. It is a real syndrome, however, and it requires appropriate treatment.[15] The most likely pathological change is ligamentous and muscular tearing. Initially, there are few symptoms

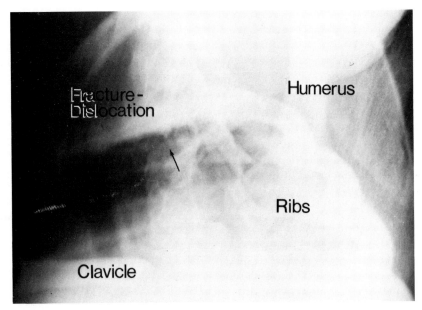

Figure 71–5   Swimmer's view of lower cervical spine. Arrow indicates fracture-dislocation.

referrable to the neck, but shortly after the accident, the patient begins to complain of neck pain and headache. Examination discloses only tenderness and muscle spasm in the posterior cervical muscles. If one examines the anterior surface of the spine by palpating deep to the sternocleidomastoid muscle and anterior to it, however, exquisite tenderness of the longus colli muscles may be found.

X-rays are usually normal, demonstrating only straightening of the cervical spine, but with more sophisticated methods such as polytomography or angled views, fractures may be demonstrated. Particular attention should be paid to the lateral masses of the articular facets, the pedicles, and the transverse processes of the cervical spine as sites for occult fractures.

With sophisticated x-ray examination, far more extensive fractures may be shown than are suspected from plain films.[6,55] The routine use of polytomography has shown it to be of value in about 25 per cent of cases, as in that number of cases the treatment was changed as the result of polytomograms. It proved to be of little value in fractures about C1 and C2 and probably should not be used in such cases.[36] Polytomography exposes the patient to significant irradiation. About 1 rad per film is the average, so polytomography should be used carefully and only with sound indications.

If a fracture is demonstrated, the patient should be treated with immobilization in a cervical brace until the fracture has healed. If no fracture is seen, he should be treated with analgesics and brief immobilization. Four to five days usually is adequate.[35] Muscle relaxant drugs may be helpful. Their use, however, should be brief. A major mechanism of their action is sedation, so it is unwise to persist more than a week with them. If muscle spasm is severe during the acute phase, intravenous methocarbanol (Robaxin) is helpful. Traction, preferably intermittently with about 7 lb of weight is used to relieve muscle spasm.[15] The neck should be moderately flexed. Ice packs and heat to the neck should be alternated to find the more effective one. The physician should remember that reassurance is a major part of the treatment of this injury.[35] Further discussion of this subject is given in Chapter 72.

Bony Injury

There are several points to be considered in regard to the bony injury. The first is whether it involves a major portion or a minor portion of the cervical vertebra. The second, which may prove quite vexing, is whether or not the fracture or dislocation or fracture-dislocation is stable. The first matter is relatively easily discovered, as x-rays show fractures of the spinous process, pedicle, vertebral body, and the like in a high percentage of cases. If only those parts of the vertebral body that are minor are involved, as in fractures of laminae or spinous processes only, only immobilization is required. Unless the patient has other injuries, hospitalization is short and limited to the time of resolution of symptoms. Patients can be made comfortable with appropriate analgesic drugs and treated with a mild external support, such as a four-poster cervical brace or a firm cervical collar.

Fractures that involve major parts of the vertebral body, or in which dislocation is present, are another matter. Here the question of stability arises. The treating physician must be aware of the anatomical structures responsible for stability of the cervical spine. These are predominantly the ligamentous structures, particularly the interspinous ligament, the anterior and posterior longitudinal ligaments. If two of these major supporting ligaments are torn, the fracture and dislocation is likely to be unstable.[7,72]

Similarly, stability is dependent upon the integrity of the articular facets. When these are broken, displaced, or dislocated, then instability becomes a potential problem. The question of the degree of stability has many dimensions. Stable for what? is one, clearly; a fracture may be stable if the patient is in bed and unstable if he is up without support. The incidence of unstable cervical fractures is in the range of 25 to 30 per cent.[11,27,52] White, Southwick, and Punjabi have published an excellent review of the various aspects that render a fracture stable or unstable.[72]

C1 or Jefferson Fractures

Fracture of C1, the so-called Jefferson fracture, is traditionally treated as a stable fracture. Rarely is there associated neurological deficit, and the principal goals of treatment are simply immobilization and relief of pain until healing occurs.[23,28,75] In general, these fractures may be considered as healed at the end of six weeks of immobilization, so immobilization should be continued for at least this period of time. These patients, if having a great deal of muscle

spasm, may be treated by skeletal traction for a few days. The spring-loaded Gardner skull tongs have changed the approach to the use of skeletal traction.[17] The ease of application, patient comfort, and safety of these new tongs allow their use where, in the past, halter traction would have been used. Generally patients are more comfortable in skeletal traction.

Odontoid Fractures

Fractures of the odontoid process present a complicated problem. There are three types. The first is a fracture through the tip of the odontoid. This has to be carefully differentiated from the os odontoideum, a congenital anomaly. Usually the congenital anomaly is a diamond-shaped fragment of a bone with smooth edges, while the fracture looks like the tip of a normally shaped odontoid on x-ray. The second type is a fracture through the base of the dens with separation, usually anteriorly, from the body of C2 (Fig. 71–6). The third is a fracture that extends into the body of C2. The latter type of fracture, ex-

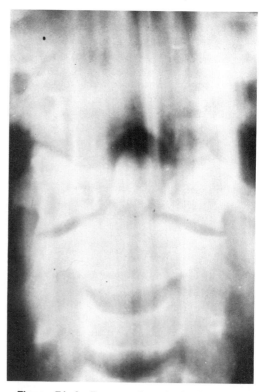

Figure 71–6 Fracture through the base of the odontoid.

tending into the marrow space of C2, requires only immobilization and analgesic treatment. This fracture will heal and prove stable. The other two fractures are a different matter.

The appropriate treatment for the fractures across the base or at the tip has been controversial for years. The traditional method has been to place the patient in skeletal traction, using about 10 to 20 lb of weight. Traction is applied in a direction that will reduce any malalignment. Usually, odontoid fractures, if displaced, are flexion in type, with the axis and the fractured tip of the odontoid being anterior to the atlas. Rarely a posterior dislocation is seen. (Usually, when the head is forced back onto the upper end of the spine, death from respiratory paralysis supervenes very promptly.) The dislocation is reduced, and the patient is kept in bed in traction for six to eight weeks. Treatment by Minerva cast fixation for three to four months follows. An additional period of immobilization by cervical brace for three to four months is generally prescribed.[42,48]

The foregoing is the classic approach to the management of such patients. With the introduction of the halo jacket device, such long periods of hospitalization are unwarranted for a number of patients. The other forms of immobilization such as the brace or the cast are far less rigid than the halo. A more modern approach to treatment of odontoid fractures includes placing the patient in skull tongs in traction for as long as necessary to effect reduction and to eliminate pain in the fracture site. Once this has been accomplished, the patient is then placed in a halo apparatus for a period of three months. Following this, the halo fixation is removed and he wears a cervical collar for an additional three-month period. Follow-up x-rays including flexion and extension films are then required.

These fractures, however, tend not to unite or to unite by fibrous union only. The question of later neurological injury arises because the union may not be solid enough to support the frequent motions of the upper cervical spine. Cases that suggest chronic instability attended by progressive neurological symptoms have been recorded.[14,36,66] Because of the hazards to the upper cervical cord, should these fractures prove unstable, Alexander and co-workers proposed treatment by posterior infusion of C1, C2, and C3 with wire immobilization to insure stability.[1] Their method of treatment is accepted widely.

Kelly and associates have reported the use of wire fixation and methyl methacrylate for stabilization.[32] McLaurin and coworkers have reported the use of simple wire stabilization of C1, C2, and C3 without an attempt at fusion.[37] McLaurin's, as well as the author's, experience with this technique indicates that fracture of the wires occurs in a high percentage of cases, requiring repeat operations or admission of failure. An attempt to obtain bony fusion is preferable, however, to relying on artificial devices to provide a lifetime of stability.

The appropriateness of advocating routine stabilization for every odontoid fracture was questioned by Munro.[42] His experience was that, when the fragments were properly immobilized, fusion occurred and no late neurological problems developed. In fact, the series of Alexander and his colleagues contained only one patient with a progressive neurological deficit, and most of their patients underwent fusion soon after the accident.[1] That the syndrome occurs is uncontrovertible. How often it occurs with adequate conservative treatment is not known. The problem has been compounded by one other fact. Until recently, no adequate form of external stabilization of the spine was available. Skeletal traction was the best, but obviously, could not be employed for six to eight months. No brace or cast can completely immobilize the cervical spine.

The introduction of the halo fixation device has changed the situation.[46] This form of immobilization is superior to any other form of external fixation, so much of what is commonly known about management of cervical spinal fracture may have to be rethought. For instance, the rigid immobilization necessary for fusion of the odontoid may well be possible. Preliminary observations in a small series of cases at Parkland Memorial Hospital indicate that operative stabilization may not be required.

In summary, it seems logical to treat type 1 and type 2 odontoid fractures by stabilization, either externally in the halo and cast or internally by wiring and fusion utilizing bone. Any odontoid fracture shown to be unstable should be fused.

Fractures at C2–C3

The hangman's fracture is a fracture occurring at C2–C3.[7,48,59,61] There is bilateral fracture of the pedicles of C2 with anterior subluxation of C2 on C3 (Fig. 71–7). This fracture is produced by extension of the spine. Neurological damage is rare and usually incomplete if present, as the spinal canal is opened by the bilateral fracture of the pedicles. This fracture has been treated in a variety of ways. It is usually considered a stable fracture. Adequate treatment includes a period in skeletal traction followed by external stabilization until union occurs.

Union is demonstrated in a variety of ways. X-ray cinematography or simple flexion and extension views may show that the fracture site does not move, indicating the presence of union. The fracture line itself becomes less distinct as time progresses and finally disappears as union occurs across it. This presence of firm bony union may be established earlier by polytomography than by plain x-rays. Recently,

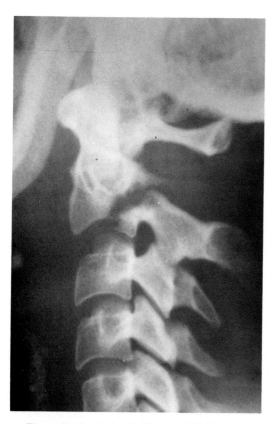

Figure 71–7 A classic "hangman's" fracture.

Seljeskog and Chou have advocated the use of halo fixation in these fractures.[61]

Fractures further down the cervical spine are treated initially according to whether concomitant dislocation does or does not exist. Without dislocation, they may be appropriately treated by a period of skeletal traction to reduce pain followed by external stabilization for six to eight weeks. Following this, a soft cervical collar should be worn for three months.[27,42]

As a general rule, simple fractures of the spine may be considered stable. Simple fractures of the spine include compression or chip fractures of the vertebral body, unilateral fractures of the facets or lateral masses, fractures of the spinous process, and fractures of the lateral mass. No dislocation or subluxation should be present, as this indicates that more severe ligamentous injury has occurred. Rarely is more than one element of the vertebral body involved. These stable fractures need only immobilization with a cervical collar until healing occurs (Fig. 71–8). Healing usually requires approximately six to eight weeks and is demonstrable by the usual x-ray findings of obliteration of the fracture line. If the patient has significant neck spasm and pain, immobilization in bed with traction for a few days may well be indicated for symptomatic relief. If that is the case, either halter traction or skeletal traction with the spring-loaded Gardner-Wells tongs is the procedure of choice. Usually, a day or two of traction and use of an intravenous muscle relaxant is adequate. Recurrence of pain after a period of ambulation in a cervical collar should alert the physician to the possibility that additional problems such as chronic subluxation have occurred. In any case, after fracture of the cervical spine, repeat x-ray examination after six months is helpful in determining the final outcome.

Schneider and Kahn called attention to the small chip fracture on the posterior lip of the vertebral body. As motion occurs in this fracture site, callus develops and ultimately may cause spinal cord compression. In their view, such a fracture was an indication for stabilization.[57]

When dislocation occurs, it is usually in flexion (Fig. 71–9). Reduction of the dislocation is mandatory and is best accomplished by the insertion of the Gardner spring-loaded skeletal tongs and application of traction in the appropriate manner.[17]

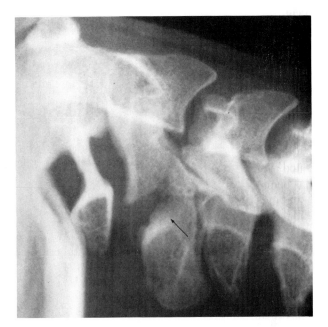

Figure 71–8 Fracture of the posterior elements of C2 (*arrow*). Probably an extension injury, but the laminae may be fractured by ligamentous pull during flexion.

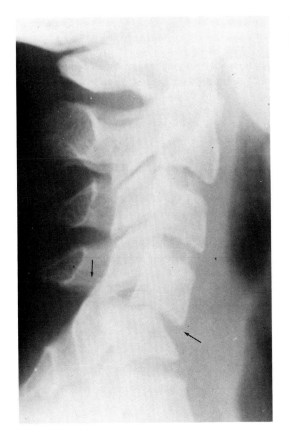

Figure 71–9 Flexion injury with complete dislocation of C4 on C5 with bilateral locked facets (*arrows*).

This should be done in the x-ray department so that frequent check films can be taken.

The usual treatment is to insert Gardner-Wells tongs. Then the patient is placed in the appropriate position on the x-ray table. Approximately 15 lb of weight is applied. The exact amount is increased or decreased, depending on the physical habitus and muscular state of the patient. After approximately 20 to 30 minutes, a lateral x-ray is obtained, checking for distraction and reduction of the fracture-dislocation. If this has not occurred, additional weight in increments of 10 lb is added, and the x-rays are repeated at 20- to 30-minute intervals. The patient should be carefully observed during this maneuver, and his neurological status should be carefully evaluated as the reduction occurs. The direction of traction should produce extension of the neck.

Reduction should be accomplished within the first six hours postinjury, traction being applied in the direction to effect reduction of the dislocation. Weight up to 60 to 80 lb may be used when the procedure is properly monitored by x-ray. If there has been substantial disruption of the ligaments of the cervical spine, however, excess weight may distract the spine and produce neurological deficit by ischemia.

The patient should be sedated with a mild muscle relaxant such as diazepam. During the procedure, the use of analgesic medication such as meperidine or morphine, given intravenously in small increments, may prove helpful. Traction should be applied in a direction to obtain distraction of the dislocated vertebral bodies. After distraction has been effected, usually reduction occurs spontaneously. If it does not, the fracture should be distracted and the neck manipulated in the appropriate direction. No attempt at manipulation should be made if distraction has not occurred. It should be done gently and stopped at any production of pain, particularly radicular pain. For instance, in a flexion fracture-dislocation, traction with 15 lb initially would be applied in extension. Increments of weight by 5 lb would be added until either reduction occurred or a maximum of 60 to 80 lb, depending on the muscular build of the patient, was reached. X-rays should be obtained after addition of each increment. The patient should be conscious and should be monitored carefully for any change in neurological status.

Other authors have recommended postural change for reduction of dislocation of the cervical spine.[16,19,21,65] This can be accomplished by appropriate positioning with pillow or bolster, as advocated by Guttmann for many years.[16,19,21] The patient is positioned with the spine supported by pillows, usually with the head in extension. Reduction is accomplished by a combination of direct force applied by the pillows to the fracture area and gravity.

An alternative way is to use two mattresses, the one on top being shorter than the one below. If the patient is placed on this bed so that the shoulders rest on the upper edge of the top mattress, the head hangs down. The top mattress should be placed no higher than the point of the shoulders. This allows the head to fall backward. This technique has been used at Parkland Memorial Hospital for the treatment of flexion fracture-dislocations of the cervical spine for over 20 years. It remains an extremely useful technique despite the addition of other mechanical devices such as circle electric beds.

Reduction is accomplished by gravity, although traction may be employed as well.[65] This bed has proved useful, as it affords a way to turn a patient through an arc of about 60 degrees while in skull tongs and still maintain extension. Once reduction has occurred, the patient may be placed on a conventional bed and traction may be maintained, an anterior cervical fusion may be performed, or the patient may be placed in a halo or brace. The technique allows for all these options.

The only complication from reduction by this technique arises if the nature of the injury is misdiagnosed and the patient has a hyperextension injury of the cervical spine. This procedure will then lead to rapid worsening of the neurological condition. If the patient requires a great deal of weight on the traction apparatus to maintain reduction, it may be difficult to keep the two mattresses and the patient in the appropriate position for reduction.

When reduction has been accomplished, the traction should be reduced to approximately 20 lb. The patient should be followed by x-rays of the cervical spine for several weeks to be sure that dislocation does not recur. If recurrent dislocation does occur, the fracture clearly is unstable, and internal fixation and stabilization are indicated.

If redislocation does not occur, management in bed in skeletal traction for a period of six to eight weeks is the time-honored approach. Following this, external stabilization by cast or brace is used for three to four months. On removal of the brace, flexion and extension films of the cervical spine should be taken to verify that recurrent dislocation does not occur.[11,27] Patients who have been treated for fracture-dislocations of the cervical spine should have flexion and extension films of the neck taken three months after the discontinuation of treatment and again one year after the discontinuation of treatment. About 20 per cent will develop recurrent dislocation and require fusion for stability.[11]

This concept of bed rest and a period of external fixation may be undergoing change. The introduction of the halo fixation device affords a new approach. In relatively simple fracture-dislocation with no neurological deficit, the halo allows the patient to be ambulatory very quickly after injury. If the halo is applied one week after injury, and the patient is monitored by follow-up x-rays, discharge from the hospital may be within 10 days of the accident.[46] The author's experience indicates that management in halo cast fixation is an excellent alternative. The chief problem with the apparatus is its weight, which limits its use in the very young, the very old, and patients with mild motor deficits. The halo device is applied by attaching the halo to the skull by four-point fixation. One of the disadvantages of the halo is that the anterior pins are placed in the forehead and may cause scarring. It is not necessary to shave the entire head to insert the two posterior pins. Only a small area where they are actually to be inserted needs to be shaved. Once the halo has been applied, a cast is applied over the shoulders, upper thorax, and even to the hips. The cast incorporates in it the strut supports of the halo. These are adjusted to maintain the appropriate amount of flexion or extension of the head.

More recently, the halo brace, which is a lighter-weight plastic jacket that fits over the shoulders and thorax, has become available. This is easy to put on and is attached to the cranial fixation device in the same way by laterally placed strut bars. The principal disadvantage of halo cast fixation, its weight, has been partially overcome by the utilization of the lightweight plastic jacket. An additional disadvantage is that occasionally the supporting lateral rods from the head to the thorax lie over the cervical spine, making it difficult to see the area of injury. It must be borne in mind that it is possible, particularly in children and the elderly, for the pins to penetrate the skull, leading to such complications as abscess or spinal fluid leak. Another complication is loosening of the halo, which makes it necessary to have the patient return to have the bolts and the skull pins tightened. A wrench is provided by the manufacturer for this purpose. If the device is allowed to loosen, the fixation of the fracture site will be compromised.

An alternative form of therapy is an anterior discectomy and fusion after reduction of the fracture-dislocation.[47] The rationale for this approach is that the intervertebral disc has been destroyed and will not heal. Therefore, the patient is subject to the likelihood of either recurrent dislocations, fibrous union, or perhaps bony union. In any event, either the spine spontaneously fuses, or the patient requires fusion because of recurrent dislocation. In the meantime, there is economic cost in keeping the patient without serious neurological deficit in the

hospital, in bed for six weeks, and immobilized in some form of external fixation for an additional long period of time. The argument for the procedure is that it permits early immobilization and return to work with a stable, painless neck. This argument is persuasive, and the method has been adopted by many.[26,30] But one has to weigh the potential complications of an open operation in each individual case.[11,33,70] It is best to individualize the treatment. An anterior discectomy and fusion in young patients without neurological deficit who need to return to work at an early date seems reasonable. Halo fixation may, however, accomplish the same result without operation. If reduction cannot be accomplished, then open reduction is the treatment.

In most cases, a trial of traction, as outlined, for six to seven hours is sufficient to effect reduction. Occasionally, reduction is possible by an anterior approach, but it is far more likely to be accomplished by a posterior approach. Following open reduction, stabilization by interlaminar wire fixation plus the addition of bone grafts to the area for fusion is indicated. If stabilization from the posterior cannot be done because of extensive fractures, an anterior fusion should be done at that time. In either case, the patient should be kept in bed, in traction with 5 to 7 lb of weight, for six to eight weeks. This should be followed by external stabilization, preferably with a halo cast, for three months.

It is important to recognize that the dislocation may recur and that, following any form of treatment, the patient should be followed closely for one year after injury. Flexion and extension films of the neck are important and should be obtained in every case.

Unilateral dislocations are more difficult to recognize. Careful attention to the appearance of each pair of facet joints is required to avoid error (Figs. 71–10 and 71–11). If a question is present, polytomography is indicated.

Reduction of the unilateral dislocation is more difficult than that of the bilateral. It can be accomplished by rotation of the head after distraction. The surgeon should try rotation in both directions. When failure of closed reduction and manipulation occurs, open reduction from the posterior is indicated. At operation, the cause for failure is usually found; a piece of cartilage

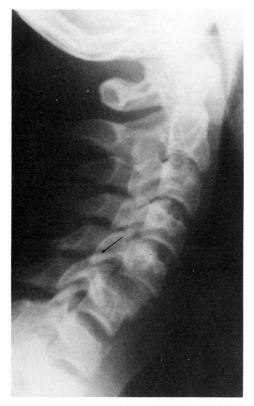

Figure 71–10 Dislocation of the cervical spine at C5–C6 with a unilateral locked facet (*arrow*).

or bone is lying in a location to block re-alignment. Usually, this fragment is free and unattached.

Unilateral dislocations are stable after reduction unless they are associated with other forms of injury. If operation is performed, an opportunity to evaluate stability is offered. If the joint seems unstable, the surgeon should perform a posterior stabilization and fusion.

Hyperextension Injuries

Hyperextension injuries of the cervical spine usually occur in falls.[55] The elderly are more likely to be involved, and in them neurological deficit is more likely to be present. The spinal cord is more vulnerable to injury by hyperextension when the canal is congenitally narrow or is narrowed by spondylosis.

With hyperextension of the head, the anterior longitudinal ligament ruptures at one segment, allowing for acute angulation at that point. Alternatively, or in combina-tion, hyperextension causes infolding of the yellow ligament, which produce cord compression over several segments.

The neurological picture of a hyperextension injury is typical. The upper extremities are most affected, in both motor and sensory function. Hyperextension and hyperpathia may be present in the hands and arms. The neurological loss is most severe in the hands. The lower extremities are less affected.[58]

Extension injuries of the spine require skeletal traction to insure fixation. Since the anterior longitudinal ligament is torn, these injuries are unstable in extension. If the neck is extended, neurological deficit will appear or will worsen.

Treatment by traction should be continued for six weeks. Then immobilization for another six to eight weeks in a cervical brace with the neck in flexion is required. After this period of time, flexion and extension films should be obtained to check for instability. Again, repeat examinations at six months and at one year, with flexion and extension films, are required. Halo fixation is an alternative treatment. For the patient who has enough motor power in the legs for ambulation, it is a very good alternative to prolonged hospitalization.

Injuries to the cervical spine are rare in infants and children. Usually, in infants they are due to birth injuries, and in young children, to falls or diving accidents. Penetrating wounds do happen; the author's experience with six children with gunshot wounds attests to this fact.

In infants, injury is usually associated with breech delivery. The aftercoming head is markedly extended, and the spine gives way. The neurological injury is usually complete transection. X-rays are of little value, as the spine is immature, making the details of injury difficult to define. Treatment is supportive. Respiratory function is the critical factor, and management by tracheal tube is preferred over tracheotomy. The prognosis in infancy is very poor. Since asphyxiation of the baby rarely occurs during breech delivery, there is little excuse for haste to deliver the head. Prevention of this injury is nearly always possible.[2]

Cervical spine injuries in children are usually due to falls and are flexion in type. Neurological injury may or may not be present, and if present, it may be incom-

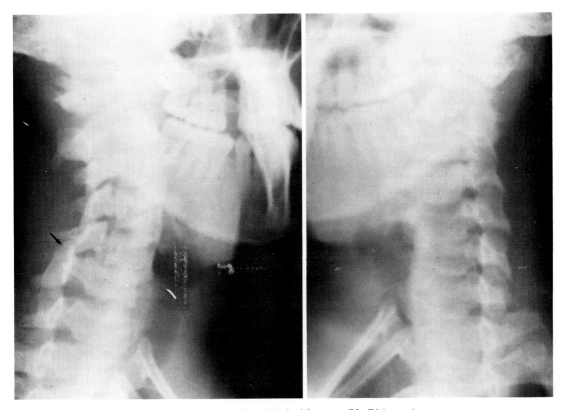

Figure 71–11 Unilateral locked facets at C5–C6 (*arrow*).

plete.[10] In general, management of children parallels that of adults with few exceptions. X-rays may not be as helpful in children because of the immaturity of the spine; details are not visible as they are in adults. Skull traction is difficult to apply in children, as their skulls are thin. Reduction of dislocation should be attempted by external traction and gravity. If this method fails, open reduction is required.[2] If the reduction is by open operation or the dislocation recurs, a fusion of the affected segment is warranted. This may be done anteriorly or by posterior means; little limitation of motion occurs, and there is little interference with bone growth.[39,54,73] Skull traction may be applied in children by placing two burr holes about 2 cm apart on each parietal bone. A stainless steel wire is passed between the holes and used as the traction handle. Prognosis for recovery of neurological deficit in children seems better than in adults.[10]

Patients with neurological deficit should be handled from the standpoint of both their bony injury and the particular type of deficit they possess. The neurological injury suffered ranges from total, complete quadriplegia, to quadriparesis, to radicular signs and symptoms. Unfortunately, 50 per cent of the patients with neurological injury have complete transections.[4,41]

Complete quadriplegia is a great burden. Recovery from a complete transection does not occur. If the patient has been completely paralyzed without feeling from the time of the accident and has no residual function below the level of injury, the chance for recovery is very slim. Priapism is an ominous sign. Similarly, if the plantar reflex is flexor but very slow, a poor prognosis is likely.[41] The other parameter that determines prognosis is the level of spinal cord injury; the higher the injury, the worse the prognosis. Lesions above C3 are usually fatal, as the patient is rendered apneic and dies from cardiorespiratory arrest prior to arrival at a hospital. The author has, however, had the opportunity to see two patients with injuries at occiput–C1, and one with injury at C1–C2, who survived because of immediate mouth-to-mouth resuscitation. These patients remained alive for months, being maintained with respirators.

Injuries that are total and complete at the level of C4 and C5 allow the patient a 50 per cent chance of surviving for one year. The incidence of survival is higher in those whose lesions are below this level. It is dependent, however, on several other factors, including age, general physical condition, pre-existing disease, and associated injuries.[41] Patients with lesions at C6 or at C7–T1 have a good chance of surviving for at least one year unless they are elderly, debilitated, or have serious associated medical problems or associated injuries.

The respiratory problem in quadriplegic patients is complex. There is an inability to fix the chest, so cough is ineffectual. The inability to fix the chest also allows for paradoxical motion of the chest wall. As the diaphragm descends, the chest wall moves inward, so total tidal volume is decreased. This also leads to unequal inflation of the lungs, so diffusion problems arise.[5,22]

The initial care of the respiratory problems should be by endotracheal tube. This should be inserted through the nose without moving the head and neck. The use of a fiberoptic bronchoscope may be very helpful in obtaining a less traumatic intubation. Respiratory assistance by a volume ventilator may be required. Monitoring of arterial oxygen and carbon dioxide tensions and pH is mandatory. Most often, management can be continued with a T bar and 40 per cent oxygen. After a few days, and with arterial blood gas monitoring, a trial in humidified room air should be done. If he tolerates this, the patient can be extubated. The important point is to try to avoid tracheostomy. The incidence of infection of the lung, tracheal stenosis, and erosion of major blood vessels is reduced by this method. Patients will tolerate nasal intubation for several days with ease.

Death in the quadriplegic patient is usually due to respiratory failure. The second most frequent cause of death is urinary tract infection leading to septicemia or kidney dysfunction. A peculiar complication of quadriplegia is automatic hyperreflexia —a symptom complex of headache, apprehension, hypertension, and sweating above the level of transection. This occurs with manipulation of the urinary tract and can be fatal. It is treated with hypotensive drugs.[3,24]

Complete quadriplegia induces a number of other complex problems. Urinary incontinence is best managed by intermittent catheterization.[21] Bowel emptying is best done by enemas, and stool softeners are very helpful. Skin care to prevent decubiti is mandatory and best accomplished in the short term by using a turning frame of some type. Should skin breakdown occur, it should be vigorously treated with debridement and closure. Split-thickness grafts may be used initially, but should be replaced by full-thickness pedicle flaps.

Muscle mass is markedly lost in quadriparesis. The negative nitrogen balance is sustained and may be life-threatening. Maintenance of nutrition by augmented feedings, either by mouth or by vein, may be required. Severe cachexia may produce a syndrome of distention and vomiting when the patient is in the supine position. This syndrome is due to obstruction of the duodenum by the superior mesenteric artery.[50]

Quadriplegia produces many psychological problems. Gentleness and repeated supportive interviews, indicating reasonable and reachable goals and if necessary deferring them, are important. Probably the greatest help is obtained from other quadriplegic patients who are further along in their rehabilitation.[45]

Incomplete Spinal Cord Injuries

The presence of the anterior spinal cord syndrome is an indication for myelography.[50] Either gas or oil myelography may be done. There are strong arguments for air myelography, as air is a medium that demonstrates ventral, dorsal, and lateral aspects of the cord well.[53] The technique is difficult, however, and polytomography is required for optimum results.

As an alternative, the patient may be placed in a turning frame and turned face down. A lateral C1–C2 puncture is performed, and 6 ml of Pantopaque is instilled (Fig. 71–12). This will fill the normal lordotic curve of the cervical spine to indicate the presence of a block. If a block is demonstrated, anterior discectomy and removal of the offending bone or vertebral disc should be done. Raynor has recently reported a series of such patients, indicating that decompression was of questionable benefit.[51] In such a desperate situation, however, decompression seems to afford

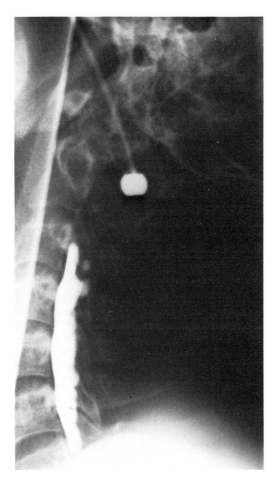

Figure 71–12 Pantopaque myelogram done through a lateral C1 puncture.

the best possibility of recovery. Return of function of significant degree occurs in approximately 50 per cent of such cases.

When a central cervical cord syndrome due to a hyperextension injury of the cervical spine exists, the treatment should be the insertion of skeletal traction that maintains the patient's neck in about 30 degrees of flexion. The anterior longitudinal ligament has been torn, making the neck unstable in a position of extension. Recovery of neurological function after a hyperextension injury follows the pattern of injury. The lower extremities recover first and best, and the hands last and least. Permanent defect may be confined to the intrinsic muscles of the hands.

Incomplete injuries to the cervical spinal cord include a Brown-Séquard lesion. This is usually due to laceration of the cord by bony fragments or in penetrating wounds.

Treatment is expectant in such conditions, and a large number of such patients will recover significant neurological function.

Incomplete lesions may show disparity between the degree of motor loss and that of sensory loss. In general, the consensus is that if motor loss is greater, the prognosis for functional recovery is only fair. When the reverse is true, i.e., more sensory than motor loss, the outcome seems more favorable.

Severe pain and paresthesias in the distribution of one cervical nerve should be considered as possible evidence of a bony spicule or herniated disc. Myelography is indicated. The presence of a filling defect at the appropriate level is an indication for anterior discectomy and fusion.

Laminectomy as a treatment for spinal cord injuries seems to be used less frequently today than in the past. There are several reasons for this. The first lies in the nature of the pathological changes in spinal injuries. Bony or disc compression of the spinal cord occurs in a very small percentage of cases. Three per cent is the figure given by Karulas and Bedbrook in a large autopsy series.[31] Tarlov reported experimental and clinical evidence that relief of compression must be very rapid if it is to be effective; in fact, it must occur within minutes.[67] Extradural and subdural hemorrhages are usually rare, and in some opinions, never cause spinal cord compression unless huge, as in cases of hemophilia. Second, spinal cord injury always extends longitudinally over several segments of the cord, and therefore the lesion is much greater than appreciated on neurological examination.[31] Third, the nature of the nervous tissue is such that disruptive injury to it is instantaneous and complete. Newer forms of therapy may prevent damage experimentally, but in their application to man, it is difficult to prove.[13] Fourth, laminectomy in itself may do harm. There may be additional neurological damage inflicted by the operation. In one series of 42 patients, 22 showed neurological worsening after laminectomy.[8] Results in other series, including 60 cases observed by the author, are not so dismal. In that series, only one patient worsened. Braakman and Penning achieved similar results in a smaller series of 21 patients.[7] By removal of posterior elements and ligaments, laminectomy may make the cervical spine unstable. This, in turn, produces pain and gibbus deformity.[19,38]

The question might be asked another way. Is there a role for laminectomy in the management of cervical spinal injury? There have been many advocates for it in the past. Schneider and co-workers have given a masterful summary of the case for laminectomy.[59] Even they, however, would limit it to cases of progression or worsening of deficit, or for compound wounds. Many surgeons have begun a career as advocates of laminectomy for spinal cord injury. Yet, as experience mounts, virtually all have moved toward increasing use of nonoperative management. Naffziger, for instance, in a nine-year period, went from a position of advocacy to a much more conservative one.[43,44] Today, laminectomy should be reserved for those patients whose neurological injuries progress and get worse despite adequate reduction and stabilization. It should be used only for such injuries and only when the offending lesion is intramedullary or posterior.[29,30,62,71]

Compound Wounds

Management of compound wounds of the cervical spinal cord and column should be treated according to good surgical principles. Penetrating wounds entering anteriorly present the problem of associated injuries. Angiography should be done to determine whether arterial injury is present. Exploration of the wound should be done in the presence of proved arterial injury or major venous injury. When perforations of trachea, esophagus,' or pharynx occur and the wound continues into the spine, the wound should be considered potentially infected (Fig. 71–13). It should be explored, and any fragments of bullet should be removed from disc or vertebral body.

Formerly, when spinal cord injury was due to posteriorly entering gunshot or stab wounds, laminectomy and exploration of the spinal cord were advocated.[8,26] Recent review of the author's experience in over 200 such cases indicates the futility of such explorations, particularly in the face of com-

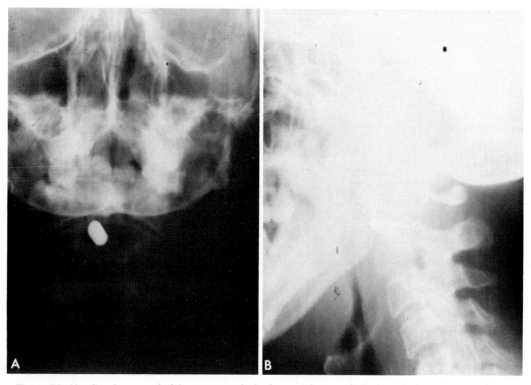

Figure 71–13 Gunshot wound of the upper cervical spine entering anteriorly through the hypopharynx but not penetrating into the spinal canal. Such missile wounds may well be infected. *A*. Anteroposterior view. *B*. Lateral view.

plete and total quadriplegia. In patients who suffer an incomplete lesion from a stab wound, return of function is just as prompt and as complete without operation as it is with operation.[34] The patient is therefore saved an operation and a potential deformity that accompanies laminectomy in the cervical region.[38,74]

REFERENCES

1. Alexander, E., Forsythe, I. T., Davis, C. H., and Nashold, B. S.: Dislocation of the atlas on the axis. J. Neurosurg., *15*:353–371, 1958.
2. Allen, J. P.: Spinal cord injury at birth. *In* Vinken, P. J., and Bruyn, G. W., eds.: Handbook of Neurology. Vol. 25, Part 1. New York, American Elsevier Publishing Co., 1976, pp. 155–173.
3. Arieff, A. J., Tigay, E. L., and Pyzik, S. W.: Acute hypertension induced by urinary bladder distension. Headache and its correlates in quadriplegic patients. Arch. Neurol. (Chicago), *6*:248–256, 1962.
4. Barner, R.: Paraplegia in cervical spine injuries. Proc. Roy. Soc. Med., *54*:365–367, 1960.
5. Bengofsky, E. H.: Mechanisms for respiratory insufficiency after cervical cord injury. Ann. Intern. Med., *61*:435–477, 1964.
6. Binet, E. F., Moro, J. J., Marangola, J. P., and Hodge, C. J.: Cervical spine tomography in trauma. Spine, *3*:163–172, 1977.
7. Braakman, R., and Penning, H. Injuries of the cervical spine. *In* Vinken, P. J., and Bruyn, G. W., eds.: Handbook of Neurology. Vol. 25, Part 1. New York, American Elsevier Publishing Co., 1976, pp. 227–380.
8. Brav, E. A., Miller, J. A., and Bouzard, W. C.: Traumatic dislocation of the cervical spine, Army experience and results. J. Trauma, *3*:569–582, 1963.
9. Brunon, J., Goutelle, A., Felman, D., Brit, P., and Ravon, R.: Results and indications for posterior osteosynthesis with metallic plates in fractures of the spine: 40 cases. Neurochirurgie, *19*:199–213, 1973.
10. Burke, D. C.: Injuries of the spinal cord in children. *In* Vinken, P. J., and Bruyn, G. W., eds.: Handbook of Neurology. Vol. 25, Part 1. New York, American Elsevier Publishing Co., 1976, pp. 175–196.
11. Cheshire, D. J.: The stability of the cervical spine following the conservative treatment of fractures and fracture-dislocations. Paraplegia, *7*:193–203, 1969.
12. DeAndrade, J. R., and McNab, I.: Anterior occipito-cervical fusion using an extrapharyngeal exposure. J. Bone Joint Surg., *51-A*:1621–1626, 1969.
13. Ducker, T. B.: Experimental injury of the spinal cord. *In* Vinken, P. J., and Bruyn, G. W., eds.: Handbook of Neurology. Vol. 25, Part 1. New York, American Elsevier Publishing Co., 1976, pp. 9–26.
14. Elliott, G. R., and Sachs, E.: Observations on fracture of the odontoid process of the axis with

15. Fleming, J. R.: The neurosurgeon's responsibility in "whiplash" injuries. Clin. Neurosurg., *20*:242–252, 1973.
16. Frenkel, H. L., Walsh, L., Michealis, J., Melzack, D., Hyslop, C., and Ungar, J.: The value of postural reduction in the initial management of closed injuries of the spine with paraplegia and tetraplegia. Paraplegia, *7*:179–192, 1969.
17. Gardner, W. J.: Principle of spring loaded points for cervical traction. Technical note. J. Neurosurg., *39*:543–544, 1973.
18. Gaufin, L. M., and Goodman, S. J.: Cervical spine injuries in infants. Problems in management. J. Neurosurg., *42*:171–184, 1975.
19. Guttmann, L.: Initial treatment of traumatic paraplegia and tetraplegia. *In* Harris, P., ed.: Spinal Injuries. Edinburgh, Royal College of Surgeons, 1963, p. 165.
20. Guttmann, L.: Spinal deformities in traumatic paraplegics and tetraplegics following surgical procedures. Paraplegia, *7*:38–58, 1969.
21. Guttmann, L.: The conservative management of closed injuries of the vertebral column resulting in damage to the spinal cord and spinal roots. *In* Vinken, P. J., and Bruyn, G. W., eds.: Handbook of Neurology. Vol. 26, Part 2. New York, American Elsevier Publishing Co., 1976, pp. 285–306.
22. Haas, H., Lowman, E. H., and Bergofsky, E. H.: Impairment of respiration after spinal cord injury. Arch. Phys. Med., *46*:399–405, 1962.
23. Han, S. Y., Wilden, D. M., and Musselman, J. P.: Jefferson fracture of the atlas, report of 6 cases. J. Neurosurg., *44*:368–371, 1976.
24. Head, H., and Riddock, C.: Autonomic bladder, excessive sweating and some other reflex conditions in gross injuries of the spinal cord. Brain, *40*:188–263, 1917.
25. Heiden, J. S., Weiss, M. H., Rosenberg, A. W., Apuzzo, M. L. J., and Kurze, T.: Management of cervical spinal cord trauma in Southern California. J. Neurosurg., *43*:732–736, 1975.
26. Heiden, J. S., Weiss, M. H., Rosenberg, A. W. Kurze, T., and Apuzzo, M. L. J.: Penetrating gunshot wounds of the cervical spine in civilians. J. Neurosurg., *42*:575–579, 1975.
27. Holdsworth, F.: Fractures, dislocations and fracture-dislocations of the spine. J. Bone Joint Surg., *52-A*:1534–1551, 1970.
28. Jefferson, G.: Fracture of the atlas vertebra. Report of four cases and a review of those previously recorded. Brit. J. Surg., *7*:407–422, 1920.
29. Johnson, R. M., and Southwick, W. O.: Surgical approaches to the spine, Part 1, Surgical approaches to the cervical spine. *In* Rothman, R. H., and Simeone, F. A., eds.: The Spine. Vol. 1. Philadelphia, W. B. Saunders Co., 1975, pp. 69–132.
30. Judet, R., Judet, J., Roy-Camille, R., Rose, B., Feghali, C., Bedoisean, M., and Saillant, T.: Tetraplegia due to fracture-dislocations of the cervical spine treated with emergency reduction and osteosynthesis. J. Chir. (Paris), *101*:249–258, 1971.
31. Kakulas, B. A., and Bedbrook, G. M.: Pathology of injuries of the vertebral column with em-

intermittent pressure paralysis. Ann. Surg., *56*:876–882, 1912.

phasis on the macroscopic aspects. *In* Vinken, P. J., and Bruyn, G. W., eds.: Handbook of Neurology. Vol. 25, Part 1. New York, American Elsevier Publishing Co., 1976, pp. 27–42.

32. Kelly, D. L., Jr., Alexander, E., Jr., Davis, C. H., Jr., and Smith, J. M.: Acrylic fixation of atlantoaxial dislocation: Technical note. J. Neurosurg., *36*:366–371, 1972.

33. Kewalrsanni, L. S., and Riggins, R. S.: Complications of anterior spondylodesis for traumatic lesions of the cervical spine. Spine, *2*:25–38, 1977.

34. Lipschitz, R.: Stab wounds of the spinal cord. *In* Vinken, P. J., and Bruyn, G. W., eds.: Handbook of Neurology. Vol. 25, Part 1. New York, American Elsevier Publishing Co., 1976, pp. 197–208.

35. MacNab, I.: The whiplash syndrome. Clin. Neurosurg., *20*:232–241, 1973.

36. Maravilla, K., Cooper, P. C., and Sklar, F.: The influence of thin section tomography on the treatment of cervical spine injuries. Radiology, *127*:131–139, 1978.

37. McLaurin, R. H., Vennal, R., and Salmon, S. H.: Treatment of fractures of the atlas and axis by wiring without fusion. J. Neurosurg., *36*:773–780, 1972.

38. McSweeney, T.: Deformities of the spine following injuries to the cord. *In* Vinken, P. J., and Bruyn, G. W., eds.: Handbook of Neurology. Vol. 26, Part 2. New York, American Elsevier Publishing Co., 1976, pp. 159–174.

39. McWhorter, J. M., Alexander, E., Jr., Davis, C. H., Jr., and Kelly, D. L., Jr.: Posterior cervical fusion in children. J. Neurosurg., *45*:211–215, 1976.

40. Michaelis, L. E.: Epidemiology of spinal cord injury. *In* Vinken, P. J., and Bruyn, G. W., eds.: Handbook of Neurology. Vol. 25, Part 1. New York, American Elsevier Publishing Co., 1976, pp. 141–143.

41. Michaelis, L. S.: Prognosis of spinal cord injury. *In* Vinken, P. J., and Bruyn, G. W., eds.: Handbook of Neurology. Vol. 26, Part 2. New York, American Elsevier Publishing Co., 1976, pp. 307–312.

42. Munro, D.: Cervical cord injuries—a study of 101 cases. New Eng. J. Med., *229*:919–933, 1943.

43. Naffziger, H. C.: Treatment of fractures of the spine with cord injury. Northwest Med., *20*:9–12, 1927.

44. Naffziger, H. C.: Neurological aspects of injury to the spine. J. Bone Joint Surg., *20*:444–448, 1938.

45. Naughton, J. A. L.: Psychological readjustment to severe physical disability. *In* Harris, P., ed.: Spinal Injuries. Edinburgh, Royal College of Surgeons, 1963, pp. 135–137.

46. Nickel, V. L., Perry, J., Garrett, A., and Heppenstall, M.: The halo. J. Bone Joint Surg., *50-A*:1400–1409, 1968.

47. Norrell, H., and Wilson, C. B.: Early anterior fusion for injuries of cervical portion of the spine. J.A.M.A., *214*:525–530, 1970.

48. Norrell, H. A.: Fractures and dislocations of the spine. *In* Rothman, R. H., and Simeone, F. A., eds.: The Spine. Vol. 2. Philadelphia, W. B. Saunders Co., 1975, pp. 529–566.

49. Osgood, R. B., and Lund, C. C.: Fractures of the

odontoid process. New Eng. J. Med., *198*:61–71, 1928.

50. Raptou, A. D., LaBau, M. M., and Johnson, E. W.: Intermittent arteriomesenteric occlusion of the duodenum in a quadriplegic patient. Arch. Phys. Med., *45*:418–423, 1964.

51. Raynor, R. B.: Cervical cord compression secondary to acute disc protrusion in trauma. Spine, *2*:39–43, 1977.

52. Rogers, W. A.: Fractures and dislocations of the cervical spine. An end-result study. J. Bone Joint Surg., *39-A*:341–376, 1957.

53. Rossier, A. B., Berney, J., Rosenbaum, A. E., and Hacken, J.: Value of gas myelography in early management of acute cervical spinal cord injuries. J. Neurosurg., *42*:330–337, 1975.

54. Roy, L., and Gibson, D. A.: Cervical spine fusions in children. Clin. Orthop. *73*:146–151, 1970.

55. Russin, L. D., and Guinto, F. G., Jr.: Multidirectional tomography in cervical spine injury. J. Neurosurg., *45*:9–11, 1976.

56. Schneider, R. C.: The syndrome of acute anterior spinal cord injury. J. Neurosurg., *12*:95–122, 1955.

57. Schneider, R. C., and Kahn, E. A.: Chronic neurological sequelae of acute trauma to the spine and spinal cord (Part 1). The significance of the acute-flexion or "tear drop" fracture-dislocation of the cervical spine. J. Bone Joint Surg., *38-A*:985–997, 1956.

58. Schneider, R. C., Cherry, G., and Pantek, H.: The syndrome of acute central cervical spinal cord injury with special reference to the mechanism involved in hyperextension injuries of the cervical spine. J. Neurosurg., *11*:546–577, 1954.

59. Schneider, R. C., Livingston, K. E., Cave, A. J. E., and Hamilton, G.: "Hangman's fracture" of the cervical spine. J. Neurosurg., *22*:141–154, 1965.

60. Selecki, B. R., and Williams, H. B. L.: Injuries to the Cervical Spine and Cord in Man. Glebe, N.S.W., Australasian Medical Publishing Co. Ltd., 1970, p. 191.

61. Seljeskog, E. L., and Chou, S. N.: Spectrum of the hangman's fracture. J. Neurosurg., *45*:3–8, 1976.

62. Sicard, A., and Lavarde, C.: Is early surgical treatment of traumatic paraplegia and tetraplegia justified? J. Chir. (Paris), *102*:7–20, 1971.

63. Siebens, A. A., Kirby, N. A., and Poulos, D. A.: Cough following transection of spinal cord at C6. Arch. Phys. Med., *45*:1–8, 1964.

64. Skrago, C. C.: Cervical spine injuries: Association with head trauma. Amer. J. Roentgen., *118*:670–673, 1973.

65. Stookey, B.: The management of fracture-dislocation of the vertebra associated with spinal cord injury. Surg. Gynec. Obstet., *64*:407–419, 1937.

66. Stratford, J.: Myelopathy caused by atlantico-axial dislocation. J. Neurosurg., *14*:97–104, 1957.

67. Tarlov, I. M.: Spinal Cord Compression. Springfield, Ill., Charles C Thomas, 1957.

68. Tarlov, I. M., and Herz, E.: Spinal cord compression studies IV. Outlook with complete paralysis in man. Arch. Neurol. Psychiat., *72*:43–59, 1954.

69. Taylor, A. R.: The mechanisms of injury of the

spinal cord injury in the neck without damage to the vertebral column. J. Bone Joint Surg., *33-B*:543–547, 1951.

70. Tew, J. J., Jr., and Mayfield, F. H.: Complications of surgery of the anterior cervical spine. Clin. Neurosurg., *23*:424–434, 1976.

71. Verbiest, H.: Anterolateral operations for fractures and dislocations in the middle and lower part of the cervical spine. J. Bone Joint Surg., *51-A*:1489–1530, 1969.

72. White, A. A., Southwick, W. O., and Punjabi, M. M.: Clinical instability in the lower cervical spine. Spine, *1*:15–27, 1976.

73. Wickboldt, J., and Sorensen, N.: Anterior cervical fusion after traumatic dislocation of the cervical spine in children and adolescents. Child's Brain, *4*:120–128, 1978.

74. Yashon, D.: Missile injuries of the spinal cord. *In* Vinken, P. J., and Bruyn, G. W., eds.: Handbook of Neurology. Vol. 25, Part 1. New York, American Elsevier Publishing Co., 1976, pp. 209–220.

75. Zimmerman, E., Grant, J., Vise, W. M., Yashon, D., and Hunt, W. E.: Treatment of Jefferson fracture with a halo apparatus. Report of two cases. J. Neurosurg., *44*:372–375, 1976.

72

HYPEREXTENSION AND HYPERFLEXION INJURIES OF THE CERVICAL SPINE

With the increased use of the automobile during the second half of this century, larger numbers of acute flexion and extension injuries of the cervical spine have occurred. They have been a source of pain, paresthesia, persistent symptoms, and unfortunately, litigation. Evaluation of these patients is difficult, and their treatment is even more troublesome because their injuries are characterized by an abundance of symptoms with a paucity of objective findings. Unfortunately, the term "whiplash" was introduced by Crowe to describe those injuries.[8] It is a picturesque term conveying the mechanism of injury, which is the uncontrolled flinging of the head, but it is not a medical diagnosis, it does not give a picture of the pathological condition, and it should be discarded.

MECHANISM OF INJURY

Severy and co-workers studied the movement of anthropomorphic dummies during automobile collisions. Collisions at 15 mph produced head acceleration with a force 10 times that of gravity (10 G).[11] Wickstrom and his associates studied hyperextension and hyperflexion injuries to the heads and necks of primates by placing them on accelerating sleds with and without head restraints. His studies demonstrated that 75 per cent of the smaller primates, which weighed from 8 to 10 lb, sustained injuries to the head and neck when they were subjected to head velocity changes greater than 33 ft per second (22.5 mph). The larger primates with heavier necks had neck injuries at lesser velocity changes. These studies also showed that if head restraints completely immobilized the head and neck they would protect the animals against brain and nerve damage at high velocities.

Patrick performed studies of extension and flexion injuries with volunteers and human cadavers. As expected, injuries occurred when an external force of acceleration (or deceleration) was applied to the torso of the occupant of a vehicle and was transmitted to the head through the neck, producing a rotational movement. The strength required to prevent this relative motion was often greater than that of the muscles, and with a great enough force, the limits of resistance to stress of bones, ligaments, and other soft tissues were exceeded.[9]

The most common situation in which this can be seen is a rear-end automobile collision (Fig. 72–1). It is easiest to picture a striking car hitting a stationary one. The struck car is accelerated forward, and the striking car is decelerated. At low speeds, there is an elastic impact in which the struck car tends to approach the velocity of the striking car and the striking car tends to stop. At higher speeds, there is a plastic impact; the struck car tends to reach a velocity of half the initial velocity of the striking car. The most severe injuries generally occur at speeds at which the force applied

S. B. DUNSKER

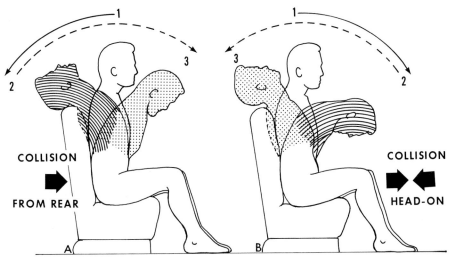

Figure 72–1   Sketches showing: *A*, the hyperextension injury caused by rear-end collision, and *B*, the hyperflexion injury caused by head-on-collison. (After Jackson, R.: The Cervical Syndrome. 3rd Ed. Springfield, Ill., Charles C Thomas, 1956. Reprinted by permission.)

to the seat back by the torso is just less than that required to break the back of the seat. At higher speeds, when the seat back itself rotates, the torso and head move together, the head and neck are more in line with the long axis of the body, and injury is prevented. Without question, extension injuries produce more damage than flexion injuries (Fig. 72–2). Also, in flexion, often there is the limiting factor of the chin hitting the chest, which prevents some tearing of soft tissues.

The location of the occupant in the automobile also determines his predisposition to injury.[8] At speeds less than 15 mph the right front passenger is at greater risk than the driver, who can brace himself on the steering wheel. When collisions occur at speeds in excess of 20 mph, the pelvis of the right front passenger will slide forward, causing the trunk to recline at an angle and preventing a hyperextension injury to the head and neck. The pelvis of the driver is prevented from sliding forward, and therefore he is at greater risk of developing an extension injury of the neck at higher speeds.

If the individual injured is in a stationary car, one must consider the weight and speed of the striking vehicle.[8] For example, a train traveling at 2 mph can impart the same angular momentum to the head as a

Figure 72–2   *A*. Sketch showing the spinal canal elongated in hyperflexion; the spinal cord and nerve roots stretch to conform to the new dimensions. *B*. The spinal canal shortened in hyperextension; the ligaments, dura, spinal cord, and nerve roots slacken accordingly. (After Vakili, H.: The Spinal Cord. New York, Intercontinental Medical Book Corp., 1967. Reprinted by permission.)

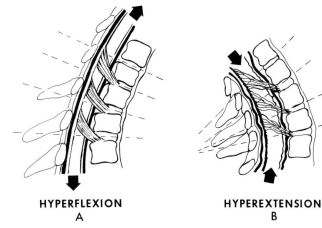

HYPERFLEXION
A

HYPEREXTENSION
B

small vehicle traveling at 40 mph. The acceleration of the struck car will also be determined by its own inertia, which is influenced by such items as the weight of the car, whether it has automatic or regular transmission, whether the brakes are on, and the road conditions.

In summary, the primary determinant of injury is the rate of acceleration of the struck car. That will determine the rate of acceleration of the head and neck, which in turn will determine the degree of angular displacement of the head. Hyperextension injuries are usually more serious and lead to clinical symptoms more often than hyperflexion injuries. Either injury can probably be prevented by physically limiting the relative angular displacement of the head. If the hyperextension could be limited to less than 80 degrees and preferably less than 60 degrees, injury would be unlikely.[9,12] Extension alone is not the only determining factor in the production of cervical spinal injury. Equally important is the position of the head with respect to the torso. With the neck rotated 45 degrees on its vertical axis, normal extension is only half as great as with the head in a neutral position. Therefore if the head is rotated 45 degrees at the time of the accident, injury to the posterior joints is more likely to occur.

PATHOLOGY

Although it is not entirely appropriate to apply conclusions from animal experiments to clinical situations, the experimental injuries produced have been impressive.[9,11,12] Sudden acceleration or deceleration forces could produce damage to the brain with hemorrhage and edema. In addition, there were sprains of the apophyseal joints and the subchondral facets, and there was often rupture and hemorrhage involving muscles. There were tears of the longus colli muscles that produced retropharyngeal hematomas and, occasionally, damage to the cervical sympathetic plexus. There were even occasional tears of the anterior longitudinal ligament, but these never occurred without a corresponding tear of the anterior cervical muscles. In all instances, the severity of the pathological changes was directly related to the degree of acceleration.[9,11,12]

SYMPTOMS

Many factors alter the patient's injury. When evaluating the severity of injury it is helpful to learn the details of the accident: acceleration, direction and force of impact, type of vehicle, position of the patient's head, use of restraint belts and head supports. The more severe injuries are associated with the immediate onset of pain. If patients are seen shortly after the accident the pain is often associated with tenderness in the anterior part of the neck.

Commonly, severe pain is delayed for 24 to 48 hours. With this pain, patients often have swollen tender sternomastoid muscles from muscular hematomas. Later, the pain radiates into one or both shoulders and often into the interscapular region. Frequently it spreads up the neck to the occiput, almost as though it were following the course of the trapezius fibers. The occipital pain commonly radiates to one or both retro-orbital areas. Occasionally dysphagia develops from a retropharyngeal hematoma. All these symptoms fluctuate in severity and may become chronic.

When patients are initially examined weeks after the accident they may exhibit the whole constellation of Barré's syndrome: headache, tinnitus, vertigo, pain in the ears, transitory obscurations of vision, and vasomotor disturbances of the face.[6] Headaches have been found to be more common in individuals who have suffered the more severe extension injuries, and irritation of the upper cervical nerves has been implicated.[2] The pathogenesis of the otological and ocular symptoms has not been determined. They may be due to secondary vasomotor responses. These symptoms are more prone to develop in patients with cervical spondylosis. Chrisman and Gervais demonstrated that ocular and otological symptoms developed in 6 of 29 patients with cervical sprain and in 13 of 33 with cervical spondylosis.[1]

Patients who continue to complain of pain in the neck and shoulder with motion of the head tend to have symptoms that are different from those of an acutely herniated cervical disc. It should be noted that it is rare to find an acute disc herniation developing after a hyperextension injury to the head and neck. The individual with an acutely herniated cervical disc tends to have pain in the neck and arm that is aggravated by lateral flexion of the head toward the side of the pain because that motion diminishes the size of the involved intervertebral foramen and probably increases root compression. The pain of the patient suffering from symptomatic hyperextension injuries in the neck usually is worsened by stretching the affected muscles. For example, the right trapezius and sternomastoid region is painful and tender. That pain is usually aggravated by lateral flexion of the head to the left, which stretches the painful muscles. In both individuals, usually, the pain is increased by extension of the head. Individuals with symptomatic cervical spondylosis may find the pain partially relieved by assuming a position of partial head flexion.

PROGNOSIS

The clinical difficulty with evaluating hyperextension acceleration injuries is the chronicity of symptoms that may develop. As stated before, the illness is characterized by an abundance of symptoms and a paucity of objective findings. The high incidence of personal injury suits probably increases the difficulty of analyzing the severity of symptoms. Gotten's report is cited often. He analyzed the effect of litigation on the clinical course of 100 cases of "whiplash injury" after settlement of the litigation. Eighty-five of the eighty-eight patients who had recovered at the time they were interviewed had liability claims. Of the 85 patients with liability claims, 49 were satisfied and 36 were not satisfied with their legal settlements. Of the 49 patients who were satisfied with their legal settlements, 29 had no significant symptoms, 11 had occasional discomfort, and 4 had enough trouble to sleep in traction. The outcome for 5 patients in this group is not reported by the author. Of the 36 patients who were not satisfied with their legal settlement, 9 had no symptoms, 20 had minor symptoms, and 7 had enough difficulty to cause them to sleep in traction.[3] It was Gotten's conclusion that patients used the injury as a lever for personal gain, either consciously or unconsciously. There have been implications that many of the individuals who have suffered these accidents have also experienced insults to their personality structure, and the emotional disturbances that follow these injuries are an integral part of the "whiplash injury."[2,7]

Hohl followed-up or reviewed 146 patients for an average of seven years after the acceleration injury. None had had preexisting degenerative changes of the spine. At the time of his follow-up, 39 per cent had such changes, which is six times as many as the expected frequency of 6 per cent for that age group. He noted that degenerative changes were seen in 60 per cent of those patients who had been unconscious at the time of the accident, who showed restricted range of motion at one segment on initial flexion and extension lateral x-rays, or who required a cervical collar for symptom control for more than 12 weeks after the injury. His work suggested that there was an increased incidence of disc degeneration in individuals who suffered a severe extension injury of the spine.[4]

The most careful analysis was presented by Macnab, who followed the clinical course of 575 patients after hyperflexion-hyperextension neck injuries. Many of them had associated injuries, such as sprained ankles and wrists, but only their necks remained painful. Therefore, he concluded that it is difficult to implicate litigation as a source of neck pain when it did not cause ankle pain. Similarly, traumatic flexion and lateral flexion of the neck were not associated with the problem of chronic pain, only the cervical extension injuries. The flexion and lateral flexion were probably better tolerated because the chin and shoulders provided a limit to the movement of the head. In Macnab's series, 266 patients obtained a satisfactory conclusion of the court settlement, but in contrast to Gotten's previously cited analysis, 45 per cent continued to have symptoms. The majority of these patients did learn to live with their symptoms, but overall, 12 per cent continued to have significant symptoms.[8]

It is not correct for a physician to ascribe to litigation or psychoneurosis (or both) a continued pain of which he is unable to relieve the patient. As Macnab poignantly stated,

. . . If neck pain following acceleration injuries is purely neurotic in origin, it is difficult to understand why patients commonly get neurotic if the head is thrown backwards and rarely get neurotic if it is jolted forward or sideways.[8]

X-RAY CHANGES

Radiological changes must be interpreted with care. Loss of the cervical lordosis does not indicate muscle spasm, because it can be demonstrated in normal subjects by just lowering the chin. Therefore, except for occasional evidence of retropharyngeal hemorrhage, the x-rays are usually normal.

TREATMENT

If the patient appears to have suffered significant injury, as indicated by pain and tenderness of the sternocleidomastoid and trapezius muscles and perhaps by pain and tenderness in the anterior soft tissues of the neck, the neck can be splinted by wearing a soft collar. It may be necessary to keep the patient at bed rest for a week in order to remove the weight of the head to achieve complete rest of the neck. If the patient has improved within 12 to 24 hours, increased activity may be allowed as tolerated. Traction can be useful in eliminating some muscle spasm, but its use should be encouraged only if it is successful in relieving pain. At the end of one week the patient should be encouraged to return to work but should avoid extension of the head and neck. Sleep may be helped by wearing a collar during the night. Any form of emotional tension or muscular tension produced by drugs such as caffeine may increase the symptoms. Often wet heat will help relieve aching muscles, and the modes of deep heat, including ultrasound, may also give increased symptomatic relief.

If the patient's problems are severe enough to warrant putting him to bed for a week, he will probably have daily discomfort for at least six weeks. If, at the end of six weeks, the patient is still conscious of some measure of discomfort all day long, then he may well have intermittent discomfort for 6 to 12 more months.

Often patients are not seen until several months after the injury, at which time the cause of the continued discomfort becomes more difficult to determine. Nevertheless, treatment is directed at encouraging the patient to perform mild range of motion exercises and to use deep and superficial heat and traction. Prolonged use of collars to immobilize the neck at this late date may well lead to a chronically restricted range of motion and, thereby, increased pain.

Operative treatment has been used after failure of conservative measures in patients who complained only of pain in the neck. The patients usually have continued to have pain, and their operative treatment has been unsuccessful. Because of the low success rate of this form of treatment, the author does not believe that it should be used in patients who have neck pain only and do not have radiculopathy pain.

SUMMARY

The hyperextension acceleration injury to the cervical spine often results in definite pathophysiological changes. The clinical picture presents a varying mixture of symptoms dependent upon the degree of soft-tissue injury, as influenced by a patient's own emotional stability as well as by the presence of pre-existing spinal changes. Although the presence of pending litigation may affect the symptoms, it is necessary to disassociate this confusing element in order to attempt to treat the patient with these disturbing and sometimes incapacitating symptoms.

REFERENCES

1. Chrisman, O. D., and Gervais, R. F.: Otologic manifestations of the cervical syndrome. Clin. Orthop., 24:34–39, 1962.
2. Gay, J. R., and Abbott, K. H.: Common whiplash injuries of the neck. J.A.M.A., 152:1698–1704, 1953.
3. Gotten, N.: Survey of 100 cases of whiplash injury after settlement of litigation. J.A.M.A., 162:865–867, 1956.
4. Hohl, M.: Soft tissue injuries of the neck in automobile accidents. J. Bone Joint Surg., 56-A:1675–1682, 1974.
5. Hunter, C. R., and Mayfield, F. H.: Role of the upper cervical roots in the production of pain in the head. Amer. J. Surg., 78:743–761, 1949.
6. LaRocca, H.: Acceleration injuries of the neck. Clin. Neurosurg., 25:209–217, 1978.
7. Leopold, R. L., and Dillon H.: Psychiatric considerations in whiplash injuries of the neck. Penn. Med. J., 63:385–389, 1960.
8. Macnab, I.: Acceleration extension injuries of the cervical spine. In Rothman, R. H., and Simione, F. A., eds.: The Spine. Philadelphia, W. B. Saunders Co., 1975, pp. 515–528.

9. Patrick, L. M.: Studies of hyperextension and hyperflexion injury in volunteers and human cadavers. *In* Gurdjian, E. S., and Thomas, L. M., eds.: Neckache and Backache. Springfield, Ill., Charles C Thomas, 1970, pp. 108–117.

10. Raney, A. P., Raney, R. B., and Hunter, C. R.: Chronic post-traumatic headache and the syndrome of the cervical disc lesion following head trauma. J. Neurosurg., 6:458–465, 1949.

11. Severy, D. M., Mathewson, J. H., and Bechtol, C. P.: Controlled automobile rear-end collisions and investigation of related engineering and medical phenomena. Canad. Serv. Med. J., 11:727–759, 1955.

12. Wickstrom, J. K., Martinez, L. J., Rodriguez, R., Jr., and Haines, D. M.: Hyperextension and hyperflexion injuries to the head and neck of primates. *In* Gurdjian, E. S., and Thomas, L. M., eds.: Neckache and Backache. Springfield, Ill., Charles C Thomas, 1970, pp. 108–117.

73

MANAGEMENT OF THORACIC SPINAL COLUMN INJURIES

The thoracic spine is designed to provide a mechanical base for the thorax and its contents—a rigid structure between the mobile cervical and lumbar spines. Although it is capable of flexion, extension, and rotation, the degree of motion occurring in the thoracic segment, either in its entirety or in an isolated segment, is less than in other parts of the spine. This rigidity is due to its internal structure and to the supporting ribs and sternum. The thoracic spinal column is rarely the focus of minor sprains or strains, as are the more mobile parts of the spine. The rigidity is demonstrated by the extreme rarity of thoracic intervertebral disc herniations. While this rigidity limits injury to the thoracic spine, it also means that when injury occurs, a large amount of force has been applied. Because of this requirement, neurological injury, except in cases of penetrating injuries due to low-mass, low-velocity missiles, is likely to be a complete transection of the spinal cord.

Injuries to the thoracic spine are caused either by a closed mechanism or by penetrating wounds such as gunshot or stab wounds. The mechanisms of closed injury to the thoracic spine are the same as those that act elsewhere in the spine: flexion, extension, compression, and rotation. Similarly, it is the combination of bony and ligamentous injury that determines the end result of injury. As already mentioned, it takes considerable force to damage the thoracic spine. This means that injuries are usually more extensive than revealed by examination or by routine x-rays. This fact should be borne in mind in planning therapy.

Closed injuries of the spinal cord in the thoracic region are usually flexion injuries in which either lower part of the body is fixed and the upper part moves sharply across a fulcrum, or the reverse, with the upper body in contact with an unyielding surface and the aftercoming bodily parts flexing acutely on the fixed upper part (Fig. 73-1).[42]

Compression fractures of the thoracic spine occur when the force is exerted in an axial direction. This fracture occurs in falls in which the patient lands on the buttocks, or in accidents while the patient is seated, as in a crash landing in an airplane. Often, compression fractures are at the thoracolumbar junction. If the amount of force is very great, the intervertebral disc may be driven into the vertebral body, producing a bursting fracture. Similarly, if a slight degree of flexion is present, the disc may be driven into the spinal canal.[34]

The thoracic spine may be injured by rotatory movement if either the upper or the lower part of the body is fixed and the opposite end is twisted violently. Sometimes, rotation of the fracture site occurs after the initial fracture has occurred. This set of circumstances produces greater injury, particularly to the spinal cord. It also results in gross displacement of the fractured segments. On occasion, the spinal cord will be injured by direct compression from posterior elements that are fractured and pushed inward against it.

When dislocation of the thoracic spine

K. CLARK

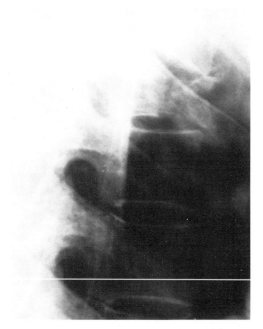

Figure 73–1 Compression fracture of thoracic vertebral body. This wedge shape is typical for a flexion injury.

occurs, there has been fracture of both the anterior and posterior elements. Usually the intervertebral disc is destroyed. Most often, fracture-dislocation of the thoracic spine produces immediate and total paraplegia.

Because of the length of the thoracic spine, injuries would be expected to be more frequent there than in the cervical or lumbar regions. Fortunately, this is not the case. Because of the greater mobility of the ends of the spinal column, the greater percentage of injuries occurs there rather than in the midsection. When an injury does occur in the thoracic area, however, the neural contents are far more likely to be involved than at the extremities of the column.[29] There are three reasons for this fact. First, the spinal cord occupies a greater percentage of the spinal canal in the thoracic region than it does in the cervical or lumbar spine. Second, the blood supply to the spinal cord is most tenuous in the upper part of the thoracic spine, which is nourished by an anastomotic network at this level rather than directly by a radicular artery. Third, the amount of force required to injure the thoracic spine produces greater destruction and displacement at the fracture site. Because of the length of the

column in the thoracic region, there may be multiple areas of bony injury. Polytomograms of the thoracic spine may show more than one level (Fig. 73–2).

CARE AT ACCIDENT SITE AND DURING TRANSPORTATION

All personnel involved in emergency medical care should be fully instructed in recognition and transportation of patients with thoracic spinal fractures. They should always ask the patient, before attempting to move him, about back pain and about sensation and motion in the legs. Movement of a patient who has back pain or complains of neurological loss in the legs should be carefully done, avoiding any motion of the spinal column. The patient should be placed on a spine board before he is moved and kept on the board until a definitive examination is done.

INITIAL EVALUATION

Emergency evaluation of the patient must include questioning about back pain and paresthesias in the lower extremities, and evaluation of motor and sensory power in the legs. Palpation of the thoracic spine by slipping a hand under the back is useful, as point tenderness or a grossly abnormal configuration may be found. A brief but thorough neurological examination is next. Evaluation of motion of the legs, sensation in the legs and trunk, and deep tendon reflexes is done. The findings of this initial examination must be carefully noted to serve as a baseline guide to further deterioration or improvement in neurological function. If the motor and sensory levels are marked on the patient's body, a graphic record is available for subsequent observations and examinations.

As soon as possible, depending on the overall condition of the patient, x-rays of the spine are obtained. The emergency room stretcher should have a film holder to allow anteroposterior films to be taken. Only after adequate films have been obtained to insure that no fracture exists, or that it is a simple and stable one, should the spine board be removed.

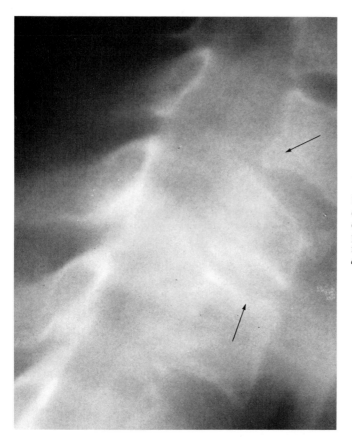

Figure 73–2 An example of multiple bony injuries. A fracture-dislocation is present at the upper part of the polytomographic cut (*upper arrow*), but an unsuspected compression fracture of one side of a lower thoracic body is seen at the bottom (*lower arrow*).

DEFINITIVE MANAGEMENT

Associated Injuries

The management of a patient with a thoracic injury requires considerable skill. For this part of the spine to sustain a fracture or fracture-dislocation implies substantial trauma to the individual, so the first issue to be resolved concerns potential other injuries that may be life-threatening. Injuries to the intra-abdominal organs or to the great vessels in the mediastinum and the retroperitoneal space must be ruled out by careful and appropriate physical, radiographic, and laboratory examination. With injuries in the upper thoracic spine, one should consider the possibility of myocardial contusion, transection of the ascending aorta, or injuries to the pulmonary parenchyma. Again, careful attention to physical examination is indicated. Careful but rapid selection of laboratory and x-ray procedures should be done.

In cases of injury to the upper thoracic spine, an algorithm, or flow sheet, like that

shown in Figure 73–3A is useful. An algorithm for lower thoracic spinal injury would be slightly different (Fig. 73–3B). For use of these algorithms, the upper thoracic spine may be arbitrarily considered as above the T6 level.

The treatment of intra-abdominal associated injuries is simplified for obvious reasons. The likelihood of pancreatic injury, small bowel injury, or great vessel injury must be borne in mind for several days after the initial evaluation. Peritoneal lavage may have to be repeated. Aortography or even exploratory laparotomy may be needed when the cause of persistent troubles is not clear. It must be remembered that in severe neurological deficit, the usual physical manifestations of peritoneal irritation are lost. Therefore, the physician is forced to rely on laboratory and radiological findings to a much greater degree than in a neurologically intact individual.

If there is any question about injuries to the aorta, an aortogram should be performed. If there is any question of injuries to the chest, pneumothorax or hemothorax,

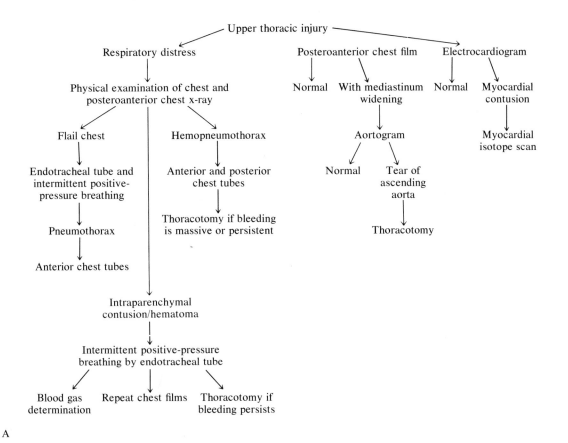

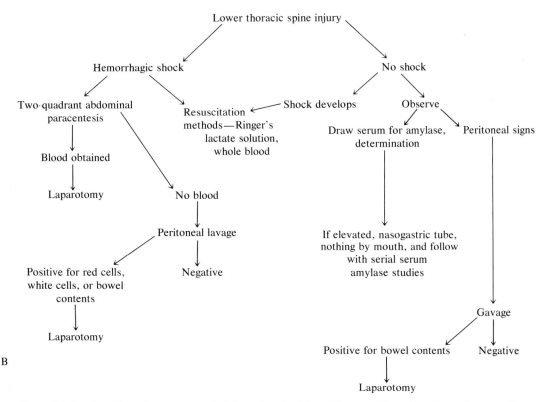

Figure 73–3 Algorithms for management of thoracic spine injury. For use of these algorithms, the upper thoracic spine may be arbitrarily considered as above the T6 level.

the appropriate treatment is proper placement of chest tubes for drainage. Myocardial contusion will be evidenced by changes on the electrocardiogram and by myocardial scan. Muscle enzyme determination may be confusing, as the muscle of the spine is contused and lacerated by the injury. A 40 per cent cross reaction between skeletal muscle creatine phosphokinase (CPK-MM) isoenzyme and cardiac muscle enzyme creatine phosphokinase (CPK-MB) can be expected. This is a high enough level to produce a false positive test of myocardial damage.

Abdominal paracentesis is a useful and easily done test to determine whether blood is being lost into the peritoneal cavity. An 18-gauge needle is introduced into the lateral aspect of the abdomen at the level of the umbilicus on both sides. The needle is gently aspirated with a syringe. If nonclotting blood is obtained, bleeding is occurring intraperitoneally and a laparotomy is indicated.

Failure of paracentesis to reveal abnormality, however, does not rule out significant intraperitoneal injury. If the shock state cannot be explained, or recurs, peritoneal lavage with 1 liter of Ringer's lactate solution through a small catheter placed just below the umbilicus in the midline is used. Gross blood is readily appreciated in the returned perfusate and indicates solid-organ injury. Peritoneal lavage can detect lesser degrees of injury to the liver and spleen than can paracentesis with a needle. It is also capable of determining injury to the bowel. For these reasons, it is preferred over paracentesis. Analysis of the cellular content of the perfusate return gives indication of the presence of intra-abdominal bleeding due to solid-organ injury, or of bowel transection.

If a life-threatening or even serious injury is uncovered by these maneuvers, it must be treated in a manner to protect the integrity of the spinal cord. Haste may be required, but not carelessness. All personnel involved in the care of the patient must be made aware of the thoracic spinal injury and the neurological state of the patient. They should carefully guard against making the deficit worse because of an inappropriately applied sense of urgency.

Once life-threatening injuries have been managed, the first goal of treatment of thoracic spinal injuries is to avoid creating or worsening neurological deficit. The second goal is to realign the spine, and the third is to insure that the spine is stable and painless.

Nonoperative Management

Treatment of the spinal column injury itself ranges from simple conservative therapy to intensive and complicated operative intervention.[8,15,33,45,46] Simple compression fractures of the thoracic spine without displacement are best treated by immobilization in hyperextension in bed. Bed rest should last for four to six weeks. After this period, a form-fitted plaster jacket should be applied in extension. The cast has the advantage of being cheap, and it cannot be removed by the patient.

Following three months of immobilization in plaster, the patient should be fitted with an extension brace for an additional 3- to 4-month period. After removal of these external stabilizing devices, further follow-up includes repeat x-rays of the fracture site. Persistent pain at the level of the fracture site indicates that abnormal motion is occurring. Either further immobilization or posterior spinal fusion to obtain stability should be considered.

Spinal Column Injury

Management of dislocations of the thoracic spine involve manipulation, either by pillow positioning as advocated by Guttmann, by reduction using pin traction in the lower extremities, or by operation.[15,17,31,39] In severe injuries in which there is gross dislocation of the spine, reduction is best accomplished by open methods.[10] Older techniques included open reduction with wiring or plate fixation of the spine after manipulation under anesthesia to restore alignment. If no neurological deficit is present, it is prudent to reduce the fracture-dislocation under direct vision. Greater care can be taken in an open operation than in closed manipulation. Spinal fusion is usually considered as an integral part of such operative technique.

Recently, the introduction of the Harrington rod apparatus has opened a new era in the management of thoracic spinal injuries. This device is introduced over a long segment of the spine with great mechanical advantage. The fracture is easily reduced, and the spine is relocated and rendered stable by the device itself. Fusion over the involved segments can then be done. The rods may be removed later if necessary (Fig. 73–4).[11]

When Harrington rods are used, there is some question about how soon the patient should be allowed to be ambulatory. Experience indicates that patients may be up and about within a few days of the procedure, as the fixation device maintains position. The benefits to the patient of early ambulation seem to outweigh any potential hazard. A plaster cast should be applied for additional support. This instrumentation is equally useful in the management of injuries in children.[4]

When neurological deficit is present, several questions must be answered. The first is the question of whether the neurological deficit is potentially reversible,

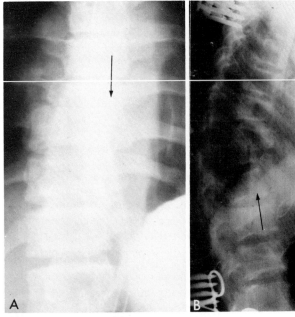

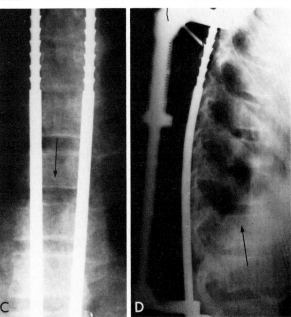

Figure 73–4 Fracture-dislocation of thoracic spine. *A* and *B*. Films of the spine before distraction. *C* and *D*. X-rays illustrate the reduction obtained with Harrington instrumentation.

being due to some remediable cause.[27] The second is how best to insure patient survival while treatment is going on. This is particularly true in the young, the aged, and those with high thoracic lesions.[28] The third is how to insure that the deficit is not made worse by inappropriate or ill-conceived treatment. The fourth concerns a reasonable prediction about ultimate outcome, so treatment may be directed toward that end.

The usually mentioned cause of a potentially reversible lesion is an object compressing the spinal cord. This diagnosis presents two problems. The first is to demonstrate such a lesion. Plain x-rays are not adequate for this. Polytomography may show the offending piece of bone but will not show an extended disc or cartilaginous plate. Myelography would seem to afford an answer. Larson and Whitesides have demonstrated the value of gas myelography with polytomography in the management of such cases.[22] They have shown bony or cartilaginous intrusion into the spinal canal. Unfortunately, this technique is difficult and time-consuming. Pantopaque myelography is even harder to do and may be misleading, as it may prove difficult to get the contrast material precisely over the affected area. A water-soluble contrast material offers hope for an easier method of investigation of the thoracic spine.

Even if a compressive lesion is found, doubt persists that its removal will affect the outcome.[41] These are rare lesions.[19] Compressive lesions in the thoracic spine tend to be associated with complete transection of the cord. Larson and co-workers report that 12 of 56 patients studied by gas myelography and polytomography had a subarachnoid block.[23]

As might be expected, in the course of procedures to determine whether cord compression exists, complicating facts may appear. If myelography is done for diagnosis or because of a worsening neurological deficit, it shows a swollen cord. The question is whether this is hematomyelia or edema of the cord. Statistically, true hematomyelia is very rare, so the surgeon may be reassured that it is edema. Should the patient have an operation? and Should the cord be opened? are two old and troublesome questions. Experimental evidence with graded spinal cord trauma indicates that myelotomy is the most effective form of treatment for the contused cord. This,

however, is graded trauma in a controlled experimental state, whereas the human victim has ungraded trauma and, many times, much more severe trauma than the animal model. The author's experience would indicate that in the human, myelotomy is not useful in cases of spinal cord injury.

Recently, other methods of handling spinal cord edema and contusion have been undergoing evaluation. Cooling of the spinal cord has been advocated, as has the use of corticosteroids. Proof of the efficiency of these methods is lacking. Cooling the cord by recirculating cold saline solution requires equipment not easily available to most neurosurgeons. Furthermore, it requires laminectomy and entails the problems inherent in that procedure.[8]

The use of high-dosage steroids, in the range of 40 to 80 mg of dexamethasone in divided doses over a 24-hour period, is promising but unproved. Similar problems exist with the use of mannitol or furosemide. While some beneficial effects can be shown in experimental spinal cord trauma, proof of efficiency in the clinical setting is lacking.[10]

Operative Management

The single clear-cut indication for investigation of the spinal column and canal in the patient with thoracic injury is worsening of neurological deficit.[39] When this is noted, the patient should undergo myelography to identify the reasons for the worsening. If a remediable lesion is found, operation through the appropriate route is indicated. If it is a thoracic disc or a fragment of bone that is encroaching on the cord from the anterior, the approach should be transthoracic, transpleural, or by costotransversectomy. While the traditional neurosurgical approach to the spine is by laminectomy, these other approaches must be considered when there is an indication for operation.

Laminectomy

The question of laminectomy in thoracic cord injuries is an old one.[31] There is extensive literature indicating the appropriateness, the inappropriateness, the success, and the failure of laminectomy in patients with spinal cord injuries.[8,29,31,32,39] Laminectomy is, however, not without its risks.[8,25]

When laminectomy is elected by the surgeon, it must be recognized that the operative procedure for spinal trauma differs substantially from laminectomy performed for disc disease or tumor. The bony injury is often far more extensive than is visualized by x-ray; therefore, the surgeon must have a much longer incision than the usual two- or three-space laminectomy used for other diseases. Second, the surgeon should recognize at the outset that removal of the laminae further endangers the stability of the spine. Preparation should be made to stabilize the spine by internal fixation at the time of the initial operative procedure. This may be accomplished by Harrington rod instrumentation or bilateral mass fusion or both.

The procedure itself should be done by sharp dissection. The paraspinous muscles should be cut away from the spinous processes and laminae with a knife. A periosteal elevator will plunge through the fractured laminae, producing additional or new neurological deficit.

If a bony spicule that seems to be penetrating through the dura and into cord substance is found, this spicule should be left alone until the full exposure has been accomplished. The dura is then opened around the spicule, and the exact extent of damage to the cord can be estimated. Then the spicule may be grasped and carefully removed from the cord substance.

The questions of whether the dura should be opened if it has not been violated by a bony fragment is a perplexing one. It has been the author's practice to open the dura if laminectomy is indicated. Once the decision to operate has been made, it is thought that inspection of the cord is worthwhile, even though it is well known that a spinal cord may appear normal to inspection and still remain completely functionless.

The question of opening the spinal cord to relieve hemorrhage and edema within it is, again, an old and controversial one. If the cord is to be incised, it should be done under the operating microscope, with a No. 11 bayonnet-pointed Bard-Parker blade. The incision through the pia must be made in the exact midline of the dorsal columns. The cord should be incised to the depth of the central canal. The necrotic pulped material is largely gray matter and lies, therefore, in the center of the cord. When the myelotomy is done, either nothing emerges

or a great deal of pulped cord extrudes. The extruded material is pulped, functionless cord tissue, and this material has not been produced by the myelotomy. Closure of the laminectomy is done in layers. It is the author's practice to close the dura in all cases, using a dural graft if necessary.

Laminectomy poses the additional problem of subsequent stability of the spine. The posterior elements, if they are uninjured or if they are injured in such a way as to remain stable, are likely to be the sole source of stability. Angulation with gibbus formation has been frequently noted after a laminectomy in the thoracic region for trauma.[26]

In addition to the foregoing reasons for not using laminectomy, there are other more compelling reasons. In most thoracic cord injuries, the offending lesion is anteriorly located. It simply cannot be handled effectively from the posterior approach in which it can be seen poorly and must be dealt with under, and around, the spinal cord. If the cord is already damaged by the accident, operative manipulation will certainly make it worse. Current opinion is against the use of laminectomy as management of thoracic spinal trauma, particularly in the presence of complete paraplegia. Consideration then should be given to the other approaches.

Transthoracic Approaches

When the spinal cord is compressed from the anterior, several approaches other than laminectomy may be used. Larson and co-workers have used a transthoracic extrapleural approach to remove the offending fragment.[23] The lateral side of the spine may be reached by resecting the head of the appropriate rib. An interesting variation of this approach is the use of a T incision. A conventional midline laminectomy incision is made and carried down to the lamina. Another incision is made through the skin and paraspinous muscles along the rib at the appropriate thoracic level, joining the laminectomy incision as a T. The head of the rib is then resected along with the transverse process. Splendid access to the intervertebral disc and to the vertebral body is obtained by this approach. Closure is done in layers, and the wound heals surprisingly well with little disfigurement.

The highest levels of the thoracic spine

may be reached by splitting the sternum.[33] The mid levels may be approaches antero-laterally through a transpleural incision.[20] The lowest levels may be approached trans-pleurally and by opening the diaphragm to gain access to the vertebral column.[34] By way of the transthoracic and transpleural route, much more of the thoracic spine may be seen. Removal of offending vertebral bodies and disc material has been reported with the use of this approach.[9,35]

Special Problems

Injuries at the thoracolumbar junction are particular problems. These injuries are frequently associated with a combina-tion of vertically directed force acting along the spinal column plus flexion of the spine with the pelvis fixed. For instance, these fractures occur in a person who is working on his knees when a weight falls on his shoulders. This forces flexion of the thora-columbar spine on the fixed pelvis, produc-ing this type of injury. More severe forms are the slice fracture of the vertebral body occurring with seat belt injuries in high-speed automobile accidents. The slice in-jury, named the Chance fracture, is a rela-tively severe injury.[2] Associated with a fair number of Chance fractures are injuries to the serosal surface of the small bowel or to the terminal aorta. The possibility of these injuries should be carefully investigated.

Many of the injuries of the thoracolum-bar region are without neurological deficit and are basically compression fractures of the spine. These should be managed as such. More severe fractures, such as the Chance fracture, are unstable and require some form of fixation. The classic manner of fixation with posterior plates along the spinous process has proved to be not totally satisfactory.[33] More recently, efforts have been directed toward insuring stability and have, thus, moved toward more radical types of operation. The transthoracic trans-diaphragmatic approach to the fracture with removal of the vertebral body and in-tervertebral discs has been advocated, fu-sion being accomplished by rib grafts.[41] Some authors have advocated both an ante-rior transpleural, transdiaphragmatic ap-proach with removal of the fractured body and posterior fixation and fusion as well.[12] In cases in which an intervertebral body graft has been placed, patients should be

kept in bed for three months at a minimum until the graft has become well solidified. Following whatever forms of stabilization and fusion that are done, it is wise to keep these patients in some sort of external fixa-tion as well. This can be a plaster jacket, a chair-back brace, or halo fixation.

The Harrington rod has offered another method of stabilizing these fractures. This technique has the great advantages of re-quiring only one operative incision, of not requiring the removal of a large amount of bone and cartilage, and of affording instant stability of the spine so that early mobiliza-tion is possible.[10]

Neurological injury, when it occurs in the region of the thoracolumbar spine, is a complex matter. The injury is both to the spinal roots in the cauda equina and, many times, to the conus medullaris itself. This produces a complex pattern of sensory and motor loss. The motor loss is a combination of upper and lower motor neuron loss. The injury to the control of the urinary bladder is particularly difficult to manage, as a flac-cid bladder without sensation is the result. Furthermore, the injury to the conus pro-duces mostly sacral and lower lumbar loss. Function is preserved in the upper lumbar segments, so ambulation and stability of the pelvis are present. An anesthetic heel and sole of the foot are, however, formidable problems to the patient. The buttocks may be rendered anesthetic, so the patient will spend a lifetime worrying about pressure sores over the ischial spines.

Penetrating Wounds

The management of penetrating wounds of the thoracic spine has changed dramati-cally in the past few years.[38] Since penetrat-ing wounds can be separated into those from high- or medium-velocity missiles, contrasted with low-velocity ones, and can also be categorized as entering from the an-terior or from the posterior, and again, as complete as opposed to incomplete lesions of the spinal cord, no single therapeutic for-mula will fit.

Complete Spinal Cord Transection

Complete spinal cord transections will not be improved by an open operation, so other indications for exploration must exist before it is justified.[46] Wounds that traverse bowel or contaminated viscera are one such indication. This in essence limits explorations to those anteriorly entering injuries that go through the peritoneal cavity. Laminectomy may not be the most appropriate neurosurgical approach to debridement. Exploration from the anterior, transabdominally, as an extension of the laparotomy, may be more proper. If not, then laminectomy of a limited type should be done. Stabilization of the spine should be considered at the same time.

Paraplegia produces many serious and vexing problems to the patient. The most pressing of these is management of the urinary tract.[11] Intermittent catheterization seems to be the best method. A paraplegic can be taught self-catheterization. Bowel incontinence can be managed by stool softeners and regular enemas. Respiratory problems, similar to those in quadriplegia may arise in patients with high thoracic lesions.[16] Skin breakdown should be preventable, but if it occurs, should be treated with debridement followed by grafting with full-thickness pedicle flaps. Sexual function may be interfered with, and reproduction difficult. Both of these produce great psychic distress, as most paraplegics are young adults at the time of their accidents.[32] Rehabilitation is a difficult but not impossible goal in the management of the paraplegic patient.

Incomplete Spinal Cord Lesions

Stab wounds, entering posteriorly, with incomplete spinal cord lesions, may represent an indication for posterior operation. In man, it is very difficult to show any change in the course of stab wounds of the cord treated either by operation or without it.[24] The route of entry into the spinal column may not be through the interlaminar space, but rather by the laminar arch, fragmenting the arch and carrying bone against the spinal cord or pushing tiny fragments of bone into the canal. Operation may be considered to remove any compressive force from a fractured lamina and to remove subarachnoid or intramedullary bone. If left, these bone fragments produce intense arachnoiditis and possibly lead to progressive delayed neurological deficit.

A word of caution is in order, however. In the face of improvement of the neurological deficit with posteriorly entering stab wounds, exploration should be delayed or not done. The chance of harm in such cases probably outweighs the advantages. In summary, the degree of neurological recovery a patient will make is not dependent upon whether the patient undergoes an operation. Since penetrating wounds of the thoracic spine rarely produce instability, fusion is not indicated.

Three rather special types of injury to the thoracic spine and cord occur. The first is in children and in infants. The infant, at breech delivery, may be made paraplegic by too vigorous attempts to deliver the head. The baby is extended over the mother's symphysis, the spine dislocated or fractured, and the spinal cord compressed. Occasionally, the baby is simply stretched, and ischemic damage is done to the cord. Such infants rarely survive very long, as respiratory problems, urinary tract difficulties, and skin breakdown with sepsis occur.[1] Since there is no indication for such vigorous extraction of the head, this injury is a preventable one.

In older children, injuries occur in the same manner as in adults. The usual ones are falls or automobile accidents.[6] Management of children is just like that of adults, but the difficulty of evaluating bony injury in nonossified spines must be realized.

On occasion, the physician may see a patient, usually a young adult, with a thoracic cord level lesion without evidence of bony injury to the thoracic spine. The patient has suffered a trivial injury and is thought hysterical. Over the next few hours, the patient recovers. Sensation usually returns before motor function. This has been called spinal cord concussion. The underlying process is probably transient ischemia of the cord produced by the injury.

REFERENCES

1. Allen, J. P.: Spinal cord injury at birth. *In* Vinken, P. J., and Bruyn, G. W., eds., Handbook of Neurology, Vol. 25, Part 1. New York, American Elsevier Publishing Co., 1976, pp. 155–173.
2. Armstrong, C. D., and Johnson, D. H.: Stabilization of spinal injuries using Harrington instrumentation. J. Bone Joint Surg., *56-B*:590, 1974.
3. Bedbrook, C. M.: Injuries of the thoracolumbar spine with neurological symptoms. *In* Vinken, P. J., and Bruyn, G. W., eds.: Handbook of Neurology. Vol. 25, Part 1. New York, American Elsevier Publishing Co., 1976, pp. 437–477.

4. Benners, B., Moiel, R., Dickson, J., and Harrington, P.: Instrumentation of the spine for fracture-dislocations in children. Child's Brain, 3:249–255, 1977.

5. Bors, E., Engle, E. T., Rosenquist, R. C., and Holliger, V. H.: Fertility in paraplegic males. J. Clin. Endocr., 10:381–398, 1950.

6. Burke, D. C.: Injuries of the spinal cord in children. In Vinken, P. J., and Bruyn, G. W., eds.: Handbook of Neurology. Vol. 25, Part 1. New York, American Elsevier Publishing Co., 1976, pp. 115–196.

7. Chance, G. O.: Note on a type of flexion fracture of the spine. Brit. J. Radiol., 21:452–453, 1948.

8. Comarr, A. E., and Kaufman, A. A.: A survey of the neurological results of 858 spinal cord injuries. J. Neurosurg., 13:95–106, 1956.

9. Cook, A., Shaw, R. R., Webb, W. R., Clark, W. K., and Shah, H. H.: Transthoracic evacuation and anterior spinal fusion in Pott's paraplegia. Ann. Thorac. Surg., 4:821–824, 1967.

10. Dickson, J. H., Harrington, P. R., and Ervin, W. D.: Harrington instrumentation in the fractured unstable thoracic and lumbar spine. Texas Med., 69:91–98, 1973.

11. Ducker, T. B.: Experimental injury of the spinal cord. In Vinken, P. J., and Bruyn, G. W., eds.: Handbook of Neurology. Vol. 25, Part 1. New York, American Elsevier Publishing Co., 1976, pp. 9–26.

12. Erickson, D. L., Leiden, L. L., Jr., and Brown, W. E.: One stage decompression-stabilization for thoraco-lumbar fracture. Spine, 2:53–56, 1977.

13. Guttmann, L.: Initial treatment of traumatic paraplegia and tetraplegia. In Harris, P., ed.: Spinal Injuries. Edinburgh, Royal College of Surgeons, 1963.

14. Guttmann, L.: Spinal deformities in traumatic paraplegics and tetraplegics following surgical procedures. Paraplegia, 7:38–58, 1969.

15. Guttmann, L.: The conservative management of closed injuries of the vertebral column resulting in damage to the spinal cord and spinal roots. In Vinken, P. J., and Bruyn, G. W., eds.: Handbook of Neurology. Vol. 26, Part 2. New York, American Elsevier Publishing Co., 1976, pp. 285–306.

16. Haas, A., Lowman, E. W., and Bergofsky, E. H.: Impairment of respiration after spinal cord injury. Arch. Phys. Med., 46:399–405, 1968.

17. Harris, P. Some neurosurgical aspects of traumatic paraplegia. In Harris, P., ed.: Spinal Injuries. Edinburgh, Morrison & Gibb, Ltd., 1965, pp. 101–112.

18. Harris, P., and Whatmore, W. J.: Spinal deformity after spinal cord injury. Paraplegia, 6:232–238, 1969.

19. Holdsworth, F.: Fractures, dislocations and fracture-dislocations of the spine. J. Bone Joint Surg., 52-A:1534–1551, 1970.

20. Johnson, R. M., and Southwick, W. O.: Surgical approaches to the spine, Part 2. Surgical approaches to the thoracic spine. In Rothman, R. H., and Simeone, F. A., eds.: The Spine. Vol. 1. Philadelphia, W. B. Saunders Co., 1975, pp. 133–149.

21. Kakulas, B. A., and Bedbrook, G. M.: Pathology of injuries of the vertebral column with emphasis on the macroscopic aspects. In Vinken, P. J., and Bruyn, G. W., eds.: Handbook of Neurology. Vol. 25, Part 1. New York, American Elsevier Publishing Co., 1976, pp. 27–42.

22. Kelly, R. P., and Whitesides, T. E., Jr.: Treatment of lumbodorsal fracture-dislocations. Ann. Surg., 167:705–717, 1968.

23. Larson, S. J., Holst, R. A., Hemmy, D. C., and Sances, A., Jr.: Lateral extracavitary approach to traumatic lesions of the thoracic and lumbar spine. J. Neurosurg., 45:628–637, 1976.

24. Lipschitz, R.: Stab wounds of the spinal cord. In Vinken, P. J., and Bruyn, G. W., eds.: Handbook of Neurology. Vol. 25, Part 1. New York, American Elsevier Publishing Co., 1976, pp. 196–208.

25. Mayfield, F. H.: Complications of laminectomy. Clin. Neurosurg., 23:435–439, 1976.

26. McSweeney, T.: Deformities of the spine following injuries to the cord. In Vinken, P. J., and Bruyn, G. W., eds.: Handbook of Neurology. Vol. 26, Part 2. New York, American Elsevier Publishing Co., 1976, pp. 159–174.

27. Michaelis, L. S.: Epidemiology of spinal cord injury. In Vinken, P. J., and Bruyn, G. W., eds.: Handbook of Neurology. Vol. 25, Part 1. New York, American Elsevier Publishing Co., 1976, pp. 141–143.

28. Michaelis, L. S.: Prognosis of spinal cord injury. In Vinken, P. J., and Bruyn, G. W., eds.: Handbook Neurology. Vol. 26, Part 2. New York, American Elsevier Publishing Co., 1976, pp. 307–312.

29. Morgan, T. H., Wharton, C. W., and Austin, G. N.: The result of laminectomy in patients with incomplete spinal cord injuries. J. Bone Joint Surg., 52-A:822, 1970.

30. Naffziger, H. C.: Treatment of fractures of the spine with cord injury. Northwest Med., 20:9–12, 1927.

31. Naffziger, H. C.: Neurological aspects of injury to the spine. J. Bone Joint Surg., 20:444–448, 1938.

32. Naughton, J. A. L.: Psychological readjustment to severe physical disability. In Harris, P., ed.: Spinal Injuries. Edinburgh, Royal College of Surgeons, 1963, pp. 135–137.

33. Norrell, H. A.: Fractures and dislocations of the spine. In Rothman, R. H., and Simeone, F. A., eds.: The Spine. Vol. 2. Philadelphia, W. B. Saunders Co., 1975, pp. 529–566.

34. Paul, R. L., Michael, R. H., Dunn, J. E., and Williams, J. P.: Anterior transthoracic surgical decompression of acute spinal cord injuries. J. Neurosurg., 43:299–307, 1975.

35. Ransohoff, J., Spencer, F., Siew, F., and Gage, E. L., Jr.: Transthoracic removal of thoracic discs. J. Neurosurg., 31:459–461, 1969.

36. Roberts, J. B.: Stability of the thoracic and lumbar spine in traumatic paraplegia following fracture or fracture-dislocation. J. Bone Joint Surg., 52-A:1115–1130, 1970.

37. Schneider, R. C.: Surgical indications and contraindications in spine and spinal cord trauma. Clin. Neurosurg., 8:157–183, 1962.

38. Schwartz, H. C., Coxe, W. S., and Goldring, S.: Definitive treatment. In Mierowsky, A. M., ed.:

Neurological Surgery of Trauma. Washington, D.C., Office of the Surgeon General, Dept. of the Army, 1965.

39. Sicard, A., and Lavarde, C.: Is early surgical treatment of traumatic paraplegia and tetraplegia justified? J. Chir. (Paris), *102*:7–20, 1971.
40. Talbot, H. S.: The sexual function in paraplegia. J. Urol., *73*:91–100, 1955.
41. Tarlov, I. M.: Spinal Cord Compression. Springfield, Ill., Charles C Thomas, 1957.
42. White, R. J., and Yashon, D.: Dorsal and lumbar spine injuries. Youmans, J. R., ed.: Neurological Surgery. Vol. 2. Philadelphia, W. B. Saunders Co., 1973, pp. 1085–1088.
43. Whitesides, T. E., and Shah, S. C. A.: On the management of unstable fractures of the thoraco-lumbar spine. Spine, *1*:99–107, 1976.
44. Wilcox, N. E., Stauffer, E. S., and Nickel, V. L.: A statistical analysis of 423 consecutive patients admitted to the Spinal Cord Injury Center, Rancho Los Amigos Hospital, 1 January, 1964 through 31 December, 1967. Paraplegia, *8*:27–35, 1970.
45. Yashon, D.: Missile injuries of the spinal cord. *In* Vinken, P. J., and Bruyn, G. W., eds.: Handbook of Neurology. Vol. 25, Part 1. New York, American Elsevier Publishing Co., 1976, pp. 209–220.
46. Yashon, D., Jane, J. A., and White, R. J.: Prognosis and management of spinal cord and cauda equina bullet injuries in 65 civilians. J. Neurosurg., *32*:163–170, 1970.

74

INJURIES TO THE
LUMBAR SPINE

The lumbar spine and the cervical spine are the two most mobile segments of the vertebral column. Therefore, they are injured in similar ways.

The incidence of fractures of the lumbar spine is less than that of the cervical spine. The reason for this lies in the greater strength of the muscles and ligaments supporting the lumbar spine. This very fact, however, makes muscular strains and sprains more common in the low back, and there is a greater total number of injuries to the low back. Also, the apparently lower incidence of fracture may be, in part, spurious. Polytomography of the cervical spine is frequently done, but this study is not done in the lumbar region. Most injuries to the lower part of the back occur in young people of childbearing age, and the radiation exposure to the gonads is too great for routine use.

The experience at Parkland Memorial Hospital in Dallas indicates that the most common cause of serious lumbar spinal injuries is vehicular accidents, followed by gunshot wounds, followed by falls and assaults. Automobile accidents and motorcycle accidents far outweigh the other two causes, accounting for approximately 75 per cent of lumbar spinal fractures alone.[10] Less serious injuries such as sprains occur about 10 times as frequently as fractures. The usual mechanism is a twisting motion during exertion such as lifting or carrying a heavy object.

Injuries may be either closed or open in type. Closed injuries result from flexion, extension, rotation, or axial force.

FRACTURES OF LUMBAR VERTEBRAE

Compression Fractures

Axial forces characteristically produce compression fractures at the upper end of the lumbar spine where the transition from lumbar to thoracic kyphosis occurs. L1 and L2 are the most frequent sites of compression for this reason (Fig. 74–1).

Patients who suffer compression fractures of the lumbar spine should be treated in a position of extension, given appropriate analgesics and muscle relaxants, maintained at bed rest for a period of six to eight weeks, and then begun on ambulation in a plaster jacket.[7] A laminectomy is contraindicated in uncomplicated compression fractures of the lumbar spine, as it will make the spine unstable by removing the intact posterior supporting elements.

The plaster jacket should be worn for a period of three months. An extension-type back brace for an additional three months should follow.

Persistence of back pain at this time indicates abnormal motion in the fracture site, and further investigation should be done. Polytomography and, in the presence of neurological deficit, myelography should be included. Patients who continue to complain of pain in the lumbar spine, when there are appropriate physical or x-ray findings, are candidates for spinal fusion. This should be a lateral mass fusion, as successful fusion is more likely with this technique. For example, if for any reason a

K. CLARK

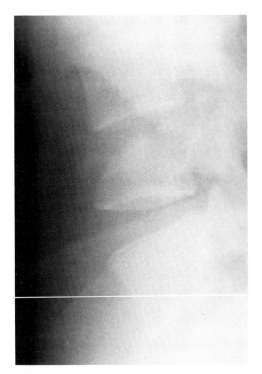

Figure 74–1 Compression fracture of a lumbar vertebra.

laminectomy is required after a compression fracture, internal stabilization and fusion at the time of laminectomy are mandatory. The best way to accomplish this is with the Harrington rod, as it affords a means of producing reduction, realignment of the spine, and stabilization at one procedure.[1,3] Ambulation, after the addition of a cast, can be started within a few days of operation.

Compression fractures may be complicated if either they are "burst" fractures or the body is pushed backward into the spinal canal. A "burst" fracture occurs when the intervertebral disc is driven into the body, causing its disruption. These fractures are usually stable and require no special treatment.[12] A longer period of bed rest may be advisable, however, because of the greater separation of the fragments.

If neurological deficit is present and there is compromise of the spinal canal by bone or disc fragments, an operation may be indicated, as is outlined later. If the malalignment of the spine is great and the patient has an obvious gibbus deformity, an indication for open reduction exists (Fig. 74–2). A word of caution is required about the op-

erative exposure of the fractured area. The dissection should be performed by sharp dissection, as described in Chapter 73. When there is little angulation of the spine, i.e., less than 15 degrees forward, open reduction to correct malalignment is not necessarily required. Lateral displacements of the spine do occur in this type of injury. If the offset is greater than one fourth of the width of the vertebral body, open reduction is indicated.

The Harrington rod device comes with both a distracting set and a compression set. In management of these fractures of the spine, it is the distraction that is most useful.

In cases with either malalignment or neurological deficit, or both, open reduction and fixation may be accomplished by a plate on the spinous processes, an anterolateral approach with interbody fusion, or a retroperitoneal approach and interbody fusion. The ideal form of treatment is with Harrington rods.[1,3] This apparatus allows reduction and internal stabilization in one procedure, and when combined with lateral mass fusion, it affords long-term stability. Laminectomy is rarely useful in such cases, as it affords less effective reduction and makes the spine less stable.

The exposure for insertion of the Harrington rod apparatus should be a generous one. The cautions for performing operative exposure of the fractured spine should be observed. The dissection should be done sharply, and use of the periosteal elevator to remove muscle from the spinous processes and laminae should be avoided. The best results seem to be obtained when the Harrington rod is placed over a long segment of the spine at least two and preferably three segments above and below the level of injury. The distraction device of the Harrington instrumentation is used to distract the spine, the intact ligaments of the spine serving as the retaining forces to effect realignment. X-rays in the lateral and anteroposterior projections should be obtained, and the distraction rods are then inserted in place of the distraction apparatus. The spine should then be fused over either the laminae and spinous processes or the lateral masses. The fusion should be short, involving only the injured segments. The wound is closed in anatomical layers. The patient may be ambulatory within a short period of time or, if paraplegic, may begin

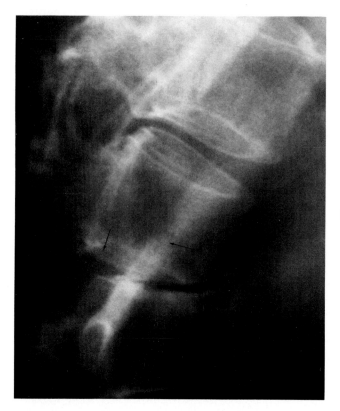

Figure 74–2   A typical thoracolumbar fracture-dislocation (*arrow*).

to transfer quite early. External support for the Harrington rods is best obtained in the thoracic and lumbar spines by the use of a close-fitting body cast.

Another fracture of the lumbar spine is that of the transverse process, or the lateral mass fracture (Fig. 74–3). This is another example of an axial force being applied to the spine. The fracture occurs when an individual sharply contracts the iliopsoas muscle in a protective movement. If the hip is fixed so that the force of the iliopsoas muscle is transmitted to the transverse process, the process is pulled off the spine. Treatment of fractures of the transverse process of the lumbar spine is symptomatic. The patient should be made comfortable by appropriate medication. Bed rest followed, when ambulation is begun, by mild support such as the corset with four rigid steel splints, front and back, is sufficient.

Rotation Injuries

Rotatory injuries of the lumbar spine occur when the pelvis is fixed and the body is able to move on the pelvis. Seat belt frac-

tures are examples of this type of injury. Such fractures should alert the surgeon to the possibility of intraperitoneal or great vessel injury. Degloving injuries with avulsion of the serosal surface of the small bowel, bladder injury, or even injury to the terminal aorta may occur.

Fractures of the vertebral body produced by this rotatory mechanism may be unstable. If there are disruption of the interspinous ligament and a slice fracture through the body, it is an unstable fracture.[15] The disruption of the ligament may be palpable. These fractures should be treated by stabilization, usually by internal means.

Extension Injuries

Extension injuries are quite rare in the lumbar spine, but they do occur. Fractures involving the posterior elements, pedicles, and facets are indications usually of sharp hyperextension injuries. Usually, hyperextension injuries occur in falls in which the body strikes a narrow object and the trunk and legs are bent sharply over a fulcrum. The anterior longitudinal ligament is torn

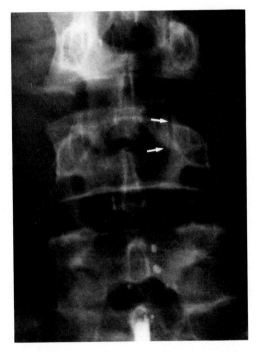

Figure 74–3 Fracture of a compression-type of the lateral mass of L4. This fracture occurs with lateral bending.

by the extension of the lumbar spine, and the spinous processes and laminae may be broken by direct injury.

Penetrating Wounds

Penetrating wounds of the lumbar spine are usually due to gunshot wounds, rarely due to knife wounds or other types of missiles.[16,17] The policy at Parkland Memorial Hospital, in contradistinction to that regarding penetrating wounds elsewhere in the spinal column, has been to explore lumbar spinal compound wounds. The rate of recovery of the patient is markedly improved. Removal of bone fragments from the subarachnoid space reduces the scarring, thereby enhancing recovery. Ransohoff has expressed a similar view.[13]

Neurological Deficit in Lumbar Fractures

Neurological deficit in lumbar spinal fractures may be due either to a single root lesion or to multiple root lesions.[15] Injuries at the T11–T12–L1 region may involve the conus medullarus, depending on the precise

level where the spinal cord ends. This injury involves both the cord and nerve roots. It usually has a devastating effect on bladder function. In males, sexual dysfunction is common.[6]

Usually neurological deficit is due to encroachment on the spinal cord by bone fragments, disc particles, or a penetrating missile. Because of the size of the canal in the lumbar region and the mobility of the cauda equina, this deficit is not severe as a usual thing. It is far more likely to recover than deficit higher up the spinal column.[13]

Because of the mobility of the lumbar spine, the possibility that neurological deficit is due to extrusion of an intervertebral disc into the canal exists. In the absence of a fracture due to compressive force, the suspicion that the neurological deficit is due in part or in toto to a complete extrusion of one disc must arise. Polytomography will rarely define the lesion. Because the cauda equina is involved and there is substantially greater possibility for recovery, such a patient should undergo myelography, preferably with radiopaque contrast material. Unlike a lesion in the thoracic spine, a filling defect is best visualized with this material rather than gas.

A intervertebral disc that has herniated into the spinal canal as a result of acute trauma presents a surgical problem different from the usual disc herniation.[12] The common herniated disc problem familiar to all neurosurgeons is dealt with in Chapter 78. The disc herniation due to trauma involves a normal disc, may include the endochondral plates, and is inevitably massive. It cannot be safely removed by the usual interlaminar exposure. Usually, a bilateral laminectomy is required. Care in extracting the mass from under the cauda equina is required. Removal of the pedicle on the side of the greatest herniation may allow the surgeon to slip the mass out of the canal laterally and effect its removal. After laminectomy, a lateral mass fusion should be done. Again, Harrington rod fixation is very helpful in maintaining alignment and stability.

SPRAINS

Most patients who have injuries to the lumbar spine do not have massive fracture or neurological deficit. They have a sprain or strain of the lumbar muscles and ligaments. Physical examination reveals only mechanical signs in the lumbar spine. Tenderness that may be diffuse or focal is universally present. Limitation of the normal range of motion is also a frequent finding. Motion of the spine may be abnormal in that splinting may occur, and segments of the spine may not move. One or the other, this can be confirmed by lateral bending films taken in the anteroposterior plane. In bending, motion to one side and not to the other at a particular level is strong objective evidence of injury at that level.

Muscle spasm is also present. It is both a sign of injury and a presenting symptom. It must be relieved promptly, as it produces pain, and pain in turn incites more spasm.

The patient may state that the pain runs up the back or down into the buttocks and thighs. If it is sharply unilateral, focal injury to the facet joint, to the lateral ligament, or to the anulus fibrosis must be suspected. If radicular symptoms and signs are present, the injury has been severe enough to produce a herniated intervertebral disc.

Treatment of a patient with lumbar sprain is conservative. Bed rest in flexion on a firm, unyielding mattress is the keystone. Traction, if used, should be in flexion and should use about 25 lb of weight. Pelvic traction is the only effective means. Buck's traction is helpful only in keeping the patient in bed. The weight is diffused by the knees and hip joints, so it has little effect on the lumbar spine.

Medications should include muscle relaxants, preferably intravenous methocarbamol (Robaxin). Most muscle relaxants are sedative, and this action is important in alleviating the stress of enforced bed rest. Pain medication, as opposed to sedative or hypnotic drugs, should be used in appropriate strengths and frequently. A standing order for pain medication should be given rather than a PRN order. Neither the patient nor the nurse should be required to decide when medication is needed. With a standing order it can be given regularly, thus avoiding erratic medication and cycles of recurrent pain. The dose, frequency, and choice of drug should be continuously evaluated by the surgeon.

Indomethacin (Indocin), phenylbutazone (Butazolidin), and steroids have a significant role in the management of chronic back pain. In the acute phase, however, they play little part. The same applies to focal injections of anesthetics. Physical measures such as heat or cold may be very helpful. Massage, if gentle, may accelerate recovery. If the problem has been severe enough to warrant hospitalization, the physical therapist may be very helpful. If the patient is managed at home, however, the value of such treatment is outweighed by the loss of bed rest in transit to the hospital or treatment center.

As recovery occurs, and it should in a week to 10 days, the patient should be allowed up for progressively longer periods of time. He should be started on an exercise regimen, the Williams exercises being one of the better-known ones.

A brace or corset should not be prescribed unless the episode has been unusually long and severe, or is one of a recurring series. These devices produce some immobility of the spine, with associated muscle weakness. This muscle weakness, in turn, may lead to recurrent attacks.

Finally, the patient should be counseled about the use of the back and the importance of good muscle tone in the back, abdomen, legs, and buttocks. The significance of recurrent episodes should be pointed out. Weight reduction or control is an important aspect of preventing recurrence.

SACRAL FRACTURES

Pure sacral fractures are rare, but they do occur. Usually, the sacrum is fractured transversely across its body as the result of a fall. Penetrating injuries may occur. These are managed in the same way as penetrating injuries in the lumbar spine. Missiles that traverse the abdominal cavity and end in the sacrum without producing neurological deficit do not require removal, although, of course, the intra-abdominal tract must be explored. Posteriorly entering penetrating wounds may require exploration if the object penetrating the sacrum is contaminated. If neurological deficit is present after a penetrating wound, the sacrum should be explored to insure that the deficit is not due to compression by a bony fragment.

Transverse fractures without neurological deficit are treated with bed rest for a period of six to eight weeks. The patient should be flat in bed during this time and should not sit or be in a Fowler's position. These place more stress on the sacrum, produce increased pain, and may cause neurological deficit.

In the case of closed fractures of the sacrum with neurological deficit, the sacrum should be explored. This lesion is one of the spinal root, and prompt decompression is helpful in insuring recovery.

REFERENCES

1. Armstrong, C. D., and Johnson, D. H.: Stabilization of spinal injuries using Harrington instrumentation. J. Bone Joint Surg., *56-B*:590, 1974.
2. Chance, G. O.: Note on a type of flexion fracture of the spine. Brit. J. Radiol., *21*:452–453, 1948.
3. Dickson, J. H., Harrington, P. R., and Erwin, W. D.: Harrington instrumentation in the fractured unstable thoracic and lumbar spine. Texas Med., *69*:91–89, 1973.
4. Guttmann, H.: Initial treatment of traumatic paraplegia and tetraplegia. *In* Harris, P., ed.: Spinal Injuries. Edinburgh, Royal College of Surgeons, 1963, p. 165.
5. Guttmann, L.: Spinal deformities in traumatic paraplegics and tetraplegics following surgical procedures. Paraplegia, *7*:38–58, 1969.
6. Guttmann, L.: The conservative management of the vertebral column resulting in damage to the spinal cord and spinal roots. *In* Vinken, P. J., and Bruyn, G. W., eds.: Handbook of Neurology. New York, American Elsevier Publishing Co., 1976, pp. 285–306.
7. Holdsworth, F.: Fractures, dislocations and fracture-dislocations of the spine. J. Bone Joint Surg., *52-A*:1534–1551, 1970.
8. Johnson, R. M., and Southwick, W. O.: Surgical approaches to the spine: Part 3, Surgical approaches to the lumbar spine in Rothman, R. H., and Simeone, F. A., ed.: The Spine. Vol. 1. Philadelphia W. B. Saunders Co., 1975, pp. 150–156.
9. McSweeney, T.: Deformities of the spine following injuries to the cord. *In* Vinken, P. J., and Bruyan, G. W., ed.: Handbook of Neurology. Vol. 26, Part 2. New York, American Elsevier Publishing Co., 1976, pp. 159–174.
10. Michaelis, L. S.: Epidemiology of spinal cord injury. *In* Vinken, P. J., and Bruyn, G. W., ed.: Handbook of Neurology. Vol. 25, Part 1. New York, American Elsevier Publishing Co., 1976, pp. 141–143.
11. Naughton, J. A. L.: Psychological readjustment to severe physical disability. *In* Harris, P., ed.: Spinal Injuries. Edinburgh, Royal College of Surgeons, 1963, pp. 135–137.
12. Norrell, H. A.: Fractures and dislocations of the spine. *In* Rothman, R. H., and Simeone, F. A., eds.: The Spine. Vol. 2. Philadelphia, W. B. Saunders Co., 1975, pp. 529–566.
13. Ransohoff, J.: Lesions of the cauda equina. Clin. Neurosurg., *17*:331–344, 1970.
14. Schneider, R. C.: Surgical indications and contraindications in spine and spinal cord trauma. Clin. Neurosurg., *8*:157–183, 1962.
15. Smith, W. S., and Kaufer, H.: Patterns and mechanisms of lumbar injuries associated with lap seat belts. J. Bone Joint Surg., *51-A*:239–254, 1969.
16. Yashon, D.: Missile injuries of the spinal cord. *In* Vinken, P. J., and Bruyn, G. W., eds.: Handbook of Neurology. Vol. 25, Part 1. New York, American Elsevier Publishing Co., 1976, pp. 209–220.
17. Yashon, D., Jane, J. A., and White, R. J.: Prognosis and management of spinal cord and cauda equina bullet injuries in 65 civilians. J. Neurosurg., *32*:163–170, 1970.

75

ACUTE INJURIES OF PERIPHERAL NERVES

The surgeon operating upon and caring for patients with peripheral nerve injuries must be conversant with the microscopic and macroscopic anatomy of the nerve. He should know its metabolic requirements, its physiological response when injured, and in addition, the function of other structures in the extremity surrounding that nerve and of the end-organs innervated by it. Judgment concerning whether to operate, when to operate, and what to do once the lesion is exposed is extremely critical and must be based upon not only a firm understanding of the physiology of the repair but also some acceptance of the limitations for neural regeneration in terms of practical functional recovery.

PATHOPHYSIOLOGY OF NEURAL INJURY AND REGENERATION

The Neuron's Response to Injury

When an axon is interrupted the cell body, which is located either in the anterior horn of the spinal cord, in the posterior root ganglion, or in an autonomic ganglion, undergoes chromatolysis.[11] Histologically, the neuronal swelling is accompanied by displacement of the Nissl substance to the periphery of the cell and is usually regenerative rather than degenerative in nature.[22,85] Exceptions are found in severe proximal injury to neural elements, particularly the brachial plexus or the lumbosacral plexus, which can result in severe enough retrograde damage to the neuron to be incompatible with its survival. When chromotolysis is regenerative in nature, the neuronal cytoplasm increases in volume, owing primarily to an increase in ribonucleic acid (RNA) and associated enzymes.[50] Ribonucleic acid changes from large particles to submicroscopic particles, and this change results in an *apparent* loss of Nissl substance. From 4 days after injury until a peak is reached at 20 days, the amount of RNA increases, as does its metabolic rate. Ribonucleic acid appears necessary for reconstruction of axons, since it provides amino acids that in turn combine to provide polypeptides that constitute the proteins necessary for replenishment of axoplasm. Its role as the central ingredient in regeneration has, however, been questioned by some. The argument has been advanced that the increase occurs only if regeneration is already proceeding successfully, the RNA serving only as a marker for regeneration rather than heralding it.[51] In any case, it has been clearly shown that increased ribonucleic acid volume and activity persist until axon regeneration and maturation cease. The closer the injury is to the spinal cord, the more hypertrophic are the neuronal changes, while with distal lesions the changes are less marked. Since a proximal injury requires a lengthier regeneration of the axon than a distal one, it is almost as if the neuron were able to anticipate the job ahead. In a healthy axon-to-neuron relationship, metabolic building blocks for axoplasm are circulated from the nerve body down the axon and back up again. The axo-

D. G. KLINE and F. E. NULSEN

plasmic flow of these metabolites may be supplemented along the axon's course by local exchange of both metabolites and waste products. Thus, some of the elements necessary for survival of the axon may be provided by the axon's local environment rather than by the neuron itself.[155]

Despite these metabolic alterations, resting-potential spike and after-potential spike do not change.[18,49] There is, however, a disturbance in the neuron's central synaptic function. Longer latency and increased temporal dispersion of the reflex discharge evoked by afferent stimulation of the neuron occur.[48] Degenerative changes in synaptic vesicles have been shown by electron microscopy and may relate to interference in synaptic function.[118] If the axon is freshly resected proximal to the previous transection site, new regenerative activity on the part of the neuron results and a new thrust of axoplasm occurs (Fig. 75–1).[7,46]

Axonal Response to Injury

Although classification of gradations of injury can be useful, it must be recognized that nerves are composed not only of thousands of axons with differing fiber diameter and degree of myelination but also of a variable amount of perineurial and endoneurial connective tissue and differing fasicular arrangements. In addition, there may be a variety of forces or vectors of force in a given injury such as a gunshot wound. Thus, axons may have different degrees of vulnerability to a given injury, with the result that although the whole nerve is involved, multiple grades of injury may be represented. Seddon has recognized that individual axons can respond to trauma in three basic but different ways.[126,129] He defines neurapraxia as a physiological block in conduction without anatomical axonal interruption. Axonotmesis represents anatomical interruption of axonal continuity without serious disruption of the endoneurial and perineurial framework of the nerve. Neurotmesis indicates interruption of the connective tissue support, or skeleton, of the nerve as well as of the axons and their myelin sheaths. Since many peripheral nerve injuries leaving the nerve in gross continuity exhibit varying proportions of each of these grades of injury, more sophisticated but more difficult to remember grading methods have been proposed by Sunderland and used by some.[143]

Neurapraxia

Neurapraxia represents a concussion or shocklike injury to the nerve and is brought about by blunt injuries, high-velocity missile injuries adjacent to the nerve, mild compression or ischemia, or excessive stretching of the nerve. As with most diseases, an accurate history of what transpired is important in making this diagnosis. Mild degrees of compression or contusion are usually responsible for neurapraxia. A common example of a neura-

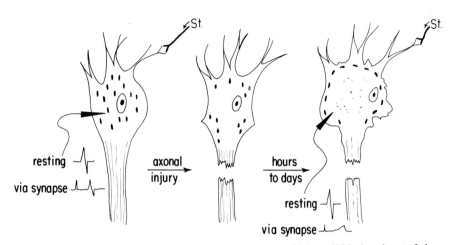

Figure 75–1 Schematic summary of cell body's response to axonal injury. With the advent of chromatolysis, the resting potential is unaffected, but the response via synapse is altered by an increased latency and temporal dispersion of the discharge related to changes in synaptic vesicles. St., stimulus site.

praxic lesion is partial peroneal palsy, which can result from a prolonged crossed-leg position; another is "Saturday night palsy" involving the posterior cord of the plexus or the radial nerve due to draping an arm over a chair or lying on the arm for a prolonged period. The cause of the lack of conduction past the point of injury probably is biochemical in nature and may involve the myelin sheath. To gross inspection and palpation, a neurapraxic nerve usually appears normal. Microscopically it may be normal. At worst it will have segmental demyelination with preservation of continuity of the axis cylinder. Experimentally, Denny-Brown and Brenner found that the large-fiber myelin sheaths close to the point of injury become swollen and with time show degenerative changes.[42] Distally the nerve is normal and does not have wallerian degeneration. Therefore, in some instances stimulation of the nerve distal to the injury will produce a conducted impulse and distal muscle function. Stimulation of the nerve above the injury will give either a partial distal response or no response if the block to conduction is complete.[13,127] Atrophy does not occur, and electromyography should show normal insertion potentials, since the muscle is not denervated. On the other hand, attempts at voluntary contraction of distal musculature may produce no evoked muscle action potentials. It must be kept in mind that more severe degrees of compression can lead to less reversible loss. A few fibrillations are frequently seen with a preponderantly neurapraxic lesion, since a few fibers have undergone axonotmesis.[84] Any early partial preservation of function favors neurapraxia. Motor loss predominates and sensory loss, when present, is greatest for the large fibers serving touch and proprioception, and least for fine fibers mediating pain and temperature. Loss of sweating is rare. Return of motor and sensory function occurs by six weeks, at a time too early to be consistent with wallerian degeneration and subsequent regeneration.

Axonotmesis

Axonotmesis involves loss of axon and myelin continuity with preservation of the supportive connective tissue framework of the nerve. Epineurium, perineurium, and endoneurial tubes are preserved, but de-generating axons are interspersed with macrophages and there is a proliferation of Schwann cells at and distal to the injury site. Associated with the injury and the distal wallerian regeneration that occurs is a retrograde decrease in diameter of axons and myelin sheaths that may extend one or more centimeters proximally, depending on the force of the injury.[6,38,61] Conduction velocity along the segment just proximal to the axonotmetic injury is slowed in relation to the decrease in axon and myelin diameter.[38] Fibrillations begin two or three weeks after loss of innervation, and denervation muscle potentials are seen shortly thereafter. Muscle action potentials are absent when voluntary movement is attempted. Stimulation causes no distal movement. Nevertheless the distal portion of the nerve can remain electrically conductive to muscle for several days.[60] The clinical picture is one of total motor and sensory paralysis. Since connective tissue structure at the injury site is preserved, regenerating axons are relatively unimpeded in their course toward the distal stump, and there is minimal straying of the axons. Although function returns almost as slowly after axonotmesis as after suture, quantitatively it is so much better that resection of the site of injury and suture of the nerve would be an error in judgment.

Neurotmesis

Neurotmesis implies partial or complete severance of a nerve that disrupts the continuity of not only the axons and their myelin sheaths but also the connective tissue elements. Severance of the neural elements can be total despite a gross appearance of continuity, since a severe contusion or stretch can result in internal neurotmesis with disruption of all the elements of the nerve. Indeed, in civilian as well as wartime practice, lesions in continuity with a predominant element of neurotmesis are as frequent as completely transected nerves. The signs of denervation are identical to those described for axonotmesis, but with the striking difference that there is no capacity for regeneration. If the nerve is severed completely, a proximal stump neuroma develops. It is composed of whorls of disorganized and branching fine axons mixed with a proliferation of connective tissue and Schwann cells. In this situation, the perineurium does not accurately reconstruct itself. New axons leave the more normal fascicular structure proximally and take a wandering course through the neuroma. The distal stump forms a glioma, or swelling, due to proliferation of Schwann cells and connective tissue. Occasionally, instead of a bulbous proximal neuroma, the proximal stump sends out a thin strand of connective tissue and axons along a tissue plane to meet the distal stump glioma. There may or may not be a gap between the proximal neuroma and the distal neuroma. If there is a small gap between the stumps, a blood clot forms and is subsequently organized by connective tissue and an ingrowth of Schwann cells. Regenerating axons push into the area of disorganization in clusters.[69] Obstruction of their regenerative pathway by scar tissue, and the disorganized fascicular pattern lead to useless branching and rerouting. Axons seem to regenerate by "contact guidance," growing along connective tissue planes.[153,154] A tortuous pathway may be provided to the distal stump, but only rare axons grow down the cell-lined endoneurial tubes. Depending on the time it takes for axons to reach a distal innervational site, the endoneurial pathways will be expanded or small in diameter. Usually more than one fiber grows down a tube, but only those reaching a distal receptor and reinnervating it go on to mature and take on myelin, while others either degenerate or fail to mature.[132]

Regenerating axons may not function even after reaching distal end-organs unless they arrive close to their original site.* Regenerating fibers can induce some, but unfortunately not complete, change in end-organs not innervated by them prior to injury. In addition, cutaneous fibers do not cross certain boundaries, and regeneration of ulnar or median fibers into the fine hand muscles seldom produces normal function. The ability of the central nervous system to readjust to new end-organ contact on the part of the axon is limited in both the sensory and the motor spheres but does occur, although usually with less than optimal results.[125,135] This is readily illustrated by the synkinesis seen with facial nerve regeneration, particularly that associated with hypoglossal- or accessory-facial anastomosis.

_____
* See references 23, 27, 66, 141, 168.

In many partial lesions there is a spectrum of injury to fibers. If there is preservation of function or partial recovery of function by six weeks, the injury that permitted some axons to suffer only neurapraxia will usually have involved the remaining axonal population in axonotmesis, thus permitting their regeneration. With no evidence for neurapraxia at six weeks, the existing proportion of axonal involvement by axonotmesis versus neurotmesis remains undetermined. It can be determined early only by combining operative inspection with electrophysiological testing (Fig. 75–2).

When denervated, the structure of muscle begins to change histologically by the third week. The muscle fibers kink, and their cross-striations decrease. With continued denervation, and particularly if this is accompanied by a lack of activity and movement, fibrosis replaces the muscle so that by two years after denervation the muscle can be totally replaced by scar tissue.[145] Intervals of denervation beyond 18 months begin to impose major limitations on the motor function that can follow subsequent reinnervation.

Grade of Injury and the Mechanics of Trauma

Laceration and Contusion

Laceration of an extremity, when total paralysis follows injury, usually has severed the nerve.[104] But a penetrating stab wound or an external blow (e.g., to the unprotected ulnar nerve at the elbow) can cause a focal contusion with gross neural continuity but an undetermined grade of axonal injury. Thus, some 12 to 15 per cent of civilian lacerating injuries to an extremity involving nerve leaves the nerve in gross continuity.

Unfortunately, even in civilian practice, a frequent source of contusion to nerve is that secondary to gunshot wound. As shown by Puckett and others, nerve explodes away from the missile as it approaches and then implodes back as the missile passes by.[116] This may result not only in an area of severe focal contusion but also in internal disruption of both axons and their connective tissue framework, including important intraneural vasculature over a varying length of the nerve. This

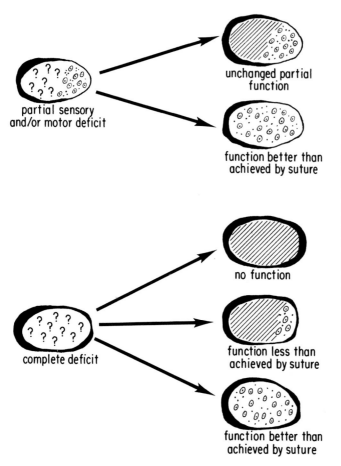

partial sensory
and/or motor deficit

unchanged partial
function

function better than
achieved by suture

complete deficit

no function

function less than
achieved by suture

function better than
achieved by suture

Figure 75–2 Schematic representation of the graded injury problem: (1) Partial nerve function (initially, or by six weeks) could theoretically fail to improve; but there will usually be a degree of regeneration through areas of axonotmesis certain to exceed the regeneration achieved by suture. (2) Complete nerve dysfunction, persisting past six weeks, can both in theory and in practice reflect a complete anatomical lesion, or a partial anatomical lesion that *may* or *may not* yield regeneration better than that achieved by suture. Gross anatomy of the lesion on operative inspection will often settle the question. Major gross continuity of the nerve requires electrophysiological testing to determine (soon after injury) whether resection and suture will provide a better result than preserving the lesion (neurolysis).

mechanism is surprisingly frequent in gunshot wounds, since many fragments responsible for paralysis do not strike the nerve itself.

Approximately half the nerves that are totally paralyzed by missile wounds will regain some degree of useful function, while only 20 per cent of neural contusions due to closed fracture involve neurotmesis severe enough to require resection and suture.[72] For these reasons, correct nonoperative as well as intraoperative management of these lesions in continuity is difficult to accomplish. The details are covered later in this chapter.

Stretch

Stretch or traction injuries most commonly result from extremes of movement at the shoulder joint, with or without actual joint dislocation or fracture, which can also involve the clavicle. Either upper or lower elements of the plexus may suffer the predominant injury. All grades of damage are possible. Roots can be avulsed from the spinal cord or a trunk that remains in continuity, or the stretch may cause only neurapraxia or axonotmesis or both. Each plexus element may suffer from a different grade of change. The important point is that the lesion is not focal, but instead, the damage extends over a great length of the nerve.[65,159] A clavicular fracture attests to the disruptive force applied to the shoulder joint but may or may not imply a focal injury to underlying plexus. The peroneal nerve can be stretched in accompaniment with fibular head avulsion, and the peroneal component of the sciatic nerve can be stretched with hip dislocation or fracture. A stretch mechanism may be responsible for occasional long segmental damage to nerves displaced by high-velocity missiles.

Occasionally, even the lumbrosacral plexus may sustain a stretch injury resulting in distraction of a lumbrosacral root, as evidenced by meningocele at that level on myelography. Distal intraneural damage to the plexus can occur in association with some extensive pelvic fractures or more rarely with severe hyperextension of the thigh.

Birth palsies due to difficult deliveries are shrinking in number because of improved obstetrical training and practices, but still occur. The most common is Erb's palsy involving upper as well as middle trunk, due usually to forcible depression of the shoulder during delivery of the infant. Klumpke's paralysis involves damage to the lower trunk or roots and occurs because the arm remains caught in the pelvis and is held abducted while traction is applied to the body. Like stretch injuries in adults, some improve and some do not.[39,162]

The important point with stretch injuries is that although some may improve, there is often no definitive operative answer for the many that do not. When the major injury is neurotmetic, it involves so long a segment of the neural complex that the only operative method for replacing the resulting lengthy neuroma is use of lengthy grafts, which at these proximal levels may fail.

Compression-Ischemia

Ischemic nerve injury occurs in a variety of situations. During either general or spinal anesthesia for an operation or during the abnormally deep sleep of the drugged or intoxicated individual, external pressure or extremes of posturing can compress nerves to produce ischemic damage. The relative roles of structural changes in axons versus ischemic damage remain difficult to resolve, although experimental evidence suggests that changes in paranodal myelination with invagination of the myelin and subsequent segmental demyelination are associated with milder degrees of compression, and wallerian degeneration with more severe compression.[3,120] A mild entrapment syndrome may first manifest itself because the individual is "too deep" to move in response to discomfort. Tourniquet paralysis is another example of ischemic injury. Clearly, the key in management is prophylaxis—and this becomes vitally important when a perforating wound provides a mechanism for extension or progression of neural injury.

Formation of an aneurysmal sac or arteriovenous fistula as a result of damage to major vessels can compress a nearby nerve and cause an injury where none existed or convert a partial injury into a complete and irreparable one (Figs. 75–3 and 75–4). Increasing pain, a pulsatile mass, and a bruit over the mass serve as warning signals for this condition. The usual vessels that are involved are the brachial, axillary, and subclavian arteries, but extension of injury from hematoma formation is possible in many loci. In the British World War II experience, the diagnosis was usually made at the operating table, and 41 arterial lesions were repaired at the same time as the definitive nerve repair.[127] Ten axillary artery aneurysms were described in the Veterans Administration monograph *Peripheral*

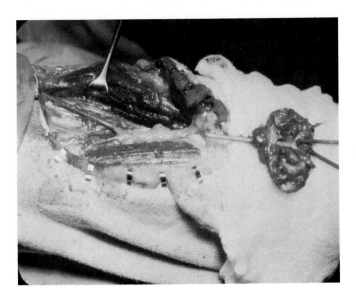

Figure 75–3 An aneurysmal sac, resulting from brachial artery laceration in the axilla, has been lifted from the neurovascular bundle where it compressed median and ulnar nerves in a closed compartment. Patient first noted numbness and inability to use fingers four days postinjury. Only partial recovery from the total median and ulnar paralysis existed at 10 days when patient was operated on. (Attention had been centered on abdominal wounding with intestinal perforation.)

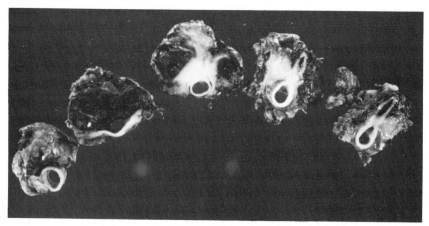

Figure 75–4 Multiple cross sections of false aneurysm of the axillary artery secondary to gunshot wound. Partial plexus injury was converted to a more complete one by expansion of this lesion, and in addition the patient had onset of burning pain in the hand and paresthesias in the distribution of both the median and the ulnar nerves.

Nerve Regeneration.[164] In three of these cases, an initial partial deficit progressed, while in the remaining seven, paralysis was present from the time of wounding. Operative findings in all patients suggested, however, that the aneurysms caused major damage to the nerve, superimposing neurapraxia upon an initial partial neurotmetic or axonotmetic lesion. Hence, whenever progressive paralysis occurs, or there is an expanding mass in the limb or a bruit, the diagnosis of aneurysm or fistula should be considered. Injury to major vessels can result in expanding blood clots, which if they occur in potentially tight spaces such as beneath the gluteal musculature, between hamstring muscles in the thigh, or beneath lacertus fibrosis and pronator teres fascia at the elbow level, can result in acute compression of nerve requiring urgent operative decompression.

Fractures also may be responsible for progression of the nerve injury. The nerve may be caught between the bony fragments as attempts are made to manipulate the fracture into alignment or if the fragments move because of inadequate immobilization (Fig. 75–5).[129] A thorough baseline examination of the extremity and frequent repetitive testing are necessary to detect the onset of such a neural injury. Occasionally, rupture of the vasa nervorum due to a traction injury to a nerve results in a hematoma large enough to cause progressive compression of the nerve. Severe torsion fractures of the tibia and fibula associated with skiing accidents may be accompanied by a delayed and progressive peroneal palsy caused by stretching and formation of a hematoma.[105]

Volkmann's contracture is a serious example of ischemic paralysis. Paralysis can follow manipulation and cast immobilization of a closed fracture near the elbow that is associated with severe muscle swelling and hemorrhage into the anterior compart-

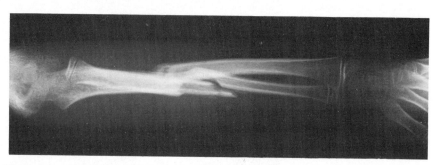

Figure 75–5 Severe comminuted fractures of radius and ulna at midforearm level associated with combined median and ulnar nerve palsy.

ment of the forearm. Actual infarction of volar forearm musculature can occur. In most cases, there is injury to the brachial artery along with diffuse segmental damage to the median nerve and muscles. The large median nerve fibers serving motor and proprioceptive function are more severely involved than the smaller pain fibers. The electromyogram may aid in diagnosis by showing temporary but repetitive and spontaneous motor discharges from muscles most distal to the injury site.[127]

Ischemia of a sufficient magnitude to produce Volkmann's contracture results in severe endoneurial scarring over so long a segment of the median nerve as to make regeneration unlikely. Bunnell felt that Volkmann's contracture was sufficiently explained by closed-space compression of the brachial vessel between the fracture and the lacertus fibrosus at the level of the elbow.[30]

Swelling of the forearm resulting in a painful paresthetic hand must alert the physician to a tight-space syndrome long before more obvious signs of vascular compromise are apparent.

Section of the damaged segment of the brachial artery may be necessary. Anticoagulation alone may not suffice and may even be deleterious; the authors have seen one patient whose syndrome progressed shortly after heparinization, probably owing to hemorrhage into already ischemic musculature.

In addition to the median nerve, the radial and even, occasionally, the ulnar may be involved because of a severely swollen elbow and forearm, particularly when associated with multiple contusive injuries at these levels. Immediate fasciotomy is in order, since remedial operation for the more severe degrees of Volkmann's contracture is disappointing.[149] Compression of the median nerve must be relieved by operation, especially in the region of the pronator teres and flexor digitorum sublimus muscles.[56] It must be kept in mind that closed-space swelling of this type can be aggravated by a tight-fitting cast or by fixation of the elbow in acute flexion. Emergency treatment at the first signs of ischemia is necessary if irreversible neural damage and contractures of the extremity are to be prevented.

In summary, extension of neural injury by compression and ischemia is a serious possibility when an aneurysm or hematoma forms in a closed neurovascular compartment. These lesions are particularly apt to occur with perforating wounds that involve arteries and with fractures. Neural damage usually is preventable, but becomes irretrievable when severe ischemic change involves a long segment of nerve.

Electrical Injury

Electrical injury by passage of a large current through a peripheral nerve usually results from accidental contact of the extremity with a high-tension wire.[5] If the individual does not succumb to respiratory or cardiac arrest, diffuse nerve and muscle damage result.[43,52] Pathological reports of peripheral nerve damage are sparse, and there are no good guidelines for treatment, although conservative management of the nerve injury itself and early orthopedic reconstruction of the extremity seem to be best. Surgical experience with four such cases involving one or more peripheral nerves indicates that some of these lesions will improve with time, but others, unfortunately, will not, and resection of a lengthy segment of damage and repair by grafts may be necessary (Fig. 75–6). Histologically, the segment of the nerve is virtually replaced first with necrosis and then with reaction to that necrosis including a severe degree of both perineurial and endoneurial scar tissue. Fascicular outline may be preserved, but intrafascicular damage may be severe enough to prevent any but fine axon regeneration. Unfortunately, the accompanying severe skin burns and necrosis of bone frequently thwart reconstructive efforts. The muscle in the extremity often is extensively coagulated, leading to severe contractures, which further decreases the likelihood of reinnervation.[83]

Drug Injection

Drug injection into or close to a nerve may cause a major injury that leaves the nerve in continuity.[24,37] The two most frequent sites for injection injury are low and medial in the buttock for the sciatic nerve and at the lateral midhumeral level for the radial nerve. The sciatic nerve lies in a trough beneath the piriformis muscle and on top of the gemelli, quadratus, and obturator internus muscles and between the

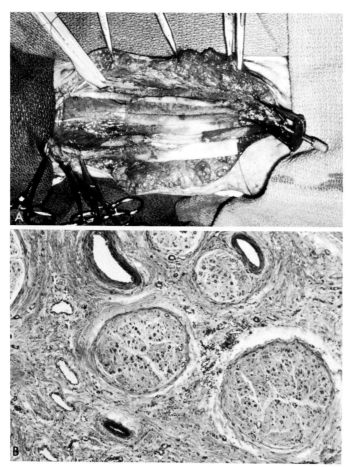

Figure 75-6 *A.* Median nerve injured at wrist level by electrical burn involving volar wrist and hand. The patient was holding onto a steel cable on a crane that struck a 13,000-volt electric line, and sustained severe distal upper extremity burns. Areas of soft-tissue loss were covered by abdominal flap transfers, but a median and ulnar neuropathy failed to improve, and exploration revealed extensive lesions in continuity. Since stimulation elicited no distal motor function and a nerve action potential could not be transmitted through either lesion at nine months postinjury, they were resected and the gaps bridged by sural interfascicular grafts. *B.* Histological examination of the resected specimens showed heavy connective tissue proliferation at both the endoneurial and perineurial levels. Axons had attempted regeneration but were fine in caliber, and areas containing infiltrates of small inflammatory cells could still be seen scattered throughout the perineurium (Masson, 100 ×).

bony boundaries of the ischial tuberosity and the greater trochanter. Drugs not injected directly into nerve may pool in the trough and bathe the nerve to produce neuritis. Intraneural damage is similar to the changes seen with antibiotic injection into the brain.[81] Although the deficit in neural function usually is due to intraneural neuritis and scar tissue rather than to extraneural scarring, some authors feel that external neurolysis for this complication can be of benefit.[34,94] Sedatives and narcotics can also cause injection neuropathy.[115] If the complication is noted immediately, 50 to 100 ml of normal saline could be placed in the region of the injection site in the hope of diluting the drug and avoiding permanent neuropathy. Open operative irrigation might be even more logical. If the nerve deficit is partial, expectant treatment is best, but if the deficit is complete, exploration becomes warranted. The authors' policy with injection injuries has been to ex-

pose the nerve that shows no function after eight weeks and to attempt to evoke a nerve action potential through the injury. If no response is recorded, the lesion has to be resected. The gross appearance of the nerve lesion is quite deceiving in many of these injuries. Segments that appear to inspection and palpation as minimally injured may have such extensive axonal disruption as to preclude useful functional regeneration (Figs. 75-7 to 75-9). In these cases, only resection and repair and not further time will provide any hope for recovery. As a result, a severe palsy secondary to injection injury should be followed for only two to three months and then, if there is no significant recovery, electrically or clinically, explored so that direct stimulation and evoked nerve action potential studies can be made.[68a] Neuropathy from drug injection must be prevented by proper education of nurses and ancillary personnel as well as of physicians.

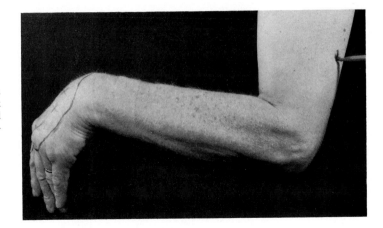

Figure 75–7 Pencil indicates point of antibiotic injection that produced a total loss of wrist and finger dorsiflexion through damage to the radial nerve.

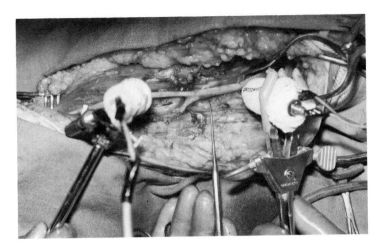

Figure 75–8 Operative picture of the exposed radial nerve (five months postinjury). The instrument indicates a nerve segment firm to palpation but normal in appearance. There was no transmission of action potentials through this area of damage. Resection and suture were done, with subsequent recovery of useful extensor function.

Figure 75–9 Cross section from center of resected segment showing complete loss of axons with replacement by connective tissue (Masson 60 ×). Antibiotic injection must have been made directly into the nerve.

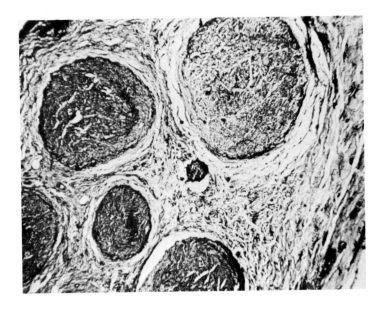

Neuromas in Continuity

Before considering the information to be gained from clinical examination and electrodiagnostic aids, it is appropriate to consider the problem of the neuroma in continuity. In the absence of any evidence of recovery of an injured nerve, the surgeon will properly elect early exploration of the lesion. The finding of gross anatomical discontinuity readily determines the need for resection and suture; and here the prompt establishment of an environment for axonal regeneration is so necessary as to justify the dictum: "When in doubt, look!" Nonetheless, 60 per cent of all civilian injuries involving nerve leave the nerve in gross continuity, and here the decisions whether to explore and what to do once the lesion is found are not easily made.

Neuromas in continuity commonly result from focal contusions and especially from passage of a high-velocity missile close to the nerve. They are encountered most frequently in military and in urban practice. To gross inspection, the "neuroma" appears swollen, and when palpated, it usually is lumpy and firm, even rocklike (Fig. 75–10). Yet, after resection and histological examination, a profusion of relatively well-oriented axons may be seen at the center of the injury. Such inappropriately resected lesions may show regenerative axons well distal to the neuroma or even preservation of some distal axons that are suffering neurapraxia only. The bulk of this type of "neuroma" is caused by proliferation of scar tissue instead of by disorganized axons. On the other hand, the neuroma may appear benign, but intrinsic connective tissue proliferation and axonal disorganization may be so extensive as to preclude adequate regeneration (Figs. 75–11 and 75–12). Thus, in the absence of gross loss of continuity, it can be most difficult to judge the regenerative capacity of the neural lesion.[107,110]

A sutured or repaired nerve also becomes a neuroma in continuity whose size, firmness, and histological appearance will depend on the interval since suture, the thoroughness of resection of damaged tissue prior to suture, and the accuracy of coaptation of the stumps. Variable portions of the lesion will be composed of scar tissue that is derived primarily from epineurial proliferation. The scar that usually thwarts successful axonal regeneration, however, derives from endoneurium and perineurium. With an excellent suture, the repair site will show occasional sworls of connective tissue and lost axons. Some axons may spread outside the fascicles and go into the thickened epineurium, while others remain intraneural but are interspersed with a disorganized proliferation of connective tissue. Nevertheless, an amazing quantity of axons do reach the distal stump, where they increase in caliber.[141] How, then, can the surgeon decide whether an average yield of regenerating axons is progressing distally or whether an anastomosis that appears technically good is simply coapting inert scarred nerve ends? Unfortunately, with sutures and with primary neuromas in continuity, one "cannot judge the book by its cover."

Nerve stimulation directly at the operating table provides objective evidence of axonal preservation (neurapraxia) or regeneration (axonotmesis) when distal muscular contraction occurs. This type of evidence

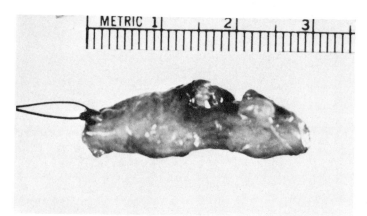

Figure 75–10 An ugly-appearing but unjustifiably resected "neuroma" of the ulnar nerve, removed three months postinjury near the elbow level. The surgeon disregarded preoperative electrophysiological evidence for partial function and did not test the nerve at operation. Histological study showed a profusion of preserved and regenerating axons distally. The uniquely poor results of ulnar nerve suture at the elbow were unfortunately imposed on this patient.

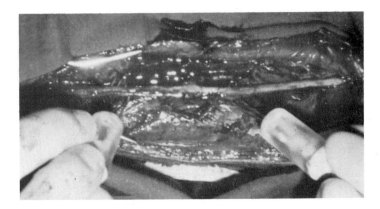

Figure 75-11 In contrast to the one shown in Figure 75–10, this lesion of the ulnar nerve (evidenced as a slight swelling at the center of picture) appeared benign. A bullet had passed nearby. But at three months postinjury no nerve action potentials were transmitted.

may antedate clinical return by as long as a month. This observation can be made without surgical exposure by percutaneous nerve stimulation, employing surface electrodes or needle electrodes inserted close to deep-lying nerve trunks.[108] If stimulation yields no response, then there is strong evidence of a complete lesion or lack of regeneration, provided enough time has elapsed to permit adequate regeneration to the first target muscles. At the operating table, the distal nerve can also be stimulated with the patient awake to see whether sensory fibers have regenerated through the injury. Since only a few regenerating axons can permit a positive response, only a negative response is important. Failure to find sensitive axons 2 cm below the lesion by six weeks after injury assures the operator that the intrinsic pathological change above is inconsistent with recovery.

If, at eight weeks postinjury, the exposed lesion is grossly consistent with neural continuity and there is some sensory perception from distal stimulation but no motor response, the capacity for recovery is undefined. The best choice is not to resect the neuroma at this time unless there is no nerve action potential. Later events (see discussion of time and distance in axonal regeneration) may define whether this lesion will permit better regeneration than would a suture.

Since many of these lesions can require six to eight months to define their potential, there is interest in studying in vivo evoked nerve action potentials as a method that can be used early to assess a neuroma in continuity.[74,75,78,148] After the surgeon inspects and palpates the exposed neuroma in continuity, bipolar stimulating and recording electrodes made of stainless steel or platinum alloy and shielded wire can be placed proximal to the lesion in continuity. Unless

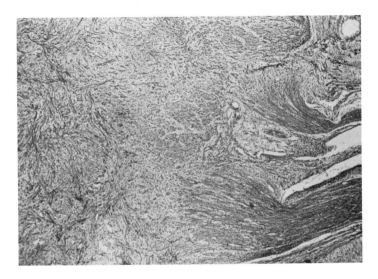

Figure 75-12 Histologically, this correctly resected lesion in continuity shows an intrinsic failure of axons (*on the right*) to penetrate a total cross-sectional segment of injury so severe as to result in permanent replacement of neural architecture by connective tissue proliferation.

there has been an element of stretch or in-continuity damage proximal to the area of focal and more apparent damage, a nerve action potential should be recordable. A stimulator that provides a stimulus of variable voltage and duration and that is also used to trigger the oscilloscope trace is necessary. Each stimulus will produce a trace on the oscilloscope and a shock artifact at the beginning of this trace. The duration of the stimulus must be brief or the shock artifact will encompass the evoked response, since distances used between stimulating and recording electrodes at the operating table are usually relatively short. One gradually increases voltage until an evoked response is apparent and then moves the more distal recording electrodes into the area of the lesion and watches the screen for change in the evoked potential. Electrodes are then moved distal to the lesion to see whether evoked potentials can be obtained. Ability to record potentials distal to the injury depends on the presence of moderate- to large-diameter fibers in the distal stump. Regenerated axons of this size usually produce functional return, and thus a potential recorded eight or more weeks postinjury suggests an excellent prognosis (Fig. 75–13).

If the injury was partial, that is, if it included a large element of neurapraxia, evoked responses may be recorded early. If the potential cannot be evoked through a neuroma in continuity after eight weeks, regeneration after axonotmesis is ruled out. With this evidence for neurotmesis, the lesion should be resected. But if a potential of good amplitude and velocity is obtained, the lesion should be left alone. If, on the other hand, many months have elapsed since the injury, ability to record an evoked potential alone may not be enough. Six or more months postinjury, the nerve action potential should be of good amplitude, and conduction and stimulation both proximal and distal to the lesion should produce function by muscles innervated by branches distal to the lesion itself if adequate regeneration is occurring. If these findings are not present, then resection and suture may still be necessary. This type of evaluation depends on a firm understanding of the timetable necessary for regeneration. Thus, the method is of most but not exclusive value at the time when distal targets could not possibly be reinnervated effi-

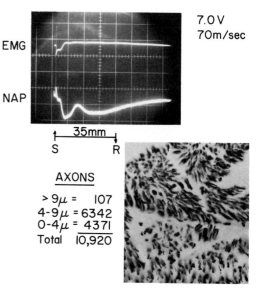

7.0 V
70m/sec

EMG

NAP

|← 35mm →|
S   R

AXONS

>9μ =   107
4-9μ = 6342
0-4μ = 4371
Total 10,920

Figure 75–13 The rationale for the method of electroneurography or nerve action potential (NAP) recording on exposure of primate tibial nerve 10 weeks after experimental crush injury. Although the electromyogram (EMG) shows no response in the gastrocnemius to nerve stimulation, the action potential response 35 mm below the injury indicates that excellent regeneration is under way. The microscopic picture in the lower insert (a cross section at the recovery site—Bodian × 100) samples the regenerating axon population; the total cross-sectional counts of axons show that most are moderate in size, to correspond with the action potential quantitation of good distal neuronal activity.

ciently enough to produce function. Evoked potentials provide semiquantitative information about the viable nerve fiber population at each recording site in the distal stump. The method must be used in conjunction with inspection, palpation, and stimulation, but is valuable at a time when distal neural targets cannot reflect the degree of regeneration upstream (cf. Figs. 75–8, 75–11, and 75–12).

The problem posed by the neuroma in continuity can be minimized by those who believe its dissection (i.e., neurolysis) will release the scar that impedes regeneration and hence solve the problem. But there is good theoretical and empirical evidence that subsequent regenerative events are already predetermined by the intrinsic configuration of the nerve lesion in relation to the grade of initial injury. If this is so (and this question of neurolysis is further considered later), complete operative exposure of a nerve lesion will not change the degree of axonal growth. To date, those lesions having an evoked potential in the early months following injury have fared well with external neurolysis alone. We have reserved internal neurolysis for partial lesions in which a portion of the nerve undergoes neurolysis and a portion undergoes direct suture or graft repair and for patients with noncausalgic pain associated with a lesion in continuity that does not require resection. Subsequent claims for the value of internal neurolysis in lesions that are complete and then recover following such a procedure should now be capable of substantiation by recording at the operating table.[77] If no nerve action potential is obtainable before internal neurolysis, and then recovery occurs before one could expect it by regeneration, this would prove that internal neurolysis can promote functional recovery.

At the time of the operation, the appearance of the lesion may not enable the surgeon to decide whether to resect a lesion that is in continuity. As a result, before beginning the operation the surgeon must know each nerve's function, the evidence for regeneration, and when this evidence developed. With this knowledge he can better predict what can be expected of the lesion if it is left undisturbed or if it is resected and sutured, with the inevitable imperfect regeneration that occurs after suture.

Time and Distance in Axonal Regeneration

The point has already been made that positive evidence for some significant nerve function, either initially or by six weeks postinjury, implies a favorable result. Except in partial lacerations, the nerve trunk is usually diffusely damaged throughout a cross-sectional segment, and intact as well as damaged motor and sensory axons are diffusely scattered through the area of maximal involvement. When a significant proportion of axons has escaped initial dysfunction or has suffered only neurapraxia, a major proportion of remaining axons will not have suffered the totally disruptive injury of neurotmesis. Rather, there will later evolve a degree of spontaneous regeneration, consistent with axonotmesis, that far exceeds what the best nerve suture can yield.

A problem in management arises in the more frequent situation of total nerve dysfunction in which either the lesion has not been operatively inspected or inspection has revealed a neuroma in continuity, or in which suture has been performed under uncertain circumstances. On the one hand, total transection or a degree of neurotmesis inconsistent with recovery can exist. Even with dysfunction that is total at six weeks, however, it is equally possible to have a lesion in which so large a proportion of the nerve is involved only in axonotmesis that spontaneous regeneration will far exceed the regeneration that can be predicted with even an ideal suture. The delay before the end result can be predicted is related to the slow progression of axonal regeneration. The same delay is encountered whether regeneration occurs spontaneously after axonotmesis at the time of injury or begins afresh after a nerve anastomosis.

In focal lacerating or contusive injuries, the earliest physical sign of regeneration of the nerve will occur in the most proximal muscles that can be reinnervated. Stretch injuries and ischemic injuries may permit sensory preservation despite total motor loss. In this case, however, there is usually no reason to elect to use operative treatment.

It is helpful to recognize that, despite the slow rate of axonal growth and maturation of motor function, regeneration proceeds at a definite rate if at all. Therefore, one may establish accurate deadlines in relationship to time of injury or suture for expecting signs of reinnervation. If the first target muscle begins to show function at the expected time and improves quantitatively in the next month or so, so as to parallel or exceed the expectancy after ideal suture, the decision against operative intervention is clear. If the expected time schedule is not met, or the subsequent early quantitative extent of motor activity in this first target muscle does not match the expectancy after suture, radical intervention is indicated even though the lesion appeared to have a favorable prognosis or the early suture appeared to be satisfactory.

The time for regeneration involves these considerations:

1. There is a delay before regenerating axons reach nerve distal to either injury or suture repair. This delay may amount to two weeks with axonotmesis and extend to

four weeks with suture. Most injuries cause an area of retrograde degeneration proximal to the injury site itself; this must be overcome, and then there is usually a delay of one or two weeks before axons can penetrate the injury or repair site and reach the distal stump.

2. Once the fibers have reached the distal stump, regeneration proceeds at an average rate of 1 mm per day or 1 inch a month. If the exact level of the nerve injury is known, one may calculate the time it will take for fibers to reach the muscle. There is variability in the level at which the branch of the nerve enters a particular muscle. This is true not only from patient to patient but also from one side of the patient to the other.[139] Sunderland has published a useful set of tables for calculating these regenerating distances; his work should be consulted for these values.[140,143]

3. There is a terminal delay of weeks to several months between the time when axons reach their distal targets and when sufficient maturation of the axons and their receptors occurs to permit maximal function (Fig. 75–14).[62,79]

Again, it is not enough for axons to reach distal targets, for they must do so in sufficient number and with enough caliber and myelination to produce acceptable function. In addition, as pointed out earlier, regenerating axons, in order to be effective, probably have to regenerate close to their original destination.[168]

It is of interest that injured nerves appear to regenerate more rapidly in children than in adults. Also, the rate of axonal growth decreases as the distance of the injury from the neuron increases. For example, regeneration through an ulnar nerve injured at the level of the axilla may proceed as fast as 3 mm per day, while regeneration through the same nerve with a lesion located at the level of the wrist may proceed at only 0.5 mm per day. The decrease in rate with the more distal lesion is probably due to increased distance from the feeding neuron in the spinal cord and not due to endoneurial scarring.

These theoretical considerations do not prevent the use of a guideline that clinical experience has shown to be useful: motor response on nerve stimulation always develops, if at all, by a deadline calculated on the overall growth rate of 1 inch per month. Visible movement on voluntary effort can take longer, and the development of maximal recovery of function continues for months after this beginning.

Early Proof of Adequate Regeneration

Up to this point, the discussion has concentrated upon the function of the most proximal muscles that are served by the injured nerve as being the first and best index of regeneration. Clinical motor testing is

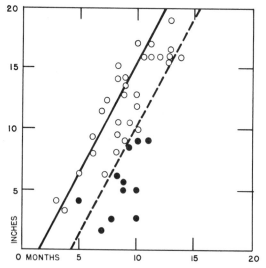

Figure 75–14   This table plots distance in inches from the point of ulnar nerve suture to the abductor digiti quinti muscle vs. time elapsed before this muscle first visibly contracts with nerve stimulation, this objective test being used at weekly intervals. The regeneration time is remarkably consistent with distance except where the ulnar nerve was transplanted (*black dots*). Here, a further delay occurs, as if regeneration had to start near the elbow even though the suture was performed in the distal forearm.

Rate=4.2 cm (1.7 inches) per month or 1.4 mm per day
"Lag"=1.2 months or 42 days

described under specific nerve lesions and is sufficient by itself when recovery is obvious. Clinically observed voluntary motor function must, however, be confirmed by motor response to nerve stimulation in situations in which anomalous innervation is possible or when "trick movements" using uninvolved muscles can simulate the action ascribed to the involved nerve. Absence of motor function on voluntary effort must be similarly confirmed by nerve stimulation because of the frequent delay between physiological motor recovery and the patient's capacity to activate and utilize the newly acquired function.

Nerve Stimulation

The technique of nerve stimulation is easily learned.[107,108] Unipolar or bipolar skin electrodes can be used for subcutaneously located nerve trunks (Fig. 75–15). Activation of deep nerves, like the radial and sciatic, requires that so much current be delivered to the surface electrodes that nearby muscles are stimulated directly and the stimulus causes discomfort. A stimulus of low intensity can be delivered to any nerve trunk by inserting two hypodermic needles close to its locus separated by 1 cm. A negative result should be checked by needle replacement. Also an adequate nerve stimulus proximal to the lesion will cause appropriate paresthesias in the areas

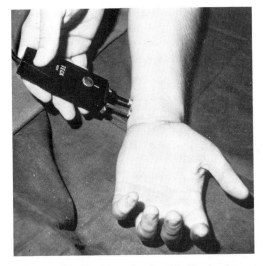

Figure 75–15 Use of a hand-held stimulator to stimulate the ulnar nerve at the level of the wrist. In this instance the examiner looks for hypothenar and adductor pollicis muscular function.

of sensory supply. Single shocks of short duration (1 msec or less) are the most comfortable, but the simple make-and-break shock of a 1.5-volt flashlight battery is an adequate stimulus for needle electrodes that are close to the nerve.

Nerves can also be stimulated at the operating table (Fig. 75–16). There are a number of disposable stimulators available, but if one is dealing with a regenerating nerve, the voltage supplied by such a stimulator may not be sufficient to evoke muscle contraction distal to the lesion. In this case, a stimulator that will provide a wider range of voltage and duration is necessary. One must be careful about mistaking muscle contraction due to stimulation of adjacent intact nerves or muscles for response in the distribution of the nerve being tested. To avoid this error it is helpful to elevate the nerve away from surrounding soft tissue when stimulating it. One also must be certain that the muscles contracting are distal to the lesion in question, for stimulation can, of course, be conducted retrograde as well as anterograde. Stimulation distal to an injury in continuity is less likely to produce proximal or retrograde conduction.

Electromyography

Electromyography, particularly if done in a serial fashion, can be a valuable adjunct to the management of peripheral nerve injuries. There will be no electromyographic activity immediately after total injury, but two to three weeks later fibrillations and denervation potentials can be recorded from denervated muscles. In addition, insertional activity on placement of the electromyographic needle will be reduced with denervation. With regeneration, insertional activity will begin to return, and the fibrillations and denervation potentials will decrease in number and sometimes be replaced with occasional nascent motor action potentials. Owing to the variable distance they have to travel, all regenerating nerve fibers do not reach motor end-plates simultaneously. As a result, individual muscle fibers discharge asynchronously, giving a nascent motor unit of multiphasic form and low voltage. These findings are the earliest electrical changes with muscle reinnervation. Unfortunately, they tell nothing of the eventual extent or quality or regeneration. When decreased fibrillations

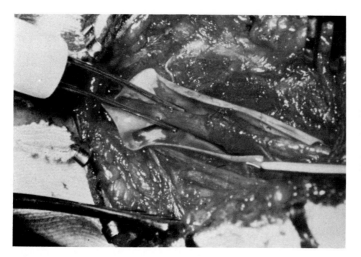

Figure 75–16 Operative stimulation proximal to pediatric radial lesion in continuity secondary to DPT injection by an automatic injector. At three months postinjury there was no brachioradialis contraction in response to operative stimulation, so lesion was correctly resected. (Courtesy of Dr. Glenn Meyer, Milwaukee, Wisconsin.)

and nascent potentials are found in the muscles innervated by an injured nerve, however, a *short* interval of further conservative management is suggested.

The electromyogram is important because it can give evidence of regeneration weeks or months before voluntary motor function is detectable.[36,84] Nevertheless, most patients who have enough regeneration to produce recordable nascent motor units also have contraction of that muscle upon direct stimulation of the nerve. Thus, in one group of 300 patients, most of whom had upper extremity nerve lesions, only 6 showed nascent potentials at a time when contraction could *not* be seen with simple nerve stimulation. Contraction and response to nerve stimulation occurred two to four weeks later in four of these six patients.[164] The electromyogram can detect retained motor units to indicate a partial lesion early after injury.[59,77] It is a sampling method whose value depends upon the thoroughness of the sample and the perseverance of the examiner. At best, it does not greatly enchance the ability to predict the adequacy of regeneration.

The presence of electromyographic changes suggesting reinnervation does not guarantee recovery of function, and as a result, the test must be weighed in conjunction with clinical and other electrical data. The test is of invaluable help in sorting out anomalous innervation such as occurs quite frequently in the hand. The authors' own experience with intraoperative stimulation and nerve action potential studies compared with electromyography indicates that

the latter is reliable if done by a well-trained, well-motivated examiner, but that it cannot provide absolute evidence for or against functional regeneration.

Electroneurography or Recording of Nerve Action Potentials

Electroneurography, or the recording of those nerve action potentials transmitted through a lesion, has already been described. This study involves operative exposure of the nerve trunk on either side of the lesion. Since ideally, one seeks to decide whether to suture a nerve by eight weeks after the injury, it becomes an important definitive test when the gross appearance of the neuroma in continuity is equivocal and the first target muscle is more than 3 inches downstream. It is an even more important diagnostic aid in lower extremity nerve lesions in which the first target muscle lie 6 to 8 inches below the lesion and neither nerve stimulation nor electromyography can settle the issue for six months or more (see Fig. 75–13). The test is of great help in sorting out brachial plexus lesions and also provides a useful index of how much of the proximal stump of the lesion in continuity to resect. The technique has been thoroughly described under Neuroma in Continuity and can be used for all such lesions regardless of the time interval between injury and exploration.

Experience over the last five years with computed nerve action potential recordings done at the skin level by summating hundreds of evoked responses has indicated that the technique is feasible though not as reliable as intraoperative nerve action potential recording (Fig, 75–17).[77] Electroencepholographic electrodes are placed along the dipole of the nerve at the skin level, and an attempt is made to stimulate the nerve distal to the lesion and to record an evoked response proximal to the lesion. More importantly, musculature distal to the lesion that does not contract voluntarily may do so to percutaneous nerve stimulation. The technique can provide early evidence of regeneration by showing an evoked response in the absence of distal muscle contraction with nerve stimulation. This noninvasive technique may pick up evidence favoring regeneration weeks to months before distal musculature will show reinnervational changes either electrically or clinically. Such computed nerve action potential recording depends on having two sites, one for stimulating and one for recording. These sites should be located along the dipole of the nerve relatively close to the skin surface, since there is a large decrement in evoked responses from level of nerve to level of skin.[41,54]

Tinel's Sign

False evidence for adequate regeneration can be obtained from the Tinel's sign. If paresthesias are obtained by distal nerve percussion, some continuity of sensory axons from the point percussed through the lesion to the central nervous system is suggested. If the response moves distally with time, and particularly if this movement is associated with diminished paresthesias in response to tapping over the injury site, evidence for continued sensory fiber regeneration down the distal stump is present. A positive Tinel's sign implies only fine-fiber regeneration, however, and tells the examiner nothing about the quantity or eventual quality of the new fibers. Some 75 per cent of the World War II soldiers who ultimately required resection and suture of nerve injuries had earlier shown an advancing Tinel's sign.[164] Henderson studied a large group of nerve injuries in a concentration camp where operation was not permitted. He found the Tinel's sign to be useful as long as it advanced rapidly along the distal stump and was not confined to the injury alone.[64] On the other hand, if no response is obtained and sufficient time has elapsed (four to six weeks) for fine-fiber regeneration to occur, then the absence of Tinel's sign is such strong evidence against regeneration as to constitute a significant negative finding.[107] In other words, the positive Tinel's sign is comparable to the finding of paresthesias on electrical stimulation of the distal nerve. It has no quantitative significance, but an absence of distal sensory response strongly suggests total neural interruption.

Sweating

Autonomic fibers are fine in caliber and, thus, regenerate rapidly. Return of sweating in an autonomous zone signifies regeneration. Sweating can be qualitated by a Ninhydrin test or by viewing small beads of sweat directly by means of the +20 lens of the ophthalmoscope.[8,70] As pointed out by Kahn,

. . . sebaceous material due to contact of the hands with the face or other areas of the body secreting sebum may be mistaken for sweat. However, the sebum appears as a fine silver substance which is not under the control of the sympathetic nervous system.[70]

Return of sweating may antedate sensory or motor return by weeks to months, but a return of sweating does not necessarily mean that sensory or motor function will

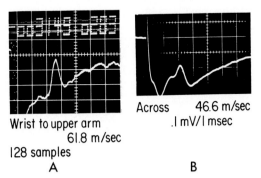

Across   46.6 m/sec

.l mV/l msec

Wrist to upper arm

61.8 m/sec

128 samples

A   B

Figure 75–17 *A.* Computed trace from median nerve made by stimulating at wrist and recording from upper arm. Conduction velocity and appearance of nerve action potential were normal. *B.* However, operative recording across small lesion in continuity complicated by pronator level entrapment due to contusion associated with a brachial arteriogram shows abnormal action potential with slowed conduction. Patient improved with section of pronator fascia and neurolysis, and did not require resection for relief of pain and ultimate recovery of satisfactory median nerve function.

follow. A test that is probably related to the presence or absence of sweating is the O'Rian wrinkle test. Normally innervated fingers, immersed in tepid water, will wrinkle after 5 to 10 minutes. With denervation, the fingers will no longer wrinkle, while with reinnervation, wrinkles will once again be seen.[114]

Sensory Recovery

True sensory recovery is a useful sign, but its evaluation can be difficult. One must be certain that observations are made in autonomous zones where the likelihood of overlapping innervation from adjacent uninjured nerves is minimal.[89,100,101,151] Autonomous zones for the ulnar nerve include the volar and dorsal surfaces of the forefinger and the volar surface of the thumb. The radial nerve does not have a reliable autonomous zone, but if there is sensory loss at all it will usually be found over the region of the anatomical snuffbox. Autonomous zones for the tibial nerve include the heel and a portion of the sole of the foot, while a less autonomous zone for the peroneal nerve exists over the dorsum of the foot (Figs. 75–18 and 75–19). In addition, sensory return in an autonomous area is a late development that follows the earliest motor return in a local contusion treatable by suture. Nevertheless, in the case of median nerve injury, sensory recovery can be the primary concern from the standpoint of practical function. The arrival of new sensory axons in a hand area short of the confined autonomous zone at fingertips can be recognized by sensory displacement. With initial testing, the patient sharply localizes the stimulus to another point within the median sensory area but often far removed from the actual stimulus site. This does not occur with overlapping innervation by neighboring nerves or with recovery from neurapraxia. Sensory displacement indicates that a regenerating axon has strayed into a sensory receptor that is remote from the one that the brain is accustomed to having it supply.

Two-point discrimination in the normal adult finger pad should span 3 to 5 mm. This can be tested simply with a bent paper clip or a pair of calipers. Values for return of good two-point discrimination for the palm as well as the sole of the foot are usually 6 to 10 mm, while those for the dorsal surfaces of the hand and foot are 7 to 12 mm.[112]

In summary, beginning neural recovery is proved by returning motor activity. Nerve stimulation may be required to be certain that motor function has returned. Definite sensory recovery in autonomous zones with sensory displacement can be important early evidence in distal lesions of major sensory nerves such as the median and tibial. Sensory recovery usually occurs relatively late and can be very misleading, particularly in the case of radial and peroneal nerves. An equally valid early proof for adequate regeneration is the ability to obtain nerve action potentials across the nerve lesion. In order to be absolutely certain, however, operative exposure is usually necessary, although experience with computed skin level recordings suggests that, in the future, reliable information might be obtained noninvasively in this way. Other qualitative evidence for neural regeneration is provided by Tinel's sign, electrical sensitivity of the distal nerve, and electromyography. If each of these sources fails to give even a slight bit of evidence favoring regeneration, then the negative evidence must be regarded as important. The same is true for failure to develop muscle contraction on nerve stimulation by the deadline that has been calculated after consideration of such factors as the distance that regeneration must cover. When this deadline is too far in the future, operative exploration will be necessary. Should a neuroma in continuity be found, the sur-

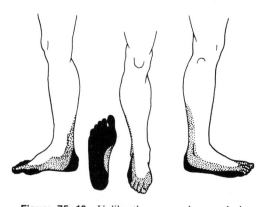

Figure 75–18 Unlike the peroneal nerve lesion, the complete tibial nerve lesion is associated with a major autonomous zone of absolute sensory loss that includes all the weight-bearing surfaces of the foot and toes. Prevention of a lifetime propensity to trophic ulceration is therefore the rationale for tibial nerve repair, even when no motor gain can be expected.

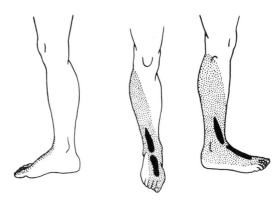

Figure 75–19 High peroneal nerve transection causes some sensory change through the large stippled area. Absolute or total sensory loss may be confined to the areas shown in solid black. The peroneal, however, like the radial, has sufficient inconsistency in its autonomous zone to negate attributing sensory improvement to its regeneration.

geon is best guided with regard to resection and suture by electroneurography (i.e., nerve action potential studies).[73a,73c] A final decision that the nerve injury is recovering as rapidly as it would after suture (or resuture) is possible when the first target muscle has developed motor action that is as strong as could be provided by suture. This quantitative judgment is possible by two months after the muscle first shows visible contraction on nerve stimulation. The importance of using several methods of electrical evaluation for lesions in continuity is demonstrated by Figures 75–20 and 75–21, while available electrical tests are shown in Figure 75–22.

Limitations of Regeneration in Time

The discussion thus far has implied that a nerve lesion showing inadequate evidence for regeneration or a disrupted nerve should be subjected to resection and suture. It therefore becomes important to define when the time for useful recovery through spontaneous regeneration has passed and also when nerve suture has little to offer. This is necessary so that if the nerve is not going to function again, the best ancillary procedures can be planned for rehabilitation. Although some nerves and muscles recover better than others and

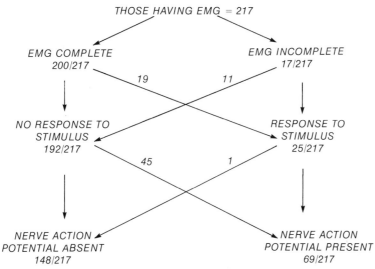

Figure 75–20 An illustration of the importance of several types of electrical tests. Note the transitions from complete to incomplete lesions and vice versa. Electromyograms (EMG) were performed in 217 of 295 lesions in continuity that appeared to be *complete* on physical examination and were subsequently operated upon. Seventeen were felt to be incomplete by electromyography. Of these, however, 11 had no distal response on operative stimulation. On the other hand, 200 of 217 in which electromyography was done had complete denervation in distal muscles, and yet 19 nerves responded to stimulation. Of the 192 having no response to stimulation, 45 had a nerve action potential across the lesion, indicating early regeneration. In all, 69 had an action potential, and as a result most of these subsequently had neurolysis rather than resection and suture.

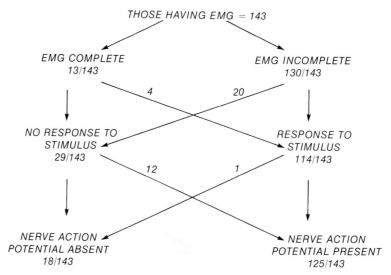

Figure 75–21 Transitions from incomplete to complete and back again are demonstrated as multiple electrical tests are used to evaluate lesions felt to be *incomplete* on physical examination. Of the 143 lesions in which electromyography (EMG) was done, 18 had no nerve action potential (NAP) and thus were felt not to be regenerating. These patients had resection and suture rather than neurolysis.

the percentage of strength required to make a muscle useful for practical function will vary, all are subject to virtually absolute, or "no-go," limitations when the duration of total muscle denervation exceeds 18 months.

The implications of this virtually absolute limitation on possible motor recovery are discussed later for each specific nerve injury at specific levels. A few examples at this point will help to clarify the use of this 18-month guideline. A peroneal suture in the thigh at a level more than 12 inches above the fibular head and delayed for 6 months or more cannot achieve a degree of motor recovery that will permit walking

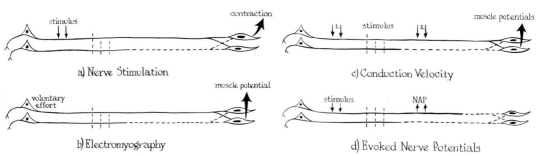

Figure 75–22 Summary of electrophysiological testing:

a. Nerve stimulation is one of the best tests for innervation distal to the injury. Muscle contraction suggests either a partial lesion or sufficient regeneration to reinnervate the motor end-plate. In either case, useful clinical function will usually follow in a few weeks.

b. Electromyography records muscle potentials upon voluntary efforts or upon stimulation of the nerve. Absence of muscle potentials coupled with fibrillations provides good evidence for denervation, while nascent muscle potentials or a decreased number of fibrillations is an early qualitative sign of reinnervation.

c. Conduction velocity can be obtained incident to studying electromyographic response to nerve stimulation at different levels. This is useful in recognizing the segment of nerve involved (by slowed conduction at that segment) where two sites of wounding or nerve entrapment can be responsible for partial dysfunction.

d. Evoked nerve action potentials (NAP) are recorded by stimulating proximal and recording distal to the neuroma in continuity. When done in the early weeks following injury, this test provides evidence for or against a partial lesion. When done 8 to 10 weeks or longer after injury, the evoked nerve action potential provides quantitative evidence for regeneration. This requires surgical exposure and guides choice of management of the lesion in continuity. (From Kline, D. G., and Hackett, E. R.: Value of electrodiagnostic tests for peripheral nerve neuromas. J. Surg. Oncol., 2:301, 1970. Reprinted by permission.)

without a lower leg brace or an ankle fusion to hold the foot in dorsiflexion. Similarly, if the peroneal nerve is transected only 6 inches above the fibular head but suture is delayed for 12 months after injury, the same result of 18 months of total muscle denervation will usually prevent useful recovery. In each instance, progression of Tinel's sign, appearance of motor signals on the electromyogram, and a barely visible muscle contraction on nerve stimulation may all occur on schedule, but the development of motor strength to a degree that will be useful will not occur.

When the site of injury is a long distance from an important muscle it is essential to perform the suture as early as possible. For example, when the radial nerve is injured in association with a closed midhumeral fracture, the probability for good spontaneous recovery is high. On the other hand, exploration should be undertaken if there is no recovery by three months, since if the radial nerve is seriously damaged between the fracture fragments, suturing it later than three months after the injury would begin to yield a less satisfactory result with motor function.

Exceptions to the 18-month rule may occur in a few lesions that have maintained some distal continuity. If some fibers are coming through the lesion, even though they are not enough to produce useful function distally, they may keep enough of the distal stump architecture relatively preserved so that very late suture after resection of the lesion can occasionally produce function. Thus, the authors have had experience with several patients who had sustained their injury years before but who nonetheless gained some recovery after greatly delayed suture because of partial reinnervation of the distal stump prior to suture repair. It must be stressed, however, that these cases are the exception rather than the rule.

By contrast, the surgeon must recognize when the distance between the nerve injury and the muscle to be reinnervated is such that nerve suture, early or late, will not accomplish the goal of a useful degree of motor recovery. Suture of the ulnar nerve near the axilla can accomplish little, as can suture of the peroneal nerve above the midthigh. Other high sutures may be indicated, either because there are proximal muscles whose recovery would be useful

(like the triceps muscle in the case of the radial nerve) or, as is discussed later, because sensory recovery would be valuable.

It should be understood that motor recovery from spontaneous regeneration (occurring without suture) has similar limitations in time. Even when a high lesion is of a severity that involves very little neurotmesis, but instead permits a major number of axons, suffering only axonotmesis, to regenerate, these will fall on barren soil if the muscle is over 18 inches downstream and is totally denervated by the injury. The slightest evidence for recovery of motor function, even if detectable only by the electromyogram, will greatly improve the prognosis, but the evidence for neuronal preservation must be evident by six weeks postinjury. Therefore, in terms of practical management, measures to compensate for lost motor function can be taken quite early. Tendon transfers or joint fusions can be done without awaiting the magical effect of a possible late regeneration from the high nerve lesions.

Sensory recovery is not subject to such severe limitations in time and may be falsely downgraded in many surveys of late results because the patient has not been followed long enough to gain maximal skin reinnervation. This is an important consideration in favor of suture of the median nerve as high as the axillary level even though it may only contribute minimal motor function at the forearm level. A high suture of the median nerve is particularly important if a mechanically useful hand can be provided by substituting the ulnar and radial motor function that does exist. Similarly, suture of the tibial component of the sciatic nerve at levels as high as the gluteal crease is indicated primarily for the protection to weight-bearing plantar areas that can be given by even a low-grade recovery of sensory function.

Implications for Management

Timing of Operation

Urgent need for prompt operative intervention in peripheral nerve injuries is unusual. The exceptions are an enlarging hematoma or an aneurysmal sac that converts a partial nerve injury into a complete and, with time, irreversible lesion unless the mass is removed. Certainly, a severely contused forearm or a distal humeral fracture associated with brachial artery injury predisposing to Volkmann's ischemic contracture constitutes another notable exception. Early fasciotomy, treatment of the vascular injury and associated spasm, and in some cases neurolysis of one or more nerves are necessary. A similar syndrome can involve the anterior compartment of the lower leg, and a similar degree of urgency is indicated if irreversible neural as well as muscular changes are to be avoided. In addition, a few cases have been encountered in which a missile or shell fragment has been embedded in nerve and has produced a severe noncausalgic pain syndrome, and in these cases considerable amelioration of pain has been produced by prompt operation and removal of the missile fragment. Injury to nerve in areas of potential entrapment may require relatively early release of the nerve and section of the offending connective tissue structure if less reversible changes are to be avoided.

Anastomosis of transected nerve ends at the time of wound closure can be considered in certain clean lacerations. These arguments favor primary repair:

1. The nerve stumps are easy to locate, since they are not bound down in connective tissue and their relationship to other injured structures usually is preserved.

2. The nerve stumps are minimally retracted. It is not necessary to mobilize the fresh stumps as widely as in the delayed repair, since the nerve ends will not have retracted as much.

3. The single operative procedure is definitive and may be the only operation that is necessary to repair soft-tissue as well as nerve injuries.

There are also strong arguments favoring a delayed or secondary repair:

1. Damage to the proximal and distal stumps has had time to define itself by visible intraneural scarring on cross section. The surgeon can be sure that he has resected back to normal neural tissue.

2. Associated injuries have had a chance to heal, infection has been eliminated, and the patient has learned to use his extremity before being subjected to immobilization and fresh discomfort.

3. The epineurium has thickened so as to permit a technically better suture.

4. The operation is elective and can be performed leisurely and accurately with trained personnel.

5. The distal stump is cleared of degenerating axoplasm and myelin. Also there may be some metabolic advantage to delay, since the neuron's regenerative activity becomes optimal in 10 to 21 days.

The argument for primary repair is valid in the case of simple, clean lacerating injuries.[57,75,129,143] The procedure, however, has to be managed as patiently and meticulously as an elective procedure and by an experienced surgeon who is willing to resect the contused nerve ends adequately before suturing them. As a result of the extensive experience in each of the major wars, the pendulum has swung toward secondary repair of most nerve injuries. Certainly, whenever there is any doubt about the nature of the injury or when there are complications of soft-tissue, vascular, or bony injuries, a delayed repair is best.*

Experience with civilian injuries has indicated that primary repair is best for sharply transected supraclavicular and axillary level brachial plexus and sciatic nerve injuries, for immediate exploration provides the best opportunity for both accurate identification of the elements involved and end-to-end repair without the need for grafts.[73a] This is especially so with sharp plexus injuries in which there is vascular damage that must be repaired at once. If the neurosurgeon explores such a wound site some weeks later, he is usually confronted by heavy scar that makes dissection and preservation of the vascular repair and identification of the involved neural elements difficult.

This is not to say that all transecting injuries at these levels merit primary repair. If the ends are ragged or contused, then delay is preferable, since in the short term, the surgeon will not know how much of either stump to resect to get back to what will eventually be a healthy neural cross section. The same argument can be used for proximal sciatic nerve transections. These rare guillotine-like transections involving musculature and other soft tissues as well as nerve can be readily repaired primarily; delay not only leads to a scar in the area but, inevitably, to stump retractions making end-to-end repair without the use of grafts difficult. Again, the surgeon must

---

* See references 47, 107, 123, 158, 164, 167.

make sure that the transection is a sharp, clean one. The authors' present philosophy with glass or knife wounds involving nerve is to inspect the lesion at once whenever they have the opportunity.[75,123] If the transection is a clean one, a primary repair can be done with at least as good results as with delayed secondary repair, provided the surgeon has the time, the necessary patience and help, good lighting, and proper instruments. On the other hand, if on immediate inspection, the stumps are contused or the epineurium is severed in a ragged fashion, then delay is in order. In this case, the stumps are tacked down to adjacent soft-tissue planes, the proximal stump being kept at a somewhat different plane than the distal stump. This maneuver will maintain length so that when secondary repair is done, a large gap will not have to be overcome.[73a]

Most military injuries are contusions or ragged lacerations. They should have a delayed repair.[138,157] Statistical analysis of World War II injuries indicated that a delay of three to four weeks between injury and repair had no adverse effect on the final outcome of the repair. Indeed, half of the repairs done on war-wounded nerves during the initial days after injury had to be resected and sutured again at a later date.[164]

When the nerve is not known to be transected, but is without function, especially following high-velocity missile wounding, secondary repair (i.e., delayed exploration) is strongly recommended. A delay of several months is in order, since this will permit any element of neurapraxia to resolve, associated injuries to heal, and most importantly, the surgeon to evaluate the lesion at the operating table in a physiological fashion. If adequate regeneration is occurring spontaneously, then activity can be picked up by means of nerve action potential recording techniques by 8 to 10 weeks postinjury. If a nerve action potential is present, the nerve will fare well with simple neurolysis, and resection and suture with all its limitations is not in order. By contrast, if a nerve action potential is not present and eight weeks have elapsed, then it is clear that recovery will not occur unless section back to healthy neural tissue and suture are performed.[73a]

Unfortunately, one of the major causes of delayed suture is delay in referral of the patient to a surgeon who has been trained to evaluate the lesion properly and to recognize that recovery is unlikely to occur without resection and suture. Relatively early referral requires education of not only the physicians with whom you consult but also as much of the medical community as possible. On the basis of the time limitations on motor regeneration, it can be argued that when a nerve suture is necessary it should be performed as early as possible; however, there is no conclusive evidence that sutures that are delayed up to three months after injury show a significant downgrading of motor recovery. In the case of high proximal lesions, exceptions may exist when an extra month's delay could make the difference in reinnervating an important muscle within the 18-month deadline.

Causes for Delayed Suture

Having defined the importance of securing anastomosis of transected nerves by no later than two months, it is worth reviewing the causes of excessive delay. Most important is the presence of extensive complicating injury to the extremity, which may require primary attention to clearing infection, to improving circulation, to resurfacing a large skin defect, or to securing healing of a fracture. While the extensiveness of an injury and the multiplicity of injuries to soft tissues and bone can downgrade the best possible result in a given situation, there are combinations of injury that downgrade the result purely because the nerve suture is left for last. For example, unless the management of the bony fracture unduly delays nerve exploration, it does not reduce the capacity for a sutured nerve to recover.[164] Therefore, it is desirable for the orthopedist and the neurosurgeon to work together, often in a combined operative procedure. If the injury involves the midhumerus and radial nerve, and a perforating wound prevents stable bony healing by six or eight weeks, the radial nerve can be readily sutured at the time of open reduction and fixation of the fracture. And if there is considerable loss of both bone and nerve substance, humeral shortening can be accepted as an aid in overcoming an extensive defect between the nerve ends. Similarly, the plastic surgeon and the neurosurgeon can work together when nerve suture is being delayed by an extensive skin defect that requires grafting. The nerve can be sutured much earlier if a combined operation is used. The anastomosis of the nerve should be covered with soft tissues as the plastic surgeon goes on to cover the defect with a split graft or a pedicle that has been prepared for transfer. The occasional occurrence of superficial infection after grafting procedures does not appear to disturb the progress of the underlying nerve that is regenerating through the suture.

The neurosurgeon himself is often to blame for delay in suturing the nerve because he has given weight to false evidence for nerve regeneration. For instance, the use of the hand may be improving only because the patient is compensating better for total dysfunction of one nerve. Anomalous motor supply, trick movements, or spotty electromyographic activity can falsely suggest neural recovery, as can Tinel's sign or shrinkage of an anesthetic area. Furthermore, the surgeon can be misled by his operative exploration when it discloses a neuroma in continuity that does not seem to be "too bad." He may disregard the absence of electrophysiological evidence for useful regeneration that should be manifest at this point in time and hope that his neurolysis will alter the course of events. Of course, it is impossible for neurolysis to help if the intrinsic architecture of the nerve segment is disrupted. When there is doubt about the need to section and resuture the nerve at the injury site, it is better to rely on such poor neural continuity as may exist when the suture is at a level so proximal or would be done at a time so delayed that this maneuver clearly has nothing to offer. The limitations on recovery with high proximal sutures and with combined nerve injuries are further discussed later for specific nerves.[28,143,164]

Technical Considerations

Unquestionably, failure to gain the average regeneration that should be predicted and expected after suture relates to overconservatism on the part of the surgeon. He is reluctant to resect scarred nerve ends back to normal nerve segments when this creates an extensive gap to be bridged. The gaps created before mobilization and suture were carefully recorded by neurosurgeons in World War II. It is important to recognize that downgrading of recovery did not occur with increasing gap until this exceeded 8 cm for most nerves and 10 cm for the ulnar nerve.[164] This analysis should therefore relieve the cautious surgeon's concern about the effects of extensive mobilization and transplantation of nerve segments and, short of causing a subsequent distraction of the repair, even the occurrence of some tension on the suture line itself. Clearly, suturing of a nerve will yield the best results when there is no cross-sectional area of inert scar to block a maximum downgrowth of axons from above or to prevent the maximum availability or receiving tubules distally. Both in concept and actual clinical experience, the need for apposition of healthy nerve ends far outweighs concern about the requirements for extensive dissection or mobilization and casting that may be required to achieve the ideal anastomosis.

On the other hand, the second leading cause of failure of suture repair to nerve is distraction. This makes skillful mobilization, transposition, and accurate but firm suture of the nerve stumps all the more important. If the repair is under too much tension, distraction is likely to occur, particularly if overflexion of the extremity is needed to gain end-to-end apposition. In this case, the surgeon should resort to short interfascicular nerve grafts utilizing an autologous nerve such as the sural, which can be sacrificed with minimal deficit.[98a,124] Experience with several hundred cases previously operated on by other surgeons has indicated that other factors leading to failure probably include manipulation of tissues that is not gentle, sacrifice of longitudinal vessels deep to the epineurial level, and intraoperative or postoperative stretch of the nerve. Poor repair or inability to achieve repair at all can also sometimes be traced to short incisions limited to the immediate injury site and dissection restricted to the immediate area around the injury.

SPECIFIC NERVE INJURIES

Median Nerve

Injury at Wrist

The most frequent site of median nerve injury is at the level of the wrist. The only motor loss is that of the intrinsic hand muscles. Therefore, any motor difficulty with finger flexion is likely to be due to tendon laceration and not to median nerve damage. The patient will have difficulty abducting and opposing the thumb owing to loss of function of the abductor pollicis brevis and opponens pollicis. Flexion of the proximal phalanx of the thumb is preserved, since the flexor pollicis brevis has usually a dual innervation from the ulnar as well as the median nerve.[103] In addition, the muscles of the thumb can readily "trick" the examiner into believing that opponens function is present. The abductor pollicis longus, which is innervated by the radial nerve, may institute an opposition-like movement, while the flexor pollicis brevis can give some flexion and a slight roll to the thumb. The movement of the thumb will be completed by the adductor pollicis, which is innervated by the ulnar nerve and in wrist level median nerve lesions by the flexor pollicis longus, which receives innervation in the forearm. Unless the examiner is observant and palpates the muscles and tendons as they contract, these movements of the thumb may trick him into believing that there is preservation of median nerve function.

A median nerve lesion at the wrist may also give loss of lumbricales function in the index and long fingers. Thus, when these two fingers are held in extension at the metacarpophalangeal joint, the patient will be unable to extend the second phalanx of the finger against resistance. A complete lesion of the median nerve at the wrist will give sensory loss in the median distribution, which includes the radial half of the palm, the palmar surface of the thumb and index and middle fingers, the radial half of the ring finger, and a variable portion of the dorsal surface of these fingers. Because of

overlap from both the ulnar and radial nerves, sensory loss usually is less than this classic pattern. The autonomous zone for median nerve innervation includes the volar surface of the terminal two phalanges of the index finger and the very tip of the thumb (Fig. 75–23). Sensory loss in the autonomous zone means median denervation, while return in that region provides hard evidence in favor of median nerve regeneration rather than overlap from another nerve.[89] Loss of autonomic fiber function will also give loss of sweating in at least the autonomous zone.

False judgment regarding retained function in the median nerve after wrist injury is likely to occur in nearly one third of cases. Opposition of thumb to fingers is so well managed (as just described) that the examiner is convinced some median function is preserved even though the sensory loss is complete. Despite reasonable opposition function, it should be evident that the thumb cannot be abducted perpendicular to the plane of the palm and that the most radial fibers of the thenar mass do not contract as this movement is attempted. The abductor pollicis brevis serves as an excellent marker muscle for the median nerve, since it receives its innervation distal to the wrist level and since it is invariably innervated by only the median nerve. One tests this muscle by placing an object such as a pen or pencil in the patient's palm and then asking him to raise his thumb against resistance and by keeping the thumb at right angles to the plane of the object. When the median nerve is not contributing to thenar muscle activity, final proof is given by nerve stimulation at the wrist. In this case no contraction of these muscles occurs on median nerve stimulation. All of the thenar

Figure 75–23 Initial sensory loss from median nerve transection usually follows the anatomical textbook pattern (*shown in dots*). But, very rapidly, total sensory loss becomes confined to the autonomous zone (*shown in black*). This shrinkage of sensory loss may falsely suggest median nerve regeneration, although the nerve remains transected.

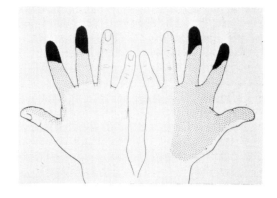

mass that the patient can contract with voluntary effort can be activated by ulnar nerve stimulation at the wrist. In this situation the individual is fortunate in having major flexor pollicis brevis innervation via the ulnar nerve.

If the median nerve is injured at the wrist, it is easily exposed where it lies between the tendons of the flexor carpi radialis and palmaris longus. It is separated from the lower end of the radius by the flexor pollicis longus and flexor digitorum profundus. After crossing the wrist level, it enters the carpal tunnel beneath the transverse carpal ligament. At the operating table, tendon injuries can be readily confused with injury to the nerve, and suture of a nerve stump to a tendon stump can occur all too readily. Use of a stimulator, if the injury is partial or fresh, may be helpful, as is the use of evoked potentials if one is dealing with a partial lesion or one that is in continuity. When operating upon injuries at or close to the wrist level, the transverse carpal ligament should be sectioned well down into the palm, for swelling of the nerve or tissues around it can, in this setting, lead to a secondary entrapment. Occasional wrist level lesions that cannot be repaired by an end-to-end technique may be candidates for a cross-anastomosis of the dorsal cutaneous branch of the ulnar nerve to the distal median nerve.[144] The technique seems possible, although Sunderland does not as yet cite any experience with patients who have had such a cross-union.

The interval between repair and recovery will depend upon the level of the injury to the nerve. After neurorrhaphy at the wrist level, sensory return may require four months. By four to five months, one should see some return of function of the abductor pollicis brevis or opponens pollicis muscles; however, visible contraction on nerve stimulation should begin by three months. Sensory loss is associated with a median nerve injury at any level. Reinstitution of sensory function is the primary reason for repairing the nerve, since this is essential for good hand function. The ability to use the thumb and fingers for fine mechanical tasks without visual aid involves re-education to overcome mislocalization of sensation on the fingers. Usually the re-education is acquired by well-motivated individuals, especially if the dominant hand is involved. Restoration of adequate thumb opposition is usual. When recovery is inadequate, opposition of the thumb can be achieved by a tendon transfer.

Injury at Elbow

Elbow level injury of the median nerve often will spare pronation of the forearm, since branches to the pronator teres muscle originate above the elbow. The forearm muscles that are innervated by the median nerve will be paralyzed, however. Of diagnostic, but not functional, importance is the fact that the flexor carpi radialis and palmaris longus will not tighten on attempts at voluntary wrist flexion. Attempts at making a fist will demonstrate flexor paralysis of the terminal index and long-finger phalanges (flexor profundus muscle) and middle phalanges (flexor superficialis muscle) and metacarpal phalangeal joints (both muscles). At times, however, the long finger will flex normally along with the ring finger, whose flexor profundus is supplied by the ulnar nerve and which may share a slip of tendon with that of the long finger. Flexion of the tip of the thumb is also lost (flexor pollicis longus muscle). These deficits lead to a so-called violin, or prelate, hand. In addition to the loss of flexor function of the forearm muscles, the same intrinsic hand muscle and median distribution sensory loss will occur as in more distal lesions of the median nerve.

In median nerve injuries at the elbow level, the proximal nerve may be readily located in the groove between the biceps and triceps muscles along the medial surface of the upper arm. At this point the nerve is in close relationship to the brachial artery and follows it across the flexor surface of the elbow beneath the lacertus fibrosus. Nerve branches to the pronator teres muscles are given off either high in the forearm or low in the upper arm, and these branches sometimes have to be sacrificed in order to gain enough length to perform a resection and repair of the nerve. As with wrist level lesions, relatively mild injury to the median nerve at the level of the elbow may be complicated by entrapment of the nerve beneath lacertus fibrosus and pronator teres fascia, and either or both of these structures may need to be sectioned to permit a swollen nerve to regenerate adequately.

As the median nerve passes beneath and sometimes through the pronator teres it

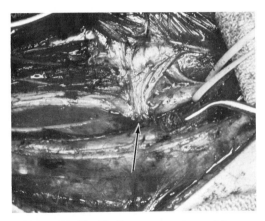

Figure 75–24 Median nerve entrapped by scar and callus secondary to fracture of radius at mid-forearm level sustained six months earlier. Exposure was gained by identifying the nerve at elbow level, transecting the pronator fascia, and tracing the nerve beneath the flexor superficialis, some of whose fibers were split. A nerve action potential could be recorded across the lesion despite a complete distal median palsy. Neurolysis with reduction of the callus and removal of scar, and further time led to significant sensory and motor recovery.

gives rise to the anterior interosseous nerve, which supplies the long flexor of the thumb (flexor pollicis longus) and the flexor digitorum profundus to the index and long fingers. Entrapment at this level gives the anterior interosseous syndrome, characterized by weakness in the flexor pollicis longus and the flexor profundus to the forefinger, resulting in a characteristic "pinch attitude" of the hand.[137] Since there may be a connection between the anterior interosseous nerve and the ulnar nerve, or a Martin-Grüber anastomosis, paralysis of some of the intrinsic muscles of the hand such as the interossei and lumbricales may also result. The syndrome is usually due to the tendinous origin for the deep head of the pronator teres, which can crease the anterior interosseous nerve at its origin from the median nerve trunk. Distal to the antecubital fossa of the forearm, the median nerve dives deep between the superficial and deep flexors of the forearm, and although mobilization distal to this point is possible, it is limited by the tethering effect of the branches going to these muscles. When repairing the median nerve at the level of the elbow, it is best to gain length by mobilizing the nerve toward the axilla. Transposition of the median nerve is not a useful way to make up length. In the upper half of the forearm the median nerve is situated deep

in the soft tissues. It is best to explore it by using more easily exposed proximal and distal nerve trunks as a guide to dissection through muscle planes and bridges (Fig. 75–24).

The first motor function to return after repair of the median nerve at the level of the elbow will occur in the flexor carpi radialis and the palmaris longus muscles. This return of function occurs about two months following suture. Flexion of the index finger should return by four months and flexor pollicis longus muscle function should come by six months, but abductor pollicis brevis and opponens pollicis function as well as return of sensation will require 10 to 12 months. Because of the irreversible effects of prolonged denervation, many patients with an elbow level injury of the median nerve may require tendon transfers to obtain thumb opposition. Sensory function can still be satisfactory.

Injury at Axilla

Injury to the median nerve at the level of the axilla is frequently associated with injuries to the brachial artery and to the ulnar and radial nerves. A complete injury of the median nerve at the axilla gives a loss of function of the pronator teres muscles in the forearm as well as the deficit described for an injury at the elbow level. Since the median nerve originates from the medial and lateral cords of the brachial plexus, total injury to one of these cords may mimic a partial median nerve deficit. Lateral cord damage results in a median distribution sensory loss but also is often accompanied by biceps loss, and thus it may be differentiated from a partial lesion to the median nerve at the level of the axilla. By comparison, medial cord injury can give a partial median nerve motor deficit that affects the intrinsic muscles innervated by the median nerve, all the ulnar-innervated intrinsic muscles of the hand, the forearm muscles innervated by the ulnar nerve, and ulnar sensory loss as well. Thus it can be readily differentiated from a partial median nerve lesion.

The median nerve may be traced proximal to its location in the groove between the biceps and triceps muscles along the medial surface of the middle third of the upper arm. As one dissects proximally, the nerve is adjacent to first the brachial artery and then the axillary artery.

Results with repair of median nerve injuries at the level of the axilla are quite poor, since it takes at least 6 months after suture for contraction to develop in the flexor carpi radialis and 15 months for sensation to return in the median nerve distribution of the fingers and palm. Reinnervation of the thenar eminence muscles is never adequate, and tendon transfers usually are necessary to provide some degree of thumb opposition.[111,136] Exceptions occur primarily because of generous ulnar nerve supply to thenar muscles. Nonetheless, injury to the median nerve at this level should be explored and repair should be attempted because this provides the best chance for sensory reinnervation of the hand as well as a chance for thumb and index finger flexion. Undue delay in repairing median nerve lesions compounds the already existing delay imposed by distance for regeneration.

Functional results following suture of the median nerve can be related to the level of the repair. In the World War II experience of the British, useful abductor pollicis brevis function returned in 32 per cent of patients who had a repair of the median nerve at the wrist level, but in only 19 per cent of patients with a repair at the axillary level.[127] Sensory return occurred in a little over 50 per cent of patients. In a comparable American series, return was recorded as averaged percentage of normal function and was approximately 59 per cent for motor and sensory return in the entire group who had repair of the median nerve.[164] The clinical suggestion of return of hand muscle function in high lesions was disproved by nerve stimulation.

Ulnar Nerve

Injury at Wrist

At the wrist level, the ulnar nerve is often injured where it lies just radial to the flexor carpi ulnaris tendon. It divides into superficial and deep branches as it passes the pisiform bone. The superficial branch innervates the motor muscles of the hypothenar eminence and carries sensation to the ulnar half of the hand, whereas a deep palmar branch runs beneath the flexor tendons to reach the adductor pollicis and the first dorsal and palmar interosseous muscles. The usual wrist laceration results in injury proximal to these branches and causes sensory loss over the hypothenar eminence, the volar and dorsal surfaces of the little finger, and the ulnar half of the ring finger. The autonomous zone for the ulnar nerve includes the palmar surface of the distal one and one half phalanges of the little finger (Fig. 75–25). Although anomalous innervation of hand muscles occurs frequently, this lesion will almost always cause weakness of the hypothenar eminence muscles, which is characterized by loss of abduction and opponens function of the little finger. In addition, there will be paralysis of the first dorsal interosseous and the adductor pollicis muscles. The first dorsal interosseous muscle abducts the index finger from the long finger, while the adductor pollicis brevis muscle adducts the thumb against the radial side of the palm. With dysfunction of the ulnar nerve, on attempted adduction of the thumb, the flexor pollicis muscles will move the thumb toward the palm, and the resultant flexion of the phalanges of the thumb provides the basis for a positive Froment's sign. The major deficit with ulnar nerve injury at this level is inability to extend the phalanges of the ring and little fingers, which causes a claw deformity (Fig. 75–26). This apparently paradoxical situation results because the ulnar-innervated intrinsic muscles (lumbricales) are unable to stabilize the metacarpal phalangeal joint. Because of this instability, the extensor muscles that are innervated by the radial nerve pull the metacarpal phalangeal joints into extension so that their action is wasted in extending the more distal phalanges.

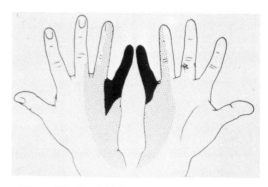

Figure 75–25 Initial sensory loss from ulnar nerve transection usually follows the anatomical textbook pattern (*shown in dots*). But, very rapidly, total sensory loss becomes confined to the autonomous zone (*shown in black*).

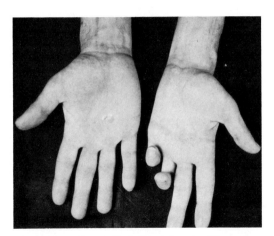

Figure 75–26 Typical claw deformity. The patient is attempting to extend all fingers, as he is doing with the normal hand. Until contractures develop, the fourth and fifth fingers can be voluntarily extended if the metacarpophalangeal joints are passively held in mild flexion.

Thus, the claw deformity results. Before fixed contractures occur, the patient can fully extend his fingers if the metacarpal phalangeal joints are held in mild flexion by the examiner or by a dorsal splint that is designed to prevent a fixed contracture.

With obvious ulnar nerve dysfunction, the existence of some function is best established by preservation of sensation in the fifth fingertip or by visible contraction in the belly of the abductor digiti quinti or first dorsal interosseous muscle. Nerve stimulation will settle any uncertainty as to muscle action and will define the occasional situation in which muscles that are presumed to be supplied by the ulnar nerve are controlled by fibers passing through the distal median nerve. This situation is suggested by a discrepancy between motor and sensory findings. The degree of claw hand formation is variable, and even the experienced examiner cannot discern whether buried muscles, such as the adductor pollicis, are functioning partially.

Exposure of the nerve in the distal forearm near the wrist is not a simple matter, for it lies deep to the flexor carpi ulnaris tendon and is closely approximated to the ulnar artery. Nerve and artery then emerge from beneath the tendinous attachment of the flexor carpi ulnaris to the pisiform bone. Both vessel and nerve pierce the deep fascia and cross the flexor retinaculum and the pisohamate ligament lying between pisiform bone medially and the hook of the hamate bone laterally. They pass beneath the superficial volar carpal ligament and the palmaris brevis, which must be sectioned to expose the nerve in the palm of the hand. It is at this level that both nerve and artery divide into superficial and deep divisions. Guyon's canal is formed by these anatomical structures, and entrapment of the nerve may occur at this level and may stimulate a more proximal or cubital tunnel level of involvement. Some length may be gained by mobilizing the nerve up the forearm where it travels between the two heads of the flexor carpi ulnaris. Gaps of over 5 cm at the level of the wrist, however, generally require mobilization of the proximal nerve to above the elbow and its transposition so as to gain length with elbow flexion. Gaps of nearly 10 cm can be overcome in the lower forearm or wrist level by a combination of mobilization, transposition, and flexion at both wrist and elbow.

Motor recovery after suture is unpredictable in terms of whether it solves the problems of mechanical function. When the nerve must grow 2 inches from a wrist suture, the abductor quinti muscle will have visible contraction on nerve stimulation by three months, and the first dorsal interosseous muscle will recover by six months. Yet, it is not certain whether the patient will regain the ability to set just his lumbricales to permit extension or unclawing of the fourth and fifth fingers. Ultimately, if needed, metacarpal phalangeal joint stabilization can be provided by tendon transfers, and the patient will have a useful hand for grasping objects after opening all fingers (and will have retained good thumb opposition to the long and index fingers). Graded separation and adduction of all fingers, as is needed for typing or piano playing, will remain a problem. These functions are assisted by tendon transfers also. Sensation to the little finger returns adequately, beginning by three months.

Injury at Elbow

At the elbow, the ulnar nerve has left the median nerve and brachial artery to enter the olecranon notch behind the medial epicondyle. After passing through the notch, the nerve enters the forearm between the two heads of the flexor carpi ulnaris, which is the first muscle that it innervates. Injury at this level may or may not result in flexor carpi ulnaris paralysis, since branches supplying this muscle frequently arise in the distal upper arm. With flexor carpi ulnaris paralysis, there is slight radial deviation of the wrist with attempted flexion of the hand on the forearm, and one cannot detect tightening of the tendon. Paralysis of flexion of the distal phalange of the little finger also results. In addition, flexion of the distal phalange of the ring finger may be weak, although seldom completely absent, since the tendon to this finger usually shares a slip with the median-innervated tendon to the adjacent long finger. There is no evidence of the functional deficit when making a fist, and careful testing is required to show that only the flexor profundus to the fourth and fifth fingers is not operating. In addition, there is sensory and intrinsic hand muscle loss, as was described for lesions at the level of the wrist.

It is necessary for the operating surgeon to understand the usual anatomical relationships of the ulnar nerve at the level of the elbow, since transposition of the nerve is frequently necessary. As the nerve descends into the distal upper arm, it separates from the brachial artery and median nerve to pass into the posterior compartment, where it lies beneath the medial intermuscular septum. This structure must be divided before the nerve is transposed volar to the elbow. In addition, in some patients, there is a connective tissue connection running between the medial intermuscular septum and the medial head of the triceps called the arcade of Struthers. This arcade can be responsible for either median or ulnar nerve entrapment, but even if this is not the case, the connection must be sectioned when transposition is done. As the ulnar nerve approaches the level of the elbow, branches running to the proximal flexor carpi ulnaris usually arise and can be spared by gently splitting them away from the parent trunk by using magnification and microdissection. Arteries and veins are in close approximation to nerve at this level, and judicious use of a bipolar coagulator is necessary to avoid direct trauma to the ulnar nerve as it is moved out of the cubital canal. If a graceful transposition without tension is to be gained, branches to the joint need to be sacrificed as well as an occasional lone distal branch to the flexor carpi ulnaris. Vasculature between the floor of the olecranon notch and the nerve itself

must also be handled with the bipolar coagulator. Distal to the notch, the ulnar nerve runs beneath the two heads of the flexor carpi ulnaris, and these must be transected, care being taken to spare flexor profundus branches arising from the lateral and deep aspect of the nerve. In the authors' experience, there is no substitute for deep burial of the ulnar nerve beneath the pronator teres muscle if a transposition is to be done. This requires sectioning of pronator teres fascia and muscle and hollowing out of a canal to place the nerve in. By releasing pronator fascia laterally as well as over the medial epicondyle, closure of pronator musculature over the nerve can be gained. At the conclusion of the procedure, one should be able, with the arm extended, to gently tug on either the proximal or distal portion of the ulnar nerve and move it back and forth through the transposition site with ease.

When resection results in two stumps, transposition can be achieved by sacrificing some of the articular branches and branches to the flexor carpi ulnaris and transposing the longer segment of nerve beneath the pronator teres muscle. The muscle must be sectioned and resutured if the nerve ends meet beneath it. With transposition, care must be taken to split the connective tissue raphe of the intermuscular septum of the upper arm. If this is not done, the nerve will buckle around this raphe and further injury will occur.

As with ulnar nerve lesions at the wrist, it is important to realize that, although innervation will readily occur, it is difficult to obtain from suture the type of reinnervation that will permit fine finger and hand movement in a synergistic, coordinated fashion. Nearly all patients will need tendon transfers to supply extension of the fourth and fifth fingers.

Injury at Axilla

In the axilla, the ulnar nerve arises from the medial cord of the brachial plexus; injury at this level gives a complete ulnar palsy much like a lesion at the elbow level and often includes a partial median nerve dysfunction, as described earlier. It is in close relation to the brachial artery and median nerve, for which the operative exposure has been described.

Owing to the distance from axilla to

hand, regeneration is poor. Reinnervation of ulnar-innervated forearm muscles alone means little functionally, since the intrinsic hand muscles will not be reinnervated and sensory return to the fifth finger is of minor importance. Nonetheless, some high ulnar repairs, particularly in children, have fared remarkably well, and there is little to lose, provided the procedure is done carefully enough not to injure other neural or vascular structures. Tendon transfer to prevent clawing of the fingers is the most important operative procedure for a high ulnar nerve injury. Suture should be undertaken, for what it is worth, only in situations of total discontinuity of nerve ends.

Following ulnar repair at all levels, restoration of some function was achieved in an average of 73 per cent of patients in the American series of World War II, which compares favorably with functional motor return at five years in the British series.[127,164] The strength of muscles that could be tested does not reflect the practical handicap, however, for only 16 per cent of the patients regained independent and coordinated finger movement. If some degree of extension of the ring and little fingers can be provided by a tendon transfer, the functional ability of the hand will be increased greatly.

Median and Ulnar Nerves Combined

This example of combined nerve injury is presented in detail because the combination of nerves is the one most frequently injured and because the resulting hand dysfunction presents unique problems. There are excellent discussions of the problem of multiple nerve injuries available.[104,122] In addition to the neural deficit, extensive soft-tissue, vascular, and bone damage is a much more likely accompaniment than with single nerve injury. In the World War II experience, an injury to the median nerve was associated with an injury to another nerve in 58 per cent of cases, whereas with injury to the ulnar nerve, the association was 40.2 per cent, and with the radial nerve, 32.8 per cent.[164] Owing to a difference in severity of wounding agents, civilian incidence of combined neural injuries is not as high, but when seen is equally disastrous.

Combined median and ulnar nerve injury commonly occurs with an extensive laceration across the wrist. In addition, the two nerves are in close proximity throughout the upper arm. Even with the distal wrist lesion, a virtually useless hand results from their combined dysfunction. All fingers share in loss of ability to open and show the same clawing deformity that affects only the fourth and fifth fingers with ulnar nerve lesions. If reinnervation can be achieved only by suture of both nerves, this serious deficit will not be corrected and will be manageable only by tendon transfers or fusions that stabilize the metacarpal phalangeal joints. Equally disabling is the total absence of intrinsic thenar muscle control. Not only is thumb opposition lost, but the thumb cannot be swept across the palm with either the short flexor or the adductor pollicis. Useful opposition is far less likely to occur after suture of both the nerves than after repair of one of them because the necessarily incomplete recovery of opponens and abductor pollicis brevis can be aided only by an equally imperfect flexor pollicis brevis. The probability of a hand with good practical function resulting after such a combined injury is only 5.3 per cent. Suture of both nerves at the wrist is nevertheless worthwhile in providing sensation and some useful thenar muscle function. Tendon transfers may provide a hand that can grip and that can pick up objects between the thumb and first two fingers.[86,117]

At higher levels of injury, the end results become increasingly dismal, but even axillary level suture of both nerves is worth undertaking, since there is the possibilty of a degree of sensation in fingertips and a degree of thumb-to-finger action (usually requiring supplementary tendon transfers and fusions) that can make the hand as functional as a prosthesis.

It should be mentioned that multiple lesions to the same nerve also carry a poor prognosis. Even when two separate lesions are in continuity and a fair degree of spontaneous regeneration is possible, there is a permanent axon dropout at each site. If the regeneration must occur through two suture lines at different levels, the total axonal loss is so great that useful motor recovery is unlikely, although sensory recovery remains possible. In addition, those axons that manage to span multiple levels of injury seldom take on enough caliber or myelination to produce useful function. This experience makes it less likely that lengthy nerve grafts to mixed nerves will provide adequate function, since in addition to the transit time required through the graft, new axons are subjected to the same limitations as the nerve that must be sutured at two different levels.

Radial Nerve

In striking contrast to median and ulnar nerve injuries, sensation is of no functional and of limited diagnostic importance with radial nerve injuries. There is no autonomous zone for radial sensation, although there may be loss over the anatomical snuffbox and the dorsum of the hand with such an injury. Even total transection of the nerve may cause no sensory deficit, owing to overlap from the median and ulnar nerves. Since radial sensation is of no functional importance, the transected superficial sensory radial injury at forearm or wrist level should usually not be repaired, for this may lead to a neuroma and painful parethesias in the back of the hand. Rather, such an injury should be treated by wide resection of the superficial sensory nerve, as should lesions in continuity that may produce painful paresthesias.

Injury at Elbow

Near the elbow, the radial nerve is susceptible to injury by deep lacerating and penetrating wounds. Furthermore, more distally it becomes closely associated with the head of the radius, where fractures commonly involve it. All forearm extensor function is lost. There is usually a complete wrist-drop, but occasionally patients are able to utilize the brachioradialis muscle to achieve some wrist extension. It is clear to the examiner that only a single radially located extensor tendon is acting and that none of the forearm muscles are contracting to assist in this movement (over the long term many patients are able to achieve quite strong wrist extension using only this muscle). Second, there is inability to extend the fingers at the metacarpal phalangeal joints owing to loss of extensor digitorum function. The distal phalanges of the fingers can be straightened by intrinsic hand muscles, and some passive metacarpal phalangeal joint extension can be achieved by flexing the wrist. But if the ex-

aminer holds the wrist in neutral position, it becomes obvious that the extensor tendons in the dorsum of the hand are not tightening actively and that the proximal phalanges of the fingers are not being extended. Third, loss of the long abductor to the thumb makes it impossible to abduct the thumb in the plane of the hand, although it can still be abducted forward of the palm by the abductor pollicis brevis. At the same time, the extensor pollicis longus cannot extend the distal phalanx of the thumb, but this can be extended passively by abducting the thumb at right angles to the palm with the normal short abductor. Accordingly, in many total radial nerve injuries, it is incorrectly believed that there is retained function in the extensor pollicis longus. The examiner must hold the thumb in the plane of the hand; it then becomes clear that neither is active extension of the thumb tip possible, nor tightening of the dorsal thumb tendons. As already mentioned, sensory preservation in the anatomical snuffbox should not prevent a conclusion that the radial lesion is a total one when there are no signs of forearm extensor muscle function.

Operative exposure above the elbow involves discovering the nerve deep between the brachioradialis and the biceps and brachialis muscles after it has penetrated from behind the lateral intermuscular septum to reach the lateral anterior compartment of the distal upper arm. Because of its depth, surface electrical stimulation of the radial nerve is technically difficult. On the normal arm, the part that best activates finger extensors can be discovered in a line directly lateral to the humerus and about 4 inches above the lateral epicondyle. If no response is obtained on the injured side, needle electrodes should be inserted close to the humerus at this point. Proximal nerve activation that causes no motor response is presumed to have been adequate only if paresthesias into the dorsal part of the thumb attest that the nerve has been stimulated. A deep, confined stimulus may be necessary to detect the earliest forearm extensor activity because to be adequate a surface stimulus must be so intense as to produce direct stimulation of brachioradialis and biceps, making it difficult to recognize weak distal motor response. The surgeon who is unaccustomed to exposing the deep radial nerve at this level is well advised to prepare his patient prior to induction of general anesthesia by locating the nerve by needle insertions so that he can make the exposure by following the needle. Moving distally, the nerve continues deep to cross the capsule of the elbow joint, where it lies beneath the brachioradialis muscle and divides into a superficial radial sensory and a posterior interosseous motor branch. The latter nerve penetrates between the heads of the supinator muscle and promptly divides into a shower of multiple small branches to all extensors. The posterior interosseous nerve can be injured at supinator level by soft-tissue contusion, fractures of the radius, or on rare occasions, a ganglion arising from the elbow joint or from spontaneous entrapment. Sensation over the dorsum of the hand will be spared, as will usually some degree of wrist dorsiflexion, but finger and thumb extension will be absent. Suture repair distal to this level is most difficult, but neurolysis, if necessary, for the rare entrapment occurring on the dorsum of the forearm is possible. The search for distal twigs to suture to a branching central nerve trunk is an exercise in frustration that rarely pays off. A better alternative is to wait the few months needed to define the extent of spontaneous motor recovery with these distal lesions and then to provide missing movements by tendon transfer. A gap of 4 to 5 cm can be overcome by flexing the elbow after mobilization of the nerve segments.

Sutures of the entire radial nerve trunk, at any point above this site of branching near the head of the radius, yield outstanding functional recovery. The radial has the least sensory component of the major mixed nerves, so a greater number of motor axons find distal tubules destined for muscle receptors. "Shuffling" of motor reinnervation is not a problem because it is functionally useful to initiate action in all the wrist and finger extensors at the same time.

Except for wrist dorsiflexion, nearly normal strength is not required; there is little handicap if all fingers can be extended with only 20 per cent strength. Wrist extension should begin by six months; thumb extension can require nine months. These may be inadequate but are remediable by tendon transfer. Ironically, this nerve is of no sensory importance, and the motor deficits can be most readily overcome by tendon transfers; but at the same time, the yield from suture of the main radial trunk is so good that its repair deserves first choice except at the forearm level of multiple branching distal to the supinator.

Injury at Midhumeral Level

Midhumeral injuries deserve special consideration, both those resulting from perforating wounds and those resulting from the nerve's involvement in fractures of the humerus, to which it is closely applied. The special situation of high likelihood of spontaneous recovery after total paralysis with humeral fracture has been previously described, but a failure at six weeks to detect any evidence for neurapraxia in terms of forearm extensor function on voluntary effort or on nerve stimulation or by electromyogram suggests that a major proportion of the nerve may well be involved in neurotmesis due to entrapment in the fracture. The clinical findings are identical to those described for injuries at the elbow level, except that the brachioradialis is usually totally involved (and in this case its beginning recovery at six weeks would speak for further watching).

Operative exposure of the radial, or musculospiral, nerve at this point does not require transecting the triceps muscle to follow its spiral course. Rather, the proximal and distal nerve trunks should be exposed by separate high medial and low lateral incisions. The medial neurovascular bundle is exposed near the axilla (stimulation being used for nerve identification), and the radial nerve is discovered deep to and behind the ulnar nerve. This medial incision plane is developed vertically and as far distally in the mid–upper arm as it can assist in pursuing the radial nerve as it spirals laterally and posteriorly between humerus and triceps. Then, a midlateral incision is developed in the distal upper arm to disclose the distal radial trunk between brachioradialis and biceps and brachialis, as described earlier. The dissection is carried proximally by vertically extending the lateral incision until the two fields of dissection meet in a plane behind the midhumerus and in front of the triceps.

In some cases, neural continuity may be discovered, and if direct stimulation or evoked potential recording provides evidence of early return of function, only a neurolysis is necessary. More often, when there has been no recovery after closed fractures, the proximal medial portion of the radial nerve disappears into the fracture site and the distal lateral nerve emerges from it with at least a 6-cm gap to be overcome. Direct deep wounding of the nerve at this point also usually involves a considerable loss of nerve substance. If the nerve ends, after adequate section, cannot be easily approximated for suture in this locus behind the humerus, mobilization of proximal nerve through the axilla to yield length on shoulder adduction, and mobilization of distal nerve beyond the elbow to yield length on elbow flexion, may solve the problem. If not, the distal nerve can be freed down to its passage through the supinator and redirected just anterior to the distal humerus beneath the biceps to oppose the proximal nerve end in the medial incision, effecting a 5-cm gain by this anterior transposition. A further alternative occurs when a high-velocity missile has destroyed a segment of the humerus along with the radial nerve. Here it is reasonable to accept humeral shortening with apposition of healthy bone ends as a means of also securing apposition of healthy nerve ends in which an extra 3 to 5 cm can permit a good suture. The tendon transfer alternatives for radial motor paralysis are so effective, however, as to contraindicate shortening of an intact humerus to secure radial suture (unless median or ulnar nerves are also involved).

The results after midhumeral suture of the radial nerve are good and are not too different from the excellent recovery that can be expected with more distal sutures. Function of the brachioradialis should return early (unless its branches were sacrificed for transposition). The extensor carpi muscle complex should begin to function by four months, and finger extension by six to nine months. A further delay (up to 9 to 12 months) required for reinnervation of thumb extensors and abductors makes their inadequacy more probable.

Injury at Axilla

At the axillary level, the triceps will be almost or entirely denervated in addition to the motor loss that was defined previously. Multiple nerve injury and brachial artery involvement are likely accompaniments. Diagnostically, the possible preservation of slight triceps function from high branches should not, by itself, argue against the probability of nerve transection or a total neurotmetic lesion.

Operative exposure of the radial nerve near the axilla has already been described. Extra nerve length to achieve suture is obtained by both mobilization beyond the axilla to gain length by shoulder adduction and distal mobilization past the elbow (possibly to include transposition).

An average radial nerve suture at the axillary level should provide excellent triceps muscle function by three months but will take over six months to reinnervate forearm extensors. A useful result after this long interval of denervation is possible but unpredictable (and more so after delayed suture). It becomes a matter of waiting up to a year and a half to define how much substitutive tendon work is required. Sutures at the axillary level are worthwhile both in triceps function and in the probability that reinnervation will at worst make a major contribution to the strength of wrist extension.

Results with suture of the radial nerve are excellent. Seventy-eight per cent of the American series and 89 per cent of the British series had a good return of function.[25,164] In the few patients who do not regain dorsiflexion of the wrist or finger and thumb extension, tendon transfers work satisfactorily.

Brachial Plexus

The brachial plexus originates from the C5, C6, C7, C8, and T1 spinal roots. Each root divides to go into two divisions; they then recombine to form three trunks, the upper trunk (C5, C6), the middle trunk (C7), and the lower trunk (C8, T1). These trunks divide and recombine to form three cords (Fig. 75–27).

The lateral cord derives chiefly from C5 and C6, gives rise to the musculocutaneous and the lateral half of the median nerve (median sensory). The medial cord, which is derived chiefly from C8, and T1, gives rise to the ulnar nerve and the medial half of the median nerve (median-innervated hand intrinsic muscles). The posterior cord is derived from C5, C6, and C7 and gives rise to the axillary and the radial nerves.

An upper trunk (C5, C6) injury involves

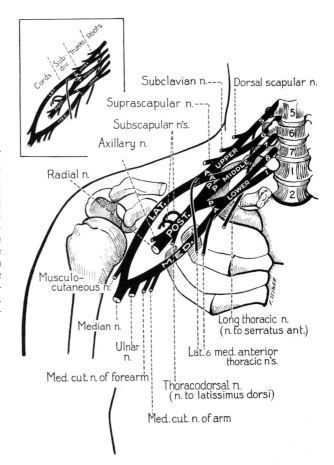

Figure 75–27 Schematic drawing of brachial plexus from its formation by roots to its distribution to peripheral nerves. The deficit resulting from section of a proximal root or cord element of the plexus is not nearly as predictably defined as the deficit resulting from peripheral nerve injury. Accordingly, motor recovery following suture of an element of the plexus can often be the result of spontaneous regeneration through lesions in continuity in other elements of the plexus. (From Haymaker, W., and Woodhall, B.: Peripheral Nerve Injuries. 2nd Ed. Philadelphia, W. B. Saunders Co., 1953. Reprinted by permission.)

virtually all shoulder muscles except the multiply innervated pectoralis major. If the suprascapular nerve and supraspinatus muscle have escaped, the lesion is either in the distal trunk or lateral cord. If the long thoracic nerve to the serratus anterior muscle is involved, the lesion must be very close to the spine. More distally, the biceps and brachialis will be lost and there is major sensory impairment in the thumb and index finger. Still more distal involvement of the lateral cord will cause a similar motor and sensory loss below the shoulder, except that the brachialis is spared to permit elbow flexion despite biceps loss, and there is the added loss of all forearm supplied by the median nerve, since these derive primarily from the lateral half of the median nerve.

Middle trunk (C7) injury produces major but incomplete triceps loss as well as some involvement of all forearm flexors and extensors, the extensors suffering more than do the flexors. The posterior cord receives input from upper and middle trunks as well as some from the lower trunk. The first

branch from the posterior cord is the thoracodorsal nerve innervating the lattissimus dorsi or "cough muscle." Proximal posterior cord injuries at its junction with the divisions will involve loss of this function. More distally, in the posterior cord, upper trunk fibers are collected that supply the axillary nerve and deltoid muscle and all of the triceps, brachioradialis, and forearm extensor muscles. After giving rise to the axillary nerve, the posterior cord continues as the radial nerve.

The lower trunk (C8, T1) is concerned primarily with forearm muscle flexors and intrinsic hand muscles, but by the time there is reshuffling into the medial cord more distally, only the ulnar forearm flexors are represented along with all the intrinsic hand muscles. Both inferior trunk and medial cord involvement cause sensory loss in the ulnar portion of the hand. More distally this medial cord provides the medial half of the median nerve, concerned primarily with median-supplied intrinsic hand muscles. The remainder constitutes the ulnar nerve, except for unimportant sensory branches to the forearm.

A neurosurgeon is first of all concerned with total focal transection of brachial plexus elements whose suture could contribute to useful function. This is considered further in the discussion of results. Axons regenerating after high-level suture have the capacity to usefully reinnervate only proximal muscles such as the supraspinatus, the deltoid, the biceps, the triceps, the brachioradialis, and possibly some forearm level muscles. No forearm muscles could receive axons from even a distal plexus lesion near the axilla in less than 10 months. Hence, in theory, little motor function below the elbow will occur as the result of a suture at the plexus level. Exceptions are provided by sharply transected lateral and posterior cords that are repaired relatively early and some complete lesions in continuity that regenerate without suture. The low-grade sensory recovery that is ultimately possible is chiefly important for the thumb and first two fingers, and this sensory supply derives from the same plexus elements that can give useful motor recovery. In other words, the potentially useful sutures involve these structures: the superior trunk, the middle trunk, the lateral cord, the musculocutaneous nerve, the posterior cord, and the axillary nerve. With disabling forearm and intrinsic hand muscle paralysis, one can only hope that spontaneous recovery, after neurapraxia or axonotmesis, will occur through inferior trunk or medial cord, since suture of these elements will accomplish little.

With these considerations in mind, evaluation of the early plexus lesion must be done carefully to determine whether there is total dysfunction that is consistent with a complete division of an upper trunk or cord and to have an accurate baseline assessment. In other words, if proximal muscles such as the supraspinatus or deltoid are paralyzed initially but begin to function by six weeks, there is great probability that this recovery will go on to include biceps and triceps. Beginning function in these muscles that are easily visualized can often be detected by simple surface stimulation of upper plexus elements close to the lateral border of the sternocleidomastoid. Electromyography can also assist in early prognosis when these same muscles can be found to harbor active motor units on vol-

untary effort as proof for a low grade of nerve trunk injury that has permitted some neurapraxia. In the face of total dysfunction in these proximal muscles that continues for several months, operative exploration of the upper brachial plexus should be strongly considered. Even if the distal musculature is involved and does not recover in time, a hand prosthesis that can be controlled by active elbow and shoulder movement will be a distinct gain.

Operative exposure of the brachial plexus, as of the radial nerve, should not be achieved by incising directly over the course of the nerve elements, which produces axillary scarring. An incision should be outlined that can permit total exposure of the plexus from roots to neurovascular bundle below the axilla.[71] This is necessary since a suture that requires extensive nerve trunk mobilization may become feasible. Only part of this exposure need be developed if favorable lesions in continuity are discovered. Starting distally for high axillary lesions, an incision to expose the neurovascular bundle in the upper arm should deviate laterally 3 inches short of the axilla to approach the cap of the shoulder and then return to the midclavicular level. This allows exposure of the cephalic vein, which demarcates the plane between deltoid and pectoralis major muscles. Separation of the distal pectoralis major permits dividing its humeral insertion so as to unroof the nerve cords above the axilla. Both ends should be tagged to permit later resuture. More proximal visualization requires sectioning of the pectoralis minor at its insertion. Proximal exposure requires extending the clavicular incision close to the sternoclavicular junction and then directing it vertically upward to follow the posterior margin of the sternocleidomastoid muscle. The higher roots (C5, C6, C7) are very easily exposed, as both the nerve trunks and the transverse processes behind them become easily palpable beneath the deep cervical fascia. Stimulation will help to identify each nerve element unless the wound is close to the spine. The joining of C5 and C6 into a single large superior trunk is a dependable anatomical aid. The structures can usually be followed under the strut of the clavicle without transecting it, provided soft tissues are dissected free on either side of the clavicle. Lesions at or close to the clavicular level may require clavicular transection, and following neural repair the clavicle should usually be pinned back in place. After suture, immobilization of the shoulder in adduction and of the elbow in flexion may be necessary.

The brachial artery is a useful guide for more distal orientation. The lateral and medial cords come to lie on either side of it, while the posterior cord is deep to it. Branches of the medial and lateral cords come together to make up the median nerve and in so doing form a bridging Y in front of the artery.

Functional results following suture are highly variable. Fortunately they often are aided by postoperative motor recovery through spared elements that are not involved in the suture. The inch a month growth rate applies to the plexus. An upper trunk suture can begin to provide deltoid function by five months. A lateral cord suture can begin to supply biceps function in four or five months. If biceps function should begin three months after an upper trunk suture, it is obvious it is receiving an anomalous contribution from the middle trunk, which was regenerating spontaneously from the date of injury instead of from the date of the suture. Accordingly, one must be very critical in considering recovery solely dependent upon regeneration through the suture; detailed follow-up data is necessary to derive such conclusions. Only proximal muscles can benefit from nerve suture at the plexus level. Brooks reported on 170 brachial plexus injuries in the British experience.[127] It was possible to repair the injury in only 11 patients, and then recovery occurred only in the proximal muscles. In the American World War II experience reported in the Veterans Administration monograph by Nulsen and Slade, sutures were possible in 76 of 89 patients selected for operation.[109] There were enough examples of recovery that could only be attributed to the suture to indicate that the supraspinatus, deltoid, biceps, and rarely triceps muscles can benefit from this procedure. Again it must be emphasized that occasional excellent results after brachial plexus exploration and limited suture occur when the lesion was not nearly as bad as it was thought to be initially. Many neural elements were subject to lower grades of injury with long periods of dysfunction before a minimum of sparing by neurapraxia became enhanced

by the delayed spontaneous regeneration of those axons suffering axonotmesis. But even in this situation, muscles below the elbow fare poorly when they must remain denervated for 10 months or more. Campbell reported a favorable result following autogenous nerve graft to the upper and middle trunks of the plexus.[32] Three years after insertion of the grafts, motor function had returned to the proximal muscles of the arm, and sensation to the median and radial innervation of the hand. Although there was some flexion and extension of the wrist, hand motor function did not return, and it is unlikely that it will because of the limitations in muscle reinnervation after several years of denervation. A few other authors have also reported some favorable grafts to the plexus.[91,98,123,124]

Operative experience with stimulation and stimulation and recording studies on a series of 45 patients with brachial plexus injuries in continuity operated upon between 1969 and 1975 by one of the authors (D.G.K.) showed 92 major plexus elements to be involved by injury. Of these, 53 underwent neurolysis and 44 improved significantly. On the other hand, 34 elements had either end-to-end suture repair or graft repair, and only 12 of these had significant improvement after follow-up ranging from two to eight years. Exploration of plexus lesions that may have an element of continuity requires the use of stimulating and recording techniques to sort out those lesions involving the plexus that need resection and repair from those that can be left alone with some hope for recovery (Fig. 75–28). Unnecessary resection of a plexus element renders the patient a disservice just as surely as does leaving alone one that requires resection and suture. Such a tactic requires a waiting period of two to three months after injury so that enough time has elapsed for potential regeneration to occur.

Immediate exploration is indicated when a plexus injury is due to glass, a knife, or another sharp object, for here distal deficit indicates that the likelihood of focal transection is great and the possibility that such can be repaired at once with some degree of useful return is good. Delay means the surgeon will face a scarred bed, particularly if an earlier vascular exploration and repair has been carried out. In addition, plexus elements may retract, making delayed end-

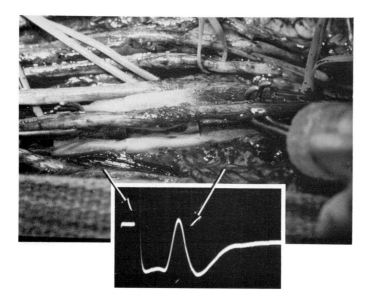

Figure 75-28 Operative nerve action potential recording from medial cord of brachial plexus. Since a nerve action potential was seen (*inset*) neurolysis rather than resection and suture was done and achieved an eventual acceptable result. Electrical techniques are especially important for sorting out brachial plexus injuries.

to-end repair difficult and the need for grafts great. Such an approach is borne out by a small series of axillary level plexus transections associated with radical mastectomy. When the insult has been recognized by the operating surgeon and help has been obtained immediately, the results with primary suture far outdistance those with secondary suture in which grafts are invariably necessary. Another small series of acutely transected *supraclavicular* plexus injuries has been repaired primarily, and results when compared with those repaired secondarily are favorable.

Traction or stretch injuries are responsible for a major proportion of brachial plexus involvement, both in military and civilian life. In the latter situation, the injury usually occurs in vehicular accidents. Even when there is a shoulder or a clavicular fracture, the mechanism of neural involvement is not focal contusion.

Neural recovery after stretch injury is seldom improved by operative intervention, although at times exploration can assist in establishing the prognosis and directing rehabilitative management. Occasional exceptions are provided by distraction at root to upper or middle trunk levels and more distal distractions, usually at the level of the clavicle. Experience with several patients requiring 3-inch interfascicular grafts to all elements at the clavicular level was favorable, with shoulder and upper arm recovery and some forearm flexor re-

turn evident by three years after repair (Figs. 75-29 and 75-30).

Traction injuries present special features that can assist in their evaluation. Often there is sensory preservation despite total motor loss. If present, it is a favorable early finding, although optimism is justified only when a three-month interval after injury has demonstrated significant motor recovery from neurapraxia.[10] Severe traction injuries usually involve avulsion of two or more roots from the spinal cord, which will be demonstrated by myelography (Fig. 75-31).[44,102,119] In addition the remaining roots may have suffered total damage by stretch force that was just short of producing an avulsion. If so there will be a total loss of function in them. The axon reflex test helps to determine when the lesion is central to the dorsal root ganglion.[16] Involvement of the most proximal innervation also favors root avulsion. The finding of a Horner's syndrome strongly suggests avulsion of at least T1 and C8. The loss of long thoracic nerve supply to the serratus anterior muscle similarly suggests proximal avulsion of the upper plexus roots. In addition, denervation of paraspinal or rhomboid muscles, or both, documented by electromyographic studies, suggests a root level and thus a less likely reversible lesion.

In conclusion, no two brachial plexus injuries are alike. Any general statements concerning their management must involve oversimplification. There is justification for

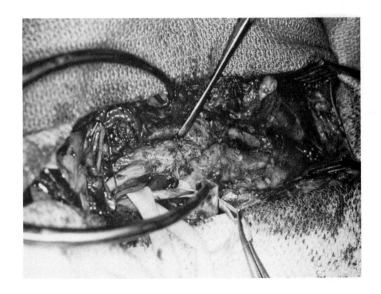

Figure 75–29 Distraction of entire brachial plexus at midclavicular level. This 14-year-old girl had been thrown from a horse and had landed on her shoulder. There were no fractures but a complete brachial plexus palsy. Loss of function of the deltoid and of the entire arm persisted for a six-month period. Myelograms were negative on two occasions. The middle segment of the clavicle was resected to make this exposure, and retractor blades are seen placed in the lateral and medial thirds of the clavicle.

direct operative intervention when focal wounding involves a division of upper or middle plexus elements that may gain useful regeneration after suture. Usually after wounding or stretch injury there is not as much permanent dysfunction as the initial picture would suggest. While regeneration is slow in all cases, useful recovery usually does not occur in muscles that do not begin to show function by 18 months. Assuming increasing strength in only those muscles that are working, and with some sensation in the thumb and finger part of the hand, it is then possible at this time to consider (1) whether there is enough working to permit achievement of a functioning hand with tendon transfers and fusions or (2) whether a

prosthesis is the better alternative and at what level it should be carried. Clearly, a major disservice is done a patient when false optimism delays inevitable amputation and prosthesis training for years after the point at which permanent dysfunction becomes clearly defined.

Peroneal Nerve

This extensor nerve is in some ways comparable to the radial extensor nerve for the forearm in that its sensory function is unimportant and its distal or lower leg involvement does not become clinically important until a point just below the knee,

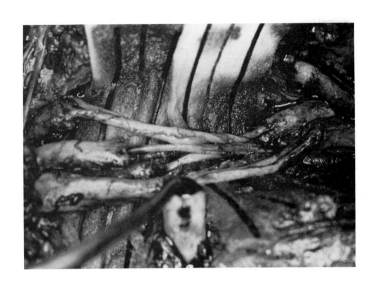

Figure 75–30 After scar and neuroma were resected from the stumps of the distracted plexus, multiple sural interfascicular nerve grafts were placed. The patient has had recovery of shoulder and upper arm muscles as well as forearm flexor movement but no intrinsic hand muscle return over a five-year period of follow-up.

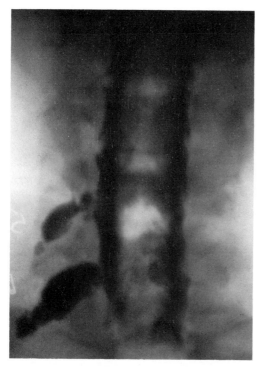

Figure 75–31 Myelogram demonstrating pouches where Pantopaque has diffused into the root sleeves of C5 and C6 roots, avulsed by a stretch injury. (The root sleeves of C7, C8 and T1 appeared normal but their dysfunction also remained permanent in this case.)

where it crosses the head of the fibula. Loss of extensor function from more distal leg injuries becomes a question of muscle and tendon damage. Unfortunately, recovery after peroneal suture is not as assured as it is after radial suture, and thus the similarities must end at this point. In injuries involving the sciatic nerve, the peroneal division almost invariably is the most severely involved. Its tendency to be selectively and more severely injured may be due to its oblique course through the thigh and its relative tethering about the head of the fibula. Other factors cited by Sunderland include the fact that peroneal fascicles are surrounded by less perineurium than those of the tibial nerve.[143] In addition to the relatively lateral and thus exposed position of the peroneal nerve in the sciatic complex, blood supply may be inferior to that to the tibial.

Injury at Knee

The nerve is very susceptible to lacerating and contusive injuries as it crosses the lateral popliteal space and the head of the fibula anteriorly. The segment of the nerve just below the knee is also uniquely susceptible to stretch injury by any dislocating force to the knee.[159] The greater incidence of stretching may relate in part to the partial attachment of the nerve sheath to the periosteum of the fibula. The nerve at this point below the knee is also susceptible to tourniquet paralysis, and even sitting in a cross-legged position or prolonged squatting can occasionally cause transient paralysis from compressive ischemia.

The nerve first supplies the peroneal muscles that evert the foot. With beginning recovery after an injury, muscle quivering can be noted for the first time just in front of the fibula, and the tendon behind the lateral malleolus can be seen to tighten. The disabling deficit is the foot-drop from loss of anterior tibial muscle function. This muscle and the consequent foot-drop recover somewhat later. Contractions are perceived just lateral to the midline ridge of the upper tibia, and the tendon can be perceived to tighten over the dorsum of the ankle joint. Next, extensor function may begin in all the toes; however, in most instances, because the extensor hallucis longus has a still more distal innervation, the large toe will recover last. The peroneal nerve has a more consistent autonomous zone than does the radial nerve. The autonomous area is a small ovoid area on the middorsum of the foot. After a peroneal nerve injury, initial sensory loss includes a wide area over the lateral anterior calf and dorsum of the foot; however, it shrinks so rapidly with time, even in the face of total nerve transection, that careful sensory evaluation gives little clue to potential recovery. Patients can be made ambulatory very quickly with a spring brace. It stabilizes the foot in dorsiflexion but permits stepping off with plantar flexion from normal use of the gastrocnemius in walking.

Nerve stimulation is of especial value in early recognition of adequate peroneal recovery and avoidance of a needless operative exploration. Patients appear to have an apraxia in that they are unable to initiate voluntary action in peroneal and anterior tibial muscles for weeks after physiological recovery has been demonstrated by strong muscle contraction on stimulation. Except in very obese persons, the nerve trunk is easily excited by a surface electrical stimulus over its course just behind the head of the fibula or just inside the lateral hamstring, where the trunk can be readily palpated.

Operative exposure involves an incision over the course of the superficial nerve. The skin incision should be kept lateral to the popliteal crease. The nerve is discovered just medial to the lateral hamstring tendon and is readily followed distally to the point of injury. The distal segment is most easily exposed as it crosses the head of the fibula. If the injury is at this point, the normal distal deep and superficial peroneal nerves usually can be exposed in healthy tissues underneath the peroneus longus muscle. Some 2 cm beyond the point, where the peroneal nerve divides into two major trunks, multiple branching occurs in both trunks and a suture becomes unfeasible. Five- to six-centimeter gaps between nerve ends can be overcome by flexing the knee if there has been mobilization beyond the fibula distally and well above the popliteal space. A further length-gaining device is to shorten the course of the distal nerve by resecting the underlying fibular head. With longer gaps, another 2 cm of length can be gained by dissecting the nerve free in the proximal direction up to a point beyond the gluteal muscle. If there is tension on the suture line after flexion of the knee and proximal and distal mobilization of the nerve, care should be taken to insure that flexion of the hip will not further increase the tension. With the patient on the operating table, the hip should be flexed and the suture line observed. If this maneuver increases tension on the suture, a spica cast should be applied to prevent hip flexion. Whether or not the spica is needed, a cast must be placed over the knee to prevent extension during the healing phase. Avulsions of the suture line occur more frequently with the peroneal than with any other nerve. This complication is often related to failure to recognize the traction that can be generated by full hip flexion.

Following peroneal nerve suture at the midpopliteal level, peroneus muscle function should begin by three to four months, and tibialis anticus muscle function should begin by six months. Recognition of beginning function by nerve stimulation will considerably antedate the establishment of voluntary function in many patients. Later recovery of toe extensors is not of great

functional importance. The important question is whether the foot can be automatically held in the dorsiflexed position, as needed during walking, so that the "foot-drop brace" can be discarded. Even with the injury at this low level on the nerve, an adequate result is obtained after an early and technically good suture in only about 50 per cent of cases. With some functional return in eversion and in dorsiflexion of the foot, an adequate assist may be provided by transferring the strong posterior tibial tendon to the dorsum of the foot. This is not effective in providing dorsiflexion by itself, so with continuing total foot-drop, reliance on the brace can be eliminated only by an ankle fusion to stabilize the foot in dorsiflexion. This procedure may be of value in lightweight patients but can break down in heavier ones. With traction injuries to the peroneal nerve at the knee, lesions still functionally complete at three months are apt to remain so, and direct operative intervention has little to offer, although White reported a favorable experience with a few cases.[159]

Injury in Thigh

At high levels, transection of the peroneal nerve (or the peroneal component of the sciatic nerve) will cause the additional minor deficit of loss of part or all of biceps femoris (lateral hamstring) function in addition to the loss of lower leg extension and eversion of the foot. The major branch of the peroneal nerve that goes to the biceps branches off at variable levels below the upper thigh. The chief difference involved in peroneal lesions at progressively higher levels is the increasing limitation that exists for any functional recovery requiring axonal regeneration. At points more than 8 inches above the head of the fibula the chances for useful ankle dorsiflexion recovery by suture become increasingly poor. With any possibility of sufficient neural continuity to permit spontaneous regeneration, as determined by direct operative inspection, nerve stimulation, and nerve action potential recording, it is far better to be conservative in not resorting to resection of the lesion with suture. With a peroneal nerve lesion above midthigh, even with mostly axonotmesis that will permit spontaneous regeneration, the axons will usually not arrive downstream in sufficient time to reverse the effects of prolonged distal denervation.[35]

It should also be mentioned that the peroneal component of the sciatic nerve usually is selectively involved in hip dislocation or fracture. Direct operative intervention has little to offer and, unless slight function in leg muscles begins by several months, a permanent peroneal deficit is likely. On the other hand, immediate reduction of the dislocation may be of value and has, the authors believe, aided in reversing one case of sciatic palsy under their care. In one series, close to 80 per cent of patients with this type of traction injury eventually required either ankle fusion or a permanent brace in order to walk.

Tibial Nerve

Injury at Ankle

Wounding behind the medial malleolus will involve the tibial nerve. The primary deficit is the sensory loss involving the sole of the foot. With time, the area of sensory loss will shrink, but unfortunately, the autonomous zone for the tibial nerve continues to involve the weight-bearing surfaces where sensation is most needed to prevent trophic ulceration. Both the heel and the ball of the foot will remain insensitive if the tibial nerve does not recover. All the intrinsic foot muscles are paralyzed, but because humans use these muscles so little, it usually is hard to recognize a deficit during voluntary effort. Some clawing of the toes may become evident, and if so it is comparable to the clawing of the hand with an ulnar nerve deficit but less disabling. With this deficit the patient may not be able to straighten his toes on the affected side as well as he does on the normal side. Occasional individuals can abduct the large toe on the normal side. Loss of this function on the injured side is a useful clue in diagnosis of a lesion of the nerve. Tibial nerve stimulation is the only adequate noninvasive means of determining whether the patient has distal motor innervation and of recognizing its recovery at early stages (which has important implications for later adequate sensory recovery). Some authors have advised against distal tibial nerve suture for the sole purpose of regaining sensation because this sensory return can cause

such unpleasant hyperesthesia and pain on weight bearing. This is just a stage in recovery, however, a temporary situation that is still worth enduring in order to prevent increasing problems in later life. These later problems include trophic ulcerations that may cause osteomyelitis and even require amputation. At best the patient with an insensitive sole is likely, despite perfect motor function, to have to return to crutches for weeks in each year to permit healing of skin ulcers on weight-bearing surfaces.

The tibial nerve is readily accessible, both well above the medial malleolus and distally below it, as it curves forward superficially to branch into lateral and medial plantar nerves. Mobilization of the nerve down to these branches and up to the midcalf will permit overcoming a gap of 3 to 4 cm by posturing the foot in marked plantar flexion. Occasionally, it becomes necessary to gain additional length by mobilizing the proximal segment beyond the popliteal space to gain length with knee flexion. This maneuver entails freeing the nerve in its deep course beneath the gastrocnemius and soleus muscles.[130]

Such an extensive operation may seem radical merely to regain sensation in the foot, but for a young and active person its protection through a lifetime of weight bearing clearly deserves this major effort. The long-term problems of the insensitive foot provide a rationale for attempting tibial nerve repair even to high levels at which its sciatic component is damaged.

Injury at Knee

Injuries at the popliteal level often are complicated by involvement of the popliteal artery and vein. The motor deficit includes a loss of plantar flexion of the foot (gastrocnemius and soleus muscles), loss of inversion of the foot (posterior tibial muscle), and loss of flexion of all toes in addition to the unimportant paralysis of intrinsic foot muscles and the important plantar sensory loss. In contrast to the patient with peroneal nerve involvement, the one in this situation naturally effects voluntary action in these flexor muscles just as soon as he acquires the physiological mechanism to do so. It is unusual to find calf muscle contractions on nerve stimulation that are not already evident on clinical testing. Recovery of plantar flexion by two to three months after injury or even slightly earlier recovery in the visible gastrocnemius after neurapraxia speaks for a good functional end result. Total tibial nerve transections occasionally are judged incomplete because the patient can set his normal anterior tibial and peroneal muscles in a fashion that will produce inversion of the foot. Careful inspection will show that the posterior tibial tendon behind the medial malleolus remains slack during the performance of this movement.

Operative exposure of the tibial nerve above the popliteal space is straightforward. Overcoming large gaps can occasionally require its proximal mobilization as high as the gluteal crease. Maintenance of the hip in a neutral position may also be necessary. The natural division between the tibial and peroneal components of the sciatic nerve may require dissection more proximally to achieve this mobilization. Distal to the popliteal space the nerve dives beneath the soleus muscle and is somewhat tethered by its motor branches, but ordinarily it can be freed sufficiently so that a 4- to 5-cm gap can be overcome by knee flexion.

Better than 60 per cent of patients with tibial nerve sutures at the popliteal level regain a degree of plantar flexion that assists in ambulation. Recovery of plantar sensation to protect weight-bearing surfaces may require as long as a year. When it occurs, it results in a remarkable reduction in susceptibility to skin breakdown and ulceration. Even at higher levels, nearly to the gluteal crease, suture of a tibial component can result in a useful degree of plantar flexion, and the hope for securing protective plantar sensation exists. Surgical dissection of the nerve at this level is considered next.

Peroneal and Tibial Nerves Combined: Sciatic Nerve

The sciatic nerve usually has such a distinct anatomical division of its peroneal and tibial nerve components that it is useful to evaluate and consider these two components separately. The level at which the sciatic divides into separate tibial and peroneal nerves varies in each patient and can occur as high as the gluteal crease.[73] Thus, what appears as a partial sciatic nerve injury, because one division's func-

tion is out and the other's is in, may in actuality be a complete injury to one nerve and little or no injury to the other. Retention of partial intrinsic function in the calf or its early recovery following injury does not carry the same good prognosis for recovery of all its function as exists when there is injury to only a single nerve trunk. For example, after an injury to the sciatic nerve at the midthigh level with initial total paralysis and sensory loss, function may begin by six weeks in the peroneus longus and tibialis anticus muscles. This would suggest a partial sciatic injury with good prognosis. Actually, the tibial half of the sciatic can be totally involved in such cases, and only its exploration and suture will provide, with good probability, a useful degree of plantar flexion and ultimately a protective degree of sensation to the sole of the foot. The converse situation is not as important. Failure to recognize total peroneal component involvement at a high level is not as serious an error, since the yield from suture is low.

Because the motor functions of the peroneal and tibial components are separate, an injury to them carries no surprises such as occur with combined injury to median and ulnar nerves, which share functions. Motor branches to the medial hamstrings remain separated from the sciatic trunk right up to the sciatic notch, and only rarely will a high injury include the deficit of complete inability to flex the knee.

The sensory loss from the section of both components is somewhat more extensive than might be anticipated, but the proneness to foot ulceration on weight bearing is not much greater than that which exists in pure tibial nerve injury. It is remarkable how well the individual with total sciatic transection can function with a proper footdrop brace and shoe designed to guard against pressure ulcerations.

The operative exposure of the sciatic nerve in its trough between the hamstrings offers no problem unless it is necessary to expose a proximal trunk above the gluteal crease or higher. Then the midline posterior incision should be extended laterally at the gluteal crease to permit reflection of the gluteus maximus muscle in its entirety (Fig. 75–32). In this region, the sciatic nerve runs beneath the piriformis muscle, crossing transversely toward the greater trochanter. The nerve then passes superficial to the obturator internus, gemelli, and qua-

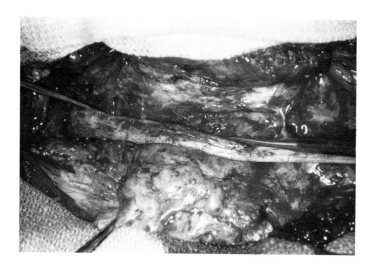

Figure 75–32 Contusive injury to sciatic nerve at buttocks level. This injury was approached by a lateral buttocks incision and reflection of gluteus maximus and medius medially. The sciatic notch is to the left. The patient was operated upon because of pain and paresthesias in the sciatic distribution.

dratus femoris muscles to reach the thigh. Care must be exercised not to damage medial branches passing to the medial hamstrings. Additional length can be gained by mobilizing the nerve past the popliteal space, then holding the knee in flexion and the thigh in neutral or slightly extended position in a cast. It is helpful to develop a plane of cleavage between the peroneal and tibial components, regardless of whether both require suture or one is in continuity. This can be begun in or proximal to the popliteal space, depending on the site of bifurcation of the sciatic nerve. By judicious use of microdissection, saline irrigation, and the bipolar forceps, each division can be safely separated up to the gluteal level if necessary (Fig. 75–33). In this fashion, each division can also be evaluated separately by stimulation and evoked nerve action potential techniques, and a separate decision made for either resection and suture or neurolysis for each division (Fig. 75–34).[73]

It is important to recognize how little can be expected from suture of both the peroneal and tibial components (total sciatic repair). In 43 cases of sciatic nerve suture in the *upper* thigh studied by Bateman, there was return of lower leg muscle function in only 27 per cent and sensory return to the foot in only 39 per cent.[12] If one considers the behavior of the tibial component alone, the World War II American experience indicated some motor recovery in 60 per cent, with strong useful plantar flexion resulting in 50 per cent. By contrast, none of the wartime peroneal component sutures above midthigh provided sufficient strength of foot dorsiflexion to permit function with-

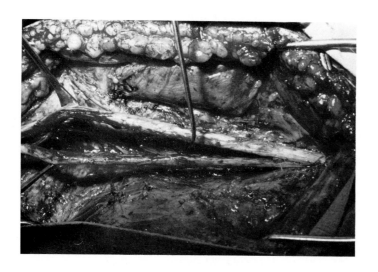

Figure 75–33 Split of sciatic complex after removal of heavy scar secondary to gunshot wound. The upper element (tibial) had a nerve action potential, while the lower (peroneal) did not and required resection and suture.

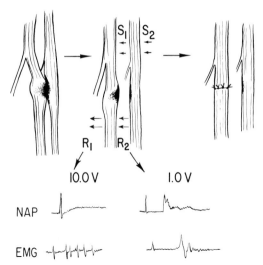

Figure 75–34 In this clinical situation, a gunshot wound involving the sciatic nerve in midthigh, the peroneal and tibial components were easily separated by surgical dissection eight weeks postinjury. The *peroneal* component (on the right) presented both a good nerve action potential (NAP) and electromyographic (EMG) response to stimulation, whereas the *tibial* component yielded no response. (The two nerves did not appear that different to the surgeon.) The resected tibial lesion in continuity showed no neural preservation and its suture yielded motor recovery. The preserved peroneal lesion permitted excellent spontaneous recovery from foot-drop. S_1 and S_2, stimulus sites for tibial and peroneal nerves respectively; R_1 and R_2, recording sites for tibial and peroneal nerves.

out a brace or an ankle fusion. In summary, it would appear that repair of the tibial component has the possibility of providing motor function from levels as high as the gluteal region and a probability of ultimately providing a degree of plantar sensation that will be protective. By contrast, yield from peroneal nerve suture above the midthigh level is low enough so that it seems contraindicated to explore it for possible suture at high thigh levels unless the tibial component also requires exploration. As in other nerves, the more focal the lesion, e.g., as caused by transection by glass or knife or some gunshot wounds, the more likely that suture repair will yield results, especially in youngsters.[73b]

Femoral Nerve

The most distal level at which femoral nerve involvement becomes important is close to the inguinal ligament, where it supplies all knee extension function via the quadriceps and also supplies the sartorius muscle, which is not essential to ambulation. One to two inches distal to the inguinal ligament, the nerve divides into superficial and deep branches. The lateral circumflex femoral artery passes between these divisions. The superficial branches provide sensation over the anterolateral thigh, while the deeper posterior division provides branches to the quadriceps muscles and also forms the saphenous nerve. The pattern of sensory loss secondary to injury to the femoral nerve is variable, owing to frequent overlap by the lateral femoral cutaneous, genitofemoral, and obturator nerves. Quadriceps loss, the most reliable index of injury, is evidenced by inability to extend the knee and a decrease in or absence of knee jerk. Sartorius weakness suggests a high lesion, since superficial branches supplying this muscle originate proximal to the inguinal ligament.

The motor supply to the important quadriceps muscle involves an abrupt division of the main trunk into many fine branches. This usually occurs at a point 1 to 3 inches below the inguinal ligament. Partial function with injury below the ligament implies that some branches have been spared and that the surgeon will be unable to discover and resuture those nerve twigs that are divided. Electromyography may be of great help, since it may show partial denervation of the quadriceps, suggesting that some of the branches rather than the main trunk of the nerve have been injured. In this case, conservative management probably is warranted, since operation can add little to the recovery. Total quadriceps loss with injury close to the ligament does warrant exploration on the chance that the main trunk is divided and can be sutured at a point where branching has not rendered a repair impossible. Regrettably, injuries rarely involve this short segment of the nerve that is available for operative repair. During wartime, injury at this level often lacerates the femoral artery, with loss of limb or even life, and thus further limits clinical experience with femoral nerve repair.[121] The authors' own case experience indicates also that the main femoral trunk can be injured during hernia repair when it is inadvertently transfixed by suture, during stripping and ligation of the saphenous vein for treatment of varicosities, or during arterial bypass procedures.[73b]

Operative approach involves locating the

femoral nerve below the inguinal ligament, where after the iliacus fascia is opened, it can be identified as part of the neurovascular bundle and traced beneath the inguinal ligament and into the pelvis if need be. In the neurovascular bundle, the femoral artery and vein lie medial to the nerve. The nerve can be traced into the femoral triangle by way of a vertical incision curving medially so that the distal femoral nerve and its branches can be identified. The nerve can also be followed intra-abdominally by splitting the inguinal ligament. Skin incision is then curved laterally over the iliac crest toward the flank, and abdominal muscles are separated obliquely. If needed, this proximal exposure can be used to gain length to overcome a gap for a distal suture. Positioning of the lower extremity is important in making up length and preventing undue tension on the suture line. Relaxation of the tension on the nerve may be achieved by hip flexion and the use of a hip spica cast.

Useful recovery of quadriceps function should follow suture of the femoral nerve trunk and has been observed. Indeed in several cases even graft repair spanning the pelvic brim has, in the author's experience and that of others, led to some degree of useful quadriceps function. Although the majority of femoral nerve explorations do not result in suture of the main trunk, even in this circumstance late recovery may occur in some cases. If so, that recovery can be attributed to sparing of some branches to the quadriceps. Fortunately, graded exercise and resulting hypertrophy of the spared muscle bundles can yield enough strength to set the knee when only a fraction of the quadriceps recovers. Inadequate function of the quadriceps requires support of the knee with a brace that can be locked for walking and unlocked for sitting. Use of this type of brace seems preferable to fusion of the knee in fixed extension. Sensory recovery is unimportant.

More proximal retroperitoneal injury of the femoral nerve usually occurs in combination with lower pelvic plexus injuries that involve the sciatic outflow as well, but can be iatrogenic and associated with resection of neurofibromas or other tumors in the infrarenal and pelvic regions. In this area the nerve can be approached in the retroperitoneal area much as one would develop the exposure for a lumbar sympathectomy. It is the largest branch of the lumbar plexus and receives the large posterior divisions from second, third, and fourth lumbar roots. Its proximal portion lies between the iliacus and psoas muscles. Suture of the femoral nerve at this level is technically feasible, but only a few documented cases of useful recovery of quadriceps function are known to the authors.

Pelvic Plexus

Injuries to the pelvic plexus are fortunately rare. Suture of the sciatic nerve components at this high level has little to offer. Often, it is important to recognize when leg paralysis results from extraspinal rather than from intraspinal neural involvement. Causes include trauma, pelvic cancer, and lumbar plexopathy due to medical complications.[53] For instance, repair of extensive pelvic plexus injury may not be possible, but release of an intraspinal compression or suture repair of some partial cauda equina lacerations can lead to useful recovery. Occasionally, benign tumors, particularly schwannomas or neurofibromas, will involve the pelvic plexus. The authors have had experience with one woman who presented with dyspareunia and who on examination had an area of tenderness on one vaginal wall that when tapped gave pain and paresthesias in the region of the inner thigh. She had previously had a mediastinal tumor removed. Exploration revealed a schwannoma involving the lower pelvic plexus that was removed with relief of pain. In addition, several schwannomas involving the mesentery of the small bowel were found.

The plexus is formed from the anterior rami of the spinal nerves of L4, L5, S1, S2, and S3. These roots cross the front of the sacroiliac joint and form the plexus. The roots then converge toward the lower part of the greater sciatic foramen and terminate as the sciatic nerve. The superior gluteal nerve forms the highest branch of the plexus and leaves the pelvis through the sciatic foramen, superficial to the piriformis, to supply the gluteus minimus and medius; while the inferior gluteal nerve leaves below the piriformis and supplies the gluteus maximus. Injuries to the pelvic plexus usually can be differentiated from those to the sciatic nerve when the examiner realizes that the gluteals, quadriceps, adductors, and abductors of the hip may be involved in the motor deficit along with the muscles that are innervated by the sciatic nerve. Sciatic injury will not give sensory loss in the perianal region, whereas such loss may occur in a pelvic plexus injury. Cauda equina lesions are more likely to produce bilateral lower extremity loss. Both pelvic plexus and cauda equina injuries can involve bowel and bladder function. Ability to sweat is lost with extraspinal lesions, while autonomic function is spared with cauda equina lesions below L2. Electromyography may be of definite help in differentiating intraspinal from extraspinal injury, since if there is evidence of paraspinal musculature denervation, an intraspinal lesion is suggested.

Fortunately some plexus injuries are reversible, as illustrated by the following example:

A 29-year-old man was shot in the left lumbosacral region. Emergency celiotomy demonstrated a laceration of the descending colon, free peritoneal blood, and a left retroperitoneal hematoma. Postoperatively, the patient was noted to have weakness of the left leg. Gluteal, quadriceps, and hamstring muscle weakness was present, as was complete loss of dorsiflexion and eversion of the foot with decreased inversion and plantar flexion. There was sensory loss in the L5–S1 distribution of the foot and also in the left perianal region in the distribution of S2 through S5. Anal sphincter tone was preserved, and the patient remained continent. At three months there was good return of function in the gluteal, hamstring, quadriceps, plantar flexor, and foot invertor muscles with partial return of dorsiflexion and eversion of the foot. By six months the patient had functional use of the entire lower extremity with excellent dorsiflexion and eversion of the foot as well as plantar flexion and inversion. Apparently, the plexus was compressed by a hematoma that caused a temporary dysfunction, primarily on a basis of neurapraxia.

Miscellaneous Nerves

While this discussion is concerned primarily with injuries to peripheral nerves that affect the function of the extremities, a discussion of the indications for and the results of certain cranial nerve sutures seems to be indicated. The important motor nerves that respond to operative repair are the facial and the hypoglossal nerves and occasionally the accessory nerve. Because these nerves are almost purely motor nerves, one would expect far less loss with regeneration through the suture by the useless downgrowth of motor axons into sensory channels. At any rate, this theoretical explanation can be used to account for the remarkable motor recovery that follows adequate suture in some. There does remain the usual time limitation on regeneration.

Facial Nerve

There are a few reliable reports of facial motor recovery following intracranial suture of the facial nerve immediately after its transection during the removal of a tumor. With intracranial suture, the distance to grow is perhaps 8 inches and the muscle denervation limit is not violated. Provided the interval between nerve division and suture is not excessive, a technically good suture performed on any part of the nerve short of the break-up of the main trunk into the pes anserinus will yield a useful recovery of facial motor function. This is also a nerve in which grafting has been quite successful. Large segments of the nerve have been replaced with success after loss due to wounds in the mastoid area. The unique success of a nerve graft in this area may relate to a greatly reduced loss of motor axons at each of the two suture interfaces (to nonexistent sensory channels) as well as to the fact that the graft is of much smaller caliber than is required to match the ends of a mixed nerve in an extremity. Finally, it should be remembered that when excessive proximal facial nerve damage cannot be repaired, its healthy distal stump readily receives adequate reinnervation from an anastomosis with the central stump of another pure motor nerve such as the hypoglossal or the spinal accessory. Synkinesis, which is the involuntary contraction of a muscle other than the one the patient is trying to contract or in addition to it, occurs frequently. This type of mass action usually detracts from the cosmetic result, whether it follows spontaneous regeneration after the axonotmesis of Bell's palsy, regeneration through a direct facial-to-facial suture, or a hypoglossal-facial anastomosis. The patient cannot use the muscles of expression individually. When he tries to smile he grimaces with the entire side of the face, squints his eye, and contracts his platysma. When he attempts to close his eye, he smiles sardonically, With time, more isolated muscle function, and therefore more normal expression, is learned by some individuals, usually women. This mass action is presumably the same problem that causes the contrast between good motor recovery and poor functional recovery in the case of the ulnar nerve, specifically in the intrinsic hand muscles that were designed to work separately. Despite these limitations, even partial facial muscle reinnervation is a major gain to the patient, both cosmetically and in giving the eye the protection provided by closure of the lid.

Hypoglossal Nerve

The hypoglossal nerve regenerates remarkably well after suture, both to itself following transection and as a transfer and suture to the distal facial nerve, as already mentioned. Its use as a graft for the facial nerve correctly implies that a patient rapidly learns to speak normally with a barely detectable slur of sibilants and to manage his food easily in the presence of unilateral hypoglossal nerve paralysis. By contrast, bilateral hypoglossal nerve paralysis is devastating. It should be possible to get a good result from suture of hypoglossal nerves. Certainly, at least, recovery of tongue protrusion after suture of one nerve when the other has been partially damaged has been rewarding.

Accessory Nerve

Unfortunately, accessory nerve injury is usually iatrogenic and secondary to removal of a lump or mass from the posterior triangle of the neck. In the course of excision, the accessory nerve or its distal branches, particularly those running to the trapezius, are injured or divided, leading to trapezius paralysis and a drooped and sometimes painful shoulder. Oftentimes the lump, which may have been nothing more than matted lymph nodes or may have been a lesion such as a neurofibroma, is mistaken for a potential malignant tumor and a modified radical neck dissection is done through a short incision, resulting in injury. Experience with six such injuries indicates that they can be repaired, provided the divided stumps can be located, but oftentimes scar from the prior operation as well as injury either at branch level or at multiple points along the main trunk makes repair impossible. One can then only hope for spontaneous regeneration and institute a regimen of shoulder exercises for the patient.

Digital Nerves

Digital nerve injury usually falls into the province of the hand surgeon. A finger retaining one normal digital nerve will usually regain sensation of adequate degree at its tip, but a major sensory handicap exists with palmar lacerations that totally denervate one or more fingers. If needed to aid in the suture, length can be obtained by mobilizing the median nerve proximally. Regeneration through the suture of these purely sensory twigs is excellent. By the same token, this is another situation in which nerve grafting is feasible when the defect to be bridged is not too long, probably because all penetrating sensory axons will reach distal sensory channels and the nerve graft can be small in caliber.

TECHNIQUE FOR NERVE LESION EXPLORATION, EVALUATION, AND REPAIR

The operation should be planned so that a total evaluation of the denervated muscle can be made. Also, if a long gap is encountered between the nerve ends, it must be possible to make a lengthy dissection that will aid in nerve lengthening to take the stress off the suture line. Freedom in positioning the extremity requires the use of stockinette after full skin preparation. If appropriate, the hand should be gloved to observe finger movement and intrinsic muscle action.

Exposure and Evaluation

Incisions for exposure of the lesion should either avoid flexor creases or course in them. One should always work from the normal proximal and distal nerve segments toward the abnormal or injured area. This is particularly important in old wounds in which major vessels as well as a nerve may be embedded in heavy scar tissue and may be lacerated if great care is not used by the surgeon.

A tourniquet should not be used because it may mask significant bleeding points, not only in the soft tissues but also in the nerve itself. In addition, use of the tourniquet by the uninitiated can cause the surgeon to confuse tendons with nerves and to suture one to the other. If, in spite of this, a tourniquet is used, it should be deflated for 15 to 20 minutes before any electrical studies are carried out, since prolonged inflation of the tourniquet (beyond an hour) at a high pressure will suppress conduction even if such is present prior to the use of the tourniquet. Such loss of conduction will reverse if the tourniquet is let down for a 15- to 20-minute period. In order to achieve the best results, soft-tissue hemostasis must be meticulous. Either local or general anesthesia can be used. With general anesthesia, motor stimulation and evoked nerve action potentials can be assessed but not sensory stimulation. Therefore it may be advisable, with early exploration of a lesion in continuity, to keep the patient awake for exposure of the distal nerve segment to evaluate its sensitivity. Early knowledge that there is no neural continuity to be preserved greatly speeds the operative dissection.

The evaluation of a lesion in continuity has already been discussed (see Neuromas in Continuity). If its gross appearance does not permit a clear decision between resection and preservation, physiological data become important. Absence of neural sensitivity just distal to the lesion attests to discontinuity; motor response to nerve stimulation is important positive evidence, but there may not have been time for it to develop. Then the recording of nerve action potentials becomes an important guide to the degree of regeneration that is under way. Bipolar stimulating and recording electrodes are placed proximal to the lesion 4 to 6 cm apart and a nerve action potential is recorded by using stimuli of brief duration—.01 to.08 msec. The more distal recording electrodes are then moved through the region of the injury and on to the distal stump, and the nerve action potential's course is followed down the nerve. One may have to increase the stimulator's voltage and also the amplitude setting of the differential amplifiers once the electrodes are over and distal to the lesion itself. If a nerve potential can be recorded and two or more

months have elapsed since injury, then the lesion will do well with just a simple neurolysis, but if a potential cannot be recorded after this time interval, resection is necessary. In early exploration when some regeneration is suggested but its adequacy is uncertain, a final decision may not be possible. The lesion must be given more time and, failing development of proof for adequate regeneration, be re-explored after two months. Finally, the surgeon must always be aware of the probable results of the suture he would substitute for the lesion in continuity.

Neurolysis

Neurolysis usually implies the careful dissection required to expose a neuroma in continuity and to free it of extrinsic scar tissue. By definition, neurolysis should mean freeing the nerve through 360 degrees around its circumference as well as dissection both proximal and distal to the lesion itself. When scarring is dense, the surgeon may feel his dissection has therapeutic value in decompressing or freeing the nerve from constricting scar. And if his decision to preserve this neuroma in continuity was correct, he may credit subsequent neural recovery to his operative intervention. Indeed, many surgeons with wide experience feel that recovery can be enhanced by neurolysis.[123,143] Yet, paradoxically, all agree that a nerve showing partial function need not be dissected, and there are few well-documented examples of subsequent regression of partial nerve function, except when the lesion is affected by an associated aneurysm, a hematoma, or a complicating entrapment. Finally, recovery after neurolysis, when good serial data are available, will usually have followed a schedule relating to the date of injury, with no relationship to the time of dissection.[107]

Dissection of the nerve from its bed of scar, or external neurolysis, can be combined with internal neurolysis. Some surgeons favor internal neurolysis by saline injection to loosen the nerve fascicles from the scar tissue. This mechanism is difficult to visualize. Further, if one records evoked potentials during such a procedure in the laboratory animal, the potentials may disappear, suggesting that saline injection can damage the axons. Thus, the authors do not favor saline injection as a therapeutic procedure.

Internal neurolysis involves resection or division of scar tissue away from the nerve fascicles. Theoretically, partial internal resection of scar tissue decompresses otherwise intact fascicles and improves the chances for nerve regeneration. Brown believes that early recovery will follow neurolysis. He reported improvement in 34 of 53 patients within 10 days of the neurolysis.[25] Yet, it can be argued that these lesions in continuity, operated on within four to six weeks of injury, could have fared equally well without operative intervention. If two or more months have elapsed since injury and an internal neurolysis is done despite absence of a nerve action potential, one can argue that the procedure has validity if subsequent significant recovery occurs. At the present time the authors reserve internal neurolysis for those lesions that have either distal response to stimulation or a nerve action potential, in which resection and suture is not necessary, and in which noncausalgic pain is a prominent portion of the syndrome. In such cases, a carefully done internal neurolysis will sometimes improve the pain syndrome. Internal neurolysis is also certainly of value in partial nerve lesions in which some of the fascicles conduct and require only a neurolysis, whereas others do not conduct and require section and either end-to-end repair or, more commonly, interposition of a fascicular or interfascicular graft.

As pointed out previously, if injury to nerve is close to a potentially tight area such as the carpal tunnel at the wrist or the olecranon notch at the elbow, a properly done external neurolysis will divide these possibly offending structures and may be of help.

For the most part, neurolysis is done when the surgeon decides the lesion will permit better regeneration if it is left alone than if it is resected and sutured. The surgeon hopes that such additional maneuvers will improve the regenerative capacity of the nerve. World War II statistics comparing neurolysis to suture showed neurolysis to be consistently superior in restoring good practical function. These statistics were 47.6 per cent versus 23.3 per cent for the median nerve, 87.5 per cent versus 50.0 per cent for the radial nerve, and 65.9 per cent versus 41.2 per cent for the ulnar nerve. Actually, these statistics are simply a reflection of the good judgment that was used by the surgeons who decided that these particular lesions should not be resected and sutured. Civilian experience in which nerve action potential recording is used to identify lesions in continuity that need only neurolysis and not suture gives results close to the 90 per cent level.[75]

Clearly, it is always correct to explore a nerve lesion in which the nerve's functional capacity is in doubt and to perform a neurolysis to aid in evaluating its appearance and consistency. But if there is clear physiological evidence that this lesion in continuity is not regenerating to a degree that is appropriate to the time that has elapsed, the surgeon will not have improved the intrinsic axonal disruption by his dissection.

Mobilization of Nerve Segments

This measure is necessary to overcome the gap that results from retraction of the stumps and resection of the damaged nerve ends. It can be done after resection, but the conservative surgeon may want first to establish how much he can resect. Maximal nerve length is obtained by dissecting beyond the distal and the proximal joints. The nerve segment must be so well freed that its end moves 3 to 4 cm toward the planned suture site with joint movement. The proximal segment can be advanced distally by meticulously splitting muscle branches from the main trunk without disrupting their continuity. Muscle branches that restrict proximal advancement of the distal segment by their tethering effect may have to be sacrificed. For example, a long median nerve gap at the elbow level may be overcome by sacrifice of branches to the pronator teres when this will permit a suture that is needed to provide more important distal motor function and sensation. The techniques for gaining further length by transposition of ulnar and radial nerves and by resecting the fibular head for the peroneal nerve have been discussed earlier.

Neurophysiological studies have shown that extensive mobilization does not affect the subsequent function of a normal nerve. As long as the longitudinal subepineurial vessels are preserved, the anastomotic vessels can be interrupted without reduction in function.[1,9,14] Some have argued, however, that mobilization that kills collateral blood supply is deleterious to successful regeneration.[90,133] Neurophysiological studies in the authors' laboratory show that the anastomotic or collateral vessels may be interrupted prior to repair of an injured nerve, and regeneration will proceed at the same rate and with the same eventual result as that of a nerve that is repaired without mobilization (Fig. 75–35).[80] While mobilization should be only as extensive as is necessary to get the job done, the risks to function are less important than those of inadequate resection of the injury or excessive tension on the repair. As stated previously, downgrading of end results of suture does not begin until gaps of over 8 cm must be overcome for most nerves and of over 10 cm for the ulnar nerve.[164] Others disagree with this concept, believing that any gap over a few centimeters in length should be corrected by grafts rather than mobilization or positioning of the extremity.[99,124] Recently, the authors have used nerve grafts rather than risk distraction from excessive tension on an end-to-end anastomosis.

Resection and Suture

The extent of resection that is needed to insure good proximal and distal stump tissue is estimated by inspection and palpation of the lesion. Before the injury is resected, a marking suture should be placed on each side of the nerve within the sheath of normal segments above and below the

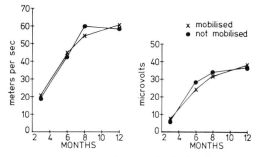

Figure 75–35 Amplitude and velocity of nerve action potentials distal to suture site at intervals of two months to one year after suture of primate sciatic nerve. Nerve on one side was mobilized for suture, while that on the other was not. In these experiments, mobilization before injury and repair did not make any difference in the eventual result. (Graph constructed by R. W. Gilliatt, M.D., London, England. Data from Kline, D. G., et al.: Effect of mobilization on the blood supply and regeneration of injured nerves. J. Surg. Res., *12*:254–266, 1972.)

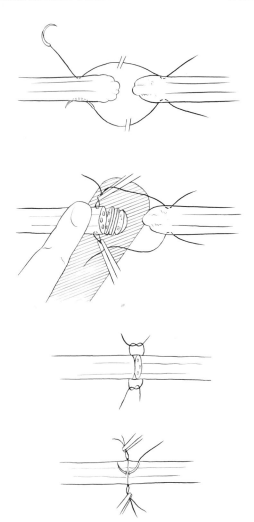

Figure 75–36 Steps in the repair of a completely severed nerve. Swedged-on sutures of fine nylon or other low-reactive suture are preplaced to prevent rotation of the stumps and to obtain optimal realignment. Stumps are then placed on a moist tongue blade and are sharply sectioned back to good fascicular structure. The resected stumps are then drawn together by the preplaced lateral sutures. Multiple epineurial sutures are closely placed anteriorly and then posteriorly. This can be accomplished by partially rotating the nerve by the preplaced lateral sutures.

neuroma (Fig. 75–36). These two preplaced lateral sutures minimize rotation of the nerve stumps after resection of the neuroma. Each lateral suture begins just distal to where the major portion of the injury ends and then is looped over and placed just proximal to the injury and under slack so that it can be tied after resection of the neuroma. Thin 1- to 2-mm serial slices are then made through each stump with a sharp razor blade. Clean section requires that the nerve be stabilized on either side of the advancing razor cut, and this can be done by holding or clamping the preplaced lateral sutures. The cuts must be made with minimal pressure on a firm surface such as a tongue blade. Resection is adequate only when good proximal and distal stump fascicular structure is encountered, perineurial connective tissue scar is minimal, and both ends bleed freely (Fig. 75–37). Magnification, either with an operating microscope or loupes, is of help in identifying normal neural architecture and in placing the sutures through the epineurium (Fig. 75–38).

The appearance of healthy nerve ends usually coincides with brisk bleeding. Neural hemostasis must be gentle and is usually obtained by the temporary tamponade afforded by Gelfoam or a piece of muscle. Firm pressure on the end of the stump is often necessary for a prolonged period to achieve hemostasis. The tamponading material must then be fully freed from the stump by irrigation, and the whole procedure repeated if bleeding resumes. Any residual clot will interfere with good repair.

The time necessary to achieve hemostasis can be utilized to begin closure of either end of the soft-tissue wound. Then the two preplaced lateral sutures should be drawn together and a series of epineurial sutures placed, using a fine nonreactive suture material such as nylon, Merceline, or silk with a swedged needle (Fig. 75–39).

Since recovery after nerve suture may be decreased by poor fascicular matching and subsequent axon regeneration into perifascicular spaces, fascicular suture has merit, although it is usually not practical. One of the difficulties with fascicular repair of other than very sharp lesions is that after nerve stumps have been trimmed back to healthy or potentially healthy tissue, the fascicular pattern has changed substantially. The fascicle previously located at one o'clock is now at three o'clock, and the one that was at three o'clock is at six or one o'clock. It then may no longer be possible to match fascicles accurately. In addition, the trade-off that occurs between fascicles is limited by a fascicular suture. An unexpected advantage of an end-to-end repair, which admittedly results in a disorganized

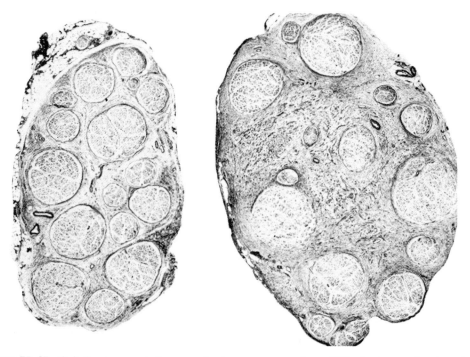

Figure 75–37   Only 2 mm separate these proximal nerve cross sections. With simple magnification, the surgeon can easily recognize that too much of the cross-sectional area on the right is occupied by perineurial connective tissue. Further resection to obtain the appearance on the left is needed to get a good yield from suture, even if this increment in nerve loss demands further nerve trunk mobilization beyond another joint.

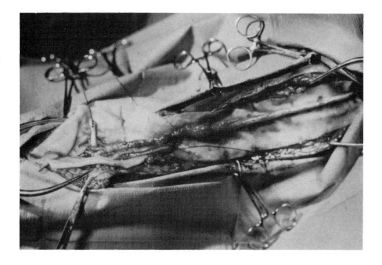

Figure 75–38 This picture of re-exploration of a nonregenerating median nerve suture reveals a frequently encountered error (the proximal nerve on the right has been sutured to the palmaris longus tendon on the left). Clearly, the original surgeon did not inspect the distal "nerve end" for a normal fascicular pattern or demand that it bleed freely on transection.

repair site, is that regenerating axons are permitted to remix and perhaps to resecure old pathways down the distal stump and are not limited by fascicular boundaries, which are at least theoretically insured by fascicular repair. Fascicular suture works best with high median and sciatic injuries and occasionally with ulnar injuries at the level of the wrist.[63,113,142,163]

Tension on the suture line will detract from the results only when actual separation occurs. If the surgeon fears distraction due to extensive tension, both nerve segments should be further mobilized to provide more length. Occasionally, with full measures to provide length such as transposition, sacrifice of branches, mobilization, and positioning of the limb, the suture line remains under tension. When such tension is unavoidable, the use of reinforcing stain-less steel sutures may prevent disruption of the stumps. The position of the metallic sutures and thus of the stumps can be followed postoperatively by x-rays. Even when reinforcement is not necessary, tagging sutures of fine stainless steel should be placed through the sheath of each stump at a measured distance from each other so that any subsequent disruption of the anastomosis can be detected by x-ray.[156] Another solution to excessive tension, after the usual measures to reduce it have been taken, is to use short interfascicular grafts, which, when correctly placed and short in length, will work.[22a,77]

A partial suture is indicated in instances in which close to half of a nerve trunk is severely damaged while the other half has escaped, especially when this can be proved by electrophysiological testing.

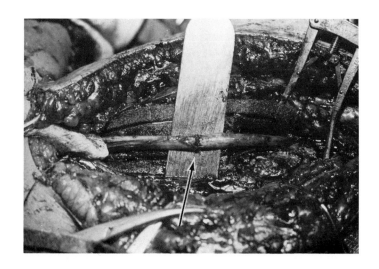

Figure 75–39 Radial nerve injection injury at level of lateral upper arm. No nerve action potential could be recorded at three months postinjection, and in addition there was no brachioradialis contraction in response to stimulation of the nerve. After resection of the injection site, epineurial suture of the radial nerve was accomplished.

This type of injury can occur with sharp lacerations of the median or ulnar nerve at the wrist. Use of interfascicular grafts to repair the portion of the injury that is neurotmetic and neurolysis of the remaining more intact nerve is probably preferable to direct suture and formation of a relatively redundant loop of intact nerve.[163]

Closure of soft tissues and fascia is contrived, when possible, to contain the nerve in an environment of healthy, unscarred tissue and in a locus that protects the sensitive new neuroma in continuity. This must be done in a way that does not increase tension on the suture and does not angulate or compress the nerve trunk. Subcutaneous tissues and skin should be sutured in routine fashion. Certain portions of the closure may be more comfortably accomplished before nerve suture, since from this point onward, the extremity must be held in its final position for immobilization, often requiring the full attention of an assistant.

Proper immobilization of the limb after repair is vital in the management of nerve injuries.[29] A plaster of Paris cast remains the best method. Early after the suture, it can be converted to a half shell that restricts extension. Campbell has suggested fashioning the cast preoperatively, then splitting it and reapplying it immediately after the operation.[32] In the authors' experience, however, the proper position for immobilization of the limb is determined before wound closure while tension on the repair can be palpated. Extension at each joint must be prohibited at that point just short of producing tension on the suture line. Especially important is the recognition that hip flexion can avulse a sutured peroneal nerve despite full restriction of movement at both the knee and the ankle. The usual policy is to leave the extremity in the cast for three to six weeks.[146] This period of immobilization should permit the area of repair to develop enough tensile strength to tolerate some tension.[88] Depending upon the gap to be overcome and the tension on the suture line observed at the time of repair, the extremity is occasionally extended in stages and a new cast is applied at each stage. Usually, however, by three weeks the patient will limit overextension of the limb of his own accord because of painful dysesthesias in the sensory distribution of the nerve.

Nerve Grafts

With experience in overcoming gaps, the surgeon finds that nerve grafts rarely are necessary. Most grafts used during both World Wars were, in retrospect, not needed, since the gaps that they filled could have been overcome if the surgeon had been experienced in making up length in these injuries.[128] Heterogenous grafts have been uniformly unsuccessful, and the usual freeze-dried homografts have also failed.[110] Both Campbell and Marmor have had some success with freeze-dried homografts that have been irradiated.[31,92] Long-term results, however, do not appear to be as encouraging as some initial reports indicated.[93] Irradiated freeze-dried grafts have worked best in making up short gaps, which limits their application.

A nearly absolute limitation on regeneration already exists when a major mixed nerve trunk requires suture at two levels, even with what should be the most ideal graft segment interposed. As discussed before, the twice compounded loss of motor axons into sensory channels and of sensory axons into motor channels at two nerve suture interfaces presents by itself a major barrier to useful reinnervation. The only exception may be the low-grade sensory recovery in the median nerve area that can result from bridging a median nerve gap by "walking" an already divided ulnar nerve segment over in two stages. Perhaps the freeze-dried irradiated homografts can work better, but with only this limited goal of sensory recovery to be expected.

A more realistic question is whether these homografts will conduct axonal regrowth as well as, or better than, autogenous grafts in those situations in which the latter are unquestionably of value. An example of such a situation is the bridging of a short gap for a pure motor or a pure sensory nerve of small caliber. This has been successful in the case of gaps up to 4 cm for facial, hypoglossal, and digital nerves. Recent experimental work has shown that the Schwann cells are much more adaptable than was previously believed and, in an autogenous graft segment, not only survive but are capable of making myelin.[2,4] Apposition of several cables to proximal and distal nerve ends usually requires interfascicular suture. The plasma glue technique of Tarlov is, however, uniquely suitable for achieving coaptation of several cables to a single nerve face. To learn the technique, the surgeon should spend a few hours practicing grafting the nerves of a cat and following Tarlov's excellent instructions.[147] One of the authors has used this method in two cases for cable grafts to facial nerve and has obtained a useful motor recovery. Grafts should be 10 to 20 per cent longer than the gap to allow for shrinkage.[31,40] The contribution of a graft to a good result must be proved either by muscle response to nerve trunk stimulation for motor nerves, or by sensory evoked potentials or absence of sensation in the appropriate area when the nerve is blocked by lidocaine injection (Fig. 75–40). Current neurosurgical thinking would include making up most of the gap by judicious mobilization, sacrifice of unimportant nerve branches, transposition of the nerve where possible, and proper positioning of the limb. Any residual gap can then be made up by use of interfascicular grafts.

Millesi and co-workers have argued that any tension on a repair can downgrade the eventual result and advise the use of interfascicular grafts for any nerve repair where the gap between stumps before mobilization or any other relaxing maneuvers is 2 cm or more.[98,98a] To date, such a concept has not been supported by the authors' own laboratory or clinical experience.[22a] Since it can be said that *short* interfascicular grafts do work, however, their current approach is to reduce as much of the gap as possible by utilizing classic maneuvers and then if a gap still persists to interpose interfascicular grafts. They do not advise use of grafts to make up small gaps that can be readily closed by proper mobilization and end-to-end repair.

It is apparent, however, that multiple small fascicular or interfascicular grafts work better than whole nerve grafts, whether they be freeze-dried or irradiated homografts or even whole-nerve autografts. The sural nerve remains the best donor for interfascicular grafts and may be readily located with an incision lateral to the gastrocnemius-Achilles tendon and proximal to the lateral malleolous. Twenty to thirty centimeters of the nerve can be taken by tracing it up to the popliteal fossa and sectioning it proximally in such a way that the sural stump is left at a deep and somewhat protected level. Sharp dissection is used to clean the sural nerve of excessive epineurial connective tissue and to section it into cables, which can then with a few sutures be used to span relatively short gaps with some hope of success.

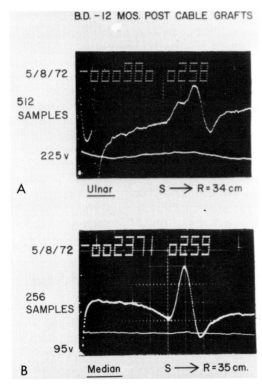

Figure 75–40 *A.* Computer tracings made by stimulating ulnar nerve at wrist distal to 4-inch interfascicular grafts and recording proximally from upper arm. A trace indicates conduction along the graft. Patient recovered hypothenar muscular function but little interosseus and no adductor pollicis and only weak lumbricales function. *B.* Trace from adjacent and presumably normal median nerve for comparison. Bottom trace in each inset represents single sample, while top one represents summated samples (in the case of the ulnar nerve, 512).

Sleeves or Wrappers

The use of a wrapper around the suture site has been advocated for many years.[68] The rationale for such a device is that it prevents connective tissue invasion of the repair site and that it shields the repair from the constrictive effects of external scar tissue. Furthermore, advocates of a sleeve state that it promotes longitudinal axonal regeneration by restricting expansion of the neuroma at the repair site.[82] To date, however, there has been no objective evidence that the use of a sleeve or wrapper will provide either earlier or more complete return of motor function than repair accomplished without such a device. A slightly positive note was sounded to the effect that when Silastic cuffs are used, sensory regeneration in the sutured and wrapped nerve occurs earlier and is more complete than with suture alone.[45] Experience with tantalum sheaths during World War II suggested the same type of improvement in sensory regeneration, but there was no improvement in motor function. Both tantalum and Millipore have in the past been widely used as sleeves because they are relatively inert.[33,152,160] With time, however, both of these materials fragment.[164] When fragmentation occurs, many surfaces are presented to surrounding tissues, including the nerve, and connective tissue proliferation results. Thus, there develops the very complication of extensive scarring that these otherwise inert materials were designed to prevent, often requiring reoperation for their removal. Silastic does not seem to disintegrate and has been in place for several years in a number of patients with no reports of complications to date.[32] Even Silastic can crinkle, however, especially if placed around nerve passing over joints. For this reason, Silastic, on occasion, may also have to be removed. Any type of wrapper, whether resorbable or not, does not reduce either perineurial or endoneurial connective tissue proliferation, and it is scar at these levels that thwarts effective axonal growth.

An ideal wrapper would be one that would be resorbable after shielding the repair site for a period of six to eight weeks until axons span the repair site and enter the distal stump. Unfortunately, resorption is accompanied by a proliferation of inflammatory cells and connective tissue. To date a suitable absorbable cuff has not been found.[76]

REHABILITATION FROM INJURY TO RECOVERY

Functional Use Despite Deficit

All too often, the physician is so preoccupied with neural events or so impressed with the patient's complaints of pain that he does not guide him toward the practical use of his hand or foot that is possible despite the neural handicap. If, both before delayed nerve suture and in the long interval of awaiting regeneration, the patient is using his extremity instead of nursing it, his whole attitude will be directed toward maximal rehabilitation. Also, a significant disability from pain is far less likely to develop. The patient with total sciatic nerve injury can be ambulatory immediately after the injury if there is no accompanying fracture, and in this event, he will be much happier than if he is immobile. By contrast, the patient with the same nerve injury and a femoral fracture will more often than not begin to require narcotics for leg pain during the long interval of immobilization in traction. Despite excellent healing of the fracture, this patient's original concept of a useless and painful leg that needs to be nursed may cloud subsequent efforts directed toward rehabilitation. In general, the physician does the patient a great favor by firmly directing him in use of his limb and giving him the conviction that it is through use that he can solve his problem of discomfort.

The patient with a median nerve injury can use his fingers for grasping and can learn to pick up objects between side of thumb and base of index finger. The patient with ulnar nerve injury retains good use of his thumb and first two fingers. He must be instructed to stretch the curled fourth and fifth fingers so that neither flexor muscle shortening nor fixed joint changes occur. Part of the time, he can wear a light dorsal splint to stabilize the fourth and fifth metacarpal phalangeal joints in mild flexion so that he can actively extend the distal phalanges of these fingers. After a radial nerve injury, a light splint can be used to hold the wrist in dorsiflexion. Fixed splinting of the metacarpal phalangeal joints in extension too often results in joint stiffness. With the wrist properly splinted, the patient quickly learns to use the thumb with the fingers to pick up small objects as well as to drape his fingers around large objects so as to grasp them actively. Failure to support the wrist in dorsiflexion most of the time may decrease the ultimate function of reinnervated extensors that have been overstretched. Dual nerve injuries present a much more difficult problem. Dynamic splinting is indicated if there is reasonable expectation for the ultimate rehabilitation of a useful hand (Fig. 75–41).

The leg and foot present usually a far simpler problem than do the arm and hand. With good hip and knee function, one has only to brace the foot in a stable position of dorsiflexion to permit good ambulation. If the sole lacks sensory innervation, the brace should be fitted to an oversized shoe (two sizes longer; two sizes wider) that is generously padded with foam rubber.[21] The patient (and the physician at first) must watch the foot as carefully as does the patient with diabetes. The slightest blister demands a return to crutches with discontinuance of shoe and weight bearing plus redesign of the padding to prevent recurrence. The effort is worthwhile, for a man with total sciatic paralysis who can play 18 holes of golf a month after injury is unlikely to have psychological problems.

Physical therapists and occupational therapists can be of tremendous help in motivating and training the individual to use his hand or to walk at these early stages. Once the limb begins to be an asset to the patient instead of a liability, he will rarely need help to reuse muscles that become reinnervated. Later, he is functioning to some degree without them and any further recovery is a delightful bonus. At the same time, the patient may require instruction in passive stretching exercises to prevent muscle stretching exercises to prevent muscle contracture or joint fixation. Again, it is motivation to do for himself outside the physical therapy room that determines whether the effort will succeed. It is not enough to go to physical therapy daily, let alone several times a week. The patient must be persuaded to exercise and work his injured limb throughout the day at home. In addition to manipulation, the patient should be taught simple strengthening exercises that he can do himself. For example, instruction in standing next to a door or a wall and walking fingers and hand up the wall is exceedingly useful for patients with shoulder disability and upper arm weakness.

Electrical stimulation of muscles during their interval of denervation has tremendous psychological appeal to both the patient and the therapist. A carefully controlled study involved teaching alternate patients with total median or ulnar nerve transection and suture to stimulate the opponens or abductor digiti quinti for at least two hours a day in a device that required the muscle to work against resistance.[87] Muscle atrophy was greatly reduced in those who were stimulated, but on follow-up in five years these patients had developed no more muscle strength on voluntary effort than had the control group with comparable delays and levels of nerve suture. The problem is that to have even the possibility of being effective, the muscle stimulation must be applied for at least half an hour per day for each muscle and must make that muscle work against resistance. Almost invariably, this is so time-consuming for the patient and the therapist that it distracts them from the practical goals of developing and avoiding contractures.

Finally, it is very important for the patient to recognize the potential use of his still handicapped limb and to work out contractures before a nerve suture requiring extensive mobilization and a cast subjects him again to disuse and to pain. If the patient is first seen at six weeks after the injury and a nerve suture is indicated, much is to be gained in some situations by a 10-

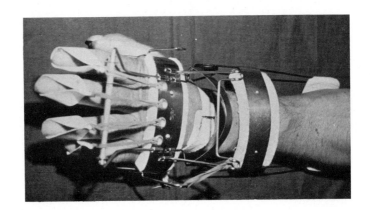

Figure 75–41 Dynamic splint for a patient with radial palsy including loss of extensor communis and extensor pollicis longus function as well as loss of wrist dorsiflexion.

day interval of intensive physical therapy before the operation.

Substitutive Mechanics

The possibilities for substituting through tendon transfer the action of normal muscles to supply movements that do not recover through nerve regeneration have been mentioned under Specific Nerve Injuries. At times, one must await the end result of neural regeneration without knowing whether a distal muscle such as the long extensor to the thumb will or will not become adequately supplied. At the same time, the limitations for nerve regeneration are so well defined in situations of proximal transection combined with a long delay in suture that the need for a tendon transfer may be apparent without waiting. If so, the tendon transfer should be accomplished without further delay. The orthopedic literature is full of excellent references on this subject.* It is important for the neurosurgeon to recognize the type of substitute mechanical help that is available and at what point it should be used. He must also recognize

---

* See references 12, 19, 30, 111, 111a, 134, 165.

those situations in which excellent repair of the nerve combined with all the substitutive mechanical procedures that are available cannot restore the slightest practical functional use to the extremity.

The most frequently useful substitutive procedures are reviewed briefly here. When median nerve regeneration fails to provide satisfactory thumb opposition, a variety of effective procedures is available.[20,55,86,117] A tendon inserted into the distal end of the thumb's metacarpal can be activated by a normal ulnar forearm muscle flexor (Fig. 75–42). The linkage usually is directed through a tendon pulley close to the pisiform bone. This gives a pulling movement that closely mimics opposition. With extensive motor loss that involves ulnar forearm muscles as well, it may be necessary to fuse the thumb's metacarpal in a fixed position of opposition.

The chief disability with ulnar nerve deficit is the inability to extend the fourth and fifth fingers. Permanence of this deficit can be predicted at an early time, and substitutive procedures can be initiated. Slips from the flexor sublimis tendons can be passed through the lumbrical canals and into the extensor expansions of the digits to give excellent finger-opening movements.[19,30] With

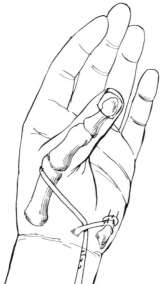

MOTOR - FLEX. CARP. ULNARIS

TENDON - GRAFT FROM PALM. LONGUS

PULLEY - PALMARIS LONGUS WITH ITS INSERTION

Figure 75–42   One device for utilizing an ulnar-supplied muscle to provide missing thumb opposition. The tendon of the flexor carpi ulnaris is prolonged with a tendon graft from the palmaris longus to be inserted into the thumb's distal metacarpal. A separate segment of the tendon graft is used to construct a pulley close to the pisiform bone.

high ulnar lesions this procedure is needed in every case and should be done early after the injury and before fixed clawing of the fingers detracts from the excellent result that this operation can offer.[161]

Tendon transfers offer the best compensation for isolated injuries of the radial nerve not correctable by suture.[122,161] Normal wrist flexor tendons are usually employed. With high radial sutures it is best to await such extensor functions as may recover by innervation, reserving the tendon transfers for and concentrating upon just those finger or thumb extensor functions that remain inadequate. If there is a paucity of good flexor muscles available for use in powering the extensors, the wrist can be fused in mild dorsiflexion. This method will save those muscles that are available for use in supplying light finger extension.

Multiple nerve injuries present more complex and often insoluble problems. There may or may not be enough power to supply the minimum for use. This minimum is thumb to finger opposition plus active separation of thumb from fingers. Moreover, these mechanical functions are useless if there is not an adequate median sensory supply to thumb and first two fingers. Occasionally, a high plexus injury will spare a good hand that requires support by fusion of a flail elbow or shoulder.[166]

Various orthopedic procedures have been recommended to permit active foot dorsiflexion in the presence of inadequate peroneal nerve recovery.[17] But even if muscles supplied by the tibial nerve are normal, dorsal transfer of the posterior tibial tendon and of the flexor hallucis longus tendon has seldom given long-term good results despite good function initially. Fusion at the ankle level generally works better in small, light individuals than in the heavier-set person, in whom it may break down or be a source of pain. The spring-action brace is surprisingly satisfactory and may be preferable to a fixed ankle fusion when the patient has active plantar flexion to assist in walking. A spring-loaded kick-up foot brace is far preferable to stabilization of the ankle and foot, since the brace will permit an almost normal walking pattern. Many patients, once they are taught to use the kick-up brace, are quite happy with it and may not even wish anything further done about their peroneal nerve palsy. But with involvement of both peroneal and tibial mus-

cles, a fixed triple arthrodesis is preferable to a brace.

Reconstructive procedures available for patients with complete femoral nerve palsy are unfortunately limited. Fusion of the knee in extension is not a very satisfactory substitute for a functional quadriceps. Similarly, braces to stabilize the knee and thigh are bulky, uncomfortable, and often expensive and seldom worn by the patient. Thus, some attempt at repair of the femoral nerve should be made.

Pain

Physicians and patients alike feel intuitively that nerve injuries should be painful. The rare condition of causalgia is so exquisitely painful that an element of causalgia may be falsely considered whenever a patient with a nerve injury complains of intractable pain and is reluctant to use his extremity. It is therefore important to define causalgia, even though it accompanies nerve injuries in less than 2 per cent of civilians and less than 5 per cent of military personnel.

Causalgia

Causalgia, as described by Weir Mitchell in 1865, presents certain well-defined characteristics, just as does true trigeminal neuralgia. Atypical causalgia does not respond to specific treatment any more than does atypical trigeminal neuralgia. Causalgia is rarely seen in association with nerve transection or in association with a major degree of motor or sensory deficit. Most commonly, it occurs with a grazing injury to the median or tibial nerve, always with some sensory preservation, and usually with all muscles functioning somewhat, at least after an interval of neurapraxia.[150] The pain begins early after the injury and is described as constant and burning by a patient who seems to be suffering intensely. A prerequisite for diagnosis of causalgia is the triggering of paroxysmal pain by the slightest external stimulus to hand or foot in a wide area far beyond the confines of sensory supply of the injured nerves. Crucial in making the diagnosis of causalgia is the patient's inability to tolerate the slightest manipulation of his extremity. The patient with a causalgia-like but not a true causalgia syndrome will permit the extremity to be manipulated, particularly if his attention is distracted. In addition, the extremity that is involved shows striking evidence of alteration in autonomic function. Mayfield has described the changes that occur over a period of time.[95,96] The hand is colder or warmer, pinker or more bluish, and almost always more moist than its mate. Ultimately, atrophic changes develop in skin, bone, joints, and muscles. Since any movement may trigger paroxysms of pain, it is difficult to judge to what extent the problem is compounded by disuse. Although almost half the patients will gradually improve spontaneously, it is important to avoid these possible dire end results and to proceed promptly with the diagnostic-therapeutic test of stellate block.

The participation of the sympathetic outflow in the mechanism for causalgic pain is difficult to understand, but Granit and coworkers' hypothesis is attractive.[58] They propose that partial injury to a nerve trunk permits efferent sympathetic discharge to activate afferent pain fibers through a breakdown in insulation at the point of injury. Although there are many objections to this theory, the fact remains that early after sympathectomy, while sympathetic axons can still conduct, stimulation of the purely efferent sympathetic chain, which is now detached from central connection, causes the patient to re-experience his diffuse burning pain. Patients who do not have causalgia and who have a sympathectomy purely to improve circulation experience no discomfort with efferent sympathetic stimulation. An alternate explanation is provided by the more recent work concerning the "gate-theory."[97] Partial injury to nerve may, under some circumstances, disturb the normal relationship between small- and large-fiber input to the spinal cord, tending to preserve proportionally more small than large fibers. Sympathectomy, since it kills some fine fibers, may restore this balance and either cure or decrease causalgia.

It is clear from most workers' experience as well as the authors' own that sympathectomy does little or nothing for the noncausalgic pain associated with many peripheral nerve injuries. Nevertheless, the necessity of sympathetic activity for the experience of causalgic pain seems so clearly a part of the mechanism that a final criterion for the diagnosis of causalgia is its dramatic relief by sympathetic block. Fortunately, this criterion is invariably met when the symptoms and the triggering of paroxysms are typical. A problem arises when stellate block relieves pain that is not typical of causalgia. It then becomes important to determine whether the improvement is due to a placebo effect and whether complete relief occurs also with sham injections or with injections that fortunately do not produce a marked warming and loss of sweating in the arm. One should always give the patient the benefit of the doubt regarding this diagnosis, however, and sympathetic block may be worth a try even in those with a less typical syndrome. The patient must not be coached as to what to expect. Rather, the physician caring for the patient must be present after the block to evaluate the limb not only for warmth and decreased sweating but also to evaluate the patient's response in terms of pain. Sometimes serial blocks will suffice; in other instances the pain will return after each period of nearly complete relief, and it will be clear that surgical sympathectomy will be needed. Clearly, injections that affect the sensory roots and cause loss of hand sensation do not prove a specific sympathetic role in the pain. With typical causalgia, which is completely relieved by stellate block, it is worthwhile to repeat the injections several times before resorting to operative sympathectomy. Often, the duration of relief will increase from hours to days after injection, and the syndrome will subside without resort to operation.

Pain that is not causalgia may respond to stellate injection when there is vascular compromise with low-grade ischemia or edema. If circulation is clearly improved or if pain is invariably partially relieved by blockade, a surgical sympathectomy would be indicated without expectation of the dramatic total abolition of pain to be anticipated in causalgia. In some patients, a partial lesion in continuity associated with a noncausalgic pain pattern will actually be a complete lesion in continuity, the apparent sparing of function being provided by overlap or trade-off with adjacent nerves. This is not uncommon with forearm and wrist level lesions of median and ulnar nerves, since anastomoses between these nerves are not uncommon. What may be needed, rather than neurolysis of a complete lesion that has fine fibers regenerating through it, is resection and suture. In some cases this has resulted in dramatic relief of the pain syndrome.

Sensory Aberration

The sensory aberration that accompanies partial loss of sensation from nerve injury is unpleasant to all patients and seriously disabling to a few. The complete numbness resulting from total section is rarely considered painful, but there is a stage in regeneration with beginning skin reinnervation that is uncomfortable. During the recovery of a nerve injury there is a stage with dysesthesia when any stimuli are mildly painful but do not produce causalgia-like pain. These situations may well be explained by the hypothesis of Noordenbos, that nonnoxious stimuli seem painful when there is more small-fiber than large-fiber sensory input.[106] Furthermore, it is true that partial nerve injuries damage large fibers selectively to a greater extent than small fibers, and that in regeneration the skin is initially supplied by a great preponderance of small fibers. Treatment is primarily reassuring the patient and persuading him to continue increasing his use of the limb despite these unpleasant feelings. It should be emphasized that this is only a stage in recovery and will not last. Patients questioned in the five-year follow-up of the American World War II series were able to look back on this interval of sensory aberration as short-lived. At the time of follow-up they noted discomfort in their extremity only when it was subjected to extremes of cold. Special padding will help to relieve the pain on weight bearing. This type of sensory disturbance is very different from the pain of causalgia.[15] It is less spontaneous and not as volatile, and hyperesthesia is confined to the area of the nerves that are involved in the sensory supply.

Neuromas

A true neuroma, that is, a proximal nerve's ending in discontinuity, can be very painful when knocked or compressed. This is especially true when it is superficially located along the side of the finger or, more importantly, when it exists at an amputation stump (finger, arm, or leg). Light percussion causes paresthesias in the distal distribution of the nerve, and use of the finger or weight bearing causes severe discomfort. Spontaneous pain in the absence of pressure or contact cannot be attributed to a neuroma. Because relief when pain is due to neuromas has so often been difficult to achieve, there is always a "new treatment" such as encasement of the nerve stump in Silastic or Millipore. More conventional methods of management have consisted in (1) burying a digital neuroma proximally in a drill hole in the phalanx; (2) ligating the stump well proximal to the point of severance and injecting formalin or alcohol below the ligature; (3) sharply sectioning the nerve well proximal to the neuroma and embedding the freshly sectioned nerve end in adjacent deep soft tissues as well as possible; (4) preserving the epineurium, sectioning the nerve subepineurially, and closing the epineurium over the end of the nerve; and (5) dissecting individual fascicles and coagulating or ligating them.[143] The authors, in the past, favored the third of these possibilities, although they had, on occasion, to reoperate and reresect a new neuroma. If the freshly sectioned nerve end is placed in a protective environment deep in the limb and surrounded by musculature, however, this is less likely. Psychological factors, including secondary gain from compensation, play a role in the pain in an amputation stump.

Phantom Limb Pain

The sensation of a phantom limb after amputation is a normal physiological occurrence, and it is unclear why in certain individuals these sensations are painful and overwhelming. Accidental loss of limb is more likely to result in phantom pain than is a loss that gains the Purple Heart or otherwise brings honor to the patient. Adaptation to a useful prosthesis early after amputation greatly reduces the probability of disabling phantom pain. Pain that is increased by pressure calls for efforts to improve the local weight-bearing situation. These measures may include resection of any localized pain-producing neuroma. When tenderness rather than spontaneous pain is the main problem, a more proximal peripheral deafferentation or even an anterolateral cordotomy may be indicated to reduce this painful input. But, more often, the discomfort seems rather to be a conceptual one in which the extremity is sensed as being in a painful position, with fingers or toes curling into the flesh. Such feelings usually are unaffected by pharmacological blockade of all conceivable sensory input. When exacerbations are caused by stress and disappointment in the life situation, a psychiatrist often can be of help. Thalamotomy can give remarkable benefit, but the benefit to a particular patient cannot be predicted in advance. Implanted dorsal column stimulators are said to have strikingly ameliorated the phantom pain, at least over a short term. It is important to recognize that elective amputation of a denervated and useless limb does not produce a more painful phantom. Rather, the patient seems far more pleased to be relieved of nursing a useless dead weight.

Pain of Disuse

For emphasis, this chapter concludes on the theme upon which it began. As anyone who has gone through a period of immobilization in a cast after a fracture knows from experience, the return to use and mobility after cast removal is a highly painful process. Joint movement, muscle contraction, muscle stretching, and even dependency of the limb may cause discomfort. Disuse is the primary basis for pain in the patient who has an injured nerve and is immobilized by a fracture. Disuse is also the most common basis for pain in the patient with nerve injury without an accompanying fracture. The patient may choose immobility for fear of pain, but more often than not a physician has advised disuse "because the nerve is injured." The disuse can involve keeping the whole arm in a sling, avoiding weight bearing, or keeping on at all times a splint that holds the fingers rigid. Early use avoids most of the pain problems that are falsely considered to be related to the nerve injury per se. Return to use after enforced disuse requires skillful management of the patient and firm rapport with and skillful direction of nurses and therapists, with rewards for increasing the activity. Nerve blocks, electrical stimulation, whirlpool, and other forms of "magic" may assist the patient psychologically in regaining use of his limb. The majority of pain problems are derived from inept management and rapidly respond to a new and thoughtful approach to the whole patient.

SUMMARY

1. Nerves in which transection is suspected can be explored at once and repaired primarily if shown to have an uncontused division. Immediate repair is especially important for brachial plexus and sciatic transections in which delay leads not only to retraction but also to severe scarring, particularly if there has been prior operation for vascular repair.

2. A focally injured nerve (not known to be transected) should be explored within 8 to 10 weeks if it remains functionless. Long delays usually are avoidable. False evidence for recovery must be recognized as such. Failure to recognize beginning recovery by stimulating the nerve trunk percutaneously *before* operation leads to needless dissection and an added interval of disuse and pain.

3. Discovery of a neuroma in continuity during an operation requires the surgeon to make a comparison between the results that should be expected from section and suture and from leaving the neuroma undisturbed and in continuity. The average result from resection and nerve suture in this specific situation is predictable. Judgment whether the lesion in gross continuity will provide better or worse function than suture requires electrophysiological evaluation. Inability to stimulate muscle function distal to the injury or to record a nerve action potential beyond it several months following injury indicates the need for resection and suture. On the other hand, positive response to one or both of these tests provides strong evidence for the type of regeneration that will eventually lead to function, and thus neurolysis rather than resection and suture. Data from stimulation and evoked nerve action potential studies must be interpreted in relation to the time that has elapsed since the injury and the distance to the muscles that need innervation.

4. Certain total and partial limitations to recovery after high-level suture are well defined and permit one to judge when the suture is not worthwhile and when the suture must be supplemented by substitutive mechanics to provide effective function. Diffuse nerve injury by traction or ischemia is usually not treatable by resection and suture, although some cases are making careful selection for operation important.

5. Overcautious, inadequate resection of scarred nerve ends is the major cause for poorer-than-average regeneration through an otherwise technically good nerve anastomosis. The second leading cause for failure of nerve suture is distraction of the repair. Thus, the surgeon must recognize that extensive nerve trunk mobilization to bridge large gaps will not lessen the benefit so surely as will anastomosis of scarred nerve ends after overcautious, inadequate resection. On the other hand, direct suture under excessive tension is equally deleterious, and when the usual measures for making up length have failed to gain approximation, then the surgeon must be ready to use short autogenous interfascicular grafts.

6. A good end result requires attention to all aspects of rehabilitation from the beginning. Overcoming disuse and pain as well as visualizing the probable end result and the operative procedures needed to achieve it is necessary. Failure to give this support to the patient will reduce the results of excellent nerve regeneration to a collection of favorable electromyographic tracings and a painful, unused extremity.

REFERENCES

1. Adams, W. E.: Blood supply of nerves. J. Anat., 76:323–341, 1942.
2. Aguayo, A., Charron, L., and Bray, G.: Potential of Schwann cells from unmyelinated nerves to produce myelin: A quantitative ultrastructural and radiographic study. J. Neurocytol., 5:565–573, 1976.
3. Aguayo, A., Nair, C., and Midgely, R.: Experimental progressive compression neuropathy in the rabbit. Arch. Neurol., 24:358–364, 1971.
4. Aguayo, A., Attiwell, M., Trecarten, J., Perkins, S., and Bray, G.: Abnormal myelination in transplanted Trembler mouse Schwann cells. Nature, January 6, 1977.
5. Aita, J. A.: Neurologic manifestations of electrical injury. Nebraska Med. J., 40:530–533, 1965.
6. Aitken, J. T., and Thomas, P. K.: Retrograde changes in fiber size following nerve section. J. Anat., 96:121–129, 1962.
7. Aleksavdrovskaya, O. V.: Degeneration and regeneration of peripheral nerves in double injury. Tr. Mosk. Vet. Akad., 10:174–188, 1956.
8. Aschan, W., and Moberg, E.: Ninhydrin fiber printing test used to map out partial lesions to nerves of hand. Acta Chir. Scand., 123:365–370, 1962.
9. Bacsich, P., and Wyburn, G. M.: The vascular pattern of peripheral nerve during repair after experimental crush. J. Anat., 79:9–14, 1945.
10. Barnes, R.: Traction injuries of the brachial plexus in adults. J. Bone Joint Surg., 31-B:10–16, 1949.
11. Barr, M. L., and Hamilton, J. D.: A quantitative study of certain morphologic changes in spinal motor neurons during axon reaction. J. Comp. Neurol., 89:93–121, 1948.
12. Bateman, J. E.: Trauma to Nerves in Limbs. Philadelphia, W. B. Saunders Co., 1962. The anatomy of reconstruction in nerve injury, pp. 19–68. Operative problems related to the individual nerves, pp. 221–260.
13. Bauwens, P.: Electrodiagnostic definition of the site and nature of peripheral nerve lesions. Ann. Phys. Med., 5:149–152, 1960.
14. Bentley, F. H., and Schlapp, W.: Experiments on blood supply of nerves. J. Physiol. (London), 102:62–71, 1943.
15. Bonica, J. J.: The Management of Pain. Philadelphia, Lea & Febiger, 1954.
16. Bonney, G.: The value of axon responses in determining the site of lesion in traction injuries of the brachial plexus. Brain, 77:588–609, 1954.
17. Bourrel, P.: Transfer of the tibialis posterior to the tibalis anterior, and of flexor hallicus longus to the extensor digitorum longus in peroneal palsy. Ann. Chir., 21:1451–1456, 1967.
18. Bradley, K., Brock, L. G., and McIntyre, A. K.: Effects of axon section on motoneuron function. Proc. Univ. Otago Med. Sch., 33:14–16, 1955.
19. Brand, P.: Tendon grafting. J. Bone Joint Surg., 43-B:444–453, 1961.
20. Brand, P.: Tendon transfers in the forearm, In Flynn, J. E., ed.: Hand Surgery. Baltimore, Williams & Wilkins Co., 1966, pp. 331–342.
21. Brand, P., and Ebner, J. D.: Pressure sensitive devices for denervated hands and feet. J. Bone Joint Surg., 51-A:109–116, 1969.
22. Brattgård, S. O., Edström, J. E., and Hydén, H.: The productive capacity of the neuron in retrograde reaction. Exp. Cell Res., 5(Suppl.):185, 1958.
22a. Bratton, B. R., Hudson, A. R., and Kline, D. G.: Experimental interfascicular nerve grafting. J. Neurosurg., 51:323, 1979.
23. Bray, G., and Aguayo, A. J.: Regeneration of peripheral unmyelinated nerves. Fate of the axonal sprouts which develop after injury. J. Anat., 117:3:517–529, 1974.
24. Broadbent, T. R., Odom, G. L., and Woodhall, B.: Peripheral nerve injuries from administration of penicillin: Report of four clinical cases. J.A.M.A., 140:1008–1010, 1949.
25. Brown, H. A.: The value of early neurolysis in contused injuries of peripheral nerves. Western J. Surg., 61:535–537, 1953.
26. Brown, H., and Smith, R.: First rib resection for neurovascular syndromes of the thoracic outlet. Surg. Clin. N. Amer., 54:1277–1289, 1974.
27. Brown, P.: Factors influencing the success of surgical repair of peripheral nerves. Surg. Clin. N. Amer., 52:1137–1155, 1972.
28. Buecker, D., and Myers, E.: The maturity of peripheral nerves at the time of injury as a factor in regeneration. Anat. Rec., 109:723–743, 1951.

29. Bunnell, S.: Active splinting of the hand. J. Bone Joint Surg., *28*:732–736, 1946.

30. Bunnell, S.: Surgery fo the Hand. Philadelphia, J. B. Lippincott Co., 1964.

31. Campbell, J. B.: Frozen-irradiated homografts shielded with microfilter sheaths in peripheral nerve surgery. J. Trauma, *3*:303–311, 1963.

32. Campbell, J. B.: Peripheral nerve repair. Clin. Neurosurg., *17*:77–98, 1970.

33. Campbell, J. B., Bassett, C. A., Husby, J., Thulin, C. A., and Feringa, E. R.: Microfilter sheaths in peripheral nerve surgery. J. Trauma, *1*:139–157, 1961.

34. Clark, K., Williams, P., Willis, W., and McGavran, W. L.: Injection injuries of sciatic nerve. Clin. Neurosurg., *17*:111–125, 1970.

35. Clawson, D., and Seddon, H.: The late consequences of sciatic nerve injury. J. Bone Joint Surg., *44-A*:1047, 1962.

36. Clippinger, F. W., Goldner, J. L., and Roberts, J. M.: Use of electromyogram in evaluating upper extremity peripheral nerve lesions. J. Bone Joint Surg., *44-A*:1047–1060, 1962.

37. Coombes, M. A., Clark, W. K., Gregory, C. F., and James, J. A.: Sciatic nerve injury in infants. Recognition and prevention of impairment resulting from intragluteal injections. J.A.M.A., *173*:1336, 1960.

38. Cragg, B. G., and Thomas, P. K.: Changes in conduction velocity and fiber size proximal to peripheral nerve lesions. J. Physiol., *157*:315–327, 1961.

39. Craig, W. S., and Clark, J. M.: Of peripheral nerve palsies in the newly born. J. Obstet. Gynaec. Brit. Comm., *65*:229–237, 1958.

40. Davis, L., Perret, G., and Carroll, W.: Surgical principles underlying the use of grafts in the repair of peripheral nerve injuries. Ann. Surg., *121*:686–699, 1945.

41. Dawson, G.: Nerve conduction velocity in man. J. Physiol., *31*:436–451, 1956.

42. Denny-Brown, D., and Brenner, C.: Paralysis of nerve induced by direct pressure and tourniquet. Arch. Neurol. Psychiat., *51*:1–26, 1944.

43. DiVincenti, F. C., Moncrief, J. A., and Pruitt, B. A.: Electrical injuries: A review of 65 cases. J. Trauma, *9*:497–507, 1969.

44. Drake, C. G.: Diagnosis and treatment of lesions of the brachial plexus and adjacent structures. Clin. Neurosurg., *11*:110–127, 1964.

45. Ducker, T. B.: Pathophysiology of peripheral nerve trauma. *In* Omer, G. E., and Spinner, M., eds.: Management of Peripheral Nerve Problems. Philadelphia, W. B. Saunders Co., 1980.

46. Ducker, T. B., and Hayes, G. J.: Experimental improvements in use of Silastic cuff for peripheral nerve repair. J. Neurosurg., *24*:582–587, 1968.

47. Ducker, T., and Garrison, W.: Surgical aspects of peripheral nerve trauma. Curr. Probl. Surg., September, 1974.

48. Eccles, J. C., Kryjevic, K., and Miledi, R.: Delayed effects of peripheral severance of afferent nerve fibers on efficacy of their central synapses. J. Physiol., *145*:204–220, 1959.

49. Eccles, J. C., Libet, B., Young, R. R.: The behavior of chromatolysed motoneurons studied by intracellular recording. J. Physiol., *143*:11–40, 1958.

50. Edstrom, J. E.: Ribonucleic acid changes in motoneurons of frog during axon regeneration. J. Neurochem., *5*:43–49, 1959.

51. Engh, C. A., and Schofield, B. H.: A review of the central response to peripheral nerve injury and its significance in nerve regeneration. J. Neurosurg., *37*:198–203, 1972.

52. Fischer, H.: Pathologic effects and sequelae of electrical accidents. J. Occup. Med., *7*:564–571, 1965.

53. Gilden, D., and Eisner, J.: Lumbar plexopathy caused by disseminated intravascular coagulation. J.A.M.A., *237*:2846–2847, 1977.

54. Gilliatt, R., and Sears, T.: Sensory nerve action potentials in patients with peripheral nerve lesions. J. Neurol. Neurosurg. Psychiat., *21*:109–118, 1958.

55. Goldner, J. L.: Function of the Hand Following Peripheral Nerve Injuries. Amer. Acad. Orthop. Surg. Instruct. Course Lectures 10. Ann Arbor, Mich., J. W. Edmonds, 1953, p. 268.

56. Goldner, J. L.: Volkmann's contracture. *In* Flynn, J. E., ed.: Hand Surgery. Baltimore, Williams & Wilkins Co., 1966, p. 1095 (see also pp. 953–977).

57. Grabb, W.: Management of nerve injuries in forearm and hand. Orthop. Clin. N. Amer., *1*:419, 1970.

58. Granit, R., Leksell, L., and Skoglund, C. R.: Fiber interaction of injured or compressed region of nerve. Brain, *67*:125–140, 1944.

59. Grundfest, H., Oester, Y. T., and Beebe, G. W.: Electrical evidence of regeneration. *In* Peripheral Nerve Regeneration. V. A. Monograph. Washington, D.C., U.S. Government Printing Office, 1957, pp. 203–240.

60. Guth, L.: Regeneration in the mammalian peripheral nervous system. Physiol. Rev., *36*:441–478, 1956.

61. Guttmann, E., and Holubar, J.: Atrophy of nerve fibers in the central stump following nerve section and the possibilities of its prevention. Arch. Int. Stud. Neurol., *1*:314–320, 1951.

62. Guttmann, E., and Young, J. Z.: Reinnervation of muscle after various periods of atrophy. J. Anat., *78*:15–43, 1944.

63. Hakstian, R. W.: Funicular orientation by direct stimulation: An aid to peripheral nerve repair. J. Bone Joint Surg., *50-A*:1178–1186, 1968.

64. Henderson, W. R.: Clinical assessment of peripheral nerve injuries. Tinel's test. Lancet, *2*:801–804, 1948.

65. Highet, J.: Effect of stretch on peripheral nerve. Brit. J. Surg., *30*:355–369, 1942.

66. Hubbard, J.: The quality of nerve regeneration. Factors independent of the most skillful repair. Surg. Clin. N. Amer., *52*:1099–1108, 1972.

67. Hubbard, J. I., ed.: The Peripheral Nervous System. New York and London, Plenum Press, 1974.

68. Huber, C. G.: Experimental observations on peripheral nerve repair. *In* Medical Department, United States Army, Surgery in World War I: Vol. XI, Part I: Neurosurgery. Washington, D.C., U.S. Government Printing Office, 1927.

68a. Hudson, A. R., Kline, D. G., and Gentilli, F.: Peripheral nerve injection injury. *In* Omer, G.

E., and Spinner, M., eds.: Management of Peripheral Nerve Problems. Philadelphia, W. B. Saunders Co., 1980.

69. Hudson, A. R., Morris, J., and Weddell, G.: An electron microscopic study of regeneration in sutured rat sciatic nerves. Surg. Forum, *21*: 451–453, 1970.

70. Kahn, E. A.: Direct observation of sweating in peripheral nerve lesions. Surg. Gynec. Obstet., *92*:22–26, 1951.

71. Kempe, L., ed.: Operative Neurosurgery. Vol. 2. New York, Springer-Verlag, 1970, pp. 149–256.

72. Kettelkamp, D. B., and Alexander, H.: Clinical review of radial nerve injury. J. Trauma, *7*: 424–432, 1967.

73. Kline, D. G.: Operative management of major lesions of the lower extremity. Surg. Clin. N. Amer., *52*:1247–1265, 1972.

73a. Kline, D. G.: Physiological and clinical factors contributing to timing of nerve repair. Clin. Neurosurg., *24*:425–455, 1977.

73b. Kline, D. G.: Operative experience with major lower extremity nerve lesion. *In* Omer, G. E., and Spinner, M., eds.: Management of Peripheral Nerve Problems., Philadelphia, W. B. Saunders Co., 1980, pp. 607–625.

73c. Kline, D. G.: Evaluating the neuroma in continuity. *In* Omer, G. E., and Spinner, M., eds.: Management of Peripheral Nerve Problems. Philadelphia, W. B. Saunders Co., 1980.

74. Kline, D. G., and Dejonge, B. R.: Evoked potentials to evaluate peripheral nerve injuries. Surg. Gynec. Obstet., *127*:1239–1248, 1968.

75. Kline, D. G., and Hackett, E.: Reappraisal of timing for exploration of civilian peripheral nerve injuries. Surgery, *78*:54–65, 1975.

76. Kline, D. G., and Hayes, G. J.: The use of a resorbable wrapper for peripheral nerve repair. J. Neurosurg., *21*:737–750, 1964.

77. Kline, D. G., and Hudson, A. R.: Surgical repair of acute nerve injuries. *In* Morley, T., ed.: Controversies in Neurosurgery. Philadelphia, W. B. Saunders Co., 1976.

78. Kline, D., and Nulsen, F. E.: The neuroma in continuity: Its pre-operative and operative management. Surg. Clin. N. Amer., *52*:1189–1200, 1972.

79. Kline, D. G., Hackett, E. R., and May, P. R.: Evaluation of nerve injuries by evoked potentials and electromyography. J. Neurosurg., *31*:128–136, 1969.

80. Kline, D. G., Hackett, E. R., Davis, G. D., and Myers, M. B.: Effect of mobilization on the blood supply and regeneration of injured nerves. J. Surg. Res., *12*:254–266, 1972.

81. Kolb, L. C., and Gray, S. J.: Peripheral neuritis as a complication of penicillin therapy. J.A.M.A., *132*:323–326, 1946.

82. Lehman, R., and Hayes, G.: Degeneration and regeneration in peripheral nerve. Brain, *90*: 285–296, 1967.

83. Lewis, G. K.: Trauma resulting from electricity. J. Int. Coll. Surg., *28*:724–738, 1957.

84. Licht, S., ed: Electrodiagnosis and Electromyography. New Haven, Conn., E. Licht, Publisher, 1961.

85. Lieberman, A. R.: The axon reaction: A review

of principal features of perikaryal responses to axon injury. Int. Rev. Neurobiol., *14*:49–124, 1971.

86. Littler, J. W.: Tendon transfers and arthrodesis in combined median and ulnar nerve paralysis. J. Bone Joint Surg., *31-A*:225–234, 1949.

87. Liu, C. T., and Lewey, F. H.: The effect of surging currents of low frequency in man on atrophy of denervated muscles. J. Nerv. Ment. Dis., *105*:571–581, 1947.

88. Liu, C. T., Benda, C. F., and Lewey, F. H.: Tensile strength of human nerves. Arch. Neurol. Psychiat, *59*:322–336, 1948.

89. Livingston, W. K.: Evidence of active invasion of denervated areas by sensory fibers from neighboring nerves in man. J. Neurosurg., *4*:140–145, 1947.

90. Lundberg, G.: Structure and function of the intraneural microvessels as related to trauma, edema formation, and nerve function. J. Bone Joint Surg., *57-A*:938–948, 1975.

91. Lusskin, R., Campbell, J., and Thompson, W.: Post-traumatic lesions of the brachial plexus. J. Bone Joint Surg., *55-A*:1159–1176, 1973.

92. Marmor, L.: Regeneration of peripheral nerves by irradiated homografts. J. Bone Joint Surg., *46-A*:383–394, 1964.

93. Marmor, L.: Nerve grafting in peripheral nerve repair. Surg. Clin. N. Amer., *52*:1177–1187, 1972.

94. Matson, D. D.: Early neurolysis in treatment of injury of peripheral nerves due to faulty injection of antibiotics. New Eng. J. Med., *242*: 973–975, 1950.

95. Mayfield, F. H.: Causalgia. American Lecture Series. Springfield, Ill., Charles C Thomas, 1951.

96. Mayfield, F.: Reflex dystrophies of the hand. *In* Flynn, J. E., ed.: Hand Surgery. Baltimore, Williams & Wilkins Co., 1966, p. 1095 (see also pp. 738–750).

97. Melzak, R., and Wall, P. D.: Pain mechanisms: A new theory. Science, *150*:971–979, 1965.

98. Millesi, H.: Microsurgery of peripheral nerves. Hand, *5*:157–160, 1973.

98a. Millesi, H.: Nerve grafts, indications, technique, and prognosis. *In* Omer, G. E., and Spinner, M., eds.: Management of Peripheral Nerve Problems. Philadelphia, W. B. Saunders Co., 1980.

99. Millesi, H., Meissl, G., and Berger, A.: The interfasicular nerve-grafting of the median and ulnar nerves. J. Bone Joint Surg., *54-A*:727–730, 1972.

100. Moberg, E.: Objective methods for determining the functional value of sensibility in the hand. J. Bone Joint Surg., *40-B*:454–475, 1958.

101. Moberg, E.: Criticism and study of methods for examining sensibility in the hand. Neurology (Minneap.), *12*:8–19, 1962.

102. Murphey, F., Hartung, W., and Kirklin, J. W.: Myelographic demonstration of avulsing injury of the brachial plexus. Amer. J. Roentgen., *58*:102–105, 1947.

103. Murphey, F., Kirklin, J. W., and Finlaysan, A. I.: Anomalous innervation of the intrinsic muscles of the hand. Surg. Gynec. Obstet., *83*:15–23, 1946.

104. Nickolson, O. R., and Seddon, H. J.: Nerve re-

pair in civil practice. Brit. Med. J., 2:1065–1071, 1957.

105. Nobel, W.: Peroneal palsy due to hematoma in common peroneal nerve sheath after distal torsional fractures and inversion ankle sprains. J. Bone Joint Surg., 48-A:1484–1495, 1966.

106. Noordenbos, W.: Pain. Amsterdam, Elsevier, 1959.

107. Nulsen, F. E.: The management of peripheral nerve injury producing hand dysfunction. In Flynn, J. E., ed.: Hand Surgery. Baltimore, Williams & Wilkins Co., 1966. pp. 457–481.

108. Nulsen, F. E., and Lewey, F. H.: Intraneural bipolar stimulation: A new aid in the assessment of nerve injuries. Science, 106:301, 1947.

109. Nulsen, F. E., and Slade, H. W.: Recovery following injury to the brachial plexus. In Woodhall, B., and Beebe, G. W., eds.: Peripheral Nerve Regeneration. V.A. Monograph. Washington, D.C., U.S. Government Printing Office, 1957, pp. 389–408.

110. Nulsen, F. E., Lewey, F. H., and Van Wagenen, W. D.: Peripheral nerve grafts. In Spurling, R. G., and Woodhall, B., eds.: Medical Department, United States Army, Surgery in World War II: Neurosurgery. Vol. 2, Part II. Washington, D.C., U.S. Government Printing Office, 1959.

111. Omer, G. E.: Evaluation and reconstruction of forearm and hand after acute traumatic peripheral nerve injuries. J. Bone Joint Surg., 50-A:1454, 1968.

111a. Omer, G. E.: Tendon transfers for the reconstruction of the forearm and hand following peripheral nerve injuries. In Omer, G. E., and Spinner, M., eds.: Management of Peripheral Nerve Problems. Philadelphia, W. B. Saunders Co., 1980.

112. Omer, G., and Spinner, M.: Peripheral nerve testing and suture techniques. American Academy of Orthopaedic Surgeons Instructional Course Lectures. Vol. 24. C. V. Mosby Co., St. Louis, 1975, pp. 122–143.

113. Orgel, M., and Terzis, J.: Epineurial vs. perineurial repair: An ultrastructural and electrophysiological study of nerve regeneration. Plast. Reconst. Surg., 60:80–91, 1977.

114. O'Rian, S.: New and simple test of nerve function in the hand. Brit. Med. J., 3:615, 1973.

114a. Osgaard, O., Husby, J.: Femoral nerve repair with nerve autografts. Report of two cases. J. Neurosurg., 47:751–754, 1977.

115. Pizzolato, P., and Mannheimei, W.: Histopathologic Effects of Local Anesthetic Drugs and Related Substances. Springfield, Ill., Charles C Thomas, 1961.

116. Puckett, W. O., Grundfest, H., McElroy, W., and McMillen, J.: Damage to peripheral nerves by high velocity missiles without direct hit. J. Neurosurg., 3:294, 1946.

117. Riordan, D. C.: Tendon transplantations in median nerve and ulnar nerve paralysis. J. Bone Joint Surg., 35-A:312–320, 1953.

118. Robertis, E.: Submicroscopic morphology and function of the synapse. Exp. Cell Res. Suppl., 5:347–369, 1958.

119. Robles, J.: Brachial plexus avulsion. A review of diagnostic procedures and report of six cases. J. Neurosurg., 28:434–438, 1968.

120. Rudge, P., Ochoa, J., and Gilliatt, R.: Acute peripheral nerve compression in the baboon. J. Neurol. Sci., 23:403–420, 1974.

121. Rukolta, G., and Omer, G.: Combat sustained femoral nerve injuries. Surg. Gynec. Obstet., 128:813, 1967.

122. Sakellorides, H.: Follow-up of 172 peripheral nerve injuries in upper extremity in civilians. J. Bone Joint Surg., 44-A:140–148, 1962.

123. Samii, M.: Use of microtechniques in peripheral nerve surgery—experience with over 300 cases. In Handa, H., ed.: Microneurosurgery. Tokyo, Igaku Shoin Ltd., 1975, pp. 85–93.

124. Samii, M., and Willebrand, H.: The technique of and indications for autologous interfascicular nerve transplantation. Excerpta Medica, International Congress Series, No. 217, 39, 1970.

125. Schemm, G. W.: The pattern of cortical localization following cranial nerve cross anastomosis. J. Neurosurg., 18:593–596, 1961.

126. Seddon, H. J.: Three types of nerve injury. Brain, 66:238–288, 1943.

127. Seddon, H. J., ed.: Peripheral Nerve Injuries. Med. Res. Council Special Report Series No. 282. London, Her Majesty's Stationery Office, 1954.

128. Seddon, H. J.: Nerve grafting. J. Bone Joint Surg., 45:447–461, 1963.

129. Seddon, H. J., ed.: Surgical Disorders of the Peripheral Nerves. Baltimore, Williams & Wilkins Co., 1972.

130. Seletz, E.: Surgery of Peripheral Nerves. Springfield, Ill., Charles C Thomas, 1951, pp. 119–137.

131. Shaw, J. L., and Sakellorides, H.: Radial nerve paralysis associated with fractures of the humerus. J. Bone Joint Surg., 49-A:899–902, 1967.

132. Simpson, S. A., and Young, J. S.: Regeneration of fiber diameter after cross-unions of visceral and somatic nerves. J. Anat., 79:48, 1945.

133. Smith, J. W.: Factors influencing nerve repair II: Collateral circulation of peripheral nerves. Arch. Surg., 93:433–437, 1966.

134. Speed, J. S., and Knight, R. A., eds.: Peripheral nerve injuries. In Campbell's Operative Orthopaedics. Vol. I. St. Louis, C.V. Mosby Co., 1956, pp. 947–1014.

135. Sperry, R. W.: The problem of central nervous reorganization after nerve regeneration and muscle transposition. Quart. Rev. Biol., 20:311, 1945.

136. Spinner, M.: Reconstruction of the hand in high median nerve injuries. Bull. Hosp. Joint Dis., 26:191–197, 1965.

137. Spinner, M.: The anterior interosseous-nerve syndrome with special attention to its variations. J. Bone Joint Surg., 52-A:84, 1970.

138. Spurling, R. G., and Woodhall, B., eds.: Medical Department, United States Army, Surgery in World War II: Neurosurgery. Vol. II. Washington, D.C., U.S. Government Printing Office, 1959.

139. Sunderland, S.: The intraneural topography of the radial, median, and ulnar nerves. Brain, 68:243–299, 1945.

140. Sunderland, S.: Rate of regeneration in human peripheral nerves. Arch. Neurol. Psychiat., 58:251–295, 1947.

141. Sunderland, S.: Function of nerve fibers whose

structure has been disorganized. Anat. Rec., *109*:503–513, 1951.

142. Sunderland, S.: Funicular suture and funicular exclusion in the repair of severed nerves. Brit. J. Surg., *40*:580–587, 1953.

143. Sunderland, S.: Nerve and Nerve Injuries. Baltimore, Williams & Wilkins Co., 1968.

144. Sunderland, S.: The restoration of median nerve function after destructive lesions which preclude end-to-end repair. Brain, *97*:1–14, 1974.

145. Sunderland, S., and Ray, L. J.: Denervation changes in muscle. J. Neurol. Neurosurg. Psychiat., *13*:159–177, 1950.

146. Tarlov, I. M.: How long should an extremity be immobilized after nerve suture? Ann. Surg., *126*:336–376, 1947.

147. Tarlov, I. M.: Plasma Clot Suture of Peripheral Nerves and Nerve Roots. Springfield, Ill., Charles C Thomas, 1950.

148. Terzis, J., and Dykes, R.: Electrophysiological recordings in peripheral nerve surgery: A Review. J. Hand Surg., *1*:52–66, 1976.

149. Tsuge, K.: Treatment of established Volkmann's contracture. J. Bone Joint Surg., *57-A*:925–929, 1975.

150. Ulmer, J. L., and Mayfield, F. H.: Causalgia: A study of 75 cases. Surg. Gynec. Obstet., *83*:789–796, 1946.

151. Weddell, G., Guttmann, L., and Guttmann, E.: The local extension of nerve fibers into denervated areas of skin. J. Neurol. Psychiat., *4*:206, 1941.

152. Weiss, P.: Technology of nerve regeneration. A Review. J. Neurosurg., *1*:400–450, 1944.

153. Weiss, P.: The nervous system. *In* Analysis of Development. Philadelphia, W. B. Saunders Co., 1955.

154. Weiss, P.: The life history of the neuron. J. Chronic Dis., *3*:340–348, 1956.

155. Weiss, P.: Neuronal dynamics and neuroplastic flow. *In* Schmidt, F., ed.: The Neurosciences (2nd Study Program). New York, The Rockefeller Press, 1970, pp. 840–850.

156. Whitcomb, B. B.: Separation at the suture site as a cause of failure in regeneration of peripheral nerves. J. Neurosurg., *3*:399–406, 1946.

157. Whitcomb, B. B.: Techniques of peripheral nerve repair. *In* Spurling, R. G., and Woodhall, B., eds.: Medical Department, United States Army, Surgery in World War II: Neurosurgery. Vol. 2, Part II—Peripheral Nerve Injuries. Washington, D.C., U.S. Government Printing Office, 1959.

158. White, J. C.: Timing of nerve suture after gunshot wound. Surgery, *48*:946–951, 1960.

159. White, J. C.: The results of traction injuries to the common peroneal nerve. J. Bone Joint Surg., *40-B*:346–351, 1968.

160. White, J. C., and Hamlin, H.: New uses of tantalum in nerve suture. J. Neurosurg., *2*:402–413, 1945.

161. White, W. L.: Restoration of function and balance of the wrist and hand by tendon transfers, Surg. Clin. N. Amer., *40*:427–459, 1960.

162. Wickstrom, J., Haslam, E., and Hutchinson, R.: The surgical management of residual deformities of the shoulder following birth injuries of the brachial plexus. J. Bone Joint Surg., *37-A*:27–36, 1955.

163. Williams, H., and Terzis, J.: Single fascicular recordings: An intraoperative diagnostic tool for the management of peripheral nerve lesions. Plast. Reconstr. Surg., *57*:562–569, 1976.

164. Woodhall, B., Nulsen, F. E., White, J. C., and Davis, L.: Neurosurgical implications. *In* Peripheral Nerve Regeneration. V.A. Monograph. Washington, D.C., U.S. Government Printing Office, 1957, pp. 569–638.

165. Wynn-Parry, C. B.: Rehabilitation of the Hand. London, Butterworths, 1966.

166. Yeoman, D. M., and Seddon, H. J.: Brachial plexus injuries: Treatment of the flail arm. J. Bone Joint Surg., *43-B*:493–500, 1961.

167. Zachary, R. B., and Holmes, W.: Primary suture of nerves. Surg. Gynec. Obstet., *82*:632–651, 1946.

168. Zalewski, A.: Effects of neuromuscular reinnervation on denervated skeletal muscle by axons of motor, sensory, and sympathetic neurons. Amer. J. Physiol., *219*:1675–1679, 1970.

76

CHRONIC INJURIES OF PERIPHERAL NERVES BY ENTRAPMENT

RELATIONSHIPS OF STRUCTURE AND FUNCTION

Entrapment neuropathies are alterations in function of the peripheral nerves due to an abnormal environment, position, or blood supply to the nerves. Since the functioning elements of peripheral nerves are the nerve fibers, a detailed discussion of these is in order (Fig. 76–1). The fibers consist of long drawn-out processes of neurons, the axons, each associated with a chain of Schwann cells. Materials synthesized in the nerve cell body are transported down the axon at various rates.[43,100,138] Neurotubules provide a mechanism of rapid transport.[29] Ochs has shown that axonal transport is a process that maintains the excitability of the membrane and supplies to the nerve terminals the components required for neurotransmission.[124]

The surface membrane of the Schwann cell is reduplicated around the larger axons, forming myelin.[11,140] The symbiotic relationship of Schwann cells and axons is complex. Schwann cells do not form myelin unless they are in contact with an axon, and Schwann cells previously associated with nonmyelinated fibers may subsequently form myelin around regenerating axons. Aguayo and co-workers have achieved major advances in the understanding of axon–Schwann cell relationships by grafting nerves from genetically abnormal strains into normal animals, and the Bunges have demonstrated the trophic effects of Schwann cells by tissue culture techniques.[5,21] Myelin lamellae are attached to the axoplasm via specialized endings at the node of Ranvier.[133] The interval between the two adjacent Schwann cells, within the basement membrane, is filled with gap substance, which plays a role in the rapid ionic exchange that accompanies electrical transmission.[95] The smaller nonmyelinated axons indent the surface membrane of a single Schwann cell, and single small axons may cross from one nonmyelinated Schwann cell chain to another.[121] Both myelinated and nonmyelinated fibers are enclosed on their outer surfaces by a continuous basement membrane (Fig. 76–2). The nerve fibers function in a peculiar environment created by the blood-nerve barrier, of which there are two anatomical sites.[127] The first is the endoneurial capillary, and the second is the perineurium (Figs. 76–3 and 76–4). This latter structure forms a stocking around the fibers and defines a tube of the greatest operative and functional importance, the fascicle.[75,82,163] Peripheral nerves are made up of groups of fascicles of varying caliber and number, bound together by a fibrofatty clothing, the epineurium.[159] The blood supply of the peripheral nerve is derived primarily from a longitudinal anastomosis of vessels.[85,86,143] The larger vessels lie in the epineurium, and their smaller branches characteristically lie immediately within the perineurium and scattered through the substance of the endoneurium. Endoneurial fibro-

A. HUDSON, H. BERRY, AND F. MAYFIELD

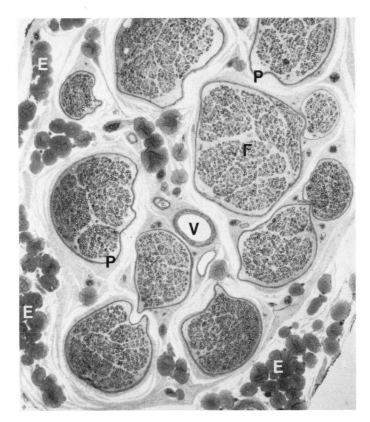

Figure 76-1 Transverse section of human peripheral nerve (100×). Compression of a peripheral nerve affects all components of that nerve. The ratio of cross-sectional area occupied by the fascicles (F) and the epineurial tissues (E) varies from nerve to nerve and also varies along the longitudinal course of a single nerve. Large quantities of epineurial tissues may protect the nerve fibers lying within the perineurial tubes (P). Blood vessels (V) are part of a rich epineurial longitudinal anastomosis and, along with the smaller intrafascicular vessels that they supply, may be compressed in entrapment neuropathies.

blasts are present within the fascicles and increase in numbers dramatically when the fascicle is injured (Fig. 76–5).[109] The transmission of the electrical impulse along peripheral nerve fibers depends upon the presence of normal axon–Schwann cell relationships existing in the peculiar environment within a nerve fascicle.[119] If pressure or ischemia alters the structure of nerve fibers or causes a breakdown in the blood-nerve barrier, the fibers will function in an abnormal manner, will delay conduction, and finally will be unable to propagate an impulse.[73,87]

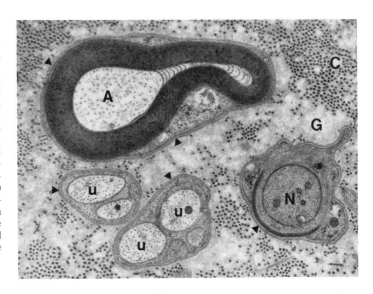

Figure 76-2 Transverse section of human peripheral nerve 12,250×). The large myelinated axons (A) are particularly vulnerable to ischemia and mechanical compression. Entrapment causes displacement of myelin lamellae. This results from movement of the axon at the node of Ranvier (N), which in turn drags the attached myelin away from the point of application of pressure. Both the myelinated and nonmyelinated fibers (u) are enclosed in basement membrane tubes (*arrowheads*), which separate the axons and the Schwann cells from the endoneurial collagen (C) and ground substance (G).

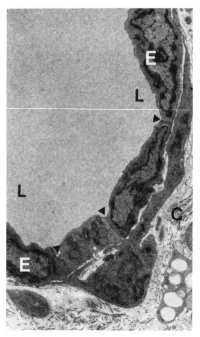

Figure 76–3 Endoneurial microvessel (6570×). The anatomical sites of the blood-nerve barrier are the endoneurial microvessel and the perineurium. Endothelial cells (E) meet at tight junctions (*arrowheads*). This biologically active barrier separates the contents within the lumen (L) of the vessel from the other tissues of the endoneurium. Collagen (C) is loosely deposited around this delicate vessel. Ischemia causes nerve fiber damage of varying severity.

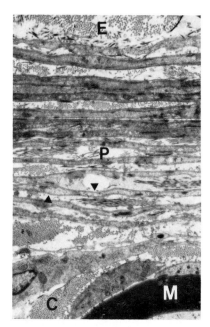

Figure 76–4 Perineurium (7810×). The flattened cells of the perineurium (P) display basement membrane (*arrowheads*) on their surfaces. The perineurial boundary, of immense biological and operative significance, is one site of the blood-nerve barrier. A myelinated fiber (M) is surrounded by collagen (C) that is of a different caliber from that observed in the epineurial tissues (E).

ETIOLOGY OF NERVE ENTRAPMENT

There are several common etiological bases for the entrapment neuropathies.[3,9,78] They derive from the anatomical relationships in which the peripheral nerves to the extremities pass to their eventual terminations through narrow and rather rigid bony, tendinous, or muscular compartments.[41] It is at these points that nerve dysfunction may result from: (1) compression by the narrowing of a compartment by local or systemic disease, or by swelling of the tissues that pass through the compartment (carpal tunnel syndrome); (2) repetitive stretching as nerves pass over anomalous structures (cervical ribs) or in direct contiguity to abnormal protuberances such as those caused by malhealed fractures (costoclavicular syndrome); (3) impingement, caused by repetitive narrowing of the normal boundaries of some of the compartments (thoracic outlet and hyperabduction syndromes); and (4) repeated dislocations (tardy ulnar paralysis).

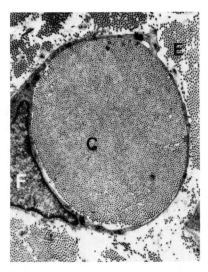

Figure 76–5 Endoneurial fibroblast (8890×). The rough-surfaced endoplasmic reticulum of both epineurial and endoneurial fibroblasts (F) synthesizes the precursors of the collagen fibrils (C). The endoneurial collagen (E) is of different caliber from the epineurial collagen. Biochemical and histological studies indicate an increase in the amount of collagen present in a damaged peripheral nerve.

None of these anomalous conditions could damage the nerves by itself. Movements combined with compression, stretching, impingement, and dislocation result in repeated episodes of pressure and ischemia.

EFFECT OF PRESSURE AND ISCHEMIA ON PERIPHERAL NERVE

Seddon coined the terms "neurapraxia," "axonotmesis," and "neurotmesis" to describe clinical situations attending nerve damage of increasing severity.[144] (This concept is discussed in Chapter 75). Sunderland expanded the concept and described degrees of nerve injury in greater detail.[158] Neurotmesis coincides with the third, fourth, and fifth degrees of injury. Application of electronmicroscopy to the study of nerve fiber injuries in experimental animals and humans has added greatly to the understanding of pathological states of the fibers. Spinner and Spencer have written an excellent review summarizing the pathological changes in nerve fiber entrapment and relating these observations to the clinical syndromes.[155] The nerve fiber abnormalities of acute and chronic nerve compression, predicted by animal experimentation, have been observed in man.*

Recurrent compression and ischemia of peripheral nerve results in changes in the nerve fiber ranging from the mildest to the most severe. The mildest form of injury probably results from a disturbance in axoplasmic flow or from disturbance of the blood-nerve barrier.[126] It is reasonable to assume that the evolution of the clinical manifestations of entrapment neuropathies occurs in the following manner: In the early stages, intermittent compression, stretching, impingement, or dislocation of nerves at points dictated by anatomical considerations constricts the axon cylinders and thus impedes the flow of axoplasm distally.[173] If the compression, stretching, or impingement is static, as might be caused by maintaining the extremity in an abnormal position for a long time, as in sleep, during operations, or in certain occupations, evanescent signs and symptoms of disordered

* See references 4, 30, 62, 67, 115, 122, 137, 161, 162.

sensory conduction could result from either distention proximally or the denial of nutritive substances and enzymes distally. If axoplasmic flow is disturbed, axonal membrane excitability is altered. Regardless of the severity of fiber damage, not all fibers within a fascicle are uniformly affected.

The next degree of injury is that which produces a polarized distortion of the internode. The myelin lamellae slip away from the site of compression and telescope through the node of Ranvier. Structural distortion appears to be the result of recurrent trauma or pressure sufficient to cause detachment of the inner myelin lamella. Ochoa and his colleagues have described the differences in the histological appearance of myelinated fibers submitted to acute, as opposed to chronic, repetitive trauma.[123] These mechanical distortions lead to paranodal and subsequent segmental demyelination (Figs. 76–6 and 76–7). In both paranodal and segmental demyelination, the axon remains intact from the cell body to its termination. Regeneration of the myelin sheath is required before the axon can resume its normal function, but as the axon and its attending Schwann cells are intact both proximal and distal to the point of injury, local remyelination at the injured site leads to a rapid return of function.[73]

If the local injury is of sufficient severity to damage the axon irreparably, the distal portion of that structure will be cut off from its cell body (its major source of nutrients) and hence will disintegrate. The chain of

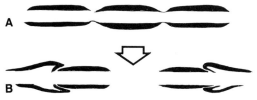

Figure 76–6 The mechanical effect of pressure on a myelinated fiber. This diagram depicts two longitudinally sectioned myelinated fibers. *A*. The axon is seen as a continuous structure surrounded by a chain of Schwann cells. *B*. Pressure has been applied at the site of the arrow, forcing axonal movement away from the site of compression. This, in turn, distorts the axon-myelin relationships at the nodes of Ranvier, which thus reduces the ability of the fiber to conduct a saltatory impulse. The details of the microhistological changes in acute compression differ from those in chronic, repetitive compression, but both abnormalities are related to the mechanical distortion illustrated here.

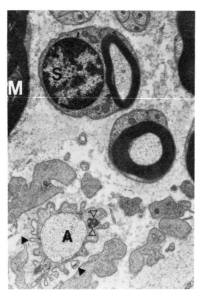

Figure 76–7 Segmental demyelination (7750×). The Schwann cell surrounding a large axon (A) has been injured by either mechanical distortion or ischemia. This Schwann cell has digested its myelin, and the remnants are visible in the Schwann cell cytoplasm (*open arrowheads*). This axon is in communication with both the cell body and the periphery, and at planes other than this would be surrounded by normal myelinated Schwann cells. The basement membrane (*closed arrowheads*) is intact. Not all fibers in this section are uniformly affected. The Schwann cell (S) of a neighboring fiber shows normal structure, as does the myelin (M) of an adjacent fiber.

Schwann cells distal to the point of injury then digest their myelin in the classic sequence of events described by Waller (Fig. 76–8).[171] The final result of this process is a band of Schwann cells containing neither axons nor myelin, enclosed in the basement membrane system of the original fiber (Fig. 76–9). Regeneration following this type of injury requires that collateral and terminal axon sprouts traverse the chain of reduplicated Schwann cells until they reinnervate and regenerate nerve endings (Fig. 76–10).[109,132] The Schwann cells subsequently remyelinate the larger axons, and function is resumed when the fibers mature in caliber (Figs. 76–11 and 76–12). Extreme fiber injury results in death and disintegration of the cell. The remnants are engulfed by macrophages, which are characterized microscopically by the absence of a basement membrane, a feature that aids in their distinction from Schwann cells (cf. Fig. 76–9).[6,72]

The authors have studied sural nerve biopsies from patients who were suffering from chronic obstructive vascular disease.[71] In a series of 15 consecutive patients who required amputation, they found myelinated nerve fiber densities ranging from normal down to 2100 fibers per square millimeter. Histograms revealed that the greatest fiber loss was in the large myelinated fiber category (Fig. 76–13). Electronmicroscopic study revealed that ischemia alone could result in the entire range of nerve fiber injury (except for the mechanical nodal distortions), confirming observations made previously by other authors.[37] *It is probable that the nerve fiber damage of varying severity seen in entrapment neuropathies is the result of both direct pressure and ischemia.*[31,157] The proportion of these injurious factors present in any single case may vary. The degree and rapidity of recovery that follows resolution of the compression depends primarily on the severity and duration of nerve fiber damage, but might also vary with the relative importance of compression and ischemia in the pathogenesis of that lesion. It is probable that the very rapid resolution of symptoms that follows decompression is in some way related to relief of ischemia.[50] The more gradual recovery of motor power and sensation is probably related to nerve fiber regeneration, the speed of which is related to the severity of the pathological process.

The role of the perineurium and epineurium in the pathogenesis of entrapment has been supported in the past. In the human cases studied, the connective tissue changes associated with enlargement of cross-sectional area did not appear to be related to the presence or absence of nerve fiber damage. The exact role of the thickened perineurial tissues remains to be resolved, but alteration in the function of this tissue alters the integrity of the blood-nerve barrier. The basis of the lateral neuromatous formation proximal to the entrapment that is seen in chronic cases appears to be the presence of regenerating axon branches that have grown between the lamellae of the perineurium and subsequently grown into the epineurial tissue. These fibers are apparently seeking alternate routes around the obstruction.[151,155] Despite the presence of a local pathological process, patients usually are unaware of the site of their nerve injury. It is most unusual for patients to identify the entrapment point in carpal

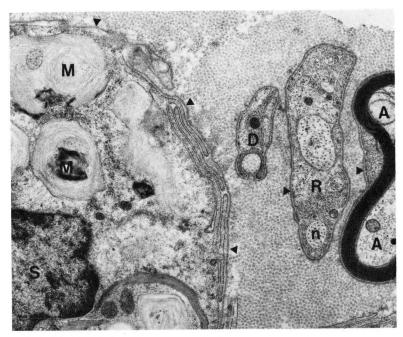

Figure 76-8   Wallerian degeneration and early regeneration (18460×). The fiber on the left has undergone a more severe injury. The axon has disintegrated and the Schwann cell (S) is digesting its myelin (M). This process occurs along the entire length of the nerve fiber distal to the point of injury (wallerian degeneration). The end result of this process is a chain of Schwann cells enclosed in the original basement membrane, devoid of both axons and myelin. This is a denervated band of Büngner (D). With the passage of time, the regenerating axon sprouts grow down this column of cells to form a reinnervated band (R). The axon sprout in this band shows prominent neurotubules (n). Not all fibers in this section are uniformly affected, as is shown by the normal myelinated fiber to the right of the picture (A). The basement membrane remains intact around all these nerve fiber systems, insuring accurate regeneration to the appropriate end organ.

tunnel or ulnar or peroneal nerve entrapment syndromes.

ELECTROPHYSIOLOGICAL INVESTIGATION IN ENTRAPMENT SYNDROMES

Although Erb introduced the use of galvanic and faradic stimulation of the motor point as tests of the "electrical reactions" of muscle in 1883, these proved to be of little assistance to the clinician; it took much time to plot the intensity-duration curves, they were of limited value, the results were inconsistent, and they did not prove useful in the detection of partial denervation.[44] Several decades later in 1929, Adrian and Bronk used a concentric needle electrode. This electrode as well as subsequent advances in electronics with the development of differential amplifiers and the cathode ray oscilloscope, provided the technical basis for the investigation of single motor units and their discharge during muscle contraction.[1] In 1938, Denny-Brown and Pennybacker described the spontaneous electrical activity of partially and completely denervated muscle, and Buchthal and Clemmeson in 1941 and Weddell and co-workers in 1944 further applied these techniques to the investigation of peripheral nerve injury and neurogenic muscular atrophy.[19,32,172] In 1947 Kugelberg recognized the difference in waveform of motor unit potentials in different types of muscle wasting, and electromyography then became useful in the distinction between neurogenic and myogenic weakness.[91]

Detection of a partial as opposed to a complete lesion is of prime importance in the operative management of peripheral nerve lesions, and until the last two decades the available electrical tests to assist in this important distinction were limited to nerve and muscle stimulation and electromyography.[69] More recently, techniques for measuring motor nerve conduction velocity in neuropathies were described by

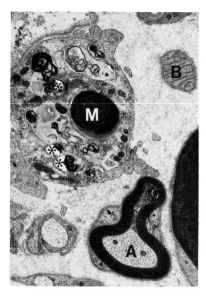

Figure 76-9 Extreme fiber injury (9480×). A nerve fiber has suffered an extreme insult, and disintegrating Schwann cell fragments have been engulfed by a macrophage. The myelin debris (M) is seen within the cytoplasm of this mobile cell. A band of Büngner (B) containing stacks of reduplicated Schwann cell processes indicates that that fiber had suffered a lesser degree of nerve injury but, as yet, shows no evidence of reinnervation. The myelinated axon (A) below is unaffected by either the mechanical or ischemic processes that have injured its neighbors.

Simpson and were applied to the measurement of sensory nerve conduction by Gilliatt and Sears.[63,148] These methods represented an important advance in the diagnosis of peripheral neuropathy, in the detection of entrapment and pressure palsy, and in some instances, in the identification of the actual site of mechanical interference with the nerve. Further refinements have been introduced with the development of quantitative evaluation of electromyographic data and the use of integrated electromyography.[20,97] The development of the digital computer as a signal averaging device has resulted in a great improvement in sensitivity and the ability to detect action potentials of very low amplitude; this has permitted the measurement and analysis of low-amplitude nerve action potentials, and has further contributed to the diagnosis and understanding of entrapment neuropathies.

These advances in electrical testing have served to clarify the mechanism and the clinical features of various forms of peripheral nerve disorder. By making it possible to demonstrate objectively the slowing of conduction in those portions of a peripheral nerve that have been subjected to entrapment or pressure, the tests offer unbiased confirmation of a clinical diagnosis.[36] Their use has led to a better understanding of previously known conditions such as palsy of the ulnar, common peroneal, radial, and other nerves. Measurement of motor nerve conduction has led to more widespread recognition of the relatively recently defined entity, carpal tunnel syndrome, which was formerly diagnosed as acroparesthesia of unknown origin or one or another form of the scalenus anticus or thoracic outlet syndrome.

Nerve conduction studies and electromyography have permitted the development of more rational methods of management of certain palsies of spontaneous onset, such as common peroneal nerve palsy and Bell's palsy.[10] For example, examinations of the facial nerve and muscles in facial nerve trauma and Bell's palsy have made it possible to determine the severity of the lesion and the indications for operative decompression in the traumatic cases or steroid

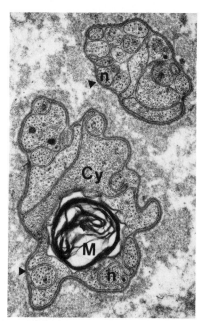

Figure 76-10 Early reinnervation of band of Büngner (17,800×). This demonstrates a later stage of reinnervation than that shown in Figure 76-8. While some myelin debris remains (M), the main features are cytoplasmic processes of reduplicated Schwann cells (Cy) and sections through regenerating axon sprouts, all confined by the original basement membrane tubes (*arrowheads*). Neurotubules (n) are clearly visible in the sections through axonal sprouts.

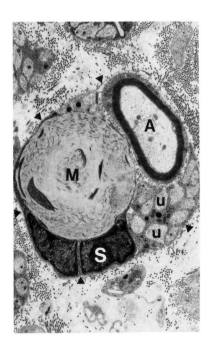

Figure 76–11 Reinnervation of Schwann cell band (7080×). With the passage of time, a larger regenerating axon sprout remyelinates (A). It is characteristically accompanied by small, unmyelinated fibers (u). In this basement membrane system (*arrowheads*), the Schwann cell (S) is still struggling to digest the myelin lamellae of the previously injured fiber. The collateral and terminal sprouts (A, u) were derived by axon sprouting from nodes of Ranvier proximal to the point of injury.

usage in the spontaneous palsies, and they have permitted a more accurate prediction of the time for recovery. In addition, the growing use of these techniques of investigation has altered the understanding of the importance and incidence of peripheral nerve disorders and has led, for example, to the recognition that carpal tunnel syndrome is a common problem, whereas the thoracic outlet and scalenus anticus syndromes are relatively rare, difficult to verify, and often incorrectly diagnosed.[66,163]

When there has been peripheral nerve trauma, pressure palsy, or entrapment, the combined investigations of motor (and occasionally sensory) nerve conduction and electromyographic detection of surviving motor units have permitted a more accurate assessment of severity and prognosis. Preserved motor conduction, as evidenced by motor unit potentials under voluntary control or on electrical stimulation of the nerve, indicates at least a degree of physical continuity and has important implications for management and prognosis.

The proper use of nerve conduction and electromyographic examination, when there are multiple causes, will help to clarify the contribution of individual conditions to the overall clinical picture. For example,

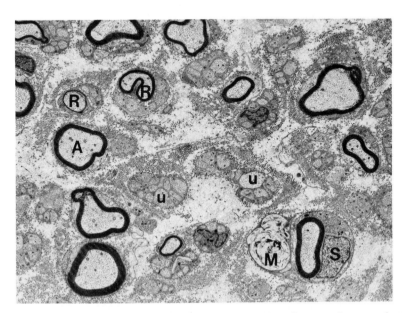

Figure 76–12 Final result of resolution of entrapment injury (3150×). Regenerating axon clusters in various stages of remyelination (R) are seen next to a normal myelinated axon that was not affected by the previous entrapment (A). Clusters of unmyelinated fibers (u) are of normal appearance. Evidence of the previous fiber damage lingers on, and the myelin debris (M), sharing a basement membrane tube with a normal Schwann cell (S), is presumably awaiting the arrival of a macrophage for its final removal from the scene.

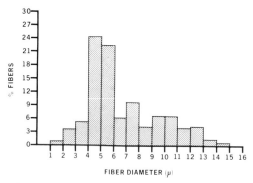

Figure 76–13 Histogram of sural nerve biopsy from a patient with chronic obliterative vascular disease in the lower limb: 955 myelinated fibers counted, myelinated fiber density 5300 per square inch. Note the flattening of the normal bimodal distribution due to loss of larger fibers. The number of large fibers recorded is artificially raised, as many of those counted were degenerating, hence of larger caliber.

the patient with cervical spondylosis and encroachment upon intervertebral foramina may have numbness involving the hands and wasting of small muscles, symptoms suggestive of cervical nerve root interference. Ulnar nerve pressure palsy or carpal tunnel syndrome may be coexistent, however, or alternatively, one of these forms of entrapment-pressure palsy, rather than cervical radicular involvement, may be responsible for the sensory motor manifestations in the hand. Such a distinction can be made with confidence only through the use of electrical testing, and these procedures have made a great contribution to the understanding and management of this type of problem.

Nerve conduction and electromyographic examinations are most useful when performed by a physician or surgeon who possesses neurological expertise. Although routine measurements of sensory and motor conduction velocity, distal latency, and evoked nerve action potentials by the signal averaging method can be accurately obtained by a trained technician, the examination of the more complex problem requires a different approach; the details of the clinical picture must be kept clearly in mind. A knowledge of the type of symptoms; the presence or absence of wasting, weakness, or sensory loss; the territories of suspected nerve involvement; the identification and electromyographic sampling of individual muscles in the case of a localized peripheral nerve injury; and an awareness

of the differential diagnosis are required in order to accomplish an exacting and useful examination.

Electromyography

In the electromyographic examination, a bipolar concentric needle electrode is inserted into muscle, and the potentials are suitably filtered, amplified, displayed on an oscilloscope, and monitored through a loudspeaker channel. A permanent record of the waveforms can be made on photographic paper by a direct-writing type of recorder. The details of instrumentation and technique are provided in standard works on this topic.[97,98]

Normal muscle in a relaxed state does not show any spontaneous activity and is electrically silent. When a recording needle electrode is first inserted into normal muscle, a brief discharge of short-duration low-amplitude potentials occurs (insertion activity), but this subsides when needle movement ceases. With voluntary contraction, the numerous individual muscle fibers that form a motor unit contract with an associated electrical discharge that can be recorded as a motor unit discharge, or action potential. These motor unit action potentials are bi- or triphasic, and their amplitude and duration vary with the muscle under examination. Values of 4 to 10 msec duration and 500 μv to 2.0 mv are common for limb muscles; the number of phases and the duration and amplitude of the action potential are altered by diseases that affect the nerve or the muscle fiber, as is discussed later. A slight contraction allows individual motor units to be inspected on the oscilloscope screen and permits an assessment of waveform, amplitude, and duration (Fig. 76–14).

As the strength of the contraction increases, there is a corresponding increase in discharge of motor units, and these summate into an interference pattern. The interference pattern is incomplete during a muscle contraction limited by volition, and it is also incomplete when the number of motor units is diminished by disease. These findings, as well as the findings in differing degrees of paralysis and in recovery, are summarized in Figure 76–15.

With denervation, after 10 to 14 days have elapsed, spontaneous electrical activ-

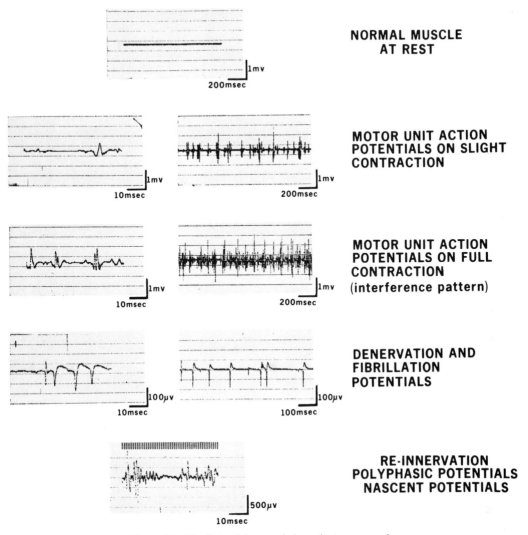

Figure 76-14   Potentials recorded on electromyography.

ity appears in muscle at rest, and fibrillation, fasciculation, and denervation potentials may be recorded. Fibrillation represents the electrical activity of a discharging individual muscle fiber, and this produces a brief, low-amplitude biphasic or triphasic potential of 1 to 2 msec duration, and 50 to 150 μv, discharging at a rate of 2 to 20 times per second. Denervation potentials are similar in voltage, but of longer duration (10 msec or more) than fibrillation potentials. They are also referred to as positive sharp waves. Fasciculation potentials are identical to motor unit discharges and represent the spontaneous discharge of an entire motor unit. It is important that the muscle be at rest, for if the patient is cold or shivering, motor unit discharges may be

misinterpreted as fasciculation potentials. When the recording needle tip is in the region of the motor and end-plate zone, low-amplitude end-plate potentials can be recorded under normal conditions and may be mistaken for the fibrillation potentials of denervation.

The waveform of a motor unit action potential is altered by disease, and this phenomenon is of value in the diagnosis of conditions such as polymyositis and muscular dystrophy as well as in the detection of reinnervation. As paralyzed muscle begins to show recovery on the basis of reinnervation, low-voltage polyphasic potentials are recorded, and these become greater in amplitude and more numerous as there is further recovery. The waveform has more

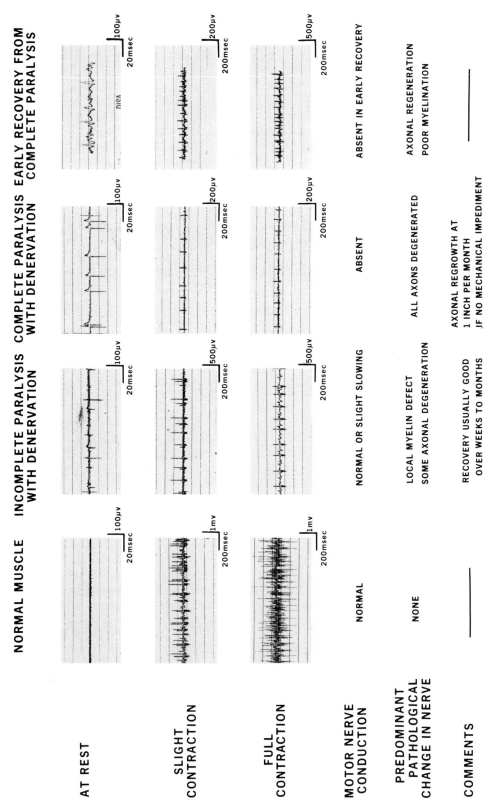

Figure 76–15   Electromyographic and nerve conduction findings in peripheral nerve injury of varying severity.

phases (four or more) than the normal motor unit action potential, and large-amplitude potentials (greater than 10 mv and referred to as giant potentials) of long duration (15 to 30 msec) are seen in long-standing neurogenic atrophy from, for example, chronic severe pressure palsy or atrophy based on anterior horn cell involvement within the spinal cord owing to syringomyelia or motor neuron disease. Muscles involved by primary muscle diseases, such as muscular dystrophy and polymyositis, also show polyphasic potentials, and these tend to be of lower amplitude than those seen in neurogenic muscle atrophy. Electromyographic examination performed under proper conditions with the patient relaxed and cooperating during willed movements, and sampling the appropriate muscle, will provide information about the integrity of the motor unit and the degree of paralysis, and evidence of denervation and of recovery through reinnervation.

With neurogenic paralysis, evidence of denervation will occur after about 10 to 14 days and will persist for a number of months, as long as there is viable muscle tissue. Weakness and a degree of wasting are usually obvious on clinical examination, and this combination of findings is commonly seen in palsies involving the common peroneal, radial, and ulnar nerves. Conversely, most patients with carpal tunnel syndrome do not have muscle wasting or weakness, and the electromyographic examination is usually normal. The use of electromyography has been extended by some to the detection of minimal nerve root compression in intervertebral disc disease when clinical signs are absent; the value of this approach is not established, and the authors have not found electromyography to be more sensitive than clinical examination in the detection of minimal nerve root compression.

In severe pressure palsy or stretch injury, paralysis is obvious and remains for some time; electromyography often provides the first evidence of recovery. Low-voltage polyphasic nascent potentials appear at rest, increase in number, and then appear on volition as an early manifestation of recovery. Serial electromyographic examinations are useful to assess the pace of recovery. When a nerve lesion has been judged to be complete but in continuity, the time and distance relationships of reinner-

vation must be considered; with a reinnervation rate of approximately 1 inch per month, recovery should appear in the muscles most proximal to the lesion after an appropriate interval. For example, a muscle normally supplied at a distance of about 4 inches from a site of injury should show evidence of reinnervation after about four months; if this does not occur, then the pace of recovery can be said to be unduly slow and the possibility of a mechanical obstacle to nerve regrowth or a complete section of the nerve must be considered. The authors have found serial electromyographic examinations under these conditions to be a sensitive indicator of the pace of recovery in patients with nerve lesions, and this is of considerable help in management. When the pace is excessively slow, the delay may indicate persisting entrapment, unsuspected section of the nerve, or some impediment to reinnervation such as excessive fibrosis or neuroma formation, and exploration may therefore be required.

It is recognized that denervated muscle will eventually undergo complete atrophy, although the exact time relationships of this phenomenon require further study. If denervated muscle can be reinnervated within a matter of a few months, a degree of function can be restored; however, if the muscle undergoes complete atrophy or if there is an ischemic complication due to an associated arterial injury, nerve regrowth is to no avail. As a practical guide, it can probably be stated that denervated muscle must be reinnervated within about six to eight months for much useful function to be restored. The timing of an operative exploration of the nerve, the verification of the nature of the lesion, or the decision to perform nerve suturing or grafting or excision of a neuroma is contingent upon an assessment of the pace of recovery and an awareness of the limited life span of denervated muscle.

The findings on electromyographic examination and the alterations in nerve conduction in the various degrees of nerve palsies are summarized in Figure 76–15. At rest, the normal muscle is electrically silent; motor unit action potentials appear during slight contraction and increase with full contraction. The findings of incomplete paralysis with denervation in a patient with paralysis of recent onset indicate a lesion in continuity and, usually, a good prognosis.

Fibrillation and denervation potentials at rest indicate that some denervation has occurred, but motor unit action potentials are present during voluntary contraction. This is the usual condition of the majority of patients who have suffered peripheral nerve trauma, such as brachial plexus stretch injuries, or have common peroneal nerve palsy due to pressure or following fracture, radial nerve palsy, the more severe degrees of ulnar nerve pressure palsy, or advanced carpal tunnel syndrome.

Complete paralysis found in conjunction with denervation is of special interest to the neurosurgeon; although it may indicate a lesion in continuity, it may also indicate that the nerve has been severed and that nerve suture or grafting is required.

When serial examinations are performed in the patient in whom complete paralysis has been established, the early signs of recovery are the appearance of low-voltage polyphasic potentials (nascent potentials) spontaneously and on attempted contraction, and these potentials gradually increase in number with further axonal regeneration. This is the earliest evidence of recovery and is seen before there is visible contraction and often long before motor nerve conduction can be demonstrated by stimulation.

Measurement of Nerve Conduction Velocity

Although in the early part of this century animal studies had demonstrated that nerve conduction was measurable, it was not until 1948 that Hodes and colleagues confirmed it in human subjects.[69] The first studies were concerned with the measurement of conduction velocity in motor nerves. When performed in conjunction with electromyographic examination, stimulation of a motor nerve at two points along its course results in an evoked potential from muscle at two different time intervals (latencies), which correspond to the two different points of stimulation (Fig. 76–16). Subtraction of the shorter from the longer latency gives the time required for the impulse to travel between the two stimulation points.[128] If an ulnar nerve is, therefore, stimulated just above the elbow and at the wrist, and an electromyographic recording is made from the abductor digiti minimi muscle, the time required (in milliseconds) for the impulse to travel from the elbow to the wrist can be determined and the velocity can be calculated by dividing this time into the distance. Any motor nerve consists of fibers of differing diameters, and as there is a relation between diameter and conduction velocity, and as the most rapidly conducting fibers require stronger stimulus, it is important to use a stimulus of an amplitude great enough (a supramaximal stimulus) to excite the most rapidly conducting fibers. The details of stimulus parameters, instrumentation, general technique, and method of measurement of specific nerves are available in standard works on this topic.

Motor nerve conduction is slowed when there is localized pressure on the nerve, and this is commonly seen in patients with ulnar neuropathy, and also with common peroneal nerve pressure palsy and with carpal tunnel syndrome. The slowing is greatest over the region of entrapment or pressure, and when the nerve has a long, relatively accessible course it is possible to demonstrate localized slowing, as, for example, at the elbow, in a pressure palsy. There are limitations to this technique, however, and errors in measurement are relatively greater when dealing with short segments of nerves.

The principle of measurement of sensory nerve conduction is similar, although there is no muscle contraction to indicate that the impulse has arrived at its destination (Fig. 76–17). Electrical potentials traveling along the sensory fibers, although of much smaller amplitude than muscle action potentials, can also be recorded. Ring electrodes, applied to the finger, permit the stimulation of purely sensory fibers; the nerve action potential can be detected at the wrist, elbow, or even more proximally, and the sensory conduction velocity can be calculated.[28] The recording of sensory nerve action potentials has proved to be of considerable value in the evaluation of peripheral nerve disorders.[63]

Motor nerve conduction velocity can be readily measured in the ulnar as well as the median, common peroneal, and posterior tibial nerves, and these techniques are widely used. Methods of measurement of conduction in the radial, femoral, and sciatic nerves have been described.[53–55] Mea-

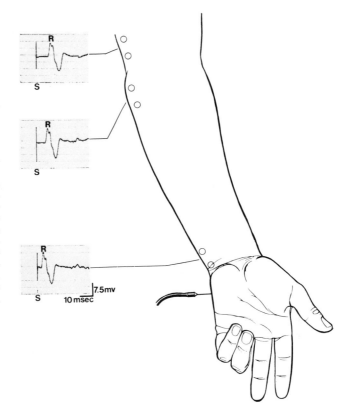

Figure 76–16 Measurement of motor nerve conduction. A stimulus (S) is applied with a bipolar electrode at the wrist and below and above the elbow, as indicated. The response (R) represents a compound motor action potential and is recorded by a needle electrode within the appropriate muscle (abductor digiti minimi for ulnar nerve motor conduction). The time required for the impulse to travel along the ulnar nerve and excite the distal muscles is indicated by the oscilloscope time base and is progressively increased as the point of stimulation becomes more proximal; that is, the latency (between S and R) is successively prolonged as the stimulus is applied farther from the recording site.

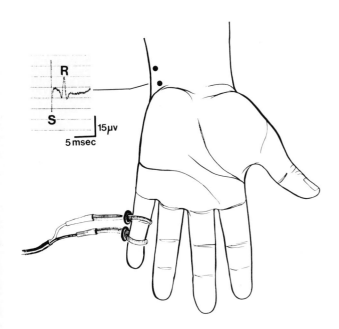

Figure 76–17 Measurement of sensory conduction. The stimulus is delivered by means of ring electrodes applied to the appropriate finger (fifth finger for ulnar nerve and middle or index finger for median nerve conduction). The response is detected over the nerve, at the wrist or at a more proximal point, by a surface electrode. In the recording, the time between the stimulus artifact (S) and the evoked sensory nerve action potential (R) represents the rate of conduction in the sensory nerve fibers. An additional recording, at the elbow or a more proximal site, allows the sensory conduction velocity to be calculated for a long segment of the nerve.

surement of terminal latency is also of value in the detection of entrapment of the ulnar palmar branch lesion.

Average values for motor nerve conduction velocity are now well established, and because of variations in technique, it is desirable that each laboratory define its own controls for each nerve and nerve segment. The normal values for several different laboratories have been noted by Downie.[36] Mean motor conduction velocities of 50 to 60 meters per second are common in the upper limbs, while 40 to 50 meters per second are usual in the lower extremities. Sensory conduction velocities are similar, and both values are influenced by factors such as limb temperature and the age of the patient.

Sensory nerve conduction can be readily measured in the ulnar and median nerves by the use of ring electrodes on the fingers. In the lower limbs, the anterior tibial and sural nerves can often be identified by palpation, and in the upper limb the sensory branch of the radial nerve also occupies a relatively constant position over the extensor pollicis longus tendon and can also be identified by palpation. Bipolar electrodes permit the recording of the evoked nerve action potentials at a more proximal site. Because of the lower amplitude of these potentials, recording can be more difficult; disc electrodes applied to the skin are usually satisfactory for the detection of sensory responses over the ulnar and median nerves at the wrist as well as the anterior tibial and sural nerves at the ankle. Monopolar recording needle electrodes are used for recording sensory responses when the nerve is deeply situated or at a more proximal position. The development of the signal averager, as a means of improving the signal to noise ratio, has made it possible to record the lower-amplitude nerve action potentials with skin electrodes.

When a mixed nerve is subject to pressure or entrapment, the earliest change involves sensory conduction, and motor conduction may remain normal. This is often the finding in mild ulnar neuritis and may also be seen in the milder cases of carpal tunnel syndrome. Electromyographic examination is also usually entirely normal at this stage. When the lesion is slightly more severe, conduction in the most rapidly conducting fibers is impaired and there is a mild slowing of motor conduction, as in a common peroneal nerve or ulnar palsy or in carpal tunnel syndrome. Sensory conduction is more conspicuously abnormal, as evidenced by a considerable reduction or loss of the sensory evoked response at the wrist to a single stimulus and by a marked slowing of the sensory conduction velocity. Changes in the waveform and duration of the sensory evoked potential and of the motor potential evoked by stimulation also occur and may be of some value in the detection of early abnormalities.

When a motor nerve or mixed nerve is completely severed at some distance from the muscle, excitability of the distal portion of the nerve is not immediately lost, and the muscle can be stimulated to contraction by an appropriate stimulus applied distal to the point of severance. Gilliatt and Taylor demonstrated that nerve fibers remain excitable within the facial nerve and conduct at a normal velocity for about four to five days following intracranial section of the seventh nerve at the time of operation for acoustic neuroma.[64] The amplitude of the evoked motor potential gradually declined over this period of time, and conduction was completely lost after about the fifth day. The process of wallerian degeneration occurs during this time and is the basis of the loss of conduction. The exact time relationships for other nerves in the human subject are not established, but it does appear that conduction in response to electrical stimulation distal to the lesion can be preserved for several days after complete severance, and may, therefore, be misleading.

If electrical studies confirm that the paralysis is complete, serial examinations are required to determine whether recovery is occurring and, if so, whether it is occurring at a satisfactory pace. Electromyographic examination of the muscles closest to the site of presumed injury must be done, as recovery will first be detectable there. For example, when the lesion is at the spiral groove level in radial nerve palsy and the rate of recovery is approximately 1 inch per month, evidence of reinnervation will first be detected within the proximal portion of the brachioradialis muscle. If this does not occur there, or within the upper portion of the forearm extensors, over a matter of four to five months (a reinnervation distance of approximately 4 to 5 inches), then operative exploration is indicated. If, on the basis of the type of injury, it is reasonable to suspect that the nerve may be transsected or that there may be some mechanical impediment to reinnervation, however, in the presence of a clinically and electrically complete paralysis, exploration should be undertaken at an earlier date.

It is well known that conduction velocity increases with the external diameter of the nerve fiber and that this is largely dependent upon the presence of myelin. Nerve conduction depends upon a wave of depolarization along the nerve, and it has been established that this process of depolarization does not travel at a uniform rate along the nerve fiber but "jumps" from node to node (saltatory conduction).[14,56] When a segment of myelin is interfered with, between such nodes, conduction is considerably slowed and approaches those values seen in unmyelinated fibers. Large myelinated fibers conduct at rates as slow as 12 meters per second. Any nerve contains fibers of different diameters, and when the nerve is stimulated with stimuli of increasing strength, the slower-conducting fibers respond first. Measurements of sensory or motor conduction velocity are based upon maximal conduction velocity, that is, the velocity of the most rapidly conducting fibers, as evoked by maximal or supramaximal stimuli. The larger-diameter fibers appear to be more sensitive to pressure and mechanical interference, presumably because of the effect on myelin. When myelin is damaged over a segment of the larger diameter, the most rapidly conducting fibers cease to conduct, and conduction now occurs through the slower fibers. If the injury to myelin is severe enough, there may be a total loss of conduction (conduction block). There may be a degree of axonal (wallerian) degeneration in entrapment pressure palsies in addition, and this serves to reduce the maximum conduction velocity. It is now established that there are two main pathological types of peripheral neuropathies, namely, a demyelinative neuropathy (segmental demyelination) in which there is marked slowing of conduction, to a value less than 70 per cent of normal, due to an interference with saltatory conduction, and the primarily axonal neuropathies (wallerian degeneration) in which conduction is slowed only slightly and is usually greater than 70 per cent of normal. Precise clinical, electrophysiological, and histological correlations are not available with respect to entrapment pressure palsies, and further work in this area is required. It can, however, be stated that there is a rough correlation between the severity of the entrapment pressure palsy and the slowing in conduction; Berry and Richardson, in a review of the clinical and electrophysiological features of common peroneal nerve palsy, noted the relationship between the severity of the palsy and the amount of slowing of conduction, and this relationship, as it involves distal motor latency, is also seen to correspond to the duration and severity of symptoms in patients with carpal tunnel syndrome.[10]

In regeneration after complete transsection of a nerve, the nerve action potential is severely diminished in amplitude and there is considerable slowing. Electrophysiologically, there is no way of distinguishing between the slow conduction in immature regenerating fibers and that in demyelinated fibers, but the speed of recovery does provide a clue; remyelination proceeds much more slowly than regeneration, and from animal experiments it is known that regenerating nerve fibers may reach 80 per cent of normal conduction, although they have a thinner axon and a thinner myelin sheath, and the internodal distances are also shorter.[27,165]

INCIDENCE

Valid information on the incidence of nerve entrapment syndromes is lacking. This is partly because, until recently, the diagnosis depended upon the correlation of the results of treatment and the surgeon's assessment of abnormalities seen at operation, both of which introduce the error inherent in subjective analysis. Furthermore, because of the multiple antecedent events and the diversity of symptoms, groups of cases tend to be treated by specialists and reported in their own literature, making it difficult to collate statistics and obscuring the basis of comparison. Mayfield and his colleagues analyzed 30,000 consecutive cases from their group neurosurgical practice and found an incidence of entrapment syndromes as reported in Tables 76–1 and 76–2. Wider use of electrical techniques will define the syndromes more sharply, and thus the true and relative incidence of certain syndromes may alter. Autopsy ma-

TABLE 76-1 ENTRAPMENT SYNDROMES, NUMBER OF CASES, AND PERCENTAGE OF TOTAL NUMBER OF CASES (30,000)

SYNDROME	NUMBER OF CASES	PER CENT OF TOTAL
Carpal tunnel	311	1.03
Cervical rib	87	0.71
Meralgia paresthetica	50	0.17
Tardy ulnar paralysis	19	0.06
Hyperabduction	14	0.05
Costoclavicular	11	0.04
Thoracic outlet	10	0.03
Total	502	2.09

TABLE 76-2 PERCENTAGE OF EACH SYNDROME OF TOTAL NUMBER OF ENTRAPMENT SYNDROME COMPLEX (502)

SYNDROME	PER CENT
Carpal tunnel	62.0
Cervical rib	17.3
Meralgia paresthetica	10.0
Tardy ulnar paralysis	3.8
Hyperabduction	2.8
Costoclavicular	2.2
Thoracic outlet	1.9

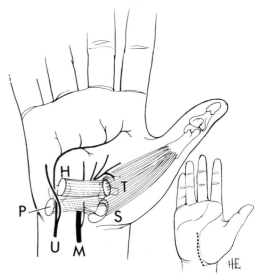

Figure 76-18 The transverse carpal ligament has four bony attachments, which are the pisiform (P) and hook of hamate (H) medially, and the scaphoid (S) and trapezium (T) laterally. The median nerve (M) runs beneath this ligament, and the recurrent branch recurves to supply the abductor pollicis and shares the innervation of the remaining thenar muscles with the deep branch of the ulnar nerve (U). The exact distribution of the two nerves in the thenar eminence varies from patient to patient.

terial should be studied at every opportunity in an attempt to delineate the incidence of the mechanical distortion of internodes described by Ochoa and his colleagues.[123]

ENTRAPMENT SYNDROMES

Median Nerve

Entrapment at Wrist

The tough flexor retinaculum has four bony attachments, which can be palpated in most patients. These are the pisiform and hook of hamate medially, and the tubercle of the scaphoid and the ridge of the trapezium laterally (Fig. 76-18).[96] It is important that this exact relationship be appreciated by the surgeon. The palmaris longus muscle, when present, passes superficial to the retinaculum and expands distally into the palmar aponeurosis. Thenar and hypothenar muscles take origin from the retinaculum, and some patients exhibit muscle fibers on the superficial surface quite close to the midline. The palmaris brevis may also extend laterally and lie superficial to

the middle of the transverse carpal ligament. The surface marking of the median nerve is the groove between the palmaris longus and flexor carpi radialis, both of which will stand out if the patient is asked to cup his hand and slightly flex the wrist. The palmar branch of the median nerve is given off proximal to the retinaculum and crosses that structure, along with the superficial palmar branch of the radial artery, just lateral to the tendon of the palmaris longus. It supplies an area of skin over the base of the thenar eminence so this area is not affected in the carpal tunnel syndrome. The median nerve passes deep to the retinaculum, where it is accompanied by the tendons passing through the carpal flexor tunnel. Normally the diameter of the tunnel allows free movement of the median nerve in response to motion at the wrist.[107] Immediately distal to the flexor retinaculum, the motor branch recurves to supply the abductor, short flexor, and opponens muscles of the thumb. This branch passes superficial to the tendon of the flexor pollicis longus. The motor branch may rarely take an aberrant course.[174] The nerve then divides into branches, which participate in the cutaneous supply of the palm of the hand and the lateral three and one half digits. The exact distribution in the hand, relative to the distribution of the ulnar nerve, varies from patient to patient, but the "autonomous zone" of the distal phalanges of the thumb and index finger is always supplied by the median nerve.

Carpal Tunnel Syndrome

Early descriptions of the carpal tunnel syndrome were made by Cannon and Love and by Brain and his associates.[15,22] It is a relatively common condition; examination by electrical studies of 3110 patients at St. Michael's Hospital in Toronto confirmed the diagnosis of carpal tunnel syndrome in 396 patients. The authors believe this condition to be the single most identifiable cause of numbness in the upper limbs. Patients with the carpal tunnel syndrome are predominantly women, and are usually between the ages of 40 and 60. Symptoms are bilateral in 20 to 30 per cent of cases and are usually of 6 to 12 months' duration. Numbness, tingling, and pain are often described, and they frequently involve the entire hand as well as the forearm. When questioned more closely, the patients will admit that mainly the thumb, index, and middle fingers are involved. Symptoms are worse at night or on awakening, and the patient will describe hanging her arm over the edge of the bed and shaking her wrist and elbow in an attempt to alleviate them. The cause of the nocturnal aggravation of symptoms is unknown, but may be related to wrist posture. If the patient has to get up frequently during the night, they seldom develop. Symptoms are often troublesome during or after manual activity such as knitting, typing, and driving an automobile ("steering wheel sign"). Occasionally, the condition may appear related to specific occupations such as those involving screwing on jar lids on an assembly line, hairdressing, butchering, or the like, but a clear occupational causation is not well established. A carpal tunnel syndrome may develop or worsen during pregnancy. It is not unusual for a woman presenting later in life to admit to having had similar transient symptoms during pregnancy many years earlier. Association of the symptoms with a phase of the menstrual cycle strongly suggests fluid retention as a pathogenetic factor. The pa-

tients rarely indicate their wrists as the site of the trouble, as there are no symptoms pointing to the carpal tunnel. Though the early reports included the clinical feature of wasting of the thenar eminence, now patients usually are seen in the earlier stages of the disease and examination does not reveal wasting: the only motor abnormality is a slight weakness of the abductor pollicis brevis muscle, and this may be difficult to assess.[52] It should be recalled that in abduction the thumb moves away, at right angles to the palm, in such a manner that the thumbnail remains in a plane at right angles to the fingernails. Sensory examination usually is normal. When the condition is more advanced, there is wasting of the abductor pollicis brevis portion of the thenar eminence with sensory loss, and symptoms in such patients usually have been present for years.[130]

In about half the patients, the clinical features are typical, and diagnosis can be made with confidence on clinical grounds alone. In the remainder, the pattern is atypical and often leads to error in diagnosis. Pain may be a troublesome symptom and may extend to involve the forearm and entire upper limb, and this raises the possibility of cervical nerve root compression. The visualization of mild or moderate degenerative changes on cervical x-ray films, a common finding in late middle age, may direct attention away from the wrist to the neck and lead to an incorrect diagnosis. Compressive radiculopathy and peripheral nerve entrapment may coexist; this combination has been termed the "double crush syndrome."[168] In some patients, although symptoms are suggestive, nerve conduction studies are normal and no cause can be established. Some patients in whom carpal tunnel syndrome is suspected have cold, sweaty hands or symptoms suggestive of Raynaud's phenomenon, and nerve conduction studies do not reveal any median nerve entrapment. In others, generalized sensory and motor neuropathy is detected by nerve conduction studies, but there is no additional evidence of median nerve entrapment.

The diagnosis is confirmed by nerve conduction studies.[160] These are particularly useful in patients with disabling symptoms but few physical findings. The electrophysiological studies are far more helpful in these cases than the use of provocative clinical tests such as forced flexion of the wrist, extension of the wrist, and the blowing up of a sphygmomanometer cuff. These clinical maneuvers are not particularly helpful. The conduction time (distal latency) is prolonged (normal latency is 2.2 to 4.6 msec over a distance of 5 to 7 cm), and the sensory evoked response (distal sensory latency of 1.8 to 3.8 msec; amplitude of 10 to 20 μv) shows a prolonged latency and is of diminished amplitude or may be entirely absent when the single sweep method is used. The authors have found that most patients with carpal tunnel syndrome have a distal motor latency greater than 5 msec, and the sensory evoked response at the wrist is absent when tested by the single sweep method. If the values are only slightly altered, it is best to postpone treatment and to re-examine the patient at a later date. If the patient has nerve conduction studies that are entirely normal, operative treatment should not be done, regardless of how suggestive the history.

Although the diagnosis of carpal tunnel syndrome can usually be confirmed on the basis of altered distal motor and sensory latency in the median nerve, it may be necessary to examine conduction in the ulnar nerve if there is reason to suspect an associated generalized neuropathy (peripheral neuritis). If ulnar nerve distal motor and sensory latencies are entirely normal, or if ulnar maximal motor conduction velocity is normal, then there is no underlying generalized neuropathy. Distal median nerve latency values may be altered along with prolongation of distal latency values of other nerves in generalized neuropathy, and although an additional median nerve entrapment (carpal tunnel syndrome) may occur in generalized neuropathy, its diagnosis becomes more difficult and depends upon a disproportionate prolongation of median distal latency.

It is unusual to delineate an obvious cause of compression. Old fractures of the wrist, rheumatoid arthritis, osteoarthritis, Paget's disease of bone, neoplasms, myeloma, acromegaly, and hypothyroidism have been cited.[99,165] Patients suffering from generalized peripheral neuropathy, as in diabetes or alcoholism, are more liable to entrapment neuropathy and pressure palsy. These diseases are usually diagnosed independently, and the carpal tunnel syndrome is an occasional complication. Analysis of

Mayfield's cases revealed that only 11 patients had a history of wrist fracture and that both these patients and the physician were aware that the wrist was the site of entrapment.[104,106]

The treatment of choice is decompression by section of the flexor retinaculum at the wrist. Various forms of conservative management may be useful in late pregnancy or if operative intervention has to be postponed for any reason.[167] These include hydrocortisone injection administered without local anesthetic (thus avoiding the nerve itself), wrist splints, and diuretic therapy. Whenever a multitude of operative approaches and techniques exist, as is the case in the carpal tunnel syndrome, it usually indicates that no one method of treatment is completely satisfactory. In fact, a simple, logical operation derived from basic surgical principles can easily be performed for this condition. More complex variations add nothing to the operation and may, indeed, endanger the median nerve itself.

The procedure can be performed on an outpatient basis in the majority of cases. A transverse subcutaneous wheal is raised in the proximal flexor wrist crease, for which a 1 per cent concentration local anesthetic and a 25-gauge needle are used. It is a mistake to use a large needle or to inject the local anesthetic too rapidly, because this causes the patient unnecessary pain. More elaborate anesthetic techniques are unnecessary and usually take more time than the operation itself. An appropriate skin crease, or combination of skin creases, running longitudinally, is then selected and infiltrated distally as far as the lower border of the outstretched thumb (cf. Fig. 76–18). A common error is to operate before the local anesthetic is fully effective; the intervening time can be profitably utilized by preparing suture material for closure, and the like. The incision is made boldly in the depths of the skin crease, starting at the wrist flexor crease and ending at the distal border of the flexor retinaculum. A self-retaining retractor is inserted, and this stems hemorrhage from any small vessels in the superficial fat of the palm. Small slips of thenar or hypothenar muscles are incised to expose the gritty, tough transverse carpal ligament. This ligament is gently divided in its full longitudinal extent. The edges spring back under the guidance of the self-retaining retractor, which has been inserted immediately superficial to the retinaculum. It is absolutely crucial that this incision be complete and that the proximal and distal borders of the retinaculum be inspected with great care to insure that no persistent fibers remain.[52] It is as well to elevate the proximal end of the incision with a small right-angle retractor to be quite certain that any fascial bands in the distal forearm are also divided. If there is any uncertainty, the incision should be extended proximally. The nerve is thus displayed in the full extent of its passage through the carpal tunnel. The recurrent branch of the median nerve is usually not seen. The median nerve should not be touched in any way.

In the majority of cases, the nerve itself will appear entirely normal. In more advanced cases, it may be obviously thinned and show some increase in caliber immediately proximal to the retinaculum. External or internal neurolysis is not performed, nor is synovectomy required. The self-retaining retractor is then removed and the fat of the palm is brought carefully together with absorbable suture material. At this stage, any small bleeding vessels are ligated with the sutures. On no account should the transverse carpal ligament be resutured. Skin is opposed in the usual manner, and a padded bandage is applied. It is illogical, and there is no need, to apply a plaster cast. The arm is placed in a sling with the hand held higher than the elbow for three days. The patient is instructed to take simple oral analgesics before the local anesthetic effect wears off. The entire operation seldom takes more than 10 minutes. The nocturnal dysesthesia disappears immediately, and the numbness and weakness improve at a rate appropriate to the regeneration of the damaged fibers over the next few months. The sutures are removed on the tenth day, but the patient must not soak her hand or return to work until the skin is completely healed—usually an additional week. The scar is painless and almost invisible with the passage of time. The operation is almost universally successful, and patients are grateful to be rid of their annoying symptoms.

Failure or early recurrence almost always indicates incomplete section of the transverse carpal ligament, a fact frequently advertised by the presence of inappropriate operation scars. More rarely, persistence of symptoms is due to an overenthusiastic operation that results in partial laceration of the median nerve or scarring from the extensive procedure. The motor branch of the median nerve is not seen in the procedure, but early failure of the operation may be attributed to section of that branch as a result of operating on the distal lateral side of the nerve. Later recurrence in a patient who has had an appropriate operation should raise the surgeon's suspicion that there is some rare underlying cause of the carpal tunnel syndrome, such as hypothyroidism. Unfortunately, the simplicity of the technique described encourages its thoughtless application, and it is not infrequent for patients suffering from cervical radicular problems to undergo carpal tunnel decompression at the hands of neurologically unsophisticated practitioners.

When the condition is bilateral, it is advisable to operate on the more troublesome hand. Conduction is often more prolonged on that side. If the second side is only mildly affected, the symptoms frequently resolve spontaneously with increased use of the hand relieved by the operation. On exceptional occasions, with recurrent pathological phenomena, a detailed microscopic dissection of the nerve and its recurrent branch may be required, but intraoperative magnification and extensive dissection are not required for the standard procedure. Repeat operations require more extensive exposure, however, and care must be given to guarding the cutaneous branch to the thenar eminence and the motor branch, as these nerves may have anomalous origins and courses.

Entrapment in Elbow Region

Anterior Interosseous Nerve

The entrance of the median nerve into the antecubital fossa is identified by the close relationship of the median nerve to the brachial artery. The bicipital aponeurosis must be incised to expose these structures. If the nerve is traced distally, the branch to the pronator teres is seen on the medial side. Short branches are given to the muscles of the common flexor origin, and the anterior interosseous nerve originates at a variable point, which may be proximal to, at, or distal to the passage of the median nerve between the two heads of the pronator teres (Fig. 76–19). If the main median nerve is gently elevated, the various branches are readily apparent. This purely motor nerve then passes down along the front of the interosseous membrane to supply the flexor pollicis longus and a portion of the flexor digitorum profundus to the index and middle fingers, ending at the pronator quadratus. Anatomical details and their variations have been discussed by Sunderland, Mangini, and Spinner.[102,153,159] Lesions of the anterior interosseous nerve are rare and have been described as isolated cases and in a small series.[92,120,150]

The nerve can be trapped as a complication of supracondylar fracture of the humerus in children as well as of a penetrating injury such as needle puncture for a retrograde brachial arteriogram, compression from a plaster cast, or carrying a weighty object over the forearm. Although a rare occurence, entrapment of the anterior interosseous nerve presents a well-defined clinical picture. There may be pain at the onset, and the patient complains of motor weakness. When he attempts to make a fist, the index finger and thumb tend to remain extended. Close analysis reveals a characteristic attitude of thumb and index finger when the patient is tested for pinch. The thumb flexes at the metacarpophalangeal joint and hyperextends at the interphalangeal joint, while the index finger flexes at the proximal interphalangeal joint and extends at the distal interphalangeal joint. Weakness may be profound, and the lack of sensory abnormality may lead to an incorrect diagnosis of tendon disease. Pronator quadratus involvement produces a loss of pronation strength of the forearm when the elbow is flexed to minimize the action of the pronator teres muscle, which is not affected in this syndrome.

Electrical studies in these patients demonstrate normal sensory and motor conduction at the median nerve distally as well as in the forearm and upper arm. Electromyographic examination reveals a diminished

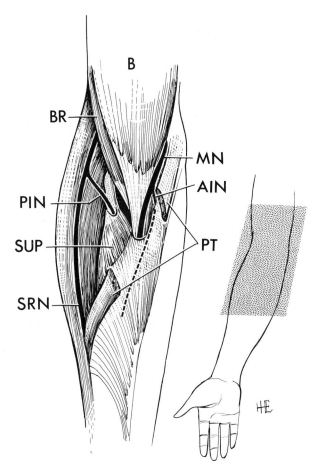

Figure 76–19 The median nerve is shown on the medial side of the antecubital fossa. All three major peripheral nerves enter the forearm by running between two heads of a muscle. The median (MN) runs between the two heads of the pronator teres (PT); the posterior interosseous (PIN), between the two heads of the supinator (Sup); and the ulnar, between the two heads of the flexor carpi ulnaris (not shown). The superficial branch of the radial nerve (SRN) enters the antecubital fossa and is easily displayed by separating the brachialis (Br) and brachioradialis muscles. Both the anterior (AIN) and posterior interosseous nerves run backward from their origins and are best displayed by gently tenting up their parent nerves. B, Biceps.

interference pattern in the appropriate muscles. From a technical point of view, it should be noted that this assessment requires accurate placement of needle electrodes into the deeper forearm muscles. This is difficult and may, therefore, limit the usefulness of the examination. O'Brien and Upton published the electrical studies in a single case, and these demonstrated normal sensory and motor conduction at the median nerve distally as well as in the forearm and upper arm. Electromyographic examination revealed a diminished interference pattern of the pronator quadratus, the median-supplied portion of the flexor digitorum profundus, and the flexor pollicis longus muscles.[120] The variations of this unusual syndrome are discussed in detail by Lake and Spinner.[92,154]

Patients who exhibit mild signs may recover quickly over a matter of weeks, while more profound abnormalities may be associated with persisting weakness. The patients are followed with repeated clinical examinations and electromyographic studies. A review of 23 cases drawn from the literature by O'Brien and Upton showed that 13 patients underwent operative exploration. Constricting fibrous bands were found in seven patients and a neuroma in one. Tendon transfer was performed in several patients.[120] If the paralysis is incomplete at the onset, or if improvement is noted over a matter of weeks, then it is reasonable to follow the patient and to expect a satisfactory outcome.[51] If paralysis is complete on clinical examination, or there is reason to suspect section of the nerve because of a penetrating injury or fracture, electromyographic studies may detect surviving motor units in the involved muscles and, therefore, provide evidence of continuity. In those patients in whom paralysis is judged to be complete (by clinical and electrical examination), there should be evidence of recovery within three to four months, and serial clinical and electromyographic examinations should be done in order to detect this. In cases in which there is significant disability of 12 weeks' duration, the nerve should be explored.

The median nerve is identified in the antecubital fossa and its relationship to the two heads of the pronator teres is identified. In the majority of limbs, the nerve passes between the two heads. The distal border of the pronator teres is defined, and dissection leads down between this muscle and the flexor carpi radialis. This reveals the median nerve running down to assume its position on the deep surface of the flexor digitorum superficialis. The origin of the anterior interosseous nerve is identified, and an external neurolysis is performed, dividing all constricting bands. The site of compression is usually close to the origin of the nerve, but the authors have experience of two cases in which the median nerve was compressed proximal to the pronator teres and the clinical presentation was that of a pure anterior interosseous nerve entrapment syndrome.

Pronator Teres Syndrome

This syndrome is rarely encountered. Entrapment of the median nerve by the upper portion of the pronator teres muscle was described by Seyffarth.[145] Also, Kopell and Thompson published a case report with operative confirmation of an anomalous fibrous band between the two heads of the pronator teres muscle that indented the median nerve.[88] Morris and Peters described the clinical and electrophysiological features in seven cases. The majority responded to steroid injection in the upper portion of the pronator teres muscle, and the patients were advised to alter their activities. There was a history of considerable activity involving the forearm and hand, including forceful pronation, and the presenting symptoms were pain and tenderness of the proximal forearm and anesthesia of the forearm, thumb, and index finger. Weakness of the flexor pollicis longus and abductor pollicis brevis muscles was almost always present, and the flexor digitorum profundus and opponens pollicis muscles were also described as weak, although it was noted that the weakness could be missed if strength was not compared with the opposite side. Sensory loss in a median nerve distribution was described in several patients, and there were tenderness over the pronator teres muscle and a positive Tinel's sign over the median nerve at that point. Slowed motor conduction of the median nerve of the elbow-to-wrist segment was usual, and the distal motor latency was normal.[108] It is doubtful whether slowing of the motor conduction in the forearm segment of the median nerve is a specific finding, as the authors have encountered this as an incidental observation in patients without any symptoms or abnormalities.

Median Nerve at Elbow

The median nerve may be entrapped by a ligament running from the medial epicondyle of the humerus to the radius. A single case report exists.[80] This syndrome, like the pronator teres syndrome, is a rarity, but possibly the condition is being missed.

Entrapment in Arm

The ligament of Struthers is a ligament running from the bony spur on the distal anteromedial aspect of the humerus to the medial epicondyle. The median nerve may rarely be entrapped and compressed by this structure.

Ulnar Nerve

Entrapment at Elbow

The ulnar nerve enters the extensor compartment of the arm by passing through the medial intermuscular septum at the level of the insertion of the deltoid muscle. Articular branches are given off proximal to the elbow joint, but it is unusual to have any significant motor branch at this point. The nerve runs behind the medial epicondyle of the humerus and gains the flexor compartment of the forearm by running between the olecranon and epicondylar head of the flexor carpi ulnaris (Fig. 76–20).

The ulnar nerve is frequently involved by pressure and entrapment; this syndrome and entrapment of the median nerve (carpal tunnel syndrome) constitute the most common pressure syndromes of peripheral nerves. In the authors' experience of 318 patients with ulnar palsy verified by electrical studies, the majority were men between the ages of 40 and 60 years. Symptoms have usually been present for a few months to one year, and the condition is usually unilateral. The patient's complaints vary according to occupation. The laborer notices a lack of grip due to weakness of the flexor digitorum profundus to the medial two fingers. The electrician notices a lack of dexterity because of weakness of the intrinsic musculature and a lack of proprioception in the hand when working where he cannot see his hands. Numbness of the fifth finger

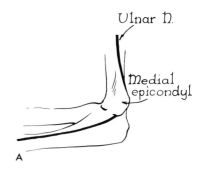

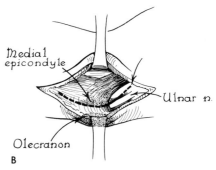

Figure 76–20 *A.* Anatomical drawing of relationships of ulnar nerve at elbow. *B.* The line of incision (*arrow*) used either for transposition of the nerve or for excision of the epicondyle. It is to be emphasized that occasionally the nerve is entrapped just distal to the elbow—posteriorly when arthritis is present or there is a valgus deformity at the elbow—in which event release of the nerve just below the elbow is sufficient.

and the adjacent surface of the ring finger, as well as of the inner border of the hand, along with a degree of weakness of the small muscles of the hand, is usual. The onset of symptoms can often be related to a period of bed rest in hospital following an operation or illness, and it is presumed that pressure on the ulnar nerve at the elbow has occurred. Characteristically, muscle wasting is present, although it may be slight in degree and detectable only by careful comparison of the first dorsal interosseous muscles of both hands. Weakness of finger abduction is readily detected, and weakness of the flexor digitorum profundus muscle action of the fourth and fifth fingers is detectable in more advanced cases when care is taken to negate the action of the flexor digitorum superficialis. In more advanced cases, there is well-defined muscle atrophy and weakness as well as sensory loss, and the diagnosis can confidently be made without the use of electrical tests.

In milder cases of ulnar neuropathy,

motor conduction may be normal over the elbow-to-wrist segment, while sensory conduction is usually impaired in such patients and the sensory evoked response at the wrist to stimulation of the fifth finger is reduced or may be lost. Motor conduction velocity of the transsulcal portion of the ulnar nerve can be obtained by stimulating above and just below the elbow and recording from the abductor digiti minimi muscle in the usual manner. Although conduction measurements over such a short segment are more prone to error, this procedure may confirm an abnormality of conduction. In the more advanced cases, slowing of conduction over the elbow-to-wrist segment is demonstrable. Electromyography reveals a degree of denervation with loss of motor units, and in the recovery stage, reveals evidence of reinnervation with polyphasic action potentials, and in the later stages, larger-amplitude action potentials.

The common site of the lesion in ulnar neuritis is at the elbow. Not all patients require operative treatment. The degree of involvement usually is mild and can be related to a period of bed rest or hospitalization during which undue elbow pressure occurs, or to an episode of trauma or other elbow pressure. Examples of activities that may cause this problem are resting the arm on the windowsill of an automobile on a long drive, habitually resting the elbow on a desk while listening to the telephone, and resting the elbow on a hard chair arm while watching television.

Although earlier reports have emphasized fracture of the humerus, arthritis, or other abnormalities about the elbow as contributing factors in tardy ulnar nerve palsy, the authors have not found any predisposing abnormality in the majority of their patients. The condition has also been said to be a slowly progressive form of palsy, but apparently this is not true.[46,58,130]

Gilliatt and Sears demonstrated the recording of nerve action potential in patients with ulnar nerve lesions at the elbow, and Gilliatt and Thomas described nerve conduction studies in 14 patients with chronic lesions at the elbow.[63,65] Payan described detailed studies of sensory and motor conduction as they could be applied to the localization of the lesion in ulnar nerve palsy. He found that three quarters of the lesions were due to unknown causes.[129] Sensory fibers were the first to be affected, and the majority of lesions could be localized, by electrophysiological means, to the elbow.[18] Investigation of a small number of patients before and after operative transposition of the nerve and after conservative management alone did not reveal any difference in outcome. The earliest electrophysiological sign of recovery was an increase in conduction velocity across the sulcus in both sensory and motor fibers. Adequate controlled observations of conservative versus operative management are required, but it does appear that operations are being performed unnecessarily.

Although most patients with ulnar nerve palsy do not have any anatomical abnormality at the elbow, Feindell and Stratford have described the presence of connective tissue bands in the region of the cubital tunnel, and these have also been noted by Wilson and Krout.[46,176]

Ulnar nerve palsy is not always a progressive condition that can only be treated by operative procedures to relieve repeated trauma at the elbow. Recovery can be detected by clinical examination as well as by electrical testing, particularly if the obvious precipitating factors are avoided. Motor conduction velocity will improve, a large number of motor units will be detected during voluntary contraction, and the compound action potential of the abductor digiti minimi muscle will also increase with recovery. When the paralysis is moderate in degree, closer follow-up assessment is required. If there is no improvement in the electrical parameters over the next months, if there is any suggestion of worsening, or if there is reason to believe that additional nerve pressure will occur because of abnormal angulation at the elbow or other deformity, then operative treatment is usually advisable.

General anesthesia is preferable for the operation in the majority of patients. Brachial plexus block also is satisfactory. If a tourniquet is used, supplementary anesthesia of the medial upper arm is required. The incision is centered between the olecranon and medial epicondyle and swung anteriorly above and below the elbow joint. The ulnar nerve is exposed proximal to, behind, and immediately distal to the elbow joint, and an attempt is made to define the abnormality in that particular case. Normally, the nerve is of slightly greater caliber in the bony groove. An obvious point of narrowing or indentation with a proximal bulb may be observed as the nerve passes between the olecranon and the medial epicondylar head of the flexor carpi ulnaris. Alternatively, the same pathological condition may be found immediately proximal to the medial epicondyle. Mobility of the nerve behind the medial epicondyle varies; the nerve may slide over the medial epicondyle with flexion of the elbow and appear to be abnormally loose, or alternatively, may be fixed overfirmly by adhesions on movement of the elbow joint. Kline has measured evoked nerve action potentials at operation and states that in the majority of his cases the slowing is within the groove itself, and in a minority is either proximal to the groove or at the cubital tunnel.[84]

The operation of anterior transposition is easy to perform, but attention must be given to certain points. The authors do not use a tourniquet but do pay particular attention to hemostasis. Incision of the skin over the anterior aspect of the common flexor origin rapidly reveals a filmy plane, which is utilized to elevate the skin flap in a lateral direction. Denser adhesions immediately above the epicondyle are divided. The nerve itself must be handled with extreme care, and surface epineurial blood vessels must be preserved. Bipolar coagulation and suction are used accurately so that there is minimal tissue damage. The ulnar nerve is elevated from its bed, posterior to the medial intermuscular septum, and followed down to the olecranon groove. Small articular branches to the elbow joint are sacrificed, and it may be necessary to split muscular branches of the ulnar nerve back into the main trunk to allow sufficient mobility of the nerve. Occasionally, there is a proximal branch to the flexor digitorum profundus, and this branch should be preserved, as the muscle plays an important role in gripping objects. The fibers of the flexor carpi ulnaris are split down in the direction of the ulnar styloid process so that the nerve can be fully mobilized. The nerve is transposed and, thus, is brought up against the sharp edge of the medial intermuscular septum. This structure is divided to the bone at the point of crossing so that there is no margin compressing the ulnar nerve. A trough is fashioned in the common flexor head, and the nerve is laid in the trough. The technique affords more protection than leaving the nerve in a subcutaneous position. The authors have had to reoperate in six cases in which the nerve was left in the subcutaneous tissues and not buried in the flexor musculature. The symptoms recurred and the patients complained of local burning pain, which was relieved by placing the nerve in the muscular trough. The procedure must be done with care so that closing sutures do not compress the nerve in the trough. This procedure is quite satisfactory, and it is unnecessary to remove the common flexor origin from the humerus and subsequently screw it back on, a practice that can cause major irreparable damage to the ulnar nerve. It would seem that the simpler conventional operation is safer. If the pathological change is obviously at the cubital tunnel, division of the entrapment point may be all that is required.

A third procedure is medial epicondylectomy. The periosteum is incised on the anterior aspect of the medial epicondyle, and the dissection is carried close to the bone around the margins of that structure. The epicondyle is then bitten off with a rongeur, and the periosteum is resutured to allow free movement of the ulnar nerve on flexion of the elbow. The ulnar nerve must be fully mobilized in the arm so that the nerve does not kink on elbow flexion.

Each of the three operations has its advocates.[116] The authors' practice has been to combine the division of the cubital tunnel with medial epicondylectomy, or to perform an anterior transposition, depending on the abnormality revealed at operation. They do not advocate wrapping the transposed nerve in anything, and have seen severe infarction of the nerve following its wrapping with gelatine sponge.

The patient should be warned that there may not be an immediate improvement. Satisfactory improvement usually occurs over a matter of months, but the outlook is poor if the condition has been neglected and there is long-standing atrophy, or if the patient is suffering from a generalized peripheral neuropathy (e.g., as in alcoholic and diabetic subjects). The patient should work the medial finger joints through a passive range at least three times a day, as fixed contractures of the interphalangeal joints may occur rapidly.

Entrapment at Wrist

The ulnar nerve crosses superficial to the transverse carpal ligament, running lateral to the pisiform bone, to enter Guyon's canal (see Fig. 76–18). This canal is roofed by an extension of the tendon of the flexor carpi ulnaris, and its sole contents are the ulnar artery and nerve. The nerve divides into superficial and deep branches within the canal. The former supplies the cutaneous distribution of the ulnar nerve in the hand, and the latter dives down into the palm. It passes between the heads of the flexor and abductor digiti minimi, winding around the hook of the hamate. The nerve runs laterally in the palm within the concavity of the palmar arch. The deep branch supplies the three hypothenar muscles, the interossei, the two medial lumbricals, and the adductor pollicis. The flexor pollicis brevis is supplied in one third of patients. It is useful to divide ulnar nerve lesions in this region into three groups according to the clinical signs and the apparent site of the lesion.[39,48,147,169,170]

Deep Palmar Branch Lesions

This is the most common variety of lesion and is usually due to a ganglion arising from the palmar aspect of one of the carpal joints and compressing the deep palmar branch of the nerve.[17] Seddon reported four such cases, and additional cases were described by Ebeling and co-workers.[38,142]

In this type of lesion, the deep palmar branch is involved after the hypothenar muscles have been supplied; the hypothenar muscles are normal in bulk and strength, and sensation is not affected. The condition occurs in men over the age of 40, and there is a history of hand trauma or unusual, excessive use of the hand in work that involves pressure on a portion of the palm. Weakness develops over weeks to a few months, and a number of patients have improved with conservative treatment alone, i.e., doing nothing other than avoid precipitating factors. If there is no improvement over the follow-up period of two to four months, or if the wasting and paralysis are unusually severe, exploration should be undertaken. A carpal synovioma is a common finding. The nerve may be of normal appearance. Thickening of the pisohamate ligament with an overhanging hook of the hamate has also been described.[38]

Electrical studies will confirm the site of the lesion. On stimulation of the ulnar nerve at the wrist, distal motor latency to the abductor digiti minimi muscle will be normal, but the latency will be prolonged to the first dorsal interosseous muscle. The electromyogram will show denervation and a decreased interference pattern for the first dorsal interosseous muscle as well as other interossei, but the electromyographic examination of the abductor digiti minimi muscle will be within normal limits. The ulnar nerve sensory evoked response at the wrist will be normal, and the wrist-to-elbow motor conduction velocity will also be normal. This combination of findings is diagnostic of a lesion of the deep palmar branch of the ulnar nerve.

Proximal Palmar Branch Lesions

In this group, the lesion is slightly more proximal and involves the branches to the hypothenar muscle but spares the superficial cutaneous branches.[76] There are weakness and wasting of the ulnar-supplied muscles of the hand, including the hypothenar eminence, but there is no sensory abnormality. Mallett and Zilkha reported two cases. Both were men over the age of 40, and there was a history of chronic occupational trauma in one and of acute wrist strain in the other. A ganglion was found on operation in both.[101]

The site of the lesion can be confirmed by electrical studies, and the changes will be identical to those described for the deep palmar branch lesion except for the additional finding of involvement of the hypothenar muscles characterized by denervation, diminished motor units, and a reduction in interference pattern and a prolonged latency to the abductor digiti minimi. Conservative management by simply avoiding the precipitating factors should be used, but if there is no improvement over two to three months, or if the wasting or weakness is severe, exploration should be advised.

Sensory and Motor Ulnar Palsy

Here the lesion is slightly more proximal and involves both motor and sensory branches. The clinical picture is one of involvement of the ulnar-supplied small muscles of the hand and sensory loss in the fifth and adjacent fourth finger and palm. Anatomically, the flexor digitorum profundus function to the fourth and fifth fingers will be spared, but although it might be expected that this clinical finding would help to distinguish this type of ulnar nerve lesion from that at the elbow, it may not. The dorsal cutaneous branch of the ulnar nerve is not involved, so normal sensation on the dorsum of the medial two fingers may provide a clue to the site of the ulnar nerve compression. Weakness of the ulnar-supplied portion of the flexor digitorum profundus muscle usually is not detectable in most patients with early ulnar nerve palsy when the lesion is at the elbow, and therefore, it is not of much value in defining when the lesion is at the wrist.

Electrical studies will allow the localization to be made; distal latency to the abudctor digiti minimi and first dorsal interosseous muscles is prolonged, and there is little or no slowing of the elbow-to-wrist ulnar motor conduction velocity and no slowing over the transsulcal portion of the nerve. The evoked sensory responses will be diminished or absent at the wrist and elbow when the fourth and fifth fingers are stimulated. With wrist fractures, a ganglion is usually found at operation, compressing the main trunk of the ulnar nerve proximal to its bifurcation into the superficial and deep divisions.

The ulnar nerve is identified lateral to the tendon of the flexor carpi ulnaris and followed lateral to the pisiform bone. Its further course is exposed by unroofing Guyon's canal. The nerve is elevated, and the branching of the two divisions is shown. The sensory branch continues in the same plane as the parent nerve, and the deep branch dives away from the operator. More distal dissection is required; the authors have followed the plan of Henry in which the pisiform bone is mobilized so that the deep branch can be followed to the opponens muscle. Entrance into the palm can be gained by the additional maneuver of elevating the sectioned opponens muscle from the fifth metacarpal bone.[68] The authors have also used an alternative exposure if there is an appropriate crease over the hypothenar eminence and have carried the skin incision down to the palm along that line. In the absence of a ganglion, an obvious indentation of the nerve by a band, usually arising from the hamate bone and running medially to compress the deep branch of the nerve, has always been found.

Posterior Interosseous and Radial Nerves

The radial nerve can be displayed in the antecubital fossa by retracting the muscles of the lateral boundary of the fossa. The nerve lies in the groove between the brachialis and brachioradialis muscles, both of which it supplies, along with the extensor carpi radialis longus (cf. Fig. 76–19). The posterior interosseous nerve then runs backward and around the neck of the radius, between the two heads of the supinator muscle.[134] Close to the lower border of that muscle, the nerve divides into numerous muscular branches to the extensor carpi ulnaris, the extensor digitorum, and the extensor indicis.[23]

The diagnosis is made by observing the characteristic posture of the hand displayed by patients when they are asked to extend all their digits.[111] Dorsiflexion of the wrist is preserved, as the extensor carpi radialis longus is supplied by the radial nerve, but is accomplished by a distinctive drift of the extended wrist. Extension of the proximal phalanges is lost, whereas extension of the distal phalanges is maintained by the intrinsic musculature of the hand. The thumb can be flexed into the palm in making a fist, but the main action of the extensor pollicus longus—retrieving the thumb from that position—is lost. There is no sensory disturbance. Electrical studies confirm the diagnosis and, in a later stage, will show evidence of denervation within the involved forearm muscles in which the motor units are reduced.[166] If the lesion is incomplete, that is, if there are surviving motor units, conservative management is indicated and recovery of strength should be looked for. If this does not occur in a matter of two to three months, or if there is obvious progression, exploration should be undertaken.

The radial nerve is found without difficulty proximally by separating the brachialis muscle from the brachioradialis and following the posterior interosseous nerve down to the supinator, where it may be entrapped at the arcade of Frohse.[152] Many small vessels surround the nerve at this point and are divided after bipolar coagulation. Attention is then turned to the proximal extensor aspect of the forearm, where the lower border of the supinator is displayed by parting the extensors, as described by Mayer and Mayfield.[103] By working alternately above and below it, the surgeon can decompress the entire nerve in its passage through the supinator muscle. Compressing bands are divided, and any ganglion, lipoma, or fibroma at the neck of the radius is dealt with appropriately.[13,93,117,146]

The posterior interosseous nerve syndrome must be distinguished from compression injury of the radial nerve itself. The most common site of involvement is at the spiral groove in a "Saturday night palsy," in which the nerve is compressed during sleep related to alcohol, or in normal sleep. It may also occur without definite precipitating cause.

In the authors' experience with 51 cases of "Saturday night palsy," patients were usually men in the middle or older age group, and a history of local pressure, often related to alcoholism, was obtained. The clinical picture is one of a variable degree of paralysis involving the outcropping muscles of the thumb (the abductor pollicis longus, and the extensor pollicis longus and brevis muscles), the extensor digitorum longus, the extensor indicis, and the brachioradialis muscles. The triceps muscle (lateral, medial, and long heads), as well as the anconeus, is supplied by more proximal branches of the radial nerve and is, therefore, spared by pressure lesions at the level of the spiral groove. The degree of paralysis within the radial nerve territory is variable and is usually incomplete. The wrist drop is symmetrical and quite different from the abnormal wrist extension (radial drift) seen with posterior interosseous nerve palsy. Sensory disturbance is usually minor and involves a small patch over the dorsal aspect of the base of the thumb. The prognosis in these cases is usually good, with improvement over weeks to a few months and ultimate full recovery.

Radial nerve palsy may be a complication of injuries such as fracture of the humerus, fracture-dislocation, or dislocation of the shoulder. Stretch or compressive forces, angulation, or injury by bone edges may be severe, and total paralysis may occur in the acute stage. Occasionally, the nerve is severed. Callus formation may interfere with recovery of function in the chronic stage of the paralysis.

Electrical studies are not definitely required when the nerve palsy is incomplete on clinical examination. In the authors' experience, some preserved muscle activity indicates that the lesion is in continuity and significant recovery will occur. When the paralysis appears complete on clinical examination, electromyographic studies should be done in order to confirm whether the lesion is or is not complete. If there are surviving motor units under voluntary control, or in response to electrical stimulation, within the forearm extensors, the outcropping muscles of the thumb, or the brachioradialis, this indicates a lesion in continuity, and usually implies a good prognosis. When such responses are found, serial examinations can be performed to assess the rate and amount of recovery.

The technique of evaluating motor and sensory conduction in different segments of the radial nerve has been described by Trojaborg and Sindrup and can be used for more detailed studies of the degree and site of involvement.[165,166] These tests, however, are not definitely required in the routine management of these patients.

The radial nerve may be involved at more proximal levels and this will produce the additional features of triceps muscle weakness and loss of reflex as well as involvement of the anconeus muscle. In a few patients, the site of the lesion is lower and the brachioradialis muscle is spared, although the forearm and thumb extensors are involved in the usual manner.

Trauma is the usual cause of radial nerve palsy; occasional cases due to lipoma, fibroma, or ganglion arising in the elbow region have been noted. The radial nerve may also be involved in mononeuritis, diabetes, rheumatoid arthritis, and other conditions.

Brachial Plexus

Cervical Rib Syndrome

The thoracic vertebrae exhibit a transverse process that is the true transverse element, or diaphysis. This carries the free rib or costal element. Fusion of these two elements is a feature of cervical vertebrae, with the costal element forming the anterior wall of the foramen transversarium as well as the costotransverse bar and the posterior tubercle. The true transverse element forms only the medial part of the posterior wall of the foramen (Fig. 76–21). The neu-

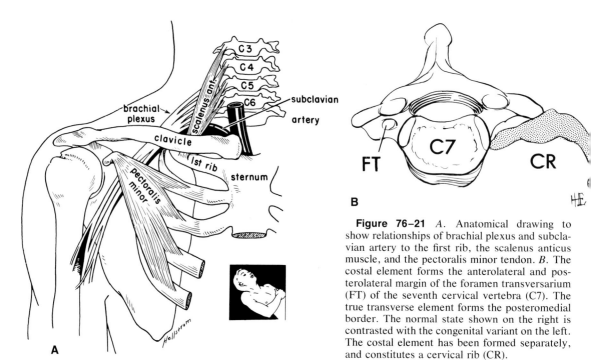

Figure 76–21 *A.* Anatomical drawing to show relationships of brachial plexus and subclavian artery to the first rib, the scalenus anticus muscle, and the pectoralis minor tendon. *B.* The costal element forms the anterolateral and posterolateral margin of the foramen transversarium (FT) of the seventh cervical vertebra (C7). The true transverse element forms the posteromedial border. The normal state shown on the right is contrasted with the congenital variant on the left. The costal element has been formed separately, and constitutes a cervical rib (CR).

ral groove is defined in front by the anterior tubercle and behind by the posterior tubercle.[49] The seventh cervical vertebra is characterized by a small foramen transversarium (the vertebral artery entering the foramen of the sixth cervical vertebra), and by the small size of the anterior and the large size of the posterior tubercles on the transverse process. The costal element may become free of the seventh cervical vertebra, forming a cervical rib. This may be of variable size and is usually connected to the upper surface of the first rib. The connection may be bony or, more frequently, a fibrous band. In either instance, the lowest trunk of the brachial plexus is tented up over this variant. Review of Mayfield's case material reveals that, while cervical ribs were verified by x-ray in 213 cases (49 bilateral and 164 unilateral), in only 87 cases (11 bilateral and 76 unilateral) was it confirmed that the ribs were the source of symptoms. Since the scalenus anticus muscle was divided with the anomalous rib, it could not be determined with certainty whether the favorable response to treatment resulted solely from rib resection, from division of the muscle, or from a combination of both.[105,106]

From the foregoing, it should be obvious that the presence of an anomalous cervical rib does not necessarily lead to an entrapment neuropathy of the overlying brachial plexus. Part of the reason for this may lie in the differences in size, configuration, and attachments of the anomalous ribs to the first rib. Variation in the anomalous rib is not the entire reason, however, as is borne out by the fact that in the authors' asymptomatic group of patients the ribs, as seen by x-ray, varied from rudimentary to large, and in the symptomatic group this same divergence was noted.

The effects of cervical ribs have been described by many authors.[16,70,139,177] Wasting of the thenar eminence was noted to be a feature of the condition. At the time, the carpal tunnel syndrome had not been recognized as an entity, but it is now known to be the most common cause of wasting of the thenar eminence. Carpal tunnel syndrome is a relatively common condition, and although cervical rib or band is often asymptomatic, it is an infrequent cause of neurological disturbance in the upper limb.

Howell described eight patients with marked weakness and wasting of the hand muscles and milder changes of the forearm muscles together with sensory loss of the inner aspect of the forearm at times involving the inner portion of the hand. The thenar muscles were usually severely involved, but there was also some involvement of the ulnar-supplied muscles.[70] In retrospect, it appears likely that some of the patients described by Howell and by Wilson had the carpal tunnel syndrome. [70, 177]

The condition is much more common in women, and presents during the adult years. In Mayfield's series, 30 per cent of the symptomatic patients were in their teens and 70 per cent were below the age of 50. In most cases, symptoms have been present for several years.[106] In the authors' experience, and in Gilliatt's cases the neurological symptoms and signs were unilateral, although the radiological changes were invariably bilateral.[61,66] The initial symptoms are intermittent ache on the inner side of the arm or forearm or diffusely throughout the limb, and at times, associated intermittent tingling of the ulnar aspect of the hand and forearm.[42] The symptoms are worsened by effort, but are not more troublesome at night. Weakness and wasting are often unnoticed by the patient, but are present on examination. The wasting may be predominantly restricted to the abductor pollicis brevis muscle and is, therefore, identical with the wasting seen in the more advanced cases of carpal tunnel syndrome. Most patients have a milder degree of weakness of the ulnar-supplied muscles of the hand, or the weakness may be evenly distributed between the median- and ulnar-supplied muscles. There may be slight thinning of the flexor mass in the forearm, with weakness of carpi ulnaris finger flexion, and slight weakness of finger extension may be noted. Reflexes and the remaining muscles are entirely normal. Pinprick sensation is usually diminished over the ulnar aspect of the forearm and, in a few patients, the ulnar fingers of the hand. Mild Raynaud's phenomenon may also be present. Patients in whom vascular symptoms and signs predominate tend to present themselves to vascular rather than neurological surgeons. The bony prominence due to cervical rib is usually not palpable in the neck, but patients with symptomatic cervical ribs are usually uncomfortable on palpation of the plexus at the posterior inferior border of the sternocleidomastoid muscle.

Motor conduction velocity in the forearm is normal, and median nerve forearm conduction velocity to the abductor pollicis brevis muscle is normal or slightly slowed.

Motor unit potentials are often diminished, but are of large amplitude (up to 10 mv). Sensory conduction is often normal, but the ulnar nerve potential may be absent or diminished. There is no prolongation of distal sensory or motor latency with respect to the median nerve, and this readily distinguishes the condition from carpal tunnel syndrome.

The characteristic radiological finding is an abnormal seventh cervical transverse process or a rudimentary or relatively well-formed rib. The x-ray changes are bilateral, and the neurological syndrome may be associated with the lesser bony abnormality. The tip of the T7 transverse process or the rudimentary rib is often pointed, suggesting that a narrow fibrous band arises there.

As has been noted, cervical ribs or abnormal transverse processes may be present without any symptoms. In some patients, symptoms are relatively mild in degree, and it is difficult to be certain whether the cervical abnormality is a factor in the production of the symptoms. Symptoms may persist following operative treatment, and it is probably best to limit operation to those patients in whom early but definite muscle changes are demonstrable. Physical therapy of the pectoral girdle muscles may restore normal posture and correct a tendency to drooping shoulders. This may relieve the symptoms as the plexus becomes less angled over the abnormal structure.

The operation is performed by making an incision immediately above the clavicle. Many surgeons fail to appreciate that the brachial plexus is in this corner of the posterior triangle of the neck and that the eighth cervical and first dorsal roots, combining to form the lowest trunk, may be well behind the arching subclavian artery. The lateral third of the sternocleidomastoid muscle is resected from the clavicle. Retraction of the skin flap reveals the omohyoid, and this muscle is incised along the lower border of both bellies. It is a simple matter to wipe the fatty pad laterally to reveal the scalenus anticus. The phrenic nerve is plastered to the anterior aspect of the scalenus anticus, and after this nerve has been mobilized by dividing the overlying fascia, the muscle is divided. The lower trunk of the brachial plexus is then defined, and arching branches of the costocervical trunk are divided. The thoracic duct on the left side must be guarded. The artery is pushed forward.[40] The sharp inner border of the first thoracic rib is palpated with the finger, and the dissection is kept superior to Sibson's fascia so that there is no danger of breaching the pleura. The particular anatomy of the patient undergoing the operation is then defined. It is easy to misinterpret fibrous bands. The surgeon's fingers can usually palpate the rounded end of the cervical rib, which may be passing through the scalenus medius, and he can then divide the band and resect the rib under direct vision. He should be certain to decompress the neural elements at both the anterior end of the rib or band and posteriorly, where the rib may angulate the root.

The authors have no experience with the transaxillary approach and have found the one just described to be satisfactory. The posterior approach to the lower brachial plexus is useful if there have been previous attempts at cervical rib resection by other routes. The disadvantage is the long incision, but a very clear view of the lower part of the proximal plexus is obtained through undisturbed tissue. In most cases, there was improvement within a few days or weeks following operation, with a subsidence of pain and paresthesia, but the muscle wasting and weakness usually remained throughout follow-up over several years.

Suprascapular Nerve

The supracapular nerve is a branch of the upper trunk of the brachial plexus. It arises from the trunk almost immediately distal to the junction of the fifth and sixth roots. The nerve transverses the posterior triangle of the neck and runs between the scapula and the transverse scapular ligament.[112] Clein describes five cases of pain around the shoulder joint in which there were appropriate motor weakness and wasting.[25] The upper trunk is characterized by the junction of C5 and C6 roots. The suprascapular nerve is easily found and is followed to the entrapment point at the suprascapular notch; the transverse scapular ligament is then divided.[112] Great care is required to distinguish this entrapment from the many causes of pain, weakness, and wasting that affect the shoulder joint.[34]

Supraclavicular Nerve

The clavicle is rarely pierced by one of the supraclavicular nerves. This is a variant of the normal situation. A single case of entrapment of a branch of the supraclavicular nerve has been reported.[59] This nerve is purely sensory in function, so the symptoms are of sensory abnormality in the area of distribution of the nerve. The inferior border of C4 abuts against the upper thoracic dermatomes, and the intervening dermatomes have been dragged out to cover the developing upper limb bud.

Hyperabduction Syndrome

The diagnosis of this syndrome is made by exclusion, and the treatment, which always must be conservative, precludes any visual confirmation of the pathological changes that might be seen at operation. [105, 106] The existence of the syndrome and the fact that it does qualify as an entrapment syndrome is confirmed by the striking similarities of arm positioning required in the occupations of Mayfield's 14 patients in whom this diagnosis was made, and the ablation of their signs and symptoms by changing occupations.

The mechanical basis underlying this syndrome was described by Wright.[179] It is compression of the brachial plexus and axillary artery and vein when the arms are held in constant abduction (Fig. 76–22).[135] The compression occurs at the point where the tendon of the pectoralis minor muscle inserts onto the coracoid process of the scapula. Indeed, the latter acts as a fulcrum around which the nerves and vascular structures are tightly constricted. Wright arrived at this conclusion by deductive reasoning and substantiated his conclusions by cadaver dissections. In his dissections, he also demonstrated that the costoclavicular space became narrowed by the rolling motion of the clavicle induced by the movements of hyperabduction. He had anticipated using ablation of the radial pulse by hyperabduction of the arms as a diagnostic test for the syndrome, but abandoned the idea when he noted bilateral ablation of the radial pulse in 82 per cent of 150 symptomless young subjects to whom this maneuver was applied. Apparently, this fact escaped Adson and Coffey's attention when they suggested the same maneuver as a diagnostic test for the then so-called "scalenus anticus syndrome."[2,126]

The hyperabduction syndrome is singular in that there are no constitutional abnormalities leading to its initiation or evolu-

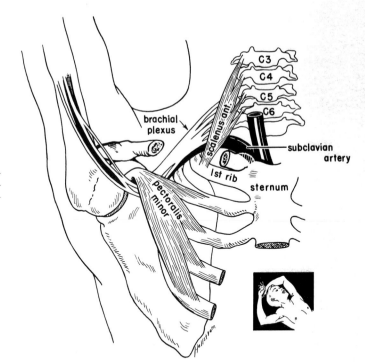

Figure 76-22 Anatomical drawing to show relationships of neurovascular bundle with arm in hyperabduction.

tion.[105] It is, rather, a matter of occupations in which unusual arm positions, maintained for varying lengths of time, cause a normal contiguous structure to impinge upon and constrict normal nerves, arteries, and veins. Although the flow of axoplasm and blood is impeded for short periods of time, there is apparently no permanent damage to the neurovascular bundle. All 14 of Mayfield's patients recovered when they were prevented from working with the arms in hyperabduction. The question of whether the signs and symptoms are caused by the impedance to the flow of blood, or to that of the axoplasm, or to a combination of both, receives a partial answer in that most of them are those of disordered nerve conduction, except for fatigability of the arms, which might be construed as being due to insufficient blood flow.[141]

Eight of Mayfield's patients were laborers who worked on ceilings as painters or plasterers, and the remainder were mechanics who regularly lay on their backs on dollies under automobiles with their arms hyperabducted as they worked.[106] All of them noted, after prolonged work of this type, fatigability of their arms accompanied by paresthesias of the thumbs and index fingers. Occasionally, the latter spread to involve the middle fingers, which perhaps

indicates involvement of the upper trunk to the brachial plexus.

Signs and symptoms rarely progressed beyond this point, were ameliorated or absent during vacation periods, and disappeared when the patients changed occupations and slept in a halter designed to prevent unconscious hyperabduction. In this group, the only diagnostic sign of any validity was the reproduction of symptoms on hyperabduction of the arm combined with percussion or deep palpation over the brachial plexus at the point where the pectoralis minor tendon inserts onto the coracoid process.

Costoclavicular Syndrome

In 1943, Falconer and Weddell noted that soldiers complained of numbness in their arms when they stood at attention wearing loaded knapsacks attached to their persons by straps that crossed the clavicles.[45] Apparently, this was not malingering, for large groups of soldiers experienced these same sensations in similar circumstances or on prolonged marches when they carried knapsacks of similar load and construction. It was the contention of these authors, which they confirmed on anatomical dissections, that weight applied to the clavicle caused it to ride down on the first rib and, in doing so, compress between them the brachial plexus and neighboring blood vessels. They also noted, in normal symptom-free subjects, that forceful backward dislocation of the shoulders would sometimes produce the symptoms and ablate the radial pulse, and that the Adson maneuver of stretching the scalenus anticus muscle would not affect this pulse when the point of compression was at the costoclavicular junction.

Their concept was apparently valid in the set of circumstances in which Falconer and Weddell studied it. It furnishes another example of abnormal positioning causing signs and symptoms due to impingement of normal structures on normal nerves and blood vessels.

The authors' material contains 15 cases of this syndrome, and in each of them a fracture of the clavicle and excessive callus formation was an antecedent clinical event. The portions of the brachial plexus that were compressed varied, the degree of compression ranged from partial to complete, and these facts dictated the extent and severity of the clinical symptoms. Because of the nature of the antecedent cause, these patients sought attention early, and the symptoms rarely had progressed beyond paresthesias and pain in the expected nerve distribution. There was little or no evidence that compression of vascular structures played any part in the evolution of the symptoms.

Treatment has consisted of wide excision of the clavicular callus, and the results have been good. In retrospect, however, it would seem that the operation of choice would be transthoracic excision of the first rib. The rib resection would release the brachial plexus and subclavian artery from compression while avoiding the skeletal instability that accompanies excision of the clavicle.

Long Thoracic Nerve

The nerve to the serratus anterior is one of three nerves that arise from the roots subtending the brachial plexus (nerve to rhomboids, nerve to subclavius, and nerve to serratus anterior). The nerve runs down the medial wall of the axilla and gains the superficial surface of the extensive thoracic origins of the serratus anterior. This muscle is attached to the medial border of the scapula, participating in rotation of that bone (with the trapezius) in shoulder abduction, and is the main muscle responsible for thrusting the shoulder girdle forward. Dysfunction of the nerve releases the medial border of the scapula from the thorax, resulting in the characteristic "winging."

Serratus anterior palsy has been attributed to pressure or stretching of the nerve while carrying a knapsack. "Pack-palsy" in soldiers has been described.[77] The condition has also been described in ceiling plaster and rope workers.[178] It may also occur after strenuous activity in sports or exercise. The lesion usually is in continuity, and gradual recovery occurs.

Electromyographic examination of the serratus anterior muscle can be done over the appropriate ribs in the midaxillary line and will reveal the degree of paralysis as well as evidence of denervation and reinnervation.

Greater Occipital Nerve

Occipital Tunnel Syndrome

The dorsal division of the second cervical nerve is much larger than the ventral division and is the largest of the cervical dorsal divisions. It emerges between the posterior arch of the atlas and the lamina of the axis caudal to the inferior oblique muscle, which it supplies. It communicates with the first cervical nerve and then divides into a larger medial branch and a small lateral branch.

The greater occipital nerve is the name given to the medial branch. It crosses obliquely between the inferior oblique and semispinalis capitis, pierces the semispinalis and trapezius muscles near their attachments to the occipital bone, and becomes subcutaneous. Interestingly, in its course through both these muscles it does not simply split the muscle fibers but traverses the muscles through a very definite fibrous canal. This canal is particularly well developed where the nerve proceeds through the aponeurosis of the trapezius, and it is here that the entrapment occurs. At this point, it is particularly vulnerable to trauma. Here, also, it joins the occipital artery.

The lymph nodes that occur in this area are well known. The lymphatic vessels of the scalp of the occipital region terminate partly in the occipital nodes and partly in a trunk that runs down along the posterior border of the sternocleidomastoid muscle to end in the inferior deep cervical nodes. The occipital nodes bear an intimate relationship to the greater occipital nerve as it traverses the fascial canal at the insertion of the trapezius. Certainly, any process that causes enlargement of these nodes could cause entrapment of the nerve. In addition, a similar situation may result from a tortuous occipital artery as it courses with the nerve through this small canal.

Patients with occipital nerve entrapment complain of pain radiating from occiput to vertex. Upper cervical pain frequently accompanies the headache. The nerve is tender on the involved side, and a palpable nodule may be present. Hypoesthesia to pinprick is present in the C2 distribution.

Mayfield has operated on 20 patients with occipital nerve entrapment, each of whom presented with hemicranial pain. In 12 cases lymph nodes related to the occipital nerve were believed to be responsible for the entrapment. Seven patients had unusually tortuous occipital arteries, and one patient had a lipoma.

The recommended treatment is decompression of the nerve and resection of lymph node or artery.

This syndrome must be carefully distinguished from the extremely common condition of extracranial muscle contraction headache. The authors believe it essential that sensory abnormality be demonstrated in the C2 anatomical distribution before the occipital tunnel syndrome is diagnosed.

It should be noted that, apart from the carpal tunnel and occipital tunnel syndromes, entrapment of peripheral nerves is usually a relatively painless condition, and although it may produce tingling and, in the case of a motor nerve, atrophy and weakness, it is not a cause of chronic or intractable pain.

Rectus Abdominis and Abdominal Cutaneous Nerve Syndromes

These syndromes are not established as clinical entities, and further studies are required.[35,89] The patients who are thought to have this problem present with sensory abnormalities in the area of supply of the ap-propriate nerve. The authors have found that ilioinguinal nerve damage has been the result of trauma, usually operative, and not the result of nerve entrapment.

Lateral Femoral Cutaneous Nerve of Thigh

This purely sensory nerve arises from the posterior divisions of the anterior primary rami of L2 and L3. It is easily seen in extraperitoneal intra-abdominal procedures, and forms a useful landmark to the uppermost root origin of the femoral nerve, which cannot be seen until the psoas muscle is retracted.[74] The nerve lies behind the fascia iliacus and is incorporated within that fascia immediately proximal to its point of exit into the thigh.[114] The nerve usually pierces the inguinal ligament immediately medial to the anterosuperior iliac spine, although this important operative relationship is variable, and the nerve may be immediately adjacent to the spine itself and may run superficial to or through the sartorius muscle. It is important to note that the nerve is deep to the investing fascia of the thigh and that it finally pierces the fascia a variable distance below the outer end of the inguinal ligament.[96] The anterior branch supplies the anterolateral aspect of the thigh, and the posterior branch (containing L2 fibers) supplies the skin over the iliotibial tract (Fig. 76–23).

The clinical picture of compression of the lateral femoral cutaneous nerve of the thigh was first described in 1895 by Bernhardt and Roth.[136] The condition presents in adult life and is slightly more common in men than in women. There is no occupational preponderance. The most usual symptoms are numbness, dull aching, burning, and increased sensitivity of the anterolateral aspect of the thigh.[156] Symptoms are usually of mild degree and often pass unnoticed. Compression of this nerve frequently is an incidental finding in patients suffering from other abnormalities and is also seen transiently in normal, healthy subjects. In younger women, the condition is often associated with pregnancy. The symptoms are often troublesome when the patient is lying down, and distressing paresthesias may be provoked by lightly stroking or touching the involved area. The only physical sign is reduction of sensation in the sen-

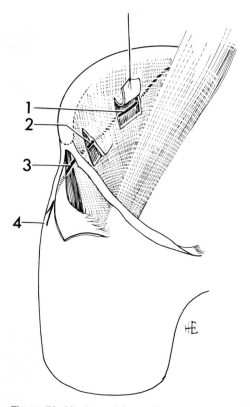

Figure 76–23 Lateral femoral cutaneous nerve of thigh. 1. The nerve is deep to the fascia iliacus. 2. The nerve is within the substance of the fascia. 3. The main entrapment point. 4. The nerve penetrates the investing fascia of the thigh.

sory distribution of the lateral femoral cutaneous nerve. The border between the affected and the normal areas is usually quite sharp, and if this is marked out with a skin pencil it will be noted that the abnormal area does not extend below the level of the knee and is characteristically within the "trouser pocket" area. The condition may be associated with obesity, local trauma, wearing of automobile seat belts in motor vehicle accidents, wearing of corsets, or altered pelvic tilt due to a variety of causes. In the anxious and hypochondriacal patient, the symptoms are often very troublesome.

The diagnosis is usually obvious, and the clinical picture is readily distinguished from femoral neuropathy, in which there is actual weakness and wasting of the quadriceps muscle with a loss of knee reflexes and some diminution in sensation on the anterior aspect of the thigh. High lumbar disc disease is relatively rare, and in it, as in other nerve root compressions, back pain is

common, with muscle weakness of the quadriceps and increased pain on hip extension in addition to the sensory loss in the appropriate dermatome.

The diagnosis can be confidently made in almost all cases on the basis of clinical assessment alone. A technique of nerve conduction studies applicable to the lateral femoral cutaneous nerve has been described, but this is not required in routine diagnosis.

In managing the condition, it is important to reassure the patient that it is benign and that it usually subsides or becomes insignificant with the passage of time. The diagnosis can be confirmed by rolling the nerve hard up against the anterior superior iliac spine, which aggravates the symptoms, or infiltrating the region with a local anesthetic, which will re-create the exact area of distribution of the patient's symptoms and also temporarily stop the discomfort. Steroid injection at the entrapment point may prolong the temporary relief gained by local anesthetic injection.

In the minority of cases in which operative treatment is required, the following points should be stressed. Cut boldly to the investing fascia of the thigh. Divide the deep fascia and pick up a branch of the main nerve, which can then be followed to the main trunk. This avoids tedious dissection, looking for the actual entrapment point with its variable location; the entrapment point is quite obvious. The scimitar band of fibrous tissue gives way to the knife, and the nerve can be followed into the pelvis until it is totally free in its tunnel of iliac fascia. The "absence" of a lateral femoral cutaneous nerve is usually related to a time-consuming superficial dissection by the inexperienced operator, but this condition may exist in reality and a search should be made more medially to find the anatomical variant of the nerve branching from the femoral nerve (this is not surprising, as both nerves arise from the posterior divisions of the anterior primary ramus of L2 and L3). Operative treatment gives relief of the symptoms in almost all cases.

Femoral Nerve

Femoral nerve palsy does occur as an isolated condition (femoral neuropathy or femoral mononeuritis). The authors have had experience with 27 cases of spontaneous onset, which they have studied electrically; about half of the patients were elderly and diabetic, and the condition was considered a form of diabetic mononeuritis. Alcoholism was an associated factor in a few, and the remainder did not have any concomitant disease. Pain was present at the onset, with numbness involving the anterior aspect of the thigh, weakness, eventual wasting of the quadriceps muscle, and a loss of the patellar reflex. Gradual improvement occurred, but several of the diabetic patients had a persisting troublesome weakness. Isolated femoral nerve involvement is also seen as a complication of anticoagulant therapy, and a recent series of cases of femoral neuropathy on the basis of trauma has been reported by Hudson and co-workers.[74,180] The nerve does not, however, appear to be involved by entrapment. Femoral nerve conduction can be tested, and the technique has been described by Gassel.[53] Electromyography will provide evidence of the completeness of the lesion, denervation, and reinnervation.

Saphenous Nerve

Branches of the saphenous nerve are frequently injured during orthopedic procedures on the knee joint. Also spontaneous saphenous nerve entrapment syndromes are thought to occur. Pain in the saphenous nerve distribution (medial aspect of knee and leg as far as the medial malleolus) is brought on by exercise, and confusion may arise as to whether these patients have true claudication from arterial insufficiency. Until detailed electrical studies and clinical experience are available in a larger number of patients, the entity should be considered to be a doubtful one.

Obturator Nerve

The obturator nerve is the nerve of the thigh adductors. It arises from the anterior divisions of the anterior primary rami of L2, L3, and L4 roots. The nerve traverses the pelvis, supplying the peritoneum immediately lateral to the ovary, and gains the obturator canal. The nerve lying against the pubic bone is here joined by the obturator artery and vein (Fig. 76–24). In the canal,

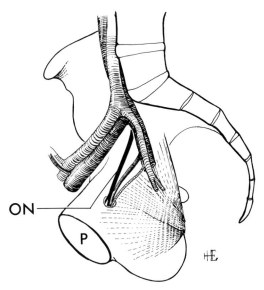

Figure 76–24 Obturator nerve. The obturator nerve (ON) runs forward and joins the obturator vessels at the obturator foramen, where it divides into its two divisions. P, Pubis.

the nerve divides into an anterior division, which passes above the obturator externus, and a posterior division, which has a variable course but usually passes through the obturator externus. Examination of a skeleton reveals that the origin of the adductor brevis lies between that of the adductor magnus and adductor longus. The anterior branch runs distally in the thigh superficial to the adductor brevis and gives a branch to the hip joint. The posterior branch runs deep to the adductor brevis and terminates in a branch to the knee joint that runs with a geniculate branch of the femoral artery in the popliteal fossa.[96] The obturator nerve supplies the pubic part of the adductor magnus—the ischial "hamstring" component is supplied by the sciatic nerve. The cutaneous distribution is to the medial aspect of the thigh, but this may vary inversely with distribution of the medial cutaneous nerve of the thigh (a branch of the femoral nerve).

A syndrome of compression of the obturator nerve has been described by Bodechtel and by Kopell and Thompson.[12,89] Compression of the nerve by callus following pubic fracture has been observed. Experience with this condition appears to be limited. The symptoms of entrapment include pain along the medial aspect of the thigh and weakness in the adductor musculature.

The diagnosis probably should not be made without convincing electromyographic evidence of denervation in the appropriate muscles. The authors advise that in most cases treatment be delayed in the hope that the condition will subside. If real disability persists, however, the area should be explored. Some authors have advised division of the obturator trunk within the pelvis via an abdominal extraperitoneal approach.[89] This maneuver, of course, results in paralysis of the adductor muscles of the thigh. A combined abdominal-inguinal approach allows complete mobilization of the whole segment of the obturator nerve within the canal.[68] During the intra-abdominal operation, the surgeon should remember the possibility of an abnormal obturator artery derived from the inferior epigastric artery.

Sciatic Nerve

The sciatic nerve is rarely, if ever, involved in entrapment.[7,60] The piriformis syndrome has been described, and it has been stated that this can be distinguished from radicular compression in intervertebral disc disease.[89] This syndrome does not appear to be an established entity. The squatting position has been implicated in unilateral sciatic nerve palsy described in 30 young adults. It was postulated that the nerve was compressed in the region of the ischial tuberosity, or beneath the piriformis muscle, or between the adductor magnus and hamstring muscles. Sciatic nerve pressure palsy has been noted in paraplegic patients, but apart from these specialized situations, sciatic nerve entrapment palsy probably is not a valid entity.

Posterior Tibial Nerve

The flexor retinaculum (laciniate ligament) is formed from the lower deep fascia and the deep transverse fascia of the leg. These two fascial layers fuse behind the ankle and effectively form a band running from the medial malleolus to the os calcis.[49] This structure forms the roof of the tarsal tunnel. The posterior tibial nerve, escaping the covering of the soleus muscle, runs distally to the tunnel immediately in front of the tendon of the flexor hallucis longus.

This latter muscle characteristically displays fleshy fibers almost to the ankle before it gives way entirely to its tendon.[96] Medial calcaneal branches are given off proximal to the flexor retinaculum, and these run down to supply the medial portion of the weight-bearing aspect of the heel (Fig. 76–25). The posterior tibial vessels lie anterior and medial to the nerve. The posterior tibial nerve divides into the medial and lateral plantar nerves within the tarsal tunnel at a point slightly distal to the division of the posterior tibial artery. The arm and leg are both pentadactyl limbs, with the medial plantar nerve being analogous to the median nerve of the upper limb. The larger medial plantar nerve becomes more anteriorly placed and winds around the os calcis and calcaneonavicular spring ligament to gain the sole of the foot. It lies deep to the abductor hallucis and reappears on the lateral side of that muscle, where it supplies the flexor digitorum brevis and abductor hallucis. The nerve to the abductor digiti minimi, a branch of the lateral plantar nerve, is usually given off deep to the flexor retinaculum. The smaller, more posteriorly placed lateral plantar nerve winds around the os calcis deep to the abductor hallucis muscle, crosses the accessorius deep to the plantar aponeurosis, and divides into a su-

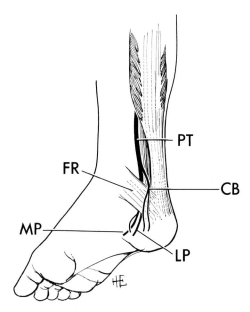

Figure 76–25 Tarsal tunnel. PT, Posterior tibial nerve; CB, calcaneal branches; MP, medial plantar nerve; LP, lateral plantar nerve; FR, flexor retinaculum.

perficial and a deep branch. Its distribution to skin and muscle is analogous, but not exactly similar, to that of the ulnar nerve.

The most striking symptom of which the patient complains is a burning pain on the sole of the foot.[94] Contact dysesthesia may be a predominant symptom. In the majority of cases, the calcaneal branches are derived proximal to the flexor retinaculum, so the heel itself is usually not involved. The sensory examination reveals a reduction in sensory appreciation. Either the medial or lateral plantar territory may be predominantly involved when the sole of the foot and the dorsal surfaces of the terminal digits are examined. In advanced cases, a pes cavus configuration with associated clawed toes is noted. In less extreme cases, there may be weakness and wasting of the small musculature of the foot. Kopell and Thompson emphasize the importance of local tenderness, either behind the medial malleolus or more distally, to distinguish posterior tibial from plantar nerve entrapments, but the authors have not found this particularly helpful in differentiating this condition from the host of conditions giving rise to the common complaint of foot pain.[89] The diagnosis may be partially confirmed by injecting local anesthetic just proximal to the flexor retinaculum and then having the patient walk on his foot for the duration of the local anesthesia. Prompt relief of the extremely irritating symptoms is usually reported.[33,57,78,94]

The incidence of spontaneous tarsal tunnel syndrome is not clearly established. Slowing of nerve conduction is seen in completely asymptomatic patients, and exploration in patients with suspicious electrical studies has given mixed results. Patients should be managed by temporizing and giving special attention to footwear. In a minority of cases, operative treatment should be undertaken.

A curved incision is made, centered one finger breadth behind the medial malleolus.[81] The deep fascia of the leg is incised, and then the transverse fascia is incised immediately in front of the flexor hallucis longus to reveal the posterior tibial nerve. The nerve is traced distally around the medial malleolus. This maneuver involves dividing the flexor retinaculum, but the structure has neither the toughness nor the thickness of the transverse carpal ligament. The medial and lateral plantar nerves are traced forward, deep to the abductor hallucis. All constricting bands are divided.

This procedure has proved efficacious in cases of nerve injury resulting from an obvious cause, e.g., chronic posterior-compartment ischemic syndromes resulting from complicated fractures, but the results of decompression in spontaneous entrapment are of questionable value.

Sural Nerve

The authors have performed electronmicroscopic evaluation of more than 100 sural nerve biopsies and have extensive experience in resecting the sural nerve for grafting procedures. In no instance has evidence of sural nerve entrapment been seen. Sural nerve entrapment has been described, but more detailed electrical and clinical studies are required before this is firmly established as an entrapment syndrome.[132]

Common Peroneal Nerve

The peroneal nerve runs downward and laterally through the popliteal fossa, forming a close medial relationship to the biceps femoris tendon, which is inserted into the head of the fibula. The common peroneal nerve winds around the neck of the fibula to gain the peroneal compartment of the leg. Applied to the bone, the nerve runs through a tunnel roofed by the peroneus longus, whose upper fibers originate from the shaft and head of the fibula. This opening is quite distinct at operation (Fig. 76–26). At this point, the nerve divides into the superficial and deep peroneal nerves and other smaller branches that are not of importance from a clinical viewpoint. The deep peroneal nerve remains applied to the fibula and runs deep to the fibers of the extensor digitorum longus, thereby reaching the interosseous membrane, where it lies between the only two muscles in the upper part of the extensor compartment, the extensor digitorum longus and the tibialis anterior.[96] The nerve descends toward the ankle joint, lying between the tibialis anticus and the extensor hallucis longus. Its terminal branches supply the extensor digitorum brevis, and the medial terminal branch runs forward on the dorsum of the

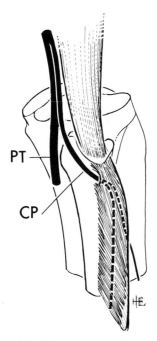

PT

CP

HE

Figure 76–26 Common peroneal nerve. The sciatic nerve separates into its two components at a variable point in the thigh. The common peroneal nerve (CP) winds around the neck of the fibula in a manner analogous to the passage of the posterior interosseous nerve in the forearm, thus gaining the lateral and anterior compartments of the leg and leaving the posterior tibial nerve (PT), which supplies the posterior compartment of the leg.

foot, lateral to the dorsalis pedis artery, to supply the first web space.

The superficial peroneal nerve runs downward within the substance of the peroneus longus. It supplies both peroneal muscles and pierces the deep fascia at the junction of the middle and lower thirds of the lateral aspect of the leg, supplying the skin of the anterolateral aspect of the leg and proximal dorsum of the foot.

Foot drop, caused by common peroneal nerve (lateral popliteal) palsy, is a common clinical condition. In a series of 75 cases of palsy, the usual causes were trauma about the knee or hip, compression, and underlying neuropathy.[10] A few palsies occurred spontaneously for no apparent reason. Large studies of military casualties are available, and a recent study of a civilian population described a number of cases due to gunshot wounds.[83] Traction injuries, ischemic peroneal nerve palsy, hematoma within the nerve sheath, and ganglia of the common peroneal nerve have also been described.[26,118]

Several peculiarities of the common

peroneal nerve make it vulnerable to injury; it is exposed over the bony prominence of the neck of the fibula and is susceptible to direct blows and lacerations. It is readily compressed at this site when the patient sits with legs crossed, when consciousness is diminished, or with fractures.[178] Nobel has noted limited longitudinal mobility of the nerve.[118] Longitudinal stretch forces applied to the nerve during posterior hip dislocation can result in a stretch injury. The nerve may also be involved by hemorrhage or swelling within the fibro-osseous tunnel below the neck of the fibula, through which it passes.[47,175]

A clinical picture is drop foot with loss of eversion and with variable paralysis of the tibialis anterior, the extensor hallucis longus, the peronei, and the extensor digitorum brevis muscles. The individual muscles are usually involved to an equal degree, but in some patients peroneal muscle function is preserved, although there is little or no function of the muscles of the anterior tibial compartment. Sensory loss is seen over the lateral aspect of the foot and lower leg, adjacent to the ankle. Pain is usually not a feature except in patients who have suffered hip trauma or undergone an operation in the region of the hip complicated by drop foot. Some of these patients have suffered injury to the sciatic nerve.

Common peroneal nerve palsy may develop in patients with underlying neuropathies (e.g., diabetic or alcoholic), and is also occasionally due to vasculitis. The clinical picture may be mimicked by lumbar intervertebral disc disease with herniation and compression of the L5 root; the pattern of muscle involvement within the common peroneal nerve territory is identical, although muscle paralysis is always incomplete. A sensory disturbance is also similar. There is, however, weakness, outside the distribution of this nerve, of the tibialis posterior muscle and hamstring muscles, and there are useful points of distinction. Back pain, sciatica, and limitation of straight leg raising are evident, and the two conditions are easily distinguishable. Motor neuron disease may begin with asymmetrical involvement of the lower extremities and present as drop foot. Bilateral progressive development of drop foot is seen in Charcot-Marie-Tooth disease and in the rare condition scapuloperoneal dystrophy.

The electrophysiological and clinical features of a large series of patients have been published.[10] Also, improved methods for localizing the lesion with sensory and motor conduction measurements have been described.[8,149] The reduction in motor conduction velocity and motor units under voluntary control roughly parallels the severity of the lesion and is a useful guide in prognosis. Nerve conduction (motor conduction velocity) and sensory evoked responses may well disclose an underlying neuropathy. When the paralysis appears to be complete, electromyographic examination may reveal surviving motor units and, therefore, imply a better prognosis. The same general principle of assessment on follow-up, in lesions that are complete clinically and electrically, applies here. Evidence of recovery should be looked for in the upper portion of the tibialis anterior muscle near the neck of the fibula (when the paralysis is complete) and should appear within two to three months. If this does not occur, exploration is advisable. Exploration should be undertaken at an earlier date if the lesion is complete by electroclinical criteria and there is reason to suspect discontinuity of the nerve.

When the palsy is incomplete, with slight to moderate weakness, the prognosis is good.[113] If the drop foot develops after diminished consciousness due to head injury, anesthesia, or other cause, there is no definite indication for any further medical or electrophysiological investigation, and the patients usually recover in a few weeks. When the condition develops spontaneously, an inquiry into general health, alcoholism, or diabetes is relevant. Rarely, progressive cases of common peroneal nerve palsy are encountered; in these underlying neuropathy should be looked for by means of electrical tests.

While the peroneal nerve and its branches may be injured by a wide variety of mechanisms, entrapment of the peroneal nerve is relatively unusual and carries a good prognosis for spontaneous recovery. The degree of muscular weakness and sensory involvement is generally less than that seen with severe common peroneal nerve injuries such as those associated with major knee injuries. The prognosis in patients with spontaneous or compressive common peroneal nerve palsy is greatly aided by electrophysiological studies, which have now been worked out in considerable detail. The patients whose electrical parameters indicate a mild disability should, therefore, not have operative exploration, as they will recover spontaneously. Patients should guard against inversion injuries to the ankle during the period of disability, as traction on the peroneal muscles, which occurs with a sprained ankle, will aggravate the condition. A light plaster foot drop splint, worn inside the shoe, is inexpensive and will facilitate walking, particularly over rough ground. Exploration is indicated in those few cases in which there is a progressively debilitating course.

The common peroneal nerve is easily identified just proximal to and behind the head of the fibula as the biceps tendon is palpated and used as a guide to the nerve. The nerve is traced to the entrapment point (see Fig. 76–26). It may show some degree of swelling immediately proximal to the arch of the peroneus longus opening or may be indented or narrowed at that point. The tough, moderately sharp edge of the arch is divided with a knife, and the deep peroneal nerve is followed forward deep to the extensor digitorum muscle to insure that it is free.

Superficial Peroneal Nerve

Entrapment of the superficial peroneal nerve as it passes through the deep fascia is an uncommon clinical entity. The patient characteristically complains of burning dysesthesia in the distribution of the superficial peroneal nerve at the end of the day after he has been standing. Conservative measures are usually successful and consist of a shoe wedge that raises the lateral border of the foot slightly so that the tissues of the lower lateral aspect of the leg are relaxed. If the problem is persistent, the nerve should be identified proximal to its division and penetration of deep fascia, and the branches should be followed to the fascia, where they are either freed or divided. The patient usually obtains relief, but the operative scars are extensive, and patients should be aware of this fact before consenting to operation.

Miscellaneous Palsies

Occasional examples of occupational palsy involving individual nerves have been described. A pressure palsy of the suprascapular nerve in the suprascapular foramen due to an unusual posture in a paraplegic patient and other isolated examples in workers who carry weights on their shoulders have been noted.[88] Pressure symptoms referable to the digital nerve and caused by excessive use of scissors or other manually held devices have been described and may produce numbness involving the sides of the digits.[89] Digits of the lower extremities may become compressed, with resulting numbness of the toes, as transiently experienced with tight shoes, but pain and disability (apart from the condition of Morton's metatarsalgia resulting from neuroma formation) do not appear to constitute a problem. Numbness of the dorsum of the foot and patchy reduction of sensation may occur. Apparently they are due to pressure on the anterior tibial and superficial peroneal nerves in their course over the dorsum, caused by tight shoes. No treatment is required other than reassurance about the nature of the condition and advice about footwear, which should be fashioned to avoid pressure on the appropriate nerves. These nerves are often palpable and visible in older patients, and sensory evoked responses can be recorded over their course.

REFERENCES

1. Adrian, E., and Bronk, D.: The discharge of impulses in motor nerve fibres. J. Physiol. (London), 67:119–251, 1929.
2. Adson, A., and Coffey, J.: Cervical rib. Method of anterior approach for relief of symptoms by division of scalenus anticus. Ann. Surg., 85:839–857, 1927.
3. Aguayo, A.: Neuropathy due to compression and entrapment. In Dyck, P. J., Thomas, P. K., and Lambert, E. H., eds.: Peripheral Neuropathy. Philadelphia, W. B. Saunders Co., 1975, pp. 688–713.
4. Aguayo, A., Nair, C. P. V., and Midgley, R.: Experimental progressive compression neuropathy in the rabbit. Arch. Neurol., 24:358–364, 1971.
5. Aguayo, A., Attiwell, M., Trecarten, J., et al.: Abnormal myelination in transplanted Trembler mouse Schwann cells. Nature, 265:73–75, 1977.
6. Asbury, A.: The histogenesis of phagocytes during Wallerian degeneration procedures. Sixth International Congress of Neuropathology. Paris, Masson & Cie, 1970.
7. Banerjee, T., and Hall, C. D.: Sciatic entrapment neuropathy. J. Neurosurg., 45:216–217, 1976.
8. Behse, F., and Buchthal, F.: Normal sensory conduction in the nerves of the leg in man. J. Neurol. Neurosurg. Psychiat., 34:404–414, 1971.
9. Behse, F., Buchthal, F., Carlsen, F., et al.: Hereditary neuropathy with liability to pressure palsies. Brain, 95:777–794, 1972.
10. Berry, H., and Richardson, P. M.: Common peroneal nerve palsy: A clinical and electrophysiological review. J. Neurol. Neurosurg. Psychiat., 39:1162–1171, 1976.
11. Bischoff, A., and Thomas, P. K.: Microscopic anatomy of myelinated nerve fibers. In Peripheral Neuropathy, Dyck, P. J., Thomas, P. K., and Lambert, E. H., eds.: Philadelphia, W. B. Saunders, Co., 1975, pp. 104–130.
12. Bodechtel, G.: Differentialdiagnose neurologischer krankheitsbilder. Stuttgart, G. Thieme Verlag, 1963.
13. Bowen, T. L., and Stone, K. H.: Posterior interosseous nerve paralysis caused by a ganglion at the elbow. J. Bone Joint Surg., 48-B:774–776, 1966.
14. Boyd, I. A., and Davey, M. R.: Composition of peripheral nerves. Edinburgh, E. and S. Livingstone, Ltd., 1968.
15. Brain, W. R., Wright, A. D., and Wilkinson, M.: Spontaneous compression of both median nerves in the carpal tunnel: 6 cases treated surgically. Lancet, 1:277–282, 1947.
16. Bramwell, E., and Dykes, H. B.: Rib pressure and the brachial plexus. Edinburgh Med. J., 27:65–88, 1921.
17. Brooks, D.: Nerve compression by simple ganglia. J. Bone Joint Surg., 34-B:391–400, 1952.
18. Brown, W. F., Ferguson, G. G., Jones, M. W., et al.: The location of conduction abnormalities in human entrapment neuropathies. Canad. J. Neurol. Sci., 3:111–122, 1976.
19. Buchthal, F., and Clemmesen, S.: Differentiation of muscle atrophy by electromyography. Acta Psychiat. (KbH.), 16:143–181, 1941.
20. Buchthal, F., Pinelli, P., and Rosenfalck, P.: Action potential parameters in normal human muscle and their physiological determinants. Acta Physiol. Scand., 32:219–229, 1954.
21. Bunge, R. P., and Bunge, M. B.: Tissue culture in the study of peripheral nerve pathology. In Dyck, P. J., Thomas, P. K., and Lambert, E. H., eds.: Peripheral Neuropathy. Philadelphia, W. B. Saunders Co., 1975, pp. 391–409.
22. Cannon, B. W., and Love, J. G.: Tardy median palsy: Median neuritis: Median thenar neuritis amenable to surgery. Surgery, 20:210–215, 1946.
23. Capener, N.: The vulnerability of the posterior interosseous nerve of the forearm. A case report and an anatomical study. J. Bone Joint Surg., 48-B:770–773, 1966.
24. Clawson, D. K., and Seddon, H. J.: The results of repair of the sciatic nerve. J. Bone Joint Surg., 42-B:205–212, 1960.
25. Clein, L. J.: Suprascapular entrapment neuropathy. J. Neurosurg., 43:337–342, 1975.
26. Cobb, C. A., and Moiel, R. H.: Ganglion of the peroneal nerve. J. Neurosurg., 41:255–259, 1974.
27. Cragg, B. G., and Thomas, P. K.: The conduction velocity of regenerated peripheral nerve fibres. J. Physiol. (London), 171:164–175, 1964.
28. Dawson, G. D.: The relative excitability and conduction velocity of sensory and motor nerve fibres in man. J. Physiol. (London), 131:436–451, 1956.

29. Davison, P. F.: Microtubules and neurofilaments: possible implications in axoplasmic transport. Advances Biochem. Psychopharmacol., 2:168, 1970.

30. Denny-Brown, D., and Brenner, C.: Lesion in peripheral nerve resulting from compression by spring clip. Arch. Neurol. Psychiat., 52:1, 1944.

31. Denny-Brown, D., and Brenner, C.: Paralysis of nerve induced by direct pressure and by tourniquet. Arch. Neurol. Psychiat., 51:1, 1944.

32. Denny-Brown, D., and Pennybacker, J.: Fibrillation and fasiculation in voluntary muscle. Brain, 61:311–344, 1938.

33. De Seze, S.: Electromyography of the tarsal tunnel syndrome. Rev. Rhum., 37:189–195, 1970.

34. Donovan, W. H., and Kraft, G. H.: Rotator cuff tear versus suprascapular nerve injury: A problem in differential diagnosis. Arch. Phys. Med., 55:424–428, 1974.

35. Doous, T. W., and Boas, R. A.: The abdominal cutaneous nerve entrapment syndrome. New Zeal. Med. J., 81:473–475, 1975.

36. Downie, A.: Studies in nerve conduction. In Walton, J. N., ed.: Disorders of Voluntary Muscle. Edinburgh, E. & S. Livingstone, Ltd., 1974.

37. Eames, R. A., and Lange, L. S.: Clinical and pathological study of ischaemic neuropathy. J. Neurol. Neurosurg. Psychiat., 30:215–226, 1967.

38. Ebeling, P., Gilliatt, R. W., and Thomas, P. K.: A clinical and electrical study of ulnar nerve lesions in the hand. J. Neurol. Neurosurg. Psychiat., 23:1–9, 1960.

39. Eckman, P. B., Perlstein, G., and Altrocchi, P. H.: Ulnar neuropathy in bicycle riders. Arch. Neurol. (Chicago), 32:130–131, 1975.

40. Eden, K.: Vascular complications of cervical ribs and first thoracic rib abnormalities. Brit. J. Surg., 27:111–139, 1939.

41. Editorial: Other tunnels, other nerves. Brit. Med. J., 2:3–4, 1976.

42. Editorial: Thoracic outlet compression syndrome. Brit. Med. J., 1:1033, 1976.

43. Engh, C., and Schofield, B.: A review of the central response to peripheral nerve injury and its significance in peripheral nerve regeneration. J. Neurosurg., 37:195–203, 1972.

44. Erb, W.: Handbook of Electrotherapy. New York, 1883.

45. Falconer, M., and Weddell, G.: Costoclavicular compression of the subclavian artery and vein: Relation to the scalenus anticus syndrome. Lancet, 2:539–543, 1943.

46. Feindell, W., and Stratford, J.: The role of the cubital tunnel in tardy ulnar palsy. Canad. J. Surg., 1:287–300, 1958.

47. Fergusson, F., and Liversedge, L.: Ischaemic lateral popliteal nerve palsy. Brit. Med. J., 2:333–335, 1954.

48. Forshell, K. P., and Hagstrom, P.: Distal ulnar nerve compression caused by ganglion formation in the Loge de Guyon. Case report. Scand. J. Plast. Reconstr. Surg., 9:77–79, 1975.

49. Frazer, J.: Anatomy of the Human Skeleton. Breathnach, A., ed. 6th Ed. Edinburgh, E. & S. Livingstone, Ltd., 1965.

50. Fullerton, P. M.: The effect of ischaemia on nerve conduction in the carpal tunnel syndrome. J. Neurol. Neurosurg. Psychiat., 26:385–397, 1963.

51. Gardner-Thorpe, C.: Anterior interosseous nerve palsy: Spontaneous recovery in two patients. J. Neurol. Neurosurg. Psychiat., 37:1146–1150, 1974.

52. Garland, H., Langworth, E. P., Taverner, D., et al.: Surgical treatment for the carpal tunnel syndrome. Lancet, 1:1129–1130, 1964.

53. Gassel, M. M.: A study of femoral nerve conduction time. Arch. Neurol. (Chicago), 9:607–614, 1963.

54. Gassel, M. M., and Diamantopoulos, E.: Pattern of conduction time in the distribution of the radial nerve. Neurology (Minneap.), 14:222–231, 1964.

55. Gassel, M. M., and Trojaborg, W.: Clinical and electrophysiological study of the pattern of conduction times in the distribution of the sciatic nerve. J. Neurol. Neurosurg. Psychiat., 27:351–357, 1964.

56. Gasser, H. S., and Erlanger, J.: The role played by the sizes of the constituent fibers of a nerve trunk in determining the form of its action potential wave. Amer. J. Physiol., 80:522–547, 1927.

57. Gathier, J. C., Bruyn, G. W., and Van Der Meer, W. K.: The medial tarsal tunnel syndrome. Psychiat. Neurol. Neurochir., 73:97–103, 1970.

58. Gay, J., and Love, J.: Diagnosis and treatment of tardy paralysis of the ulnar nerve. J. Bone Joint Surg., 29:1087–1097, 1947.

59. Gelberman, R. H., Verdeck, W. N., and Brodhead, W. T.: Supraclavicular nerve-entrapment syndrome. J. Bone Joint Surg., 57-A:119, 1975.

60. Gelmers, H.: Entrapment of the sciatic nerve. Acta Neurochir. (Wien), 33:103–106, 1976.

61. Gilliatt, R. W.: Thoracic outlet compression syndrome. Brit. Med. J., 1:1274–1275, 1976.

62. Gilliatt, R. W., and Hjorth, R. J.: Nerve conduction during Wallerian degeneration in the baboon. J. Neurol. Neurosurg. Psychiat., 35:335–341, 1972.

63. Gilliatt, R. W., and Sears, T. A.: Sensory nerve action potentials in patients with peripheral nerve lesions. J. Neurol. Neurosurg. Psychiat., 21:109–118, 1958.

64. Gilliatt, R. W., and Taylor, J. C.: Electrical changes following section of the facial nerve. Proc. Roy. Soc. Med., 52:1080–1083, 1959.

65. Gilliatt, R. W., and Thomas, P. K.: Changes in nerve conduction with ulnar lesions at the elbow. J. Neurol. Neurosurg. Psychiat., 23:312–320, 1960.

66. Gilliatt, R. W., Le Quesne, P. M., Logue, V., et al.: Wasting of the hand associated with a cervical rib or band. J. Neurol. Neurosurg. Psychiat., 33:615–624, 1970.

67. Gilliatt, R. W., Ochoa, J., Ridge, P., and Neary, D.: Cause of nerve damage in acute compression. Trans. Amer. Neurol. Ass., 99:71–574, 1974.

68. Henry, A.: Extensive Exposure. Edinburgh, E. & S. Livingstone, Ltd., 1962.

69. Hodes, R., Larrabee, M., and German, W.: Human electromyogram in response to nerve stimulation and the conduction velocity of

motor axons. Arch. Neurol. Psychiat., *60*:340–365, 1948.

70. Howell, C.: A consideration of some symptoms which may be produced by seventh cervical ribs. Lancet, *1*:1702–1707, 1907.

71. Hudson, A., and Bilbao, J.: Angiopathy in peripheral nerve surgery (Abstr.). Neurosurgery, *1*:70–71, 1977.

72. Hudson, A., and Hunter, D.: Polyglycolic acid suture in peripheral nerve II: Sutured sciatic nerve. Canad. J. Neurol. Sci., *3*:69–72, 1976.

73. Hudson, A., and Kline, D.: Progression of partial experimental injury to peripheral nerve. Part 2: Light and electron microscopic studies. J. Neurosurg., *42*:15–22, 1975.

74. Hudson, A., Hunter, G. A., and Waddell, J. P.: Iatrogenic femoral nerve injury. Canad. J. Surg., *22*:62–66, 1979.

75. Hudson, A., Morris, J., Weddell, G., et al.: Peripheral nerve autografts. J. Surg. Res., *12*:267–274, 1972.

76. Hunt, J.: Occupation neuritis of the deep palmar branch of the ulnar nerve. J. Nerv. Mental Dis., *35*:673, 1908.

77. Ilfeld, F., and Holder, H.: Winged scapula: A case occurring in a soldier from knapsack. J.A.M.A., *120*:448–449, 1942.

78. Johnson, E. W., and Ortiz, P. R.: Electrodiagnosis of tarsal tunnel syndrome. Arch. Phys. Med., *47*:776–780, 1966.

79. Karpati, G., Carpenter, S., Eisen, A. A., et al.: Familial multiple peripheral nerve entrapments. Trans. Amer. Neurol. Ass., *98*:267–269, 1973.

80. Kelly, M. J., and Jackson, B. T.: Compression of median nerve at elbow. Brit. Med. J., *2*:283, 1976.

81. Kempe, L. G.: Operative Neurosurgery. Vol. 2. New York, Springer-Verlag, 1970.

82. Kerjaschki, D., and Stockinger, L.: Zur Struktur und Funktion des Perineuriums. Z. Zellforsch., *110*:386–400, 1970.

83. Kline, D. G.: Operative management of major nerve lesions of the lower extremity. Surg. Clin. N. Amer., *52*:1247–1265, 1972.

84. Kline, D. G.: Personal communication, 1978.

85. Kline, D. G., and Hudson, A.: Early management of peripheral nerve injury. *In* Morley, T., ed.: Current Controversies in Neurosurgery. Philadelphia, W. B. Saunders Co., 1976, pp. 181–198.

86. Kline, D. G., Hackett, E. R., Davis, G. D., et al.: Effect of mobilization on the blood supply and regeneration of injured nerves. J. Surg. Res., *12*:254–266, 1972.

87. Kline, D. G., Hudson, A. R., Hackett, E. R., et al.: Progression of partial experimental injury to peripheral nerve. Part 1: Periodic measurements of muscle contraction strength. J. Neurosurg., *42*:1–14, 1975.

88. Kopell, H. P., and Thompson, W. A. L.: Pronator syndrome. New Eng. J. Med., *259*:713–715, 1958.

89. Kopell, H. P., and Thompson, W. A. L.: Peripheral Entrapment Neuropathies. Huntington, N.Y., R. E. Krieger Publishing Co., 1975.

90. Komar, J., and Varga, B.: Syndrome of the rectus abdominus muscle. J. Neurol., *210*:121–125, 1975.

91. Kugelberg, E.: Electromyograms in muscular disorders. J. Neurol. Neurosurg. Psychiat., *10*:122–133, 1947.

92. Lake, P. A.: Anterior interosseous nerve syndrome. J. Neurosurg., *41*:306–309, 1974.

93. Lallemand, R. C., and Weller, R. O.: Intraneural neurofibromas involving the posterior interosseous nerve. J. Neurol. Neurosurg. Psychiat., *36*:991–996, 1973.

94. Lam, S. J. S.: Tarsal tunnel syndrome. J. Bone Joint Surg., *49-B*:87–92, 1967.

95. Landon, D., and Langley, O.: The local chemical environment of nodes of Ranvier: A study of cation binding. J. Anat., *108*:419, 1971.

96. Last, R.: Anatomy, Regional and Applied. 6th Ed. Edinburgh, E. & S. Livingstone, Ltd., 1977.

97. Lenman, J. A., and Ritchie, A. E.: Clinical Electromyography. Philadelphia, J. B. Lippincott Co., 1970.

98. Licht, S., ed.: Electrodiagnosis and Electromyography. 3rd Ed. Baltimore, Williams & Wilkins Co., 1961.

99. Low, P. A., McLeod, J. G., Turtle, J. R., et al.: Peripheral neuropathy in acromegaly. Brain, *97*:139–152, 1974.

100. Lubinska, L.: Axoplasmic streaming in regenerating and normal nerve fibres. Progr. Brain Res., *13*:1–71, 1964.

101. Mallett, B., and Zilkha, K.: Compression of the ulnar nerve at the wrist by a ganglion. Lancet, *1*:890–891, 1955.

102. Mangini, U.: Flexor pollicis longus muscle. Its morphology and clinical significance. J. Bone Joint Surg., *42-A*:467–470, 1960.

103. Mayer, J., and Mayfield, F.: Surgery of the posterior interosseous branch of the radial nerve. Analysis of 58 cases. Surg. Gynec. Obset., *84*:979–982, 1947.

104. Mayfield, F.: Causalgia. Springfield, Ill., Charles C Thomas, 1951.

105. Mayfield, F.: Neural and vascular compression syndromes of the shoulder girdle and arms. *In* Vinken, P., and Bruyn, G., eds.: Handbook of Clinical Neurology. Vol. 7. Amsterdam, North Holland Publishing Co., 1970, pp. 430–446.

106. Mayfield, F., and True, C.: Chronic injuries of peripheral nerves by entrapment. *In* Youmans, J. R., ed.: Neurological Surgery. Philadelphia, W. B. Saunders Co., 1973, pp. 1141–1161.

107. McLellan, D. L., and Swash, M.: Longitudinal sliding of median nerve during movements of the upper limb. J. Neurol. Neurosurg. Psychiat., *39*:566–570, 1976.

108. Morris, H. H., and Peters, B. H.: Pronator syndrome: Clinical and electrophysiological features in seven cases. J. Neurol. Neurosurg. Psychiat., *39*:461–464, 1976.

109. Morris, J. H., Hudson, A. R., and Weddell, G.: A study of degeneration and regeneration in the divided rat sciatic nerve based on electron microscopy. Z. Zellforsch., *124*:76–203, 1972.

110. Mozes, M., Ouaknine, G., and Nathan, H.: Saphenous nerve entrapment simulating vascular disorder. Surgery, *77*:299–303, 1975.

111. Mulholland, R. C.: Non-traumatic progressive paralysis of the posterior interosseous nerve. J. Bone Joint Surg., *48-B*:781–785, 1966.

112. Murray, J.: A surgical approach for entrapment

neuropathy of the suprascapular nerve. Orthop. Rev., *3*:33–35, 1974.

113. Nagler, S., and Rangell, L.: Peroneal palsy caused by crossing the legs. J.A.M.A., *133*:755–761, 1947.

114. Nathan, H.: Ganglioform enlargement of the lateral cutaneous nerve of thigh. J. Neurosurg., *17*:843–850, 1960.

115. Neary, D., Ochoa, J., and Gilliatt, R. W.: Subclinical entrapment neuropathy in man. J. Neurol. Sci., *24*:283–298, 1975.

116. Neblett, C., and Ehni, G.: Medial epicondylectomy for ulnar palsy. J. Neurosurg., *32*:55–62, 1970.

117. Nielsen, H.: Posterior interosseous nerve paralysis caused by fibrous band compression at the supinator muscle. Acta Orthop. Scand., *47*:304 –307, 1976.

118. Nobel, W.: Peroneal palsy due to haematoma in the common peroneal nerve sheath after distal tortional fractures and inversion ankle sprains. J. Bone Joint Surg., *48-A*:1484–1495, 1966.

119. Noble, D.: The nerve impulse. *In* Hubbard, J., ed.: The Peripheral Nervous System. New York, Plenum Press, 1974, pp. 27–46.

120. O'Brien, M. D., and Upton, A. R. M.: Anterior interosseous nerve syndrome. J. Neurol. Neurosurg. Psychiat., *35*:531–536, 1972.

121. Ochoa, J.: Microscopic anatomy of unmyelinated nerve fibers. *In* Dyck, P. J., Thomas, P. K., and Lambert, E. H., eds.: Peripheral Neuropathy. Philadelphia, W. B. Saunders Co., 1975, pp. 131–150.

122. Ochoa, J., and Marotte, L.: The nature of the nerve lesion caused by chronic entrapment in the guinea pig. J. Neurol. Sci., *19*:491–495, 1973.

123. Ochoa, J., Fowler, T. J., and Gilliat, R. W.: Anatomical changes in peripheral nerves compressed by a pneumatic tourniquet. J. Anat., *113*:433–455, 1972.

124. Ochs, S.: Axoplasmic transport—energy metabolism and mechanism. *In* Hubbard, J., ed.: The Peripheral Nervous System. New York, Plenum Press, 1974, pp. 47–67.

125. Ochs, S.: Axoplasmic transport—a basis for neural pathology. *In* Dyck, P. J., Thomas, P. K., and Lambert, E. H., eds.: Peripheral Neuropathy. Philadelphia, W. B. Saunders Co., 1975, pp. 213–230.

126. Ochsner, A., Gage, M., and DeBakey, M.: Scalenus anticus (Naffziger) syndrome. Amer. J. Surg., *28*:669–695, 1935.

127. Olsson, Y., and Reese, T.: Permeability of vasa nervorum and perineurium in mouse sciatic nerve studied by fluorescence and electron microscopy. J. Neuropath. Exp. Neurol., *30*:105, 1971.

128. Payan, J.: Electrophysiological localization of ulnar nerve lesions. J. Neurol. Neurosurg. Psychiat., *32*:208–220, 1969.

129. Payan, J.: Anterior transposition of the ulnar nerve. An electrophysiological study. J. Neurol. Neurosurg. Psychiat., *33*:157–165, 1970.

130. Phalen, G. S.: The carpal-tunnel syndrome. Clin. Orthop., *83*:29–40, 1972.

131. Pringle, R. M., Protheroe, K., and Mukherjee, S.

K.: Entrapment neuropathy of the sural nerve. J. Bone Joint Surg., *56-B*:465–468, 1974.

132. Ramon y Cajal, S.: Degeneration and Regeneration of the Nervous system. Translated by R. M. May. New York, Oxford University Press, 1928.

133. Ranvier. M.: Leçons sur l'Histologie du Système Nerveux. Paris, F. Savy, 1878.

134. Roles, N. C., and Maudsley, R.: Radial tunnel syndrome. Resistant tennis elbow as a nerve entrapment. J. Bone Joint Surg., *54-B*:499–508, 1972.

135. Rosenberg, J.: Arteriographic demonstration of compression syndromes of the thoracic outlet. Southern Med. J., *59*:400–403, 1966.

136. Roth, V.: Meralgia Paresthetica. Berlin, S. Karger, 1895.

137. Rudge, P., Ochoa, J., and Gilliatt, R. W.: Acute peripheral nerve compression in the baboon. J. Neurol. Sci., *23*:403–420, 1974.

138. Samuels, A., et al.: Distribution, exchange and migration of phosphate compounds in the nervous system. Amer. J. Physiol., *164*:1–15, 1951.

139. Sargent, P.: Lesions of the brachial plexus associated with rudimentary ribs. Brain, *44*:95–124, 1927.

140. Schwann, T.: Microscopic Researches into the Accordance in the Structure and Growth of Animals and Plants. Translated by H. Smith. London, Sydenham Society, 1847.

141. Schlesinger, E.: The thoracic outlet syndrome from a neurosurgical point of view. Clin. Orthop., *51*:49–52, 1967.

142. Seddon, H.: Carpal ganglion as a cause of paralysis of the deep branch of the ulnar nerve. J. Bone Joint Surg., *34-B*:386, 1952.

143. Seddon, H.: Nerve grafting. J. Bone Joint Surg., *45*:447–461, 1963.

144. Seddon, H.: Degeneration and regeneration. *In* Seddon H.: Surgical Disorders of the Peripheral Nerves. Edinburgh, E. & S. Livingstone, Ltd., 1972, pp. 9–31.

145. Seyffarth, H.: Primary myoses in the m. pronator teres as cause of lesion of the n. medianus (pronator syndrome). Acta Psychiat. Neurol. Scand., suppl. *74*:251–254, 1951.

146. Sharrard, W. J. W.: Posterior interosseous neuritis. J. Bone Joint Surg., *48-B*:777, 1966.

147. Shea, J. D., and McClain, E. J.: Ulnar-nerve compression syndromes at and below the wrist. J. Bone Joint Surg. *51-A*:1095–1103, 1969.

148. Simpson, J. A.: Electrical signs in the diagnosis of carpal tunnel and related syndromes. J. Neurol. Neurosurg. Psychiat., *19*:275–280, 1956.

149. Singh, N., et al.: Electrophysiological study of peroneal palsy. J. Neurol. Neurosurg. Psychiat., *37*:1202–1213, 1974.

150. Smith, B. H., and Herbst, B. A.: Anterior interosseus nerve palsy. Arch. Neurol. (Chicago), *30*:330–331, 1974.

151. Spencer, P.: Reappraisal of the model for "bulk axoplasmic flow." Nature, [New Biol.], *240*:283–285, 1972.

152. Spinner, M.: The arcade of Frohse and its relationship to posterior interosseous nerve paralysis, J. Bone Joint Surg., *50-B*:809–812, 1968.

153. Spinner, M.: The anterior interosseous-nerve syndrome. J. Bone Joint Surg., *52-A*:84–95, 1970.

154. Spinner, M.: Injuries to the Major Branches of Peripheral Nerves of the Forearm. Philadelphia, W. B. Saunders Co., 1972.

155. Spinner, M., and Spencer, P. S.: Nerve compression lesions of the upper extremity. A clinical and experimental review. Clin. Orthop. *104*:46–67, 1974.

156. Stevens, H.: Meralgia paresthetica. Arch. Neurol. Psychiat., *77*:557–574, 1957.

157. Strain, R., and Olson, W.: Selective damage of large diameter peripheral nerve fibers by compression: an application of Laplace's law. Exp. Neurol., *47*:68–80, 1975.

158. Sunderland, S.: A classification of peripheral nerve injuries producing loss of function. Brain, *74*:491, 1951.

159. Sunderland, S.: Nerves and Nerve Injuries. Edinburgh, E. & S. Livingstone, Ltd., 1968.

160. Thomas, J. E., Lambert, E. H., and Cseuz, K. A.: Electrodiagnostic aspects of the carpal tunnel syndrome. Arch. Neurol. (Chicago), *16*:635–641, 1967.

161. Thomas, P. K.: The cellular response to nerve injury. 3. The effect of repeated crush injuries. J. Anat., *106*:463–470, 1970.

162. Thomas, P. K., and Fullerton, P. M.: Nerve fibre size in the carpal tunnel syndrome. J. Neurol. Neurosurg. Psychiat., *26*:520–527, 1963.

163. Thomas, P. K., and Jones, D. G.: The cellular response to nerve injury. 2. Regeneration of the perineurium after nerve section. J. Anat., *101*:45–55, 1967.

164. Tompkins, D. G.: Median neuropathy in the carpal tunnel caused by tumour-like conditions. J. Bone Joint Surg., *49-A*:737–740, 1967.

165. Trojaborg, W.: Rate of recovery in motor and sensory fibres of the radial nerve: Clinical and electrophysiological aspects. J. Neurol. Neurosurg. Psychiat., *33*:625–628, 1970.

166. Trojaborg, W., and Sindrup, E. H.: Motor and sensory conduction in different segments of the radial nerve in normal subjects. J. Neurol. Neurosurg. Psychiat., *32*:354–359, 1969.

167. Trimm, A., and Evans, J.: Carpal tunnel syndrome: A note on conservative treatment. Practitioner, *196*:410–412, 1966.

168. Upton, A. R. M., and McComas, A. J.: Double crush in nerve-entrapment syndromes. Lancet, *2*:359–361, 1973.

169. Uriburu, I., Morchio, F., and Marin, J.: Compression syndrome of the deep motor branch of the ulnar nerve. J. Bone Joint Surg., *58-A*:145–147, 1976.

170. Vanderpool, D. W., Chalmers, J., Lamb, D. W., et al.: Peripheral compression lesions of the ulnar nerve. J. Bone Joint Surg., *50-B*:792–803, 1968.

171. Waller, A.: Experiments on the section of the glossopharyngeal and hypoglossal nerves of the frog. Phil. Trans. Roy. Soc. (London), *140*:423–429, 1850.

172. Weddell, G., Fernstein, B., and Pattie, R.: The electrical activity of voluntary muscle in man under normal and pathological conditions. Brain, *67*:178–256, 1944.

173. Weiss, P.: The concept of perpetual neuronal growth and proximodistal substance convection. *In* Kety, S. S., and Elkes, J., eds.: Regional Neurochemistry. Elmsford, N.Y., Pergamon Press, 1961, pp. 220–224.

174. Werschkul, J.: Anomalous course of the recurrent motor branch of the median nerve in a patient with carpal tunnel syndrome. J. Neurosurg., *47*:113–114, 1977.

175. White, J.: The results of traction injuries to the common peroneal nerve. J. Bone Joint Surg., *50-B*:346–350, 1968.

176. Wilson, D. H., and Krout, R.: Surgery of ulnar neuropathy at the elbow: 16 cases treated by decompression without transposition. J. Neurosurg., *38*:780–785, 1974.

177. Wilson, S.: Some points in the symptomatology of the cervical rib with special reference to muscular wasting. Proc. Roy. Soc. Med., *6*:133–141, 1913.

178. Woltman, H.: Crossing the legs as a factor in the production of peroneal palsy. J.A.M.A., *93*:670–672, 1929.

179. Wright, J.: The neurovascular syndrome produced by hyperabduction of the arm. Amer. Heart J., *29*:1–19, 1945.

180. Young, M. R., and Norris, J. W.: Femoral neuropathy during anticoagulant therapy. Neurology (Minneap.), *26*:1173–1175, 1976.

77

PROBLEMS ASSOCIATED WITH MULTIPLE TRAUMA

The neurosurgeon must be alert to the possibility that his patients may have injuries to areas outside the brain or spinal cord, even though these injuries are typically handled by other surgical specialists. The neurosurgeon must be able to recognize them and be capable of rendering necessary, often lifesaving, treatment during the initial phase of management. Furthermore, he should have some understanding of their management so that he can intelligently participate in the total care of the patient.

In the initial evaluation of the injured patient, certain priorities must be kept in mind. Most urgently, an adequate airway must be established and satisfactory pulmonary ventilation insured. Second, hemorrhage must be controlled. This includes the management of shock and identification of sources of occult bleeding. Once these two vital steps are taken, more leisurely and thorough evaluation of other possible injuries can be made.

The most important immediate consideration is the maintenance of an adequate airway. The patient should be thoroughly examined to see that free and easy flow of air into the lungs is possible and that adequate pulmonary function is present. If the natural airway is not adequate, an artificial airway such as an oral airway, an endotracheal tube, or even a tracheostomy must be provided.

Once an airway has been obtained, the patient's cardiovascular status must be examined. Shock, if present, must be diagnosed and treated without delay. Obvious areas of hemorrhage need to be controlled.

Most injured patients will require some type of supportive intravenous fluid, in the form of either balanced salt solutions or blood. The need for such therapy may not be immediately apparent, as shock may develop at any time. It is, however, important that a means of administering this treatment be established early in the course of evaluation. Large-bore (18-gauge or larger) needles should be securely placed in extremity veins. Lower extremity veins should not be used if obvious abdominal injury is present, as extravasation of the administered fluid from a ruptured inferior vena cava is possible. Blood specimens for typing and crossmatching and hemoglobin and hematocrit determinations should be drawn at the time of the venipuncture.

If shock is present, a search must be made for its cause. Intra-abdominal organs may have been ruptured, hemorrhage may have occurred from long-bone fractures, or sympathetic tone may have been lost because of spinal cord injuries; all these conditions may produce shock. Shock secondary to head injury alone is unusual, and all other causes must be excluded before brain injury is assumed to be the cause. Rarely, serious hemorrhage from extensive scalp lacerations may produce the shock syndrome.

Once these initial steps have been performed, further measures in management are necessary. A nasogastric tube should be inserted and connected to suction. The tube will empty the stomach, reducing the chance of aspiration pneumonitis and preventing gastric distention if ileus is present. A Foley catheter is inserted into the blad-

---

C. WATTS AND M. PULLIAM

der. Injury to the urinary system may be demonstrated by the presence of hematuria. More importantly, the indwelling catheter facilitates accurate measurement of urinary output, which is important in the treatment of shock, in the regulation of fluid balance, and in the recognition of several complications of injury.

By this point in the evaluation, the physician will have obtained considerable information about the patient. He should determine what other studies, such as x-ray examinations and serum electrolyte and blood gas determinations, will be needed. It is important to obtain a history from any source that is available. If his condition will permit, the patient is the best informant. Relatives, ambulance attendants, police officials, and anyone else who may have knowledge about the injury should be questioned. As the physician examines the patient and institutes therapy, he must recognize changes that may occur in the priorities of treatment. The airway may become compromised; shock, not previously present, may develop. He must be flexible and quick to modify his management as new problems arise. The measures necessary to maintain vital functions must be accomplished immediately without the delay of further investigations. Imminent threat to life may require immediate operative intervention to accomplish these measures.

If the physician is sure no immediate threat to life exists, then he may begin the investigation and management of injuries that are severe but not life-threatening. Injuries to the abdomen, the chest, and the extremities are usually included in this category. While little time must be lost in treating them, additional information can usually be obtained by such diagnostic techniques as contrast studies and abdominal paracentesis. Other laboratory studies, e.g., blood chemistry, may be needed for accurate diagnosis.

Finally, there are those patients whose injuries are of an occult nature and require observation for proper diagnosis. A classic example is the patient with a subcapsular splenic rupture who does not develop shock for several hours or days after injury. Patients who potentially may have suffered significant injury should undergo a period of observation. A good policy is to admit all such patients to the hospital for 24 to 48 hours of observation.

MAINTENANCE OF RESPIRATORY FUNCTION

The Airway

The airway of an injured patient should be evaluated systematically from the mouth to the alveolus. A large percentage of patients with head injuries will also have facial injuries.[22] Seventy-one per cent of the victims of automobile accidents sustain injury to the head, midface, or upper airway. Sixty-four per cent of these patients die from intracranial and ventilatory complications. The principal cause of deaths from facial injuries is obstruction of the upper airway. The time that a patient survives with a partially obstructed upper respiratory tract varies inversely with the percentage of lumen obstruction and directly with myocardial reserve. Priority must, therefore, be given to the establishment of an airway.

Fractures of facial bones, particularly of the maxilla and the mandible, result in distortion of the nasal and oral pathways, producing poor ventilatory function. Certain fractures of the mandible may allow the tongue to fall posteriorly and obstruct the pharyngeal airway. This problem is most effectively managed by passing a large towel clip or safety pin through the anterior part of the tongue and exerting traction to bring both the tongue and mandibular arch forward.

The patient's mouth should be opened and carefully examined for broken teeth, dentures, and other foreign bodies, and for severe lacerations of the tongue. Generally, bleeding from the gums, lips, or tongue can be controlled by simple compression. Rarely, ligation of the facial or external carotid artery may be necessary. The oral cavity should be cleaned of all secretions and blood. The patient may be placed in the lateral or semiprone position to facilitate drainage of secretions. An oral airway should be inserted; frequent suctioning will be necessary to maintain its patency.

Endotracheal Intubation

Often the foregoing measures will not be sufficient to maintain adequate respiratory function. When this is true, a cuffed endotracheal tube should be inserted. Because of the logistics of performing a tracheostomy, an endotracheal intubation is preferable in the early management of the severely injured patient. The type of injury in the facial area will dictate the type of intubation. Generally, the orotracheal tube is the method of choice, but if the nasopharynx is intact, a nasotracheal tube may be used. A patient with adequate pharyngeal reflexes may not tolerate endotracheal intubation. In handling this problem, the use of topical anesthetics is indicated.

The technique of oral intubation is not difficult. The patient should be supine with the neck in a neutral postion and the head at midchest height for the operator, reducing the need to bend or lean over. A laryngoscope is inserted into the oral cavity in such a manner as to displace the tongue anteriorly and to the left. The type of laryngoscope used should vary, depending on the size of the patient. In general, a No. 3 MacIntosh (curved) blade will be adequate for most adults. The blade is advanced under direct vision anteriorly and inferiorly until it lies in the vallecula between the tongue anteriorly and the epiglottis posteriorly. Lifting the laryngoscope anteriorly and superiorly will open the glottis, and the vocal cords will be visualized. The endotracheal tube can then be gently passed between them. This procedure affords the opportunity for inspection of the posterior pharynx and the glottis. All foreign material, loose teeth, and blood should be removed. Due care must be exercised to avoid manipulation of the neck in any patient who may have a cervical fracture.

Some form of lubricant for the endotracheal tube, usually one containing 4 per cent lidocaine or other topical anesthetic, should be used to minimize coughing. The larynx may be sprayed with a topical anesthetic. Use of a stylet frequently aids in rapid insertion with minimal manipulation of the patient's neck. The endotracheal tube should be cuffed to reduce the chance of aspiration and make possible adequate positive ventilation of the lungs. Although tracheal intubation is used to manage immediate airway problems, the tube may be left in place for several days. Those tubes that are not to be removed immediately postoperatively should be of plastic or silicone rather than rubber. Immediately after the tube is in place, an auscultatory check should be performed to assure bilateral ventilation, as it is quite easy to advance the tube too deep, into the right main bronchus. When time allows, further evaluation of its position by x-ray is desirable. An oropharyngeal airway must be used in conjunction with an orotracheal tube to prevent the patient from occluding the latter with his teeth. The endotracheal tube should be secured with appropriately placed tape. Care must be taken at all times to keep the tube patent.

Tracheostomy

Upper airway problems likely to last more than a few days will require tracheostomy. Most patients with severe facial trauma or those who are comatose for any length of time are in this category. In general, if the physician considers a tracheostomy, the patient probably needs one. There are several major complications associated with the performance of a tracheostomy, so it should be done without hurry, with sterile techniques, with good light, and with adequate instruments.[64] If time is of the essence, the patient should be intubated and ventilated through the endotracheal tube. Use of the endotracheal tube allows the performance of an unhurried tracheostomy.

If intubation is not possible, because of the presence of laryngeal spasm or facial trauma, or because of lack of adequate experience in inserting endotracheal tubes, a cricothyreotomy (coniotomy) may be performed. This procedure is condemned by many because of the high rate of complications, including frequent subcutaneous emphysema. With experience a tracheostomy can be performed nearly as rapidly. Should the surgeon, however, elect to use it as a lifesaving procedure, the cricothyreotomy can be done by making a transverse incision through the skin and cricothyroid membrane and then securing the opening by placing a single suture in each edge of the incision. Alternatively, a 15- to 13-gauge needle (or larger) can be inserted rapidly through the cricothyroid membrane, which can be easily palpated just below the prominences of the thyroid cartilages in the midline. This latter technique, especially, is proposed as a means of providing a better field in which to perform a careful tracheostomy.[22] Although a needle will not permit full spontaneous respiration because of excessive resistance, attached to a tube from an oxygen tank, it will provide adequate oxygenation for several hours. In actual practice, the tracheostomy should be done as soon as possible (within an hour at most) to prevent excessive accumulation of carbon dioxide and resultant respiratory acidosis.

A final option available in conjunction with coniotomy is the insertion of a small tracheostomy tube (No. 6 Jackson or 32 Portex) through the incision. This maneuver allows for relatively good ventilatory exchange but should be followed by formal tracheostomy within a maximum of six hours to prevent ulceration of the vocal cords and subsequent vocal cord fusion that will compromise both airway and phonation. Coniotomy is rarely indicated.

For a careful elective tracheostomy, a transverse skin incision is preferred. This is placed halfway between the cricoid cartilage and the suprasternal notch. Skin and subcutaneous bleeders are controlled by temporarily placed hemostats or careful electrocoagulation. The use of ligatures is not necessary and should be avoided. The ligatures constitute foreign bodies in a wound that will inevitably become infected. The cervical fascia is incised in the midline from the cricoid to 1 cm above the sternal notch. The dissection is carried between the strap muscles of the neck and below the isthmus of the thyroid. It should be exactly in the midsagittal plane of the neck. Occasionally, a large thyroid isthmus will have to be clamped, transected, and suture ligated. The midline plane of dissection is imperative, as the dome of the parietal pleura may rise laterally to the level of the lower poles of the thyroid. Lateral dissection will result in pneumothorax or injury to the recurrent laryngeal nerves. The only vascular structure of note in the midline is the inconstant thyroid ima vein, which can simply be ligated and divided or retracted to one side. The pretracheal fascia is incised sharply, bringing the trachea into view. A tracheal hook is inserted beneath the first tracheal ring, and the trachea is retracted anteriorly and superiorly. If an endotracheal tube is in place the cuff is deflated. One to two milliliters of lidocaine is injected into the trachea to minimize coughing. A cruciate incision is made with one limb between tracheal rings 2 and 3 and the other dividing the rings vertically in the midline. A window of cartilage should not be removed, as this is associated with an increased incidence of post-tracheostomy tracheal stenosis.[48] This precaution is especially important in infants and small children in whom some advocate using only a vertical incision.[26] The endotracheal tube is removed, culture specimens are taken, and the trachea is suctioned. The tracheostomy tube is inserted with obturator in place. The obturator is removed, and the incision is covered with sterile gauze. The head is flexed, and the tube is secured with umbilical tape passed around the neck and tied with a square knot. A minimal number of wound sutures are used because the wounds tend to become infected.

A truly emergency tracheostomy may be necessary in some cases of severe laryngeal injury, facial fractures, and other conditions in which intubation cannot be performed. In this event the midline structures of the neck are palpated. A vertical incision is made from the cricoid cartilage to 1 cm above the suprasternal notch. The procedure is then continued as already outlined. Complications occur more frequently after emergency tracheostomies. The likelihood and results of such complications must be weighed and deemed less life-threatening than the patient's current status.

A constantly humidified atmosphere must be maintained for the patient with an endotracheal or tracheostomy tube; otherwise, drying and crusting of the trachea and tubes occur. Humidification of the atmosphere is best done with an apparatus that provides cold steam. Room air or oxygen, as appropriate, is applied by a tracheostomy mask or Briggs' adapter. Bronchodilators are used only if indicated, never routinely. The tracheostomy cuff should be used only during times when upper airway secretions are excessive, in patients who are being fed (either orally or through the gastric tube), and while positive-pressure ventilation is being used. If the cuff remains inflated too long, necrosis of the trachea may occur. Necrosis can develop as quickly as in one to two hours. Should long-term assisted ventilation be required, the cuff should be deflated for at least five minutes every hour. A plastic tracheostomy tube is preferred, as it causes less erosion than those made of metal. Information about the tube size most likely to be appropriate for patients of various sex and age is available in the references; however, most adults will accommodate a No. 36 Portex.[22,26,48,64]

In general, longer tubes are more frequently associated with such complications as innominate artery erosion. Suctioning should be performed as necessary and must be done under the most aseptic conditions possible. Should dry, thick secretions be noted, 1 to 3 ml of sterile saline may be instilled prior to suctioning. Once a stoma is well established, the cleaning, changing, and ultimate removal of the tracheostomy tube is relatively simple. The tracheostomy tube should not be "corked" as a test of the patient's ability to breathe. Should a "weaning period" be desired (especially in children), stepwise daily reduction in the size of the tube is advocated. Once the tube has been permanently removed, the wound is kept covered with sterile dressings until healing occurs. Usually the wound is airtight in 2 to 3 days and healed in 7 to 10 days.

Chest and Lung Injuries That Alter Ventilatory Function

Trauma to the chest may affect ventilatory function in many ways.[55] Roughly 25 per cent of all civilian deaths from trauma in this country result primarily from chest injuries, and in another 25–50 per cent these injuries contribute significantly to the lethal outcome; yet the relative contribution of chest injuries to mortality, once trauma victims reach the hospital ward, is small. These facts serve to emphasize the importance of appropriate action on the part of the physician who first attends these patients. If initial care is adequate, only 10 per cent or less of victims of major trauma will subsequently require thoracotomy. The trauma may be obvious, such as a gunshot or stab wound of the chest; or it may be less obvious, such as blunt trauma from steering wheel impact, which may or may not leave a telltale contusion or abrasion.

Simple rib fractures are usually of very little consequence. If only a few ribs are broken, no special treatment other than analgesics is required. Local infiltration with anesthetics is helpful to minimize the discomfort. If the pain reduces the excursion and the volume changes of the lungs and limits respiration, this technique should be used. In the case of multiple rib fractures it is possible to provide more extensive anesthesia with an indwelling epidural catheter placed by an anesthesiologist. In practice, however, such multiple fractures often result in a flail chest, which will be managed by tracheostomy and a respirator, in which case control of respiration allows more liberal use of analgesics. Adhesive strapping in rib fractures has more disadvantages than advantages.

Sternal fractures are not uncommon in association with head trauma. Simple sternal fractures require very little treatment per se. Reduction and fixation are required only for completely displaced fractures and for partially displaced fractures with false motion. It is worthwhile to recall the relatively frequent association of sternal fracture with disruption of the thoracic aorta, tracheal or brachial tears, rupture of the diaphragm or esophagus, flail chest, and contusion of the lung or myocardium. Severe ventilatory insufficiency developing *soon* after chest trauma should call to mind airway obstruction, open pneumothorax (penetrating wounds), flail chest, tension pneumothorax, and massive hemothorax.

Flail Chest

More extensive rib or sternal fractures, however, may produce softening or loss of rigidity of the chest wall, and limit respiration.[55] A flail chest, or crushed chest syndrome, is present when paradoxical motion is seen. A patient with a flail chest suffers from a specific type of respiratory deficit. During inspiration, as the intrathoracic pressure becomes negative in relation to atmospheric pressure, the greater atmospheric pressure presses the injured area of the chest inward, thus correcting the negative intrathoracic pressure. The loss of negative intrathoracic pressure results in a sharp reduction in flow of air into the lungs; if it is extensive, there may be no pulmonary ventilation. If only one side of the chest is flail, air is shunted from the normal side of the chest, which develops positive pressure during expiration, into the abnormal side, which, because it is flail, has remained at atmospheric pressure. Thus, a to-and-fro movement of air within the chest occurs. This motion was once thought to be the cause of the distress. Other factors most certainly are involved, however. A marked reduction in vital capacity and maximum breathing capacity contributes greatly to the respiratory distress.

The treatment of this condition depends upon its severity and the presence of associated conditions. Treatment is designed to minimize the derangements of the breathing mechanism. Minor degrees of flailing require only periodic suction, intercostal blocks, and intermittent positive-pressure breathing for short periods of time to prevent atelectasis. Some indications for a more vigorous approach include: (1) significant initial impairment of or deterioration of arterial blood gas tensions, including need for more than 5 to 6 liters of oxygen per minute to maintain an adequate Po_2; (2) significant mechanical interference with ventilatory exchange; (3) increasing respiratory distress, tachypnea, increased work of breathing, and signs of fatigue; (4) significant associated pulmonary contusion or pre-existing underlying lung disease; (5) the need for general anesthetic and surgical intervention for associated trauma; and (6) an uncooperative patient (e.g., one comatose from head injury). Should one or more of these be present, immediate stabilization by either external compression with sand bags or traction with 5 to 10 lb of weight attached by towel clips and a cord over a pulley must be instituted. This allows time for a careful tracheostomy. Once completed, the external stabilization is replaced by internal pneumatic stabilization employing *continuous* positive-pressure ventilation. The modern respirators that are basically volume regulated, while allowing high-pressure cutoff, are ideal for this purpose, especially in cases with coexistent wet lung.

Serial arterial blood gas analyses are essential in monitoring adequacy of therapy. Strong consideration should be given to prophylactic bilateral chest tube drainage to avoid the threat of tension pneumothorax. Unforeseen complications aside, this mode of treatment should allow for adequate healing in 10 to 14 days.

More recent evidence indicates that the major respiratory problem associated with a flail chest is the resulting pulmonary contusion and wet lung, rather than any effects of the paradoxical movement.[66] On this basis, treatment is directed primarily at the pulmonary contusion. Fluids are restricted to 1000 to 1200 ml per day. Furosemide is given intravenously in doses of 40 mg per day. Blood loss is replaced with whole blood or plasma, not crystalloids. Salt-poor albumin is given for three days at 100 gm per day. Methylprednisolone is used at a dosage of 500 mg parenterally every six hours for three days. Good pulmonary toilet and early mobilization are used along with intercostal nerve blocks for pain. Oxygen is given by mask or nasal cannula to keep arterial Po_2 above 80 mm of mercury. Endotracheal intubation and mechanical ventilation are used only temporarily when the arterial Po_2 falls below 60 mm of mercury on room air or 80 mm of mercury on supplemental oxygen. With this regimen, significant reductions of the mortality rate and the duration of hospitalization attendant on the time-honored regimen of tracheostomy and mechanical ventilation may be accomplished. Since early patient mobilization and adequate basic respiratory drive are crucial factors in the success of the newer approach, however, its applicability to patients with multiple severe trauma will sometimes be limited.

Pneumothorax and Hemothorax

Pneumothorax occurs as a result of laceration of the lungs by fractured ribs, perforating or penetrating injuries by missiles or weapons, and blunt force that injures the trachea or bronchi. Rib fractures are present in 90 per cent of adult cases of traumatic pneumothorax secondary to blunt trauma. Usually some degree of associated hemothorax is found. Air is permitted to escape into the pleural cavity; a decreased vital capacity results as collapse of the lung occurs. Small decreases in vital capacity may be tolerated well by the average adult patient; even total collapse of one lung is usually not life-threatening.[55]

A pneumothorax is readily recognized. The patient is usually dyspneic. Physical examination discloses hyperresonance to percussion over the pneumothorax, with decrease or absence of breath sounds in the same area. X-rays of the chest rapidly confirm the diagnosis. Expiratory films of good quality may be necessary to reveal minor degrees of pneumothorax. The presence of rib fractures or subcutaneous emphysema should alert the examiner to this possibility. Of course, arterial blood gas analysis will provide objective evidence of the physiological embarrassment that is present.

Appropriate treatment is the insertion of chest tubes by closed chest thoracotomy.

Needle aspiration and observation are even less defensible in ''minor'' degrees of traumatic pneumothorax than they are in spontaneous pneumothorax. A single tube is sufficient for management of a simple pneumothorax. The tube is placed in the upper anterior portion of the chest in the second intercostal space in the midclavicular line. It can be introduced through an appropriate-sized trocar. To minimize potential damage to underlying lung, however, most surgeons prefer another technique. A small incision is made in the desired location, and a tract through subcutaneous tissue and muscle is developed down to pleura by advancing a Kelly clamp in increments and spreading gently. The pleura is entered with a quick thrust of the clamp. Following this maneuver, an appropriate-sized catheter is clamped at its distal tip and introduced through the tract into the pleural cavity; then the tube is clamped proximally. The skin is closed snugly around the catheter with a heavy silk suture that can also be used to anchor the tube. An occlusive dressing may be applied but is rarely necessary if the suture is properly located. After the tube is securely connected to the drainage system (with adhesive tape) the clamp is released. Drainage may consist of either a simple water-sealed bottle system or a water-sealed system designed for and connected to constant gentle suction. Usually it employs a negative pressure of between 5 and 20 cm of water. This system provides continuous removal of air from the pleural cavity and allows the lung to expand. As normal healing occurs, the pleural leak closes. When pleural closure occurs, air no longer bubbles in the water seal; the chest tube can be removed 24 hours later, and the chest x-rays will show re-expansion of the lung to be complete.

Occasionally a tension pneumothorax will occur. It happens when a small tear in the bronchus or lung allows air to escape into the pleural cavity during inspiration, but does not allow air to escape from the pleural cavity back into the bronchial system during expiration. Air progressively accumulates under pressure within the pleural cavity on the involved side, which produces collapse of the lung. Finally, as the pressure increases, the mediastinal structures are shifted toward the opposite side, thus reducing the effective ventilation of the opposite lung. Circulatory problems occur as venous return to the heart is impaired. Arrhythmias and interference with pulmonary blood flow may also occur. The most important sign on examination, again, is hyperresonance to percussion along with decreased movement of the involved hemithorax and distention of neck veins. Tension pneumothorax demands immediate treatment. Rapid initial relief can be obtained most simply by percutaneous needle puncture of the involved hemithorax. This maneuver converts the condition into an open pneumothorax, but with a small opening that, functionally, is little worse than a simple pneumothorax. Use of the percutaneous needle provides time to insert a chest tube as already described. If the patient has progressed to the point of having failure of his respiratory drive, however, artificial ventilation with oxygen should be instituted even before placement of the chest tube. The frequent association of tension pneumothorax with rupture of a bronchus must be remembered and will be manifest by a large and persistent air leak that causes almost constant bubbling in the chest drainage bottle and difficulty in re-expanding the lung. This situation requires treatment by an efficient (low-pressure and high-volume) suction system and, in some cases, may require an immediate thoracotomy. A tension pneumothorax may be produced under general anesthesia if positive-pressure ventilation is used in patients with fractured ribs or with a simple pneumothorax. In these patients it may be wise to institute closed-chest tube drainage before operation.

Trauma to the chest may produce a hemothorax alone; in most cases, however, an accompanying pneumothorax is present. Hemothorax usually occurs with injury to the lung from fractured ribs or from penetrating trauma. The bleeding usually is minor and ceases within minutes of the injury. Continued bleeding indicates more severe vascular injury, for instance, to the internal mammary or intercostal arteries or to one of the major pulmonary vessels. A patient may become moribund from shock due to severe hemorrhage into the pleural cavity alone.

The diagnosis should be suspected if the patient is dyspneic or cyanotic. Physical findings include dullness to percussion over the posterior chest and decrease or absence of breath sounds. X-ray findings are those of lung collapse with fluid in the pleural space or in the lung. A hemothorax of less than 300 ml, however, is often not demonstrable on the upright chest film. A major hemothorax (about 25 per cent of all cases) will usually present with shock that overshadows the respiratory embarrassment.

The blood should be drained out of the pleural cavity, as it compromises the respiratory function in the same way as the air in the pneumothorax. Furthermore, blood left in the pleural cavity may serve as a culture medium for infection. Later, fibrosis and scarring may occur, restricting pulmonary function.

Initial treatment may be simple needle aspiration of the pleural cavity. The aspiration may be diagnostic, to confirm the diagnosis, or for temporary relief. If shock is present, however, restoration of blood volume should be the first therapeutic measure. Once treatment of shock is under way, more definitive treatment usually requires closed thoracotomy with continuous drainage of the blood, utilizing the water-sealed bottle system, or preferably, constant gentle suction (-20 cm of water). Usually a single chest tube in the posterior axillary line in the sixth or seventh intercostal space is adequate. It is placed in a manner similar to that for pneumothorax. Continuous drainage not only insures adequate drainage but also allows for accurate measure of the total volume and rate of blood loss. If the bleeding continues to be brisk, an open thoracotomy may be necessary.

Hemopneumothorax, being a combination of the foregoing, presents similar problems. The physical and radiological findings are a mixture of the two. Treatment with chest tube drainage is best. One tube may need to be placed anteriorly for the pneumothorax, and one tube posteriorly for the hemothorax. Open thoracotomy may be necessary to control major vascular bleeding. The judicious use of the tracheostomy, positive-pressure ventilation, and closed thoracotomy when indicated, however, will prove adequate in most instances.

Open Chest Wounds

Open chest injuries (open pneumothorax) from penetrating or perforating wounds are life-threatening. If the defect in the chest wall is greater than the diameter of the upper trachea, the disturbance in ventilatory function will be lethal in a short time without treatment. It is imperative that these open wounds be closed as soon as possible. They should be closed temporarily by an adequate dressing or permanently by an appropriate operative procedure. Immediate coverage can be obtained by using a sterile towel or a sterile gloved hand. A suitable dressing can be made of dry gauze wadding covered with petrolatum-impregnated gauze, which is air- and water-impermeable. The dressing should be of adequate size to extend at least 2 inches beyond the wound in all directions. It is placed in the defect and secured with adhesive tape. By this maneuver, the open chest injury is converted to a closed chest injury. Physiologically the patient will be left with at least a pneumothorax or hemothorax, which can be treated appropriately. Debridement and repair can be accomplished later.

Respiratory Arrest

Respiratory arrest occurring in the severely traumatized patient is a poor prognostic sign, usually indicating the presence of one or more fatal conditions.[49] A head injury may involve the respiratory centers in the medulla, and the patient can no longer respond to the physiological and biochemical stimuli needed to maintain respiration. The arrest may be the result of severe hypoxia from injuries that produce poor ventilation, or it may occur after severe profound shock when adequate cerebral perfusion is not maintained and irreversible damage has occurred to the brain stem.

Artificial ventilation must be begun immediately. Mouth-to-mouth respiration is the simplest and most basic form of artificial ventilation. The more common basic approach is bag and mask ventilation. Both methods are unsuitable for prolonged use, especially if the patient has maxillofacial injuries, and may be ineffectual from the beginning. In such cases, an oral airway or endotracheal tube, or even a tracheostomy, must be used and mechanical ventilation begun. Adequate mechanical ventilators should be available in every emergency room, operating suite, and intensive care unit.[19] These instruments are regulated by either pressure or volume. Both types are adequate for most circumstances.

Mechanical ventilatory assistance is performed in two different fashions. If, after resuscitative measures, the patient is able to initiate some ventilatory effort, then assisted positive-pressure breathing may be helpful. In this technique, the patient initiates the respiratory cycle himself, and the machine then takes over the cycle, producing deeper breathing with increased rate of exchange. Expiration is passive. This improves the patient's overall ventilatory effort while conserving his energy as well as insuring a continuous ventilatory effect. If, however, following resuscitative measures, the patient is unable to initiate respiration on his own, then controlled, or automatic, ventilation is necessary. In controlled ventilation, the machine initiates the cycle and controls the rate and depth of respiration. During this form of ventilation, hyperventilation invariably occurs as the patient's P_{CO_2} falls below levels required to drive the respiratory center.

Patients in whom automatic ventilation is being used require close observation.[50] Crude evaluation of respiration can be made by observing the expansion of the chest wall during ventilation and by auscultation of breath sounds. Respirator settings recommended initially are a tidal volume of 15 cc per kilogram of body weight, frequency of 10 to 12 per minute, and 50 to 60 per cent oxygen. If the patient has had cardiac or respiratory arrest, has aspirated, or has pulmonary edema, 100 per cent oxygen should be used initially.

The clinician must not depend solely upon excursion of the chest wall and breath sounds to determine adequacy of respiration. Measurements of the arterial pH, P_{CO_2}, and P_{O_2} are the best indices of adequacy of respiration. These measurements should be done after the patient has been on the respirator for 15 to 30 minutes. The P_{CO_2} is the indicator of adequate ventilation; carbon dioxide diffusion is so great that it is almost never affected by alveolar block. Values above or below 40 mm of mercury indicate relative acidosis or alkalosis (respectively) and signal the need for more or less ventilation. The pH and P_{CO_2} may be used in acid-base nomograms to determine buffer base excesses or deficits, as described later. The degree of oxygenation is obtained by measurement of arterial P_{O_2}. Normally, this has a value of 95 to 100 mm of mercury; however, values above 60 mm of mercury are usually satisfactory. Arterial blood gases and pH should be measured frequently to monitor the patient. Placement of an indwelling intra-arterial cannula should be considered. Control of the degree of oxygen saturation and carbon dioxide levels can be effectively done by varying the gas delivered to the respirator. Room air, 100 per cent oxygen, and mixtures of the two are the agents most frequently used.

Later Respiratory Complications

Aspiration Pneumonia

Patients with multiple injuries, including head injuries, are quite prone to aspiration pneumonia. Regurgitation and subsequent aspiration of gastric contents occur often during unconsciousness from head injuries. Some patients require prolonged nasogastric suction, which, alone, results in an incidence of aspiration as high as 54 per cent in patients undergoing operation and 25 per cent in those not having an operation.[2] The pH of gastric contents is usually 2 or lower. Entrance of this acid material into the trachea sets off an immediate spastic tracheobronchial reflex that impairs ventilation and has long-range effects also. The overall mortality rate following aspiration, even with treatment, is 62 per cent, and 79 per cent of the deaths result directly from sequelae of aspiration.[18]

The best treatment for aspiration is prevention. Constant nursing attention is essential. The patient's position in bed is crucial, especially in comatose patients. If nasogastric tubes are required, they must be functioning at all times. Tube feedings should be given with the patient elevated in bed and at a rate not exceeding gastric emptying. If a general anesthetic is required, the patient's stomach must be emptied prior to induction.

Should aspiration be suspected, certain consideration should be given to fiberoptic bronchoscopy to confirm the diagnosis.[75] When the diagnosis is confirmed, or when obvious gross aspiration is noted, treatment should begin promptly. The trachea should be vigorously suctioned. If particulate matter has been aspirated, bronchoscopy may be necessary. Tracheal lavage with saline, sodium bicarbonate, or steroids has been of little or no benefit clinically or experimentally and may, in fact, produce additional areas of involvement.[2]

After the airway has been cleaned, attention must be directed to maintaining adequate oxygenation (an arterial Po_2 above 60 mm of mercury). It may be possible to achieve this level by using only nasal or mask oxygen; however, it frequently is necessary to use prolonged assisted ventilation and even tracheostomy. If bronchospasm is noted, administration of aminophylline intravenously and of bronchodilators by nebulizer may be required. While hypotension, if present, is usually secondary to hypovolemia or hypoxia, it may indicate the need for digitalization.

Corticosteroids may help by diminishing the inflammatory response and preventing aggregation of platelets and leukocytes from obstructing the pulmonary microcirculation. A dosage equivalent to 1600 mg of methylprednisolone daily in divided doses is recommended. To have any chance of being effective it must be started as early as possible after diagnosis and continued for 48 hours.

While it is doubtful that bacteria play any significant role early in the pathogenesis of the process, antibiotics are recommended to prevent secondary infections. Studies have demonstrated that the predominant organisms in aspiration pneumonia reflect the oropharyngeal flora.[7] Anaerobes were present in 93 per cent of the patients and were the only organisms in 46 per cent. If prophylactic antibiotics are to be used, broad coverage such as would be provided by cephalothin and gentamicin or penicillin G and gentamicin is usually advocated. Some authorities, however, recommend only pencillin, 1,200,000 units every six hours.[2] If prophylactic antibiotics are not given, smears and cultures should be performed on transtracheal aspirates or empyema fluid and blood of patients who aspirate and subsequently show radiographic evidence of pneumonitis. Antiobiotics appropriate to the organisms recovered should be instituted promptly.

Pulmonary Embolism and Thrombophlebitis

Comprehensive reviews of the incidence, diagnosis, prevention, and management of venous thrombosis and pulmonary thromboembolism are listed in the references.[21,43,62] Thrombophlebitis and pulmonary embolism are rarely seen soon after trauma, but are not uncommon during the prolonged care of patients with multiple injuries. The patient immoblized during an extended period of unconsciousness or by casts or traction is at an even greater risk than usual. Advancing age further increases the incidence. Venous thrombosis is present in 26 to 36 per cent of patients examined at autopsy. On the other hand, the frequency with which pulmonary emboli are noted at autopsy is only 10 to 15 percent. As a corollary, in as many as 20 per cent of patients with pulmonary emboli at autopsy, no source is found. Most pulmonary emboli arise from the deep veins of the lower extremities and the pelvic veins, occur from the fourth to the fourteenth postoperative or postinjury day, and have a peak incidence between the fifth and ninth days.

The accuracy of the diagnosis of venous thrombosis has improved considerably in recent years. If the classic symptoms and signs of calf pain, tenderness, edema, and a positive Homan's sign alone are relied on, from 70 to 80 per cent of cases of venous thrombosis will be missed, although the presence of most or all of these findings together readily makes the diagnosis of thrombophlebitis. Less than 50 per cent of patients who die with pulmonary embolism will have premortem symptoms or signs of thrombophlebitis.

Ascending plebography remains the most reliable diagnostic procedure but has the disadvantage of being invasive. Newer methods of diagnosis are available but still not fully evaluated. Scanning with [125]iodine-labeled fibrinogen, which is incorporated into the thrombus, will demonstrate newly forming thrombi. It is simple and can even be done on the ward. While highly accurate below the iliofemoral region, however, it loses accuracy at this level. It also carries a small risk of hepatitis and gives false positive readings from hematomas in operative sites. Ultrasonic scanning based on the Doppler principle is 90 to 95 per cent accurate in detecting complete occlusion of the deep venous systems but gives false negative results in 50 per cent of partial occlusions. Impedance phlebography, which is based on changes in resistance of an electrial signal passed through the extremity with changes in blood flow, is only 50 per cent accurate.

Treatment of venous thrombosis should be directed most strongly at prevention.

Simple measures can reduce its incidence. Early and frequent ambulation is ideal, but short of this, elevation of the foot of the bed, the use of properly fitting elastic stockings, and active and passive motion of the lower extremities in the immobilized patient all decrease the duration and amount of venous stasis. A newer method of mechanical prophylaxis is a device that intermittently inflates and deflates two plastic boots with air.[20] The device has been shown to reduce the incidence of thrombi detectable by [125]iodine-fibrinogen scanning by 80 to 90 per cent. Most of the aforementioned modes of therapy would be applicable to trauma patients.

Many pharmacological means of prophylaxis have been tried. Use of platelet suppressive drugs such as aspirin and dipyrimadole have not proved effective in reducing the incidence of deep venous thrombosis. Furthermore, the efficacy of low-molecular-weight dextran remains unresolved. Studies have shown, however, that heparin administered in low dosage significantly reduces the rate of venous thrombosis in patients undergoing operation and in high-risk patients with medical problems. The usual regimen for a medical patient at high risk is 5000 units of aqueous heparin subcutaneously within 18 hours of admission and three times a day until he is mobilized. Patients having an elective operation are given 5000 units of heparin subcutaneously 2 hours preoperatively and then every 8 hours postoperatively (beginning 9 to 10 hours postoperatively) until resumption of full activity. The heparin treatment is supplemented with elastic stockings and active and passive movement of the lower extremities. The use of heparin in patients with multiple trauma must be tempered with concern for bleeding from injured sites, especially in the immediate post-trauma period.

Once venous thrombosis has occurred, other methods of treatment must be considered. Acute superficial thrombophlebitis usually responds to simple measures of limitation of activity, elevation of the affected limb, application of heat to the involved area, and anti-inflammatory agents to reduce the pain. Only in cases that are extensive or progressive are anticoagulants needed. Septic superficial thrombophlebitis may also require antibiotics and occasionally drainage.

Acute deep venous thrombophlebitis is much more serious because it places the patient at risk for pulmonary embolism and for the postphlebitic syndrome. These patients should be placed at bed rest with the involved limb elevated above the level of the heart and given anti-inflammatory agents, analgesics as needed for pain, and anticoagulants or fibrinolytic agents or both.

Heparin remains the drug of choice in acute deep venous thrombosis. If contraindications to heparin therapy such as active bleeding, heparin sensitivity, or severe hypertension do not exist, the patient should be given 500 units per kilogram of body weight intravenously as a bolus and another 500 units per kilogram by continuous infusion over the next 24 hours. After the first 24 hours the heparin infusion is adjusted to keep the whole blood clotting time at 30 minutes or the partial thromboplastin time at 100 seconds. Continuous infusion of heparin has the advantage over subcutaneous or intermittent intravenous modes. It maintains a constant heparin level and obviates the necessity of drawing blood samples for clotting analysis at prescribed times. Also, it reduces slightly the incidence of the bleeding problems seen with the latter two routes of administration. The heparin is continued for 14 days. Next, less intense anticoagulation is continued for three to six months. The less intense treatment can entail either patient-administered subcutaneous heparin at a dosage of 5000 units every 12 hours for two months, or sodium warfarin in a dosage to prolong the prothrombin time to twice the control value. The sodium warfarin is continued for three to six months.

In the absence of any risk of bleeding, fibrinolytic agents such as urokinase or streptokinase can be used and are effective in restoring venous patency. Both agents, but especially streptokinase, are associated with frequent allergic responses. When urokinase is available in a more purified form, it will become more widely used in the management of acute venous thromboses.

Operative thrombectomy rarely restores complete venous patency and rarely preserves venous valves. Few, if any, cases of iliofemoral thrombosis will not respond to vigorous heparin therapy and steep elevation of the lower extremities.

If the foregoing recommendations are not

contraindicated and are followed closely, the incidence of venous thrombosis and pulmonary embolism should be very low. When pulmonary embolism is suspected, in either acute or recurrent form, it demands prompt diagnosis and treatment.

Accurate clinical diagnosis of acute pulmonary embolism is difficult. Studies have shown that tests for pulmonary embolism identified it positively in only 41 per cent of cases and equivocally in another 15 per cent. Detailed statistics on occurrence of individual symptoms, signs, and laboratory abnormalities in acute pulmonary embolism are available in the references.[21,43,62]

Pulmonary embolism may present in at least four different ways with pulmonary infarction, acute cor pulmonale, acute unexplained dyspnea, or increasing left ventricular failure. The two most important clues from the history are the fact that patients with pulmonary embolism usually have an obvious predisposition to venous thrombosis, and that the most important symptoms are dyspnea and pleuritic pain. The most nearly universal finding (about 94 per cent of cases) in acute pulmonary embolism is tachypnea with a respiratory rate greater than 20. The most valuable laboratory findings are: (1) arterial blood gas values that show a decreased Po_2 (88 per cent of patients have a Po_2 less than 80 mm of mercury), a decreased Pco_2, and respiratory alkalosis; (2) the chest x-ray that shows an infiltrate, an elevated diaphragm, or a pleural effusion (in the majority of patients); and (3) the lung scan that shows segmental perfusion defects in normally ventilated areas. While lactic dehydrogenase (LDH) levels are elevated in nearly all cases, this is of little help in differential diagnosis. The classic triad of increased lactic dehydrogenase and bilirubin with normal serum glutamic oxalacetic transaminase (SGOT) occurs in only about 10 per cent of patients with acute pulmonary embolism.

Clearly, the lung scan is the most useful screening test for acute pulmonary embolism. A technically adequate, entirely normal lung scan excludes the possibility of symptomatic acute pulmonary embolism. If the scan shows segmental perfusion defects in normally ventilated areas, pulmonary embolism is extremely likely. In cases with equivocal scans, a pulmonary angiogram is necessary for a definitive diagnosis. There-

fore, pulmonary angiography remains the most definitive laboratory test.

Hypotension in acute pulmonary embolism is unusual. If present, it frequently is transient. When persistent hypotension occurs in the setting of pulmonary embolism, it signals massive embolism and may be followed quite rapidly by cardiac arrest. Massive embolism results in acute cor pulmonale with right-sided heart failure; therefore, a normal venous pressure in the presence of shock virtually excludes pulmonary embolism from the differential diagnosis. Thus, acute massive pulmonary embolism is a clinical syndrome characterized by severe respiratory distress with sustained hypotension or shock. In general, pulmonary arteriography shows these patients to have complete or partial obstruction of at least 50 per cent of the central pulmonary arterial bed. Many of them die within a few minutes, and an additional 22 per cent die within two hours. Therefore, these cases demand immediate medical and thoracic surgical consultation. Initial treatment must be directed at maintaining adequate oxygenation by means of intubation and mechanical ventilation when required. Circulatory support is obtained with vasopressors (metaraminol, replaced when possible with isoproterenol), sodium bicarbonate, steroids, and digoxin. Anticoagulation with heparin, 10,000 units in a bolus intravenously followed by 5000 units at four-hour intervals or by continuous drip, is given according to the schedule noted earlier. Careful monitoring of central venous pressure, urine output, and arterial pressure and blood gases (preferably by indwelling arterial catheter) is crucial. As soon as these measures are under control pulmonary angiography should be performed. In general, if the angiogram shows less than 60 per cent obstruction of the central pulmonary arteries and the patient's condition is reasonably stable, continued respiratory and circulatory support are warranted. With greater degrees of obstruction or lack of evidence of improvement of cardiac output with medical management, prompt embolectomy is indicated. Early results with urokinase as an adjunct to the medical management of massive embolism are promising, but cost and availability currently limit its practical use.

Lesser degrees of pulmonary embolism are treated with a regimen of heparin as described earlier for the treatment of deep venous thrombosis. To this is added oxygen administered in a fashion to keep arterial Po₂ above 80 mm of mercury. In the face of recurring pulmonary embolism, several procedures are available for vena cavae interruption. All are associated with a definite operative mortality rate, especially in patients with compromised cardiopulmonary reserve as a result of severe pulmonary embolism. In general, these procedures have proved no better than adequate anticoagulant or fibrinolytic therapy (or both) in reducing the incidence of recurrence.

Pulmonary Infection

Pulmonary infections are major complications in the patient with multiple injuries. The problem of aspiration pneumonitis has already been discussed. This form of pneumonitis may occur at any time during the patient's course, but other forms develop because the patient usually is severely ill. The head injuries or chest injuries often make managing pulmonary secretions and providing adequate self-ventilation difficult. The patient with a tracheostomy is very susceptible to secondary infections; organisms may be implanted during any of the processes required for its management. They may be instilled from the mechanical ventilator. Loculated pleural fluid, whether effusion, transudate, or hematoma, can become secondarily infected via closed thoracotomy tubes or by blood-borne organisms.

These "secondary" pneumonias, like the aspiration variety, may produce marked necrosis of lung tissue and abscess formation. The specific treatment will depend upon the organism involved.[35] The most common organisms involved are *Staphylococcus aureus*, especially the hospital strains, and specific gram-negative organisms of the *Pseudomonas* and *Proteus* type. Extensive cultures are necessary for adequate therapy. These will include cultures of blood and sputum and of material obtained through nasotracheal suction, percutaneous tracheal aspiration, or aspiration of pleural fluid. Once an organism is obtained, sensitivity studies should be made and the appropriate antibiotics given. Occasionally, bronchoscopy with suction to remove mucus plugs is necessary. Pleural empyemas will have to be drained, often with closed chest drainage but occasionally by open thoracotomy and decortication.

It is important in the management of all patients with multiple injuries that diligent care be given to the pulmonary system. Constant turning of the patient combined with suction and pulmonary drainage is necessary. Good pulmonary toilet should be a never-ending part of the treatment. Adequate pulmonary care includes maintaining a warm moist atmosphere in which to breathe, proper pulmonary suction and drainage, and intermittent positive-pressure ventilation to inflate poorly used sections of the lungs to prevent atelectasis.

Atelectasis

Obstructive atelectasis with collapse of the pulmonary alveolus due to bronchial obstruction is the most frequent pulmonary complication. It occurs frequently when ventilatory effort is poor. It is the forerunner of many of the secondary pneumonias. Clinically, it may be suspected when there is fever, tachycardia, rarely dyspnea; physical findings include rhonchi, rales, and decreased breath sounds. Chest x-ray is helpful. Treatment should be directed at the cause and includes suction, bronchoscopy, postural drainage, and intermittent positive-pressure breathing.

Adult Respiratory Distress Syndrome (Shock Lung)

Numerous terms have come to be associated with the adult respiratory distress syndrome (ARDS) or acute pulmonary insufficiency that may develop in critically ill or injured patients.[74] "Shock lung," "traumatic wet lung," "post-traumatic pulmonary insufficiency," and "septic lung" refer to respiratory distress associated with well-defined clinical situations.[4,5,55] "Congestive atelectasis" and hemorrhagic atelectasis" are based on pathological changes that are noted.[9]

In simplest terms the pathophysiology of shock lung consists of an increase in lung water and a decrease in functional residual capacity with a variable degree of disturbance of gas exchange and pulmonary hemodynamics. The process is based on the forces described by Starling, which regulate movement of fluid in and out of the interstitial fluid spaces at the capillary level. These forces normally result in a total net pressure of 0.5 to 1.0 mm of mercury pushing the fluid into pulmonary interstitial spaces and will gradually produce fluid accumulation in the lungs if the fluid is not rapidly removed by the pulmonary lymphatics.

It should be apparent, therefore, that movement of fluid from the capillaries into the interstitial spaces will be favored by factors increasing capillary permeability. These factors include any process that (1) increases capillary permeability, such as sepsis, (2) increases capillary hydrostatic pressure, such as congestive heart failure, or (3) decreases plasma osmotic pressure, such as cirrhosis or administration of excessive crystalloids.

A study of the pathological changes reveals four basic phases. First, swelling of capillary endothelial cells is noted and is associated with their retraction from adjoining cells, leaving enlarged intracellular spaces. Next, fluid moves through the resulting defects from the capillary space into the expanded interstitial compartment, giving edema. This interstitial edema reduces oxygen diffusion and decreases pulmonary compliance, making the lung stiffer and more difficult to ventilate. The third phase involves increasing congestive atelectasis. Usually it is at this stage that the respiratory problem first manifests itself clinically. Pulmonary capillaries dilate and fill with red blood cells, and severe diffuse microatelectasis progresses. The red blood cells leak into interstitial spaces, causing peribronchial hemorrhage. Finally, progressive damage to alveolar cells and destruction of alveolar lining are noted, and fluid moves from the interstitial spaces into the alveoli. Proteins in this fluid tend to inactivate surfactant, further increasing the atelectasis, and may, if the patient survives, form a hyaline-like membrane. In this milieu secondary bacterial pneumonitis frequently appears.

On the basis of the foregoing discussion it would be expected that certain clinical problems would frequently be associated with adult respiratory distress syndrome. These include sepsis, shock, trauma, fluid overload, massive transfusion, aspiration, pulmonary infections, fat embolism, and oxygen intoxication. Several of these conditions are particularly germane to the immediate post-traumatic period.

Severe or persistent shock results in pulmonary ischemia. The decreased perfusion present with shock, either alone or coupled with varying degrees of hypoxia, commonly occurs early in the course of patients with severe injury. The decreased perfusion appears to lead to shock lung by a mechanism that is of particular interest to neuroscientists. Animal studies have demonstrated that a centroneurogenic factor is of importance and may suffice alone to explain the pathogenesis and pathological changes.[45] It is known that cerebral hypoxemia produced experimentally can result in shock lung, even though systemic blood pressure and oxygen tension are maintained at normal levels. This work has provided evidence that the reduction in cerebral blood flow and oxygenation deranges central autonomic function, which in turn causes increased tone in the pulmonary venule, resulting in a tourniquet action that produces vascular congestion, hemorrhage, edema, and atelectasis. The lung changes could be prevented by autonomic denervation of the lung. Administration of phenytoin and, especially, methylprednisolone was protective in the animals.

The other etiological factors of particular importance in the patient with severe trauma are fluid overloading, particularly with crystalloids; massive transfusion, especially with older blood; and aspiration of gastric contents. Later in the course of severely injured patients sepsis and fat embolism may become more important.

Early clinical diagnosis is very important and relies heavily on anticipation of this problem coupled with institution of vigorous prophylactic measures. In the early phase tachypnea may be the only sign noted. If one waits for classic signs of respiratory failure such as use of accessory muscles of respiration, flaring of alae nasi, and restlessness to appear, the process will be far advanced and very difficult to reverse. Again, obvious x-ray abnormalities with confluent infiltrates and consolidation are seen only late in the course. Early x-ray findings are nonspecific and consist only of a patchy bilateral alveolar infiltration often interpreted as mild pulmonary edema.

Frequent blood gas analysis is mandatory if early diagnosis is desired. While critically injured patients frequently seem to develop adult respiratory distress syndrome rather suddenly, retrospective analysis of blood gases usually reveals that the process has been developing and progressing for 24 to

48 hours. Arterial P_{CO_2} is usually 25 to 35 mm of mercury, which reflects the hyperventilation characteristic of the syndrome. Arterial P_{O_2} should be carefully monitored—it is especially helpful to evaluate it when the patient is breathing room air followed by 100 per cent oxygen. Normally, an arterial P_{O_2} of 90 to 100 mm of mercury on room air will rise to 300 to 400 mm of mercury on 100 per cent oxygen. In shock lung, however, the greatly increased pulmonary admixture (shunting) may result in an arterial P_{O_2} of 50 mm of mercury on room air that increases to only 80 to 100 mm of mercury with 100 per cent oxygen. A more sensitive measure is the alveolar-arterial oxygen difference (AaD_{O_2}). At sea level the alveolar P_{O_2} in a patient breathing 100 per cent oxygen is about 670 mm of mercury and normally results in an arterial P_{O_2} of 300 mm of mercury, giving a difference (AaD_{O_2}) of 370 mm of mercury. With this test, a difference of more than 400 mm of mercury on 100 per cent oxygen, especially if it is increasing, is indicative of severe intrapulmonary shunting and a need for ventilatory assistance.

When the diagnosis is suspected or confirmed, appropriate therapy is urgently required. Simple measures that may prevent occurrence or progression of the problem in some cases include good nursing care with encouragement of frequent coughing, deep breathing, and position changes. If not contraindicated, some elevation of the head of the bed improves the ventilation-perfusion ratio throughout the lung. Chest physical therapy should be instituted early. Other general measures include prevention and control of infection and a search for occult infection should pulmonary insufficiency develop with no obvious cause. Reduction of abdominal distention, if present; reduction of oxygen demands by control of fever; and thoracentesis for excessive pleural fluid also are important. Gradual dehydration will aid in reducing pulmonary interstitial fluid. While dehydration is being accomplished, there should be careful monitoring of pulse, blood pressure, urine output, and serum osmolality. Serum osmolality should be kept at about 280. Use of colloids is controversial and probably best reserved for patients with plasma albumin levels below 2.5 to 3.0 gm per 100 ml. While hemoglobin levels around 10 gm per 100 ml often provide the best overall cardiac output and oxygen transport, levels of 12.5 to 14.0 gm per 100 ml have, in some studies, been found to provide a lower mortality rate and less shunting in the lung. Bronchodilators often are helpful when bronchospasm is present. Digitalis and diuretics should be instituted at the first sign of heart failure. Diuretics may also be beneficial in reducing interstitial edema, even in the absence of heart failure. Sodium bicarbonate is used as needed to correct acidosis. While its efficacy is not proved, methylprednisolone in a dose of 15 mg per kilogram probably is helpful if started early.

In the early phase, and in milder cases, intermittent positive pressure breathing with aerosols and nebulizer is indicated. Use of continuous ventilatory assistance early in the process probably offers the best hope. It has been suggested that the presence of shock coupled with injury to three or more long bones, more than seven rib fractures, head injury, massive pulmonary disease, or age of 65 or over requires immediate institution of ventilatory assistance. Laboratory indications for the more vigorous approach include: (1) an arterial P_{O_2} less than 55 to 60 mm of mercury on room air, especially if adequate improvement of gases is not seen on 40 per cent oxygen, (2) an arterial P_{CO_2} greater than 45 to 55 mm of mercury in a patient with previously normal lung function and no metabolic alkalosis, and (3) an alveolar-arterial oxygen difference on room air of more than 55 mm of mercury (calculated as $145 - [P_{O_2} + P_{CO_2}]$). Of even more importance than a single finding of one or all of these is evidence of deterioration of these parameters on serial observations.

If conservative management as outlined proves inadequate and the laboratory indications of severe respiratory insufficiency are found, continuous ventilatory assistance must be instituted promptly. Ventilatory assistance requires a cuffed endotracheal tube or tracheostomy. Use of a volume-cycled respirator is recommended, since the decreased pulmonary compliance (stiff lungs) renders the pressure-cycled machines inadequate. Assisted respiration should be started with an initial tidal volume of 10 to 12 ml per kilogram of body weight, a rate of 10 to 12 per minute, and 40 per cent inspired oxygen. If arterial P_{CO_2} remains high, tidal volume may be increased to 15 ml per kilogram, and the rate may be increased also. If possible, the peak inflation pressure should be less than 40 cm of water. If the larger tidal volume should result in hypotension by reducing venous return, tidal volume must be reduced or more fluid given, or both, to restore adequate tissue perfusion. If the arterial Po_2 remains at unacceptable levels (less than 55 to 60 mm of mercury), inspired oxygen concentration may be increased to a maximum of 60 per cent. In order to avoid oxygen intoxication, a higher concentration should not be given. If larger tidal volumes and higher respiratory rate create severe respiratory alkalosis, dead space can be added to the system to maintain arterial Pco_2 in the range of 30 to 40 mm of mercury. The respirator should be set to sigh 6 to 12 times per hour at a sigh volume of about one and a half times the tidal volume.

If prompt improvement in the blood gases is not achieved by these measures the use of positive end-expiratory pressure (PEEP) should be instituted. Positive end-expiratory pressure helps to prevent collapse of the alveoli during the expiratory phase, increases the functional residual capacity of the lung, and reduces the amount of pulmonary shunting. A pressure of 8 to 10 cm of water is recommended.

While positive end-expiratory pressure is frequently quite helpful in combating severe shock lung, it is not without hazards. At higher levels (10 cm of water and above) significant reduction in venous return can compromise cardiac output and tissue perfusion. Ideal monitoring in such cases, therefore, includes use of a balloon-type Swan-Ganz catheter to measure pulmonary capillary wedge pressure. This information will help to strike the delicate balance required to re-expand collapsed alveoli without compromising the pulmonary circulation and causing heart failure. An additional aid in evaluating adverse effects of positive end-expiratory pressure on tissue perfusion, especially in patients with marginal renal function, is the one-hour creatinine clearance. Should the creatinine clearance indicate a reduction in glomerular filtration rate below 50 ml per minute, positive end-expiratory pressure may have to be discontinued. Other notable, but generally less serious, complications include pneumothorax that can become tension pneumothorax in 5 to 20 per cent of all patients, pneumomediastinum, and subcutaneous emphysema

in 20 to 40 per cent of patients. Should pneumothorax develop, proper drainage will usually allow continuation of positive end-expiratory pressure.

Of particular importance to neurosurgeons is the development of a significant increase in intracranial pressure in some patients in whom positive end-expiratory pressure is used.[5] The patients who would sustain such rises could be accurately predicted by assessment of the intracranial volume-pressure response. If on introduction of 1 ml of Ringer's lactate solution into the ventricles, an immediate rise in intracranial pressure of 2 mm of mercury per milliliter was observed, the patient was considered to have a significant increase in cerebral elastance. When this criterion was applied, all patients manifesting an elevation of intracranial pressure with positive end-expiratory pressure (either a doubling of baseline pressure or an increase of baseline pressure from normal to levels higher than 13 mm of mercury) were those also found to have increased cerebral elastance. Half the patients sustained impairment of cerebral perfusion pressures to levels of less than 60 mm of mercury, in addition to elevation of intracranial pressure. Intracranial pressure returned to baseline levels with discontinuation of positive end-expiratory pressure.

CARDIOVASCULAR INJURIES

Peripheral Vascular Injuries

A major cause of shock in the patient with multiple injuries is hemorrhage from peripheral vascular injuries. In most instances, the source will be quite obvious, with blood flowing from a distinct puncture or laceration in the vicinity of a major extremity blood vessel. Immediate control of the hemorrhage by compression or clamping of the involved vessel should be done as emergency treatment. A tourniquet about the limb is dangerous and should be used only with great caution. When the tourniquet is applied tightly enough to occlude arterial blood flow, ischemic damage is very common because there is a tendency to leave the tourniquet in place for too long a time.

A peripheral vessel, particularly a major vessel, should not be ligated.[61] In most instances reconstruction can be accomplished by a competent vascular surgeon. Ligation may compromise the chance for repair of the vessel and endanger the survival of the limb.

Low-velocity penetrating wounds from small-caliber hand guns, fragments, or knives may be deflected during their course through the body, and an examination of the entrance and exit wounds may not give the actual course of the missile. Until proved otherwise, all injuries that are in the approximate area of a major blood vessel should be considered to involve the vessel. The presence of a pulse distal to the suspected site of injury does not exclude significant vascular injury. Even an arteriogram may be misleading. When in doubt, the vessel should be operatively exposed and inspected. A penetrating injury to the neck that violates the platysma should be explored. If possible, the exploration should be undertaken before tracheostomy is performed.

Significant arterial injury may occur with blunt trauma to areas near the vessel. Blunt injury to the neck may produce severe extracranial carotid artery spasm or intimal disruption.[13] Decreased intracranial blood flow may result in neurological signs or symptoms. The diagnosis will be confirmed by cerebral arteriography. Similarly, blunt trauma to extremities may result in arterial injury. Crushing of the extremity may cause vascular spasm severe enough to produce ischemia or thrombosis. Although operative procedures have not been successful in releasing spasm, some improvement may be brought about by dilating the artery and stripping it of all its nerve supply. If thrombosis has occurred, thrombectomy can be done. In any case, exploration of the artery is indicated.

The incidence of post-traumatic arteriovenous fistulae and aneurysms is inversely related to the successful detection and repair of injuries to the major peripheral vessels.[31]

Cardiac Injury

Major cardiac injuries, while extremely serious, are by no means universally fatal.[52] While extensive lacerations or gunshot wounds can result in rapid exsanguination and death, many small-caliber missile injuries or stab wounds can be successfully treated.

Shortly after injury the patient shows signs of cardiac tamponade and elevation of central venous pressure. The neck veins are full even in the upright position. There is a plethoric appearance over the upper portion of the chest, shoulders, neck, and face. As the pericardial sac confines the accumulation of blood within it, the venae cavae and the right side of the heart are compressed. As the tamponade becomes more complete, the cardiac output decreases progressively. There is a fall in systolic and diastolic blood pressures, the systolic more than the diastolic, producing a narrowing of the pulse pressure. The pulse rate rises and may become paradoxical. Percussion will demonstrate a widened mediastinum. Heart sounds are distant and muffled. X-rays of the chest show widening of the heart shadow. A very low pulse rate indicates that the patient is either moribund or that the penetrating injury has damaged the bundle of His, causing atrioventricular dissociation. When this happens, pulse rates below 40 may be present. An electrocardiogram will aid in the diagnosis.

Pericardial tamponade can be diagnosed by needle aspiration. In fact, this may be adequate emergency treatment. A large-bore needle, No. 16 or No. 18, is inserted just to the left of the xiphoid. It is directed at an angle 45 degrees cephalad and 45 degrees to the right. A significant "give" is noted when the pericardial sac is punctured. As much blood as possible should be removed, but the needle should not be moved about while in the pericardial sac. Pericardiocentesis can be repeated as often as required. If the patient requires three such taps, however, then open thoracotomy will probably be necessary.

The most common instrument causing blunt injury to the heart is the steering wheel in an automobile accident. Any object striking the anterior chest may produce this sort of injury. Although there is a paucity of clinical signs or symptoms that help in making this diagnosis, it should be suspected from the nature of the injury and the clinical course of the patient. The electrocardiogram may show ST segment and T wave changes, which become diagnostic only if they return to normal. A rapid pulse out of keeping with the general condition of the patient should also alert one to this possibility. Treatment is essentially the same as for myocardial ischemia or infarction. Adequate oxygen and bed rest should be given. Other trauma should be avoided, i.e., if possible, operation should be postponed. The prognosis usually is good.

Cardiac Arrest

One of the most dramatic complications of trauma or operation is cardiac arrest. In most cases, this complication is preventable and treatable. Despite the fact that the average physician will encounter this entity only a few times in his practicing life, he should be well versed in its management. More importantly, he should be aware of the underlying causes so that he may avoid them when possible.

After trauma or operation, the most common cause of cardiac arrest is hypoxia with carbon dioxide retention secondary to inadequate ventilation of the patient.[65] Decreased coronary perfusion from hypovolemia and hypotension are significant causes of this problem. This mechanism is the responsible one in most injured patients. An overdose or drug sensitivity may incite cardiac arrest. An uncommon cause of cardiac arrest occurs when large volumes of blood are given to a patient with severe trauma. Refrigerated stored bank blood tends to become acidotic and hyperkalemic. If this blood is given rapidly, as it may need to be in the severely traumatized patient, hyperkalemia with cardiac arrhythmias and arrest can result. Large volumes of cold blood can cause cardiac hypothermia and, in turn, cardiac arrest.

The diagnosis of cardiac arrest can be difficult, and valuable time may be lost trying to confirm it. Although loss of blood pressure and loss of pulse may not mean necessarily that cardiac arrest has taken place, these are its major clinical signs. Cardiac arrhythmias occurring prior to loss of blood pressure and pulse make it almost a certainty. In any case, it is best to begin treatment immediately and then confirm the diagnosis later.

The treatment of cardiac arrest revolves around three dicta: (1) Speed is of essence; (2) the pumping action of the heart should be maintained; and (3) Adequate ventilation of the lungs must be assured.

When the heart stops, about three minutes remain in which to reinstate blood flow to the various organs of the body if irreversible damage is to be prevented. The patient is placed flat in the supine position on a firm surface. Mouth-to-mouth respiration should begin immediately. An endotracheal tube should be inserted if resuscitation is not promptly obtained. As soon as possible, 100 per cent oxygen should be administered through the endotracheal tube.

External cardiac massage should be begun simultaneously. The heel of the palm of the physician's hand is placed over the lower sternal area. The palm of the opposite hand is superimposed. The arms are kept straight. A downward thrusting action of the arms is begun at the rate of 60 to 80 times per minute. The sternal area should be depressed approximately 2 inches with each stroke. This force is required to maintain good peripheral pulse and blood pressure. Failure to maintain a peripheral pulse indicates either that the operator is performing the act improperly or that some restricting element, such as cardiac tamponade, exists. Complications of closed cardiac massage include fracture of the ribs and sternum, and lacerations of the liver or spleen. The physician need not concern himself about them. He should treat the arrest, then worry about the complications.

If closed massage does not produce adequate peripheral pulses within two to three minutes, and if normal cardiac action does not begin with external defibrillation, the chest should be opened.[70] Time does not permit preparation of the chest or of the surgeon's hands. An incision is made from the left of the sternum laterally to the midaxillary line in the fourth intercostal space. As the heart is not beating, there is no worry about blood loss during this opening; it must be done swiftly in a matter of seconds. A rib spreader is inserted or, if it is not available, the ribs are fractured at the cartilaginous insertions near the sternum to give adequate room for the operator's hands to perform the massage.

The surgeon's hand is inserted into the chest cavity and, with the thumb anterior and the fingers posterior, grasps the heart. This grip allows the best position for effective massage. The pericardium need not be opened unless cardiac tamponade is present. The operator should squeeze the heart approximately 80 to 90 times per minute. Occasionally, because of the size of the patient, it may be necessary to use both hands in the chest to gain adequate control of the heart. In this situation, one hand is anterior and the other one is posterior to the heart.

When cardiac arrest is due to hypovolemia, the heart may be flaccid and poorly filled. The surgeon can fill the left ventricle with blood or isotonic fluid by direct cardiac puncture. This maneuver allows an adequate initial stroke volume. As the resuscitative measures are begun, intravenous administration of fluid and drugs must be started. A large-gauge needle should be put in a saphenous or antecubital vein, either percutaneously or by venesection. If the pericardium has been opened, the myocardium should be irrigated with 5 to 10 ml of 1 per cent lidocaine. The lidocaine may prevent undue sudden irritability and fibrillation as spontaneous heart action begins.

Approximately 10 per cent of "cardiac arrest" cases will actually be in ventricular fibrillation when the heart is observed. Cardiac massage is required to maintain coronary artery flow and adequate perfusion of the myocardium. Once the pink color has returned to the heart, defibrillation may occur spontaneously. If it does not occur in a few seconds, artificial defibrillation should be used. Usually the defibrillation is accomplished by administering an electric shock to the myocardium. One electrode is placed anterior and one posterior to the heart. The electrodes of most commercial defibrilating devices are shaped like paddles. A shock as brief as one sixtieth of a second may be all that is necessary to return normal cardiac action; the duration, however, should not exceed a tenth of a second. A 110- to 120-v 60-cycle alternating current that renders at least 1 amp of current is required. The shock may be repeated several times if normal cardiac rhythm is not restored.

Occasionally, when a cardiac monitor is being used, ventricular fibrillation may be diagnosed without thoracotomy. In these cases, external defibrillating devices may be used. One electrode is placed in the upper sternal region and the other beneath the left breast. The voltage required for external defibrillation is quite high, and the operator should wear gloves and should be grounded. For these larger doses, direct current is safer for the operator than alternating current. It will require around 480 v for an adult and 240 v or less for a child for effective defibrillation. This current should be given in less than 2.5 msec.

Several drugs can be used advantageously in the management of cardiac arrest. Following cardiac arrest, acidosis begins in the nonperfused body tissues. Forty milliequivalents of sodium bicarbonate should be given intravenously every few minutes to correct the acidosis. The use of lidocaine topically on the exposed myocardium has been suggested. In addition, quinidine or lidocaine should be used intravenously to reduce myocardial irritability as spontaneous heart action begins. Epinephrine, 1:10,000 solution, administered into the heart 1 ml at a time, may restore tone to the flaccid heart. Calcium chloride, 5 to 10 ml of 10 per cent solution, is a better agent, as it is less likely to render the myocardium hyperirritable. Once spontaneous cardiac action has begun, a continuous infusion of dopamine (5 to 10 μg per kilogram per minute), is helpful in improving the strength of the cardiac contraction without increasing myocardial irritability.[54]

Since hypothermia causes arrhythmias and fibrillations when the temperature of the myocardium is reduced below 28° C, its use in management of cardiac arrest is still controversial. It does, however, reduce the metabolic activity of the poorly perfused tissues. Hypothermia to levels of 30° C has been used in selected cases of prolonged arrest. It is accomplished either by using commercially available perfusion blankets or by packing the patient in ice. Chlorpromazine, in doses of 25 to 50 mg intramuscularly every four to six hours, is given to combat shivering. Shivering should be avoided, as it increases the metabolic activity of the body.

The physician should remember that most cases of cardiac arrest that occur after trauma or during operation are preventable. In managing these patients, steps to prevent cardiac arrest should be routine.

To prevent cardiac arrest the conditions likely to produce it should be understood and should be systematically investigated. The patient should be examined immediately for his ventilatory ability. If necessary, ventilatory assistance should be instituted. History may not be available concerning the patient's drug sensitivities. An unconscious patient or one in shock, however, will not require the same dose of a given drug as a healthy patient. Indeed, these patients rarely need any drugs, particularly opiates, sedatives, or tranquilizers, which are the ones most likely to produce cardiac arrest. The patient who has been drinking alcohol prior to his injury is extremely susceptible to the barbiturates and general anesthetics in normal dosage. The use of heavy sedation to control the behavior of the inebriated patient may set the stage for cardiac arrest.

Every effort should be made to replace blood loss prior to an operation. During the operation on a traumatized patient, blood should be replaced as it is lost. The blood should be as fresh as possible and warmed to body temperature prior to infusion. Whenever possible, properly typed and cross-matched blood should be used. Intravenous infusion of balanced salt solutions will gain time for proper blood matching to be done.

FLUID AND ELECTROLYTE MANAGEMENT

Normal Body Fluids

The understanding of daily requirements of fluids and electrolytes requires knowledge of their normal composition and distribution. Additional discussion of this subject is given in Chapter 26. Most important is an understanding of the distribution of total body water, which is approximately 50 to 70 per cent of the total body weight.[73] In the leaner adult individual, the elderly person, and the infant it approaches 70 per cent, while in the obese it is nearer to 50 per cent. Total body water comprises extracellular and intracellular water. Intracellular water totals 40 per cent of body weight, while extracellular water represents approximately 20 per cent, of which 5 per cent is in the plasma and 15 per cent in the interstitial fluid. The proportions of extracellular and intracellular water are independent of body habitus. In the body water are other substances that make up the osmolar concentration, which in the normal individual is approximately 310 milliosmoles in both the extracellular and intracellular compartments. The major osmotically active ion of the extracellular fluid is sodium, which is present in concentrations of 135 to 140 mEq per liter. Potassium, calcium, and magnesium represent the bulk of the remaining extracellular cations. The extracellular anions are represented by chloride, which averages 103 mEq per liter, with the remainder in the form of bicarbonate ions, proteins, and the ions of organic acids. The major intracellular cation is potassium, with a concentration of 110 mEq per liter, the remaining cations being largely magnesium and sodium. The intracellular anions are mainly organic acids but also include bicarbonate and protein.

The normal individual maintains the osmolar concentration by varying his fluid and electrolyte intake and output. This is done largely through the kidney by excreting the fluid and electrolytes that the body does not require. For example, a normal individual might ingest 2000 ml of water as fluid and in solid foods. The water of metabolism would contribute an additional 500 ml to the fluid intake, giving a normal daily total fluid intake of 2500 ml of water. An average of 250 ml of water is lost in the stool, and another 750 ml is insensibly lost through the skin and respiration. Approximately 1500 ml is left to be excreted in the urine to maintain total body water at its previous level. Similarly, a normal daily intake of 50 to 90 mEq per liter of sodium is balanced by a similar excretion of sodium in the urine by the normal individual.

Any alteration of these fluid and electrolyte exchanges results in changes in the composition of the body fluid. Such changes may be in volume, in concentration, in composition, or in distribution. The total volume of the body fluid can be increased or decreased by an intake or loss of fluid that has the same number of osmotically active particles as the body fluid. In other words, an isotonic loss or gain results in only a volume change in the body fluids. In this case, the fluids do not change their osmotic pressures. A patient who has undergone a volume change is considered as overexpanded or "wet" if a fluid overload is present and depleted or "dry" if short on fluid.

If, however, water alone is added to or removed from the body fluids, there is a concentration change of the osmotically active particles. An example of a concentration change is seen in a patient with a fluid restriction for diabetes insipidus. If the osmotically active particles remain unchanged, but only the relationships of the ions with each other have been changed, then a compositional change has taken place. The development of hyperkalemia in a patient with acute renal failure who loses a small amount of sodium per day from the gastrointestinal tract represents a compositional change. A switch of fluids from one compartment to another is a distributional change. The movement of interstitial fluid into the intravascular compartment in a patient in hemorrhagic shock is illustrative of this change.

Management of Fluid Abnormalities

Volume Derangements

The causes of volume deficits are innumerable. Traumatic blood loss and underestimation of loss during an operation contribute to volume deficits. Internal shifts of fluid with losses from the vascular tree can result in large volume deficits.[44] Fluid sequestration in a crushed limb or at the site of a burn is functionally a loss to the intravascular compartment. Large volumes of isotonic fluid can be sequestered in the abdominal cavity in severe peritonitis.

Clinically, the patient with a moderate isotonic fluid volume deficit will be apathetic with slow responses and anorexia. His peripheral veins are collapsed and fill poorly distal to a tourniquet. Orthostatic hypotension with tachycardia is often seen. The oral mucous membranes are sticky, and the urine decreased in volume and somewhat concentrated. With more severe deficit, the patient lapses into stupor or coma. Myotatic reflexes are decreased. Prior to coma, nausea and vomiting may develop. Cutaneous lividity and hypotension prevail in the supine position. Peripheral pulses, if present, are very weak; the eyes are sunken, and body temperature is below normal. Urine volume is further decreased. Early volume deficits do not cause significant or alarming changes in the vital signs. The blood pressure may be normal or slightly low, and pulse rates below 120 can be present without the clinical signs of shock.

Laboratory findings may be of some help. They tend to support the concept of hemoconcentration; a slight increase in the blood urea nitrogen, hematocrit, and hemoglobin is found. Serum electrolytes are normal.

In a patient with a volume deficit, the best signs to observe are the urinary output and the central venous pressure, both of which are low. If the replacement of an additional 1000 ml of isotonic salt solution results in improvement in the clinical signs, this is further evidence. Further search may be required if continuing volume loss is occurring. The treatment of volume deficit is the replacement of isotonic extracellular fluid in appropriate measured amounts; often the use of 1000 to 1500 ml of salt solution will correct the situation.

Volume excesses occur with the administration or excessive amounts of either isotonic solutions or whole blood.[60] This usually happens either during a vigorous attempt to treat shock in which the fluid loss has been overestimated or as a result of inaccurate measurements of fluid lost during the postoperative period. The normal person with normal kidneys can tolerate excess isotonic fluids for a long time. In the traumatized patient, however, kidney function may be impaired and may be inadequate to handle any excess fluid load. The earliest signs of volume overreplacement are weight gain and pitting edema. The patient becomes dyspneic on exertion; his eyelids are puffy. Urine volume is quite large if renal function is normal. The patient's mucous membranes are moist, and the peripheral veins are full. Pulmonary rales or frank pulmonary edema may be present. Central venous pressure is elevated. Monitoring central venous pressure during fluid administration will alert the physician to the presence of circulatory overload.

The treatment of volume excesses includes reduction of the volume of isotonic fluid given. This alone may be sufficient. An accurate measurement of daily fluid intake and output is required to follow the rate of loss. Daily weighing of the patient affords another check on treatment. In the case of volume excess due to overtransfusion, phlebotomy will be required. Two hundred and fifty milliliters of blood should be removed every four to six hours, and the patient's central venous pressure, his hemoglobin and hematocrit, and the clinical picture should be kept under close observation. If the volume overload from blood is in excess of 1500 ml, clinical evidence of circulatory failure with pulmonary signs of overload will develop.

Concentration Abnormalities

In the immediate post-trauma or postoperative period, it is unusual to see concentration abnormalities if fluid loss has been replaced with blood or balanced salt solutions. A person with relatively normal kidneys will excrete both sodium and water to compensate for minor water and salt differences that may occur as a result of the fluid losses and the extracellular fluid shifts during operation or trauma. After the immediate postoperative or post-traumatic period, however, concentration changes may occur if replacement of lost sodium and water is not adequate.

The most common metabolic derangement in the early postoperative or post-traumatic period is hyponatremia.[44] It occurs if water is given to replace sodium-containing fluid or if water is consistently given in excess of water losses. In the first 24 to 48 hours after stress, an antidiuretic state is produced, mediated by the antidiuretic hormone from the posterior pituitary and by aldosterone from the adrenal cortex. Both sodium and water are reabsorbed by the renal tubules. As the water reabsorption is the more efficient, the normal postoperative condition is one of relative water excess. In addition, as much as 500 ml of endogenous water is freed through metabolism. If, postoperatively, urinary losses are replaced with water only, this normal water excess is converted to overexpansion of the total body water with hyponatremia. Hyponatremia to levels of 130 mEq per liter may occur in the immediate postoperative or post-trauma period without significant clinical signs. If the condition is not recognized and no attempt is made to correct it, the serum sodium concentration will continue to decrease. Clinical symptoms begin at serum sodium levels of approximately 120 to 125 mEq per liter. These include somnolence and lethargy, progressing to coma. Convulsions may occur, particularly if an absolute water excess accompanies the hyponatremia.

This condition is relatively simple to treat. It can be prevented by understanding the shifts in electrolyte balance, as related to sodium and water, that occur normally in the immediate postoperative period. If these are taken into consideration when calculating the fluid requirements, the problem does not arise. With the sodium level above 130 mEq per liter, simple restriction of water intake is usually sufficient to correct the hyponatremic state. If the serum sodium level has fallen below 120 mEq per liter, however, or if the syndrome of inappropriate antidiuretic hormone (ADH) secretion exists, then salt-containing solutions will have to be used.

The syndrome of inappropriate antidiuretic hormone secretion causes hyponatremia because it results in an excessive retention of water that persists despite a reduction in the osmolarity of the extracellular fluid. The basic features of this disorder are hyponatremia and hypo-osmolarity of the serum, continued excretion of sodium, absence of clinical evidence of volume depletion (normal skin turgor and blood pressure), and hyperosmolarity of the urine with reference to the plasma.[8] Renal and adrenal function are normal in this entity. The pathophysiology of the syndrome is poorly understood, but there is loss of salt in excess of water loss despite the development of hyponatremia. This loss may be quite severe, and very low levels of serum sodium are common. Sodium values below 115 mEq per liter are not uncommon if the disorder goes uncorrected. Loss of deep tendon reflexes, muscular weakness, pseudobulbar palsies, stupor, and convulsive episodes may occur at these low levels, at which the hypotonicity of the body fluids is a threat to life. Death occurs at sodium levels of 100 mEq per liter. Inappropriate antidiuretic hormone secretion is seen in moderate degrees following head injury, and in lesser degrees following elective intracranial operations. It is also seen following a wide variety of disorders involving the lungs and in patients with congestive heart failure or cirrhosis. Treatment is similar to that of the postoperative hyponatremia already mentioned. In some patients, simple restriction of water intake will be adequate to correct the problem. Additional discussion of inappropriate antidiuretic hormone secretion is given in Chapter 25.

While the basic condition in hyponatremia may be one of water retention, if the hyponatremia is severe, salt losses must be replaced. The use of a hypertonic saline solution is the treatment of choice. Calculation of the amount of sodium to be given is simple. For example, a patient with a serum sodium content of 120 mEq per liter has a sodium deficit of 20 mEq per liter. If the patient weighs 75 kg and is on the lean side, his total body water will be approximately 70 per cent of his body weight. This will be approximately 52.5 liters. His total body sodium deficit then is 1050 mEq. It should now be determined whether the patient is in acidosis or alkalosis, as the choice of replacement solution depends on this fact. In an alkalotic condition, 3 per cent sodium chloride should be used, 1 liter of which contains 500 mEq of sodium. Sodium lactate as a one molar solution should be used in acidosis, as it contains 1000 mEq per liter of sodium.[15]

The time used for replacement is important. Approximately half of the calculated sodium deficit should be replaced over the first six to eight hours. Serial sodium determinations should be used to follow the rate and degree of correction. The remainder of the deficit is then corrected during the next 24 hours. Replacement of an existing deficit does not mean that routine maintenance is not also required. Adequate fluid and ions should be given to counterbalance any continuing loss that is occurring.

In this type of hyponatremia, the deficit is gradual in onset. Correction requires calculation of total body water rather than of extracellular fluid, as water tends to move out of the cell to replace extracellular loss. In acute sodium loss, such as accompanies vomiting and diarrhea, the calculation is based on extracellular fluid volume only.

Hypernatremia is present when the sodium concentration exceeds 150 mEq per liter. It is more easily produced in a person with normal renal function than is hyponatremia. It occurs when water is lost as a result of the evaporation of sweat and in patients with tracheostomies who are placed in dry environments. Three to five liters of water per day can be lost from extensive open burns. Renal water loss occurs with the diuresis associated with high-output renal failure and diabetes insipidus. Osmotic diuretics, such as mannitol and urea, or excessive sugar loads result in large-volume water losses. Hypernatremia can also result if isotonic salt solutions are used to replace pure water losses rapidly. A common cause is the use of high-caloric tube feedings in comatose patients.

The correction of hypernatremia is the use of free water in the form of 5 per cent dextrose in water, administered in appropriate amounts slowly over several hours. Theoretically, the sodium excess should be purely in the extracellular fluid, since intracellular sodium concentration is quite low. Because of the other metabolic derangements that usually are present, however, this assumption cannot be exact. To make the calculation, it can be assumed that the sodium will be distributed in equal concentration throughout the total body water. A simple way of calculating the volume needed for correction is as follows. A patient has a serum sodium value of 160 mEq per liter (normal is 140 mEq per liter). The total body water in a 75-kg lean man is assumed to be 52.5 liters. It will take approximately 7.5 liters of free water to reverse this condition:

$$\frac{52.5 \text{ L} \times 160 \text{ mEq/L}}{140 \text{ mEq/L}} - 52.5 \text{ L} = 7.5 \text{ L}$$

Half the fluid is given as 5 per cent dextrose in water during the first 24 hours. In addition, the normally required maintenance fluids are given. Then the patient's chemical balance can be reassessed. Additional corrections can be made in the next 24 hours. Too rapid correction of the hypernatremic state, particularly in elderly people and in infants, can result in severe neurological derangements, including convulsions, coma, and death.

Normal Acid-Base Regulation

Acid-base regulation by the body is basically regulation of hydrogen ion content. The normal plasma pH is approximately 7.4, but extraordinary conditions may result in pH ranges of 7.0 to 7.8. Beyond this range, in either direction, the condition is incompatible with life if it persists for any length of time. The body pH is regulated primarily by respiratory and renal functions. Respiratory control consists essentially of hyperventilation to reduce carbon dioxide in the case of acidosis, and hypoventilation with retention of carbon dioxide in the case of alkalosis. The kidneys normally serve in the maintenance of acid-base equilibrium through the excretion of nitrogenous waste products, organic acids, and chloride, and by the reabsorption of bicarbonate and sodium. The most important body buffer, the bicarbonate–carbonic acid system, is intimately connected with both respiratory and renal function. In addition to pulmonary and renal regulation of acid-base control, body buffers, including hemoglobin, protein, and the salts of certain weak acids, are present. These play only minor roles in acid-base maintenance, as they become exhausted with persistent acidosis or alkalosis.

Measurements of blood carbonic acid, base buffer, and pH are indispensable in the evaluation of the acid-base balance. Although venous measurements may be adequate, arterial measurements are preferable. Carbonic acid, being a volatile acid, is determined by the measurement of the partial pressure of carbon dioxide in the blood. This measurement is expressed in millimeters of mercury, but multiplication by the factor 0.03 converts the value to milliequivalents per liter. The normal arterial values are 40 mm of mercury or 1.20 mEq per liter. Carbon dioxide is excreted through the lung, and its arterial value is, in part, a measure of respiratory function. Bicarbonate levels, on the other hand, are regulated by metabolic functions. Total carbon dioxide content minus P_{CO_2} gives the bicarbonate level. Thus a normal carbon dioxide content of 28.2 mEq per liter minus a normal P_{CO_2} of 1.2 mEq per liter yields a bicarbonate level of 27.0 mEq per liter.

The bicarbonate level does not completely express the total base buffering capacity of the blood. Hence, the term "buffer base" was introduced by Singer and Hastings in 1948.[63] This includes the bicarbonate, hemoglobin, and protein buffering systems; therefore, it expresses the total base buffering capacity of the blood. The normal value for arterial blood is 47.5 mEq per liter. Kintner simplified the terminology by reporting the buffer base as the deviation from normal.[34] As it is deviation, the term "delta (Δ) base" was applied. The value calculated, therefore, may be positive, indicating an excess of base, or negative, indicating a deficit. Thus, an arterial buffer base value of 27.5 mEq per liter would be reported as Δ base = -20 mEq per liter. A change from the normal P_{CO_2}

(40 mm of mercury in the case of an arterial determination) may also be reported as a ΔP_{CO_2}. Similarly, positive and negative values are possible. Thus, an arterial P_{CO_2} value of 60 mm of mercury would be reported as ΔP_{CO_2} = + 20 mm of mercury.

A pH value tells only whether the blood is acidotic, alkalotic, or normal (pH = 7.4). This, in turn, fails to disclose any information as to the cause of the abnormality. Combining P_{CO_2}, Δ base, and pH on the Kintner nomogram, however, will give rapid information of a more meaningful nature.

An example is shown in Figure 77–1. The Kintner nomogram is in the form of an H. The left limb expresses the ΔP_{CO_2} in a plus or minus number of millimeters of mercury and gives information concerning the respiratory compensating mechanisms of the buffer systems. The right limb expresses Δ base in a plus or minus number of milliequivalents per liter and gives information concerning the metabolic compensating mechanisms. The normal horizontal limb indicates zero, or normal, levels of both P_{CO_2} and buffer base. Coincidentally, the ΔP_{CO_2} to Δ base ratio associated with a normal pH (7.4) can be expressed as 2/1. On the Kintner nomogram, two graduations on the P_{CO_2} scale therefore equal one graduation on the base scale, so that a horizontal limb indicates a normal (or compensated) pH of 7.4.

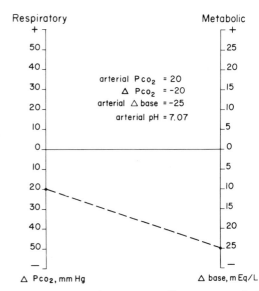

Figure 77–1 The nomogram illustrates a marked buffer base deficit in a patient with metabolic acidosis, as explained in the text.

In the example shown in the figure, the ΔP_{CO_2} is -20 mm of mercury, and the Δ base is -25 mEq per liter. Plotting these on the nomogram and connecting them with a straight line yields a sloping line downward toward the base scale. The sloping line indicates an uncompensated state. The pH is 7.07, indicating that the patient has acidosis. The largest deficit is in the base buffer, indicating that the major derangement is metabolic. Thus, the patient has uncompensated metabolic acidosis. If the acidosis is to become compensated (i.e., pH = 7.4), the sloping line must be made horizontal. This change can most easily be accomplished by bringing the Δ base value to -10 mEq per liter. Therefore, the patient will need additional base to increase the arterial base buffer. The importance of this concept cannot be overemphasized. Restoration of the blood pH to normal is not the goal. Correction of the defect, either metabolic or respiratory, is the goal, and when this is done, the pH value will automatically return to normal. The Kintner nomogram is merely a rapid means of ascertaining the cause of the derangement.

Since all buffer systems are in equilibrium, evaluation of the bicarbonate-carbonic acid system is sufficient to elucidate the acid-base status in minor derangements. Gaining this information requires the measurement of the levels of blood carbonic acid (P_{CO_2}) and pH plus bicarbonate or total carbon dioxide instead of buffer base (Table 77–1).

Acid-Base Derangements

Metabolic Acidosis

Metabolic acidosis is probably the most important clinical acid-base derangement in the post-traumatic or postoperative patient.[51] The most common form of acidosis confronting the surgeon is lactic acidosis,

which is due to poor tissue perfusion. Other causes of metabolic acidosis include diabetic keto-acidosis and excessive administration of acid anion-containing fluids. For example, isotonic saline, or 0.9 per cent sodium chloride, has 154 mEq of sodium, which is only slightly hypertonic, but it also contains 154 mEq of chloride. For each liter of normal saline given, a chloride excess of approximately 51 mEq is delivered. The excess of chloride ions, or other acid ions, such as the organic acids, results in a shift of the pH downward. The body compensates by an increase in rate and depth of respiration, which increases the excretion of carbon dioxide through the lungs and reduces the P_{CO_2}, or carbonic acid level, of the blood. In addition, the kidneys excrete the excess chloride ion and exchange hydrogen in the urine for sodium and bicarbonate ion. If the kidneys fail in this function or if the chloride load is massive, metabolic acidosis results. The major laboratory findings include low pH and bicarbonate (total carbon dioxide) levels.

The treatment of acidosis from a metabolic source requires the use of added base buffer, usually administered as lactated Ringer's solution or sodium lactate solution. For minor derangements, lactated Ringer's solution is preferable, since it approaches an isotonic salt solution. A liter contains 130 mEq of sodium, 4 mEq of potassium, and 3 mEq of calcium, balanced by 109 mEq of chloride and 28 mEq of bicarbonate. Each liter of solution furnishes approximately 100 to 150 ml of free water. Its chief disadvantage is its slight hypo-osmolarity with respect to sodium. If these facts are kept in mind in the calculation of daily sodium and water needs, however, appropriate amounts of each can be given. With more severe forms of metabolic acidosis, sixth molar sodium lactate, containing 167 mEq each of sodium and bicarbonate ion or even one molar sodium lactate, containing 1000 mEq per liter of each ion, should be used.

Metabolic Alkalosis

Metabolic alkalosis is characterized by elevated serum pH and bicarbonate levels. Its chief cause in the patient who has suffered trauma is the failure to replace the acid secretions of the gastrointestinal tract, particularly the stomach, with appropriate

TABLE 77–1 PRIMARY CHANGES IN UNCOMPLICATED ACID-BASE DISORDERS

DISORDER	PRIMARY CHANGES	
Metabolic acidosis	$HCO_3 \downarrow$	pH $\downarrow$
Metabolic alkalosis	$HCO_3 \uparrow$	pH $\uparrow$
Respiratory acidosis	$P_{CO_2} \uparrow$	pH $\downarrow$
Respiratory alkalosis	$P_{CO_2} \downarrow$	pH $\uparrow$

fluid. In the attempt to control the developing alkalotic state, carbon dioxide is retained through respiratory depression. Excretion of potassium, ammonia instead of ammonium ion, and bicarbonate ion in the urine with retention of hydrogen and chloride also results. This condition is prevented by adequate replacement of the acid gastrointestinal fluids daily. The replacement is accomplished by using salt solutions containing sodium and chloride in appropriate amounts. The stomach secretions will average 60 mEq per liter of sodium and 130 mEq per liter of chloride. If metabolic alkalosis occurs, it is usually mild in the postoperative and post-traumatic patient and is easily corrected by using salt infusions.

Respiratory Acidosis

Respiratory acidosis is most often the result of airway obstruction, respiratory failure, or drug-induced respiratory depression, either acute or chronic. There occurs a rise in arterial P_{CO_2} associated with a low pH. It is corrected by the establishment of an adequate airway and maintenance of ventilation. Rarely must one administer a buffer in managing this condition.

Respiratory Alkalosis

Respiratory alkalosis is very rarely seen in the postoperative or post-traumatic patient. It is usually the result of hyperventilation during anesthesia, and rarely occurs in the patient who is hyperventilating from severe agitation and pain. A high pH and a low P_{CO_2} are noted. This condition seldom needs any specific form of treatment except removal of the cause of the hyperventilation.

Potassium Abnormalities

Potassium abnormalities are intimately connected with acid-base metabolism. Although 98 per cent of the total body potassium is intracellular, the turnover rate is extremely rapid. Significant quantities of intracellular potassium move extracellularly in response to injury, operation, acidosis, or a catabolic state. Dangerous hyperkalemia, when serum potassium levels greater than 6.0 mEq per liter are reached,

is rarely encountered if renal function is normal. At these levels, cardiac arrhythmias and arrest may occur.

The most common potassium abnormality is hypokalemia, which may occur as a result of increased renal excretion, movement of potassium into cells, continued renal excretion of potassium after intake has been reduced to zero, or infusion of large quantities of potassium-free fluid. In either respiratory or metabolic alkalosis, potassium is in competition with hydrogen for urinary excretion in exchange for sodium. Increased potassium excretion occurs as the potassium ion is exchanged for sodium, permitting the retention of hydrogen ion to buffer the alkalosis. Similarly, hypokalemic states encourage the development of metabolic alkalosis since potassium is not available to exchange for sodium, therefore making the excretion of hydrogen ion mandatory.[53]

Potassium excretion is increased when increased quantities of sodium are present. The more sodium present in the renal tubules, the more potassium will be excreted in exchange for sodium. Therefore, potassium requirements are increased in hypernatremic states.

The normal renal excretion of potassium is small, however, compared to the gastrointestinal secretion. The major potassium loss is via the stool or gastric aspirate. This situation does not prevail if derangements of acid-base balance are present.

The treatment of hypokalemia is the infusion of a calculated amount of potassium. Since much of the body store of potassium is intracellular, calculation of deficit by the formula used for sodium is difficult. In true hypokalemic states, total body potassium is diminished, and this is not accurately reflected in serum levels. A crude calculation, as for sodium, is done, and the calculated amount is given over a 24-hour period. Serial determinations and calculations become necessary to correct the deficit.

Lactated Ringer's solution contains 4 mEq per liter of potassium, and is useful for potassium maintenance. An additional 20 to 40 mEq of potassium chloride per day, dissolved in a liter of intravenous fluids, can be safely administered to an adult who is not in severe shock or in renal failure. The rate of administration of the potassium-rich solution should be no more than 10 ml per kilogram per hour.

The treatment of hyperkalemia is almost

invariably associated with renal failure. It requires the use of exchange resins or dialysis and is considered in the section on Acute Renal Failure.

Calcium Abnormalities

Calcium abnormalities are seen less often than potassium abnormalities in the post-traumatic and postoperative patient. Hypercalcemia rarely occurs except in association with renal failure and subsequent acidosis. The levels reached, however, are usually not pathological, since associated with acidosis and renal failure, there is hyperphosphatemia, which enhances the deposition of the calcium in bones and other tissues of the body.[42]

The major calcium abnormality of the patient in the postoperative and post-traumatic period is hypocalcemia. This is seen most commonly following extensive blood transfusion. A citrate solution, which binds the ionized calcium and prevents clotting by blocking the conversion of thromboplastic factors to thromboplastin, is the usual anticoagulant for stored blood. To block the conversion of thromboplastic factors, the citrate must be in excess of ionized calcium in the stored blood. If blood transfusions are massive and rapid, the excess citrate may bind the recipient's ionized serum calcium. The administration of 1 gm calcium gluconate with every 4 to 5 units of blood will prevent the occurrence of this citrate intoxication.

Hypocalcemia may occur in patients as the result of calcium precipitation with acute pancreatitis or when large losses of calcium-containing fluids, particularly through the gastrointestinal tract, are not replaced or if fluids low in calcium are used for replacement. Treatment is with an intravenous infusion of calcium gluconate.

Practical Application of Fluid and Electrolyte Management

The average patient who requires intravenous fluids and does not have unusual fluid losses can be managed adequately with approximately 2500 to 3000 ml of intravenous fluid a day, with 500 to 1000 ml of this being a salt-containing solution (usually lactated Ringer's or normal saline). These figures include replacement for average

urine losses of 1000 to 1500 ml per day. In addition, gastrointestinal losses should be replaced. Potassium chloride, an average of 60 to 80 mEq per day, should be given.[60] Additional sodium and potassium may be required if large concentrations of these electrolytes are excreted in the urine. Blood chemistry determinations should be done daily. The determinations should include serum sodium, potassium, chloride, bicarbonate, and blood urea nitrogen if the patient is dependent upon intravenous fluids. If severe acid-base derangements are present pH, total carbon dioxide, and buffer base are indispensible daily determinations. If there is a question of abnormal renal function developing, blood urea nitrogen and serum creatinine levels should be determined. Daily intake and output charts should be kept. These charts are the key to satisfactory long-term intravenous fluid therapy of the injured patient. In the daily administration of fluid volumes and composition of fluids to be given, it is better to give what appears to be a slight excess. If the patient has normal kidneys, compensation for mild overloads of all forms of fluids and electrolytes is easy. The development of chronic deficit is best avoided by this technique. Restoration of derangements in volume or composition requires much more demanding and careful calculation.

In the fluid and electrolyte management of the patient with multiple injuries and brain trauma or recent intracranial operation, cerebral edema must be a matter of concern. The edema is aggravated by overhydration or by water retention secondary to inappropriate antidiuretic hormone secretion. The management of this condition by restricted fluid intake and by the use of steroids such as dexamethasone can further complicate the total therapeutic endeavors.[59] Careful attention must be given to daily urine and serum electrolyte, especially sodium, and osmolarity determinations. Continuous monitoring of intracranial pressure may be helpful, especially in the more complicated situations.

MANAGEMENT OF SHOCK

Definition of Terms

The successful management of injured patients requires a working knowledge of the pathology of shock. While many attempts have been made to define shock in precise terms, most definitions usually fail to encompass its many facets and are too complex to allow general adaptation. Therefore, it is expedient to define shock simply as *a generalized state of inadequate tissue perfusion that, if uncorrected, will eventually result in cellular death and failure of vital organs.*[4,56] The cardinal features of shock must be considered both in physiological, or hemodynamic, terms (low cardiac output and inadequate tissue perfusion) and in biochemical terms (cellular hypoxia and metabolic dysfunction). The etiology of these characteristics has been the subject of intensive investigative work. Obviously, the causes of low cardiac output with inadequate tissue perfusion are multiple.[11] A slight modification of this classification that is helpful in the management of the traumatized patient includes: (1) hypovolemic shock; (2) neurogenic shock, either vasogenic or spinal; (3) cardiogenic shock; and (4) septic shock.

Another classification categorizes the causes of shock according to: (1) pump failure, i.e., cardiogenic or vasogenic; (2) volume failure, i.e., hypovolemic or hemorrhagic; and (3) vascular failure, i.e., neurogenic or endotoxic (Table 77–2). It is important to realize, however, that the three most frequent causes of shock in the severely injured patient are fluid loss, myocardial failure, and sepsis, and that while they often are distinguishable in early

TABLE 77–2 CLASSIFICATION OF SHOCK

Cardiogenic shock
  Primary myocardial dysfunction
    Myocardial infarction
    Cardiac arrhythmias
    Myocardial depression from other causes
  Miscellaneous causes of impaired cardiac function
    Tension pneumothorax
    Venae cavae obstruction
    Cardiac tamponade
Hypovolemic shock
  Blood loss
  Plasma loss
  Water loss
  Any combination or blood, plasma, and water loss.
Vasogenic shock brought about by specific disorders
  Decrease in resistance
    Spinal anesthesia or spinal shock
    Neurogenic reflexes, as in acute pain
    Possible end-stage hypovolemic shock
  Septic shock
    Change in peripheral resistance
    Change in venous capacitance
    Peripheral arteriovenous shunting

shock, they may later blend one into another.

Pathological Physiology

The changes occurring in shock are multiple and include many organ systems. These changes have been and are the subject of intense investigation. To attempt a complete discussion of them would require more space than is available. To simplify these changes, they can be considered as involving the vascular tree, the body fluid compartments, the kidney, and the endocrine system.

Hypovolemic Shock

Hypovolemic shock is characterized by a decreased volume of fluid in the intravascular tree. The fluid lost may be whole blood or extracellular fluid or a combination of both. Frank hemorrhage produces whole blood loss, while thermal burns, diarrhea, or vomiting produce loss of extracellular fluid. Sequestration of fluids in the pleural space after spontaneous esophageal perforation, in the peritoneal cavity after perforation of a viscus or bowel obstruction, or in traumatized tissue after crush injuries can be large enough to precipitate hypotension.

The rate of loss and the volume lost from the effective circulation determine the cardiovascular response to hypovolemia. At one extreme is the "open artery" exsanguinating type of hemorrhage in which a profound loss of peripheral vascular resistance occurs in spite of compensating mechanisms. Hypotension is out of proportion to volume loss. While this state is rare even in trauma, it is important to recognize because prolonged efforts to treat it with only volume-expanding fluids instead of prompt operative intervention for hemostasis are futile. At the other extreme is gradual, slow volume loss that may be entirely compensated for by renal mechanisms of fluid retention coupled with repartition of body fluids without grossly detectable hemodynamic alterations.

Between these extremes is the situation that is more frequently seen in trauma. It is produced by the combination of losses from small arteries, veins, and capillaries. Unless stopped, this blood loss may lead to progressive stages of compensated hypovolemia, impending shock, hypotensive shock, and finally, refractory shock. In an otherwise healthy young patient, a gradual volume loss of 15 per cent usually produces minimal changes, a loss of 30 per cent may be compensated for without hypotension, and a loss of 40 to 50 per cent is necessary to produce progressive hypotension to a mean arterial pressure of 50 mm of mercury.

With minimal hypovolemia up to a loss of about 15 per cent the primary compensatory response is vascular. The great veins, probably as a result of neurohumoral mechanisms involving the sympathetic system, contract. The reduction in volume of this capacitance system decreases the functional vascular space to be filled by the existing blood volume. These adjustments can buffer a loss of about 10 per cent of normal blood volume. At the same time a net inflow of extracellular fluid to the vascular space begins. Oxygen consumption, cardiac output, endocrine and metabolic changes are minimal. The signs and symptoms relating to these changes are transient.

Volume loss above 15 per cent calls forth additional cardiovascular responses. Tachycardia is seen as a result of sympathetic stimulation that caused the heart to function in a new work-pressure relationship whereby a greater output is produced at a given filling pressure; however, the filling pressure may, even at this point, be reduced so that a net reduction in cardiac output occurs. Blood flow to muscle and skin is reduced by arteriolar constriction. Definite endocrine changes are seen, as manifested by elevated aldosterone and antidiuretic hormone levels with resultant salt and water retention along with decreased urinary output. Variable increases in circulating growth hormone and catecholamines occur along with, usually, elevation of the cortisol level. Metabolic responses include increased glycolysis producing mild hyperglycemia, increased lipolysis yielding additional free fatty acids, increased oxygen consumption, and slight rises in lactate levels. Some degree of hyperventilation occurs, resulting in alkalemia. Signs and symptoms become more easily discernible. They include thirst, apprehension, orthostatic hypotension, weakness, pallor, and coolness of the skin.

By the time volume loss reaches the 30 per cent mark nearly all patients will show symptoms of shock and a systolic blood pressure below 100 mm of mercury even while supine. Nearly all patients will have a significant reduction in cardiac output in spite of persistent arteriolar vasoconstriction. If it has not already done so, central venous pressure will decrease. Blood flow to the viscera, previously maintained at the expense of skin and muscle, now begins to fall to protect the heart and brain. In fact, as shock progresses the heart may come to receive as much as 25 per cent and the brain 80 per cent of the cardiac output as compared to normal levels of 5 to 8 per cent and 20 per cent, respectively. Renal blood flow decreases as renal vascular resistance increases. The previously noted endocrine responses are more marked. Lactic acid levels are significantly elevated.

With continued volume loss, the compensatory mechanisms are exceeded and, certainly at the point of 45 to 50 per cent blood loss, reduction in blood flow to the heart and brain occurs. Marked reduction in cardiac output and severe hypotension are seen. Catecholamine levels are quite high. Severe lactic acidosis appears as the result of progressive anaerobic metabolism in tissue beds coupled with reduction in liver function as a result of a critical reduction in hepatic blood flow. Severe oliguria is evident, and mixed venous P_{O_2} is 20 mm of mercury or less. Air hunger becomes marked, and the patient's level of consciousness deteriorates steadily.

A blood volume of 50 per cent of normal cannot be tolerated for an extended period. Current evidence shows that several abnormalities result from profound reduction in perfusion and the resulting reliance on anaerobic metabolism. Ischemic cells probably undergo lysosomal membrane disruption, which leads to self-destruction and more widespread harm. Better established and more important changes are those of reduction in mitochondrial efficiency of oxidative phosphorylation, which result in reduction in production of ATP and thereby of cyclic $3',5'$ AMP. These changes lead to numerous serious effects on cellular metabolism and integrity, not the least of which is malfunction of the membrane sodium — potassium ion pump.

When shock is profound and prolonged, a state of hypocoagulability may ensue as the result of extravasation of clotting factors, a decrease in their production and mobilization, and especially, disseminated intravascular coagulation. The hypocoagulability may be aggravated by an increase in fibrinolytic activity and the release of circulating anticoagulants plus the transfusion of blood deficient in clotting factors. If severe and unrecognized, this may pose a serious threat to the patient and undermine the therapeutic efforts being made on his behalf.

Vasogenic Shock

Vasogenic shock usually falls into one of two broad categories: neurogenic shock due to decrease in resistance brought about by neurogenic mechanisms, and septic shock due to change in peripheral arterial resistance and venous capacitance secondary to a primary cellular defect.

Neurogenic Shock

Neurogenic shock is seen as simple syncope following exposure to unpleasant events such as a sudden pain or an unpleasant sight. Apparently these stimuli increase vagal influence on the heart, with resulting bradycardia and decreased cardiac output. This mechanism is also believed to be, in part, responsible for some shock states seen during abdominal operations when peritoneal stimuli may result in massive vagal influences upon the heart. Atropine will block these vagal impulses. It has, however, been shown that vagal block alone may not be sufficient to prevent the syncope. The syncope still may occur because of the presence of peripheral vasodilation produced by the action of sympathetic cholinergic fibers, in particular sudomotor fibers, resulting in the release of bradykinin, a potent vasodilator.

Neurogenic shock can also be of spinal origin. During spinal anesthesia, or following spinal cord transection above T6, shock can develop secondary to loss of sympathetic tone.

The clinical picture of neurogenic shock is quite different from that of hypovolemic shock. The blood pressure may be low, but the pulse is usually not fast; in fact, it may be slow. The skin is warm and may even be flushed, because a normovolemic state is present, but the volume is pooled into the capillaries, arterioles, and venulae. The peripheral veins are full, and urinary output usually is normal. The patient is alert and mentally clear.

Septic Shock

Septic shock is a distinct clinical entity.[4,72] Infection with either gram-negative or gram-positive organisms can produce septic shock, but gram-negative sepsis seems to produce a more distinct clinical syndrome. Shock associated with gram-positive organisms is apparently due to a low-flow state secondary to hypovolemia. The hypovolemia often is associated with a local infectious process such as a profound cellulitis, fasciitis, or tissue necrosis. While some gram-positive bacteria produce diffusible endotoxins, these do not appear to directly produce a low-flow state as do those found in gram-negative bacteria.

Many gram-negative bacteria produce endotoxin. In most cases of septic shock, *Escherichia coli* is the causative organism; however, *Klebsiella, Aerobacter, Pseudomonas, Proteus, Bacteroides,* and multiple species are not uncommonly identified.

The pathophysiological and metabolic derangements that occur in septic shock are extremely complex. Initially, the problem seems to be defective blood flow caused by abnormal vasoconstriction, which is followed by vasodilatation in the microcirculation. This reduction in blood flow due to stagnation may be associated with intravascular coagulation, and in isolated instances endotoxemia has resulted in a generalized Shwartzman reaction in both experimental animal and human subjects. A combination of circulatory, metabolic, biochemical, and coagulation disorders leads to a generalized decrease in tissue perfusion and alterations in oxygen transport capacity, and perhaps in cellular utilization of oxygen and other substrates. Evidence exists for the development of substantial numbers of physiological shunts in the capillary exchange beds in both the lung and the systemic circulation. Further, a reduction in the ability of hemoglobin to release oxygen in the periphery may be present and, thereby, partially explain the reduced availability of oxygen during the bacterial shock state. Which of these or other factors is the most crucial in the ultimate disruption of cellular function remains to be elucidated.

In gram-negative septic shock the patient appears to have a hemodynamic defect. Arterial hypotension, decrease in cardiac output, and increase in peripheral resistance are seen. Unlike the state in hypovolemic shock, however, the central venous pressure and blood volume are normal. Sequestration of blood in venous pools is present. These factors can result in renal ischemia and renal failure as in hypovolemic shock.

Usually, septic shock presents with evidence that bacteremia has occurred. Patients develop a sudden hyperpyrexia, often greater than 101° F, and, frequently, have a hard shaking chill. Despite the hypotension, the skin is usually warm and dry, but if the hypotension continues, the skin will become cool, moist, and even cyanotic. Mental confusion occurs early. Tachypnea without obvious ventilatory dysfunction is common. Blood cultures taken at this time are usually positive, and leukocytosis is generally present. Tachycardia, if it does occur, is mild, particularly in older patients. Septic shock often follows a major urological or gastrointestinal procedure. It may occur with a simple insertion of a Foley catheter.

Cardiogenic Shock

In cardiogenic shock the heart fails to pump effectively. This may be due to extrinsic or intrinsic causes. Extrinsic causes such as cardiac tamponade or major mediastinal shifts with tension pneumothorax require operative intervention and have been discussed previously. Massive pulmonary embolism blocking cardiac flow is another extrinsic cause. Intrinsic problems include cardiac arrhythmias, myocardial contusions, and frank infarction. In trauma, cardiac arrhythmias are most commonly due to hypoxia and poor ventilation. Arrhythmias that persist despite adequate ventilation may respond to intravenous lidocaine or quinidine. The assistance of a cardiologist is helpful in managing persistent arrhythmias. Cardiac contusions or myocardial infarction require therapy directed at the myocardial damage.

As in hypovolemic shock, the cardiac output is depressed and the total vascular peripheral resistance is markedly increased. Prior to a fall in blood pressure,

associated metabolic acidosis always occurs, reflecting cellular anoxia. The main feature that helps differentiate cardiogenic shock from hypovolemic shock is the significant elevation of the central venous pressure, or more specifically, the pulmonary capillary wedge pressure (measured with a Swan-Ganz catheter). Differentiating the two types of shock is particularly important in the patient who has suffered multiple trauma and has a reduced cardiac output secondary to cardiac tamponade. Should this patient be deemed hypovolemic and should rapid fluid infusions be begun, a fatal outcome is likely. It must, however, be remembered that, especially in trauma patients, hypovolemia may occur in tandem with a myocardial infarction. This combination carries a mortality rate in excess of 20 per cent. When this combination exists, fluids must be given at a rate rapid enough to expand the intravascular compartment, while cardiac filling pressures are carefully monitored with a central venous pressure catheter and pulmonary artery pressure catheter.

Pharmacological agents remain a very important part of the management of patients in cardiogenic shock. These are usually drugs that increase the contractility of the heart (a positive inotropic action). Norepinephrine and dopamine fall into this category. Digitalization of these patients is generally recommended. The use of vasodilators such as phenoxybenzamine and nitroprusside to reduce the afterload on the heart secondary to peripheral vasoconstriction, while theoretically attractive, has not been evaluated adequately enough to recommend their routine use. Shock due to cardiac problems is relatively rare except as a terminal event in the patient with multiple injuries. If the shock is not due to arrhythmias and hypoventilation, the prognosis is usually poor.

Therapy

Once the diagnosis of shock is made, treatment should be begun immediately. First, a route for intravenous fluids and drugs is established (preferably two large lines). The etiology of the shock should be established as soon as possible. Once the causes are known, specific therapy can be given.

Hypovolemic Shock

The basic problem in hypovolemic shock is the volume deficit.[8] Obviously, the first therapeutic measure is to prevent further loss. If hemorrhage is occurring, it should be controlled and then the volume should be restored. Splinting of major fractures is very important; a 1-liter hemorrhage can be prevented by early use of a Thomas splint.

Several factors must be kept in mind to understand the concept of treatment of hypovolemic shock. It is of paramount importance to recognize that the rate, volume, and type of fluid loss will dictate the choice of replacement fluid. Recognition of the shifts that occur in the extracellular fluid is necessary. Finally, the changes in renal function and acid-base balance during hypovolemic shock must be considered.

To illustrate this concept of management in a neurosurgical context, true hypovolemic shock can be rapidly induced by draining the ventricles of a 4-kg hydrocephalic infant. This fluid is almost pure extracellular fluid. Its volume may be 200 to 300 ml, while the infant's total body fluid is about 2 liters and the extracellular fluid space is about 400 ml. Sudden loss of this volume percentage of the total extracellular fluid produces profound, often irreversible, shock. Transfusion of whole blood will make the situation worse. This type of fluid loss produces hemoconcentration, and transfusion will aggravate this concentration.

If an adult has a sudden hemorrhage of 500 ml of whole blood, he has lost 10 per cent of his circulating blood volume. As the loss was rapid, he will show the cardinal signs of shock with tachycardia, tachypnea, and hypotension. Infusion of a liter of balanced salt solution such as lactated Ringer's solution will promptly restore his physiological balance to normal. No whole blood replacement will be necessary.

If another hemorrhage of another 500 ml of blood occurs, another 10 per cent of the blood volume has been lost suddenly. Now, infusion of a second liter of lactated Ringer's solution may produce only a transient rise in blood pressure. In this circumstance, whole blood is required for volume replacement.

Suppose that after the initial 500-ml hemorrhage, no further acute hemorrhage of any consequence occurs. Even if there is a slow loss of an additional 500 ml of blood, the patient may not show signs of shock. Probably, maintenance of blood pressure and urinary flow can be easily accomplished by infusion of saline or lactated Ringer's solution. During or just after anesthesia, the patient might show evidence of blood pressure lability and tachycardia. These changes in blood pressure and pulse rate would indicate a significant reduction in circulating blood volume. If the symptoms or findings are marked, routine transfusion of whole blood is indicated. If not, the administration of oral iron is the recommended treatment.

In hemorrhages of more than 10 per cent of circulating volume, blood transfusion is likely to be required, and in hemorrhages of 20 per cent or more, it definitely will be required. By employing a balanced salt solution with blood, the physiological mechanism of shift of the extracellular fluid can be used to advantage, as the salt solution tends to replenish the extracellular fluid volume. Some experimental evidence indicates that a significant fraction of the extracellular fluid shifts intracellularly and cannot be used to restore intravascular volume, so a relative extracellular deficit develops during hemorrhage. More recent work, however, disputes these concepts. A more cogent reason for using cystalloids in resuscitation of trauma patients is to replace extracellular fluid sequestered in damaged tissues. Furthermore, clinical studies have demonstrated that the use of salt solutions will afford significant protection against acute renal failure from hypovolemic shock.

Clinically, one may wonder how he can estimate the percentage of total blood volume that has been lost by hemorrhage. Patients in shock should receive 1000 to 2000 ml of Ringer's solution as rapidly as possible. If the blood loss is less than 10 per cent, this will prove adequate replacement. If the loss is more than 10 per cent, or if the hemorrhage is continuing at a slow rate, a transient response will be obtained. During this response, time to obtain properly typed and cross-matched blood is gained. Then the transfusion can be given. If exsanguinating hemorrhage is occurring, infusion with type-specific whole blood is required. Unmatched type O Rh-negative blood should be used in only the most extreme circumstances, since after the patient has received several O-negative units cross-matching becomes impossible. An efficient blood bank should be able to make type-specific blood available within 10 minutes. Only in the care of mass casualties, in which overloading of a blood bank's personnel makes human error likely, should universal donor transfusions be used routinely.

In any circumstance, administration of lactated Ringer's solution will restore the extracellular fluid volume toward normal. Acute renal failure is rare with this type of resuscitation, and if it occurs, it is usually of the high-output type. The Ringer's solution also gives some protection against hemoglobinuria in case mismatched blood is given in an emergency such as exsanguinating hemorrhage.

The use of a balanced salt solution is more than just a test for degree of shock and more than a method of gaining time. The balanced salt solution (lactated Ringer's) is near the composition of the extracellular fluid and serves as a replacement for it. In traumatic hemorrhagic states, saline is essentially as useful in this regard as lactated Ringer's. Excessive use of crystalloids should be discouraged. These fluids expand the extracellular fluid space, with expansion of plasma volume resulting only as plasma constitutes a compartment of this extracellular space. To the extent that the plasma volume is expanded, its specific osmotic pressure relative to the interstitial space is reduced. The specific disadvantages of these fluids are that they flood the extracellular space and reduce plasma-specific osmotic activity, thus promoting the development of interstitial edema that can be damaging in the lungs (viz., shock lung). In large single hemorrhages or extensive continuous or repeated blood loss, whole blood must always be included in the therapy. Of the fluids available for resuscitation, only whole blood or red cell preparations have the ability to restore oxygen delivering capacity as well as a normal spectrum of plasma proteins for osmotic, immunological, and clotting effects. The blood should be as fresh as possible and be given through a filter to remove particulate matter. There are numerous disadvantages to the use of whole blood, but the most serious is one discovered only recently. Stored blood is severely depleted of 2,3-diphosphoglyceric acid (2,3-DPG), which is im-

portant in regulating oxygen dissociation from hemoglobin. The net result of this is an increase in the affinity of hemoglobin for oxygen, resulting in impairment of oxygen unloading from hemoglobin in the periphery. Obviously, this decrease in oxyhemoglobin dissociation further compounds problems already present in tissues that are inadequately perfused. Also the problem is further compounded in hemodilutional states (hematocrit below 40 per cent). This finding serves as another reason to be cautious about use of excessive crystalloid solution in proportion to whole blood in the treatment of severe hemorrhage.

To monitor the requirements of patients who are severely injured requires several techniques. An indwelling bladder catheter is needed to measure urinary output. A catheter placed in the superior vena cava or right atrium through the antecubital vein is used to monitor central venous pressure (CVP). The importance of this monitoring aid cannot be overstressed, and its position should be documented by x-ray. These two parameters, plus pulse rate, blood pressure, and the clinical state of the patient, are almost always adequate guides for fluid and blood replacement therapy. If the urinary output is below 40 to 60 ml per hour, fluid replacement has not been adequate. A central venous pressure that rises appreciably with infusion of a few hundred millimeters of crystalloid solution usually indicates a full blood volume. On the other hand, a pressure that does not change with rapid infusion of blood indicates hypovolemia or an erroneous reading.

Three errors are commonly made in the use of central venous pressure monitoring in trauma patients. The position of the catheter is sometimes not confirmed. The absolute value of the central venous pressure is too often taken as an indication of the presence or absence of hypovolemia or normovolemia; the change in pressure is more valuable than an absolute value (unless it is elevated). Finally, perhaps most often, the central venous pressure is relied upon to detect fluid overload when crystalloid solutions are being administered. Gross overloading with salt solutions can occur with a normal central venous pressure. Crystalloid solutions expand the extracellular volume primarily, and a relatively small fraction remains in the plasma space if blood loss has been extensive. The central venous pressure does not measure changes in the interstitial space, which is where flooding occurs with the use of crystalloid solutions. The central venous catheter also allows measurement of central venous oxygen tension. A mixed venous Po_2 of 40 mm of mercury usually indicates functionally adequate circulation, while a value below 30 mm of mercury is seen in clinically significant low-flow states, and a value near 20 mm of mercury denotes a system that is barely supplying enough oxygen to support life.

Careful observations of these parameters, plus frequent determination of arterial blood gases, serum electrolytes, blood urea nitrogen, hemoglobin concentration, and hematocrit afford safe guides to management.

The question arises among neurosurgeons about the intracranial pressure during fluid replacement therapy. It has been shown that a balanced isotonic solution has little, if any, effect on the intracranial pressure even when large volumes are given rapidly.[12] Ten per cent of an animal's body weight given as lactated Ringer's solution in ten minutes produces no significant rise in intracranial pressure. This volume is equivalent to giving a patient 7 liters of fluid in 10 minutes. Hypotonic solutions such as 5 per cent dextrose in distilled water or half normal saline solution, however, will produce a rapid and prolonged rise in the intracranial pressure, particularly if given at rates exceeding 200 ml per hour.

The need for fluids other than whole blood and crystalloid solutions is rare in the management of hypovolemic shock. Plasma carries a significant risk of hepatitis or antigen-antibody reactions. It contains no hemoglobin, so does not contribute toward improved oxygenation. Like dextran, it remains largely in the intravascular space and does not replenish extracellular fluid loss. Low-molecular-weight dextran avoids the risk of hepatitis, but otherwise has no advantages over plasma. It has produced some clotting defects and may have renal toxicity. Both plasma and dextran are expensive. Lactated Ringer's solution is inexpensive, is readily available, has a composition similar to the extracellular fluid, and is an adjunct in the treatment of metabolic acidosis.

During shock, an adequate airway and adequate ventilation are important. The use of 100 per cent oxygen or of oxygen under tensions higher than atmospheric pressure has not, however, been shown to be beneficial as an isolated form of therapy. Oxygen should be used only in a supportive role.

The head-down position is detrimental and should be avoided. When a patient is placed in this position, the abdominal contents press against the diaphragm, limiting its excursions and reducing the efficiency of the patient's respiratory function. Since adrenal corticosteroids are increased during hypovolemic shock, the administration of exogenous adrenal corticoids usually is not warranted. In the circumstance of the patient's having received prior treatment with steroids, however, their use is strongly indicated. Hydrocortisone, 300 mg intravenously as a slow drip, should be given each 24 hours. Hypovolemic shock is produced by volume deficit, so digitalis will have no effect unless cardiac damage is pre-existent or has been induced by the injury.

Vasopressors have no role in the treatment of hypovolemic shock. The regulatory mechanisms of the body function adequately to produce vasoconstriction. More and more experimental and clinical evidence is becoming available that vasopressors are harmful.[28] For example, when they are used, the incidence of acute renal failure is much increased.

Animal experiments have suggested that hypothermia may be beneficial in the treatment of shock, but studies in man are meager. It is quite an undertaking to institute hypothermia, and the time needed to lower the temperature significantly could be put to better use.

Occasionally, despite measures that seem adequate to control the volume loss and to replace volume, the patient does not respond to therapy. Several causes of this refractory shock exist. Undetected continued loss of blood should be the first possibility investigated. A ruptured spleen or inferior vena cava may be present. Fluid replacement, thought adequate, may not be so. Cardiac tamponade, pneumothorax, or similar injuries may have been overlooked or may have developed since resuscitation began. Septic shock, shock lung, or myocardial insufficiency may have developed. In evaluating the patient apparently in refractory shock, every means to estimate the amount of fluid available for circulation and the ability of the cardiovascular system to deliver this fluid to the peripheral tissues must be used. Because of the fluid shifts that are occurring, the hemoglobin level and hematocrit may be misleading. Central venous pressure and urinary output should be measured, as they may help to define the problem. If the central venous pressure remains low, fluid replacement has likely been inadequate and more fluid is required, either blood, a salt solution, or both. If the venous pressure is elevated at the time of initial measurement, cardiac tamponade or pneumothorax should be suspected.

If low blood pressure persists despite additional infusion of blood and fluids, the problem may be complicated by cardiogenic shock. One clinical measure of the adequacy of perfusion of tissues, and therefore the heart, is urine output, a very sensitive indicator of renal perfusion. Urinary output above 20 to 40 ml per hour indicates adequate renal perfusion. Pulmonary capillary wedge pressure measured with a Swan-Ganz catheter is an even more sensitive indicator of cardiac failure. An estimate of cardiac output can be made from arteriovenous oxygen differences or, more accurately, from dye dilution according to the principles of Fick. Operatively remediable causes of decreased cardiac output, such as cardiac tamponade, pneumothorax, or pulmonary embolism, must be treated when found.

The use of alpha-adrenergic blocking agents (vasodilator drugs) in refractory hypovolemic shock is a concept that remains controversial.[28] The use of such drugs is more often mentioned in the context of septic shock. Once other remediable causes of refractory shock have been eliminated, this form of treatment might well be used. Patients with truly refractory shock apparently have maximum peripheral constriction. Peripheral pulses are absent, and there is cyanosis of the distal extremities. Despite the systemic hypotension present, central venous pressure is elevated and will rise further with additional fluid administration. Phenoxybenzamine (1 mg per kilogram) is used to produce vasodilation. Careful monitoring of the central venous pressure as this drug is given is very important. As the central venous pressure falls because of peripheral vasodilation, additional fluids (blood and lactated Ringer's) must be given. As the intravascular space is

expanded, fluid must be added to fill this space by replacement. If the replacement is not accomplished, perfusion of organs will be further reduced. The rate of fluid administration is dependent upon the rate of central venous pressure reduction. Central venous pressure should be maintained at about 8 cm of water. The object of this treatment is to increase the volume of the vascular system to normal levels and to reduce the vasoconstriction secondary to shock. Maintaining an adequate blood volume reduces cardiac strain, decreases the central venous pressure, and increases perfusion of organs, including the kidneys. Adequate therapy is indicated by increased magnitude of the palpable peripheral pulses, disappearance of cyanosis in and warming of the distal extremities, and increased formation of urine.

The use of isoproterenol and steroids, while advocated by some, has diminished in favor in the eyes of most experts in the treatment of hypovolemic shock. Steroids can potentiate the susceptibility to infection and stress ulceration, and isoproterenol is potentially arrhythmogenic and requires a large increase in coronary flow to accomplish an increase in cardiac output. While dopamine has been shown to increase cardiac output, blood pressure, and urine flow in patients unresponsive to other agents, volume replacement is clearly the first priority and is usually all that is necessary.[23]

Neurogenic Shock

In neurogenic shock, a normovolemic state exists, but with a greatly expanded cardiovascular space. Therefore, treatment should be directed at either increasing the volume or decreasing the size of the space. Often merely correcting the cause effects a cure. Benign forms of this disease, such as simple syncope, can be treated by simply moving the patient away from the stimulus or placing him in a supine position. Acute gastric dilation can be relieved by nasogastric suction. Obviously, peripheral sympathectomy from a high spinal cord injury cannot be corrected. The basic problem is decreased peripheral vascular resistance. Treatment is not indicated in many mild cases. Others will require an infusion of a liter or more of salt solution or vasopressors. It should be stressed that, in the management of neurogenic shock, fluid replacement should be used only secondarily, and careful monitoring of the central venous pressure will be of great value in determining the relative importance of fluids versus vasopressors in this disorder.

Most vasopressors in use at this time are catecholamines, which have inotropic, chronotropic, and peripheral vasal effects. The biochemical and pharmacological basis for these effects is based on the type of adrenergic receptor sites (alpha or beta) found in the tissue in question (heart or peripheral or visceral vessels) and the relative action of the drug in question on each type of receptor. The heart has only beta receptors, which when activated by drugs with strong affinity for them (isoproterenol and epinephrine), respond by increasing the rate (chronotropic effect) and contractility (inotropic effect). Arteries of skin and mucosa have only alpha receptors and will respond to drugs having strong alpha activity (methoxamine and norepinephrine). Arteries of skeletal muscle and abdominal viscera have both alpha and beta receptors, which when stimulated, produce vasoconstriction or vasodilatation, respectively. Systemic veins, likewise, contain both types of receptors, but stimulation of either type of receptor produces constriction.

Since in neurogenic shock the predominant need is for the peripheral vasoconstricting effect, the drugs of choice are those that are predominantly vasopressors with little cardiac effect. Phenylephrine hydrochloride (Neo-Synephrine) is primarily an alpha agonist that produces little effective inotropic response and is, therefore, predominantly a peripheral vasopressor. It is the drug of choice in this disorder. Usually 50 mg in 1000 ml of 5 per cent dextrose in water or a balanced salt solution is adequate for good titration (0.5 to 1.5 ml per minute) of blood pressure in patients who have high spinal anesthesia or other forms of neurogenic shock. Drugs such as levarterenol bitartrate (Levophed) and methoxamine (Vasoxyl) produce intense peripheral vasoconstriction and should not be used. Isoproterenol hydrochloride (Isuprel), a pure beta agonist, has strong cardiac effects, produces peripheral vasodilatation, and, therefore, is contraindicated for neurogenic shock.

Septic Shock

The treatment of septic shock requires management of both the infection and the shock.[4,10,29] Therapy of septic shock is much more controversial than that of either cardiogenic or hypovolemic shock, and the mortality rate remains greater than 50 per cent in most series.

Prevention is critical and is undoubtedly possible in many patients. Long-term, indiscriminate use of prophylactic antibiotics must be avoided. Careful attention must be given to the nutrition of seriously ill patients. Prompt correction of blood volume deficits, careful sterile techniques with indwelling lines and catheters and during pulmonary care procedures, judicious use of corticosteroids and immunosuppressive drugs, and an alert infection control committee can reduce the incidence of septic shock.

The prime factor in treating septic shock is early clinical recognition. High-risk patients must be recognized and the diagnosis suspected in its early stages so that supportive measures can be mobilized to reverse the effects of inadequate perfusion. Unexplained hyperventilation, tachycardia, confusion, and fever must be interpreted as impending bacteremia and possible septic shock until proved otherwise. Appropriate monitoring and treatment should be instituted immediately. Cultures of blood, urine, sputum, and matter from all wounds must be done. The presence of an abscess or similar source of infection is an indication for drainage, removal of intravenous lines from inflamed vessels, and the like.

Once cultures have been obtained, antibiotic administration should be begun promptly. Local hospital experience should serve as a guide in the choice of antibiotics, but a combination of cephalothin and gentamicin is usually a good initial regimen. If a large bowel source is suspected, clindamycin can be added to combat *Bacteroides* species.

Pulmonary insufficiency occurs frequently and makes the administration of oxygen mandatory; intubation and mechanical ventilation are often required. Frequent monitoring of arterial blood gases and careful recording of urine output are important. Careful assessment of the hemodynamic status is obtained via a central venous line, a Swan-Ganz catheter to measure pulmonary capillary wedge pressure, and an intra-arterial needle.

Patients with gram-negative bacteremia are likely to have low arterial blood pressure associated with low cardiac output and evidence of increased arterial resistance. Central venous pressure and pulmonary capillary wedge pressure may be low initially, but infusion of crystalloids sufficient to elevate cardiac filling pressure, as evidenced by these measurements, does not restore hemodynamic stability. Lactic acidemia, reduced urine output, coagulation abnormalities, and increased oxygen consumption (manifested by widened arteriovenous oxygen differences) develop. Thus, the pathophysiological picture represents a combination of depressed myocardial function and altered venous capacitance with peripheral pooling of blood that is not fully responsive to volume infusion. This combination of findings is the presentation of hypodynamic septic shock—a primary hemodynamic defect.

Specific treatment of this form of septic shock requires appropriate measures in addition to the volume replacement. Digitalis remains an excellent inotropic drug and should be given promptly. Isoproterenol and dopamine are both beta adrenergic agents and are useful in this state when given as a constant infusion and with careful electrocardiographic monitoring. Dopamine appears to have more inotropic action and produces fewer arrhythmias and less tachycardia. Both drugs serve to dilate arterioles in muscle, kidneys, and abdominal viscera, and to constrict systemic veins, thereby improving peripheral blood flow and venous pooling. Phenoxybenzamine is also favored by many to further relieve the peripheral vasoconstrictor component by its alpha adrenergic blocking activity. An infusion of 1 mg per kilogram in 100 to 200 ml of fluid over a one-hour period is recommended.

Patients with gram-positive bacteremia, peritonitis complicated by bacteremia, or bacteremia in the presence of cirrhosis may manifest a circulatory picture that is termed hyperdynamic septic shock. It is a low-resistance type of shock associated with inflammatory vasodilatation and peripheral and pulmonary arteriovenous shunting. High cardiac output is seen; however, a serious perfusion deficit is present and results in profound lactic acidemia and depressed oxygen consumption.

Hyperdynamic shock appears to be based on a primary metabolic deficit with secondary failure of compensation by the circulatory system.

Specific treatment in this case again requires removal of the source of sepsis, administration of antibiotics, pulmonary support, and restoration of blood volume to assure adequate cardiac ventricular filling pressures as monitored by central venous and pulmonary capillary wedge pressures. Treatment of this form of septic shock usually is less successful than treatment of ordinary septic shock.

Corticosteroids are advocated by some and condemned by many others as agents to use in all forms of septic shock. They may exert a beneficial effect by stabilizing lysosomal membranes and preventing destruction in intracellular organelles. Their direct hemodynamic effects, vasodilatation and inotropism, are controversial. Considering the many undesirable side effects of steroids, their use, even in septic shock, can be recommended only when all else has been to little or no avail.

Therefore, treatment of septic shock must be based on prevention, identification of high-risk patients, early diagnosis, prompt drainage of foci of infection, antibiotic coverage after cultures have been obtained, volume replacement, pulmonary support, and use of drugs appropriate to the specific hemodynamic defects that are present.

ACUTE RENAL FAILURE

Etiology, Diagnosis, and Clinical Course

The causes of anuric renal failure in traumatized patients include ischemia from hypovolemic shock, transfusion reactions, myoglobinuria, the crush syndrome, and hyperbilirubinemia.[23,39,41] For convenience, acute renal failure secondary to trauma can be subdivided into prerenal, renal and postrenal clinical groups.

Prerenal failure can result from hypovolemia caused by hemorrhage after trauma, sequestration due to crush injuries, or post-traumatic peritonitis. A second class of prerenal failure results from cardiovascular failure secondary to myocardial failure due to infarction or tamponade, or secondary to vascular pooling, as occurs in sepsis. Regardless of cause, prerenal factors produce hypotension and a marked reduction in renal blood flow. This results in a concomitant diminution in glomular filtration rate (GFR) leading to progressive azotemia. An increased fractional resorption of the glomerular filtrate by renal tubules gives rise to marked oliguria. Early correction of the derangements that result in prerenal failure prevents ensuing renal damage; delay in recognition and treatment may result in development of acute tubular necrosis.

Renal causes of acute renal failure in trauma are several, but the final common denominator is acute tubular necrosis. This pathological entity underlies approximately 75 per cent of all cases of acute renal failure. In patients with severe injury it is most commonly a postischemic process resulting from any or all of the factors noted in the preceeding paragraph. Other causes include hemepigments resulting from intravascular hemolysis (e.g., transfusion reaction), rhabdomyolysis, and myoglobinuria, and nephrotoxins including drugs such as kanamyin and colistin that are used in injured patients. Other post-traumatic causes of primary renal damage include traumatic thrombosis of renal artery or vein and fulminant renal cortical necrosis secondary to severe renal hemorrhage, infarction, or injury. Renal cortical necrosis may be clinically indistinguishable from acute tubular necrosis but is a distinct pathological entity whose diagnosis is possible via renal biopsy.

The last category of post-traumatic causes of renal failure are classified as postrenal. These may result from obstruction of the urinary passages by extrinsic compression from hematomas and displaced bony fragments, or intrinsic blockage by massive blood clots or sloughed renal papillae. Disruption of urinary conduits, including intraperitoneal rupture of the bladder and inappropriate surgical ligation or resection of a ureter, is another postrenal cause of acute renal failure associated with severe injury.

Finally it should be recalled that in as many as 30 per cent of patients with acute renal failure, no cause may be apparent.

In spite of vigorous clinical and laboratory study, the pathogenesis of acute renal failure remains undetermined. Briefly summarized, renal ischemia is the most common precursor of acute tubular necrosis and resultant acute renal failure. Through a process of autoregulation mediated by renal arteriolar smooth muscle (probably controlled to a great extent by intrarenal release of prostaglandins) renal blood flow (RBF), total kidney glomerular filtration rate, and single nephron glomerular filtration rate tend to remain constant down to arterial perfusion pressures of about 30 mm of mercury. At pressures below this these rates decrease progressively, and by the time perfusion pressure reaches 45 mm of mercury most species become anuric. Thus, at perfusion pressures below 30 mm of mercury renal vascular resistance appears to be relatively fixed and minimal.

In postischemic acute renal failure, therefore, initial hemodynamic insufficiency (e.g., in hypovolemia or shock) directly causes renal ischemia, which in turn leads to a decrease in glomerular filtration rate and urine flow. The renal ischemia, then, somehow becomes self-perpetuating. This persistent reduction in renal blood flow appears to be the principal mechanism of renal insufficiency. In severe postischemic and in nephrotoxic renal failure, tubule cell necrosis is often prominent histologically and may cause backleak of filtrate and obstruction of tubules by cell debris. Precipitation of pigments or mucoproteins in oliguric tubules may also contribute to intratubular obstruction. Current knowledge has shifted the emphasis from tubule cell necrosis to persistent ischemia as the central feature of typical acute renal failure, but has not completely eliminated backleak of filtrate and tubule obstruction as significant mechanisms of oliguria.

While the clinical hallmarks of acute renal failure are oliguria and rapidly progressive azotemia, other presentations are possible. It is rare for a prerenal or renal lesion to result in complete anuria, and any patient presenting with anuria or severe oliguria (less than 50 ml per day) should be considered to have renal failure of postrenal etiology until this diagnosis is eliminated. Ruling out a post-renal cause is best accomplished by radiography, as discussed later in this chapter, and excluding a postrenal lesion is important because considerable improvement usually promptly follows relief of obstruction.

As a practical matter, urine flow of less than 400 ml per day (less than 20 ml per hour according to some authorities) is considered to represent oliguria. It should be recalled, however, that low urine flow of this magnitude can also result from either appropriate or inappropriate release of antidiuretic hormone in response to injury, anesthesia, or operation; or from a fluid regimen that is inadequate to match losses. "Rapidly" progressive azotemia is less rigidly defined, but with significant acute renal failure plasma creatinine levels rise at least 0.5 mg per 100 ml per day and blood urea nitrogen (BUN) at least 10 mg per 100 ml per day. It should be kept in mind that acute renal failure can present in a nonoliguric form. Further, the blood urea nitrogen level can rise because the rate of protein catabolism increases, and plasma creatinine concentration rarely may rise because of rhabdomyolysis. For practical purposes, however, progressive increase of plasma creatinine over several days is a good clinical index of acute renal failure even in the absence of oliguria. The cause of acute renal failure can usually be determined by commonly available diagnostic tests properly selected and interpreted.

While it may seem obvious, it is necessary to exclude simple urinary retention of the bladder. This may be done by a careful one-time catheterization, the catheter being removed promptly after exclusion of retention to avoid introducing infection.

A plain film of the abdomen with tomography, if necessary, aids in defining renal size and helps to exclude obstruction by calcified stones. Kidney size is normal or increased in acute renal failure, as opposed to being reduced in chronic renal failure. The diagnosis of pre-existing chronic renal disease is only occasionally possible by history alone. Modern infusion urography has proved safe even in oliguric acute renal failure and will show an immediate, dense, and persistent nephrogram in acute tubular necrosis unlike that in other forms of acute renal failure. While the kidney is not visualized, the nephrogram itself should allow detection of dilated calices and provide the diagnosis of obstructive uropathy. Retrograde studies may, however, still be vital in some patients to determine the locus of obstruction and in those in whom results of in-travenous pyelography are uncertain. Once the diagnosis of obstruction is excluded, other tests must be performed to determine the cause of the renal failure.

Careful review of the hospital record is an important initial step. It may reflect evidence of inadequate fluid administration. In assessing this possibility, critical attention must be paid to insensible losses and the possible presence of third-space losses. Fluid overloading may also be evident if it is determined that the patient is, in fact, in acute renal failure. In evaluating urine flow, it must be recalled that as many as 15 per cent of patients (33 per cent in some series of severe cases) with post-traumatic acute renal failure are nonoliguric (defined as having urine volume of over 400 ml per day).

Examination of urinary sediment can be very helpful in differential diagnosis. In prerenal failure, moderate numbers of hyaline and finely granular casts may be seen, but cellular or coarsely granular casts are unusual. If acute tubular necrosis supervenes, the sediment becomes more characteristic with "dirty" brown granular casts and epithelial cells, free and in casts. Such characteristic sediment may be appreciated in 80 per cent of oliguric and 70 per cent of nonoliguric patients. Red blood cell and hemepigmented casts are unusual except in cases of hemoglobinuria or myoglobinuria. Instead, the latter usually point to primary glomerular or vascular disease. A benign sediment should make the presence of obstruction strongly suspected.

The physiochemical composition of urine is often helpful in separating prerenal failure from acute tubular necrosis. A random urinary sodium concentration is low (usually less than 10 mEq per liter) in prerenal failure but is elevated (at least to 25 mEq per liter) in acute tubular necrosis. An exception to this rule is nonoliguric acute tubular necrosis in which urine sodium is less consistently increased. Urine osmolality and specific gravity tend to be high in prerenal failure, whereas isosthenuria is typical of acute tubular necrosis, with a specific gravity of usually 1.010 to 1.015. Urinary to plasma (U/P) osmolality ratios of 1:1 or less are characteristic of acute tubular necrosis. Patients with such ratios do not respond to volume expansion. An exception is the elderly patient who may fail to concentrate the urine with prerenal failure. This elderly patient will, however, still have the low urine sodium concentration of prerenal failure. Also of considerable help are the urine to plasma ratios of urea and creatinine. In prerenal failure the urine to plasma urea ratio exceeds 20:1, whereas in acute tubular necrosis it is usually 3:1 or less and very rarely exceeds 10:1. In prerenal failure the urine to plasma creatinine ratio is usually 40:1 or more, and rarely less than 10:1; in acute tubular necrosis, the ratio is nearly always less than 10:1.

The administration of mannitol has been advocated both as a diagnostic test and as therapy in oliguric patients. This is of value only in the first 48 hours after the appearance of oliguria; mannitol is not effective after acute tubular necrosis has developed. It is given as 20 to 25 gm of 20 per cent solution over a 20-minute period. Absence of a prompt diuresis confirms the presence of intrinsic renal damage. If diuresis ensues, usually within 30 minutes, some evidence suggests that this therapy may prevent progression to acute tubular necrosis. If there is concern about fluid overload secondary to mannitol, one may use intravenous furosemide or ethacrynic acid in the same diagnostic and therapeutic fashion, since neither produces expansion of the blood volume. If 40 mg furosemide or 50 mg ethacrynic acid produces diuresis, they can be repeated in two to four hours at the same dosage. While the efficacy of mannitol and loop diuretics is controversial, most would agree that they should be used to maintain high rates of urine flow after muscle-crushing injuries, mismatched transfusions, rapid intravascular hemolysis, or acute hyperuricemia.

Once acute tubular necrosis is confirmed it can be expected to proceed, clinically, in three phases: oliguric, diuretic, and recovery. The oliguric phase usually begins within a day of the inciting event, but may be delayed for up to a week after nephrotoxic insults. This phase commonly lasts one to two weeks but ranges from a few hours to several weeks. When it extends past four weeks, cortical necrosis, glomerulonephritis, or vasculitis must be suspected rather than acute tubular necrosis. Daily urine output averages about 150 ml but may be less in the first few days. As noted, however, anuria (less than 50 ml per day) is very rare. Azotemia, with proper management, progresses largely at a rate governed by the degree of protein catabolism to produce elevation in the blood urea nitrogen level of 10 to 20 mg per 100 ml per day and in the plasma creatinine level of 0.5 to 1.0 mg per 100 ml per day. Extensive tissue trauma or sepsis may produce blood urea nitrogen increases of as much as 100 mg per 100 ml per day; while severe muscle trauma can yield elevations of the creatinine level at a rate of 2 mg per 100 ml per day. Salt and water overload are ever-present dangers. It must be remembered that normal metabolic processes provide an endogenous source of more than 500 ml of water daily, and tissue catabolism results in decreases of weight of 0.2 to 0.5 kg per day. Hyponatremia may result from excessive water intake.

Hyperkalemia will occur even in the absence of exogenous sources of potassium. This increase in potassium level will proceed at a rate of less than 0.5 mEq per liter per day except in patients with severe tissue trauma, large hematomas, or sepsis; in these the rate may be as high as 1 to 2 mEq per liter per day. Advanced hyperkalemia may result in ventricular fibrillation or cardiac arrest. The most prominent electrocardiographic features are elevated, peaked T waves followed by prolonged QRS complexes, then prolonged P-R intervals, and, finally, complete heart block. These changes will be potentiated by hyponatremia, hypocalcemia, and acidosis. Acidosis results from metabolic production of fixed acid and will be manifested by falls in plasma bicarbonate of 1 to 2 mEq per liter per day. Hypocalcemia in the range of 6.3 to 8.3 mg per 100 ml is usual and may occur as early as two days after the onset of oliguria. Along with this hyperphosphatemia of as much as 8 mg per 100 ml is common. Even though cardiac arrhythmias and congestive heart failure are common in acute renal failure, specific cardiac intoxication is not seen.

Neurological and psychiatric manifestations of acute uremia may be quite varied. Prominent features may include lethargy, confusion, stupor, and coma; agitation; hyperreflexia, twitching, and asterixis; and abnormal behavior that includes anxiety and paranoia. Convulsions in the absence of water intoxication are infrequent. All of the foregoing are rare in appropriately dialyzed patients.

Gastrointestinal disorders are more common and frequently include anorexia, nausea, and vomiting. Erosive gastric ulcers are not uncommon and, especially when coupled with the bleeding dyscrasia of acute uremia, may produce gastrointestinal bleeding. Hematological manifestations include progressive anemia, leukocytosis, and platelet abnormalities. These last result from both qualitative defects and decreased production. They, combined with decreases in various coagulation factors, are possible causes of the bleeding disorder noted with acute renal failure. Frequent infections and poor wound healing are also associated conditions.

A progressive increase in urine volume signals beginning recovery of renal function. Typically, this is noted at a rate resulting in daily doubling of urine volume to a level of 1 liter by the third day of the diuretic phase. More rapid or less abrupt increases are not uncommon, however. Although this increase in urine volume portends impending recovery, renal function remains distinctly abnormal. The persistent reduction in glomerular filtration rate is manifested clinically by failure of the blood urea nitrogen and creatinine levels to fall, and in some cases rises may persist for several days at the beginning of this phase. Late in this phase daily urinary output may exceed 2 liters for several days. While past experience found this polyuric phase frequently resulting in major disturbances of body fluid volume and composition as a result of inadequate regulatory capacity of the kidney, the current use of regular dialysis during the oliguric phase more effectively prevents the overhydration and subsequent massive diuresis commonly reported in older series. Frequent, careful adjustment of fluid and electrolyte administration remains essential to prevent production of deficits or excesses in hydration and sodium and potassium levels while abnormalities of glomerular and tubule function persist in varying degrees. Further, infection, gastrointestinal bleeding, and cardiovascular disturbance may still occur.

A prolonged recovery phase of 3 to 12 months then ensues, resulting in renal function compatible with normal health in all but a few patients. The glomerular filtration rate, however, becomes completely normal in only a minority and may remain 20 to 40 per cent below normal for at least a year after the oliguric phase. Prolonged oliguria probably lessens the extent of functional recovery. Tubular function also usually remains below par, resulting in permanent impairment of maximum concentrating ability. Histological changes become minimal to none at all. Incidence of infection and hypertension are not significantly increased.

The major determinant of survival in patients with oliguric acute renal failure is the nature of the condition precipitating the renal insufficiency. About 60 per cent of patients developing acute tubular necrosis after operation or trauma die, whereas about 30 per cent with medical causes, such as exposure to nephrotoxins, and only 10 per cent with obstetrical complications fail to recover. Younger patients tend to fare better than the elderly. In the past poor understanding of fluid and electrolyte management that resulted in pulmonary and cerebral edema, potassium intoxication, and "uremia" were the main causes of death. Today, infections and the primary illness that precipitated the renal failure have become the chief causes of death.

A brief comment about nonoliguric acute tubular necrosis is necessary. These patients have urine volume ranging from 400 ml to 1 liter per day. Since oliguria is not present, many such patients whose blood and urine chemistry is not being closely monitored are probably missed. The absence of oliguria, the ability to excrete urine low in sodium concentration, and the less striking abnormalities in the urinary sediment indicate less severe damage to the renal tubules in these patients than in those with oliguric acute tubular necrosis. The urine to plasma osmolality ratio does not exceed 1:2 in these patients, suggesting tubule dysfunction. While nonoliguric acute tubular necrosis occurs as a consequence of all the conditions implicated in the oliguric form, the former is seen in particular in association with nephrotoxins, burns, and operations. The nonoliguric patients tend to have a more benign clinical course consistent with less severe renal disease; they less commonly require dialysis. In spite of this, careful monitoring of fluid intake is necessary, since uring output, although in the "normal" range, does not show normal response to physiological stimuli. As a result fluid loads can easily precipitate pulmonary edema. Although the renal damage is apparently less severe, 20 to 25 per cent of patients with nonoliguric acute tubular necrosis, like those with the oliguric form, die because of the underlying condition or infection. Should a nonoliguric patient become oliguric after a few days, the prognosis is particularly poor.

Prophylaxis and Treatment of Acute Renal Failure

Acute tubular necrosis usually occurs in predictable settings; anticipation is the key. Postischemic acute tubular necrosis can be prevented by prompt and sufficient replacement of blood and fluid losses in severely injured patients. Equally important is early, effective management of septic and cardiogenic shock. Cautious prescription of potentially nephrotoxic drugs is a particularly important way for physicians to reduce the incidence of acute renal failure. The use of mannitol or furosemide or both in prevention of acute tubular necrosis has already been discussed in the section on differential diagnosis.

Should prevention be unsuccessful, the first principle of good management is to identify the causes of acute renal failure that are possibly reversible by specific treatment. In traumatized patients these will most often include obstructive uropathy and renal vascular obstruction. Once it has been determined that the renal failure is caused by acute tubular necrosis, there is no specific treatment available.[39,41] The principles of management are few, but important: (1) accurate maintenance of body water, (2) correction of any change in ionic components, (3) suppression of protein metabolism, (4) maintenance of adequate caloric intake, and (5) avoidance of use of drugs that are nephrotoxic or excreted by the kidney.

Volume deficits should be corrected even if acute tubular necrosis has supervened in order to improve the circulation, but not with any hope that this will reverse the renal failure. Daily weight and serum sodium determinations are important aids in calculating total body water. Increase in weight indicates water excess, while decreasing weight and a rising serum sodium level indicate a deficit. Water loss should be calculated carefully, including the urinary output, gastrointestinal loss either by suc-

tion or diarrhea, and insensible loss through the lungs and skin. Insensible loss of water is markedly increased with fever or sepsis. Replacement of water should be based on the calculated water loss, literally volume for volume. Appropriate fluid intake is judged by a loss of about 0.5 kg per day of weight (due to tissue catabolism) and a normal serum sodium level.

The chief ionic shifts involve potassium, as it accumulates from protein breakdown. It is increased in states of hypermetabolism associated with infection, acidosis, and hypoxia. Potassium is also reabsorbed from blood in the gastrointestinal tract. Daily determination of serum potassium is mandatory. Sodium and potassium are provided only to replace losses. The patient's diet should be protein-free. Protein catabolism is controlled by giving an adequate caloric intake in the form of fats and carbohydrates so that protein breakdown is not required. Obviously, the food given should contain no sodium or potassium. Approximately 1000 to 1500 calories per day can be given in a diet of ginger ale, sugar water, rock candy, butter balls, and butter soup if the patient is able to take them orally. A minimum of 100 gm of carbohydrate should be given daily. If intravenous fluids must be used, infusions containing as much as 25 per cent glucose can be used. The volume of fluid must be carefully controlled in order not to overload the patient, and limiting the quantity of fluid often requires the use of hypertonic glucose solutions. Recent evidence suggests that infusion of a mixture of hypertonic glucose and essential amino acids decreases the mortality rate and speeds the recovery of patients with acute tubular necrosis. Androgens such as testosterone or norethandrolone may further reduce protein catabolism, particularly in women.

Slow daily increases of potassium (up to plasma levels of 5.5 to 6.5 mEq per liter) can be controlled by the use of cation exchange resins, preferably of the sodium cycle (Kayexalate), administered orally or by retention enema. An oral dose of 15 to 20 gm every 12 hours should be given with 20 ml of 70 per cent sorbitol solution. For rectal administration use 50 gm in a mixture of 50 ml of 70 per cent sorbitol and 100 ml of tap water. The sorbitol serves to prevent impactions and to remove sodium released from the resin in loose stools.

For moderate hyperkalemia (plasma levels of 6.5 to 7.5 mEq per liter and electrocardiographic findings of peaked T waves) prompt intravenous treatment, accomplished by infusion of 10 per cent glucose, is necessary. Give about 300 to 400 ml over a one-hour period and another 600 to 700 ml during the next two to three hours. Ten to fifteen units of regular insulin is suggested, particularly in diabetic patients. Effects are seen within 30 minutes. For patients with coexistent acidosis and no evidence of fluid overload, two or three ampules of sodium bicarbonate are added to the 1-liter infusion. This infusion can be repeated as needed so long as oliguric patients are not overloaded.

In patients with severe hyperkalemia (plasma levels over 7.5 mEq per liter or absence of P waves, prolonged QRS complex, or ventricular arrhythmias in the electrocardiogram), the cardiac intoxication is most rapidly managed by calcium infusion. While the electrocardiogram is observed continuously, 10 to 30 ml of calcium gluconate is given intravenously at 2 ml per minute. This treatment usually is effective within five minutes, but its results are temporary and it must be followed by the hypertonic glucose regimen just outlined.

While dialysis effectively removes potassium, it may take several hours to do so. Therefore, dialysis is primarily a prophylactic tool; immediate therapy of moderate to severe hyperkalemia requires the foregoing measures.

Other electrolytes should be administered after accurate measurements of loss. Daily or more frequent determination of serum calcium levels is mandatory. Hypocalcemia occurs regularly, but it is difficult to correct with intravenous calcium preparations. Rapid deposition of calcium in the bone and skeletal muscle occurs during uremia. The most effective measure for maintaining adequate calcium levels is to have the patient ambulatory as soon as possible.

The use of drugs in patients with renal failure needs comment.[3] The potassium and sodium content of drugs should be carefully noted so that the electrolyte management of the patient can be accurately followed. For instance, large doses of potassium penicillin can result in significant hyperkalemia. Drugs requiring renal excretion should be carefully used, as toxic levels may be rapidly reached in the absence of excretion.

The dose of streptomycin, kanamycin, or colistin, for example, in a person with acute renal failure will be approximately 25 to 50 per cent of the usual daily dose. The usual dose of tetracycline may be reduced 20 per cent. Chloramphenicol and erythromycin are exceptions in that, in large part, they are metabolized by the liver, so the daily dose is usually not changed by renal failure. Phenobarbital is excreted in part by the kidney, so the dose should be reduced; phenytoin, however, as a result of shortened half-life and reduced binding to plasma proteins offsetting one another, can usually be given in normal dosages.

The management of the patient with nonoliguric renal failure is somewhat less demanding than that of the one with oliguric renal failure. The most important aspect is to insure adequate fluid intake to replace the urinary and other measurable losses of water. Five per cent dextrose in water, volume for volume of output, is used for this purpose. A balanced salt solution such as normal saline or lactated Ringer's is used to replace electrolyte-containing fluid lost from the gastrointestinal tract or in sweat. The amount of replacement should be carefully determined, taking into account serum electrolyte levels and known losses. The blood urea nitrogen (BUN) and potassium levels should be determined serially or daily, as uremia and hyperkalemia may occur in this disorder. Although the potassium and blood urea nitrogen levels usually do not rise as high as they do in the oliguric patient, they may be high enough to require dialysis or the use of exchange resins to prevent their reaching toxic concentrations.

Although patients without complications can be managed by the foregoing conservative measures and occasional dialysis for specific indications, most nephrologists advocate a more vigorous use of dialysis, particularly in oliguric patients. The use of routine, periodic dialysis simplifies the overall management and improves the well-being of patients. Fluid and dietary intake can be more liberal, with resultant improvement in nutrition. The frequency of dialysis varies with patients. Some hypercatabolic patients require daily hemodialysis to control hyperkalemia, acidosis, and uremic symptoms. In patients who have no complications, dialysis two or three times a week may be adequate—the frequency is governed by the interval required to keep the blood urea nitrogen below 100 mg per 100 ml. As much as 20 to 40 gm of protein and 1 liter of fluid per day can be given to patients on such a regimen. Generally, in uncomplicated cases, the first dialysis is peritoneal. This method of management allows for a few days of observation to determine whether the oliguria will be of short duration. Peritoneal dialysis is inefficient, however, and the risk of peritonitis is significant. Therefore, an arteriovenous shunt for standard hemodialysis is placed at once in hypercatabolic patients and after it is clear that oliguria will not promptly resolve in others. Although patients feel better on such an aggressive regimen, no definite evidence is available to support a significant reduction in the mortality rate.

Infection and associated primary disease remain the major causes of death in most centers. Dialysis has not affected these statistics. Since the cause of the propensity for and severity of infections in acute renal failure remains obscure, prevention is the hallmark of care. Currently, control of infection depends on the usual principles: avoidance of intravenous and urinary catheters whenever feasible, good pulmonary toilet, mouth care, and careful, aseptic techniques for handling endotracheal and tracheostomy tubes. The use of reverse isolation is debatable, since any advantages it may have are usually offset by resultant decreased attention by the medical staff.

CRUSH INJURIES

The Syndrome

A patient who is admitted with an apparently relatively minor injury may die several days later from major complications of that injury. This course is not unusual in patients with major crush injuries. Although the pathophysiology of this disorder is still poorly understood, the clinical syndrome is well recognized. Bywaters, who studied several patients trapped in the debris of a bombed building in London during World War II, gives a very vivid description of this syndrome.

The patient has been buried for several hours with pressure on a limb. On admission he looks in good condition except for swelling of the limb with some local anesthesia and whealing. The hemoglobin, however, is raised and a few hours later, despite vasoconstriction made manifest by pallor, coldness and sweating, the pressure falls. This is restored to preshock level by (often multiple) transfusions of serum, plasma, or occasionally blood. Anxiety may now arise concerning the circulation of the injured limb, which may show diminution of arterial pulsation distally accompanied by all the changes of incipient gangrene. Signs of renal damage soon appear and progress even though the crushed limb be amputated. The urinary output, initially small, owing perhaps to the severity of shock, diminishes further. The urine contains albumin and many dark brown or black granular casts. These later decrease in number. The patient is alternatively drowsy and anxiously aware of the severity of his illness. Slight generalized edema, thirst, and incessant vomiting develop, and blood pressure often remains slightly raised. The blood urea and potassium, raised at an early stage, become progressively high, and death occurs comparatively suddenly, frequently within a week. Necropsy reveals necrosis of muscle and, in the renal tubules, degenerative changes and casts containing brown pigment.[17]

Originally, this syndrome was related only to a major crushing injury to an extremity. Recently, however, there have been reports of its development after arterial repair to an extremity when temporary vascular occlusion has been used, or after an embolic occlusion of a major artery to the extremity.[30] These observations have given rise to the concept that the initial episode of shock is due to rapid sequestration of large volumes of extracellular fluid and blood into the previously ischemic extremity. This is hypovolemic shock and responds to appropriate therapy. Following the initial episode, the patient recovers for 24 to 48 hours and seems to be doing well, and then a second shock phase ensues. This second phase is relatively refractory to treatment. Its cause seems to be the release of fixed intracellular acids. Probably more significant is the release of protein substances, chiefly myoglobin, which is precipitated in the renal tubules. The precipitate in the tubules effectively blocks them, producing oliguria. The renal failure that follows the episode of myoglobinemia may prove fatal.

Myoglobinuria

A patient with a crushing injury who develops oliguria and a dark-colored urine should undergo investigation to differentiate between primary renal damage and myoglobinuria. If the patient has received a recent blood transfusion, the picture may be further obscured, as renal failure after myoglobinuria is similar to that following a transfusion reaction. The differential diagnosis includes primary renal injury, transfusion reaction, and myoglobinuria secondary to crush injury.

Several simple laboratory examinations can help make the differentiation. Microscopic examination of the urine will reveal large numbers of red cells in primary renal injury. In a transfusion reaction the patient's serum will show evidence of hemolysis, while the serum of a patient with myoglobinuria is usually clear.

It is possible to identify myoglobin in the urine.[14] The screening technique is relatively simple. The urine is centrifuged, then 3 ml of 3 per cent sulfosalicylic acid is added to 1 ml of the supernatant, and the mixture is boiled. This process produces precipitation of the protein. If a red precipitate forms, it is either myoglobin or hemoglobin. At this point, the rare causes of discolored urine such as porphyria, dyes, or drugs have been eliminated. The further differentiation between myoglobin and hemoglobin is made by adding 2.8 mg of ammonium sulfate to 5 ml of the cell-free urine. The mixture is then either centrifuged or filtered. Hemoglobin is precipitated by ammonium sulfate, leaving the supernatant color-free. If no precipitation occurs, then the cause of the urinary discoloration is myoglobin. More sophisticated determinations of the exact amount of myoglobin can be made by using spectrophotometric, chromographic, or resin column techniques. These techniques are time consuming, and although they are useful for confirmation, treatment must be started before they are completed.

The object in treating myoglobinuria is to prevent acute renal failure. Therapy is directed toward combating the second shock phase of the crush syndrome that accompanies excretion of the myoglobin pigment. Prevention of intrarenal precipitation of the pigment and of further release of myoglobin from the injured limb are the foremost considerations. The involved extremity may be swollen out of proportion to the original injury. Early, the swelling might have been prevented by fasciotomy, but by the time the myoglobin appears in the urine, it is too late for fasciotomy, and

amputation must be done and should be carried out as soon as the diagnosis is made. In order to reduce the amount of myoglobin that is released, physiological amputation should precede operative amputation. Once the decision to amputate is made, the extremity is packed in ice and separated from the systemic circulation by a tight tourniquet. When the patient's condition is stabilized, operative removal of the limb is performed.

Fluid that has been sequestered into the extremity must be replaced. The volume is calculated on the basis of a general rule. If the leg is involved, 1 to 1.5 liters of balanced salt solution is given for each 1-inch increase in the circumference of the thigh. For upper extremity injuries, 500 to 1000 ml is given for each 1-inch increase in the circumference of the upper arm. This volume is adequate to replace the systemic deficits from sequestration and will promote diuresis. The diuresis dilutes the urine, reducing precipitation of the protein in the renal tubules. Diuresis is further enhanced by the administration of 20 per cent mannitol and one-sixth molar sodium lactate solution or 10 per cent dextrose in water or both. Approximately 2 liters of each may be required over the next 24 to 48 hours. The diuresis must be maintained as long as there is myoglobin in the urine.

If laboratory or clinical evidence of acidosis develops, then 40 to 80 mEq of sodium bicarbonate should be added per liter of fluid given. This serves the double purpose of combating the systemic acidosis while maintaining an alkaline urine. An acid urine increases precipitation of myoglobin in the renal tubules.

Accurate intake and output records must be kept during the administration of large volumes of intravenous fluid. While the patient is undergoing diuresis, overinfusion must be avoided. A fine balance must be maintained between overload on one hand and inadequate diuresis on the other. If renal tubule damage has already begun and renal failure is imminent, overload may be fatal. Similarly, inadequate fluid replacement may lead to renal damage.

Hyperbilirubinemia

Hyperbilirubinemia is a rare complication suffered by patients with multiple injuries when shock has been a prominent feature of the clinical course and several transfusions have been given. The hyperbilirubinemia is thought to be due to the release of hemoglobin and hemoglobin-like substances from the injured tissues, from hematomas, and from the rapid hemolysis of old bank blood.[32] The syndrome appears during the second week of injury and may last one to two weeks. Marked elevation in the serum bilirubin level is noted, with values of 30 mg per 100 ml or more being reported. Most of the bilirubin is in the conjugated form. Serum alkaline phosphatase levels are elevated. The clinical picture simulates extrahepatic obstruction. The patient is jaundiced but does not have a palpable liver. Intravenous cholangiography is normal. Careful evaluation is necessary to rule out obstruction of the biliary tree as a cause. Hyperbilirubinemia from this cause is a benign disease.

The high serum bilirubin levels help to differentiate this from primary hemoglobinemia following transfusion reactions or from the myoglobinemia following transfusion reactions or from the myoglobinemia syndrome. The pigment excretion may be quite severe and may be associated with some precipitation in the renal tubules. If significant precipitation does occur, mild forms of renal failure (including the high-output form) may be seen. The only treatment of this disorder that seems to be relatively effective is maintenance of an adequate urine output and avoidance of anesthetics and other hepatotoxic drugs that may cause liver damage. Patients who have come to autopsy as a result of other injuries have shown pathological evidence of mild renal damage and very little liver damage.

ABDOMINAL TRAUMA

Intra-abdominal injuries are either penetrating or blunt.[2] Penetrating wounds are more lethal initially; however, if the patient survives the early period and is treated properly, chances of fatal complications from tissue destruction caused by the injury are almost nil. On the other hand, although the initial survival of a patient with severe blunt trauma is good, the final mortality and morbidity rates are greater than from penetrating injury. The increased death rate and morbidity from this type of trauma are pri-

marily due to the great difficulty in diagnosis and the tremendous, often occult, tissue destruction that frequently occurs and that greatly increases the incidence of delayed trauma-related complications. This is especially true of blunt injuries involving the liver, spleen, kidney, and pancreas.

While the ultimate management of abdominal trauma will require the assistance of a general surgeon, a few points are worth noting in the present discussion. Although it should be obvious, it is necessary to reinforce the maxim that shock in association with abdominal trauma is due to the abdominal injury until proved otherwise. Head injuries in adults do not produce hypotension except in terminal stages. Children under 18 months of age have relatively large heads and small blood volume. As a result, they may have a hemorrhage into the head that is large enough to produce shock and yet not have fatal compression of the brain.

It should be noted that except in the case of a rapidly progressive craniocerebral injury, such as epidural hematoma, or similar life-threatening situations in the thorax, such as cardiac tamponade or a massive continuing hemothorax, abdominal injuries usually take highest priority. The sum of these two facts is that any seriously injured patient who, early in the course of evaluation, develops significant unexplained hypotension must have a prompt, complete evaluation for intra-abdominal bleeding irrespective of associated intracranial trauma.

Penetrating injuries are more obvious on initial examination and, therefore, will receive early evaluation by a general surgeon. Older concepts regarding the need for immediate exploratory laparotomy have been replaced with a more selective approach. Alternatives to routine laparotomy include local exploration of wounds under six hours old, exploration or sinography of wounds over six hours old, and use of abdominal paracentesis and peritoneal lavage in either group. An abdominal exploration is performed only after findings have confirmed peritoneal penetration. Indications for mandatory laparotomy include: unexplained shock, signs of peritonitis, gastrointestinal bleeding, free air in the peritoneal cavity, massive hematuria, evisceration, stab wound through the lower rib cage, and multiple stab wounds seen in the first 12 hours.

As previously noted, blunt trauma is the

more frequent and more dangerous entity in patients with multiple trauma. These patients usually present a more difficult problem than patients with penetrating injuries. Indications for prompt laparotomy are: obvious and persistent evidence of peritonitis, shock or persistent hypotension with no other obvious causes, gastrointestinal bleeding, and positive findings on abdominal paracentesis. In the absence of these, the decision for laparotomy rests on such factors as: results of cystogram or intravenous pyelogram or both in patients with hematuria, scans or angiograms in the presence of findings suggesting a specific organ injury, peritoneal lavage in patients with equivocal findings, and finally, close observation for the development of new signs and symptoms that make the need for laparotomy clear.

FRACTURES AND FAT EMBOLISM

Initial Management of Fractures

The diagnosis of fracture in an extremity may be easy or difficult. An obvious comminuted open fracture with the bone protruding through the skin can be appreciated without difficulty. However, an occult hairline or cortical fracture of an extremity bone in an unconscious patient may never be recognized. Because of the damage and disability that unrecognized fractures can cause, it is imperative that after the patient's vital functions have become stabilized the physician make a thorough examination of the multiply injured patient in a conscientious effort to identify all fractures that are present. This effort should include an x-ray examination of all suspected bones.

Fractures can be classified simply as closed or open.[25] A closed fracture is one in which the overlying tissues are intact and bacteria cannot gain access to the fracture site. An open fracture is one in which the fracture has direct access to the air and bacteria as a result of loss of integrity of the overlying skin and tissues.

The initial treatment of closed fractures involves splinting and, in some cases, traction. The agitated patient should have fractures splinted promptly to prevent damage to contiguous nerves and major vessels in the area of the fracture. The unconscious patient with pathological posturing may require more aggressive management than usual. Definitive treatment of closed fractures after the patient's condition has become stabilized should be left to an orthopedic surgeon.

The management of open fractures can be much more complicated than that of closed fractures. The surgical principles for care of open wounds should be carefully observed in dealing with these fractures. Often close examination will be enough to decide whether the laceration of the skin and the fracture of the underlying bone are continuous. Sometimes, however, this determination may only be possible in the operating room. Therefore, initially, it should be assumed that a fracture with overlying skin disruption is an open fracture, and treatment should proceed accordingly. Again, as soon as possible, the management should be left to the orthopedic consultant.

Fat Embolism

The etiology of the fat embolism syndrome is not fully known.[24] Fat embolism is most frequently seen in patients with multiple injuries that include fractures of long bones. According to the "mechanical" theory, fat droplets from the bone marrow and surrounding fatty tissue are swept into the bloodstream. They are carried to the pulmonary vascular system, where they are trapped in the lungs or swept through the pulmonary capillaries. In the systemic circulation, they become emboli to brain, kidney, and other areas. The "metabolic" theory suggests that the emboli are formed from a fusion of pre-existing tiny chylomicrons in physiological suspension within the plasma because of injury-initiated biochemical changes that are not understood. An association between pulmonary fat embolism and intravascular coagulation has been reported.[57] Since the clinical syndrome may be overlooked and the pathological findings are often scanty, the number of deaths attributable to fat embolism is unknown. Unless fresh frozen sections of tissue are stained for free fat, the diagnosis will be missed. Perhaps as many as 16 per cent of all deaths caused by trauma are related to fat embolism. Shock is a major finding in many of the patients.

The clinical syndrome of fat embolization can be roughly categorized into three types. In the fulminating form the patient, previously awake and oriented, becomes agitated and rapidly lapses into lethargy and coma and dies within a few hours after injury. At autopsy, evidence of massive fat embolism to the lungs, kidneys, brain, and other organs is found. The diagnosis of this condition prior to death is extremely difficult because the same symptoms are present in refractory shock. Often, such patients are thought to have an intracranial hematoma or cerebral edema, and many of them have undergone angiography or craniotomy on the assumption that a major intracranial lesion was present.

The classic form of fat embolization appears somewhat later, around 24 to 72 hours after injury. The symptoms are predominantly cerebral. The syndrome may be heralded by sudden elevation of temperature, often as high as 105° to 106° F, and tachycardia. The patient becomes agitated, delusional, often delirious, and may be considered to have delirium tremens. Over the next few hours, the patient rapidly becomes lethargic, stuporous, and comatose. False lateralizing neurological signs and shift of these focal signs present a confusing clinical picture. If the patient has a head injury, the differentiation between the fat embolism syndrome and a worsening of a primary intracranial process may be very difficult. Examination of the eye grounds may reveal petechial hemorrhages. The cerebrospinal fluid is usually normal. Accompanying the cerebral signs and symptoms are tachypnea and cyanosis associated with rales and pulmonary edema. These respiratory manifestations may be the result of cerebral involvement rather than of pulmonary embolization. The presence of petechiae over the upper portion of the body, including the anterior chest, the axillae and upper arms, the neck, and the lower lids and conjunctivae of the eyes, is a reliable and almost pathognomonic clinical sign. The petechial hemorrhages are small and may be present for only 24 to 48 hours and then disappear.

The incomplete form of the disorder is a fragment of the classic form of the disease with some of the symptoms and signs appearing transiently. It is benign, and the patients usually recover.

Diagnostic tests usually are of little value. The finding of fat in the urine or in the blood on microscopic examination is suggestive, but a negative examination is meaningless. Renal biopsies and biopsies of the skin petechiae have been done, but are of little value and are impractical.

The prognosis is quite variable. The patient either dies or recovers completely. Even subtle sequelae are rarely encountered and can often be attributed to associated injuries. The mortality rate, however, is quite high, particularly in the fulminating form of the disease. In general, death is related to the depth and duration of coma.

The treatment of the condition is mainly supportive with special attention being paid to ventilation, adequate fluid and nutritional replacement, and careful nursing care. The fractured extremity should be handled gently in the hope of reducing the entrance of fat into the blood. The value of tourniquets above the fracture of the extremity during manipulation has not been proved, and they should not be used. Specific treatment is based on the predominant signs and symptoms. Good pulmonary ventilation with high oxygen concentration should be provided as described earlier in the discussion of the acute respiratory distress syndrome. Hypothermia has been used, but to little avail. Several agents have been used to try to dissolve the intravascular fat that is present. Heparin, which has known fat-clearing properties, has been used, but the results are not convincing. It has the added disadvantage of enhancing bleeding. To avoid the problems of anticoagulation from heparin, 5 per cent alcohol in a solution of 5 per cent dextrose in water has been given intravenously in intermittent doses of 500 to 1000 ml. Many clinical studies have been made, but none have correlated the forms of treatment with depth and duration of coma.

BLEEDING DISORDERS

Acute Bleeding Disorders

Although somewhat uncommon, acute uncontrollable bleeding may complicate the management of the patient with multiple injuries. This can be especially unnerving if it occurs during an operation. In general, the cause is one of three processes: specific clotting factor deficiencies, acute fibrinolysis, or disseminated intravascular coagulation. While it would be wise under these circumstances to consult a physician trained specifically in the management of hematological disorders, the neurosurgeon can institute analytical and therapeutic procedures that may be lifesaving.

Although the specific clotting factor abnormalities are epitomized by classic hemophilia (congenital factor VIII deficiency), this is quite rare and the surgeon would be well advised to consider other more common conditions. The major ones are listed in Table 77–3 along with the specific tests that, if values are normal, exclude the specific entity. The treatment for the disorder will depend, of course, upon the disease state. Fresh whole blood, frozen plasma, or concentrated platelets may be administered when indicated.

Acute primary fibrinolytic states are rare and are due to an increase in plasminogen activator, which in turn converts plasminogen to plasmin, which promotes breakdown of fibrin.[36] This condition can occur during prolonged operative procedures with excessive blood loss, especially in prostatic operations in which urokinase, which is a specific plasminogen activator, is released. The disorder is characterized by the finding of normal platelets, decrease in fibrinogen levels, and increase in fibrin split products. The treatment is the administration of epsilon-aminocaproic acid, which is a specific antifibrinolytic agent that acts as a competitive inhibitor of plasminogen activation. It may also act noncompetitively to inhibit plasmin. Five to ten grams can be given intravenously in an hour followed by one to two grams per hour for the next two to three hours. During this time, fresh frozen plasma should also be administered.

Disseminated intravascular coagulation is characterized clinically by a bleeding diathesis in which a consumptive coagulopathy and an acute fibrinolytic process are combined.[37] It is seen in gram-negative septicemias, stasis (shock), and metabolic acidosis. Well documented in several non-neurological states including prostatic carcinoma operations, amniotic fluid embolization, abruptio placentae, trauma, and snakebite, it has been reported following brain injury and operations for brain tumor during which an autotransfusion of brain thromboplastin is thought to occur. It can be suspected when a generalized diathesis occurs along with the screening coaguloanalytic findings of low platelet count, low fibrinogen value, and prolongation of the prothrombin time and partial thromboplastin time. In addition, because of the acute fibrinolytic process, fibrin split products are increased. Some of these fibrin split products themselves have anticoagulant properties.

The management of disseminated intravascular coagulation will depend upon the stage of the process at the time of the diagnosis.[67] Early during the primary coagulation process, heparinization should be instituted to preserve the unconsumed coagulation factors. Approximately 2000 to 4000 units of heparin should be given intravenously every 30 to 45 minutes for two or

TABLE 77–3 BLEEDING DISORDERS

HEMOSTATIC ABNORMALITY	NORMAL TEST RESULTS THAT EXCLUDE THE DIAGNOSIS					
	Platelets	Bleeding Time	Prothrombin Time	Partial Thromboplastin Time	Thrombin Time	Blood Urea Nitrogen
Thrombocytopenia	X					
Vitamin K deficiency			X	X		
Liver disease			X	X		
Uremia		X				X
Drug-induced platelet deficiency		X				
Heparin therapy					X	
Coumadin therapy			X	X		

three doses. If the coagulopathy has progressed to the stage of being primarily fibrinolysis, then epsilon-aminocaproic acid may be instituted. Infusion of fresh whole blood or frozen plasma in order to replace the consumed clotting factors is, of course, the treatment of choice, especially if the exact nature of the process is undiagnosed.

THE INJURED CHILD

The general approach to the early evaluation and management of trauma in infants and children is not unique.[26] In infants and small children (especially those under 10 kg), however, the margin of safety in such matters as vascular and pulmonary reserve is significantly less. Thus, a much smaller loss of blood volume or a modest amount of abdominal distention (with reduction in chest volume) may have disastrous consequences. Since the young patient frequently cannot adequately communicate his symptoms and since over 80 per cent of pediatric trauma results from blunt injury, detection of subtle signs, particulary of the lack of response to ongoing treatment, is necessary. Neurological surgeons, especially, should be aware of these smaller reserves, since head injury is associated with multiple trauma relatively more often in children than in adults. It is important to remember that the smaller the patient the more rapid the evolution from health to illness and from illness to death.

Minimal hypovolemia, whether due to hemorrhage or sequestration, can be devastating to an infant or small child. Even one blood-soaked sponge may signal impending vascular instability in a neonate. Excessive heat loss due to large surface area to weight ratios and poorly developed thermal regulatory capacity make careful temperature monitoring crucial. Drugs must be used even more judiciously than in adults, with special consideration being given not only to dosage but, even more importantly, to the child's biochemical immaturity and the resultant hazards of using aspirin, atropine, vitamin K, chloramphenicol, and sulfonamides in neonates and infants.

The need for and the use of massive replacement of fluids is especially important. Precise records of intake and output are crucial. Appropriate monitoring of blood pressure (including use of Doppler techniques or, when necessary, arterial catheters) is a necessary adjunct, especially in infants. It must be recalled that the normal mean systolic pressure in a neonate is only 60 mm of mercury (by Doppler) and increases only to 90 to 100 mm of mercury by the age of one year. Monitoring of urinary output is as important in children as in adults in assessing hypovolemia and decreased tissue perfusion, but it must be noted that neonates have less ability to increase urine volume and to concentrate urine. Central venous pressure monitoring (with special attention to relative rises or falls rather than absolute values) is advised as strongly in infants and children as in adults. Infants, however, present a particular problem in this regard because there are precious few sites for cannulation to measure central venous pressure. Most clinicians favor using the basilar vein or the external or internal jugular vein, making use of a cutdown in most cases as the surer and probably safer technique of cannulation. The subclavian vein also offers an alternate route but is generally reserved as a last resort in infants with relatively less respiratory reserve than older children and adults. Temporary cannulization of the sagittal sinus through an open anterior fontanelle has been used. Brittle thermal stability makes the warming of blood or fluids mandatory in these young patients.

In addition to careful assessment of massive replacement, general care of traumatized children requires careful administration of fluids. Many good detailed charts are available to make this possible.[40] As a general guideline, children weighing less than 10 kg should be given 100 ml per kilogram per 24 hours, those weighing 10 to 20 kg can be given 50 ml per kilogram per 24 hours, and for those over this weight adult guidelines are generally safe. Use of any of several types of infusion pumps makes constant, accurate parenteral fluid administration much easier in infants. An important monitoring aid that is relatively simpler in children is frequent determination of body weight (daily or even twice daily).

Airway problems and their management are important in adults and even more critical in young children and infants. As in adults, tracheostomy is used only when necessary, but greater problems with subglottic inflammation and subsequent stenosis are common to the very young. Two to three days is the upper limit for use of endotracheal intubation. When tracheostomy is to be done in these patients, a few points are worthy of mention. The presence of an endotracheal tube during tracheostomy is mandatory. No tracheal tissue should be excised. Therefore, only a vertical incision through two or three rings is utilized, generally avoiding even the addition of a transverse incision between the the two incised rings that is commonly done in adults, as described earlier. Use of flexible, inert Silastic tubes reduces tracheal inflammation. Reduction of the caliber of the tube as a "weaning" process is recommended as is the avoidance of "corking" the tracheostomy tube to test the patient's ability to tolerate its removal. Several types of respirators are available that are specifically designed for pediatric patients.

Since smaller pulmonary reserve is common to infants and small children, gastric retention secondary to trauma or an operation is poorly tolerated. Likewise, nasogastric tubes are even more objectionable in children than in adults, again because of infringement on an already marginal airway. This problem has led many pediatric surgeons to a more vigorous use of gastrostomies for both gastrointestinal decompression in the initial stage and early tube feeding to maintain good nutrition later in the recovery stage. Short-term decompression, especially in the older child, still is best accomplished by a nasogastric tube.

Following the foregoing guidelines and precautions is an important first step in successful management of the severely injured child by the neurosurgeon. Equally important is the recognition of the small margin for error that mandates early consultation with the neonatologist, pediatrician, and pediatric surgeon for assistance in the management of even minimally complex problems in the young patient who has been injured.

STRESS ULCERS

Stress ulceration of the gastrointestinal tract is a major complication following injury. The bleeding usually occurs within the first 3 to 15 days after injury and tends to occur somewhat earlier following head injury than after injuries to other parts of the body. It is frequently associated with burns or other major trauma. Frequently, stress bleeding begins after a second stress, such as reoperation. There is no reason to believe that large doses of steroids for a short period of time, as in the management of cerebral edema, can be implicated.

Although most clinically significant ulcers are found in the stomach and duodenum, they can occur throughout the portion of the gastrointestinal tract innervated by the vagus nerve. This innervation extends from esophagus to mid-transverse colon. The ulcerative lesions are of two main types—either there are superficial multiple erosions, or more rarely, the entire wall of the viscus is involved. The latter type, termed gastromalacia, presents as an acute abdominal crisis rather than gastric hemorrhage.

The cause of stress ulcers is unknown. The major theories include an association of high levels of gastric acidity and pepsin with poor mucus formation and immotility of the gastrointestinal tract. The immotility allows pooling of the acidic contents. The mucosa, unprotected by sufficient mucus, begins to ulcerate. Other theories include ischemic infarction of the mucosa during early stress from shock and the general effect of trauma. These hypotheses are speculative, and there is very little confirmation that the mechanisms exist in man.[38]

The clinical diagnosis of stress ulcers is based on the evidence of hemorrhage with the rapid development of anemia and the finding of blood in the gastric secretions and melena in the stool. The differential diagnosis includes a previous peptic ulcer and esophageal varices.

The initial treatment consists of iced saline lavage through a nasogastric tube until the secretions are clear of blood. If the patient develops shock, lactated Ringer's solution and blood are used in appropriate quantities. After the initial hemorrhage has been controlled, antacids are used. A suitable technique is to place approximately 60 ml of antacid in the stomach through the nasogastric tube; clamp the tube for approximately 30 minutes, and follow this by 30 minutes of continuous suction drainage. This routine is repeated every hour. Blood transfusions are given and repeated when needed. Occasionally an emergency gastrectomy will be required for a severe uncontrollable gastric hemorrhage. This usually requires removal of most of the stomach. Because the ulcerations may not be limited to the stomach, a vagotomy usually is performed at the time of the gastrectomy. The mortality rate for stress ulcers that require operative treatment approaches 80 per cent, chiefly because of severe hemorrhage and complications from it. Stress ulceration occurs in very ill and debilitated patients who tolerate major operations quite poorly. The chief means of reducing the mortality rate has been early operation, particularly within three days of the onset of bleeding.

Excessive gastric acid output has been demonstrated in decerebrate patients.[68] If it is prolonged, stress bleeding is likely in this group. This excessive acid production can be blocked by intramuscular anticholinergic drugs, which will reduce the incidence of stress bleeding.[69] Use of these drugs is recommended for protection in decerebrate patients if early tube feedings cannot be instituted.

MISCELLANEOUS PROBLEMS

Total Patient Care

The management of a patient with multiple injuries involves wise, continuous, good nursing care.[27] Beds should be kept clean, dry, and free of wrinkles or hard padding. Linen changes may be needed several times a day for patients with abdominal drains. Patients should be encouraged to turn or should be turned manually every one or two hours. For a comatose patient whose legs are in plaster casts or in traction, an alternating pressure mattress should be used. The patient should be kept clean and dry. The combination of wet linen, wrinkles in the bed sheets, and immobility results in decubitus ulcers in a matter of hours. Padding should be placed around heels and elbows to prevent pressure sores.

Careful attention should be paid to the eyes, particularly in the comatose patient. The eyes should be kept moist with methylcellulose or boric acid (2 per cent) drops.

The patient in cervical traction should be closely observed for the development of occipital decubiti. Turning the patient, of course, is the best preventive measure, but occasionally this is not possible. Therefore, soft padding, such as a foam rubber pillow, placed beneath the occiput, is helpful; a doughnut-shaped pillow of foam rubber can also be used.

Unless absolutely necessary, the delirious patient should not be restrained. Instead, padded bed rails should be used, and his extremities, particularly the hands, should be covered with thick padded mittens to prevent injury or removal of dressings or catheters. Nets can be placed over the side rails in order to keep the patient, especially the pediatric patient, from going over the top of the rails.

If fractures are present, open reduction and internal fixation may be required to prevent the patient from compounding the fracture. Small doses of chlorpromazine, 25 mg every six hours intramuscularly in the average adult, can be very helpful in quieting the patient with minor head injury. Patients who are comatose or who have spinal cord injury should have the healthy limbs and joints exercised daily to prevent phlebothrombosis, tendon shortening, and contractures.

The Nasogastric Tube and Feeding Enterostomies

The initial evaluation of the patient, after stabilization of vital functions, includes introduction of the nasogastric tube and removal of all gastric contents. This maneuver is a prophylaxis against regurgitation and aspiration pneumonitis. In patients with abdominal injuries or who have had abdominal operation, the nasogastric tube is left in place to manage ileus. It is imperative that careful measurements of the secretions from the nasogastric tube be made. These secretions represent a source of significant electrolyte loss. Also, it has been shown that there is a direct correlation between gastric acidity and gastric hemorrhage in the decerebrate patient; periodic measurement of gastric acid production should be made in this group of patients.[68]

The nasogastric tube often has been used to feed the unconscious patient. For the administration of milk and crystalloid fluid, tubes as small as a No. 8 French feeding tube can be employed in the adult. Emulsified and pureed foods require larger tubes, but usually smaller than a No. 20 French. A major problem associated with tube feeding is diarrhea. The likelihood of diarrhea can be reduced by gradually increasing the number of calories per feeding. For the first two to three days after tube feeding is instituted, only routine intravenous fluids are administered. Then for the next day or two, the free water previously given as 5 per cent dextrose in water is replaced with skim milk. For example, if the patient is to receive 2000 ml of 5 per cent dextrose in water and 100 ml of Ringer's lactate in a 24-hour period, this would be given as 125 ml of lactated Ringer's plus 250 ml of skim milk every three hours. When this mixture has been tolerated for 24 to 48 hours without diarrhea, whole milk is substituted for skim milk. Eventually, the routine tube feeding diet can be given.

Youmans has suggested a tube feeding diet that rarely causes diarrhea.[76] He uses a blended mixture of the regular home or hospital diet of the day. The low incidence of diarrhea and other complications probably is due to the fact that the gastrointestinal tract is accustomed to this diet. In preparing the blended diet, only the bones and decorations are removed. The remainder is pulverized in a blender. Enough water is added to increase breakfast to 400 ml, lunch to 1000 ml, and dinner to 1000 ml. The tube feeding is begun with small amounts, 10 to 30 ml each two hours, as the intravenous fluids are decreased. Ten milliliters of water is injected in one quick bolus after each feeding. This method is used to clear the feeding tube. Gradually the feeding is increased until 200 ml is given each two hours throughout the day and night. Youmans emphasizes that it is important to give the feedings in 200 ml boluses rather than larger doses that may distend the stomach and increase the probability of regurgitation and aspiration of the gastric contents. Experience has shown that if the patient develops diarrhea on this diet, it will be found that there has been an unauthorized change in the diet by the personnel in the kitchen. In order to decrease the work of blending the diet, such items as milk, raw eggs, or emulsified fat will have been substituted for the regular hospital diet. A check with the kitchen personnel should identify and remedy the problem. A patient being fed by nasogastric tube requires the addition of sodium chloride in the same amount as a normal patient. The diet kitchen staff must be kept informed of this need. Periodic checks of the serum electrolytes are necessary to insure that adequate sodium and potassium are included in the diet.

The technique of nasogastric feeding is important. During the administration of the feeding, the patient's head should be elevated. If a tracheostomy is present, the cuff needs to be inflated. The entire feeding should be given in approximately 30 minutes, and the patient should be left in the head-up position for a least 30 minutes afterward.

A major complication of nasogastric feeding is erosion of the alimentary tract from the nasopharynx to the stomach. Often this occurs at the level of the epiglottis or larynx. A tracheoesophageal fistula results and is manifest by coughing and retching during feeding. Frequent bouts of pneumonitis occur. The treatment is operative closure of the fistula. The use of a small soft tube may reduce the incidence of this complication.

Another major complication is regurgitation that results in aspiration. This is rarely a problem if the patient's head is kept elevated during feeding and for at least 30 minutes thereafter. If aspiration occurs frequently, the location of the tube should be checked. Roentgenological evaluation with Gastrografin may demonstrate a tracheoesophageal fistula. Barium should be avoided because of tracheobronchial irritation.

Patients who require nasogastric tube feedings can be managed in the nursing home. Care should be exercised, however, that enough water is given to avoid a hyperosmolar syndrome.

The reluctance of the family about the tube or the presence of associated injuries may preclude use of this method at home. In these circumstances, feeding enterostomies may be used. These have the further possible advantage of reducing the likelihood of aspiration. Presumably, the nasogastric tube produces incompetence of the sphincter at the cardiac end of the stomach. Its mere presence is all that is required. A feeding gastrostomy, or more particularly a feeding jejunostomy, should leave this sphincter intact. The jejunostomy interposes the pylorus as an additional sphincter. Proof of this concept is difficult, however, as many other factors influence the incidence of aspiration pneumonitis. The chief one is the competence and care used by the individuals giving the tube feedings. It is not uncommon to have patients maintained at home by their family for years without the slightest trouble. On the other hand, in less desirable circumstances, aspiration, pulmonary abscess, and death are accompaniments of tube feeding.

Gastrostomy is rarely used for feeding the unconscious patient. It is no less of an operative procedure than jejunostomy, nor is the management of the feeding easier. Furthermore, it seems logical to use the pylorus as an additional protection against aspiration. Gastrostomy has been used, however. A tube type or a permanent type can be done. Institution of feeding is the same as with jejunostomy.

The major feeding jejunal enterostomies are the Witzel and the Maydl (Roux-en-Y).[16] Usually, these are performed through an incision just to the left of the midline of the abdomen in the upper left quadrant. They are both placed in the proximal jejunum, at least 6 to 8 inches distal to the ligament of Treitz. The Witzel jejunostomy is a temporary enterostomy performed over a large-caliber tube (No. 26 to No. 30 French) that is placed directly into the lumen of the jejunum. Once the need for a feeding enterostomy ceases, the tube is simply removed and the defect heals spontaneously. The problem is that once the tube has been withdrawn, it requires another operative procedure to replace it. The Roux-en-Y jejunostomy, however, is a permanent enterostomy. It involves bringing a loop of the jejunum to the surface of the abdomen with eversion of the mucosa outward. Once it has healed, feeding can be accomplished with a small feeding tube introduced into the stump of the enterostomy or with a long-necked rubber-tipped syringe. If there is no longer a need for the enterostomy, an operative procedure is required to close it.

The philosophy concerning parenteral feeding is that, with a temporary feeding problem in the patient expected to recover, a nasogastric feeding tube will suffice. If it appears that the patient's recovery may be extremely long or may never occur, then a permanent jejunostomy of the Roux-en-Y type is the procedure of choice. A temporary feeding enterostomy might be indicated between these two extremes.[15]

Normally the decision as to the type of enterostomy needed is made about the second to third week following injury. Most of the injuries that require this are head injuries, but occasionally injuries to the face, neck, and even the chest will make major diversional procedures necessary for a long time before the patient is able to resume normal eating. The technique for starting the feeding in an enterostomy is similar to that for the nasogastric tube. The chief complication is diarrhea due to a high colloid concentration in the formula. Treatment is to withhold the feeding, maintain the patient on intravenous fluid, and use antiperistaltic agents.

Catheters

Most severely injured patients will have a catheter in the bladder for some time. The catheter serves many purposes. Urine is examined for blood, which may indicate trauma to the urinary tract. Radiopaque material can be injected into the bladder in cases of pelvic fracture in which there is the probability of bladder rupture. The catheter prevents bladder distention in the comatose patient, and keeps the bed dry, should the patient be incontinent. Most vital is the assessment of urinary output for control of fluid requirements; a catheter is the best means of accurate measurement. Discussion of catheter care is given in Chapter 28, which concerns urological care of the neurosurgical patient.

Fever of Unknown Origin

The management of a patient with a fever of unknown origin can be very perplexing. A systematic search often reveals its precise cause, however.[46] Rarely does the type of fever curve aid in diagnosis of a specific condition. One exception to this is the presence of a high sustained fever, usually about 105° F, with an abrupt onset. This is fairly characteristic and denotes hypothalamic or brain stem disturbance. Frequently seen with uncal herniation and secondary pontine hemorrhages, this type of fever has an ominous outlook.

Most febrile episodes in the post-traumatic, and, indeed, the postoperative patient as well, are spiking fevers between 101° F and 104° F, alternating with periods of lowered or normal temperature. While temperatures of 101° F and 102° F are not uncommon in the first 24 hours postoperatively, elevated temperatures after the day of operation denote some pathological condition and require investigation. Low-grade temperature elevations may be the result of inadequate volume replacement.

Pulmonary tract infections are the most common cause of fever in the immediate postoperative period. Careful auscultation and chest roentgenograms are usually adequate for diagnosis. A more subtle and valuable test is the determination of arterial blood gas values. Microatelectasis is diagnosed by this examination, which will demonstrate the presence of a shunt before the physical or x-ray findings of atelectasis appear. The combination of fever, decreased level of consciousness, a normal arterial Pco_2 and a low Po_2 is almost pathognomonic of microatelectasis. Improvement will be prompt if ventilatory assistance is provided.

A companion complication of tracheostomy is pulmonary infection. The incidence can be reduced by careful aseptic care of the tracheostomy, including the use of nebulized warm mist from clean ventilating equipment. Culture of the tracheal aspirate may disclose the cause of the fever.

The second common source of fever in the immediate postoperative period is the infected urinary tract, particularly if a urethral catheter is present. The fever of urinary tract infection is usually seen a day or two later than that from pulmonary infections. Extremely high fevers and septic shock can occur shortly after urinary tract manipulation, whether by open operation or by the simple introduction of an indwelling catheter. Careful urine examination including cultures should be made. Costovertebral angle tenderness and testicular inflammation may be seen.

Careful general examination of a patient with fever should include examination for thrombophlebitis. The veins of the lower extremities, particularly, and the sites of venipuncture or venisection should be examined. Redness, tenderness, and a palpable thrombus make the diagnosis.

Any operative areas should be examined closely for evidence of loculated pus. The pus may be in the incision or in the general operative area, e.g., an intraperitoneal abscess. Incision and drainage of the abscess together with administration of appropriate antibiotics resolve the problem.

The most common type of transfusion reaction is a febrile one, sometimes associated with a chill. There is no distinct hemolysis with this type of reaction, as it is probably related to certain pyrogenic substances that may be in the blood or in the transfusing equipment.

Drug fever is a distinct entity, presenting as a low-grade fever, most prominent an hour or two after the patient receives the medication. Simply stopping the medication is sufficient treatment.

Patients on prolonged antibiotic therapy may develop bacterial overgrowth that is resistant to the agent, and fever represents sepsis engendered by inappropriate therapy. As a result of a change in the flora induced by long-term antibiotic therapy, a specific complication may herald itself initially as fever. Pseudomembranous colitis, which is the result of staphylococcal overgrowth in the gastrointestinal tract, is an example.

The general evaluation of a patient with a fever of unknown origin is a careful examination to locate physical evidence of abnormality. Appropriate cultures are made, particularly of the blood, the sputum, the urine, and any abnormal-appearing fluid from operative sites or drains.

Use of Antimicrobial Drugs

In the early initial management, the patient with multiple injuries should be given prophylaxis against tetanus. Fortunately, most individuals have been actively immunized during childhood or military service. They require only the administration of 0.5 ml tetanus toxoid intramuscularly as a booster shortly after admission. Adequate debridement of all wounds is necessary. When the wound is grossly contaminated, if there has been a long time between injury and medical attention, or if the patient has not been actively immunized, passive immunization should be carried out immediately. In the past, this has required the use of horse serum antitoxin. Now, human immune globulin is more plentiful and should be used preferentially. The dose varies from 2.3 units per pound in children under 6 years to 200 to 600 units in adults. The antibody given this way has no bactericidal effect and will only neutralize free toxin. Active immunization should be started at the same time in another extremity.

While there is no evidence supporting the use of prophylactic antibiotics in elective surgical procedures, experience with war wounds indicates that prophylactic use of antibiotics in such grossly contaminated wounds has greatly decreased the incidence of clostridial and streptococcal infections. In general, the indications for early or preoperative prophylactic antibiotics include gross soiling of the peritoneal cavity or other tissues with intestinal contents; the presence of unretrievable foreign bodies such as shotgun waddings, soil, or clothing; gangrene in an extremity from massive contusion or crush injuries; or the presence of a suitable medium for multiplication of clostridial organisms such as a hematoma.[1] The most nearly ideal combination of antibiotics to use prophylactically in the patient who has been injured is aqueous pencillin, at least 1,000,000 units every six hours intravenously, and tetracycline, 250 mg every six hours. Prior to institution of antibiotic therapy, cultures should be made of material from the contaminated area. Further discussion of the use of antibiotics in neurosurgery is given in Chapter 110.

REFERENCES

1. Altemeier, W. A., and Walsin, J. H.: Antimicrobial therapy in injured patients. J.A.M.A., *173*:527, 1960.
2. Anderson, C. B., and Ballinger, W. F.: Abdominal injuries. *In* Ballinger, W. F., Rutherford, R. B., and Zuidema, G. D., eds.: The Management of Trauma. 2nd ed. Philadelphia, W. B. Saunders Co., 1973, p. 396.
3. Anderson, R. J., Gambertoglio, J. G., and Schrier, R. W.: Fate of drugs in renal failure. *In* Brenner, B. M., and Rector, F. C., Jr., eds.: The Kidney. Philadelphia, W. B. Saunders Co., 1976, p. 1911.
4. Anderson, R. W.: Shock and circulatory collapse. *In* Sabiston, D. C., and Spencer, F. C., eds.: Gibbon's Surgery of the Chest. 3rd Ed. Philadelphia, W. B. Saunders, 1976, p. 107.
5. Apuzzo, M. L. J., Weiss, M. H., Peterson, V., Small, R. B., Kurz, T., and Heiden, J. S.: Effect of positive end expiratory pressure ventilation on intracranial pressure in man. J. Neurosurg., *46*:227, 1977.
6. Arms, R. A., Dines, D. E., and Twistman, T. L.: Aspiration pneumonia. Chest, *65*:136, 1974.
7. Bartlett, J. G., Gorbach, S. L., and Finegold, S. M.: The bacteriology of aspiration pneumonia. Amer. J. Med., *56*:202, 1974.
8. Bartter, F. C., and Schwartz, W. B.: The syndrome of inappropriate secretion of antidiuretic hormone. Amer. J. Med., *42*:790, 1967.
9. Berry, R. E. L., and Sanislow, C. A.: Clinical manifestations and treatment of congestive atelectasis. Arch. Surg., *87*:169, 1963.
10. Blair, E., Wise, A., and Mackay, A. G.: Gram negative bacteremic shock, J.A.M.A., *207*:333, 1969.
11. Blalock, A.: Shock, further studies with particular reference to effects of hemorrhage. Arch. Surg., *29*:837, 1934.
12. Bland, J. E., and Clark, K.: Experimental induction of cerebral swelling. Neurology, *18*:821, 1968.
13. Bland, J. E., Perry, M. O., and Clark, K.: Spasm of the cervical internal carotid artery. Am. Surg., *166*:987, 1967.
14. Blodhein, S. H.: A simple test for myohemoglobinuria. J.A.M.A., *167*:453, 1958.
15. Boles, T., Jr., and Zollinger, R. M.: Critical evaluation of jejunostomy. A.M.A. Arch Surg., *65*:358, 1952.
16. Brintnall, E. S., Daum, K., and Womack, N.A.: Maydl jejunostomy. A.M.A. Arch. Surg., *65*:367, 1952.
17. Bywaters, F. G. L., and Beall, D.: Crush injuries with impairment of renal function. Brit. Med. J., *1*:427, 1941.
18. Cameron, J. L., Mitchell, W. H., and Zuidema, G. A.: Aspiration pneumonia. Arch. Surg., *106*:49, 1973.
19. Ciocatto, E.: Choice of mechanical ventilators. *In* Caldwell, I. B., and Moya, F., eds.: Advances in Respiratory Care and Physiology. Springfield, Ill., Charles C Thomas, 1973, p. 238.
20. Cotton, L. T., and Roberts, V. C.: The prevention of deep vein thrombosis, with particular reference to mechanical methods of prevention. Surgery, *81*:228, 1977.
21. Davis, C. W.: Immediate diagnosis of pulmonary embolus. Amer. Surg., *30*:291, 1964.
22. Edgerton, M. T., Jr.: Emergency care of maxillofacial and neck injuries. *In* Ballinger, W. F., Rutherford, R. B., and Zuidema, G. D., eds. The Management of Trauma. 2nd Ed. Philadelphia, W. B. Saunders Co., 1973, p. 255.
23. Goldberg, L. I.: Dopamine—clinical uses of an endogenous catecholamine. New Eng. J. Med., *291*:707–710, 1974.
24. Gurd, A. R., and Wilson, R. I.: The fat embolism syndrome. J. Bone Joint Surg., *56B*:408–416, 1974.
25. Hampton, O. P., Jr., and Fitts, W. T., Jr.: Fractures and dislocations: General considerations. *In* Moyer, C. A. et al., eds.: Surgery, Practice and Principles. Philadelphia, J. B. Lippincott Co., 1965, p. 415.
26. Haller, J. A., Jr., and Talbert, J. L.: Trauma and the child. *In* Ballinger, W. F., Rutherford, R. B., and Zuidema, G. D., eds.: The Management of Trauma. 2nd Ed. Philadelphia, W. B. Saunders Co., 1973, p. 719.
27. Haynes, W. G., and McGuire, M.: Textbook of Neurosurgical Nursing. Philadelphia, W. B. Saunders Co., 1952, Chapters 7 & 8.
28. Hermrick, A. S., and Thal, A. P.: The adrenergic drugs and their use in shock therapy. Curr. Probl. Surg., July, 1968.
29. Hershey, S. G., DelGuerico, L. R. M., and

McCon, R.: Septic Shock in Man. Boston, Little, Brown & Co., 1971.

30. Horowitz, H. I.: Myoglobinuria after acute arterial occlusion. New Eng. J. Med., 262:1116, 1960.

31. Hughes, C. W., and Jahnke, E. J.: The surgery of traumatic arteriovenous fistulas and aneurysms. Ann. Surg., 148:790, 1958.

32. Kantrowitz, P. A., Jones, W. A., Greenburger, N. J., and Isselbacher, K. J.: Severe postoperative hyperbilirubinemia simulating obstructive jaundice. New Eng. J. Med., 276:591, 1967.

33. Kiley, J. E., Power, S. R., and Bube, R. J.: Acute renal failure: Eighty cases of renal tubular necrosis. New Eng. J. Med., 262:481, 1960.

34. Kintner, E. P.: The A/B ratio, a new approach to acid-base balance. Amer J. Clin. Path., 47:614, 1967.

35. Kittle, C. F., and Levin, S.: The use of antibiotics in cardiac and thoracic surgery. In Sabiston, D. C., Jr., and Spencer, F. C., eds.: Gibbon's Surgery of the Chest. 3rd Ed. Philadelphia, W. B. Saunders, Co., 1976, p. 160.

36. Kwaan, H. C.: Disorders of fibrinolysis. Med. Clin. N. Amer., 56:163–176, 1972.

37. Kwaan, H. C.: Disseminated intravascular coagulation. Med. Clin. N. Amer., 56:176–191, 1972.

38. Leonard, A. S., Long, D., French, L. A., Peter, E. T., and Wangensteen, O. H.: Pendular pattern in gastric secretion and blood flow following hypothalmic stimulation—origin of stress ulcer? Surgery, 56:109, 1964.

39. Levinsky, N. G., and Alexander, E. A.: Acute renal failure. In Brenner, B. M., and Rector, F. C., Jr., eds.: The Kidney. Philadelphia, W. B. Saunders Co., 1976, p. 806.

40. Lopez, R. I.: Fluid and electrolyte balance. In Graef, J. W., and Cone, T. E., Jr., eds.: Manual of Pediatric Therapeutics. Boston, Little, Brown & Co., 1974, p. 83.

41. Manley, C. B., and Robson, A. M.: Acute renal failure following trauma. In Ballinger, W. F., Rutherford, R. B., and Zuidema, G. D., eds.: The Management of Trauma. Philadelphia, W. B. Saunders Co., 1973, p. 123.

42. Mark, J. B. D., and Hayes, M. A.: Studies of calcium and magnesium metabolism during surgical convalescence. Surg., Gynec., Obstet., 113:213, 1961.

43. Mobin-Uddin, K., ed.: Pulmonary Thromboembolism. Springfield, Ill., Charles C Thomas, 1975.

44. Moore, F. D., and Ball, M. R.: The Metabolic Response to Surgery. Springfield, Ill., Charles C Thomas, 1952.

45. Moss, G.: Shock lung: A disorder of the central nervous system. Hosp. Prac., Aug., 1974, p. 77.

46. Moyer, C. A.: Nonoperative surgical care, Section 2, Fever. In Moyer, C. A., et al., eds.: Surgery, Practice and Principles. 3rd Ed. Philadelphia, J. B. Lippincott Co., 1965, p. 282.

47. Nelson, T. G.: Tracheotomy: A Clinical and Experimental Study. Baltimore, Md., Williams & Wilkins Co., 1958.

48. Newman, M. M.: Tracheostomy. Surg. Clin. N. Amer. 49:6, 1969.

49. Plum, F.: Respiratory failure and its management. In Beeson, P. B., and McDermott, W., eds.: Cecil-Loeb Textbook of Medicine. 12th Ed. Philadelphia, W. B. Saunders Co., 1967, p. 1487.

50. Pontoppidan, H.: Bedside pulmonary function tests and their interpretation. In Caldwell, T. B., and Moya, F., eds.: Advances in Respiratory Care and Physiology. Springfield, Ill. Charles C Thomas, 1973, p. 220.

51. Randall, H. T., and Roberts, K. E.: The significance and treatment of acidosis and alkalosis in surgical patients. Surg. Clin. N. Amer., 36:315, 1956.

52. Ravitch, M. D.: Traumatic Heart Disease. Concepts of Cardiovascular Disease, 29:615, 1960.

53. Roberts, K. E., Magida, G., and Pitts, R. F.: Relationship between potassium and bicarbonate in blood and urine. Amer. J. Physiol., 172:47, 1953.

54. Rosenblum, R.: Physiologic basis for the therapeutic use of catecholamines. Amer. Heart J., 87:527–530, 1974.

55. Rutherford, R. B.: Thoracic injuries. In Ballinger, W. F., Rutherford, R. B., and Zuidema, G. D., eds.: The Management of Trauma. 2nd Ed. Philadelphia, W. B. Saunders Co., 1973, p. 333.

56. Rutherford, R. B.: The pathophysiology of trauma and shock. In Ballinger, W. F., Rutherford, R. B., and Zuidema, G. D., eds.: The Management of Trauma. 2nd Ed. Philadelphia, W. B. Saunders Co., 1973, p. 24.

57. Saldeen, T.: Fat embolism and signs of intravascular coagulation in post-traumatic autopsy material. J. Trauma, 10:273–286, 1970.

58. Sanford, J. P., and Barnett, J. A.: Septicemia. In Conn, H. F., ed.: 1966 Current Therapy. Philadelphia, W. B. Saunders Co., 1966, p. 51.

59. Shenkin, H. A., Bezier, H. S., and Bouzarth, W. F.: Restricted fluid intake, rational management of the neurosurgical patient. J. Neurosurg., 45:432–436, 1976.

60. Shires, G. T., and Baxter, C. R.: Complications of parenteral fluid therapy. In Artz, C. P., and Hardy, J. D., eds.: Complications in Surgery and Their Management. 2nd Ed. Philadelphia, W. B. Saunders Co., 1967.

61. Shires, G. T., and Patman, R. D.: The management of civilian arterial injuries. Surg., Gynec., Obstet., 118:125, 1964.

62. Silver, D., and Harrington, M. P.: Thrombophlebitis: Prevention, recognition, and management. Primary Care, 4:585–599, 1977.

63. Singer, R. B., and Hastings, A. B.: An improved clinical method for the estimation of disturbances of the acid-base balance of human blood. Medicine, 27:223, 1948.

64. Skaggs, J. A., and Cogbill, C. L.: Tracheostomy: Management, mortality, and complications. Ann. Surg., 36:393, 1969.

65. Stephenson, H. E., Jr., Reid, L. C., and Hinton, J. W.: Some common denominators in 1200 cases of cardiac arrest. Ann. Surg., 137:731, 1953.

66. Trinkle, J. K., Richardson, J. D., Franz, J. L., Groves, F. L., Arm, K. V., and Holstrom, F. M. G.: Management of flail chest without mechanical ventilation. Ann. Thorac. Surg., 19:355, 1975.

67. Watts, C.: Disseminated intravascular coagulation. Surg. Neurol., 8:258–262, 1977.

68. Watts, C., and Clark, K.: Gastric acidity in the comatose patient. J. Neurosurg., 30:107, 1969.

69. Watts, C., and Clark, K.: Effects of an anticholinergic drug on gastric acid secretion in the coma-

tose patient. Surg., Gynec., Obstet. *130*:61, 1970.

70. Wegria, R., Frank, C. W., Wang, H., Misiahy, G., Miller, R., and Kornfield, P.: A study of the usefulness and limitations of electrical countershock, cardiac massage, epinephrine and procaine in cardiac resuscitation from ventricular fibrillation. Circulation, *8*:1, 1953.

71. Weil, M. H., and Shubin, H.: The VIP approach to the bedside management of shock. J.A.M.A., *207*:337, 1969.

72. Weil, M. H., Shubin, H., and Biddle, M.: Shock caused by gram negative micro-organisms: Analysis of 169 cases. Ann. Intern. Med., *60*:384, 1964.

73. Welt, L. G.: Clinical Disorders of Hydration and Acid-Base Equilibrium, 2nd Ed. Boston, Little, Brown & Co., 1959.

74. Wilson, R. F., and Sibbald, W. J.: Acute respiratory failure. Crit. Care Med., *4*:79, 1976.

75. Wolfe, J. E., Bone, R. C., and Ruth, W. E.: Diagnosis of gastric aspiration by fiberoptic bronchoscopy. Chest, *70*:458, 1976.

76. Youmans, J. R.: Personal communication, 1978.

IX

BENIGN SPINE LESIONS

78

EXTRADURAL SPINAL CORD AND NERVE ROOT COMPRESSION FROM BENIGN LESIONS OF THE LUMBAR AREA

THE INTERVERTEBRAL DISC

Historical Background

Recognition of the common clinical syndromes of disc disease developed slowly in medical history.[8,177] The first anatomical descriptions of the intervertebral disc are credited to Vesalius in 1555. There was an early description of sciatica by Domenico Cotugno in 1770, but the association between low back pain and sciatica was not recognized until the work of Lasègue 100 years later. In the mid-nineteenth century, Virchow and Von Luschka gave complete descriptions of discs and their abnormalities; posterior protrusion of the intervertebral disc was recognized as a clinical entity in 1858 by Von Luschka.[194] In 1895, Ribbert produced "Virchow's tumor" in rabbits by puncturing the intervertebral discs.

Probably the first report of a traumatic rupture of an intervertebral disc was made by Kocher in 1896: the patient fell 100 feet in a standing position, walked a few steps, collapsed, and died of visceral injuries. A posterior displacement of the intervertebral disc between the first and second lumbar vertebrae was found at postmortem examination.

In 1911, Goldthwait had a patient who very likely had compression of the cauda equina due to a narrow canal. In studying the problem in the anatomy laboratory, however, he concluded that compression of the dural elements could be brought about by mobility of the lumbosacral articulation or by "the crowding backward of the intervertebral disc alone."[70] Within a few years, Elsberg and others described "chondromata" causing compression of the spinal canal, and they considered this and other irritative lesions of the nerve roots to be the cause of sciatica.[41a] Schmorl, in his intensive investigation of the intervertebral disc at postmortem examinations, found a small posterior prolapse beneath the spinal ligament in about 15 per cent of the spines.[154] He believed that this was produced by degenerative changes in the anulus fibrosus from mild trauma that created fissures in the anulus, permitting escape of semifluid nuclear material. In 1929, Dandy operated on two patients with midlumbar compression of the cauda equina and he stated that "the lesion is a completely detached fragment from an intervertebral (lumbar) disc . . . the lesion is undoubtedly of traumatic origin."[34]

The modern era of definition for surgical treatment of the ruptured intervertebral disc—the most common cause of nerve root compression in the lumbar spine—was ushered in by Mixter and Barr at the annual meeting of the New England Surgical Society in September, 1933.[130] They cited the work of others and, in a note at the end of their published article, credited the detailed monograph of Mauric, whose deductions were similar to theirs. In reporting their 11 cases of herniation of lumbar discs, the authors concluded that this rupture is a com-

C. H. DAVIS, JR.

mon cause of symptoms and that, in patients who do not respond to conservative measures, "results from surgical treatment are very satisfactory if compression has not been too prolonged."

Following this, operative assault on the intervertebral disc won enthusiastic and widespread acceptance with wide swings away from and toward conservatism. An increasing but still incomplete fund of knowledge now exists about the basic etiology, modes of investigation, and treatment of disorders of the intervertebral disc.

Developmental and Functional Anatomy

Gross Anatomy and Biomechanical Function

The intervertebral disc acts as an articulation between the vertebrae and as a shock absorber or a cushion; it is composed of three parts.[8,20,30,102] The cartilaginous plate is a structure of hyaline cartilage covering the bone of the vertebra and acting as a limiting plate above and below. It functions as a barrier between the active pressure of the nucleus pulposus on the adjacent vertebral bodies and allows the nucleus pulposus to act as a hydrodynamic ball bearing. The anulus fibrosus arises from the cartilaginous plate, surrounds the nucleus pulposus, gives size and shape to the disc, and is the seat of most of its strength and tenacity. It is composed of fibrous and fibrocartilaginous lamellae in three groups: those that stream off the inner surface of the cartilaginous plates, those that pass anteriorly and posteriorly to insert into the longitudinal ligaments, and those that pass over the edge of the vertebral body and insert into the bone of the vertebrae. The anulus appears stronger anteriorly where the attachment to the longitudinal ligament is very strong, while posteriorly the attachment is much looser (and the posterior ligament is weaker than the anterior one). The nucleus pulposus is the fibrogelatinous center of the disc and, in its semigelatinous state, is subject to the laws of fluids and therefore is incompressible; it is confined to its normal shape and position by the strong and elastic anulus fibrosus. Pressure within this nucleus pulposus material in the living organism is the result of elastic tension, muscle

tone, and static forces transmitted from one vertebral body to the next. When its limiting structures are sound, the nucleus transmits these forces and functions as a hydrodynamic ball bearing or axis of motion upon which each vertebral body must work. Nachemson and Elfström have cited their work and the work of others in measuring the intradiscal pressures in human subjects as well as autopsy specimens under various conditions.[135] They noted during compression tests that autopsy discs showed great resistance to fracture or permanent change on vertical loading, but that such resistance lessened with increasing age. They further noted that, because of the relatively high internal pressure of the normal disc, the anulus fibrosus is subjected to relatively little vertical stress, but the horizontal or tangential tensile stresses will be severe and are sometimes as much as five times the vertical load applied. Significant increases in intradiscal pressure with the Valsalva maneuver and coughing, and striking increases during forward bending with lifting were noted.

Mechanical compression tests performed on freshly obtained autopsy specimens of the spine by Brown and co-workers demonstrated an axial compression load for lumbar discs ranging from 1000 to 1300 pounds, before failure occurred.[24] At those loads, failure tended to occur in the vertebral cartilaginous end-plates rather than the discs. On combined actual loading and bending tests, the discs expanded on the concave side and contracted on the convex side; portions of the disc lying 90 degrees to the plane of motion showed very little change. These authors concluded that the anulus was subjected primarily to direct compression and buckling rather than to hoop tension, as would be the case if its only function were to resist deformation of the nucleus; however, they agree that this may vary with age. They further noted during axial compression tests that the volume of the five discs tested decreased from 1 to 2.5 cc before failure. They thought that this decrease in volume was due to collapse of the fissures and spaces ordinarily present within the adult disc and the passage of fluid across the vertebral end-plates into the medullary spaces of the adjacent vertebral bodies.

In addition to compression and flexion factors, rotational stresses have been analyzed. In producing injury by slowly applying rotation in amounts within the range of normal lumbar movement, Farfan and associates concluded that torsional strains are probably more important than compressive loads in the production of anular degeneration and disc rupture.[51] Since two thirds of the resistance to torque is attributed to the articular processes (coupled with the capsules and interspinous ligaments), these investigators further concluded that impairment of function of the articular joints may result in a greater risk of disc degeneration.

Related Anatomy and Function

In addition to the changes taking place in the intervertebral spaces on movements of the spine, flexion is accompanied by an upward, forward separation of the inferior facet of a vertebra from the superior facet of the subjacent vertebra. This movement is checked by the joint capsules, posterior ligaments, and epiaxial muscles. Extension is more limited, with a posterior downward gliding movement of the inferior facet in relation to its apposing fellow. This movement is checked by the anterior longitudinal ligament and all adjacent ventral muscles; the laminae and spinous processes may also limit extension. Lateral flexion involves some rotation and is checked by the intertransverse ligaments and lateral ligaments of the spine as well as the muscles of the trunk and the buttressing effect of the articular processes. In the lumbar spine, movements of ventral and lateral flexion and extension are well performed, but the planes of the facet faces markedly limit rotation.[141] During walking, the thoracic vertebrae rotate around an axis through the disc center while the lumbar vertebrae rotate around an axis posterior to the disc, thus subjecting the lumbar disc to additional stress.

The evolutionary mechanics that have occurred as the species has gone from the horizontal to the upright position have been analyzed, and it is obvious that the lower lumbar discs carry more shock and strain than the others, and that in addition there is a shearing force as the fifth lumbar vertebra rides forward on the first sacral segment.[8,30,99,100] This is, in part, compensated for by the nearly vertical placement of the facet articulations, which serve as buttresses against this movement, and by the relative strength and thickness of the

anulus anteriorly at this level. Nevertheless, half of the motion between the lower thoracic region and the sacrum takes place at the lumbosacral joint.[70]

Other adjacent anatomy has significance.[141] In the lumbar region, the vertical diameter of the intervertebral foramina varies from 12 to 19 mm, so nerve root compression in this direction is unlikely even with complete collapse of a disc. The transverse diameter from the ligamentum flavum to the vertebral body and the disc may be as little as 7 mm, however, and since the fourth lumbar nerve root may be only slightly less than 7 mm in diameter, there is very little tolerance for pathological alteration. Furthermore, transforaminal ligaments are frequently found in the lumbar region. These ligaments may be as wide as 5 mm and are strong, unyielding cords of cartilaginous tissue that pass anteriorly from various parts of the neural arch to the body of the same or an adjacent vertebra.

Dynamic Histology and Pathology

Not only is the functional anatomy dynamic and variable, but the histological anatomy is one of constant change from early embryogenesis throughout life. In the embryo, the notochord, which is derived from the endoderm, is quickly surrounded by mesenchymal cells, and each provertebra divides horizontally, the caudad half attaching to the cephalad half of the adjacent provertebra to form the rudimentary vertebra; the future intervertebral disc thus becomes the farthest point from the intersegmental artery. By the tenth embryonic week, the notochord has become extruded into this intervertebral region and is separated from the cartilaginous vertebral bodies by a fibrocartilaginous envelope derived from the original mesenchymal intervertebral cells. At the same time, separate ossification centers for the body and each half of the vertebral arch appear, and the cells of the notochord begin their mucoid degeneration, which becomes complete so that they disappear sometime in the first decade of life.*

By the twenty-fourth week of embryonic development, the two cartilage plates have appeared and there is progressive invasion of the nucleus pulposus by fibroblasts from

---

* See references 8, 20, 30–32, 102, 140.

the outer zone of the anulus fibrosus. This anulus is strongly attached to the cartilaginous plates and to the margins of the vertebral bodies. The cartilaginous plates in turn are intimately fused to the vertebral bodies by long bony clefts and ridges that have appeared in a radial fashion in the superior and inferior margins of these bodies at the time of birth, and that increase in size in the first decade and gradually smooth out over the next 10 to 15 years. The cartilaginous plates and the epiphyseal rings are genetically one structure, comparable to the epiphyses of long bones. The epiphysis develops as a small ring of cartilage surrounding the superior and inferior rims of each vertebral body with small foci of calcium in girls aged 6 to 8 and in boys 7 to 9. These foci gradually enlarge and fuse to form a ring that is completed by the age of 12 to 15 and gradually fused into the vertebral body by the age of 21 to 25. (While Bradford and Spurling stated that the epiphyseal ring was not formed posteriorly, this is refuted by Coventry and associates, who noted a complete ring in all their patients, with the cartilaginous plate ending before it reached the posterior edge of the vertebra and abutting against a definite rim of bone.[20,30])

Within this epiphyseal ring and adjacent to the disc, the vertebral body is composed of a specialized, dense, smooth bone that is perforated by small holes corresponding to marrow cavities, apparently to permit fluid to pass from the spongy bone into the disc for nourishment. It is thought that these areas and the ossification gaps for the clefts may account for weak places in the bony plate that cause later development of Schmorl's nodes. The vertebral body itself has a biconvex appearance at birth that is gradually altered to the flattened form seen in the adult.

After birth, the intervertebral disc continues to function actively. By the age of 6 months, the anulus fibrosus is well developed and has attached itself to the newly developed anterior and posterior ligaments; the anulus is completely developed by the tenth year. The nucleus, which started as a rectangular structure, has become oval, and the notochordal elements have disappeared with progressive invasion by fibroblasts. The cartilaginous plate continues to be active, but in the second decade this activity decreases. Up to the age of 8 years, small blood vessels enter the disc by way of

the cartilaginous plate, but these channels are completely obliterated by scarring by the age of 20 to 30 years.

The epiphysis is fused to the body of the vertebra by the age of 19, and the plate ends abruptly at the end of the epiphysis rather than extending anteriorly and posteriorly to the edge of the vertebra. Fibers stream forward to insert in the longitudinal ligament and the vertebral bone, the plate becomes thinner, and retrogression crosses the curve of progression at about age 18. The anulus still progresses, but degeneration becomes evident in the late years of the second decade: the nucleus has become broken up and irregular, losing its diffuse character, and a more distinct demarcation has appeared between the nucleus and the anulus. The nucleus continues to take on fluid and is maturing, but the cartilaginous plate shows definite wear and tear with some longitudinal fissures appearing that may be the result of trauma.

It is thought that the maximum point of function is reached by the third decade. By the fourth decade, retrogressive changes in the cartilaginous plate are striking, the nucleus has gradually lost fluid and is being replaced by fibrous tissue, and the anulus shows aging by pigmentation and vascularization as well as by hyaline degeneration. Older age is accompanied by continued degeneration, ballooning of the disc into the body of the vertebra with actual erosion and protrusion into the body, frequently by posterior breaks in the anulus, calcification of the disc, and replacement of the nucleus by fibrocartilage. When ruptures of the anulus appear, they are associated with flowing out of disc material, most commonly in a posterolateral direction.

In addition to the alterations produced by age alone, many changes are the result of repetitive minor and sometimes major trauma. The relatively greater stress borne by the low lumbar disc in man has already been cited, and it is suggested that fixed lumbar lordosis may be a causative factor in producing the ruptured intervertebral disc. Levy noted that the European, who has a relatively high incidence of disc disease, can straighten his normal lumbar lordosis only on forward bending, while the African, who has a relatively low incidence, can actively flex his lumbar spine.[111] Many years earlier anthropologists noted racial differences in the sacrum, which tends to form a right angle to the lumbar spine in the European, while it continues the line of the lumbar spine in the African.[99] Experimentally, Lindblom tied rats' tails in a U and reported changes in the structure of the anulus fibrosus, proliferation of connective tissue and bone, and bulging and rupture of the disc on the concave side.[112] Other experimenters, working with dogs and monkeys, injured discs by drilling through the cartilaginous plate, producing Schmorl's nodes; by cutting into the anulus with a sharp scalpel, they produced narrowing of the interspace, kyphosis, and lipping.[102]

Other important, although less dramatic, changes take place when the disc stops performing its proper function: shock is borne directly by the vertebrae, ligaments, and facets, and there is increased mobility of the vertebral bodies on one another with increased tension on the attachment of the longitudinal ligaments above and below the disc anteriorly; tugging of these attachments stimulates the formation of new bone. Posteriorly, as the degenerated disc bulges, there is stretching of the ligament, which pulls on the periosteum and again creates new bone.

Biochemistry

The nucleus pulposus is composed predominantly of protein polysaccharide molecules. The protein core is similar to other nonstructural protein such as plasma, and more than one kind of polysaccharide (keratosulfate and chondroitin sulfate) is attached in covalent linkage to the same protein core. These proteins do not cross-react with anti–serum protein antibodies but, in experiments in rabbits, they have been shown to produce their own autoantibodies that produce an inflammatory reaction in response to vascularization of a nucleus by operative trauma.[50] While some authors differentiate the changes of the aging process from other disc degeneration, common features are depolymerization and degradation of the protein-polysaccharide molecules leading to subtle changes in the nucleus pulposus that alter the ability of the matrix to imbibe fluids against pressure, a resulting gradual decrease in water content, and the appearance or unmasking of a beta protein.[23,50] Naylor has suggested that, early on, there is an increase in fluid content causing a very high intradiscal pressure that in turn causes rupture of the anulus.[136]

In contrast to the protein-polysaccharide composition of the nucleus pulposus, the substance that makes up the anulus is primarily collagen protein. A relatively greater resistance of this substance to proteolytic enzymes has been observed during trials of chemonucleolysis.

Neural Elements Involved in Disc Derangement

Pain and other symptoms are produced by compression or irritation of sensitive structures. A recurrent nerve originates distal to the dorsal ganglion, enters the spinal canal through the intervertebral foramen, and distributes to the ligamentous structures in the anterior spinal wall, extending to two vertebrae below the point of origin as well as going to the dura. In the fetus and newborn, nerve fibers have been found in the longitudinal ligament, in peripheral layers of the anulus fibrosus, and around the vessels in the bodies, and encapsulated receptors have been found in the facet joints; the ligamentum flavum is relatively free of neural networks. In the adult, a few endings are found in the supraspinous and infraspinous ligaments, many neural fibers are found in the capsules of the facets, and plexuses of fibers in the longitudinal ligaments. Only a few fibers are seen in the outer zones of the anulus fibrosus and none in the disc or in the trabecular bone.[91,143,199]

The histopathology of spinal nerve compression has been studied at postmortem examinations in which disc protrusions were found.[114] The distal half of the spinal ganglion and the first centimeter of the spinal nerve were compressed and flattened. Histologically, flattening, deformity, and atrophy of the ganglion cells were noted as well as normal degenerating and regenerating fibers in the nerves, particularly in the ventral root bundles; connective tissue was altered and increased. There were no signs of retrograde degeneration, and there was no detectable ascending degeneration of the dorsal columns or the ventral cell columns of the spinal cord. In some instances, "secondary" compression was also found of the proximal or midspinal ganglion from enlargement of the intervertebral joint by osteoarthritis.

Symptomatic Disc Disease

With this background knowledge of the pathological anatomy of the diseased disc, one can correlate the clinical picture of the patient who has symptomatic disc disease.* Back pain is common, being present at some time in 80 per cent of the population. About one third of those with back pain are incapacitated for varying lengths of time.[134] The incidence in male and female populations is about the same, and there is no definite correlation between type of work or body build.[84,89,90] About one third of those with significant back pain will develop sciatica, and of these, 90 per cent will have recurrence. To further emphasize the importance of this disorder, findings of an industrial survey indicated that about one fourth of the days lost from work were due to low back disorders and that, if the individuals were out of work for more than six months, only half ultimately returned to work. While the average industrial disability claim was for 25.5 days, the average disability claim for back disorders was for 123 days.[148]

As already noted, symptomatic disc disease results from biochemical changes, particularly within the nucleus pulposus, from secondary mechanical stresses associated with this degeneration and from additional stresses placed on the lumbar disc by awkward posture, poor musculature, and particularly by outreach lifting with the back in a flexed or rotated position.[6,8,135] Kelsey and Hardy note that regular and prolonged driving of motor vehicles probably increases the risk of acute disc herniation.[101]

There have been unsupported allegations that common anomalies of the lumbar spine may be associated with a high incidence of disc degeneration and low back pain.[203] On the other hand, in a careful industrial survey, La Rocca and Macnab found no radiographic, developmental, or degenerative criteria that could be used to obtain a reasonable prediction of risk of subsequent lumbar spine disability.[108]

Symptoms

As a generalization, symptomatic disc disease is more common in the adult Caucasian, and more than half the patients have some history of injury before the onset of symptoms. The low back pain that is usually the initial complaint may be a dull, diffuse aching pain of gradual onset, worse on exertion and better on rest; or it may be a severe crippling pain of sudden onset following an awkward movement, associated with muscular spasm and aggravated by any type of motion. The pain is thought to be caused by stretching of the posterior anulus and the posterior longitudinal ligament involving the pain fibers of these structures. By compressing the involved ligament and anulus during operations under local anesthesia, the pain has been reduplicated in the midline of the back and lateralized pain has been produced in the back, hip, and occasionally in the groin and testicle on the involved side.[133,199]

The patient who later has typical sciatica from a ruptured disc usually has a history of previous episodes of intermittent catches in the back or attacks of soreness and weakness of the low back that have cleared after rest. The incapacitating radiating pain ordinarily starts with back pain of one of the two described varieties. Within a few days or weeks, there is some relief from the back pain, followed by a progressive boring aching pain in the buttock and posterior or posterolateral aspect of the thigh and leg, accompanied by some numbness and tingling that radiates into the part of the foot served by the sensory fibers of the affected nerve root. Pain in the foot itself is uncommon; when it is present, other causes, particularly local disease in the foot, should be considered.

Occasionally, the clinical picture is one of severe sciatic pain and cramping from the onset of the symptoms. The pain is characteristically aggravated by sitting, standing, and walking, and by coughing, sneezing, or straining. Generally, it is relieved to some degree by lying down, particularly on the unaffected side with the painful leg flexed. Back and leg pain may persist together; the relative lessening of the former apparently occurs when the disc fragment is extruded so that it no longer stretches the pain fibers in the anulus fibrosus and the posterior longitudinal ligament. Likewise, on rare occasions, severe sciatica may suddenly be relieved, but this is associated with motor weakness and numbness because of physiological interruption of the function in the greatly compressed nerve root.

In the presence of a narrow canal and a

---

* See references 8, 76, 105, 133, 137, 163, 177.

midline protruded disc, the patient may complain principally of back pain and vague leg pain alternating in intensity from side to side; in the rare sudden transverse protrusion, there is onset of cauda equina paralysis causing motor and sensory changes in the legs and dysfunction of bladder and bowel. Urinary retention has been described as the only manifestation of protruded discs in several female patients.[42]

In sciatica due to nerve root compression, frequently the patient will be able to trace the distribution of the pain. In the common L4–L5 disc protrusion, the pain characteristically is present from the posterior hip along the posterolateral thigh and leg, with numbness and tingling going into the great toe or the first two toes. In the equally common L5–S1 disc protrusion, the pain characteristically is localized in the hip, posterior thigh, and posterior calf, going into the heel, with numbness and tingling in the lateral aspect of the foot and the outer toes. In the less common L3–L4 disc protrusion, there may be some pain in the groin, extending down the anterior thigh and leg to the medial aspect of the ankle.

Signs

The characteristic stance of the patient who has a ruptured intervertebral disc is one that flattens the lumbar spine, a slight forward tilting of the trunk, and slight flexion of the hip and knee of the affected side with only the toes resting on the ground. About half the patients will have some scoliosis, which may have its lumbar convexity either toward or away from the affected side. The patient walks slowly and deliberately, frequently supporting his back with a hand. He prefers standing to sitting and he changes position in a slow, deliberate manner. Forward bending is limited to a variable degree, usually from lack of mobility in the lumbar spine, which remains splinted; the scoliosis may be accentuated. When the patient bends forward to a point at which he begins to experience pain and then rapidly drops his head, excruciating pain in the hip and leg will occur. When he straightens from the flexed position, his trunk may go through a corkscrewlike motion. Occasionally his back may be "locked" in a flexed position, although this forward-bending posture is more commonly found in camptocormia. Extension of the back, especially toward the affected side, may cause accentuation of the pain. There may be local point tenderness over the lumbar vertebral spines and paravertebral musculature, and there may be evidence of muscular tightness.

With the patient standing, jugular compression for a minute or two may cause accentuation of pain and paresthesias in the affected area of the leg (Naffziger's test). With the patient sitting, marked forward flexion of the neck will often cause reduplication of the pain, apparently because of tugging on the thecal sac. Extension of the affected leg, and often of the contralateral one, will cause accentuation of pain.

With the patient lying in the supine position, various leg-raising tests are valuable in the diagnosis of disc disease. The Lasègue test, as described by his pupil Forst, has two maneuvers: the first is a straight-leg-raising test, and the second or confirmatory movement is one of flexion of the knee and hip while sliding the heel slowly up the bed.[200] Sciatic pain is reproduced by the first and not by the second maneuver. To carry out the straight-leg-raising test, the patient is asked to lie supine while holding his knees in full extension and his ankles in plantar flexion. The examiner then raises the leg by flexing it at the hip without altering the position of the knee and ankle. Normally, it is possible to carry this maneuver to about 90 degrees, causing only some discomfort in the hamstring muscles. In the presence of nerve root compression, among other disorders, the leg raising is limited. Normally, root movement does not begin until the leg is raised to about 30 to 40 degrees, and at this point the patient with root compression usually experiences acute discomfort and reduplication of his pain. In the laterally placed disc protrusion, this limitation of leg raising is to be expected on the ipsilateral side only. A well-leg-raising test has been described in which the asymptomatic leg is raised, causing the pain to be referred into the affected hip and leg.[205] This phenomenon is attributed to the presence of a herniated disc in the axilla between the root and dural envelope, with tugging of the sensitive root against the protrusion by the contralateral maneuver. Various modifications of the straight-leg-raising test have been developed in attempts to differentiate the pain of sciatic stretch from that of the postulated pain of sacroiliac or lumbosacral movement or of compression of the nerve by a spastic pyriformis muscle.

The simplest of these modifications is to raise the leg in a straight-leg fashion until discomfort begins and to lower it an inch or two until the patient is again comfortable. The ankle is then strongly dorsiflexed so that only sciatic stretch is brought into play. The patient who has a ruptured disc will experience acute accentuation of his pain. The Kernig test is another useful variation: the patient is placed in the supine position and the leg is raised by flexing both the hip and the knee. When the hip has been flexed to 90 degrees, the knee is slowly extended. Again, the normal range is a full extension, but with nerve root irritation, the maneuver is limited because of severe pain. The "figure-four maneuver," performed by externally rotating the hip when the hip and knee are flexed, tests hip rotation and further differentiates pain caused by hip disease.

A "femoral nerve traction test" has been described and advocated as an aid in diagnosis of disc herniations that affect the upper lumbar spine.[38] The patient lies on the unaffected side with the neck and the knee and hip on that side slightly flexed. The affected lower extremity, with the knee extended, is then gently hyperextended at the hip; radiating pain in the anterior thigh is considered a sign of radiculitis of the third or fourth lumbar nerve root. The second part of this maneuver is then bending the knee while the hip is kept in hyperextension. When positive, this test will produce or intensify the pain.

Significant differences in leg length are best determined by x-rays made for this purpose while the patient is in the standing position. Abnormalities of muscular tone and bulk, however, are detected by direct observation, including circumferential measurements of the thigh and leg at measured distances below the anterior superior iliac spine. Tests of strength of the quadriceps muscle and of the extensor of the great toe can be done by having the patient sit on the side of the bed and exert his foot against the force of the examiner's hand. The relative strength of plantar flexion of the foot is best tested by having the patient stand on the toes of first one foot and then the other. The foregoing three motor groups are those principally affected by protruded discs at the levels of L3–L4, L4–L5, and L5–S1 respectively.

Similarly, the knee and ankle reflexes are of considerable value, but not infallible in localization. These reflexes are best elicited by having the patient sit on the side of the bed with his legs hanging in as relaxed a manner as possible. The knee reflexes may be reinforced if necessary by the patient's extending his leg about 3 inches at the knee to touch his toe to the examiner's outstretched hand; the Achilles reflex can be reinforced by having the patient put his toes in slight plantar flexion. Occasionally, it is necessary to have the patient kneel on a chair and grasp the back of the chair with his hands in order to bring out the ankle jerks.

A ruptured disc at the L3–L4 interspace will commonly cause definite diminution or absence of the knee jerk. Disc protrusion at the L4–L5 interspace is also associated with a diminished knee reflex in a small percentage of patients; a large protrusion at this level compressing both the L5 and the S1 roots is associated with diminution or absence of the ankle jerk. The characteristic reflex abnormality in the L5–S1 protrusion is absence of the ankle jerk. The variable responses of reflexes and motor weakness from individual to individual undoubtedly reflect differences in anatomical makeup as well as in the degree of compression by the lesion.

Sensory response to pinprick is even more variable, particularly if one tries to trace dermatome patterns over the entire leg. Characteristically, however, the protruded disc between L5 and S1 is associated with hypalgesia of the lateral aspect of the foot and ankle; the L4–L5 protrusion causes hypalgesia of the dorsal foot, perhaps extending up over the dorsum of the ankle. The more rare protrusion at L3–L4 is associated with hypalgesia along the anterior border of the shin.

Protruded discs in the higher lumbar areas are rare.[9,76] Acute herniation from severe trauma causes paralysis of the cauda equina at the involved level. Lesser herniation is often associated with a long clinical history, perhaps dating from an old injury sustained during sports. Chronic lumbar backache, accompanied by exacerbations of pain and numbness in the anterolateral thighs, may resemble meralgia paresthetica. These symptoms and weakness of the muscles of the thigh, the peronei, and particularly the quadriceps may be unilateral or bilateral because of the relative crowding of the canal by the many roots. Motor weakness is often accompanied by disturbances in micturition and sexual potency. Absence or depression of the knee reflexes is common.

Special Examinations

X-rays

After an adequate history and physical examination, x-ray examination is indicated for the patient who has significant low back and leg pain. This should include an anteroposterior erect view of the pelvis for leg length and to visualize the hips, as well as the usual anteroposterior and lateral views of the lumbosacral spine; right and left posterior oblique views are necessary to demonstrate the anatomy of the facets, the pars interarticularis, and the sacroiliac joints. Occasionally, lateral views of the back in flexion and extension are indicated.[61]

Plain x-ray examination has its particular usefulness in differential diagnosis to demonstrate such lesions as arthritis, prespondylolisthesis or spondylolisthesis, fracture, primary and secondary tumors of the bone, chronic pyogenic or tuberculous infection, congenital malformation, significant difference in leg length, osteitis deformans (Paget's disease), Marie-Strümpell arthritis, fibrous dysplasia, and hemangioma of the vertebral body.

X-ray films of the patient with a ruptured disc are usually negative, perhaps revealing some straightening of the lordotic curve or scoliosis. Some narrowing of the lumbosacral interspace is commonly seen in normal people. Narrowing of the other interspaces may be considered an indication of degenerative disc disease, particularly if there are end-plate sclerosis and adjacent osteophytic formation. These latter changes must be seen before narrowing at the lumbosacral interspace can be considered to be clinically significant.

Macnab has described the distinctive appearance of the "traction spur."[121] This is a horizontally directed osteophyte arising at the site of the outermost anular fibers about 2 mm away from the discal border of the anterior and lateral surfaces of a vertebral body. It is his opinion that this type of spur denotes segmental instability and should be differentiated from the clawlike marginal osteophyte that is related to degenerative collapse of the disc space.

The clinician must remember that in patients with back and leg pain, but with signs of upper motor neuron involvement and sensory changes over the trunk, the lesion is above the lumbar level and the appropriate area must be studied. In the lumbar region, the symptomatic narrow spinal canal cannot usually be diagnosed on plain x-ray examination. When this disorder is suspected, further useful information can be obtained from classic tomography, but the most promising recent development is that of computed tomography. With further refinement, it seems, this technique will be useful in diagnosing and analyzing stenosis and other congenital and acquired defects of the spinal canal (see section on Narrow Spinal Canal).[62,63,93,94]

Myelography

Intraspinal tumors and ruptured intervertebral discs cannot be demonstrated on routine x-ray films; therefore various contrast studies have been developed to aid in their detection. The most universally used and the most useful of these contrast procedures is myelography.* The initially used contrast medium, Lipiodol, has been discarded because of its instability and significant meningeal irritation. Thorotrast was used for a short time, but has been discontinued because of its retention and persistent radioactivity. Isotopic myelography or myeloscintography has been described, but it is considered impractical.[12,195] A technique of radioisotopic scanning of the spinal canal has outlined dural, epidural, and vertebral space-occupying lesions, but would not be directly applicable to the lesions described in this section.[52] Soluble substances such as iodopyracet (Diodrast) and meglumine iothalamate, 60 per cent (Conray), have been used in a limited fashion but are highly irritating and considered unsafe for general use in myelography.[106] Recently, meglumine iocarmate (Dimeray, Dimer-x) has been described as giving improved radiographic definition in the lumbosacral spinal canal, but again the statement is made "it cannot be used above the lumbar region, since it is too irritating to the spinal cord."[123] The hazards of these water-

---

* See references 8, 9, 35, 118, 161, 190.

soluble media may have been reduced to an acceptable level in a new medium, metrizamide (Amipaque), which has recently been made available in the United States. This medium gives good visualization of the lumbar theca and nerve root sleeves.[144] It is not as useful for thoracic and cervical myelography, can cause meningeal irritation in some patients, and can cause a seizure if inappropriately used. Areas of great potential use that are now being evaluated are computed tomography of the spine and brain stem after lumbar introduction of metrizamide, and epidurography of the lumbosacral region. Air has the disadvantage of providing a poor contrast between the air and the bony shadows, making interpretation difficult and inaccurate. At present, ethyl iodophenylundecylate (Pantopaque) is still the preferred medium for a large-volume, complete visualization of the spinal canal, although it is associated with a small risk of meningeal irritation if it is not aspirated.[125,144] The procedure itself is frequently uncomfortable and subject to some error.

Certain clinicians have argued for limited selective use of myelography and have believed surgical exploration to be a more simple and effective screening procedure. The attitude in many clinics, including the author's own, is that when a patient is being considered for operation because of back and leg pain, myelography is extremely helpful in revealing the occasional intradural malformation, neoplasm, or symptomatic "narrow canal," and in determining or confirming the level of a herniated disc.[9] It should be used as a part of the entire clinical picture, and the occasional false-negative examination does not diminish its usefulness. To balance the false-negative results, there are a number of patients with large protruded discs in the midline who have back pain, only vague complaints of leg pain, and a remarkably normal physical examination in whom the diagnosis and the plan of operative approach are greatly facilitated by myelographic studies.

Electromyography

Because of its innocuous nature, the electromyogram (EMG) takes on particular value as a screening test in the evaluation of patients with backache and sciatica, particularly when the organic nature of pain may be in question. Martins Campos and co-workers have reported that electromyography is helpful in differentiating between high and low lumbar disc protrusions but is less reliable as a test for localization of the specific interspace involved.[124] It is said that the electromyogram becomes positive after neural damage has existed for three weeks. False-positive tests have occurred, but a rate of accuracy comparable to that of myelography has been reported by many authors.*

Epidural Venography

Interosseous vertebral venography was once recommended as a valuable screening procedure.[4,155,156] It was said to be more accurate than myelography in localizing the lateral protrusion of an intervertebral disc, but the test never gained wide acceptance. In recent years, however, epidural venography via injection of the ascending lumbar veins by way of the femoral vein has been described and is advocated by some as the study of choice in patients with suspected lumbar disc herniation.[63,65,110] Miller and co-workers recommend using this test when a suspected disc herniation is not demonstrated by myelography.[129] Venography is of limited usefulness in the patient who has had a previous operation, and the number of false-negative tests in cases with midline disc protrusion is significant. These defects, and defects in the technical quality of the study, support the view of Sackett and associates that the test is not the most reliable of those available.[150]

Discography

Since its introduction in 1948, the direct injection of a contrast medium into the intervertebral disc has been widely investigated, and there have been various claims of success or failure.[27,113] The amount of contrast medium injected and its radiographic appearance have been considered to indicate normality or abnormality of the disc. Generally, the suspected disc and the one above and below are injected. Various authors have described the confirmatory radiation of pain on injection under local anesthesia. Many claims of the usefulness of discography have been refuted by Holt.[86]

---

* See references 21, 33, 56, 71, 96, 105, 127.

The wide variation between different age groups revealed by discography has been shown in anatomical specimens; in particular, it has been noted that 35 per cent of the injected discs in persons over 40 years of age showed rupture of the anulus discographically despite lack of clinical evidence for nerve root compression.[103] Against the procedure is the fact that demonstrable injury to the intervertebral disc may follow needle puncture.[64,142] It is Taveras's opinion that the use of discography should be limited to the lumbar region and its use should be "very restricted."[186] He noted that over a 15-year period, he had recommended discography on an average of not more than once or twice a year in a large neuroradiographic series. Certainly discography should not be carried out without preceding myelography to rule out neoplasm and to demonstrate lesions in areas remote from the levels at which the injections are usually made.

Treatment and Prevention

Proper posture in standing, sitting, walking, and working, good muscular support, and avoidance of flexion strains will minimize the development of symptomatic disc disease.[152,163] Nachemson provided a good general review with graphic portrayal of the intradiscal pressures with various activities and emphasized the preventive aspects of treatment, including properly fitted chairs and car seats and the trial of a structured educational approach ("The Low Back School") for certain patients and for high-risk industrial groups.[134] He and his co-workers have recently demonstrated that the distance between the weight lifted and the back is the most important factor influencing stress on the back.[6]

Conservative Treatment

Armstrong simplified the sequence of pathological change into three stages: nuclear degeneration, nuclear displacement, and fibrosis.[8] The principle of conservative treatment is to protect the abnormal disc from strain and to put the part at rest to encourage healing by fibrosis.[8,163,177] Even sequestered fragments may respond to this treatment because their high content of water will desiccate in time. The type of rest and avoidance of strain prescribed varies according to the severity of the symptoms. The patient with mild or moderate symptoms is treated by a decrease in general activity, avoidance of lifting and bending and twisting, the use of a firm bed, and the wearing of a well-fitting lumbosacral corset or a chair-back brace.

The patient with severe symptoms is treated by absolute bed rest on a firm bed with his knees elevated on a pillow, if this makes him more comfortable, and by administration of the necessary analgesics and sedatives. If his symptoms abate, his activities are gradually increased after one or two weeks and he is treated in the same way as those patients who have mild to moderate symptoms.

When the symptoms have subsided, he is started on simple tension exercises to develop the abdominal and erector spinae muscles, and he is instructed in proper posture and proper performance of activities of daily living. Maintenance of good abdominal muscle tone and the associated increased intra-abdominal pressure make the lower portion of the body a semi-rigid cylinder, strikingly reducing the compressive forces exerted on the lumbar disc.[132] Nachemson and co-workers have demonstrated the potentially harmful effect of the frequently prescribed flexion exercises and emphasize isometric abdominal muscle training in the crooked lying position.[134,135] As the abdominal muscles are strengthened, the corset is gradually discarded; it should still be worn at times of expected physical stress and as required for discomfort. Other forms of conservative treatment, such as application of superficial heat and gentle massage, may make the patient more comfortable, but have no real therapeutic value. Traction applied by attaching a weight to the leg or pelvis serves only to keep the patient in bed; forcible pelvic distraction and manipulation are potentially harmful.[39,135,189]

The pregnant patient with symptomatic disc disease is best treated by periods of bed rest and a properly fitted maternity corset. Discomfort is more pronounced during the first and last trimesters, and back rather than abdominal discomfort may be prominent during labor.

Injection of anesthetics into painful areas of the back has no therapeutic usefulness. Injection of steroids into the spinal canal or disc, while widely practiced in some areas, has not been proved to be a beneficial adjunct in treatment.[54] An enthusiasm for intradiscal injection of proteolytic substances waxed for a while, particularly in orthopedic circles. Macnab gave a review and a fair appraisal of the situation in 1973 when he emphasized that chemonucleolysis was not a panacea for all manifestations of disc degeneration but did deserve a further trial.[122] The potential hazards were emphasized by Sussman and by Shealy.[164,182] Placebo and chymopapain double-blind clinical trials were not started until December 1974; when it became obvious, on the basis of these experiments, that there was no statistical difference between the injection of chymopapain and placebo in regard to frequency or degree of pain relief, this type of treatment was discontinued and the new drug application for the material was withdrawn by the sponsoring laboratory.[53,157]

There has developed a widespread clinical trial of percutaneous radiofrequency "facet denervation" as a treatment for back pain and sciatica.[165] In a recent careful review, Lora and Long concluded that this procedure might be a useful part of a broad conservative treatment program in some patients.[115] It is suggested that the prospective candidate for the procedure have a positive response to diagnostic blocks with a local anesthetic. The long-term results are not known, and whether this procedure will prove to be of value remains uncertain.

A number of "muscle relaxants" are available, but there is no good evidence that the oral preparations are clinically effective except for their sedative and analgesic action. High intake of certain vitamins has been advocated, but here again scientific proof of their value is lacking.[72]

Various claims have been made concerning the effectiveness of conservative treatment, but a reasonable estimate is that about 20 per cent of patients are permanently relieved of all symptoms and can resume full, active lives; 10 to 20 per cent require surgical treatment; and the remainder modify their activities and learn to live with a tolerable degree of discomfort.[8]

Operative Treatment

INDICATIONS. There are three generally accepted indications for operative intervention: (1) a massive midline protrusion that causes compression of the cauda equina, resulting in motor and sensory paresis and loss of sphincter control, requires immediate operation; (2) nerve root compression associated with quadriceps paresis or footdrop should be operated on early (interestingly, however, in one reported series patients with foot extensor paralysis who were operated on in the first week did not fare better than the others, and similar findings have been reported in cases in which operation was postponed for a longer period of time[7,197]); and (3) the lack of satisfactory relief of sciatica by conservative treatment (the most common indication). To belong in this category, the patient should have had his symptoms for at least one month and have been at absolute bed rest for one week or longer without response before conservative treatment is abandoned.

A fourth indication is the recurrence of incapacitating episodes of back pain and sciatica that prevent the patient from leading a reasonably normal life. Operative exploration when the diagnosis is in doubt is rarely indicated. When the organic origin of the pain is in question, the use of graduated spinal anesthesia may be helpful in reaching a diagnosis.[119]

Psychiatric considerations in pain are not within the scope of this chapter.[17] Nonetheless, recognition of the syndromes of depression and pain neurosis too often comes only after bitter experience and several needless operations. Psychometric screening and neuropsychiatric consultation are frequently helpful but do not replace good surgical judgment.

Obviously, as in all operative procedures, informed consent of the patient is essential. This involves a frank discussion of realistically expected results as well as possible hazards.

OPERATIVE PROCEDURE. The operative procedure may be performed under local, spinal, or general anesthesia with the patient in the prone, lateral, or knee-elbow position. At this clinic, general endotracheal anesthesia is preferred. The patient is placed in the prone position, his head to the side, and long sheet rolls are extended on either side from the shoulders to the lower pelvis to eliminate compression of the thorax and abdomen. The table is flexed in a manner to flatten the lumbar curve, and the foot-piece is elevated to give partial flexion of the legs.

A midline skin incision is centered over the affected interspace (this localization is facilitated by the presence of the puncture wound for the myelography). The incision is carried down to the level of the deep fascia, hemostats are applied to the superficial fascia, and self-retaining retractors are inserted. The fascia over the spinous processes is then incised in the midline; if the disc protrusion is clearly lateralized, the paraspinous musculature is stripped subperiosteally on that side only. This is done with a sharp periosteal elevator, starting at the lowermost spinous process, packing in a gauze section sponge as the dissection proceeds to facilitate the dissection and to control oozing from the muscle.

The laminal arches are exposed laterally to the articular facets, care being taken to identify the sacrum positively as a check in localization. Bleeding is controlled by electrocoagulation, and a Taylor or similar retractor is inserted. It is usually necessary to remove a portion of the caudal lip of the rostral laminal arch at the affected interspace. This is done with a bone rongeur or a Kerrison punch, and the bleeding is controlled with bone wax.

The ligamentum flavum is picked up with a sharp hook and cut through in the midline. A cottonoid patty with a string attached may be inserted through this opening to push away the extradural fat and the dura while the ligamentum flavum is being excised. The opening is enlarged with a Kerrison punch, particular attention being given to removal of the lateral extent of this ligament. This is done under direct vision, and extreme care is exercised to avoid damaging the root, which may be pushed up from its normal position by the protruded disc. The lateral edge of the dural envelope and of the nerve root must be identified; this may require a more extensive removal of the bone and ligament. An attempt is made not to damage the articular facet, but in some instances of extreme lateral herniation or an unusually tight foramen from congenital stricture or spondylosis, or both, partial or even complete removal of the facet may be indicated.[1,166,181] Insertion of cottonoid patties with marking strings up and down the lateral recess of the spinal canal will aid in exposure and in control of bleeding.

With a nerve root retractor, the root is then gently displaced medially to expose the interspace. Occasionally, a large sequestered fragment of disc presenting in the axilla between the nerve root and the dura must be removed before the root can be mobilized. Careful inspection and insertion of an angled probe across the canal anterior to the thecal sac, as well as probing and inspection of the foramen, may reveal fragments that would otherwise be missed. The presence of a rent or hole in the disc space indicates extrusion of a fragment. More commonly, one sees a shining, localized bulging at the interspace or over the adjacent posterior border of the body where a fragment has dissected up or down from the interspace between the posterior longitudinal ligament and the vertebral body. When this ligament is touched with a knife, there is a spontaneous extrusion of degenerated disc material. Less often, the interspace merely seems soft on palpation, but the disc will bulge perceptibly when the table is straightened. This latter state assumes particular significance in the patient who has a small canal.

A circular opening is made into the interspace with a small knife, and using variously angled pituitary rongeurs and curets, an attempt is made to remove the entire disc and cartilaginous plate, leaving only a firm horseshoe of anulus anteriorly and on the two sides.[163] Extreme caution is exercised to avoid passing through the anterior ligament and damaging the adjacent vessels.

Bleeding from the venous plexus in the spinal canal is usually not troublesome and can be controlled by brief tamponade with cottonoid. Electrocoagulation is occasionally necessary, and at times Gelfoam is useful. After brief application, this substance often can be removed without resumption of bleeding. When hemostasis is complete, the wound is irrigated and inspected to make certain that all foreign material has been removed. A Gelfoam membrane is then placed over the exposed dura.[120] If available, free fat from the subcutaneous tissue may also be used to obliterate dead space and, it is hoped, reduce epidural scar formation.[107] Extradural instillation of 40 mg of methylprednisolone acetate seems to reduce the discomfort of the immediate postoperative period. The deep fascia, subcutaneous fascia, and skin are closed in layers with interrupted sutures without drainage.

Discomfort during the postoperative period may vary from insignificant to severe pain. Narcotics are used freely if needed during the first 72 hours, but only simple analgesia is necessary after that period of time. Much ritual and dogma exists about the degree of activity permitted in the immediate postoperative period, varying from immediate ambulation and early flexion exercises to protracted bed rest for several weeks. The end-results seem to be the same. A reasonable practice is to encourage walking within the first few days, as soon as comfort permits, but to avoid flexion exercises.

The patient is discharged from the hospital within a week following the operation to continue bed rest and house activities for the next two weeks with minimal sitting and thereafter to gradually increase activities that involve walking. He can generally return to office work within two to six weeks after discharge and to physical work, avoiding unnecessary lifting and bending, about three months after discharge. Isometric exercises to strengthen the abdominal and erector spinae muscles are resumed. A corset or brace is worn only if there is appreciable persistent back pain that is relieved by rest and support.

RESULTS. There are a number of recorded results of operative treatment of disc disease.* The percentages vary, but roughly two thirds or more can be considered good to excellent, half of the remaining are improved, and half are not. The poorest results were in patients who had primarily back pain, while the best results were in patients whose symptoms were principally those of root compression.

Recurrence of pain leading to reoperation occurs in about 5 per cent of patients.[73,188] This may be due to extrusion of more disc material at the same level or on the opposite side, or it may be the result of rupture of another disc.[75,206] The decision for reoperation is based upon the criteria already outlined. The prognosis is reasonably good if there has been a significant pain-free interval since the previous operation.

In these patients, myelography is particularly useful in demonstrating dural compression as well as arachnoiditis, if present.[128,169] The operative procedure is carried out in a similar manner, but more bone is removed above and below the area of the previous laminotomy to find the edge of the dural envelope in an area unobscured by scar. By sharp and gentle blunt dissection, preferably under some magnification, the root and dura in the scarred area are dissected and mobilized. On rare occasions of persistent radicular pain associated with scarring, a dorsal rhizotomy may be helpful.†

It is now generally accepted that the results from simple removal of discs in patients with sciatica are as good as or superior to those from treatment with a combination of disc removal and spinal fusion.[57,147,198] The presence of neural arch defects coincidental with disc disease (except in the elderly), instability created by bilateral facet joint removal, and certain cases of chronic disc degeneration with significant back pain in which the degeneration is limited to one or two disc levels are considered indications for fusion after nerve root decompression.[148] In selected cases, fusion by a number of routes may remove a reasonable number of patients from the category of failure.‡

Complications

Aside from recurrences, complications are related to trauma to the nerve roots and dural envelope, trauma to adjacent structures in the retroperitoneal space and abdominal cavity, infection, and the rare occurrence of mechanical instability of the lower back.

DIRECT INJURY TO NEURAL ELEMENTS. This complication should be extremely uncommon if reasonable technical skill is employed. During removal of the lateral extent of the ligamentum flavum and overlying laminal arch with a Kerrison punch, accurate visual placement of this instrument is required, particularly if the subjacent nerve root is displaced upward by a protruded disc. Careful viewing, properly sized instruments, and the use of a sharp punching rather than a wrenching technique will minimize the danger of laceration or avulsion of the underlying root. Careful identification of the lateral border of the dural envelope and nerve root with gentle and intermittent traction, the occasionally needed decom-

---

* See references 8, 74, 76, 139, 163, 171, 179.

† See references 73, 76, 139, 159, 168.
‡ See references 8, 26, 28, 69, 95, 163, 177, 178.

pression of the area by extracting an extruded disc fragment through the axilla of this root, and in the case of reoperation, the exposure of a normal area above and below the scarred area before dissection will decrease the likelihood of damage to the exposed root. On occasion, rents occur in the dural envelope with pouching of the arachnoid or extravasation of cerebrospinal fluid and perhaps protrusion of a nerve root. The herniation must be reduced and the dural tear closed to prevent the complication of a traumatic arachnoid cyst.[58] The possibility of thermal injury to the nerve root secondary to electrocoagulation of extradural vessels can be minimized by the use of bipolar coagulation.

INJURY TO GREAT VESSELS AND VISCERA. In removing the disc, one must be aware that the anulus along the anterior border may be defective, thinned, or perforated.[109] A number of authors have described injury to the great vessels, consisting of damage to the aorta or vena cava or both, or to the iliac vessels, causing associated fall in blood pressure and shock.[37,180,204] A disaster can be prevented by the realization that in these accidents bleeding does not ordinarily flow back into the wound and that a sudden drop in blood pressure and shock may be indication for an immediate laparotomy. In addition, arteriovenous fistulae, injuries to the ureter, bladder, ileum, and appendix have all been described.[85,174] These dangerous complications can be averted by having good exposure and lighting, by exercising particular care in using the pituitary rongeur, introducing it into the interspace with the jaws open, and by making sure that the curet is against bone and that the cutting movement is toward rather than away from the operator.[15] Some authors have advocated the use of depth markers on interbody instruments; these are probably not dependable because of anatomical variations and might introduce a false sense of security. Generally, visceral injuries have been an accompaniment of vascular injury, but the development of signs of peritoneal irritation in a patient recovering from a discectomy must suggest the possibility of isolated visceral injury.

SPASM. Postoperatively there is generally moderate discomfort in the back and an altered aching pain in the affected leg; this requires only routine care. Postopera-

tive abdominal discomfort and urinary retention (particularly in the older man) are also minor problems that are dealt with in a routine manner. On occasion, the postoperative period is marred by severe spasms of the back that respond only to narcotics and to sedation, but that do recede within a few days.[163] In the past, long-acting curare preparations were used; the presently available oral preparations of "muscle relaxants" do not seem to be useful except for their sedative effect.

INFECTION. Major infections of the wound seldom occur, but there is the occasional occurrence of severe, persistent low back pain accompanied by abdominal and groin pain and muscle spasm, coming on five days to several weeks following removal of a disc. Frequently, this is associated with an elevated sedimentation rate, but without other signs of infection. After about 30 days, a progressive destructive change of the opposing surfaces of the vertebrae is seen at the affected interspace, followed by eventual fusion. On reoperation, often a negative culture is obtained from the disc space, although on occasion gram-positive and gram-negative organisms have been incriminated. Unless obvious sepsis is present, characterized by fever, a draining wound, and a positive culture, the effective treatment is usually that of immobilization, and eventual cure may be expected.[153,179,187]

MECHANICAL INSTABILITY. While certain authors have been so bold as to suggest facetectomy and foraminotomy, it is generally maintained that the facets should be preserved to prevent postoperative spinal dislocation or instability with pain.[166]

CHRONIC ADHESIVE ARACHNOIDITIS. Less obvious is the cause of postoperative chronic adhesive arachnoiditis.[175] This is thought to be related to trauma at operation and, in the past, to reaction to the contrast medium; but in the author's experience it has been confined to large midline protrusions with severe compression of the entire spinal canal. Time and occasionally reoperation for removal of the extradural scar seem to benefit most patients. It has been suggested that a dural patch is helpful.[126]

UNRECOGNIZED OR ACQUIRED SPINAL STENOSIS. Significant spinal stenosis may not be recognized preoperatively unless an adequate myelogram has been performed. In such instances a limited interlaminal approach may increase the likelihood of direct damage to or inadequate decompression of the neural elements. In cases with moderate stenosis, operative intervention with an incomplete laminectomy may be associated with the development of later symptomatic stenosis. This is particularly true in some cases in which a posterior fusion has been done; the subsequent stenosis of the spinal canal may become quite marked.

FAILURES. A few patients will remain in the failure category despite all reasonable therapeutic effort. Both organic and functional factors must be reconsidered.[87] Multidisciplinary pain clinics are currently in vogue, but the principles of a combined approach of physical therapy, occupational therapy, superficial psychotherapy, nonaddicting pharmacotherapy, and perhaps external electrical stimulation can be practiced in most settings. Secondary gain factors, when present, should be eliminated. As a general rule, invasive destructive or ablative procedures such as cordotomy are strongly contraindicated; they merely compound the problem. A bonus for an older surgeon is to see many of these "failures" return years later for other reasons after having done quite well in the intervening years.

Disc Disease in Childhood and Adolescence

In one series of 565 patients operated on for ruptured disc, 14 were 18 years of age or under.[116] In another series of 6500 patients, 60 were 18 or younger, but only 5 were less than 16 years old.[196] Generally, reports of confirmed intervertebral disc disease in this age group concerned even fewer patients.*

Usually, the child who has a ruptured disc will have a syndrome similar to that of the adult except that the signs are often more striking than the symptoms. Known trauma is the precipitating factor in about one third of the patients. Backache alone is the earliest symptom and may be associated with a peculiar gait or gait change, limping, and inability to stoop normally, relieved by rest and aggravated by sitting or coughing. Others will have low back pain that is later relieved at the onset of sciatic pain. Walking difficulty, scoliotic posture, and inability to bend forward are often

---

* See references 19, 36, 43, 55, 149.

more pronounced than in the adult counterpart. Lack of response to conservative treatment is indication for myelography; a massive transverse protrusion is found frequently at the lower two interspaces and less often at other levels. At operation, one is struck by the firm, spongy consistency of the massively dislocated disc. Lowrey described three cases of slipping of the vertebral epiphysis along with the disc into the spinal canal (three similar cases have been reported in older patients).[116,170] The results from operative treatment are ordinarily better than those in the adult patient.

While calcification of the intervertebral disc has been noted to be a common accompaniment of aging, there are a number of reports that tabulate over 75 cases of intervertebral disc calcification in childhood.[81,184] In most of these the cervical or thoracic region has been affected, but some instances of lumbar or sacral interspace involvement have been reported. Patients with multiple disc-space involvement may be asymptomatic, but when there is one affected interspace there is usually evidence of an acute illness, sometimes preceded by trauma or a nonspecific upper respiratory infection, and accompanied by a relatively short period of pain and fever and subsequent development of radiographic evidence of disc calcification. Neurological abnormalities are rare, and prognosis is generally excellent with conservative treatment. The principal differential diagnosis is probably spontaneous disc space infection or spondylarthritis. This latter condition is predominantly lumbar, and usually has more evidence of sepsis; there will be progressive radiographic changes, and antibiotic treatment may be necessary.[92,176]

Disc Disease in the Elderly

It has already been noted that as age advances there are progressive desiccation of the disc, increasing degeneration of the cartilaginous plate, and fractures of the anulus with subsequent attempts at healing and calcification. It has also been noted that frequent defects appear in the cartilaginous plate with protrusion of the disc into the bone, and that sometimes there is actual erosion of the cartilage by fragments of marrow and bone. The elderly patient may have a typical herniated disc; progressive spondylosis and secondary changes at the interspace and in the facets may develop because of the loss of normal function, or a transvertebral rupture of the intervertebral disc may develop with spinal compression occurring away from the interspace.[172,173] This may lead to the erroneous preoperative impression of a malignant tumor.

Obviously, in the elderly one is more concerned with the differential diagnosis of possible metastatic neoplastic disease, but the presence of these atypical manifestations of benign correctible disease makes absolute histological diagnosis even more imperative. Reported results from operative intervention are good.[47,183] Radicular pain resulting from foraminal compression in elderly patients with lumbar scoliosis has also been successfully treated by lateral decompression and facetectomy.[46]

Differential Diagnosis

A number of important diseases causing similar symptoms of back and leg pain can be differentiated or at least suspected on the basis of the routine history and physical examination.[8,76,163,177]

In chronic degenerative disc disease associated with osteoarthritis, there is generally a dull aching pain and increasing stiffness and discomfort when the patient is immobile for a period of time, but it is at least partially relieved by mild to moderate activity.

The patient with Marie-Strümpell disease will show a striking decrease in expansion of the chest.

If there is a tumor of the cauda equina, the patient characteristically will complain of intractable low back or sciatic pain or both, which is not relieved by bed rest and usually is worse at night. He may state that he can obtain relief and sleep only by sitting up in a chair.[158]

Vascular insufficiency may be suspected from the history and by palpation and auscultation over the abdominal, inguinal, and peripheral vessels.[66]

The history and a pelvic examination will help to differentiate endometriosis and pelvic neoplasm in women; laparoscopy is useful in some cases to establish the diagnosis of endometriosis.[59,79] The rectal examination permits evaluation of the prostate gland in men.

Disease of the hip may be suspected from the history and the findings on rotation and x-ray examination of the hip. The rare peripheral neural tumors may be found on careful palpation over the course of the peripheral nerves.

Less likely to cause confusion are diabetic neuropathy and sciatic neuropathy due to injection.

Other causes that require additional study for differentiation have been listed in the section on x-ray examination; spondylolisthesis and the narrowed spinal canal are described in more detail in a following section.

In addition, intrasacral meningocele is a rare cause of back and leg pain, as are such conditions as congenital absence of the lumbar articular facets and diastematomyelia.[10,98,162] Malformations of the lumbar spinal roots and sheaths and redundancy of the nerve roots have been described as causes for low backache and sciatica.[49,60] Here, the diagnosis can be made only by operative exploration. It is thought that the symptoms develop as the result of acquired narrowing, and the results from operative decompression are reasonably good.

In epidural exploration, the epidural vein complex may seem small or on occasion may seem unduly large. Often this latter state is caused by abdominal compression and problems with anesthesia, but the surgeon may be tempted to consider a vascular anomaly within the spinal canal. Such anomalies have been described in which relief of symptoms was obtained by coagulation.[68] This condition should not be confused with the symptomatic vertebral hemangioma. This latter diagnosis should be made by the finding of characteristic vertical striation of the involved vertebral bodies on plain x-ray examination. When there is evidence of an intraspinal mass, it has been suggested, preoperative spinal angiography and perhaps embolization should be used.[117]

Another reasonably rare cause of extradural nerve root compression simulating the clinical picture of disc extrusion with radiographic evidence of spondylosis, occasionally intact arch spondylolisthesis, and a dorsolateral filling defect on myelography is a synovial cyst (ganglion) originating from the facet joint.[14]

Tarlov is mainly responsible for suggesting that cysts of the sacral nerve roots be considered as a cause for pain when herniated intervertebral disc or other adequate cause is not found.[185] In the presence of large cysts, the diagnosis can usually be made by careful inspection of plain x-ray films of the sacrum. These large cysts and smaller ones may be demonstrated at the time of myelography, showing slow filling when the patient stands for a period of time. Subsequent x-ray films may reveal that retained oil has filtered into a sacral cyst. Treatment by unroofing the sacrum and obliterating the cyst has been advocated. The experience in this clinic and in others has been that the complaints often have not been relieved by this procedure.

Obviously, when there has been a history of primary malignant disease, one is suspicious of recurrence when the patient begins to complain of back pain and sciatica. It must be remembered, however, that symptoms may not be related to a recurrence but rather to a benign second disease, such as a ruptured intervertebral disc, and appropriate treatment will provide a particularly gratifying response.

SPONDYLOLISTHESIS*

Spondylolysis

Incidence and Etiology

Spondylolysis occurs in about 5 per cent of the adult population, but its presence has never been demonstrated in fetal specimens. There is a case report of a child with a back deformity noted after an uncomplicated birth in whom spondylolisthesis was diagnosed roentgenographically at four months of age.[18] The consensus is that the etiology of spondylolisthesis in children is related to congenital factors of predisposition associated with stress.[5,82] While there are now a number of reports of this disorder occurring in infants and young children, its recognition is unusual before the age of 7 or 8 years. From this age on, it is recognized progressively more frequently; 20 per cent of patients with symptomatic spondylolisthesis are under 20 years of age. Cases have been cited that showed that spondylolysis and spondylolisthesis can be acquired in later life from repeated stress over a long period of time.[13] The average age of the patient seeking treatment is 35 years with a history of symptoms for about 7 years.[25]

Symptoms and Signs

While the defect is found in 5 per cent of cadaver specimens, the clinical incidence is less. Many people go through life with an asymptomatic spondylolysis, but following trauma, usually extension injuries or those incurred when a strong force is exerted vertically downward upon the spine, symptoms may develop.

The clinical manifestations are pain and deformity. The pain is of two varieties. Midline low lumbar pain is thought to be due to instability of the vertebrae and the mechanical stresses caused by this mobility. It is accentuated by weight bearing, lifting, and moving, and is relieved by recumbency and rest. It is frequently aggravated by extension movements. Often it commences insidiously early in life, gradually increasing in severity, or it may appear suddenly associated with an injury. Leg pain is caused by pressure on the roots of the spinal canal and is less common than backache; it occurred in one series in only 36 of 100 cases. Various authors have pointed out that the pain results from nerve root compression from degenerative and proliferative changes about the pseudarthrosis and less commonly from an associated herniation of a disc or distortion of the neural groove.[2,67,80,160]

At the level of the steplike deformity between the vertebrae, the dural envelope makes a double bend and is often densely adherent, but in most instances the cauda equina is not actually compressed; however, cauda equina compression can occur, especially in cases with an intact neural arch. Some authors have postulated that stretching and adhesions may account for some of the sacrococcygeal pain.

On examination, the deformity of the back may not be noticed, but in severe cases there is a steplike change in the alignment of the tips of the spines at the lumbosacral level. Characteristically, the pelvis is rotated forward so that the sacrum becomes more vertical in an attempt to realign the weight of the body for more adequate support. In extreme cases, the hips and knees will be slightly flexed, the trunk tilted forward, and some scoliosis may be present. In extremely severe deformities, the

---

* See references 2, 8, 11, 78, 193.

trunk cannot be held erect over the legs and settles down into the pelvis so that the lower ribs touch the iliac crest and folds appear about the waist.

Intact Neural Arch

Spondylolisthesis with intact vertebrae can occur.[2,48] This is usually seen at the L4–L5 level in patients past middle life who have considerable osteoarthritis of the spine and degenerative changes of the articular cartilage of the facets that allow forward displacement and subluxation; it may occur at the L5–S1 level in the elderly from degenerative changes alone. Recently, however, the case of an 11-year-old girl has been reported.[131] When the vertebral arches are intact, slipping is limited by the impingement of the displaced inferior facet against the body of the vertebra below. The displaced facet thus comes into close relationship with the nerve root, which passes toward the pedicle and the intervertebral foramen of the segment below, while the intact isthmus compresses the nerve root posteriorly. In addition, the superior facet of the subjacent vertebra may add to the compression. In severe deformity, the entire cauda equina may be greatly compressed by the intact neural arch.

Special Examinations

The diagnosis is confirmed by radiological examination, and oblique views are particularly helpful in revealing defects of the pars interarticularis. Lateral views will reveal the degree of forward slippage, which is arbitrarily divided into four grades depending on the quartile of relative forward slippage. Flexion and extension lateral views will give additional information. If operative intervention is being considered, myelography performed with a large amount of contrast medium may be useful, particularly a horizontal-beam study made in flexion and extension.

Treatment

Conservative treatment, consisting of immobilization and flexion exercises, is the first choice unless a severe neurological deficit is present. Continued conservative treatment is generally recommended in children, but children in grade 3 and 4 categories may require lateral fusion.[83] Recently, reduction of severe spondylolisthesis by internal distraction procedures and stabilization has been reported.[77] As the patient grows older and if conservative measures have failed to halt the symptoms, it is generally agreed that operative intervention is indicated. In cases in which radicular symptoms predominate, this operation will consist of exploration and decompression, removal of the mobile unit and pseudarthrosis, and a complete decompression of the nerve root.[67] Discectomy is performed if indicated. In operating upon patients whose back pain is a significant factor, decompression should be combined with stabilization of the spine by fusion. Indications for fusion diminish in patients over 50 years of age and are rare after age 60. A review of 216 cases operated on at the Mayo Clinic (mostly adult patients with grade 1 or 2 spondylolisthesis) suggests that in these cases the best results were obtained from removal of the loose dorsal elements combined with fusion using iliac bone.[80] The author noted that 46 patients had protrusion or extrusion of intervertebral discs as well. Not enough patients had decompression alone to evaluate the effect of this procedure properly. This and other reviews cited in the article suggest that satisfactory clinical results can be expected in from 65 to 90 per cent of the cases treated by operation.[80]

In pseudospondylolisthesis (intact neural arch), liberal laminal decompression including foraminotomy and medial or total facetectomy gives good to excellent results.[48] Rothman and Simeone further note that in some individuals the nerve root will still be tightly tethered around the pedicle, which has undergone movement during this disc degeneration, and in these individuals the pedicle must also be excised.[148]

NARROW SPINAL CANAL

Recent years have brought increasing recognition of and interest in evaluation and treatment of symptom-producing strictures of the lumbar vertebral canal. While an incidence of occurrence is not known, a recent article described 33 cases diagnosed by myelography from a total of about 2000 myelograms performed in a three-year period.[145]

Congenital Strictures

Sarpyener described symptom-producing congenital strictures of the spinal canal.[151] While noting the frequent association of narrowing in spina bifida occulta, he reported 10 cases of congenital stricture not associated with this deformity. All his patients were children who had enuresis and variable degrees of paralysis and atrophy of the lower extremities. Some of his patients had a ringlike stricture at one or more levels in the lumbar region, some strictures involved the entire lumbar canal, and some had local constrictions associated with what was probably diastematomyelia. Two patients who had clefts of the cord and dura mater also had tumors (probably myelomeningocele) and died. The remainder were improved by laminectomy. It is interesting that he notes that the anteroposterior x-ray views did not show narrowing between the pedicles.

Achondroplasia

Another congenital narrowing that becomes symptomatic because of acquired changes is seen in patients with achondroplasia.[3,43] The predisposing factors are a narrow shallow spinal canal with shortened pedicles, incomplete straightening of the vertebral column during fetal life, unusually thick wedge-shaped intervertebral discs, and, in the adult, thickening of the laminae and development of marginal exostoses. Thus the pronounced dorsal kyphosis becomes associated with large osteoarthritic spurs and an occasional herniated disc causing severe constriction of an already small canal. The generalized constriction is most prominent from T11 downward with progressive terminal lumbar stenosis. Naturally, the symptoms of compression will vary according to the area involved; for example, compression of the cervical cord causes spastic paresis of the arms and legs, but low dorsal compression is manifest by spastic paraparesis and bladder and bowel disturbance. If the lower lumbar region is primarily involved, paresthesias and pain (particularly on standing), weakness, and a foot-drop will develop.

Lumbar puncture is difficult because of crowding of the nerve roots; myelography by cisternal or lateral cervical puncture will demonstrate the area of constriction. Widespread decompressive laminectomy should halt the progression of the neurological deficit and, it is hoped, relieve pain and lead to some improvement in the neurological status. Stabilization of the spine may be indicated in some patients. Hazards of operation and a high complication rate, including an increase in neurological disability and spine instability, have been emphasized by Roberts and co-workers.[146]

Two patients with acromegaly have been described who had bone forming in the cartilaginous end-plates, widening of the vertebral bodies by subperiosteal osteogenesis, and increasing kyphosis.[138] They had protruded discs at the conus and were improved by operation.

Spondylosis and the Small Canal

While protruded discs are the common cause for nerve root compression in the middle years, the fifth and sixth decades are marked by dehydration and collapse of the nucleus and bulging in all directions of the anulus, which becomes calcified or ossified; new bone forms along the adjacent vertebral margins, creating lips or spurs. With collapse of the disc, there is subluxation of the corresponding intervertebral joints and narrowing of the intervertebral foramina, which may be further compromised by osteophytic formation at the articular processes.[22]

Foraminal compression of the spinal nerves is less common in the lumbar than in the cervical region, but the incidence increases in the older age group, particularly in the seventh and eighth decades and especially in diabetic patients. The syndrome may be indistinguishable from that of a ruptured intervertebral disc, although the pain is usually less severe than the sciatic pain of disc protrusion, and it is less likely to be exacerbated by coughing or sneezing. Clinical involvement may be of one or more roots, and it may be unilateral or bilateral. Dysesthesias without pain may be prominent, and, if several roots are involved, conspicuous muscular weakness, wasting, and reflex changes may be present.

Considerable interest has been focused in recent years on the small but otherwise normal spinal canal that has had its already borderline lumen further compromised by spondylosis. Myelopathy resulting from the narrow spondylotic cervical canal is well known; pseudoclaudication, or a more profound neural dysfunction of the lower extremities resulting from spondylotic embarrassment of the small lumbar canal, is just beginning to get wide recognition.

Of historic interest, Goldthwait, in 1911, described the case of a 39-year-old man who gave a previous history of back pain and a recent exacerbation accompanied by leg pain.[70] After responding once to manipulation, the pain recurred; after repeated manipulation and immobilization in a cast, the patient became paraplegic. Harvey Cushing performed a lumbar laminectomy on him and on intradural exploration found only a narrowed canal at the lumbosacral interspace. Following this decompression, the patient made a slow and incomplete recovery.

Several authors have reported cases of cauda equina compression from hypertrophy of the laminae, hypertrophic arthritis, and thickened yellow ligaments, but Ehni has stressed the additive compression of the entire spondylotic syndrome.[41]

Standard measurements of the lumbar canal were made in 1951.[88] It was found that the important sagittal diameter varies in normal adults from a minimum of 14 mm at L1 to 11 mm at L4 to a maximum of 20 mm at L2 to 27 mm at L3. Unfortunately, these measurements cannot be made on routine x-rays as they can in the cervical spine, and the measurable interpedicular distances have been found to be of little importance in clinical evaluation. These measurements were made at the request of Verbiest, who described a series of patients, all men, whose symptoms began between the ages of 37 and 67 years and produced a characteristic syndrome of disturbance of the cauda equina on walking and standing, manifested by bilateral radicular pain, disturbance of sensation, and impairment of motor power in the legs that disappeared immediately when the patient lay down, and associated with a normal neurological examination.[191,192] He stated that the symptoms could be misinterpreted as intermittent claudication of vascular origin. No anomalies were seen on the plain x-ray films, but myelographic studies showed gradual narrowing of the lumbar canal with a block. At operation, only narrowing of the canal was found, and the symptoms were relieved by decompressive laminectomy.

After further study, Verbiest concluded that developmental narrowing of the lumbar canal caused by an abnormally short anteroposterior diameter does exist and that additional slight deformity, such as posterior lipping or a small protruded disc, can produce symptoms of compression, especially when the back is in the standing lordotic position.

Others call attention to the relative importance of variations in the shape of the canal, particularly the triangular canal with a narrow lateral recess in which a small protruded disc or osteophyte can cause considerable compression of the overlying nerve root.[8,44,45,76]

Subsequent contributions have pointed out the dangers of acute extension of the back, especially when the patient is under anesthesia, and the fact that two forms of intermittent claudication of the cauda equina may exist, namely, the postural variety producing symptoms of compression from hyperextension of the lumbar spine and the ischemic variety resulting from impaired blood flow through constricted radicular arteries.*

The diagnosis may be suspected from the clinical picture and principally must be differentiated from intermittent claudication due to arterial insufficiency.[202] Polytomography may reveal narrowing of the anteriorposterior diameter of the canal; computed tomography may prove to be of diagnostic value, but at this time the diagnosis can be confirmed only by myelography or by intraoperative measurement of the canal. Myelography can usually be accomplished only by introduction of the contrast medium through the cisternal or the lateral cervical approach. Treatment includes wide laminectomy and partial facetectomy well above and below the stenotic areas delineated on the myelogram. Some authors routinely remove the inferior articular processes and their facets.[167] Postoperative instability has not been a problem in these patients. When extensive neural damage has not already occurred, dramatic relief has been described.[104]

REFERENCES

1. Abdullah, A. F., Ditto, E. W., III, Byrd, E. B., and Williams, R.: Extreme-lateral lumbar disc herniations: Clinical syndrome and special problems of diagnosis. J. Neurosurg., *41*: 229–234, 1974.

---

* See references 16, 29, 40, 97, 201, 202.

2. Adkins, E. W. O.: Spondylolisthesis. J. Bone Joint Surg., *37-B*:48–62, 1955.

3. Alexander, E., Jr.: Significance of the small lumbar spinal canal: Cauda equina compression syndromes due to spondylosis. Part 5: Achondroplasia. J. Neurosurg., *31*:513–519, 1969.

4. Amsler, F. R., Jr., and Wilber, M. C.: Intraosseous vertebral venography as diagnostic aid in evaluating intervertebral disk diseases of lumbar spine. J. Bone Joint Surg., *49-A*:703–712, 1967.

5. Amuso, S. J., and Mankin, H. J.: Hereditary spondylolisthesis and spina bifida. Report of a family in which the lesion is transmitted as an autosomal dominant through three generations. J. Bone Joint Surg., *49-A*:507–513, 1967.

6. Andersson, G. B. J., Örtengren, R., and Nachemson, A.: Quantitative studies of back loads in lifting. Spine, *1*:178–185, 1976.

7. Andersson, H., and Carlsson, C-A.: Prognosis of operatively treated lumbar disc herniations causing foot extensor paralysis. Acta Chir. Scand., *132*:501–506, 1966.

8. Armstrong, J. R.: Lumbar Disc Lesions. 3rd Ed. Baltimore, Williams & Wilkins Co., 1965.

9. Aronson, H. A., and Dunsmore, R. H.: Herniated upper lumbar discs. J. Bone Joint Surg., *45-A*:311–317, 1963.

10. Baker, G. S., and Webb, J. H.: Intrasacral meningocele causing backache and sacral nerve pain. Report of a case. Proc. Mayo Clin., *27*:231–234, 1952.

11. Barr, J. S.: Spondylolisthesis. An editorial. J. Bone Joint Surg., *37-A*:878–880, 1955.

12. Bauer, F. K., and Yuhl, E. T.: Myelography by means of I¹³¹. The myeloscintigram. Neurology (Minneap.), *3*:341–346, 1953.

13. Beller, H. E., and Kirsh, D.: Spondylolysis and spondylolisthesis following low back fusions. Southern Med. J., *57*:783–786, 1964.

14. Bhushan, C., Hodges, F. J., III, and Wityk, J. J.: Lumbar spine synovial cyst (ganglion) simulating extradural space-occupying lesion. Read before the American Association of Neurological Surgeons, San Francisco, Calif., April 4, 1976.

15. Birkeland, I. W., Jr., and Taylor, T. K. F.: Bowel injuries coincident to lumbar disk surgery: A report of four cases and a review of the literature. J. Trauma, *10*:163–168, 1970.

16. Blau, J. N., and Logue, V.: Intermittent claudication of cauda equina. An unusual syndrome resulting from central protrusion of a lumbar intervertebral disc. Lancet, *1*:1081–1086, 1961.

17. Blumer, D.: Psychiatric considerations in pain. *In* Rothman, R. H., and Simeone, F. A., eds.: The Spine. Philadelphia, W. B. Saunders Co., 1975, chap. 18.

18. Borkow, S. E., and Kleiger, B.: Spondylolisthesis in the newborn: A case report. Clin. Orthop., *81*:73–76, 1971.

19. Bradford, D. S., and Garcia, A.: Lumbar intervertebral disk herniations in children and adolescents. Orthop. Clin. N. Amer., *2*:583–592, 1971.

20. Bradford, F. K., and Spurling, R. G.: The Intervertebral Disc with Special Reference to Rupture of the Annulus Fibrosus with Herniation of the Nucleus Pulposus. 2nd Ed. Springfield, Ill., Charles C Thomas, 1945.

21. Brady, L. P., Parker, L. B., and Vaughen, J.: An evaluation of the electromyogram in the diagnosis of the lumbar-disc lesion. J. Bone Joint Surg., *51-A*:539–547, 1969.

22. Brain, R.: Spondylosis—the known and the unknown. Lancet, *266*:687–693, 1954.

23. Brown, M. D.: The pathophysiology of disc disease. Orthop. Clin. N. Amer., *2*:359–370, 1971.

24. Brown, T., Hansen, R. J., and Yorra, A. J.: Some mechanical tests on the lumbosacral spine with particular reference to the intervertebral discs: A preliminary report. J. Bone Joint Surg., *39-A*:1135–1164, 1957.

25. Caldwell, G. A.: Spondylolisthesis. Ann. Surg., *119*:485–497, 1944.

26. Cloward, R. B.: Treatment of ruptured lumbar intervertebral discs by vertebral body fusion. I. Indications, operative technic, after care. J. Neurosurg., *10*:154–168, 1953.

27. Collis, J. S., Jr., and Gardner, W. J.: Lumbar discography. An analysis of one thousand cases. J. Neurosurg., *19*:452–461, 1962.

28. Connor, A. C., Rooney, J. A., and Carroll, J. P.: Anterior lumbar fusion. Technic combining intervertebral and intravertebral body fixation. Surg. Clin. N. Amer., *47*:231–237, 1967.

29. Cooke, T. D. V., and Lehmann, P. O.: Intermittent claudication of neurogenic origin. Canad. J. Surg., *11*:151–159, 1968.

30. Coventry, M. B., Ghormley, R. K., and Kernohan, J. W.: The intervertebral disc. Its microscopic anatomy and pathology. Part I. Anatomy, development, and physiology. J. Bone Joint Surg., *27*:105–112, 1945.

31. Coventry, M. B., Ghormley, R. K., and Kernohan, J. W.: The intervertebral disc. Its microscopic anatomy and pathology. Part II. Changes in the intervertebral disc concomitant with age. J. Bone Joint Surg., *27*:233–247, 1945.

32. Coventry, M. B., Ghormley, R. K., and Kernohan, J. W.: The intervertebral disc. Its microscopic anatomy and pathology. Part III. Pathological changes in the intervertebral disc. J. Bone Joint Surg., *27*:460–474, 1945.

33. Crue, B. L., Pudenz, R. H., and Shelden, C. H.: Observations on the value of clinical electromyography. J. Bone Joint Surg., *39-A*:492–500, 1957.

34. Dandy, W. E.: Loose cartilage from intervertebral disk simulating tumor of the spinal cord. Arch. Surg. (Chicago), *19*:660–672, 1929.

35. Davis, C. H., Jr., and Martin, J. F.: Ordering x-rays and performing contrast studies. Problems, pitfalls, and practical points. *In* Toole, J. F., ed.: Special Techniques in Neurologic Diagnosis. Philadelphia, F. A. Davis Co., 1969, pp. 49–69.

36. Day, P. L.: The teen-age disk syndrome. Southern Med. J., *60*:247–250, 1967.

37. DeSaussure, R. L.: Vascular injury coincident to disc surgery. J. Neurosurg., *16*:222–229, 1959.

38. Dyck, P.: The femoral nerve traction test with lumbar disc protrusions. Surg. Neurol., *6*:163–166, 1976.

39. Editorial. Physiotherapy or psychotherapy? Lancet, *2*:1483, 1973.

40. Ehni, G.: Significance of the small lumbar spinal canal: Cauda equina compression syndromes

due to spondylosis. Part 4: Acute compression artificially-induced during operation. J. Neurosurg., *31*:507–512, 1969.

41. Ehni, G.: Significance of the small lumbar spinal canal: Cauda equina compression syndromes due to spondylosis. Part 1: Introduction. J. Neurosurg., *31*:490–494, 1969.

41a. Elsberg, C. A. (Cited by Armstrong, J. R., see ref. 8).

42. Emmett, J. L., and Love, J. G.: Urinary retention in women caused by asymptomatic protruded lumbar disk. Report of 5 cases. J. Urol., *99*:597–606, 1968.

43. Epstein, J. A., and Lavine, L. S.: Herniated lumbar intervertebral discs in teen-age children. J. Neurosurg., *21*:1070–1075, 1964.

44. Epstein, J. A., and Malis, L. I.: Compression of spinal cord and cauda equina in achondroplastic dwarfs. Neurology (Minneap.), *5*:875–881, 1955.

45. Epstein, J. A., Epstein, B. S., and Lavine, L.: Nerve root compression associated with narrowing of the lumbar spinal canal. J. Neurol. Neurosurg. Psychiat., *25*:165–176, 1962.

46. Epstein, J. A., Epstein, B. S., and Lavine, L. S.: Surgical treatment of nerve root compression caused by scoliosis of the lumbar spine. J. Neurosurg., *41*:449–454, 1974.

47. Epstein, J. A., Lavine, L. S., Epstein, B. S., and Carras, R.: Herniated disks and related disorders of the lumbar spine. Surgical treatment in the geriatric patient. J.A.M.A., *202*:187–190, 1967.

48. Epstein, J. A., Epstein, B. S., Lavine, L. S., Carras, R., and Rosenthal, A. D.: Degenerative lumbar spondylolisthesis with an intact neural arch (pseudospondylolisthesis). J. Neurosurg., *44*:139–147, 1976.

49. Ethelberg, S., and Riihede, J.: Malformation of lumbar spinal roots and sheaths as causation of low backache and sciatica. J. Bone Joint Surg., *34-B*:442–446, 1952.

50. Eyring, E. J.: The biochemistry and physiology of the intervertebral disc. Clin. Orthop., *67*:16–28, 1969.

51. Farfan, H. F., Cossette, J. W., Robertson, G. H., Wells, R. V., and Kraus, H.: The effects of torsion on the lumbar intervertebral joints: The role of torsion in the production of disc degeneration. J. Bone Joint Surg., *52-A*:468–497, 1970.

52. Fazio, C., Agnoli, A., Bava, G. L., Bozzao, L., and Fieschi, C.: Demonstration of spinal tumors with intravenously injected ^{99m}Tc-pertechnetate. A new diagnostic technique. J. Nucl. Med., *10*:508–510, 1969.

53. FDA Drug Bulletin, Feb.–March, 1976, p. 20.

54. Feffer, H. L.: Therapeutic intradiscal hydrocortisone. A long term study. Clin. Orthop., *67*:100–104, 1969.

55. Fernstrom, U.: Protruded lumbar intervertebral disk in children. Report of a case and review of the literature. Acta Chir. Scand., *111*:71–79, 1956.

56. Flax, H. J., Berrios, R., and Rivera, D.: Electromyography in the diagnosis of herniated lumbar disc. Arch. Phys. Med., *45*:520–524, 1964.

57. Foltz, E. L., Ward, A. A., and Knopp, L. M.: Intervertebral fusion following lumbar disc excision. J. Neurosurg., *13*:469–478, 1956.

58. Ford, L. T.: Local complications of lumbar-disc surgery. J. Bone Joint Surg., *50-A*:418–428, 1968.

59. Forrest, J. S., and Brooks, D. L.: Cyclic sciatica of endometriosis. J.A.M.A., *222*:1177–1178, 1972.

60. Fox, J. L.: Redundant nerve roots in the cauda equina. J. Neurosurg., *30*:74–75, 1969.

61. Friberg, S., and Hirsch, C.: Anatomical and clinical studies on lumbar disc degeneration. Acta Orthop. Scand., *19*:222–242, 1950.

62. Gargano, F. P.: Transverse axial tomography of the lumbar spine. *In* Rothman, R. H., and Simeone, F. A., eds.: The Spine. Philadelphia, W. B. Saunders Co., 1975, chap. 9, part 2.

63. Gargano, F. P., Meyer, J. D., and Sheldon, J. J.: Transfemoral ascending lumbar catheterization of the epidural veins in lumbar disk disease. Clinical application and results in the diagnosis of herniated intervertebral disks of the lumbar spine. Radiology, *111*:329–336, 1974.

64. Gellman, M.: Injury to intervertebral disks during spinal puncture. J. Bone Joint Surg., *22*:980–985, 1940.

65. Gershater, R., and Holgate, R. C.: Lumbar epidural venography in the diagnosis of disc herniations. Amer. J. Roentgen., *126*:992–1002, 1976.

66. Gilfillan, R. S., Jones, O. W., Jr., Roland, S. I., and Wylie, E. J.: Arterial occlusions simulating neurological disorders of the lower limbs. J.A.M.A., *154*:1149–1152, 1954.

67. Gill, G. G., Manning. J. G., and White, H. L.: Surgical treatment of spondylolisthesis without spine fusion. J. Bone Joint Surg., *37-A*:493–520, 1955.

68. Gloor, P. P., Woringer, E., Schneider, J., and Brogly, G.: Lombo-sciatiques par anomalies vasculaires épidurales. Contribution à l'étude de la pathologie du plexus veineux intrarachidien, Schweiz. Med. Wschr., *82*:537–542, 1952.

69. Goldner, J. L., Urbaniak, J. R., and McCollum, D. E.: Anterior disc excision and interbody spinal fusion for chronic low back pain. Orthop. Clin. N. Amer., *2*:543–568, 1971.

70. Goldthwait, J. E.: The lumbosacral articulation. An explanation of many cases of "lumbago," "sciatica," and paraplegia. Boston Med. Surg. J., *164*:365–372, 1911.

71. Goodgold, J.: Letter to the editor. J. Bone Joint Surg., *51-A*:1451, 1969.

72. Greenwood, J., Jr.: Optimum vitamin C intake as a factor in the preservation of disc integrity. Med. Ann. D. C., *33*:274–276, 1964.

73. Greenwood, J., Jr., McGuire, T. H., and Kimbell, F.: Study of the causes of failure in the herniated intervertebral disc operation. An analysis of sixty-seven reoperated cases. J. Neurosurg., *9*:15–20, 1952.

74. Gurdjian, E. S., Ostrowski, A. Z., Hardy, W. G., Lindner, D. W., and Thomas, L. M.: Results of operative treatment of protruded and ruptured lumbar discs based on 1176 operative cases with 82 per cent follow-up of 3 to 13 years. J. Neurosurg., *18*:783–791, 1961.

75. Haft. H., and Shenkin, H. A.: Herniated lumbar intervertebral disks with unilateral pain and midline myelographic defects. Unilateral or bilateral excision? Surgery, *60*:269–273, 1966.

76. Hanraets, P. R. M. J.: The Degenerative Back. Amsterdam, Elsevier Publishing Co., 1959.

77. Harrington, P. R., and Tullos, H. S.: Reduction of severe spondylolisthesis in children. Southern Med. J., 62:1–7, 1969.

78. Harris, R. I.: Spondylolisthesis. Ann. Roy. Coll. Surg., 8:259–297, 1951.

79. Head, H. B., Welch, J. S., Mussey, E., and Espinosa, R. E.: Cyclic sciatica. Report of case with introduction of a new surgical sign. J.A.M.A., 180:521–524, 1962.

80. Henderson, E. D.: Results of surgical treatment of spondylolisthesis. J. Bone Joint Surg., 48-A:619–642, 1966.

81. Henry, M. J., Grimes, H.A., and Lane, J. W.: Intervertebral disk calcification in childhood. Radiology, 89:81–84, 1967.

82. Hensinger, R. N., and MacEwen, G. D.: Congenital anomalies of the spine. In Rothman, R. H., and Simeone, F. A., eds.: The Spine. Philadelphia, W. B. Saunders Co., 1975, chap. 5.

83. Hensinger, R. N., Lange, J. R., and MacEwen, G. D.: Surgical management of spondylolisthesis in children and adolescents. Spine, 1:207–216, 1976.

84. Hirsch, C., Jonsson, B., and Lewin, T.: Low-back symptoms in a Swedish female population. Clin. Orthop., 63:171–176, 1969.

85. Holscher, E. C.: Vascular and visceral injuries during lumbar-disc surgery. J. Bone Joint Surg., 50-A:383–393, 1968.

86. Holt, E. P., Jr.: The question of lumbar discography. J. Bone Joint Surg., 50-A:720–726, 1968.

87. Hubbard, J. H.: The management of chronic pain of spinal origin. In Rothman, R. H., and Simeone, F. A., eds.: The Spine. Philadelphia, W. B. Saunders Co., 1975, chap. 17.

88. Huizinga, Heiden, and Vinken (Cited by Verbiest, H., see ref. 191).

89. Hult, L.: Cervical, dorsal and lumbar spinal syndromes. A field investigation of a non-selected material of 1200 workers in different occupations with special reference to disc degeneration and so-called muscular rheumatism. Acta Orthop. Scand., Suppl. 17:1–102, 1954.

90. Hult, L.: Munkfors Investigation. Acta Orthop. Scand., Suppl. 16:32–57, 1954.

91. Jackson, H. C., II, Winkelmann, R. K., and Bickel, W. H.: Nerve endings in human lumbar spinal column and related structures. J. Bone Joint Surg., 48-A:1272–1281, 1966.

92. Jacobs, G. B., Rubin, R. C., Cooper, P. R., and Mazzola, R.: Disc space infection in children. Read before the American Association of Neurological Surgeons, San Francisco, Calif., April 4, 1976.

93. Jacobson, R. E., Gargano, F. P., and Rosomoff, H. L.: Transverse axial tomography of the spine. Part 1. Axial anatomy of the normal lumbar spine. J. Neurosurg., 42:406–411, 1975.

94. Jacobson, R. E., Gargano, F. P., and Rosomoff, H. L.: Transverse axial tomography of the spine. Part 2. The stenotic spinal canal. J. Neurosurg., 42:412–419, 1975.

95. Johnson, R. M., and Southwick, W. O.: Surgical approaches to the spine. Part III. Surgical approaches to the lumbar spine. In Rothman, R. H., and Simeone, F. A., eds.: The Spine. Philadelphia, W. B. Saunders Co., 1975, chap. 4.

96. Kambin, P., Smith, J. M., and Hoerner, E. F.: Myelography and myography in diagnosis of herniated intervertebral disk. J.A.M.A., 181:472–475, 1962.

97. Kavanaugh, G. J., Svien, H. J., Holman, C. B., and Johnson, R. M.: "Pseudoclaudication" syndrome produced by compression of the cauda equina. J.A.M.A., 206:2477–2481, 1968.

98. Keim, H. A., and Keagy, R. D.: Congenital absence of lumbar articular facets. Report of 3 cases. J. Bone Joint Surg., 49-A:523–526, 1967.

99. Keith, A.: Hunterian lectures on man's posture: its evolution and disorders. Given at the Royal College of Surgeons of England. Lecture II. The evolution of the orthograde spine. Brit. Med. J., 1:499–502, 1923.

100. Keith. A.: Man's posture. Notes on its evolution. In Ellis, J. D., ed.: The Injured Back and Its Treatment. Springfield, Ill., Charles C Thomas, 1940, chap. 1.

101. Kelsey, J. L., and Hardy, R. J.: Driving of motor vehicles as a risk factor for acute herniated lumbar intervertebral disc. Amer. J. Epidem., 102:63–73, 1975.

102. Keyes, D. C., and Compere, E. L.: The normal and pathological physiology of the nucleus pulposus of the intervertebral disc. An anatomical, clinical and experimental study. J. Bone Joint Surg., 14:897–938, 1932.

103. Kiefer, S.A., Stadian, E. M., Mohandas, A., and Peterson, H. O.: Discographic-anatomical correlation of developmental changes with age in the intervertebral disc. Acta Radiol., 9:733–739, 1969.

104. Kirkaldy-Willis, W. H., Paine, K. W. E., Cauchoix, J., and McIvor, G.: Lumbar spinal stenosis. Clin. Orthop., 99:30–50, 1974.

105. Knutsson, B.: Comparative value of electromyographic myelographic and clinical-neurological examination in diagnosis of lumbar root compression syndrome. Acta Orthop. Scand., suppl. 49, 1961.

106. Knutsson, F.: Lumbar myelography with water-soluble contrast in cases of disc prolapse. Acta Orthop. Scand., 20:294–302, 1951.

107. Langenskiöld, A., and Kiviluoto, O. Prevention of epidural scar formation after operation on the lumbar spine by means of free fat transplants. A preliminary report. Clin. Orthop. 115:92–95, 1976.

108. La Rocca, H., and Macnab, I.: Value of pre-employment radiographic assessment of the lumbar spine. Industr. Med. Surg., 39:253–258, 1970.

109. Leavens, M. E., and Bradford, F. K.: Ruptured intervertebral disk. Report of a case with a defect in the anterior annulus fibrosus. J. Neurosurg., 10:544–546, 1953.

110. LePage, J. R.: Transfemoral ascending lumbar catheterization of epidural veins. Exposition and technique. Radiology, 111:337–339, 1974.

111. Levy, L. F.: Lumbar intervertebral disc disease in Africans. J. Neurosurg., 26:31–34, 1967.

112. Lindblom, K.: Technique and results of diagnostic disc puncture and injection (discography) in the lumbar region. Acta Orthop. Scand., 20:315–326, 1951.

113. Lindblom, K.: Intervertebral-disc degeneration

considered as pressure atrophy. J. Bone Joint Surg., 39-A:933–945, 1957.

114. Lindblom, K., and Rexed, B.: Spinal nerve injury in dorsolateral protrusions of lumbar disks. J. Neurosurg., 5:413–432, 1948.

115. Lora, J., and Long, D.: So-called facet denervation in the management of intractable back pain. Spine, 1:121–126, 1976.

116. Lowrey, J. J.: Dislocated lumbar vertebral epiphysis in teenagers. Read before the American Academy of Neurological Surgery, Colorado Springs, Colo., Oct. 7, 1968.

117. McAllister, V. L., Kendall, B. E., and Bull, J. W. D.: Symptomatic vertebral haemangiomas. Brain, 98:71–80, 1975.

118. MacCarty, W. C., Jr., and Lane, F. W., Jr.: Pitfalls of myelography. Radiology, 65:663–670, 1955.

119. McCollum, D. E., and Stephen, C. R.: The use of graduated spinal anesthesia in the differential diagnosis of pain of the back and lower extremities. Southern Med. J., 57:410–416, 1964.

120. Macnab, I.: Personal communication. (Cited by Gargano, F. P., see ref. 62).

121. Macnab, I.: The traction spur. An indicator of segmental instability. J. Bone Joint Surg., 53-A:663–670, 1971.

122. Macnab, I.: Chemonucleolysis. Clin. Neurosurg., 20:183–192, 1973.

123. McNeill, T. W., Huncke, B., Kornblatt, I., Stiehl, J., and Khan, H. A.: A new advance in water-soluble myelography. Spine, 1:72–84, 1976.

124. Martins Campos, J. A., Pratas Vital, J., and Céu Coutinho, A.: Electromyelography in the diagnosis of lumbar disc protrusion. Read before The Society of British Neurological Surgeons, Southwick, U.K., Oct. 7, 1976.

125. Mason, M. S., and Raaf, J.: Complications of Pantopaque myelography. Case report and review. J. Neurosurg., 19:302–311, 1962.

126. Mayfield, F. H., and O'Brien, M.: Segmental adhesive arachnoiditis (or pachymeningitis), postoperative. A method of surgical treatment. Read before the American Association of Neurological Surgeons (Harvey Cushing Society), St. Louis, Mo., April 20, 1966.

127. Mendelsohn, R. A., and Sola, A.: Electromyography in herniated lumbar disks. Arch. Neurol. Psychiat. (Chicago), 79:142–145, 1958.

128. Meredith, J. M.: The vagaries and peculiarities of studies with subarachnoid oil in cases of protruded disc. A plea for early study with oil after negative or even "positive" surgical exploration for protrusion of lumbar and cervical discs with persistent postoperative symptoms. Southern Med. J., 52:322–329, 1959.

129. Miller, M. H., Handel, S. F., and Coan, J. D.: Transfemoral lumbar epidural venography. Amer. J. Roentgen., 126:1003–1009, 1976.

130. Mixter, W. J., and Barr, J. S.: Rupture of the intervertebral disk with involvement of the spinal canal. New Eng. J. Med., 211:210–215, 1934.

131. Moiel, R., and Ehni, G.: Cauda equina compression due to spondylolisthesis with intact neural arch. J. Neurosurg., 28:262–265, 1968.

132. Morris, J. M., Lucas, D. B., and Bresler, B.: Role of the trunk in stability of the spine. J. Bone Joint Surg., 43-A:327–351, 1961.

133. Murphey, F.: Sources and patterns of pain in disc disease. Clin. Neurosurg., 15:343–351, 1968.

134. Nachemson, A. L.: The lumbar spine. An orthopaedic challenge. Spine, 1:59–71, 1976.

135. Nachemson, A., and Elfström, G.: Intravital dynamic pressure measurements in lumbar discs. A study of common movements, maneuvers and exercises. Scand. J. Rehab. Med., suppl., 1:1–40, 1970.

136. Naylor, A.: Intervertebral disc prolapse and degeneration. The biochemical and biophysical approach. Spine, 1:108–114, 1976.

137. Norlen, G.: On the value of the neurological symptoms in sciatica for the localization of a lumbar disc herniation. Acta Chir. Scand., suppl. 95, 1944.

138. O'Connell, J. E. A.: Involvement of spinal cord by intervertebral disc protrusions. Brit. J. Surg., 43:226–247, 1955.

139. O'Connell, J. E. A.: The indications for and results of the excision of lumbar intervertebral disc protrusions. Review of 500 cases. Ann. Roy. Coll. Surg., 6:403–412, 1950.

140. Parke, W. W.: Development of the spine. In Rothman, R. H., and Simeone, F. A., eds.: The Spine. Philadelphia, W. B. Saunders Co., 1975, chap. 1.

141. Parke, W. W.: Applied anatomy of the spine. In Rothman, R. H., and Simeone, F. A., eds.: The Spine. Philadelphia, W. B. Saunders Co., 1975, chap. 2.

142. Pease, C. N.: Injuries to the vertebrae and intervertebral disks following lumbar puncture. Amer. J. Dis. Child., 49:849–860, 1935.

143. Pedersen, H. E., Blunck, C. F. J., and Gardner, E.: The anatomy of lumbosacral posterior rami and meningeal branches of spinal nerves (sinuvertebral nerves). J. Bone Joint Surg., 38-A:377–391, 1956.

144. Peterson, H. O.: Commentary on myelography: Defense of Pantopaque. In Morley, T. P., ed.: Current Controversies in Neurosurgery. Philadelphia, W. B. Saunders Co., 1976, chap. 2.

145. Roberson, G. H., Llewellyn, H. J., and Traveras, J. M.: The narrow lumbar spinal canal syndrome. Radiology, 107:89–98, 1973.

146. Roberts, M., Collias, J. C., Gahm, N. H., Dunsmore, R. H., and Whitcomb, B. B.: The treatment of spinal stenosis associated with achondroplasia. Read before the Congress of Neurological Surgeons, Atlanta, Ga., Oct. 21, 1975.

147. Rothman, R. H.: Indications for lumbar fusion. Clin. Neurosurg., 20:215–219, 1973.

148. Rothman, R. H., and Simeone, F. A.: Lumbar disc disease. In Rothman, R. H., and Simeone, F. A., eds.: The Spine. Philadelphia, W. B. Saunders Co., 1975, chap. 9, Part 1.

149. Rugtveit, A.: Juvenile lumbar disk herniations. Acta Orthop. Scand., 37:348–356, 1966.

150. Sackett, J. F., Damm, M. G., and Javid, M. J.: Unreliability of epidural venography in lumbar disc disease. Surg. Neurol., 7:35–38, 1977.

151. Sarpyener, M. A.: Congenital stricture of the spinal canal. J. Bone Joint Surg., 27:70–79, 1945.

152. Schein, A. J.: Evolution and pathogenesis of discogenic spine pain and associated radiculitis as seen in the New York City Fire Department. J. Mount Sinai Hosp., 35:371–389, 1968.

153. Scherbel, A. L., and Gardner, W. J.: Infections

involving the intervertebral disks. J.A.M.A., *174*:370–374, 1960.

154. Schmorl (Cited by Mixter, W. J., and Barr, J. S., see ref. 130).

155. Schobinger, R. A.: Intra-Osseous Venography. New York & London, Grune & Stratton 1960, chap. 9.

156. Schobinger, R. A., Krueger, E. G., and Sobel, G. L.: Comparison of intra-osseous vertebral venography and Pantopaque myelography in diagnosis of surgical conditions of the lumbar spine and nerve roots. Radiology, *77*:376–398, 1961.

157. Schwetschenau, P. R., Ramirez, A., Johnston, J., Barnes, E., Wiggs, C., and Martins, A. N.: Double-blind evaluation of intradiscal chymopapain for herniated lumbar discs. Early results. J. Neurosurg., *45*:622–627, 1976.

158. Scott, M.: Relief of nocturnal intractable low back and sciatic pain by "chair sleep." J.A.M.A., *196*:738–739, 1966.

159. Scoville, W. B.: Extradural spinal sensory rhizotomy. J. Neurosurg., *25*:94–95, 1966.

160. Scoville, W. B., and Corkill, G.: Lumbar spondylolisthesis with ruptured disc. J. Neurosurg., *40*:529–534, 1974.

161. Scoville, W. B., Moretz, W. H., and Hankins, W. D.: Discrepancies in myelography. Statistical survey of 200 operative cases undergoing Pantopaque myelography. Surg. Gynec. Obstet., *86*:559–564, 1948.

162. Seaman, W. B., and Schwartz, H. G.: Diastematomyelia in adults. Radiology, *70*:692–696, 1958.

163. Semmes, R. E.: Ruptures of the Lumbar Intervertebral Disc. Springfield, Ill., Charles C Thomas, 1964.

164. Shealy, C. N.: Dangers of spinal injections without proper diagnosis. J.A.M.A., *197*:1104–1106, 1966.

165. Shealy, C. N.: Percutaneous radiofrequency denervation of spinal facets: Treatment for chronic back pain and sciatica. J. Neurosurg., *43*:448–451, 1975.

166. Shenkin, H. A., and Haft, H.: Foraminotomy in the surgical treatment of herniated lumbar disks. Surgery, *60*:274–279, 1966.

167. Shenkin, H. A., and Hash, C. J.: A new approach to the surgical treatment of lumbar spondylosis. J. Neurosurg., *44*:148–155, 1976.

168. Sicard, A., and Leca, A.: La place de la radicotomie dans le traitement chirurgical des sciatiques. Presse Méd., *62*:1737–1739, 1954.

169. Silver, M. L., Field, E. A., Silver, C. M., and Simon, S. D.: Postoperative lumbar myelogram. Radiology, *72*:344–347, 1959.

170. Skobowytsh-Okolot, B.: "Posterior apophysis" in fourth lumbar vertebra. Cause of neuroradicular disturbance. Acta Orthop. Scand., *32*:341–351, 1962.

171. Slepian, A.: Lumbar disk surgery. Long followup results from three neurosurgeons. N.Y. Med. J., *66*:1063–1068, 1966.

172. Smith, F. P.: Transvertebral rupture of intervertebral disc. J. Neurosurg., *19*:594–598, 1962.

173. Smith, F. P.: Experimental biomechanics of intervertebral disc rupture through a vertebral body. J. Neurosurg., *30*:134–139, 1969.

174. Smith, R. A., and Estridge, M. N.: Bowel perforation following lumbar-disc surgery. J. Bone Joint Surg., *46-A*:826–828, 1964.

175. Smolik, E. A., and Nash, F. P.: Lumbar spinal arachnoiditis. A complication of the intervertebral disc operation. Ann. Surg., *133*:490–495, 1951.

176. Spiegel, P. G., Kengla, K. W., Isaacson, A. S., and Wilson, J. C.: Intervertebral disc-space inflammation in children. J. Bone Joint Surg., *54-A*:284–296, 1972.

177. Spurling, R. G.: Lesions of the Lumbar Intervertebral Disc. Springfield, Ill., Charles C Thomas, 1953.

178. Stauffer, R. N., and Coventry, M. B.: Anterior interbody lumbar spine fusion. Analysis of Mayo Clinic Series. J. Bone Joint Surg., *54-A*:756–768, 1972.

179. Stern, W. E., and Crandall, P. H.: Inflammatory intervertebral disc disease as a complication of the operative treatment of lumbar herniations. J. Neurosurg., *16*:261–276, 1959.

180. Stokes, J. M.: Vascular complications of disc surgery. J. Bone Joint Surg., *50-A*:394–399, 1968.

181. Sugar, O.: Editorial comment. *In* Year Book of Neurology and Neurosurgery. Chicago, Year Book Medical Publishers, 1976, pp. 390–391.

182. Sussman, B. J.: Inadequacies and hazards of chymopapain injections as treatment for intervertebral disc disease. J. Neurosurg., *42*:389–396, 1975.

183. Swan, S. D., Silver, C. M., and Litchman, H. M.: Lumbar disk surgery in the elderly (over the age of 60). Clin. Orthop., *41*:157–162, 1965.

184. Swick, H. M.: Calcification of intervertebral disc in childhood. J. Pediat. *86*:364–369, 1975.

185. Tarlov, I. M.: Sacral Nerve-Root Cysts. Another Cause of the Sciatic or Cauda Equina Syndrome. Springfield, Ill., Charles C Thomas, 1953.

186. Taveras, J.: Is discography a useful diagnostic procedure? (Editorial). J. Canad. Ass. Radiol., *18*:294–295, 1967.

187. Thibodeau, A. A.: Closed space infection following removal of lumbar intervertebral disc. J. Bone Joint Surg., *50-A*:400–410, 1968.

188. Törma, T.: Postoperative recurrence of lumbar disc herniation. Acta Chir. Scand., *103*:213–221, 1952.

189. Traction for neck and low back disorders. The Medical Letter, *17*:16, 1975.

190. Trowbridge, W. V., and French, J. D.: The "false positive" lumbar myelogram. Neurology (Minneap.), *4*:339–344, 1954.

191. Verbiest, H.: A radicular syndrome from developmental narrowing of the lumbar vertebral canal. J. Bone Joint Surg., *36-B*:230–237, 1954.

192. Verbiest, H.: Further experiences on the pathological influence of a developmental narrowness of the bony lumbar vertebral canal. J. Bone Joint Surg., *37-B*:576–583, 1955.

193. Verbiest, H.: Spondylolisthesis. Value of radicular signs and symptoms. A study based on surgical experience and treatment. J. Int. Coll. Surg., *39*:461–481, 1963.

194. Von Luschka (Cited by Coventry, M. B., Ghormley, R. K., and Kernohan, J. W., see ref. 32).

195. Wachenheim (Cited by Mackay, R. P.: Neurology: Diagnostic and therapeutic methods. Yb. Neurol. Psychiat. Neurosurg., 1966–1967, p. 260).

196. Webb, J. H., Svien, H. J., and Kennedy, R. L. J.: Protruded lumbar intervertebral disks in children. J.A.M.A., *154*:1153–1154, 1954.

197. Weber, H.: The effect of delayed disc surgery on muscular paresis. Acta Orthop. Scand., *46*:631–642, 1975.

198. White, J. C.: Results in surgical treatment of herniated lumbar intervertebral discs. Investigation of the late results in subjects with and without supplementary spinal fusion—a preliminary report. Clin. Neurosurg., *13*:42–54, 1966.

199. Wiberg, G.: Back pain in relation to nerve supply of intervertebral disk. Acta Orthop. Scand., *19*:211–221, 1950.

200. Wilkins, R. H., and Brody, I. A.: Lasègue's sign. Arch. Neurol. (Chicago), *21*:219–221, 1969.

201. Wilson, C. B.: Significance of the small lumbar spinal canal: Cauda equina compression syndromes due to spondylosis. Part 3: Intermittent claudication. J. Neurosurg., *31*:499–506, 1969.

202. Wilson, C. B., Ehni, G., and Grollmus, J. Neurogenic intermittent claudication. Clin. Neurosurg., *18*:62–85, 1971.

203. Wiltse, L. L.: The effect of the common anomalies of the lumbar spine upon disc degeneration and low back pain. Orthop. Clin. N. Amer., *2*:569–582, 1971.

204. Wood, J. P.: Lumbar disk surgery: Complications. J. Amer. Osteopath. Ass., *74*:234–240, 1974.

205. Woodhall, B., and Hayes, G. J.: The well-leg raising test of Fazersztajan in the diagnosis of ruptured lumbar intervertebral disc. J. Bone Joint Surg., *32-A*:786–792, 1950.

206. Wycis, H.: Contralateral recurrent herniated disks. Arch. Surg. (Chicago), *60*:274–278, 1950.

79

EXTRADURAL SPINAL CORD AND NERVE ROOT COMPRESSION FROM BENIGN LESIONS OF THE DORSAL AREA

Herniated thoracic discs are a rare cause of spinal cord compression and are the reason for only 0.15 to 1.7 per cent of all disc operations.[2,30,35,36] Possibly the true incidence of thoracic disc herniation is higher than these figures would indicate, since an autopsy study by Haley and Perry revealed two small thoracic disc herniations in 99 cases.[20] These lesions occur predominantly between the ages of 30 and 55, but have been reported to occur in children.[28,29,38]

The condition seems to affect the two sexes with equal frequency, but some report a slight male preponderance.[15,28,31]

Although thoracic disc protrusions occur at every level of the thoracic spine, protrusions between T9 and T12 account for approximately two thirds of cases.[7,15] Herniations affecting the middle four thoracic vertebrae rank next, and least common are those in the upper thoracic spine. Several reports indicate that the eleventh is the single interspace most frequently involved.[16,31,48] Most herniations are single, but multiple protrusions have been reported.[1,46,49] The disc tends to protrude in the midline rather than to either side.

PATHOGENESIS

Like disc herniations elsewhere, thoracic disc protrusion is a consequence of disc degeneration. Sometimes other predisposing conditions exist, such as Scheuermann's disease, which causes excessive fragility of the disc, or kyphosis.[34,42,49] Both occupation and trauma appear to be related only incidentally in most cases, though trauma sometimes seems to be an important precipitating and aggravating factor.[9,28,31] The lower incidence of disc protrusions of the thoracic, as compared with the lumbar and cervical, area has been attributed to the limited motion in the thoracic spine, which is a consequence of the small size of the thoracic intervertebral discs, the restraints of the rib cage and sternum, and the anterior-posterior direction of the apophyseal joints.[12]

PATHOPHYSIOLOGY

An understanding of the anatomical relationships in the thoracic spine helps to explain the clinical symptoms due to ruptured thoracic disc. The thoracic spinal canal is small, and little leeway exists between the thoracic disc and the spinal cord. The cord is restrained from backward displacement by the dentate ligaments.[25] Circulation to the lower dorsal and lumbar segments of the spinal cord is precarious, since these regions may be supplied largely or entirely by a single unilateral medullary artery, the arteria radicularis magna, or the artery of Adamkiewicz, which usually arises

---

E. ARBIT and R. H. PATTERSON, JR.

between T8 and L4 and is on the left side in over 60 per cent of cases.[13] Occasionally the artery may originate as high as T5, as reported by Fauré and co-workers.[17]

Mechanical trauma and vascular compression, either separately or combined, can damage the thoracic spinal cord. Neurological deficit due to vascular compromise has been reported in the monkey by Yoss and by Doppman and Girton.[14,50] In three patients, Caron and associates observed indirect signs of ischemia of the cord caused by protruded discs that compressed the artery of Adamkiewicz.[7]

A myelopathy arising from compression of the cord between a modest protrusion of the disc in front and a buckled and hypertrophic ligamentum flavum behind has been reported.[9,31] The combination of mechanical and vascular damage to the cord may account for the severe neurological symptoms that sometimes seem out of all proportion to the size of the protrusion and also for the poor recovery that sometimes follows complete removal of the ruptured disc.[41] Vascular damage may account for symptoms that seem inappropriately rostral for the level of the rupture.[2,21,23]

CLINICAL SYMPTOMS

Most patients with thoracic disc rupture can give no history of a precipitating event. A few patients, however, associate exacerbation of symptoms with trauma. Occasionally a patient gives a history of a fall on the buttock, parachute jumping, weight lifting, or awkward rotational strains.[2,9,48]

Patients with herniated thoracic discs present with a variety of symptoms. Complaints vary greatly from patient to patient and often seem poorly correlated with the location and size of the rupture. The most common presenting symptom is poorly localized back pain. The pain can be unilateral or bilateral, and generally is mild to moderate in intensity rather than severe. It generally is aggravated by movement and is relieved by rest. When the pain is unilateral, the clinical picture tends to have a slowly progressive course, whereas patients with bilateral pain tend to progress rapidly toward a transverse myelitis. Pain may, however, be absent, so the symptoms can simulate a demyelinating disease such as multiple sclerosis.[5,9,30]

Sensory symptoms, particularly numbness, are common. Although the numbness may be segmental, unilateral, or bilateral, it usually begins peripherally in the lower extremities and gradually ascends. Some patients complain of a girdlelike band of tightness around the trunk at the level where sensory loss begins. Decreased pain and temperature sensations as well as hyperesthesia and paresthesias are common. Kuhlendahl and Carson and co-workers have emphasized that pronounced subjective sensory changes in association with minimal motor deficit are highly suggestive of thoracic disc herniation.[9,27]

Sensations of unsteadiness and complaints of a stiff or staggering gait are common. Flexor spasms trouble some patients. Others are bothered by dysuria, frequency, incontinence, urinary retention, and abnormal bowel function. Impotence, decreased sensation during intercourse in women, absence of sweating of the feet, and trophic ulcers at the tips of the toes may occur as well. The duration of symptoms varies greatly; some patients quickly develop an acute transverse myelitis, whereas others may have symptoms for many years.[9,30] The majority, however, give a history of two to four years. Commonly the symptoms are progressive and not remittent, but in some a period of exacerbations and remissions precedes the time when the symptoms become progressive.

DIFFERENTIAL DIAGNOSIS

Pain in the thoracic spine with or without radiation to the chest or abdomen can be caused by thoracic disc herniation as well as by a number of other pathological entities. The infrequency of thoracic disc rupture and the wide spectrum of symptoms that it produces often results in a delayed or erroneous diagnosis. Other diseases affecting the spine, such as rheumatoid or ankylosing spondylosis, malignant or benign tumors, disc space infections, fractures, and dislocations must all be considered, as they may mimic a herniated thoracic disc. Costovertebral syndromes have been described as producing dorsal spinal pain with segmental radiation.

A number of intrathoracic and intra-abdominal disorders can be confused with thoracic disc herniation. Posterior penetrating ulcers, pancreatitis, retroperitoneal tumors, gallbladder disease, ischemic conditions of the myocardium, urinary tract disorders such as renal colic, and aortic aneurysms all can produce similar symptoms. Herpes zoster also needs to be included on the list.

Sometimes a ruptured thoracic disc will produce a compression myelopathy without pain.[2,12,31] The clinical picture that results is easily confused with multiple sclerosis or other degenerative conditions. After careful questioning, such patients may disclose a history of pain induced by coughing, sneezing, straining, or laughing that suggests the proper diagnosis.

PHYSICAL FINDINGS

There are no typical neurological findings for thoracic disc herniation. Limitation of motion, paravertebral muscle spasm, and scoliosis are consequences of the back pain. Sensory findings are quite common and are absent in only a distinct minority of patients.[5,31,48] Hyperalgesia, hypalgesia, analgesia, and hypothermalgesia are all possible and usually are bilateral.[5] Not infrequently a Brown-Séquard syndrome is present.[3,28,31] The sensory level may be typically one or two levels lower than the level of the lesion.[9] Ataxic gait and a positive Romberg test may be observed if spinocerebellar or posterior column function is impaired. Abnormal motor findings are common and are due to involvement of the lateral corticospinal tracts.[31] The deficit may range from mild monoparesis to paraplegia. Most patients have increased muscle tone, exaggerated knee and ankle reflexes, extensor plantar responses, absence of abdominal reflexes, and perhaps a Beevor's sign.[34] Disturbances in bladder, bowel, and sexual function are late manifestations. As with other intraspinal tumors, pain is often the first symptom, to be followed by sensory disturbances, weakness, and finally visceral abnormalities.

Some interesting and unusual findings have been described in patients with ruptured thoracic disc. A fragment of disc may erode into the anterior part of the spinal cord, causing loss of pain and temperature sensation on one or both sides of the body. Hematomyelia with a dissociated sensory loss has been described, as has posterior infarction of the cord with loss of position sense. The cord may be stretched or deformed over the protrusion, and areas of necrosis and edema may result, producing confusing neurological signs.[19,30,31,37]

ROENTGENOGRAPHY

Roentgenograms may reveal disc space narrowing, osteophytic spurs, or evidence of calcified disc material either in the interspace or within the canal. Striking collapse of the disc space is rare. Osteophytic lipping, though present in the majority of cases, is nonspecific. On the other hand, disc space calcification is highly suggestive of thoracic disc herniation and is present in 20 to 70 per cent of cases, as opposed to an incidence of only 4 per cent in the normal population.[15,28,31,33] Two patterns of disc calcification may occur: a fine linear type, probably arising in the anulus fibrosus; and a more dense, central calcification involving the nucleus pulposus. Calcified material in the spinal canal, probably representing extruded nucleus pulposus, is an important radiological feature and was present in 55 per cent of cases in McAllister and Sage's series.[33]

Myelography

The diagnosis ultimately rests on positive-contrast or gas myelography.[1,28,31,33,47] Most authors recommend that on the order of 25 to 30 ml of iodized oil be used to visualize the defect. If anteroposterior and lateral views are unrevealing, then right and left decubitus and oblique views should be obtained to exclude lateral defects. Partial myelographic blocks to the flow of contrast agent are frequent, but complete obstruction is rare and is seen predominantly in advanced cases.

Central protrusions yield a quite characteristic picture. The anteroposterior view may be confused with either an intra- or extramedullary tumor, as a rounded or semilunar filling defect is present, often associated with an increase in the transverse diameter of the cord. On the lateral projection in the prone position, however, the posterior extradural displacement of the dye column opposite the disc space establishes the diagnosis (Fig. 79–1). Anterolat-

Figure 79–1 An almost complete obstruction due to an anterior extradural mass centered over a calcified T7–T8 intervertebral disc with an apparent intradural component. Silver clip represents site of previous laminectomy. *A*. Frontal projection. The black arrow marks the level of the block. *B*. Lateral projection. The black arrow identifies calcification within the disc, and the white arrow marks the abnormal disc.

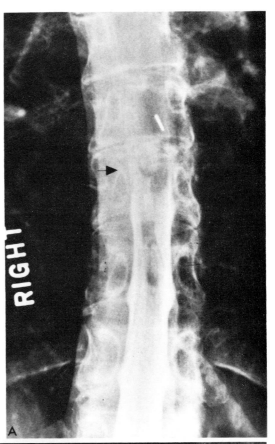

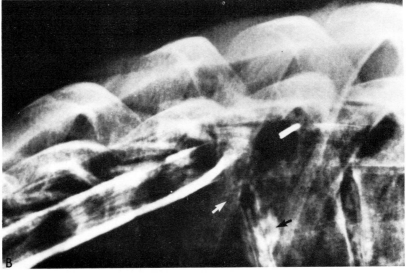

eral protrusions show evidence of lateral displacement of the cord in association with posterior displacement of the dye column at the level of the disc space. In lateral films, a double contour is often seen because part of the contrast material runs over the convexity of the prolapse and part runs in a lateral gutter. In lateral disc protrusion the anteroposterior and lateral myelographic views may be normal, or they may show lateral impression on the dye column associated with lateral displacement of the cord. In such cases, oblique and lateral decubitus films are diagnostic. Occasionally a protruded thoracic disc may erode the dura and become intradural or even intramedullary, as shown in Figure 79–1. These cases are often misdiagnosed as intradural extramedullary or intramedullary tumors. Changes noted on plain films may be helpful in differentiation. Some authors emphasize the importance of gas myelography or myelotomography, especially when a diagnosis is questionable.[5,24,26] Myelography may be followed occasionally by rapid neurological deterioration in cases of thoracic disc herniation, just as may happen in patients with an intraspinal neoplasm. Consequently, myelography is best not performed unless facilities for an operation are available. As far as the newer techniques of transaxial tomography and computed tomography are concerned, their role remains to be defined.

Angiography

Angiography can be helpful, particularly in identifying the artery of Adamkiewicz if rib resection and a lateral or anterior approach to a disc below T8 is contemplated.[7,40] The artery, being single, may be the only blood supply to the lower thoracic cord, and thus it will be important to spare it during operation. Sometimes division of an intercostal artery will be required to expose the interspace adequately, and prior angiography is necessary to assure that the spinal cord will not be infarcted as a consequence.

ELECTROMYOGRAPHY

There are a few isolated reports in the literature attesting to the fact that electro-

myography may be of value in making the diagnosis, particularly if a myelogram shows no abnormality.[32] The presence or absence of electromyographic evidence of anterior root compression can be quite helpful in the differential diagnosis of herniated thoracic disc and various degenerative conditions of the spinal cord.

TREATMENT

Prompt operation is the appropriate treatment for herniated thoracic disc with spinal cord compression. Temporizing measures are risky because the neurological state of the patient may deteriorate suddenly, and the sooner the cord compression is relieved the better the quality of recovery is likely to be. Patients with thoracic disc herniation have a progressive course, and a patient not operated upon can only get worse. One should not be influenced by an apparent remission, since chances are great that it is only temporary.

Operative Treatment

An approach to a herniated thoracic disc by routine laminectomy has been attended with great risk in most hands. Of Müller's four patients, three were paraplegic after operation.[34] Perot and Munro collected 91 cases from various sources in 1969. Forty of the patients were not improved by laminectomy, and sixteen were rendered paraplegic as a result of the operation. Central disc herniation and an advanced preoperative neurological deficit carry the most ominous prognosis for laminectomy.[39] Despite the bad experience reported by most, some surgeons report that a carefully performed laminectomy is safe in their hands.[45] This is not the general experience, however.

The dismal results of laminectomy in a benign disease have stimulated interest in alternative approaches. In 1960, Hulme treated four cases through a lateral approach by costotransversectomy. His results were encouraging. Three of the patients were cured and one showed improvement.[22] In 1969 Perot and Munro, and Ransohoff and associates reported success in, respectively, two and three patients operated on by a transpleural approach utilizing an ordinary thoracotomy.[39,40] A constant

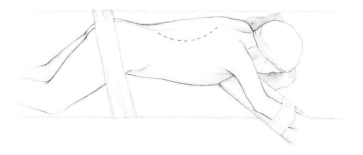

Figure 79–2 Lateral costo-transversectomy approach: positioning and incision. (From Simeone, F. A., and Rashbaum, R.: Transthoracic disc excision. *In* Schmidek, H. H., and Sweet, W. H., eds.: Operative Neurosurgery. New York, Grune & Stratton Inc., 1977. Reprinted by permission.)

trend toward simplification of the approach to thoracic disc herniation has yielded two newer operations, the posterolateral operation described by Carson, Gumpert, and Jefferson, and the transpedicle operation described by Patterson and Arbit.[9,37]

Costotransversectomy or Lateral Approach

The patient is placed in the partial lateral decubitus position with a 30-degree elevation, thus slightly tilted away from the surgeon (Fig. 79–2). A pad is placed under the chest to curve the spine. The interspace is approached from either the right or the left side, depending upon the presence of lateralizing features in the clinical presentation. If the surgeon has to deal with a central disc, a right-sided approach seems to be more appropriate, as the artery of Adam-kiewicz usually arises from the left lower intercostal vessels. Care must be taken to identify the interspace accurately by roentgenographic means; otherwise the wrong interspace may be operated on. A long curved paraspinal incision is made that extends at least three intervertebral bodies above and below the protruded disc. Then either the trapezius is incised in line with the skin incision and retracted medially along with the paraspinal muscles or the muscle mass can be transected over the rib to be removed and the muscles retracted in cephalic and caudal directions. The rib is identified, and the intercostal neurovascular complex is separated from its inferior surface (Fig. 79–3). The periosteum is stripped from the rib, the costal transverse and capsular ligaments are divided, and the head and neck of the rib are removed along with perhaps 20 cm of the shaft (Fig. 79–4).

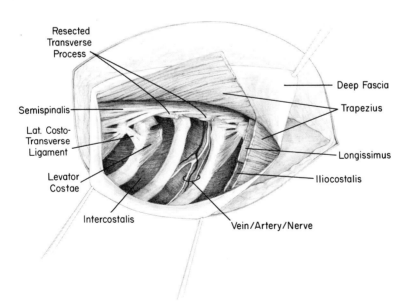

Resected Transverse Process

Semispinalis

Lat. Costo-Transverse Ligament

Levator Costae

Intercostalis

Deep Fascia

Trapezius

Longissimus

Iliocostalis

Vein/Artery/Nerve

Figure 79–3 Lateral approach: exposure of the neurovascular bundle. (From Simeone, F. A., and Rashbaum, R.: Transthoracic disc excision. *In* Schmidek, H. H., and Sweet, W. H., eds.: Operative Neurosurgery. New York, Grune & Stratton Inc., 1977. Reprinted by permission.)

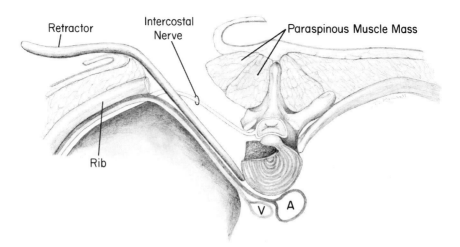

Figure 79–4 Lateral approach: exposure after rib resection. (From Simeone, F. A., and Rashbaum, R.: Transthoracic disc excision. *In* Schmidek, H. H., and Sweet, W. H., eds.: Operative Neurosurgery. New York, Grune & Stratton Inc., 1977. Reprinted by permission.)

Once the rib has been removed, the intercostal vein and arteries can be preserved and followed to the nerve root foramen. The parietal pleura then is separated from the adjacent ribs and spinal column and is reflected forward and laterally away from the spine. The segmental vessels along the side of the vertebra are identified and preserved. Parts of the pedicles are then removed with bone instruments and the high-speed air drill. Some surgeons recommend using the operating microscope at this point, as it provides excellent illumination and magnification of the important neural structures.[4,44] Once the pedicle has been removed, the dura and the disc are identified. The interspace is entered laterally and emptied by curettage. Parts of the posterolateral margins of the vertebral bodies may have to be separated carefully from the dura, pushed into the previously prepared cavity in the interspace, and removed laterally. Prior to closure of the wound the lungs are inflated to expel air from the chest cavity. In most cases a chest tube will not be necessary, but a chest x-ray should be taken in the recovery room to look for a pneumothorax.[8,10,22,44]

Transthoracic Transpleural Approach

A standard right posterior thoracotomy incision is made, usually on the right side because the artery of Adamkiewicz usually arises on the left side and because the heart and aorta are out of way (Fig. 79–5). In older patients it usually is wise to remove a rib, but in young patients adequate exposure often can be obtained without taking a rib. The intercostal neurovascular bundle is followed to the appropriate intervertebral foramen, which must be positively identified by x-ray. The pleura is resected from the vertebral bodies and the head of the rib, exposing the sympathetic chain (Fig. 79–6). Usually it is necessary to ligate the segmental artery and vein to gain access to the interspace. For this reason, preoperative angiography to identify the artery of Adamkiewicz is advisable for herniations at

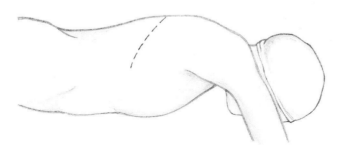

Figure 79–5 Transthoracic approach: positioning and incision. (From Simeone, F. A., and Rashbaum, R.: Transthoracic disc excision. *In* Schmidek, H. H., and Sweet, W. H., eds.: Operative Neurosurgery. New York, Grune & Stratton Inc., 1977. Reprinted by permission.)

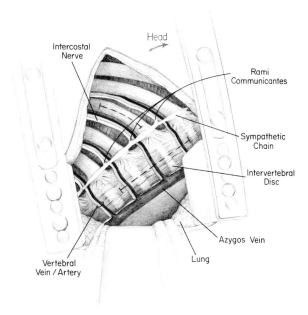

Figure 79–6 Transthoracic approach: exposure of vertebral bodies after reflection of the pleura. (From Simeone, F. A., and Rashbaum, R.: Transthoracic disc excision. *In* Schmidek, H. H., and Sweet, W. H., eds.: Operative Neurosurgery. New York, Grune & Stratton, 1977. Reprinted by permission.)

T8 and below. The intercostal nerve is followed to its foramen and gently retracted to expose the pedicle above and below. The pedicles are then removed with a high-speed drill and bone instruments to expose the dura (Fig. 79–7). An operating microscope may be helpful at this stage. The intervertebral disc is then incised, and the anterior two thirds of the contents is removed with pituitary rongeurs and curets (Fig. 79–

8). No attempt is made to remove the extruded fragment initially. By flexing the table or using a vertebral body spreader, the interspace may be opened further. Once the intervertebral disc space has been emptied the posterior fragments of bone and disc may be removed. One must search carefully for sequestered fragments, and it may be appropriate to remove the anulus fibrosus and its associated ligaments. The

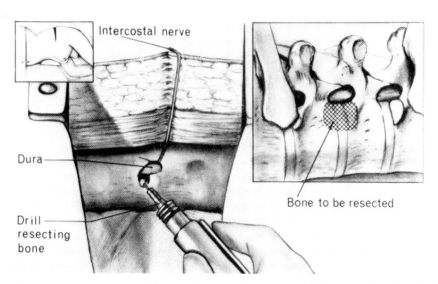

Figure 79–7 Transthoracic approach: bone to be resected. (From Perot, P. L., and Munro, D. C.: Transthoracic removal of midline thoracic disc protrusions causing spinal cord compression. J. Neurosurg., *31*:452–458, 1969. Reprinted by permission.)

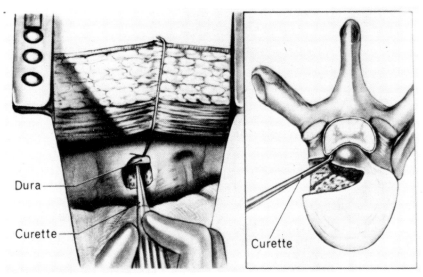

Figure 79–8   Transthoracic approach: curetting the protruded disc away from the spinal cord. (From Perot, P. L., and Munro, D. C.: Transthoracic removal of midline thoracic disc protrusions causing spinal cord compression. J. Neurosurg., *31*:452–458, 1969. Reprinted by permission.)

parietal pleura then is sutured over the vertebral body, chest tubes are placed, and the chest is closed.[8,11,39,40,44]

Posterolateral Approach

In 1971, Carson, Gumpert, and Jefferson described their experience with 14 patients who were operated upon through a lateral approach. This approach combines laminectomy, complete excision of the ligamentum flavum, and the extradural removal of protruded disc. They favor a knee-chest position to reduce epidural bleeding. After exposure of the spines and lamina through a midline incision, laminectomy is performed with the high-speed air drill, first by thinning the lamina and then by removing the residual bone with a rose-ended burr. The technique makes it possible for a laminectomy to be performed without inserting any instruments under the lamina. Once the lamina has been removed, the ligamentum flavum is excised and the original midline skin incision is converted into a T-shaped incision by adding a horizontal limb through skin and underlying paraspinal muscles. The horizontal incision is placed at the level of the disc. Since its purpose is to provide a lateral approach to the lesion, removing part of the transverse process may be advisable. Thereafter a portion of the lateral wall of the spinal canal is drilled away. The epidural venous plexus is coagu-

lated and divided to clear the posterior aspect of the vertebral body. A space is drilled out from the vertebral body so that hard fragments of disc may be pulled anteriorly away from the cord. These authors suggest that a calcified intradural lesion adherent to the dura may be removed en bloc with its dural attachment. The dura is opened only if an intradural fragment is present. The nerve root emerges from the spinal canal at a sufficient distance from the interspace that it need not be divided.[9,23]

Transpedicle Approach

Patterson and Arbit described an approach to a thoracic disc through the pedicle. The spine is exposed through a midline incision, and the paravertebral muscles are reflected on one side far enough to expose the facet joints. The facets and the pedicle of the vertebra caudal to the disc are removed with an air drill (Fig. 79–9). This creates a cavity as deep as the diameter of the spinal canal and exposes the disc space. The interspace is entered, and disc material is removed from the center of the disc (Fig. 79–10). After a cavity has been created in the center, posterior disc material is removed, progressing from laterally under the root toward the midline under the spinal cord. A down-biting curet is helpful in this maneuver, and the curet can be hammered with a mallet to knock off posterior bone

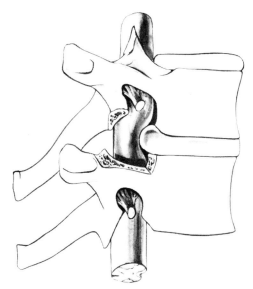

Figure 79–9 Transpedicle approach: area of initial bone removal. (From Patterson, R. H., Jr., and Arbit E.: A surgical approach through the pedicle to protruded thoracic discs. J. Neurosurg., *48*:768–772, 1978. Reprinted by permission.)

spurs. If laminectomy seems appropriate, it is easy enough to complete after the cord has been decompressed anteriorly (Fig. 79–11). Usually the dura need not be opened. If an intradural or an intrameduallary fragment is suspected, however, the dura should be opened and the cord gently displaced to allow inspection of the anterior surface of the spinal cord and dura. This maneuver is not risky, since the spinal cord has already been adequately decompressed, and it may be safer to extract any intradural fragments under direct vision

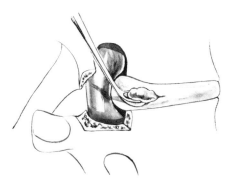

Figure 79–10 Transpedicle approach: curetting the disc. (From Patterson, R. H., Jr., and Arbit E.: A surgical approach through the pedicle to protruded thoracic discs. J. Neurosurg., *48*:768–772, 1978. Reprinted by permission.)

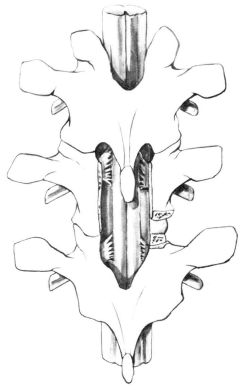

Figure 79–11 Transpedicle approach: extent of bone removal after evacuation of the disc and completion of the laminectomy. (From Patterson, R. H., Jr., and Arbit, E.: A surgical approach through the pedicle to protruded thoracic discs. J. Neurosurg., *48*:768–772, 1978. Reprinted by permission.)

than to remove them blindly from the extradural space.[37]

COMMENTS

The transthoracic transpleural approach can provide access to the vertebral bodies and intervertebral spaces from T2 to T12. It is, however, most suitable for exposing the midthoracic interspaces because exposure is obtained with difficulty at the most rostral and caudal interspaces. It also would seem that the risk of overlooking a fragment of disc embedded within the dura might be greater with the transpleural transthoracic approach. Besides this, there may be some risk to the circulation of the spinal cord if an intercostal artery is sacrificed. For these reasons the authors regard it with less favor than the other lateral approaches to the interspace. The postero-lateral extrapleural approach gives better

TABLE 79-1   RESULTS OF VARIOUS APPROACHES IN OPERATIONS ON THORACIC DISCS

RESULT	LAMINECTOMY*		TRANSTHORACIC APPROACH†		LATERAL EXTRAPLEURAL APPROACH‡	
	No. of Patients	Per Cent	No. of Patients	Per Cent	No. of Patients	Per Cent
Cure	41	43	7	88	24	59
Improvement	21	22	—	—	12	29
No improvement	10	11	1	12	5	12
Paraplegia	16	17	—	—	—	—
Death	7	7	—	—	—	—
Total	95	100	8	100	41	100

* Data from references 1, 2, 6, 16, 18, 19, 28, 30, 34, 41–43, 45, 48, 49.
† Data from references 7, 11, 39, 40.
‡ Data from references 4, 7, 9, 10, 22, 23, 36, 37.

access to the spinal canal than the approach by thoracotomy, but it shares with the transpleural approach both the risk of vascular complications and the possibility of a cerebrospinal fluid fistula into the pleural cavity if the dura is opened. The authors prefer the transpedicle approach because of its simplicity, but any one of these approaches seems safer than laminectomy (Table 79–1).

Regardless of the operative technique employed, several important points deserve emphasis. Operating on the wrong interspace is a common pitfall and can be avoided by proper identification of the interspace by means of roentgenograms. In the course of the operation, the spinal cord commonly is damaged when instruments are inserted between the lamina and dura. There is no space for an instrument in the presence of a herniated thoracic disc, and this maneuver must be avoided.

Sometimes the cord is damaged because a disc herniation has not been diagnosed preoperatively and a routine laminectomy is performed. A herniated thoracic disc should be considered in any patient with an anterior mass at the level of a disc interspace. With the proper preoperative diagnosis, an operation for thoracic disc should carry no great risk for the patient.

If the preoperative diagnosis is incorrect, and a thoracic disc is encountered unexpectedly after laminectomy, then removal of the disc provides the best chance of helping the patient. This goal can be accomplished by removing the pedicle caudal to the nerve root and entering the disc space laterally, as described earlier.[37]

REFERENCES

1. Abbott, K. H., and Retter, R. H.: Protrusions of thoracic intervertebral disks. Neurology (Minneap.), 6:1–10, 1956.
2. Arseni, C., and Nash, F.: Thoracic intervertebral disc protrusion. A clinical study. J. Neurosurg., 17:418–430, 1960.
3. Arseni, C., and Nash, F.: Protrusion of thoracic intervertebral discs. Acta Neurochir. (Wien), 11:1–33, 1963.
4. Benjamin, V., and Ransohoff, J.: Thoracic disc disease. In Rothman, R. H., and Simeone, F. A., eds.: The Spine. Vol. 1. Philadelphia, W. B. Saunders Co., 1975, p. 435–442.
5. Benson, M. K. D., and Byrnes, D. P.: The clinical syndromes and surgical treatment of thoracic intervertebral disc prolapse. J. Bone Joint Surg., B-57:471–477, 1975.
6. Borghi, G.: La hernie discale dorsale. Minerva Neurochir., 5:123–128, 1961.
7. Caron, J. P., Djindjian, R., Julian, H., Lebrigand, H., and Comoy, J.: Les hernies discales dorsales. Ann. Med. Intern. (Paris), 122:675–688, 1971.
8. Caron, J. P., Julian, H., Lebrigand, H., Comoy, J., and Caruel, N.: Discussion sur les voies d'abord des hernies discales dorsales et leurs résultats. Neurochirurgie, 14:171–182, 1968.
9. Carson, J., Gumpert, J., and Jefferson, A.: Diagnosis and treatment of thoracic intervertebral disc protrusions. J. Neurol. Neurosurg. Psychiat., 34:68–77, 1971.
10. Chesterman, P. J.: Spastic paraplegia caused by sequestrated thoracic intervertebral disc. Proc. Roy. Soc. Med., 57:87–88, 1964.
11. Crafoord, C., Hiertonn, T., Lindblom, K., and Olsson, S. C.: Spinal cord compression caused by a protruded thoracic disk. Report of a case treated with anterolateral fenestration of the disk. Acta Orthop. Scand., 28:103–107, 1958.
12. De Palma, A. F., and Rothman, R. H.: The Intervertebral Disc. Philadelphia, W. B. Saunders Co., 1970, pp 171–180.
13. Doppman, J. L., and DiChiro, G.: The arteria radicularis magna. Radiographic anatomy in the adult. Brit. J. Radiol., 41:40–45, 1968.

14. Doppman, J. L., and Girton, M.: Angiographic study of the effect of laminectomy in the presence of acute anterior epidural masses. J. Neurosurg., *45*:195–202, 1976.

15. Dreyfus, P., Six, B., Dorfmann, H., and Desezi, H.: La hernie discale dorsale. Sem. Hop. Paris, *48*:3045–3052, 1972.

16. Epstein, J. A.: The syndrome of herniation of the lower thoracic intervertebral discs with nerve root and spinal cord compression. A presentation of four cases with a review of the literature, methods of diagnosis and treatment. J. Neurosurg., *11*:525–538, 1954.

17. Fauré, C., Debrun, G., and Djindjian, R.: La vascularisation artérielle normale et pathologique du renflement lombaire de la moelle épinière chez l'enfant: l'artère d'Adamkiewicz. Ann. Radiol. (Paris), *10*:129–140, 1967.

18. Feiring, E. H., Extruded thoracic intervertebral disc. Arch. Surg. (Chicago), *95*:135–137, 1967.

19. Fisher, R. G.: Protrusions of thoracic disc. The factor of herniation through the dura mater. J. Neurosurg., *22*:591–593, 1965.

20. Haley, J. C., and Perry, J. H.: Protrusions of intervertebral discs. Study of their distribution, characteristics and effects on the nervous system. Amer. J. Surg., *80*:394–404, 1950.

21. Hawk, W. A.: Spinal compression caused by ecchondrosis of the intervertebral fibrocartilage with a review of the recent literature. Brain, *59*:204–224, 1936.

22. Hulme, A.: The surgical approach to thoracic intervertebral disc protrusions. J. Neurol. Neurosurg. Psychiat., *23*:133–137, 1960.

23. Jefferson, A.: The treatment of thoracic intervertebral disc protrusions. Clin. Neurol. Neurosurg., *78*:1–9, 1975.

24. Jirout, J., and Kune, Z.: Traumatic herniation of the thoracic intervertebral disc. Acta Neurochir. (Wien)., *8*:88–93, 1960.

25. Kahn, E. A.: Role of dentate ligaments in spinal cord compression and syndrome of lateral sclerosis. J. Neurosurg., *4*:191–199, 1947.

26. Komaki, S., and Komaki, R.: Diagnosis of thoracic and lumbar disc diseases by gas myelography. Wisconsin Med. J. *75*:29–31, 1976.

27. Kuhlendahl, H.: Der thorakale Bandscheibenprolaps als extramedullärer Spinaltumor und in seinen Beziehungen zu internen Organsyndromen. Ärztl. Wschr., *6*:154–157, 1951.

28. Logue, V.: Thoracic intervertebral disc prolapse with spinal cord compression. J. Neurol. Neurosurg., Psychiat., *15*:227–241, 1952.

29. Lombardi, G., and Passerini, A.: Spinal Canal Disease: A Radiological and Myelographic Analysis. Baltimore, Williams & Wilkins Co., 1964.

30. Love, J. G., and Kiefer, E. J.: Root pain and paraplegia due to protrusions of thoracic intervertebral disks. J. Neurosurg., *7*:62–69, 1950.

31. Love, J. G., and Schorn, V. G.: Thoracic-disc protrusions. J.A.M.A., *191*:627–631, 1965.

32. Marinacci, A. A.: Applied Electromyography. Philadelphia, Lea & Febiger, 1968.

33. McAllister, V. L., and Sage, M. R.: The radiology of thoracic disc protrusion. Radiology, *27*:294–299, 1976.

34. Müller, R.: Protrusion of thoracic intervertebral disks with compression of the spinal cord. Acta Med. Scand., *139*:99–104, 1951.

35. O'Connel, J. E. A.: Involvement of the spinal cord by intervertebral disc protrusions. Brit. J. Surg., *43*:225–247, 1955.

36. Otani, K., Manzoku, S., Shibasaki, K., and Nomachi, S.: Surgical treatment of thoracic and thoracolumbar disc lesions using the anterior approach. Spine, *2*:266–275, 1977.

37. Patterson, R. H., Jr., and Arbit, E.: A surgical approach through the pedicle to protruded thoracic discs. J. Neurosurg., *48*:768–772, 1978.

38. Peck, F. C., Jr.: A calcified thoracic intervertebral disc with herniation and spinal cord compression in a child. J. Neurosurg., *13*:105–109, 1957.

39. Perot, P. L., and Munro, D. C.: Transthoracic removal of midline thoracic disc protrusions causing spinal cord compression. J. Neurosurg., *31*:452–458, 1969.

40. Ransohoff, J., Spencer, F., Siew, F., and Gage, I. Jr.: Transthoracic removal of thoracic disc. Report of three cases. J. Neurosurg., *31*:459–461, 1969.

41. Reeves, D. L., and Brown, H. A.: Thoracic intervertebral disc protrusion with spinal cord compression. J. Neurosurg., *28*:24–28, 1968.

42. Roth, G.: Double hernie discale thoracique et maladie de Scheuermann, à propos d'un cas. Rev. Méd. Suisse Rom., *85*:296, 1965.

43. Scharfetter, F., and Twerdy, K.: Der thorakale Diskusprolaps. Ther. Umsch., *34*:412–418, 1977.

44. Simeone, F. A., and Rashbaum, R.: Transthoracic disc excision. *In* Schmidek, H. H., and Sweet, W. H., eds.: Current Techniques in Operative Neurosurgery. New York, Grune & Stratton, 1977, pp. 323–333.

45. Singounas, E. G., and Karvounis, P. C.: Thoracic disc protrusion. Acta Neurochir. (Wien), *39*: 251–258, 1977.

46. Svien, H. G., and Karavitis, A. L.: Multiple protrusions of intervertebral disks in the upper thoracic region. Report of a case. Proc. Mayo Clin., *29*:375–378, 1954.

47. Thomson, J. L. G.: Myelography in dorsal disc protrusion. Acta Radiologica, 7th Symposium Neuroradiologicum, New York, pp. 1140–1146, 1964.

48. Tovi, D., and Strang, R. R.: Thoracic intervertebral disc protrusion. Acta Chir. Scand. suppl., *267*:1–41, 1960.

49. Van Landingham, J. H.: Herniation of thoracic intervertebral disc with spinal cord compression in kyphosis dorsalis juvenilis (Scheuermann's disease). J. Neurosurg., *11*:327–329, 1954.

50. Yoss, R. E.: Vascular supply of the spinal cord. The production of vascular syndromes. Univ. Mich. Med. Bull., *16*:333–345, 1950.

80

EXTRADURAL SPINAL CORD AND NERVE ROOT COMPRESSION FROM BENIGN LESIONS OF THE CERVICAL AREA

Cervical joint disorders affected man and lower animals in the remote past just as today. Indeed, 4500 years ago, the Egyptians knew that certain neck lesions produced paraplegia.[18] Historical and literary sources indicate that a rich variety of diagnoses and etiologies, some correct and others fanciful, were entertained.[32,113]

In 1838, Key described instances in which firm ventral ridges across cervical disc spaces encroached on the spinal cord.[50] Gowers made similar observations in 1892.[40] In that same year, Horsley operated on this type of lesion with success.[104] In 1893, VonBechterew described a form of spinal disease producing pain, weakness, paresthesias, and pathological spinal curvature; but lacking necropsy proof, his views were ridiculed.[87,112] Bailey and Casamajor deserve notice for their 1911 observation that arthrosis is capable of compressing the spinal cord and its roots just as is a tumor.[6] In 1928, Stookey described several cervical syndromes due to what he called "ventral chondromas."[100] The next year, Dandy removed the chondroid material from two patients with sciatica.[27] He identified it as normal disc tissue rather than neoplastic material. A confirming report on the nature of the chondroid material came from France the following year.[1]

The strongest confirmation of the identity of ventral chondromas or enchondromas and disc tissue came from Mixter, Barr, and Kubick of Boston. In 1932, Mixter became the first surgeon to remove a preoperatively diagnosed ruptured intervertebral disc.[32] In the 1934 report of their experiences with these lesions, Mixter and Barr described four patients with cervical disc disease, three of whom were operated upon and benefited.[67] The significance of this report was that it showed that spine and extremity pains were sometimes and perhaps often due to simple nerve root compression rather than to infection or other pathological change. Further, it confirmed that the compression could be accurately diagnosed and that operative removal of the displaced cartilage could relieve the pain and other disabilities. Half their patients had arthrosis shown in the x-rays. Routine differentiation between disc ruptures and arthrotic compressions was 15 years in the future, however. Mixter and Barr called these lesions "ruptured" discs, while others favored such adjectives as "prolapsed," "herniated," or "protruded."[57,96]

The principal influence of Mixter, Barr, and Kubick's discoveries was on treatment of disorders in the lumbar area. As a result of their work, increasing numbers of operations were done to treat herniated lumbar disc. In the cervical area, however, section of normal scalenus anticus muscles continued because patients with herniated cervical discs had been given erroneous diagnoses of scalenus anticus syndrome. Eventually, the syndromes of cervical root compression were defined, and differentiation from myocardial ischemia with referred pain, brachial neuritis, thoracic outlet syndromes, and neuropathy of the median nerve in the carpal tunnel became ever more certain.* Aided by the new contrast material Pantopaque, surgeons were able to diagnose an increasing number of cervical disc lesions.[99] Those surgeons, still ignorant of spondylotic cervical myelopathy and the significance of the smaller than normal spinal canal, encountered two problems. First, some cervical discs were soft detached or ruptured fragments of cartilage similar to the ruptured lumbar discs that were being so effectively treated. Other abnormal discs were firm or almost completely osseous. Sometimes they extended across the cervical spinal canal, quite unlike anything seen in the lumbar spine. The question was raised whether the firm bony disc abnormality represented an end-stage of soft disc disease. Second, paraplegia was a too frequent result of attempts to remove these "hard discs" by employing chisels and curets of various design.

After Brain, Northfield, and Wilkinson, and others defined the cervical myelopathic syndromes due to arthrosis, it became apparent that there were two cervical disc abnormalities rather than one.[17,113] It also became apparent that failure to recognize the differences between disc rupture and arthrosis, and treatment of one as though it were the other, would give poor results. Before cervical spondylotic myelopathy was recognized, the diagnosis of primary lateral sclerosis often was made to explain pure spastic-paretic states. Amyotrophic lateral sclerosis without bulbar involvement and prolonged survival was diagnosed to explain arm and hand atrophy and fasciculation with spastic and paretic legs. The diagnosis of combined system disease without pernicious anemia (but usually treated with crude liver injections anyway) was given in cases of spastic-paraparesis with dorsal column sensory deficits. Chronic unremitting pure spinal multiple sclerosis was said to account for spastic-paretic states with the Brown-Séquard type of sensory changes. In addition, there were special forms of spinal syphilis for other patterns of disease. Nearly all patients with

such manifestations are now found to have spondylotic cervical myelopathy.

Payne and Spillane's demonstration of a shallower than normal spinal canal in myelopathic patients explained why in some instances severe and obvious arthrosis failed to produce myelopathy, while other patients with relatively little abnormality shown on the x-rays became severely affected.[79] The premorbid capacity of the spinal canal, particularly its depth, or anteroposterior dimension, was shown to be of extreme importance in determining whether myelopathy would result from arthrosis. The blood supply of the spinal cord, apart from the local ischemia produced at the site of direct arthrotic compression, is probably of equal importance.[54,103,108] How malfunction of the intraspinal neural elements can cause such varied symptoms remains a puzzle. Sometimes there is pain, but often there is none. Sometimes there are Lhermitte's phenomenon and other paresthesias. There may be predominantly gray matter involvement. Usually bladder and sexual function is undisturbed. There is almost always early corticospinal tract involvement.

Even before the frequency of cervical myelopathic syndromes was recognized, Kahn speculated on how the spinal cord could be deformed or stressed by a hard anterior ridge to cause corticospinal tract involvement that produced a syndrome that was given the name of primary lateral sclerosis.[48] Although it was never confirmed by experimental demonstrations in an animal model, there was wide acceptance of his hypothesis implicating the denticulate ligaments in the generation of internal cord stresses. The harmful effects of these stresses were said to be concentrated in the corticospinal tracts. After spondylotic myelopathy came to be diagnosed and operations of various sorts were being devised for it, intradural exploration with section of denticulate ligaments was widely employed in North America. It still enjoys a certain popularity despite lack of proved efficacy over decompression alone.[34] Europeans, and especially the English, were not attracted to this singular notion of etiology and described a variety of mechanisms for the production of myelopathy. These mechanisms entailed direct neuronal compression by a bony spur; rubbing or compression by invagination of the yellow

---

* See references 13, 14, 20, 58, 71, 93, 94, 97.

ligament; root sleeve fibrosis; obstruction of flow in the draining veins; and reduced flow in the anterior spinal artery, the radicular arteries, and the larger intramedullary derivatives of the arteries on the surface of the cord.*

Kaplan and Kennedy found that extension of the neck of the patient with cervical arthrosis and myelopathy could produce obstruction of the spinal subarachnoid space in Queckenstedt's test.[49] They did not make further studies of the biomechanical mechanisms at work nor a detailed correlation with clinical symptoms. In this omission, they appear to have missed an opportunity to pioneer the study of biomechanics of the cervical spine in relation to neurological disease and to become known as the discoverers of spondylotic myelopathy. Allen's 1952 observation of blanching of the operatively exposed spinal cord on flexion of the neck was one of the first of a large number of clinical and experimental observations on the influence of dynamic mechanisms at work in the neck that could increase or decrease the room available to the roots, the spinal cord, and their nutrient vessels.[2,19,82,90] All these structures are dangerously vulnerable in a small canal when it is further reduced in size by pathological encroachments of the disc or posterior articulations and ligamentous enlargements and invaginations.

FREQUENCY OF OCCURRENCE

Cervical spine disorders produce pain, which may be local or referred to other areas. The pain may arise from a herniated disc or malfunctioning joints. Pain, paresis, spasticity, and reflex and sensory disturbances due to compression or other forms of irritation or interference with the roots or spinal cord are common. These disorders account for 1 to 2 per cent of the admissions to large general hospitals.

During 1974 and 1975, the Saint Luke's Hospital, Houston, with a very large cardiovascular patient population, owing to inclusion of the Texas Heart Institute, recorded 53,556 discharges. Four hundred forty of these patients had diagnoses of cervical spondylosis, cervical myelopathy,

cervical herniated disc, cervical radiculopathy, cervical radiculitis, cervical syndrome, or cervicobrachial syndrome. Thus, they represented 0.82 per cent of the discharges from a hospital that does not emphasize neurology or neurological surgery. During the same years, The Methodist Hospital, Houston, also with a large cardiovascular patient population but with a greater emphasis on neurosurgery as well, had 74,652 discharges, 1.6 per cent of which were in the aforementioned categories. One hundred seventy nine patients had cervical disc displacements causing radiculitis, while 91 had myelopathy. A recent report on neurosurgical operations performed over a five-year period on residents of Olmstead County, Minnesota, whose access to neurosurgical care of high quality is optimal, suggests that approximately eight cervical disc removals or decompressions are required per annum per 100,000 population.[38] In this same population, brain tumors were operated upon with equal frequency and intracranial aneurysms somewhat less frequently. During the entire five-year period, only one primary intraspinal tumor was encountered. The ratio of lumbar to cervical disc disease is estimated to be six to one.[69]

OVERVIEW OF PROBLEM

From decade to decade in this century, one diagnostic entity has replaced another to explain difficulties of the cervical area. The great popularity enjoyed by the scalenus anticus syndrome as an explanation of shoulder and arm pains (replacing earlier syndromes of focal infection and neuritis) faded in the late 1940's with realization of the frequency of occurrence of cervical root compression by abnormalities of the discs. At present, there may be overdiagnosis of this condition and neglect of diagnoses such as diabetic mononeuropathy, Spillane's neuritis, neuropathy of the median nerve in the carpal tunnel, thoracic outlet syndrome, sprains, and traumatic arthritis of posterior articulations. Primary care physicians and patients themselves have long seemed willing to accept "pulled muscle" and other speculative myopathies as legitimate causes. This has been harmless, for the most part, since most of these conditions prove to be self-limited or be-

---

* See references 8, 16, 37, 41, 59, 77, 102, 103.

come subject to more accurate diagnosis before harm has been done. It seems likely that muscles themselves are not primarily at fault except in a minority of cases.

Most patients with cervical disc herniation, arthrosis, or cervicobrachial syndromes will have self-limited conditions. Manifestations are chiefly subjective; however, neck motion may be limited, and minimal reflex inequalities and paresthesias may be present. These patients usually respond to heat, traction, reduced activity, and salicylates over a period of time. Exceptions occur when the syndrome was provoked or aggravated by trauma for which an employer or other blameworthy person is believed to be responsible. In these latter cases, magnification of the intensity of pain, the constancy of pain, the frequency of complaint, and the incapacity for work cause impatience in the patient and spouse, the employer, the insurance company, and the lawyers. In these circumstances, the stage is set for performance of ill-conceived operations that, at large monetary cost to society, fail to produce satisfactory results.

Inaccurate diagnosis and poor judgment in choice of therapy account for far more unsatisfactory results than faulty operative technique. Skill in performance of one or another cervical operation is not an indication for its routine employment over the wide range of syndromes to be discussed. Common judgmental errors accounting for disappointing results include: (1) fusion of one or more motion segments when decompression was preferable; (2) intradural exploration and denticulate ligament division to deal with a theoretical pathophysiological mechanism; (3) fusion or decompression for hyperextension neck sprain; (4) fusion of multiple motion segments in series after an ill-advised initial operation fails to provide relief, as shown in Figure 80–1; (5) fusions predicated on the belief that discography or intranuclear injections of anesthetic solutions or saline helps to identify a painful joint; (6) operations for neck and occipital pains due to anxiety and depressive reactions; (7) attempts to remove stable arthrotic processes (spurs) through the posterior approach; and (8) paraplegia-risking techniques for removal of disc fragments and spurs from shallower than normal spinal canals intolerant of the introduction of footed rongeurs of the Ker-

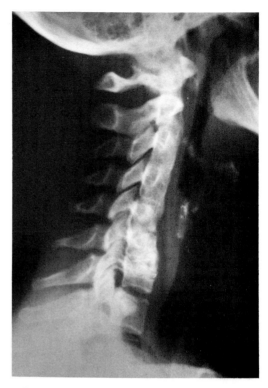

Figure 80–1 Lateral radiograph of the cervical spine of a victim of a galaxy of judgmental errors that may be made in treating cervical disc disease. 1. The complaints originated in a litigated accident. 2. There were no radicular or myelopathic organic manifestations. 3. The myelogram was normal. 4. A one-level fusion was performed after what was thought to be an abnormal discogram. 5. When complaints continued, additional interspaces were fused in three subsequent operations until the entire spine from C2 through C7 had been so treated. 6. Iatrogenic miseries were added to those initially present. 7. The surgeon did not appreciate the fact that anterior interbody fusion is not proper treatment for neck pain whose exact origin cannot be specified.

rison type until wide decompression has been provided.

Investigations beginning in the mid 1930's on radiculopathies and in the late 1940's on myelopathies have provided a large body of information. Large gaps in our knowledge remain, however. Chronically developing spondylotic cervical myelopathy seen in humans has not been duplicated in an animal model, although a combination of radicular artery interruption and mechanical compression of the cord of dogs has produced a similar condition.[39] The subtle pathophysiological aspects, particularly the factor of ischemia of the spinal cord resulting from reduced flow through the radicular and anterior and posterior spinal arteries, are only beginning to be appreciated.[53,107] Unfortunately, methods are not available to determine the adequacy of the cord circulation and the effect on it of root and radicular artery compression. When a compromised cord circulation is present, operative maneuvers may be used that critically interfere with the already endangered blood supply. The occasional case of intraoperative worsening of myelopathy or the production of myelopathy during the course of an apparently uncomplicated decompressive or fusion procedure may be explained by this mechanism.

Except for occasional misfortunes, proper selection of patients and wise choice and skillful performance of the procedure will afford relief of almost all pain and recovery of most of the lost strength and some of the sensory loss in a high percentage of patients suffering from root compression by disc herniations or bony spurs. Myelopathy that has been diagnosed early should be arrested and perhaps improved, especially in the younger patient. Only myelopathic patients who are treated early and before severe impairments develop can be expected to become nearly normal. Without strict diagnostic criteria and an understanding of the pathophysiological changes and how they may be most effectively modified, good results will not be produced regularly.

ETIOLOGY OF DISC RUPTURE AND ARTHROSIS

The simplistic view that disc rupture is caused by a single major injury and arthrosis by the additive effect of countless smaller and forgotten or unnoticed traumatic events fails to explain many well-known features of these disorders. Ninety per cent or more of cervical disc ruptures occur without recognized trauma having occurred.[34,69] Divers into shallow water may fracture bone without rupturing a cervical disc, and football players violently stress their necks but sustain relatively few cervical injuries despite the frequency of opportunity for an injury. Though certain evidence suggests that repeated stress produces or aggravates arthrosis, it is not uncommon to see patients of very indolent disposition with severe arthrosis and lifelong athletes without it.[52,89] Clearly, other factors must be involved.

Disc rupture following minimal trauma may have various explanations. One or more discs of certain individuals may have defects in physical or chemical composition akin to the weaknesses that lead to fallen arches, inguinal hernias, varicose veins, and hemorrhoids.[66] Internally generated stresses due to involuntary paraspinal muscle contractions and other factors, may be greater than realized. Regaining balance after a slip or misstep and suddenly turning the neck in response to alerting signals from behind are examples of this sort of strain. It appears reasonable to regard the anterior and posterior longitudinal ligaments as unimportant in determining whether a disc will rupture. The longitudinal ligaments are always incomplete and flimsy structures insufficient to bolster the annulus and contain the nucleus should the former be stressed to the point of being breached under conditions of acutely rising intranuclear pressure. The nucleus pulposus is an incompressible passive substance that is gelatinous in youth but more fibrous with age. It has no tensile or other strengths except resistance to volume reduction when compressed. A more important feature of the nucleus appears to be its disposition to take on water and swell under certain conditions.[72]

The anulus fibrosus, composed of sheets of lamellae or collagen that crisscross one another like a cat's cradle, is subject to a variety of inherent weaknesses and defects (Fig. 80–2). The bonding where the lamellae cross one another may be a weak link in annular microanatomy that permits fissuring and the development of pathways for nuclear migration and eventually herniation. Through the cartilaginous end-plates of the bodies must come all of the nourishment and maintenance of the avascular annulus. These functions deteriorate with age and no doubt earlier in some patients than in others.[3]

The water content of the disc is highest in utero. At birth the water content is higher in the nucleus than in the annulus. Desiccation occurs throughout life in both structures. During the fifth decade, however, the nucleus begins to dehydrate at a faster rate than the annulus.[73] Disproportionate desiccation with reduction of volume of the nucleus probably changes the stress to which the annulus is subjected. In youth, when the nucleus is turgid because of high water content, the annular lamellae are under ten-

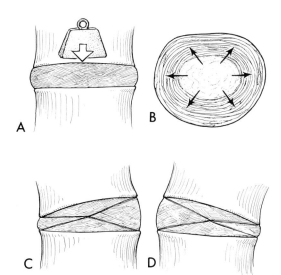

Figure 80–2 Diagram of the obliquely crossing lamellae of the anulus fibrosus. *A*. Direct compression tending to force the annulus of a desiccated disc out of the interspace and loosen its osseous attachment. *B*. Tension stresses placed on annular fibers by a turgid nucleus under compression. *C* and *D*. Shearing stresses acting on weak bonds between the fibers of the annular lamellae as the spine is bent.

sion similar to the tension on the fibers of the fabric or cord of an inflated vehicle tire. With nuclear dehydration, a flat tire situation develops, and instead of the annular fibers being under tension, they come under grinding compression forces. Such an annulus may be more vulnerable to compressive detachment from the vertebral bodies as a consequence of minimal trauma.[55]

Another mechanism predisposing to disc rupture has been proposed by Naylor and Smare, who believe that degradation of the protein polysaccharide complexes of the nucleus results in an *increase* in its fluid content much as a subdural hematoma is supposed to acquire fluid and enlarge as the number of osmotically active particles in it increases.[74] The increased fluid produces increased intradiscal pressure so that trauma, either trivial or severe, becomes the precipitating factor that triggers rupture at a particular moment. Whether this happens in consequence of nuclear desiccation or nuclear swelling, the precipitating trauma that is remembered by the patient is less important etiologically than the underlying predisposition. Once the predisposing circumstances are present, eventually trauma or strain will be encountered to cause the symptoms.

Finneson likens the acute disc abnormality to subarachnoid hemorrhage from rupture of an aneurysm because, in both diseases, a predisposing cause exists that is unknown to the patient.[35] With aneurysms, the straining at stool, the orgasm, the argument, or the other event precipitating the hemorrhage is merely the provocation. Had it not occurred when it did, another provocation would have been certain to come along and bear responsibility. In litigated cases, the provocative cause of the disorder becomes all-important to the patient, his attorney, and the court, while the predisposing factor or factors usually are ignored or depreciated.

The origin and progression of arthrosis are similarly clouded. Some individuals seem destined to suffer degenerative joint disorders, though mendelian transmission is unproved. Wide variation in severity of arthrosis exists among individuals in the same age group who have similar histories in which there has been no trauma. Severely affected patients do not usually beget children destined to have the same problem, but exceptions are known.[21,68] Occupational and internally generated stresses probably play significant but unquantifiable roles. Victims of spasmodic torticollis are likely to have more cervical arthrosis than others. Congenital lack of vertebral segmentation and antecedent spinal fusion increase stress in adjacent motion segments and accelerate degenerative change in them (Fig. 80–3). The protuberant annulus at a narrowing disc space appears to stimulate marginal spurring as an expression, perhaps, of the wisdom of the body at work shoring up a failing articulation.[80] Since the pathogeneses of disc rupture and arthrosis are quite dissimilar, it is unlikely that the spurring is an end-stage of a ruptured disc. Spurring at vertebral motion segments exhibits strong predilection for certain sites. Usually they are anterior and intraforaminal; to a somewhat lesser degree they are posterior in the cervical region. In the lumbar area, they are almost exclusively anterior and lateral, and seldom encroach on the spinal canal posteriorly or into the intervertebral foramina.

The yellow ligament has attracted considerable attention. Some authors describe it as having a special pathology of its own that causes it to fibrose and thicken.[98,109] Others regard it as a passive structure that fibroses and loses its elasticity with age and

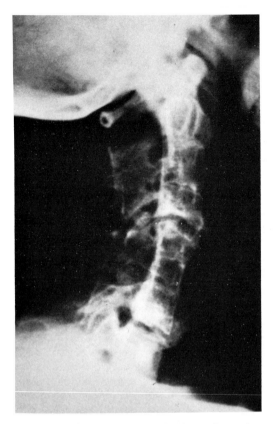

Figure 80–3 Severe arthrotic change in motion segments C4–C5 and C6–C7 as a consequence of abnormal stress due to congenital "fusion" or defective segmentation of C2–C3–C4 and C5–C6. Operative fusion and stresses generated by the excessive motion associated with spasmodic torticollis have similar effects. This patient's myelogram was abnormal at C4–C5 only.

causes harm only when the laminae approach one another in extension, causing it to invaginate, or when the posterior articulations enlarge and depress it into the spinal canal.[29,102,110] Arthrotic changes in the posterior articulations are pathologically no different from degenerative change in other diarthrodial joints such as the metacarpophalangeal and interphalangeal joints that are undergoing change through the influences of age, familial predisposition, and stress. These changes are part of the spondylotic process, but sometimes they are much more advanced than changes in the disc.

The posterior longitudinal ligament was dimissed earlier as being of little consequence in relation to disc rupture. Occasionally it undergoes great thickening and calcification independent of arthrotic change in the discs and posterior articulations. Further, it may produce a clinically significant mass ventral to the spinal cord and dura as it bridges several vertebral bodies and discs (Fig. 80–4). Calcification in such a thickened posterior longitudinal ligament may be insufficiently dense to be identified in plain radiographs. This situation illustrates the need for laminagraphy and myelography in the diagnosis of myelopathy and radiculopathy.

Production of pain by encroachment of a spur or disc fragment on a nerve root probably is not due simply to direct mechanical irritation of pain fibers in the root. Some patients whose myelograms show severe flattening of one or more roots have no pain or even sensory loss or paresthesias. They develop only muscle paresis, atrophy, and fasciculation.[56] Other patients have relatively small root deformations associated with severe radicular pain. Neurophysiological studies indicate that constant compression of axons in a root does not give rise to the repetitive firing presumably necessary to produce chronic pain. Recent evidence does indicate that chronic inflammatory changes in a root confer on it the capability of repetitive firing in response to a constant stimulus.[47] The cells in a normal dorsal root ganglion appear to be capable of repetitive firing in response to constant compression. Alternate explanations of how direct pain fiber stimulation causes chronic pain have been suggested. Ischemia or direct neuronal compression may cause ablation of function of the larger fibers in the root that normally modulate the pain experience at the gate in the substantia gelatinosa or higher centers. A breakdown of myelin and other insulation of root axons, may permit ephaptic conduction to take place at an artificial synapse so that nerve impulses generated in efferent systems and destined for muscles or skin organs cross over and are felt as pain. Relevant to an inquiry into how small disc herniations can cause pain is the discovery that nuclear cartilage is antigenic.[10] Possibly this antigenic material, separated from the root only by its thin sleeve, could generate pain through its inflammation-producing potential. This factor may also account for those instances in which a previously untreated disc herniation is found to be accompanied by marked hyperemia and fibrosis surrounding the root.

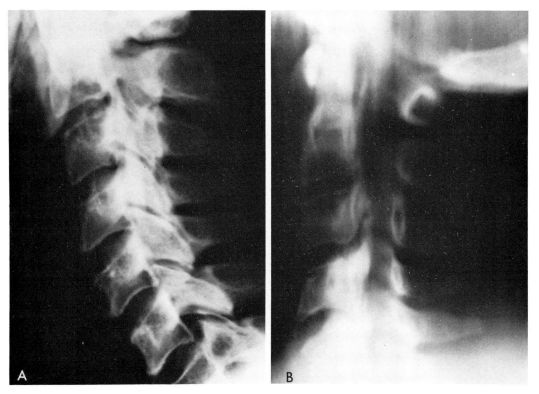

Figure 80-4 *A*. Normal lateral roentgenogram of a patient with clinical evidence of myelopathy affecting mid-cervical segments. *B*. Midline laminagram showing significant encroachment on the anterior spinal canal opposite the lower body of C2, C3, and C4 and the intervening discs. There is thickening and calcification of the posterior longitudinal ligament. Myelography revealed severe deformation of the spinal cord in this area.

Developmental Shallowness of the Canal and Foramina

Axons thrive and transmit impulses normally, and radicular blood vessels remain patent, whether curved or straight. The function of neither is impaired by being draped or gently bent over a spur or a ridge any more than the ulnar nerve or the cervicomedullary junction of the neuraxis is inconvenienced by flexion and extension of the elbow or neck under normal circumstances. Ruptured disc fragments and arthrotic joint enlargements are incapable of harming the roots or spinal cord without help from cooperating structures in the posterior wall of the intervertebral foramen or spinal canal. This statement applies even to the occasional patient with a canal of normal depth who harbors a high transverse ridge across an interspace producing myelopathy where, it is likely, the cord is pressed down upon the ridge by the inelastic posterior dura, which "bow strings" to-

ward the anterior wall of the spinal canal in neck flexion.[19]

To produce radiculopathy, abnormal discs and spurs require help from the superior facet of the inferior vertebra, which constitutes the posterior wall of the intervertebral foramen (Fig. 80–5). For them to produce myelopathy, help is required from the laminae and yellow ligaments, which constitute the posterior wall of the spinal canal. How effectively these surrounding structures participate with a herniated disc or spur to cause neural compression depends on the premorbid size of the foramen and the spinal canal. For example, the patient whose spine is displayed in Figure 80–5 is highly unlikely to develop radiculopathy or myelopathy due to disc disease. Thus, the developmental premorbid configuration of the spine has importance equal to that of the pathological changes that are popularly perceived to be the cause of the problem. The spine with which a person is born determines whether there will, in later

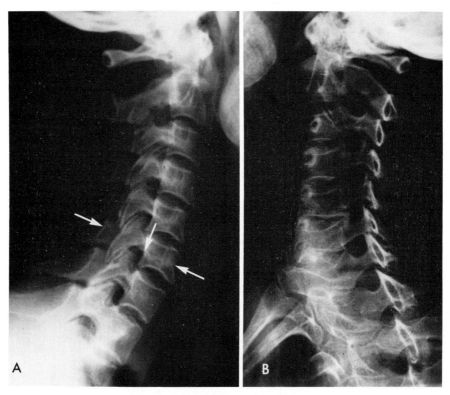

Figure 80–5   *A*. Lateral radiograph of a cervical spine whose canal is 25 to 30 per cent deeper than the antero-posterior dimension of the body at all mid and lower cervical levels. Verification can be made by comparing the distances between the points of the arrows. The pedicles are of such generous length that the images of the posterior articulations are projected far back of the posterior line of the bodies and entirely within the projected image of the canal itself. This technique permits a "look" in one intervertebral foramen and out the other at several levels. Note that the superior facet at each level constitutes the posterior wall of the foramen. *B*. Oblique view of the same spinal canal displaying long pedicles and large circular intervertebral foramina.

life, be room for its neural contents and enough in reserve for a degree of harmless encroachment by motion segment abnormalities or whether these encroachments will cause symptoms. Thus disc herniations and arthrotic spurs and ridges produce symptoms and signs earlier in individuals with spinal canals that are developmentally small in one or more dimensions. It has been suggested that certain cases of developmental shallowness may be hereditary, apart from its prevalence in achondroplasia, but in most instances, cases are sporadic and parental transmission is not demonstrable.[68] Almost all instances of cervical myelopathy depend on shallowness and arthrosis in the mid and lower cervical spine, since the canal normally enlarges considerably as it passes through the neural arches of C2 and C1.[114] Occasionally, myelopathy may be due to developmental shallowness at a high level, while

the middle and lower cervical spinal canal maintains average depth (Fig. 80–6). Reports of myelopathy and radiculopathy resulting from developmental shallowness alone without participation by changes dependent on motion, stress, and aging must be rejected because these patients, including the achondroplastic, enter adult life without evidence of neural impairment. Failure to demonstrate interspace narrowing and ridges or spurs only means that the radiographic techniques are insufficiently sensitive to detect the first stages of motion segment degeneration.

Discs and other joint enlargements invading space designed for the neural elements have an important difference from neoplasms and granulomas in that they do not relentlessly enlarge by arithmetic or geometric progression. There are limits to the amount of cartilage that can herniate from a cervical disc and to the size attainable by

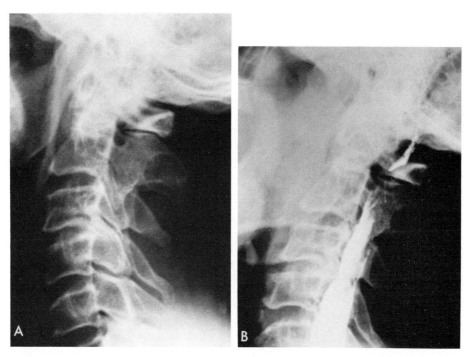

Figure 80–6 *A*. Lateral radiograph of a cervical spine responsible for severe myelopathy at a high level. Note the unusually short interval between the posterior arch of C1 and the dens, though the anterior arch of C1 seems to be in normal position. At C3, C4, and C5 the pedicles are so short and so laterally directed as to cause the projected images of the posterior articulations to overlap the posterior line of the bodies (compare with Figure 80–5). The laminal angle is obtuse, but the overall depth of the spinal canal is marginally adequate at C4 and below, owing to massiveness of the facets, which make a larger than usual contribution to the neural arch. *B*. Lateral myelogram confirming severe encroachment on the spinal subarachnoid space beneath the posterior arch of C1 and the aberrant C1–C2 articulation.

the intraforaminal spurs and intracanalicular ridges. No canal or foramen can be so capacious as to accommodate, without the neural elements being progressively affected, the bulk that tumors can attain. Canals and foramina of average and larger than average size, however, regularly accommodate arthrotic encroachments without effect on the neural elements. Accordingly, many, perhaps most, intraforaminal and intracanalicular spurs and ridges are unimportant and incidental findings. Attention to the depth and anatomical configuration of the canal and foramina in plain films and to certain other changes, such as retrolisthesis, shown in Figure 80–7, permits recognition of those patients in whom pathological processes are of great significance despite their mild appearance.[81]

The depth of the cervical spinal canal, from C4 through C7 as seen in lateral radiographs made with the x-ray tube at 1.5 meters distance, has an average depth of 18.5 mm with a range of 14.2 to 23 mm.[11]

The depth of the canal in each individual is constant through this region. Sufferers from spondylotic myelopathy have shallower canals that measure 14 mm or less in depth.[79] Measurement from the midpoint of the back of a body to the nearest point of that segment's lamina reflects the premorbid depth of the spinal canal. Measurement from the apex of the most prominent transverse ridge to the nearest lamina is relevant also. An average depth of 10.9 mm has been reported in myelopathic patients.[75] Thus, arthrotic disease such as spurs and retrolistheses may effect a further reduction, approximating 25 per cent, in the room needed by the spinal cord in a developmentally shallow canal. Although canal shallowness predisposes to myelopathy, should arthrotic encroachments occur, this does not necessarily mean that the foramina will be small and that there will be increased liability to radiculopathy.[45] The severity of myelopathy is dependent upon the severity of the morbid change in the spine, not shal-

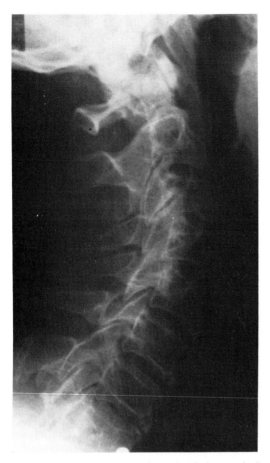

Figure 80-7 Lateral radiograph of the cervical spine of a patient with severe paresis and spasticity due to spondylotic myelopathy, read as "essentially normal except for anterior hypertrophic spurring at several levels." This canal is one quarter to one third shallower than the midbody dimension. Of equal importance is the retrolisthesis at the C3–C4 motion segment. The interval on the original film between the lower edge of the body of C3 and the upper edge of the lamina of C4 was only 9 mm.

lowness of the canal alone. In the absence of degenerative changes the shallowness does not necessarily forecast later myelopathy, its progression, or eventual disablement of the patient.[76] Interpediculate distance is irrelevant to myelopathy, since it is twice the anteroposterior dimension of the canal.[22]

Estimation of the true depth of the spinal canal by use of conventionally made radiographs is difficult, since anode to spine to film distances vary among radiographic departments. Some inconstant factors produce less variation than might be expected. For instance, if a canal measuring 16 mm in depth on a film 72 inches from the anode is

re-examined on a film 40 inches from the anode, the increase is only 2.37 mm. Shoulder widths varying between 7 and 11 inches are inconsequential on films made at 72 inches.[22] A reliable reference from which to judge the normal depth of a canal is the area encompassed by the lower cervical bodies and the intervening discs as seen in the lateral radiograph. This measurement should equal the area encompassed by the spinal canal through the same segments (Fig. 80–8).[23] The use of this comparison obviates the need for correction for magnification or resorting to tables of normal measurements. Patients with myelopathy have canal areas that are smaller in relation to body areas than do those without myelopathy. Since, in lateral x-rays, the areas encompassed by the canal projection and

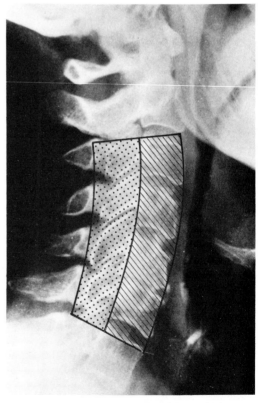

Figure 80-8 Lateral radiograph of a patient (not myelopathic) in whom the area encompassed by the canal (stippled) equals or exceeds the area encompassed by projections of the bodies (hatched). A ratio of canal area to body area approximating or exceeding unity is normal, while ratios well below unity (0.85 or below) indicate significant shallowness and disposition to myelopathy. This patient had no symptoms attributable to the C5–C6 arthrosis. She had a severe C7 radiculopathy due to a ruptured disk at C6–C7.

by the body projection have equal cranio-caudad length, the actual determinant of the area ratio is the ratio between the anteroposterior depth of the canal and the anteroposterior dimension of the lower cervical bodies. Both these measurements are uniform through the mid and lower cervical spine.[11] Thus, the lateral projection of the cervical spine contains within it a reliable standard, the body depth, with which to compare canal depth for normality or shallowness. Since the body and the canal are in the same plane parallel with the film and are equally magnified, it is unnecessary to know anode to target to film distances or to correct for magnification. The midpoints of the front and the back of the body and the crescentic line marking the midpoint of the lamina are easily seen in good films. Three pencil marks on a card or a millimeter rule suffice to determine whether the canal to body ratio is near unity. If the canal is 15 to 25 per cent smaller than the body measurement, vulnerability to myelopathy increases in patients who develop spondylosis. On the contrary, if canal depth is as large or larger than the body measurement, it is unlikely that even severe arthrosis will be found the cause of myelopathy or deformation of the cord on myelography (see Fig. 80–5).

Among 28 patients whose canals were as large as or larger than the body measurement, only 2 had myelopathy and 10 had radiculopathy, whereas 16 had neither (Fig. 80–9). Among 21 patients whose canals were from 1 to 3 mm shallower than the body measurement, 2 had myelopathy, 5 had radiculopathy, and 14 had neither. Among the 29 patients whose canals were 4 mm or more shallower than the body measurement, 8 had myelopathy, 16 had radiculopathy, and only 5 had other conditions. On films made at 72 inches (1.8 m), a measurement between the midpoint of the posterior body and the nearest point of the lamina of the same vertebra of 14 mm or less proclaims developmental shallowness and disposition to myelopathy. If such a patient has a ridge or spur, the interval between this ridge and the nearest lamina may be much smaller and will be the site of greatest cord deformation. The cervical spinal cord is 10 to 11 mm in anteroposterior dimension on these films and, with its investment, requires 11 or 12 mm of canal depth. Since these measurements are magnifications of

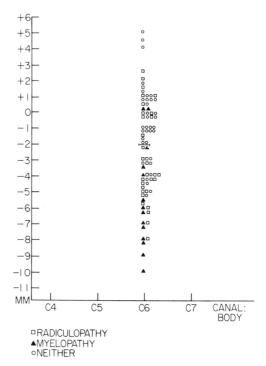

Figure 80–9 Spinal canal depth compared to vertebral body depth in 78 patients with cervical ailments. Canals deeper than the body are represented on the vertical scale by + millimeters above zero and the smaller canals by − millimeters below it. Only differences at C6 are depicted for simplicity. The median is at − 2 mm. Note the concentration of myelopathic disease in those patients whose canals are 2 mm or more shallower than the bodies.

reality, and the dynamic encroaching processes such as disc bulging and yellow ligament infolding in extension increase cord deformation further, any measurement from a ventral ridge to the closest lamina of 12 mm or less will correlate well with the presence of spondylotic myelopathy at that level (see Fig. 80–7).

Valuable additional information about the cervical spine may be gained from inspection of plain radiographs. The depth of the canal is a function of several observable variables, such as the length and obliquity of direction of pedicles, the size of the facet contribution to neural arch design, and the angle at which the right and left halves of the lamina meet in the midline. If the pedicles are short or if they are more laterally directed than usual, the posterior articulations will, in lateral view, be projected tangent to or even overlying the posterior aspects of the bodies (Fig. 80–10). It is simple to observe where the posterior articulations are projected with respect to the posterior

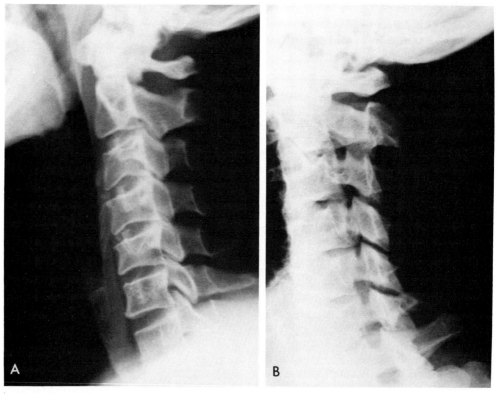

Figure 80–10 *A*. Lateral radiograph of a cervical spine showing facets hugging and overlapping the posterior line of the vertebral bodies owing to the shortness or lateral direction of the pedicles (compare with Figure 80–5). Observe the depth of lamina that may be seen between the cortical bone of the posterior facets and the cortical bone of the midline of the lamina because the right and left halves of this patient's laminae meet at an acute angle, perhaps approaching 90 degrees. The acute laminal angle tends to increase overall depth of the spinal canal and compensates for pedicle shortness. *B*. Oblique view of the same spine confirming shortness of the pedicles and shallowness of the intervertebral foramina. These measurements favor the early development of radiculopathy should small encroachments by the discs develop.

line of the bodies. The length of the pedicles may be measured in oblique views, but the degree of lateral direction of pedicle takeoff from the body is not easily discerned and, when sufficient, draws the facets close upon the back of the bodies, though the pedicles may be amply long to provide for generous-sized intervertebral foramina. The canal depth component contributed to by facets is difficult to estimate, but the amount of laminal contribution to canal depth is easily observed or measured. In some cases, the right and left halves of the lamina meet at an obtuse angle with no foreshortened lamina visible posterior to the posterior articulations. This type of canal will be shallow because of this feature, but the shallowness may be compensated for by good length and posterior direction of pedicles (Fig. 80–11).

Dynamic Factors in Cervical Radiculopathy and Myelopathy

The prominence of the discs, arthrotic spurs and ridges, and the shallowness of intervertebral foramina and cervical spinal canal are static factors in the production of radiculopathy and myelopathy. They are relatively unvarying from day to day, week to week, and in some instances, year to year. Retrolisthesis has a static aspect (see Fig. 80–7). After it has arisen at a particular motion segment, it will remain as an unfavorable encroachment on the spinal canal with the neck in neutral position. It may also, however, be a dynamic factor. It can vary with reduction and aggravation of the displacement on neck flexion and extension because of the action of the inclined plane of motion of the posterior articulations. The

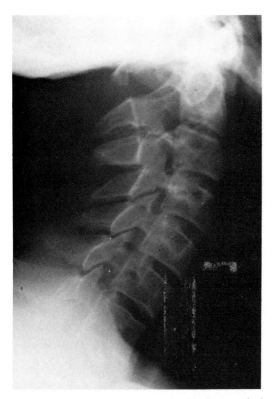

Figure 80–11 Lateral radiograph of a cervical spine with a very obtuse laminal angle (perhaps 180 degrees). A crescentic line of cortical bone concave to the rear normally marks the midpoint of the lamina. It cannot be identified at C4–C5–C6–C7 because the laminae, which extend straight across from side to side, are obscured by the overlying posterior articulations. The crescentic cortical bone line that is seen at C4–C5–C6–C7 is the cortical bone of the inferior facet at each level, whose curve is convex to the rear and thus the reverse of the midline laminal indicator. An obtuse laminal angle of this type favors shallowness of the canal. In this patient, there is compensation in the generous length of the pedicles, which causes the facets to be projected well posterior to the posterior line of the bodies.

factors that contribute to radiculopathy and myelopathy by coming into effect innumerable times daily as a consequence of ordinary neck motion may be regarded as the dynamic factors in production of these disorders.

At any one motion segment, the fulcrum on which the superior vertebra moves on the one inferior to it on flexion and extension is well ahead of the facets and somewhere in the posterior half of the disc itself. A variety of effects are produced by going from a neutral position to extension: (1) The anterior longitudinal ligament is tightened and, with the anterior part of the an-

nulus, acts as a check on widening of the anterior interspace. (2) The posterior longitudinal ligament and the posterior portion of the annulus constituting the anterior wall of the spinal canal slacken, while the transverse prominence across the disc increases as the distance between the posterior vertebral surfaces is reduced. (3) The inferior facet of the upper vertebra of a motion segment descends on the inclined plane of the superior facet of the inferior vertebra and draws the superior vertebra posteriorly. Also, retrolisthesis, if it exists, is increased. (4) The pedicles of each vertebral pair come closer together to reduce the height of the intervertebral foramen. This effect is further enhanced if the head is tilted to the same side. (5) The laminae come closer together and even tend to overlap so that the yellow ligament, attached to the undersurface of the superior lamina and to the upper edge of the inferior one, bulges into the spinal canal. If the spinal canal is critically shallow, the bulging ligament may compress the spinal cord against a prominent spur or herniated disc.[102] Presumably, these dynamic effects account for the increased radicular pain and paresthesias produced by neck extension and ipsilateral inclination and the relief of symptoms produced by movement in an opposite direction or by cervical traction. Also body tingling of the Lhermitte variety and blocking of the subarachnoid space when the neck is extended probably are the result of these dynamic changes.[49]

When the neck is flexed, opposite effects occur. (1) The anterior longitudinal ligament and the anterior annulus slacken. The anterior aspects of the vertebral interspaces narrow slightly. (2) The posterior longitudinal ligament and the posterior annulus draw tight. The prominence of the discs as palpable ridges is reduced. (3) The inferior facet of the superior vertebra of a motion segment slides forward and rises on the inclined plane of the superior facet of the inferior vertebra. This motion reduces the retrolisthesis and increases the height of the intervertebral foramen. (4) The interval between the adjacent laminae and spinous processes increases to tighten the interspinous ligament and the ligamentum flavum. The surface of the posterior wall of the spinal canal is made flatter and smoother.

The effects of dynamic movements of the

spine can be demonstrated by tracing from lateral radiographs the position of each vertebra with the spine in flexion and extension. The tracing may be based on a line drawn through the lower surface of the C7 vertebra and intersecting the midpoint of its lamina. The upper reference line is drawn across the lower margin of the foramen magnum (Fig. 80–12). In a representative patient going from flexion to extension, the anterior aspects of the five intervertebral discs between C2 and C7 widen by 13.5 mm. The anterior wall of the spinal canal measured from the foramen magnum to the lower corner of C7 loses 4.5 mm because of a slight narrowing of the discs at each interval posteriorly. This movement is also accompanied by an increased prominence of the discs that is not shown on the diagram.

The most striking change in going from flexion to extension occurs in the posterior wall of the spinal canal. In flexion, the length from the foramen magnum to the middle of the lamina of C7 is 139 mm. In moving to full extension, there is a loss of 40.5 mm due to approximation of the laminae. Interlaminal spaces occupied by ligamenta flava total 62 mm in the flexed configuration and

only 21.5 mm in the extended configuration. Since the volume of the ligamentum flavum does not diminish and the ligament must occupy space somewhere, it is easy to appreciate how it is driven into the spinal canal by the pistonlike effect of the inferior lamina moving up under the inferior edge of the superior lamina at each motion segment. When the volume of the cervical spinal canal is calculated by using its mean lengths in the flexed and extended configurations and assuming its cross section to be circular, it is found that the canal has a capacity of 31.3 ml in the flexed position and 26.3 ml, or 5 ml less, when the neck is extended. In extension, the spinal cord does not lose volume commensurate with the reduced capacity of the extended canal. In fact, each segment of the cord shortens and actually increases slightly in cross-sectional area. The end result is that although the cord actually needs more space in the extended as opposed to the flexed position, the dynamic effects of extension force it to accommodate to a smaller space.

It might appear that flexion of the neck is helpful to the myelopathic cord, but this is not necessarily so. The spinal dura has strong collagenous fibers that are predominantly vertically oriented. It is quite inelastic and is firmly attached to the posterior margin of the foramen magnum. Its only inferior attachments are the root sleeves themselves, and these attachments are susceptible to only a small amount of cephalad and caudad motion in the intervertebral foramen.

When the neck is flexed, the posterior dura is drawn tight and adopts the shortest line between the foramen magnum and a point beneath an upper thoracic lamina. In the taut position of flexion, the dura presses the spinal cord down on the anterior wall, which may harbor a ridgelike elevation. This movement accounts for Lhermitte's phenomenon in neck flexion and for some cases of myelopathy (Fig. 80–13).

In extension, the root sleeves and nerve roots lie slack. They are relaxed against the upper aspect of the inferior pedicle at a foramen. In flexion, the root sleeves are also drawn upward and the roots are drawn obliquely upward and tightened.[82] The flexed position is unfavorable for exploration ventral to a root by the posterior approach, which is a strong argument for avoiding the maximal degrees of neck flex-

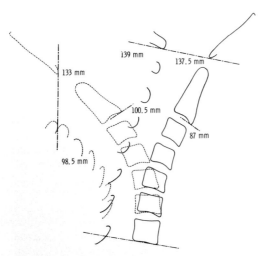

Figure 80–12 Action diagram prepared by tracing lateral cervical spine radiographs in flexion and extension. Both tracings are based on a line drawn through the lower surface of the C7 vertebra and measurement from this line cephalad to the plane of the foramen magnum and lower anterior corner of C2. The various measurements shown here demonstrate the changes in the dimensions of the spinal canal that take place in going from flexion to extension, as explained in the text.

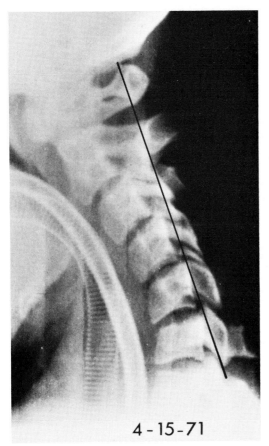

4-15-71

Figure 80–13 Lateral radiograph of a patient positioned upright with maximum neck flexion in preparation for cervical laminectomy. The operation was for a syndrome featuring largely subjective complaints. Following the operation, the patient was found to have myelopathy. There was no hematoma or other wound complication. Because of his young age, arteriosclerosis was ruled out. A straight line drawn from the posterior margin of the foramen magnum to the undersurface of the lamina of C7 describes the position that the inelastic posterior dura tries to take when the neck is so sharply flexed. Only the spinal cord and the posterior wall of the spinal canal prevent it from doing so.

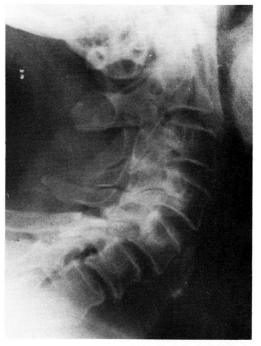

Figure 80–14 Lateral cervical radiograph of a patient with cervical myelopathy. The spinal canal depth is not notably shallow, and there is minimal interspace narrowing or spur formation. The two most striking abnormalities are the hyperlordosis with consequent approximation of the laminae in a neutral position of the neck and intense multilevel posterior articulation arthrosis. Very probably there is enlargement of the posterior articulations, although they are not seen on this film.

ion that can be achieved in the sitting position.

Some patients with myelopathy seem to have had their problems caused more by the dynamic than the static factors. They have no significant interspace narrowing, spurring, disc bulging, retrolisthesis, or striking shallowness of the canal. They do, however, have significant myelographic blocks. These blocks may be accompanied by paresthesias and electric sensations increased by neck extension (Figs. 80–14 and 80–15). Presumably, myelopathy and also some of the chronic forms of radiculopathy result from constant squeezing and massaging of the neural elements uncounted times in ordinary daily activity. These movements produce a chronic ischemia that varies in severity from time to time and irreversible pathological alterations in the spinal cord.[59]

Vertebra, Nerve Root, Spinal Cord, and Blood Vessel Relationships

The cervical nerve roots and spinal nerves are so related to the seven cervical vertebrae that each root and nerve bears the same number as the vertebra inferior to it. The C1 root leaves the spinal canal between the skull at the foramen magnum and the atlas. The C7 root departs at the C6–C7 motion segment cephalad of the C7 pedicle. The C8 root, for which there is no correspondingly numbered vertebra, passes through the C7–T1 foramen. The middle

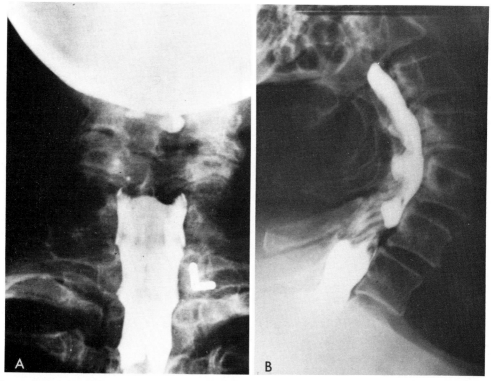

Figure 80–15 *A.* Anteroposterior myelogram of the patient depicted in Figure 80–14 showing a complete block at C6–C7 with the neck in moderate extension. Note also the severe posterior articulation arthrosis. *B.* Lateral myelogram after flexing the neck to allow Pantopaque to pass the C6–C7 block. Observe again the lack of interspace narrowing or posterior disc spurring. Multiple yellow ligament indentations are evident, the largest at C6–C7, where the spinal cord is pressed firmly down on the disc. The subarachnoid space ventral and lateral to the cord is obliterated. This patient's myelopathy was due to arthrotic enlargement of posterior articulations, especially at C6–C7, with intracanalicular depression of the subjacent yellow ligament. The problem is aggravated by yellow ligament infolding in extension.

and lower cervical roots have a constant relationship to the underlying discs, resting upon and in contact with them (see Fig. 80–5). In neutral posture, the lower cervical nerve roots lie in contact with or very close to the pedicle bearing the same number and are less close to the superior pedicle.

The relationship of nerve root and pedicle in the cervical area is unlike that in the lumbar region, where the departing root hugs the inferior aspect of the superior pedicle. Lumbar vertebrae have greater height than the cervical vertebra, and since pedicles arise from the upper part of the centra, the emerging lumbar root occupies a cephalic position in the foramen with bone of the lower body, rather than the disc, directly ventral to it. Ordinarily, a ruptured lumbar disc impinges on the root crossing it vertically in order to depart just beneath the

pedicle inferior to the disc in question, whereas a cervical disc prominence most commonly impinges on the root making its exit at the foramen that the disc bounds anteriorly. Thus, a disc abnormality at C5–C6 affects the C6 root rather than the C7, whose filaments of origin, still contained within the subarachnoid space and dura, are crossing the C5–C6 disc and are being organized into a cylindrical bundle to emerge at the foramen below (C6–C7).

The individual filaments that will make up the motor root spring from a zone on the surface of the anterolateral quadrant of the cord, while the sensory filaments emerge along the line of the posterolateral sulcus. The Bell-Magendie law, assigning purely afferent function to dorsal roots and purely efferent function to ventral roots, has been shown to be invalid by the discovery of unmyelinated axons that have their cell bodies in the ganglia and that enter the cord via anterior roots.[25] In light of this new information, ganglionectomy may be more effective than rhizotomy in the treatment of inflammatory, traumatic, and mechanical affections of the spinal nerves that are not amenable to treatment dealing with their primary causes.

Except at the highest levels in the spine, spinal cord segments do not correspond to and overlie vertebral segments having the same number. The mismatch is due to the shorter length of the spinal cord as compared with the spinal canal. The disproportion increases from cephalad to caudad. In the lower cervical region, the C6–C7 disc is overlain by the emerging C7 root and also by the C8 segment of the cord. The cord segment giving rise to the C7 root lies higher, at the C5–C6 level. Thus, an encroachment that is strategically situated may affect not only the emerging root but also the gray matter and other intramedullary systems of the next lower segment, producing a picture of multilevel herniation or spondylotic encroachment when such is not the case. The emerging spinal nerves are directed not only laterally but also ventrally and caudally. Because of this position, they are held snugly against the underlying disc and inferior pedicle. The articulations posterior to the root in normally large foramina and lateral to the cord in a normally deep canal probably contribute little to holding the roots or the cord against ventral excrescences.

All intraspinal epidural blood vessels are veins in which the pressure is low. This fact explains the ease with which hemorrhage from them is controlled. Outside the foramen, the vertebral artery lies ventral to the dorsal root ganglion and the spinal nerve. From C6 upward, the artery threads the beads of the foramina transversaria. The anterior tubercle of the transverse process of C7 cannot be palpated, since it is far posterior and is overlain by the vertebral artery. The tubercle of Chassaignac, the anterior tubercle of the transverse process of the C6 vertebra, is the lowest one that can be palpated. It is a reliable guide to identification of the cervical interspace via the anterior approach. Occasionally, the vertebral artery enters its lower transverse process at a level higher than C6. In this circumstance, radiographic identification of the anterior interspace is desirable. Only the anterior and lateral operative approaches bring the operative procedure near the vertebral artery.

The blood supply to the cervical spinal cord comes from the downward coursing anterior spinal artery. This artery is derived from the vertebral arteries and a few arteries that accompany nerve roots within their dural sleeves.[107,108] None of these arteries is seen in any extradural decompressive procedure. The arterial supply to the cord is highly irregular axially and is asymmetrical. Usually, only one or two radicular arteries augment the supply of blood descending in the anterior spinal artery. A three dimensional network of longitudinal, circumferential, and penetrating arteries on and within the cord distributes the arterial blood to the cord segments. The gray matter receives a much richer circulation than does the white. Should the predominant source of supply to one or more segments become inadequate, supplementation via anastomoses within the distribution network becomes critical.[53]

Interruption of flow in the radicular arteries is important for the segments they supply primarily or through the anastomotic network. Little is known about the effects of aging, genetic inheritance, root compression by disc disease, or intraradicular fibrosis on flow in the radicular arteries and veins. Nevertheless, there is a growing belief that impaired circulation to the spinal cord due to such factors plays a part, perhaps as great as or greater than that of direct neuronal compression, in causing myelopathy.[39,53,59] Mechanical effects such as flattening and other deformations of the cord and roots can be demonstrated and roughly quantitated in myelograms and on direct inspection at operation. However, a method for appraising the adequacy of the circulation of the cord is not available for clinical application. When a safe reliable method does become available, spontaneous intraoperative and postoperative myelopathies of unknown causation probably will yield some of their mystery and grief.

RADICULOPATHY

Although the explanation that "a nerve is pinched" is acceptable to most patients, the intimate pathophysiology of production of pain, paresthesias, and motor and sensory deficits is not completely understood. As a rule, compression of a nerve root produces pain that is proximal in the dermatome and paresthesias that are distal. The sensory and motor deficits usually are in proportion. Sometimes, for reasons that remain obscure, a differential vulnerability among the sensory and motor components of the root is manifested. There may be pure motor deficit without pain, paresthesias, or sensory loss. Conversely, there may be severe pain, paresthesias, and sensory deficits unaccompanied by paresis or other motor system deficit. Examples of the former are seen in those patients who have either trivial or no cervical or arm pains but who have progressive weakness and atrophy. So widely known is amyotrophic lateral sclerosis and the fate that befell Lou Gehrig that such patients are quickly subjected to elaborate diagnostic study including muscle biopsy. Clues that are helpful in recognizing the motor radiculopathy are its unilaterality or extreme asymmetry and the absence or paucity of fasciculations, muscles innervated by the cranial nerves remaining normal and pathological electromyographic activity being limited to the weak and atrophic muscles. Confirmation lies in appropriate radiographic examination of the cervical spine.

An unfavorable evolution that may seem to be favorable sometimes occurs in the symptoms following severe cervical root compression by a herniated disc. Initially there may be severe pain proximally, paresthesias distally, and appropriate motor and reflex deficits. Under conservative treatment, the pain may begin to abate, leading both the patient and the physician to believe that the treatment has been effective and recovery is under way. This is not necessarily the case. A nerve root subjected to compression of sufficient severity will transmit pain for a time, but eventually its function will be abolished. In this situation, the pain ceases but without a corresponding improvement in sensory and motor deficits. Whenever paresthesias and sensory and motor deficits are either not improving or worsening, lessening of pain is an indication for myelography. The myelogram will help to determine whether the nerve root compression is trivial or no longer exists or there is need for operative relief. If such a situation occurs at the C4–

C5 level affecting the C5 root, the rather early disappearance of pain with persistent or increasing atrophy and paresis of the supraspinatus and infraspinatus and deltoid muscles may lead to confusion with Spillane's neuritis.[58,94]

The recent literature contains highly divergent and seemingly irreconcilable opinions concerning the value of myelography in the diagnosis of root lesions produced by discs and spurs.[34,44,69] Some authorities believe that myelography is not only unnecessary but unreliable, especially in the differentiation between C5 root compression and brachial neuritis. Others maintain that it is nearly always or invariably diagnostic. It appears safe to state that the overwhelming majority of neurosurgeons in the United States find Pantopaque myelography invaluable in the management of disc and spondylosis problems. Currently European and some American neurosurgeons extoll the use of metrizamide, a water-soluble contrast agent. They claim that it not only improves definition of pathological changes but also has less potential for causing arachnoiditis. That Pantopaque is toxic to humans and is likely to produce arachnoiditis is not unequivocally established. Almost all patients with arachnoiditis develop it in the lumbar region where they have preexisting disease or where they have had one or more operations, perhaps attended by inadvertent opening of the dura and unusual bleeding. The author does not believe that lumbar arachnoiditis is seen as a consequence of Pantopaque myelography undertaken for cervical disc disease when the lumbar region is normal.

Whether or not radiculopathy produced by disc herniation has the same manifestations as that produced by spondylotic spurs is disputed.[69] Some surgeons find that osteophytes rarely produce classic findings of radiculopathy unless a small herniated disc fragment is present. Other equally experienced surgeons appreciate little difference between disc herniation and spondylotic compression of a root except that spondylotic spurs occur more frequently and have a more innocent-seeming onset and a chronic course.[34,44] Also, the spurs usually can be identified in plain x-rays. In 90 per cent of the cases there is no history of initiating injury.[69] Further, there is general agreement that root compression and irritations due to impingement by disc prominences rarely result from hyperextension ("whiplash") injury.

Differential vulnerability of the various ascending and descending white fiber tracts of the spinal cord is one of the hallmarks of myelopathy. The corticospinal tracts are especially vulnerable, and spastic paraparesis is the single most frequent mode of expression of myelopathy. If this type of disability continues for a long time and is unaccompanied by other deficits, the diagnosis of primary lateral sclerosis may be made. In many patients, the corticospinal tract abnormality is accompanied by impairment of dorsal column function or of the anterolateral quadrants, producing combined system disease or the Brown-Séquard type of dissociated sensory loss.

An interesting group of patients with myelopathy are those who recognize their illness by inability to feel pain or temperature differences on one side of the body. An example is the patient who was only mildly concerned about deterioration in his handball game due to increasing fatigue of his legs until one morning in the shower he found that he could not feel the warmth of the water as well with one leg as with the other. Another patient who gave no clear history of any motor impairments came to medical attention after he had stumbled over a fork-lift truck loaded with pipe. Twenty minutes later, he discovered himself to be bleeding from a laceration from which he had no pain. The reasons for such variability of manifestation are not known but may be variations in intimate circulatory arrangements within the cord and slight differences in geometric configuration of the stenotic canal.

A severe single motion segment arthrosis in a shallow canal usually is manifested by a combination of gray and white matter malfunction. An example is the accompaniment of weak and spastic legs by weakness of triceps and pectoralis muscles, loss of triceps reflex, normally active finger flexor reflexes, and finger flexor clonus. Clearly, such a patient has myelopathy of both white and gray substances at the C7 cord segment occupying the C5–C6 motion segment of the spine. Incorrect identifications of level due to pre- or postfixation of the plexus should not occur. Rarely the gray matter lesion may be strongly expressed by

weakness, flaccidity, fasciculation, and reflex loss while long-tract signs are minimal. Primary muscular atrophy or amyotrophic lateral sclerosis may be diagnosed when the motor fibers are differentially injured in radiculopathy.[56] In all instances of myelopathy or radiculopathy, the possibility of spondylosis in a shallow canal should be actively entertained and a search made for the confirming shallowness and motion segment arthrosis.

Clinical Diagnosis of Radiculopathy

With the exception of the first cervical root, which usually has no sensory component, and the C2 root, which has no disc ventral to it, all the cervical roots are susceptible to encroachment by spondylosis and herniation of the disc. In a series of 684 patients there were no instances of C3 or C4 involvement.[69] Frequencies of involvement by a ruptured cervical disc at lower levels were C5, 26; C6, 171; C7, 393; C8, 50; and T1, 4. In only four instances were the disc ruptures multiple, thus casting doubt on the frequently heard assertion that a patient had two or even three or four ruptured discs. Spondylotic compression of roots is two or three times as frequent as compression by a ruptured disc. Moreover, it is frequently present at more than one site. The distribution of spondylotic compression is probably about the same as for disc rupture, with compressions of the C6 and C7 root accounting for the great majority of the occurrences.

The *C2 root* has a large sensory component distributed to the dermatome bordering the trigeminal skin field rostrally and running from near the vertex through the external auditory canal across the angle of the mandible to just beneath the chin. Its caudal border with the C3 dermatome is indistinct at the high collar level. Its motor fibers supply nuchal and strap muscles. There is no disc at an appropriate level to impinge on the C2 root. Yet, it and the greater occipital nerve have been targets of many operations seeking to relieve "occipital neuralgia" in patients with ill-defined post-traumatic and tension headache syndromes. Many of these operations probably were not indicated. There is, how-

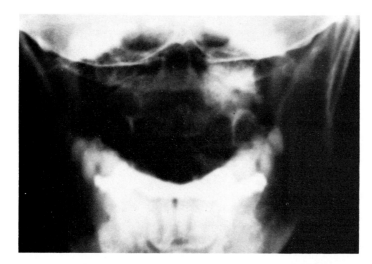

Figure 80–16 Open mouth view of severe and painful arthrosis of the atlantoaxial articulation on the right. The myelogram is normal in this condition.

ever, one easily recognized and operatively treatable condition at the C1–C2 motion segment that has received little notice (Fig. 80–16). Sufferers from unilateral painful arthrosis of the atlantoaxial joint have ipsilateral suboccipital pain with point tenderness over the area of abnormality and marked limitation of neck motion. If typical findings of atlantoaxial arthrosis are seen in an open mouth radiograph, temporary relief may be given by deposition of 5 ml of 0.5 per cent lidocaine lateral to and on the posterior aspect of this joint. Since this articulation is supplied by an articular twig of the sensory root of C2, lateral rhizolysis or intradural C2 rhizotomy will give relief. Because of overlap from bordering dermatomes, dorsal rhizotomy of C2 produces only a small area of sensory loss that is well tolerated in most instances.

The *C3* and *C4 roots* pass respectively through the C2–C3 and C3–C4 motion segments. The joints of these motion segments may be affected by arthrosis. If C4 is the affected root, there will be pain along one side of the neck running to the point of the shoulder. Though the C3 and C4 roots contribute motor fibers to the diaphragm, nuchal, and strap muscles, single root lesions cause no detectable loss of function. In certain instances, a root may be squeezed in an intervertebral foramen that is occluded by disc disease or by arthrotic spurring of the posterior articulation (Fig. 80–17). In either case, the myelogram may be negative or uninformative. In other instances, a disc herniation or spur ventral to the C4 root will be well displayed in myelograms (Fig.

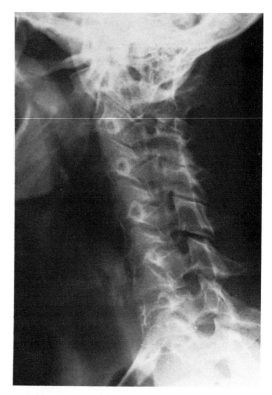

Figure 80–17 Oblique view of the cervical spine of a patient suffering from C4 radiculopathy due to arthrotic occlusion of the C3–C4 intervertebral foramen by spurs from the disc ventrally and arthrotic enlargement of the posterior articulation as well. The myelogram was normal.

80–18). A lesion of this sort is to be suspected whenever a patient places his hand along the side of his neck, moving it out toward the point of the shoulder, to indicate the site of pain that is aggravated by neck

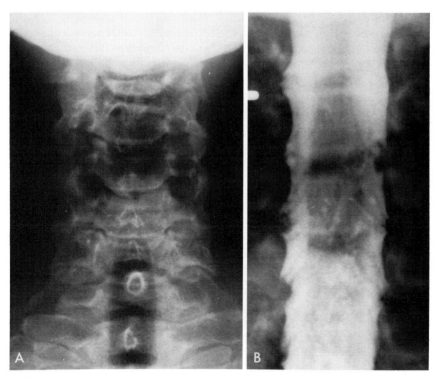

Figure 80–18 *A*. Uncovertebral process spurs on the right at C3–C4 foramen. The right side of the patient is on the left in this view. *B*. Anteroposterior myelogram showing right C4 root compression by intraforaminal arthrotic spurs.

motion but does not go down into the area of the deltoid or lower arm nor into the upper interscapular or rhomboid region.

Cervical roots 5, 6, 7, and 8 and the first thoracic root supply the arm and hand via the anterior primary divisions of the spinal nerves and the brachial plexus. The paraspinal muscles are innervated by the posterior primary divisions of the spinal nerves. Compression or other irritation of any of the lower cervical roots produces almost identical pain in the base of the neck, posterior scapular region, and shoulder. The precise level of involvement cannot be determined by distribution of the proximal pain, tenderness of muscles, limitation of neck motion, or abnormal neck posture. A lesion affecting the C6 root is more likely to cause pectoral pain simulating that of angina pectoris, but this pain is not a reliable localizing feature. Paresthesias and numbness usually accompany severe root compression and are appreciated distally in the dermatome. Rarely will a patient with index and adjacent finger paresthesias also complain of any similar feelings above the elbow.

An accurate description of the distribution of paresthesias and numbness usually is of help in determining which root is affected, but muscle power and reflex deficits are more accurate indicators. Nevertheless, if the index finger is predominantly affected, other evidence can be expected to confirm the suspicion that C7 is at fault.

A *C5 root* lesion causes paresis of the supraspinatus and infraspinatus muscles, the deltoid muscles, and one or more of the flexor muscles of the elbow. Also there is diminution of the biceps reflex, and pain and possibly mild paresthesias over the deltoid muscles.

Rarely is numbness and tingling complained of with a C5 root lesion. Presumably this lack of paresthesia is because the dermatome has no distal extension to the forearm or hand. The biceps and brachialis muscles are difficult to examine separately. Palpation of the biceps belly or its tendon may show the affected side to be weaker. Palpation of the muscle belly during an attempt to pull the flexed elbow straight is the best test of brachioradialis function. An important point in differentiating C5 root compression from paralytic brachial neuritis lies in examination of the elbow flexors. In the latter condition, the biceps, brachialis, and brachioradialis are not weakened.

Compression of the *C6 root* gives rise to paresis of all three muscle groups that flex the elbow and the extensor carpi radialis. There is diminution or absence of the biceps and brachioradialis reflexes. Paresthesias are felt in the thumb and index finger and may extend a short way up the radial forearm. The most distal distribution of pain from a C6 root usually is in the anterior aspect of the upper arm down to the antecubital fossa.

The *C7 root* deficit includes paresis of the triceps, latissimus dorsi, pectoralis major, and wrist and finger extensor muscles, and diminished triceps and pectoralis reflexes. Paresthesias are most intense in the index and middle fingers. They may be felt in the thumb also. The pain extends down the back of the upper arm and a short way into the forearm. The reliability of latissimus dorsi and pectoralis major muscle weakness as an indication of C7 root involvement and the tests for these muscles are not widely appreciated. The latissimus is a powerful accessory muscle of respiration. If the examiner stands behind the patient, grasps the bellies of these muscles in each hand, and asks the patient to cough, strong symmetrical contractions will be felt. If the muscle is weakened on one side, the contractions will be unequal. The pectoralis major is a strong adductor of the humerus, whether projected dependently or forward. This muscle may be tested by inspection and palpation of its belly under the anterior axillary fold while the patient presses his palms against his trochanters or one palm against the other while the arms are extended forward. A more elegant test is to employ the principle underlying Froment's sign for weakness of the adductor pollicis muscle. The test works because the pectoralis major functions on the humerus just as the adductor pollicis does on the metacarpal of the thumb. If the pectoralis major muscle is weak, the flexors of the elbow, acting in the same way as the flexors of the terminal phalanx of the thumb, will produce elbow flexion. The test for pectoralis major strength is made by having the patient hold a book between his palms with elbows extended while the examiner tries to pull the book from between the palms (Fig. 80–19). If the pectoralis muscle is weak, the elbow on that side will flex in compensation.

Nonfunction of the *C8 root* causes weakness of the triceps, the extensor carpi ulnaris, wrist and finger flexors, and intrinsic hand muscles. The triceps and finger flexor reflexes will be reduced. Froment's sign for weakness of the adductor pollicis will be positive.

The *T1 root* lesion produces weakness of intrinsic hand muscles and one or more components of the Horner's syndrome. It is unusual for this root to be compressed.

Neurological Examination Versus "Tests"

Refinement and precision in history taking and neurological examination have not been made superfluous by myelography, electromyography, discography, polytomography, and other ancillary diagnostic methods. Unsuitable operations and unsatisfactory results are the inevitable consequences of a surgeon's ignorance of or lack of appreciation of the value of clinical neurological examination. An illustration is the problem presented by the patient who had neck and arm pain of sudden onset that was aggravated by neck extension. He also had ill-defined paresthesias and weakness of several muscle groups due, in part, to inhibition by pain and slight asymmetry of reflexes. He had C5–C6 interspace narrowing and intraforaminal spurs of modest dimension. Electromyography gave minimal indication of abnormality that was not clearly attributable to one root. The physician's options were to advise traction and other conservative modalities in the belief that the condition was sufficiently understood, to recommend myelography seeking additional information about the condition of the root over the C5–C6 spurs, and to recommend discography as a preliminary to anterior interbody fusion at one or more levels. The answer came in tests for pectoralis major and latissimus dorsi paresis that require no conscious effort by the patient to cause the muscles to contract with equal strength and little liability to weakness due to inhibition by pain. This test told the examiner that it was the C7 rather than the C6 root that was causing the difficulty. Further, the lesion was likely to be a disc

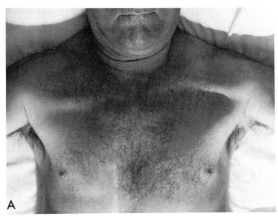 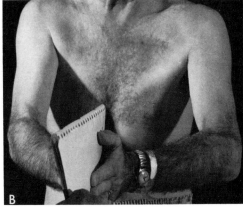

Figure 80–19 *A*. Pectoralis muscle atrophy and weakness due to C7 root compression is visible on inspection. *B*. The "book test" for pectoralis muscle weakness. Note that the left humerus is not maintained in adduction and that involuntary elbow flexion is attempting to compensate.

rupture at a radiographically normal interspace. The surgeon knows that if he is to relieve this patient, he must find free cartilaginous fragments underlying the C7 root regardless of what myelography or discography reveals at C5–C6 (see Fig. 80–8).

SPONDYLOTIC MYELOPATHY

The modes of clinical expression of myelopathy have been discussed, but certain features of therapeutic importance deserve special attention. Patients who develop this disorder do not acquire it full blown. They begin with mild manifestations that may not be given sufficient attention by the patient or the physician. The symptoms develop at a variable rate that may be rapid or quite slow. Gradually the patient descends to a level of moderate disability and often, perhaps as a result of mild hyperextension injury or just the passage of time, becomes severely disabled.

Early in the course the patient has only mild impairments, and the changes in his spinal cord are reversible. Patients in this mild category are those who complain of weakness, slowness, or undue fatigue of the legs on fast walking, stair climbing, or running on sand or in shallow water. They may have mild paresthesias or electricity-like body tingling on neck motion, but they are free of any motor, reflex, or sensory deficits on examination. Such patients will gain the most benefit from a proper opera-

tion. A return to normal or nearly normal can be expected.

The examiner must be cognizant of the fact that the tests he employs in clinical examination in a relatively small room, where the patient walks back and forth and hops and walks on heels without difficulty, are not as sensitive as the patient's own appreciation of impairments in the course of daily living. A patient who complains of leg weakness but has none detectable by the examiner should not be regarded as hypochondriacal. Rather, because of the frequency of spondylotic myelopathy, the cervical spine should be radiographically examined even if it is entirely comfortable and pain-free. By the time the patient has become severely affected with paraparesis, scissoring gait, and obvious sensory losses, the time has passed for decompression or any type of operation to promise great improvement, though stabilization of the condition and prevention of further worsening may be rewarding.

In view of the underlying mechanical causation and pathologic changes, it is surprising that Lhermitte's phenomenon, the production of electric-like shocks in the lower body by neck flexion or extension, is not seen more often in cervical spondylotic myelopathy. Physical deformation of the cord produced by disc bulging and yellow ligament infolding in extension, and a taut posterior dura bearing down upon the cord in flexion have already been described. Each of these mechanisms is at work in the production of myelopathy. Occasionally a patient is seen who has only Lhermitte's phenomenon as a symptom of his myelopathy. This type of patient experiences body shocks every time he puts his chin on his chest and also when stepping down heavily from a curb. If the patient has a spinal canal of generous size with no hint of arthrosis, a ventral midline meningioma should be suspected. An exception is the patient in a younger age group in whom multiple sclerosis is a reasonable possibility.

Another feature of myelopathy deserving comment is the infrequency with which micturition is affected and its unfavorable prognostic indications.[42] In contrast, urinary retention is one of the early manifestations of spinal cord compression by metastatic epidural tumor.

OTHER HEAD AND NECK SYNDROMES

Some patients with one or more levels of arthrosis in a shallow canal will not have the usual clear-cut evidence of myelopathy or radiculopathy. Instead they may have neck and suboccipital pain that extends as far forward as the eyes. Often, the pain is related to extension or other activity of the neck. Possible explanations are that pain is referred from the arthrotic processes or that there is irritation of the dura or other meninges or of the dorsal root filaments as they arise from the back of the cord. Another mechanism may incorporate nuchal muscle spasm based on a pain referral circuit involving afferent input through the cervical roots, the descending trigeminal tract, and the sensory innervation of intracranial dura.

Representative of this problem was a middle-aged woman with suboccipital neck and arm pains, but minimal evidence of motor impairments attributable to radiculopathy or myelopathy. Myelography revealed significant broadening of the cord at the C4–C5 and C5–C6 levels. Neck extension produced a block at the C5–C6 level. Laminectomy of C6, C5, and the lower edge of C4, together with thorough removal of intervening yellow ligaments, produced relief of the arm discomfort and some improvement in neck and head pain. Although she remained neurologically normal, the pain worsened over several years. Repeat myelography revealed a normal appearance at the C5–C6 motion segment. There was ventral displacement of the cord shadow against the anterior dura (Fig. 80–20). The intervening yellow ligaments and the sensory rootlets were unusually prominent on the back of the cord beneath the unremoved laminae of C4, C3, and C2. Clearly this patient had had an insufficient first laminectomy. After the remaining laminae and yellow ligaments were removed, all her head and neck complaints disappeared.

TREATMENT OF CERVICAL PAIN SYNDROMES

General Considerations

Treatment should not be based on oversimplified concepts of the disease process since the problem may be complex. There are three articulations at each motion seg-

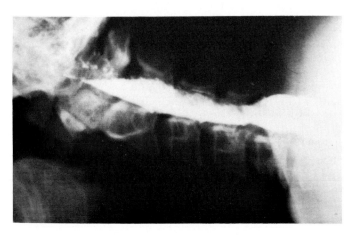

Figure 80–20 Lateral myelogram of a patient performed several years after laminectomy of C6, C5, and the lower edge of C4. Pains in the arms were relieved by the operation, but pain the the upper neck extending into the head continued and gradually became worse. The unremoved laminae at C4, C3, and C2 with the intervening yellow ligaments are pressing the cord ventrally against the anterior dura. There may be irritation of the posterior root filaments, which are prominent. Extension of the laminectomy upward to include the rest of C4 together with C3 and C2 relieved all the head and neck complaints.

ment and six motion segments between the C2 and T1 centra, a total of 18 joints to evaluate by tests that are quite fallible.

Fusion of a motion segment that is abnormal on x-ray and thought to be responsible for pain may have no effect. A joint that is normal by all tests usually employed may be the source of the pain. Fusion of a motion segment, whether painful or not, increases stresses on adjacent unfused joints and accelerates arthrosis in them. Fused spines with shallow canals or foramina may develop clinically significant disease at new levels. The treatment of cervical segment abnormalities can not be sterotyped to use of one technique only, whether it be posterior fusion, posterior decompression, or one of the anterior or lateral approaches with or without interbody fusion. The type of disease process, the characteristics of the spine in which it is occurring, its course and manifestations all must be taken into account to choose the most appropriate treatment.

Simple situations do exist. An example is a detached cartilaginous fragment that suddenly causes disability accompanied by clear clinical and myelographic evidence. Its extraction by any method gives relief. Many radicular pains are more complex, however, and nearly all cases of myelopathy are more complex. Also, all cases of head and neck pain accompanied by arthrosis, but without clinical evidence of cord or root compression or myelographic abnormality, are more complex. Most clinical situations feature important but unquantifiable factors that are critically important in determining the treatment and prognosis. For example, a myelopathic patient with paresis, spasticity, and sensory loss is unlikely to become completely normal regardless of the treatment. The prognosis is poor because the spinal cord has undergone irreversible pathological changes. The pathological process is poorly understood. ''Pressure'' on the cord may be relieved, and its accommodations made more spacious and comfortable, but the myelopathy may remain unchanged. Usually it ceases to worsen.

The indications for operation must take into account the patient's employment and social situation, his expectations, and his understanding of the problem as well as its straightforward medical features. Illustrative of patients at one end of the spectrum

is a 35-year-old spacecraft pilot preparing for a voyage to the moon. Three days prior to being seen he noticed his right leg to be less sensitive than the left in perception of warmth while showering. He also remembered that his legs had been less quick and more easily fatigued during handball for the past two or three months. All motor function was normal. Reflexes were normal. There was reduced ability to distinguish between warm and cold objects below D8 on the right and greater tolerance of strong Achilles tendon squeeze on the right. Cervical spine x-rays revealed the canal to be 20 per cent shallower than normal and the C6–C7 motion segment to be arthrotic. Spondylotic myelopathy was strongly suggested by this combination of findings. Myelography confirmed the diagnosis and operative treatment was accepted.

Exemplifying an opposite situation is a 64-year-old banker nearing retirement. He had not played golf for several years because nine holes fatigued his legs too much and he enjoyed gardening just as much. There had been no further deterioration in his leg function for at least two years. He gave a history of heavy smoking and emphysema. On testing, he performed well on his feet. The leg reflexes were brisk with unsustained clonus. Perception of vibration was diminished. There was moderate adductor pollicis atrophy. X-rays revealed shallowness of the spinal canal with multiple-level arthrosis. By history his myelopathy was stationary. The examination suggested that it was mild to moderate in severity. Neither myelography nor discussion of an operation was in order. An operation to halt the advance of something already halted could hardly be proposed even if it entailed no risk. Since he was vulnerable to traumatic cervical hyperextension that could produce hematomyelia, posterior decompression might be offered as prophylaxis. It was necessary to reassure him that he did not have amyotrophic lateral sclerosis. Further, it was prudent to arrange for electromyography to back up the opinion that amyotrophic lateral sclerosis was not the diagnosis.

Conservative Treatment

The patient's expectations of treatment, the settings in which he works, his functions in society, the system of medical care under which he is being treated, geographic latitude, and political philosophy all influence the choice of therapy. It may be acceptable to treat a northern European with myelopathy or radiculopathy by having him wear a collar, cast, or brace 24 hours a day. Several factors are pertinent to this choice of treatment. The climate is cool and less frequent bathing may be acceptable. The state will support the patient while he is incapacitated for work. Further, the medical profession is traditionally more conservative in managing conditions that do not threaten life. In contrast, in the United States, more aggressive treatment is likely to be chosen. This is especially true if the patient resides in a warm and humid region where a collar or brace would be uncomfortable. The patient would be impatient to return to work. His pay for work would be much more than the compensation he would receive while he was ill. Through payroll deductions or fringe benefits, the operative procedure that could put him back to work with the least delay has already been paid for. This patient is more likely to have an operation recommended to him and is likely to accept it. He is unlikely to accept weeks or months of nonoperative treatment willingly if he realizes that its outcome is unpredictable and it may not produce the result he desires. Thus, under one set of circumstances an operation that promises quick relief is considered desirable and even necessary; in other circumstances, it may be viewed as unnecessary.

Conservative treatment modalities for acute disc problems are numerous. The author's preference is for head halter traction in the recumbent position. Five to eight pounds of weight is attached over a pulley placed 8 to 12 inches above the plane of the surface on which the head rests. This position will produce a minor vector of neck flexion. If the use of traction during alternate two hours while the patient is awake fails to reduce pain within 24 to 48 hours, there is little reason for its further use. Manual traction for a few moments by the examiner gives a good clue to whether traction will be worthwhile and how it will be tolerated by the patient. Some authorities see little logic in the use of traction and find it to be ineffective.[69]

The use of deep heat generated by short-wave electromagnetic or sonic energy for 15 to 30 minutes twice daily appears to be superior to infrared lamps and heating pads. Immersion in warm water for similar periods is quite useful also. The warm water has the advantage of being almost universally available and inexpensive. Combinations of aspirin and its compounds with 30 mg codeine added and diazepam (Valium), methocarbamol (Robaxin), or carisoprodol (Soma) are usually adequate to deal with the pain. Exceptions are found in the patient who is hyperemotional or has a truly acute radicular compression that merits immediate operative relief. Not infrequently patients depreciate the analgesic effects of agents requiring prescriptions and prefer alcohol. Some physicians and many patients have faith in exercises. Since the development of myelopathy and possibly of radiculopathy are dependent on motion, however, it is difficult to understand how increasing such motion may be beneficial. Furthermore, nothing known about pain, paresthesias, weakness, or other accompaniments of radiculopathy suggests that weak or toneless muscles bear primary responsibility. Exercise of muscles weakened by denervation will not reverse the primary disease even though motor units that remain functional may be made hypertrophic. Rest and avoidance of the activity that initiates pain and paresthesias combined with antispasmodic and pain-relieving medication and deep heat appear to be more rational treatments. If the patient has severe pain, significant paresis, or increasing sensory loss, it is inappropriate to insist that conservative measures be used for any specific number of days or weeks. When conservative treatment is not giving some improvement in the first four to seven days, it probably will not help. As stated earlier, conservative treatment should be questioned for those patients whose pain diminishes while motor deficits and sensory losses remain unchanged or worsen. Such changes suggest that the root is compromised to such a degree that pain transmission is no longer possible.

The genesis and progression of myelopathy requires: (1) a shallow canal; (2) static (arthrotic) encroachment; (3) dynamic invasions of the canal by discs, ligaments, or retrolisthesis; and probably, (4) marginal circulatory inadequacy. None but the dynamic encroachments appear to be modified by nonoperative treatment. Wearing a collar for 24 hours a day and other forms of external immobilization favorably influence myelopathy and radiculopathy by halting the dynamic effects.[17] The wearing of a collar for myelopathy, however, is infrequently advocated by physicians and poorly accepted by patients.

Operative Treatment

Static and dynamic factors that combine to affect the cervical neural elements unfavorably may be excised, negated, or modified by a large number of procedures. These procedures include laminectomy and yellow ligament removal, sometimes combined with section of denticulate ligaments; removal of herniated disc masses by the posterior route; foraminotomy for decompression of roots; posterior fusion; and disc or spur removal by anterior or lateral approaches with or without interbody fusion. Particular procedures have certain advantages and disadvantages, depending on the result that needs to be obtained. No one procedure is best for all radiculopathies and myelopathies.

Anesthesia

In the opinion of most surgeons, general anesthesia with intubation is preferable, but some prefer local anesthesia.[69,93] With the patient awake, most surgeons cannot accomplish the procedure quickly enough not to feel hurried by the patient's indications of discomfort. Also, the awake patient is likely to misinterpret any teaching discussion or to view it as prolonging his ordeal. Blood should be needed infrequently for cervical laminectomy, foraminotomy, or disc removal. Nevertheless, the expense of having one or two units cross-matched is justified if the surgeon is concerned that blood loss may exceed 200 to 500 ml.

Position of the Patient

For a posterior approach to a cervical operation, the sitting or prone position of the patient should be chosen by what is safest for the patient rather than what is convenient for the surgeon. A surgeon should not, without understanding the other factors involved, use the sitting position simply because there may be less blood loss.

Negative venous pressure is a poor substitute for accurate hemostasis aided by sharp dissection of muscle attachments from spinous processes and laminae.

If the sitting position is preferable because of reduced ventilatory capacity or obesity, a number of precautions are in order. Care must be taken to maintain the neck in neutral position. It must not be allowed or caused to be flexed strongly. As noted earlier, excess flexion tenses the posterior dura and the root sleeves, reducing their slackness and mobility, causing difficulty with the exposure of the disc ventral to them. Even worse is the ischemia of the cord produced when the tight straplike posterior dura presses it down upon a ventral ridge or the anterior wall of the canal.[2] Flexion may be made so extreme in the sitting position that midline opening of the dura causes the dural edges to slip ventrally on either side of the cord. The cord appears to herniate through the dural opening as though propelled by an immense pathological process ventral to it. An ischemic cord, pressed upon by the posterior dura, or one that has herniated through the dural opening, is in danger of infarction, and restoration of the neck to neutral position should be made without delay (see Fig. 80–13).

Air embolism has long been recognized as a special hazard of the upright position. It may occur in the prone position as well, but with far less frequency than in the upright position.[61] It occurs more frequently during intracranial than during cervical spinal operations. A report from the Mayo Clinic indicates that 7 of 29 patients undergoing cervical laminectomy in the upright position had 10 episodes of air embolism.[63] Other investigators detected intracardiac air in 26 per cent of 200 operations performed in the sitting position.[60] Formerly, treatment of air embolism was to force the wound edges together hurriedly, flood the wound with saline, straighten the table, and turn the patient onto the left side so the heart could clear itself of air and regain its efficiency as a pump. Many neurosurgeons who have had an encounter with clinical air embolism when the upright position was used have decided to have the patient face down or in the lateral recumbent position whenever possible, in the belief that avoidance of the problem is more sensible than treatment of incipient catastrophe. Other surgeons appear to believe that air embolism is a vastly overrated risk of the upright position because they have never encountered or at least never recognized it. Most episodes of air embolism go undetected unless sensitive monitoring methods are employed. Hypotension, the commonest clinical manifestation of air embolism, often is attributed to postural or other benign causes.[60,63,64]

The sitting position should not be avoided in all circumstances; there are definite indications for its use. When it is used, multimodal monitoring and provision for immediate aspiration of air from the heart should also be used. It is not acceptable, after positioning a patient in an upright position and raising the feet to head level, to simply monitor the heart by electrocardiography and auscultation and intermittently check the blood pressure by sphygmomanometry. Additional discussion of the diagnosis and treatment of air embolism is given in Chapter 30.

In the upright position, little of the head's own weight is borne by the forehead or malar eminences. When the face-down position is used, great care must be exercised to prevent loading on the globe of the eye. Blindness has resulted from lack of attention to this detail. Also care must be taken to prevent pressure on a too-small area of skin, lest necrosis develop in the forehead, bridge of the nose, or malar eminence. The headrest that features three sharp pins that engage the skull obviates these risks, but a well-padded, old-fashioned horseshoe may be safely used provided attention is devoted to details. The entire forehead must rest upon the toe of the horseshoe, while the malar eminences make only slight contact with the heels. The eyes should be closed and should not come in contact with anything. Before the head is positioned, the patient's body must be fixed by a footboard and an oblique strap supporting the buttocks to prevent movement in a caudal direction. Caudal movement of a few centimeters can bring the orbits over the heels of the horseshoe and cause blinding pressure on the globes. The never-to-be-violated rule is: Position the body and make it fast *before* making the final adjustment of the headrest to the head.

The Incision

Care should be taken to insure that a laminectomy incision is straight. It should be exactly in the midline and no longer than required. To the layman, a scar is visible and permanent testimony to the surgeon's skill or lack of it. Off-center, slanting, and jagged scars proclaim haste, carelessness, or mediocre proficiency. Asymmetry of the wound area caused by a slight twist of the neck, tilting the table to one side for the operator's convenience, or asymmetrical tension on the towels or drapes may distort the midline. The true midline should be marked prior to making the incision. Pens made for this purpose are barely adequate and do not leave enough color at crosshatches to aid in closure. Gentian violet on a splintered applicator stick used as a pen is better. A light scratch made with an inverted scalpel tip is suitable only for those surgeons whose first stroke will be correct, since superficial scars may remain to mark misguided efforts. It is better to depend on skin wrinkles to match the sides of the incision at closure, since scratch marks may remain visible. No pressure for hemostasis or skin stabilization should be used on either side of the line to be incised, for distortion will result. The incision is best made perfectly straight and on the predetermined line by putting the skin under tension along the line proposed.

Laminectomy and Flavectomy for Myelopathy

Posterior decompression for myelopathy has several important advantages: (1) Spondylosis in a shallow canal is often a multilevel process in which two, three, or more motion segments are affected. Decompressing two or more levels by the posterior approach requires little more time for the surgeon or trouble for the patient than treating a single level. (2) Posterior decompression increases the space available to the spinal cord. (3) The procedure does not stiffen the motion segments that are treated and therefore does not accelerate spondylotic degeneration at adjacent levels. Disadvantages are said to be greater postoperative discomfort than accompanies operations from the anterior approach and the need for more skill. The face-down position requires attention to hemostatic detail, and the penalties for mediocre performance are more severe than those that occur with the sitting position or the anterior approach. When all sources of patient discomfort are taken into account, decompressive laminectomy, which requires only one wound, may be less disagreeable than operations that entail a donor site wound and the wearing of a collar or brace postoperatively. Dexamethasone is highly effective in diminishing postoperative laminectomy wound pain. Most patients who have posterior operations are able to go to the toilet the first postoperative evening and begin sitting and walking the next day. They do not require braces and should be able to leave the hospital in seven to nine days.

Accurate clinical and myelographic determination of the interspace responsible for the patient's disorder may not be translated into a good result unless the surgeon knows how to find his target. Occasionally the surgeon will expose the wrong interspace. No harm is done if there is prompt recognition of the error. Failure to recognize the error may result in excessive exposure with destruction of facet integrity, unneeded retraction, exploration ventral to the dura, and even intradural exploration.

The spinous process of C2 is much longer and bulkier than those of C3 and C4. It is easily recognized by palpation with a finger placed up the midline through an incision in the nuchal ligament. Since C1 has no palpable spinous process, only the occiput lies superior to the C2 spine. If attention to bifidity, relative length, and slenderness of spinous processes is not sufficient to identify the motion segment sought, a count of spinous processes from C2 should help. The C3 spinous process is so much smaller than that of C2 and may be so close beneath it that it may be missed unless the tip of each spinous process is felt to be separable from those adjacent to it by the tip and nail of the operator's index finger.

Plain spine films or myelograms taken previously always reveal identifying and distinctive features of the vertebrae in the field of interest. Careful attention to these features as seen in the wound usually will obviate the need for taking x-rays during the operation. Cervical spines 2, 3, and 4 are almost invariably bifid; C5 is usually bifid; C6 is infrequently so and usually is shorter and slenderer than C7, which most often is identical in construction to T1. The most reliable means of identifying the interspace to be operated upon is to mark a spinous process or interspinous ligament with a needle or towel clip and take a lateral radiograph.

The technique of separation of muscle from spinous processes, laminae, and pos-terior articulations accounts for most of the blood loss that may be avoided. Muscles should be separated from bone by relatively *sharp* dissection. The surgeon should deepen the dissection progressively along the length of the wound rather than diving deeply down to the laminae at certain sites, while leaving muscular attachments bridging to bone at others. A sharp Adson laminectomy chisel or a large stiff B-D No. 22 rib-back blade allows clean sharp subperiosteal separation of muscular attachments from bone. The dissection should begin with an incision in the midline through the cartilaginous cap of each spinous process down to bone. There are few vessels bridging from bone and interspinous ligament to muscle, and none cross the midline. Vessels responsible for most blood loss and air embolism are those in the muscles that are exposed, stretched, and torn by dull periosteal instruments and gauze stuffing. The subperiosteal separation should proceed in an upward direction, because the muscle attachments to spinous processes insert obliquely from below, making an acute angle with the midline as viewed from below. The cutting instrument should work into this acute angle so that the muscle insertions tend to direct the edge against the bone; working from above onto the obtuse side of the angle, the muscle attachments tend to carry the instrument out into muscle.

The cutting current delivered to a slender needle effects a relatively bloodless dissection. It, however, converts what may be kept equally bloodless by the technique first described into a superficial burn on both sides of the exposure. Such heat-divided tissues seem to heal as satisfactorily as those divided by sharp dissection. Perhaps the odor produced and the appearance of the burned surfaces are more offensive than the micropathological effects.

The number of laminae to be exposed will depend on the linear extent of the myelopathy and the surgeon's disposition toward relatively limited or relatively radical decompressions. Some surgeons advocate a radical laminectomy from T1 up through C2 in almost every instance, even in those cases in which myelopathy and myelographic abnormalities are principally at one level.[34] In support of this approach it is reasoned that the presence of myelopathy, though currently limited, heralds future extension, since a shallow canal is shallow at more than one level and spondylosis is by nature a multilevel process. Further, it is logical to treat the entire cervical spine at one operation. Certainly if the canal is generally shallow and the spondylotic defects are multiple, removal of the upper edge of C7, all of C6, C5, C4, and C3, together with all the intervening ligaments, appears to be appropriate. The canal through C2 is generally much larger than at lower levels, and in most cases there is no need for further enlargement. Except in those cases in which the C7–T1 motion segment is shown to encroach on the canal, removal of the upper half of C7, together with all of the ligament, will be adequate at the lower end of the decompression. In patients with canals of average or nearly average size with myelopathy due to spondylotic encroachments of unusual magnitude at one or two levels, the decompression may be safely confined to those levels.

The lower edge of the superior lamina overlaps the upper edge of the inferior lamina. As a result, it is necessary to begin laminectomy at the lower edge of the lowest lamina to be removed and to work upward. Bone must be removed without introducing footed rongeurs of the Kerrison type into the spinal canal. The cord is already compromised by insufficient space, and any further encroachment by an instrument will produce an acute worsening of myelopathy. The Leksell rongeur with one shallow jaw, the straight Adson rongeur, the narrow-jawed Stookey rongeur, and a small angled curet of the Lempert type are safe and sufficient to do the procedure. The small curet permits separation of the yellow ligament from the undersurface of the lamina so efficiently that a multilevel laminectomy may be accomplished without removal of yellow ligament, or in some cases, even exposure of the dura. Since the meningorachidian veins lie deep to the yellow ligaments, the operation up to this point is relatively bloodless. After the laminae have been removed, the yellow ligaments may look so delicate and innocent that it may appear appropriate to leave them in situ, thus preserving the venous drainage system intact. One patient treated in this manner experienced an early recurrence of myelopathy. At reoperation, the yellow ligaments were found to be incorporated in a dense band of fibrotic scar that had replaced the removed laminae. Perhaps yellow ligament tissue ex-

posed in this manner stimulates formation of more scar tissue than would otherwise occur. Complete flavectomy should accompany the laminectomy. The resection should go well lateral to remove all flakes and shreds of the ligament from beneath posterior articulations. Unless radiculopathy accompanies the myelopathy, foraminotomies need not be done.

Because the lamina slants downward and away from the operator, removal of the upper half of one that does not need to be totally removed may pose a problem. Temptation to use the forbidden Kerrison rongeur should be resisted. The upper half of the lamina may be thinned with an air-driven or electric burr until the cortical bone on the underside of the lamina can be removed with the Lempert curet. Another effective method is to flatten the lamina by ronguering away the upper half of the attachment of the spinous process to the midlamina into the cancellous bone. Next, the upper edge far laterally on each side may be nibbled away with the Stookey rongeur.

Bleeding from meningorachidian veins is easily controlled by accurate placement of small pea-sized fragments of Gelfoam under strips of cotton felt. Clipping of veins and cautery should not be necessary. The secrets of Gelfoam hemostasis of intraspinal veins are precise identification of the bleeding point and application of the gelfoam to this point so that pressure is exerted laterally against the pedicle rather than downward upon the root or the anterior wall of the canal. When a vein is bleeding near the dorsal midline where application of any pressure is forbidden, the vein-bearing tissue should be divided and separated from dura so that each cut end may be held laterally under Gelfoam.

In former years, intradural exploration of arachnoid adhesions and denticulate ligament division usually accompanied laminectomy for decompression.[34,48] The intradural procedures do not improve the quality of the results and are less frequently employed at this time. Opening the dura increases the hazards and should not be done routinely in the treatment of a disease whose cause is wholly extradural.

Duraplasty for Myelopathy

When a patient with myelopathy has an unusually prominent transverse spondy-

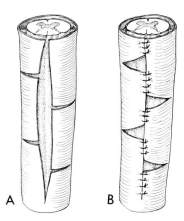

Figure 80–21 A method of simple duraplasty to lengthen the cervical spinal dura posteriorly. *A.* A vertical midline opening and two staggered side incisions to the denticulate ligament on each side have been made. The arachnoid is not opened. *B.* The midline opening is closed, leaving triangular gaps with arachnoid intact under each.

lotic ridge and Lhermitte's phenomenon on neck flexion, it may be desirable to lengthen the dura posterior to the cord. Lengthening the dura will decrease its propensity to force the cord down upon ventral ridges when the neck is flexed (see Fig. 80–13). The dural lengthening may be accomplished without employing foreign substances or making a second wound to secure fascia lata by making a long midline dural opening and two staggered lateral cuts on each side down to the level of the denticulate attachments. The lateral incisions will gape to produce triangular apertures when the dural midline is closed and will significantly lengthen the posterior dura (Fig. 80–21). The bulging arachnoid at each triangular aperture may be supported by a small patch of Gelfoam prior to closure of the muscle. If the arachnoid was opened, the dural apertures should be closed with fascial grafts or a suitable substitute.

Foraminotomy for Root Decompression or Disc Removal

Most patients have myelopathy or radiculopathy but not both. Only occasionally will one or more roots need to be exposed as an adjunct to laminectomy and flavectomy for decompression of the cord. More often a root or roots must be exposed in the foramen in the absence of any indication for laminectomy, except as the initial step in foraminotomy. In order to expose a root,

the medial side of the facet at the faulty motion segment must be removed. Total extirpation of the inferior facet of the superior vertebra will expose only the articular cartilage of the superior facet of the inferior vertebra, but not the root. It is not necessary to remove the entire inferior facet of the upper vertebra in order to gain access to the medial half of the underlying superior facet. Total facetectomies, though advocated by some surgeons, are not widely regarded as necessary or desirable, since they may contribute to instability if the disc is ruptured and the annulus is incompetent to maintain alignment.[91,92] This is unlikely if the motion segment is already spondylotic and stiffened.

A sharp burr in a hand-turned Hudson brace is favored by some surgeons for thinning the medial aspect of the posterior articulation enough to permit removal of the remainder with a small curet.[34] Other surgeons prefer a small motor-driven steel or diamond burr to remove the lower edge of the superior lamina, the medial side of the inferior facet, the medial side of the superior facet of the inferior vertebra, and the upper edge of its lamina.[92] The author's preference is to use a sharp narrow-jawed Stookey rongeur and straight and curved Lempert curets. Occasionally a small thin footed 40-degree slant-ended rongeur of the Cloward-Hooper type will prove useful. The curets cleanly separate the yellow ligament from laminal edges. Small bites with the Stookey rongeur progressively remove the edge of the superior lamina, the medial aspect of the inferior facet of the same vertebra, the upper edge of the inferior lamina, and finally the medial half of the superior facet of that vertebra. The curets, a No. 15 blade, and Love-Gruenwald forceps are used to remove the yellow ligament from the upper edge of the inferior lamina and from beneath the superior lamina. The Stookey single-action rongeur's jaws open so widely that the point of one jaw may be placed lateral to a facet while the other engages the bone to be removed from the medial side of either the inferior or superior facet. Movement of the gently closed handles away from the midline will remove bone from the medial side of the facet in a precisely controlled fashion without damaging the functional integrity of the facet (Fig. 80–22). If the spinous process is a hindrance it should be removed. No im-

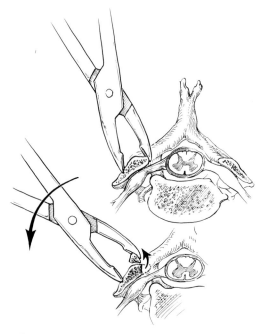

Figure 80–22 A method of employing a narrow-jawed wide-opening rongeur of the Stookey design to decompress a root in the foramen. The lateral jaw engages bone laterally on the facet and acts as a pivot. The medial jaw pulls bone up and away from the root when the lateral movement of the gently closed rongeur handle is translated into a vertical movement of the medial jaw of the rongeur.

provement in the results of foraminotomy for spur compression or removal of the ordinary ruptured disc fragment results from total laminectomy, however.

With the neck in a neutral posture, the root is closer to the inferior than to the superior pedicle. It lies in direct contact with the posterolateral aspect of the disc and is directly overlain posteriorly by the superior facet of the inferior vertebra. Regardless of the technique used, removal of the medial side of the superior facet of the inferior vertebra flush with the inner aspect of the pedicle is critical. This permits easy palpation and direct visualization of both superior and inferior pedicles and allows the probe or curved Lempert curet to pass along the root into and lateral to the foramen. This exposure affords good access for exploration ventral to the root from above or below.

During exposure of a root, the temptation to place a footed rongeur, however small, into the foramen should be resisted. Even the end of a blunt hook forced into a tight foramen may further injure the root and

possibly its accompanying radicular artery. If veins beneath the yellow ligament are opened, very small pledgets of Gelfoam should be placed and held laterally against the pedicles above and below the root.

If preoperative studies revealed an intraforaminal spur that is confirmed by palpation as a stony hard prominence, it is necessary only to make sure the path of the root out of the foramen accepts the passage of a curved Lempert curet or a ball-ended nerve hook. If the ventral prominence is soft, however, or the preoperative studies suggested the possibility of a ruptured disc, the pararadicular meningorachidian vein-bearing soft tissue must be divided by cutting it with scissors in the direction of the root while the latter is held aside by a hook. This procedure permits visualization of the underlying disc from both above and below the slack and easily mobilized root. A rotating motion with the end of a blunt hook or Adson aneurysm needle that has been manipulated toward the medial side of the soft prominence can be used to milk it or sweep it laterally to the upper or lower aspect of the root, where the edge of the free fragment may be seen and gently extracted. Three or more separate fragments should always be expected. Unless they are quite large, single fragments are infrequent. The surgeon should repeatedly sweep and press laterally and downward around the base of the soft prominence until no further fragments remain and the root is free of any mass ventral to it.

The fissure in the annulus through which the fragments came need not be searched for. Further, there need be no attempt to enter the disc to remove material from within it. Unlike ruptured lumbar discs, cervical discs do not extrude more cartilage at a later date.[34,92] The recurrence rate of cervical disc rupture at the same site has been reported to be less than 1 per cent.[69] If, at a later date, the same root is again found to be compressed by cartilaginous material, the probability is that all of the extruded fragments of the ruptured disc were not found and removed at the initial operation.

Early's Technique

The usual posterior midline incision for foraminotomy detaches the trapezius, rhomboid, and levator scapulae muscles from the spinal axis, which supports the shoulder girdle and upper appendage much as a suspension bridge supports a roadway. Regardless of the manner of closure, this wound has certain weaknesses. Five to six weeks are required for normal tensile strength to be regained so that lifting and carrying heavy loads are safe and free of risk of subcutaneous dehiscence. Early's approach to a single root does not entail division of muscle attachments or require a number of weeks' abstinence from heavy lifting.[31] He employs a muscle-splitting technique similar to McBurney's for appendectomy. The posterior articulation overlying the root to be decompressed is identified by placing a spinal needle down to it, under local anesthesia, through a cutaneous puncture 3 cm lateral to the midline. Verification of its position is made by anteroposterior and lateral radiographs. Once the needle tip is correctly placed, a small amount of indigo carmine is injected as the needle is withdrawn, producing a track of stained tissue to serve as a guide to the desired area. The skin incision along a line approximately 45 degrees from the sagittal plane is centered on the needle puncture. The muscles encountered are opened parallel with their fibers, and no muscle is detached from the nuchal ligament or a spinous process. Two self-retaining retractors placed at right angles to one another maintain exposure. The remainder of the operation is performed as described earlier. At the conclusion of the procedure, the muscles come together without need for suture. Postoperative discomfort is decreased and there is little danger of wound disruption even by immediate heavy lifting.

The Anterior Approach

The indications for, the advantages and disadvantages of, and the technique for using the anterior approach are discussed in Chapter 81.

Complications

The difficulty in knowing the complication rate may be judged by comparing the rarity of reports of serious intraoperative and postoperative spinal cord and root impairment with a report given at the American Association of Neurological Surgeons in 1976.[36] The latter report concerned complications of anterior operations. Of the surgeons who responded to a questionnaire, 132 had produced one or more permanent neurological deficits. The intraoperative complications numbered 240; the postoperative, 102. The cause of 129 myelopathies was trauma by a surgical instrument. Although the true incidence of this type of complication may be low, published reports falsely lead one to believe it to be almost nonexistent.

Wound infections, hematomas, operations at wrong interspaces, injury to the spinal cord or nerve root, and immediate and delayed quadriplegias of unknown causation occur with both anterior and posterior procedures. They are caused by misdirected bone grafts and slipped drills, chisels, curets, and rongeurs. Myelopathic patients with severely compromised cord space and mechanical deformation of the cord are at particular risk of intraoperative worsening.

When a significant postoperative impairment is recognized, it is mandatory to distinguish at the earliest possible moment between extradural compression by hematoma or other mass and cord swelling that may follow infarction or trauma. Queckenstedt's test may give guidance during the hours when myelography is not available. The cell count and total protein level may be of minimal importance if the operation entailed opening the arachnoid. Myelography should be performed at the earliest opportunity. If extradural compression exists, the wound must be opened promptly.

As mentioned earlier, laminectomy and foraminotomy done in the upright posture carry substantial risk of air embolism. Subcutaneous wound dehiscence may be a complication of posterior operations that require separation of muscles supporting the weight of the arm and shoulder girdle from the spine. Inadequate sutural repair and heavy lifting before adequate healing are responsible. The skin does not open, but the muscles pull away from the spine, causing discomfort and instability as well as an unfavorable appearance due to the depression along one side of the spinous processes. This complication should be repaired as soon as it is recognized.

Occasionally radical posterior operations in which facet integrity is destroyed will be followed by postoperative kyphosis. This complication may be due to imcompetence of the annulus. Stabilization, preferably by the anterior interbody fusion method, is corrective. Narrowed, stiffened, and arthrotic interspaces are less subject to this complication. One group reports reflex sympathetic dystrophy as a postoperative complication.[69] Presumably, it would yield to repeated sympathetic blocks or cervical sympathectomy.

Postoperative Results

Radiculopathy should readily respond to any type of operation that permits removal of the ruptured disc fragment or spur or decompression of the root without removing the spur. Overall success rates appears to be somewhat higher for surgeons using the posterior approach.[34,69,92] Apparently they are more strict in limiting their operations to genuine radiculopathic syndromes. In contrast, many surgeons who favor the anterior operative approach use it in patients with only chronic neck pain. Use of the anterior operative approach for neck pain only is understandable, since that is the problem for which the operation was originally devised.[85] Such use of the procedure for neck pain, however, does lead to poorer results than when radiculopathy or spondylosis is present.

Multiple-level myelopathies, treated by extensive posterior decompression, and one- or two-level myelopathies treated by anterior interbody fusion seem to do equally well initially if the operation is done early in the course of the disease before permanent intramedullary changes develop.

One of the earlier reports on the favorable effect of posterior decompression is that of Spurling.[95] In patients with a mixture of radiculopathy and myelopathy, he had 73.7 per cent excellent results, 16.7 per cent good results, and 10 per cent poor results. The last group included several patients who had irreversible cord damage before they were subjected to laminectomy. Knight reported the use of posterior operations in 25 patients with radiculopathy, 22 of whom were relieved of their pain. Seven had had paresthesias, and all of them were relieved. Ten of the twelve who had sensory loss and five of the nine who had paresis were relieved.[51] Murphey and co-workers reported on over 600 posterior operations for cervical root compression by

rupture of the disc.[69] They claimed excellent, or 100 per cent, relief in 37.3 per cent and 90 per cent relief in 47.6 per cent, and stated that not a single patient received less than 50 per cent relief. Only 4 per cent of their patients changed jobs because of postoperative difficulties with the neck or arm. A corroborative report on the efficacy of posterior operations has recently been provided by Scoville and associates.[92] Three hundred eighty-three cervical disc operations done by Scoville since 1941 were studied. No patients were operated upon for subjective neck complaints alone. Of the 297 who were followed up, 208 had been operated upon more than four years before the study. Eighty-three patients had had lateral disc prominences, mainly soft ruptures of the disc. In this group, not a single patient suffered a recurrence, but 19 per cent developed disc lesions at other sites. Most of the patients returned to their regular jobs in just over a month. Sixty-six per cent were judged as receiving 100 per cent relief, and 29 per cent had somewhat lesser results, but only 2 per cent were judged fair and 2 per cent were not benefited. No patient was made worse or died. Eleven of Scoville's patients had had soft central herniations interfering with spinal cord function, and all but one of these derived a good to excellent result from posterior removal.

From the foregoing it appears appropriate to assure a patient with radiculopathy from a herniated disc or bony spur that there is a 90 to 95 per cent probability of a highly satisfactory outcome and a 2 to 5 per cent risk of gaining less than satisfactory relief. The probability of serious complications or death is less than 1 per cent.

The outlook for myelopathy treated by posterior decompression is reasonably satisfactory. Rothman and Simeone reported on a collected series of patients treated for myelopathy by laminectomy.[86] They found 56 per cent to be improved, 25 per cent to be unchanged, and 19 per cent to be made worse. Scoville and co-workers had 39 patients with transverse spondylotic ridges that produced myelopathy. They obtained relief in 10 per cent and substantial benefit in 54 per cent; the remainder had their disease process arrested.[92] Of the 39 patients, 5 suffered minor deficits from the operation. Gregorius and co-workers reported on 25 patients with myelopathy who appear to have been more severely affected than those reported in other series.[42] Nineteen of them underwent laminectomy by a series of surgeons. Twelve operations entailed dorsal grafting, and in nine the denticulate ligaments were sectioned. There were a few gratifying improvements, but later on progressive deterioration was the rule. They concluded that the 15 patients treated by Cloward's technique fared somewhat better than the 18 with disease of similar severity treated by laminectomy. They decline, however, to recommend one operation in preference to the other because of the small size of the sample and other variables.

REFERENCES

1. Alajouanine, T., and Petit-Dutaillis, D.: Le nodule fibrocartilagineux de la face postérieure des disques inter-vertébraux. Presse Méd., 2: 1657–1662; 1749–1751, 1930.
2. Allen, K. L.: Neuropathies caused by bony spurs in the cervical spine with special reference to surgical treatment. J. Neurol. Neurosurg. Psychiat., 15:20–36, 1952.
3. Armstrong, J. R.: Lumbar Disc Lesions. 3rd Ed. Baltimore, Williams & Wilkins Co., 1965, p. 15.
4. Arnold, J. G.: The clinical manifestations of spondylochondrosis (spondylosis) of the cervical spine. Ann. Surg., 141:872–889, 1955.
5. Aronson, N. I.: The management of soft cervical disc protrusions using the Smith-Robinson approach. Clin. Neurosurg., 20:253–258, 1973.
6. Bailey, P., and Casamajor, L.: Osteoarthritis of the spine as cause of compression of the spinal cord and its roots with reports of five cases. J. Nerv. Ment. Dis., 38:588–609, 1911.
7. Barnes, R.: Paraplegia in cervical spine injuries. J. Bone Joint Surg., 30-B:234–244, 1948.
8. Bedford, P. D., Bosanquet, F. D., and Russell, W. R.: Degeneration of the spinal cord associated with cervical spondylosis. Lancet, 2:55–59, 1952.
9. Bethune, R. W. M., and Brechner, V. I.: Detection of venous air embolism by carbon dioxide monitoring. Anesthesiology, 29:178, 1968.
10. Bobenchko, W. P., and Hirsch, C.: Autoimmune response of the nucleus pulposus in the rabbit. J. Bone Joint Surg., 47-B:574–580, 1965.
11. Boijsen, E.: Cervical spinal canal in intraspinal expansive processes. Acta Radiol., 42:101–115, 1954.
12. Boldrey, E. B.: Anterior cervical decompression without fusion. Presented to American Academy of Neurological Surgery. Key Biscayne, 1964.
13. Booth, R. D., and Rothman, R. H.: Cervical angina. Spine, 1:28–32, 1976.
14. Bradford, F. K., and Spurling, R. G.: The Intervertebral Disk. 2nd Ed. Springfield, Ill., Charles C Thomas, 1945.
15. Bradshaw, P.: Some aspects of cervical spondylosis. Quart. J. Med., 26:177–208, 1957.
16. Brain, W. R.: Some aspects of the neurology of the cervical spine. J. Fac. Radiol., 8:74–91, 1956.
17. Brain, W. R., Northfield, D., and Wilkinson, M.: The neurological manifestations of cervical spondylosis. Brain, 75:187–225, 1952.
18. Breasted, J. H.: The Edwin Smith Surgical Papyrus. Chicago, University of Chicago Press, 1930.
19. Breig, A., Turnbull, I. M., and Hassler, O.: Effects of mechanical stresses on the spinal cord in cervical spondylosis. A study of fresh cadaver material. J. Neurosurg., 25:45–56, 1966.
20. Bucy, P. C., and Chenault, H.: Compression of seventh cervical nerve root by herniation of an intervertebral disk. J.A.M.A., 126:25–27, 1944.
21. Bull, J., El Gammal, T., and Popham, M.: A possible genetic factor in cervical spondylosis. Brit. J. Radiol., 42:9–16, 1969.
22. Burrows, E. H.: The sagittal diameter of the spinal canal in cervical spondylosis. Clin. Radiol., 14:77–86, 1963.
23. Chrispin, A. R., and Lees, F.: The spinal canal in cervical spondylosis. J. Neurol. Neurosurg. Psychiat., 26:166–170, 1963.
24. Cloward, R. B.: The anterior approach for removal of ruptured cervical discs. J. Neurosurg., 15:602–617, 1958.
25. Coggeshall, R. E., Applebaum, M. L., Fazen, M., et al.: Unmyelinated axons in human ventral roots, a possible explanation for the failure of dorsal rhizotomy to relieve pain. Brain, 98:157–166, 1975.
26. Connolley, E. A., Seymour, R. J., and Adams, J. E.: Clinical evaluation of anterior cervical fusion for degenerative cervical disc disease. J. Neurosurg., 23:431–437, 1965.
27. Dandy, W. E.: Loose cartilage from intervertebral disk simulating tumor of the spinal cord. Arch. Surg., 19:660–672, 1929.
28. Dereymaeker, A., and Mulier, J.: La fusion vertébrale par voie ventrale dans la discopathie cervicale. Rev. Neurol. (Paris), 99:597–616, 1958.
29. Dockerty, M. D., and Love, J. G.: Thickening and fibrosis (so-called hypertrophy) of the ligamentum flavum: A pathologic study of 50 cases. Proc. Staff Meet. Mayo Clin., 15:161–166, 1940.
30. Dohn, D. F.: Anterior interbody fusion for treatment of cervical disk conditions. J.A.M.A., 197:897–900, 1966.
31. Early, C. B.: Muscle splitting approach to cervical disc excision. Presented to Neurosurgical Society of America, Marco Island, 1976.
32. Ehni, G.: Effects of certain degenerative diseases of the spine, especially spondylosis and disk protrusion, on the neural contents, particularly in the lumbar region. Mayo Clin. Proc., 50: 327–338, 1975.
33. Epstein, J. A., and Davidoff, L. M.: Chronic hypertrophic spondylosis of the cervical spine with compression of the spinal cord and its nerve roots. Surg. Gynec. Obstet., 93:27–39, 1951.
34. Fager, C. A.: Rationale and techniques of pos-

terior approaches to cervical disk lesions and spondylosis. Surg. Clin. N. Amer., *56*:581–592, 1976.

35. Finneson, B.: Psycho-social considerations in low back pain. Presented at the meeting of the International Society for Study of the Lumbar Spine, Bermuda, June 1976.

36. Flynn, T. B.: Complications of anterior cervical fusion. Presented at meeting of American Association of Neurological Surgeons, San Francisco, 1976.

37. Frykholm, R.: Cervical nerve root compression resulting from disk degeneration and root sleeve fibrosis: A clinical investigation. Acta Chir. Scand., Suppl. 160, 1951.

38. Glista, G. G., Miller, R. H., Kurland, L. T., and Jereczek, M. L.: Neurosurgical procedures in Olmsted County, Minnesota, 1970–1974. J. Neurosurg., *46*:46–51, 1977.

39. Gooding, M. R., Wilson, C. B., and Hoff, J. T.: Experimental cervical myelopathy. Effects of ischemia and compression of the canine cervical spinal cord. J. Neurosurg., *43*:9–17, 1975.

40. Gowers, W. R.: Diseases of the Nervous System. 2nd Ed. Vol 1. London, Churchill, 1892, p. 260.

41. Greenfield, J. G.: Malformations et dégénérescences des disques intervertébraux de la région cervicale. Rev. Méd. Suisse Rom., *73*:227–250, 1953.

42. Gregorius, F. K., Estrin, T., and Crandall, P. H.: Cervical spondylotic radiculopathy and myelopathy. A long-term followup study. Arch. Neurol., *33*:618–625, 1976.

43. Hacuba, A.: Trans-unco-discal approach. A combined anterior and lateral approach to cervical discs. J. Neurosurg., *45*:284–291, 1976.

44. Hankinson, H. L., and Wilson, C. B.: Use of operating microscope in anterior cervical diskectomy without fusion. J. Neurosurg., *43*:452–456, 1975.

45. Hinck, V. C., and Sachdev, N. S.: Developmental stenosis of the cervical spinal canal. Brain, *89*:27–36, 1966.

46. Hirsch, C., Wickhom, I., and Lidstrom, A.: Cervical disc resection. A followup of myelographic and surgical procedure. J. Bone Joint Surg., *46-A*:1811–1821, 1964.

47. Howe, J. F.: Mechano-sensitivity of dorsal root ganglia in chronically injured axones: A physiological basis for radicular pain of nerve root compression. Presented at Meeting of American Academy of Neurological Surgeons, Charleston, S.C., 1976.

48. Kahn, E. A.: The role of the dentate ligaments in spinal cord compression and the syndrome of lateral sclerosis. J. Neurosurg., *4*:191–199, 1947.

49. Kaplan, L., and Kennedy, F.: The effect of head posture on the manometrics of the cerebrospinal fluid in cervical lesions: A new diagnostic test. Brain, *73*:337–345, 1950.

50. Key, C. A.: Guy Hosp. Rep., *3*:17, 1838. (Cited by Wilkinson, ref. 112).

51. Knight, G.: Neurosurgical treatment of cervical spondylosis. Proc. Roy. Soc. Med., *57*:165–168, 1964.

52. Lane, W. A.: Some points in the physiology and pathology of changes produced by pressure in the bony skeleton of the trunk and shoulder girdle. Guy Hosp. Rep., *43*:321–434, 1886.

53. Lazorthes, G.: Pathology, classification and clinical aspects of vascular diseases of the spinal cord. *In* Vincken, P. J., and Bruyn, G. W., eds.: Handbook of Clinical Neurology. Vol 12. New York, American Elsevier Publishing Co., 1972, pp. 492–506.

54. Lazorthes, G., Poulhes, J., Bastide, G., et al.: Recherches sur la vascularisation artérielle de la moelle; applications à la pathologie médullaire. Bull. Acad. Nat. Med. (Paris), *141*:464–477, 1957.

55. Lindblom, K.: Intervertebral disc degeneration considered as a pressure atrophy. J. Bone Joint Surg., *39-A*:933–945, 1957.

56. Liversedge, L. A., Hutchinson, E. C., and Lyons, J. B.: Cervical spondylosis simulating motor neurone disease. Lancet, *2*:652–659, 1953.

57. Love, J. G.: Protrusion of the intervertebral disk (fibrocartilage) into the spinal canal. Proc. Staff Meet. Mayo Clin., *11*:529–535, 1936.

58. Magee, K. R., and DeJong, R. N.: Paralytic brachial neuritis. J.A.M.A., *174*:1258–1263, 1960.

59. Mair, W. G. P., and Druckman, R.: The pathology of spinal cord lesions and their relation to the clinical features in protrusion of cervical intervertebral disks. Brain, *76*:70–91, 1953.

60. Maroon, J. C., and Albin, M. S.: Air embolism diagnosed by Doppler ultrasound. Anesth. Analg. (Cleveland), *53*:399–402, 1974.

61. Marshall, B. M.: Air embolus in neurosurgical anesthesia, its diagnosis and treatment. Canad. Anaesth. Soc. J., *12*:255–261, 1965.

62. Martins, A. N.: Anterior cervical discectomy with and without interbody bone graft. J. Neurosurg., *44*:290–295, 1976.

63. Michenfelder, J. D., Miller, R. H., and Gronert, G. A.: Evaluation of an ultrasound device (Doppler) for the diagnosis of venous air embolism. Anesthesiology, *36*:164–167, 1972.

64. Michenfelder, J. D., Martin, J. T., Altenburg, B. M., et al.: Air embolism during neurosurgery: An evaluation of right atrial catheters for diagnosis and treatment. J.A.M.A., *208*:1353–1358, 1969.

65. Mitchell, J. K.: On a new practice in acute and chronic rheumatism. Amer. J. Med. Sci., *8*:55–64, 1831.

66. Mitchell, P. E. G., Hendry, N. G. C., and Bilewicz, W. Z.: The chemical background of intervertebral disk prolapse. J. Bone Joint Surg., *43-B*:141–151, 1961.

67. Mixter, W. J., and Barr, J. S.: Rupture of the intervertebral disk with involvement of the spinal canal. N. Eng. J. Med., *211*:210–215, 1934.

68. Moiel, R. H., Rasso, E., and Waltz, T. A.: Central cord syndrome resulting from congenital narrowness of the cervical spinal canal. J. Trauma, *10*:502–510, 1970.

69. Murphey, F., Simmons, J. C. H., and Brunson, B.: Ruptured cervical discs. 1939–1972. Clin. Neurosurg., *20*:9–17, 1973.

70. Murphy, M. G., and Gado, M.: Anterior cervical discectomy without interbody bone graft. J. Neurosurg., *37*:71–74, 1972.

71. Nachlas, I. W.: Pseudoangina pectoris origi-

nating in the cervical spine. J.A.M.A., *103*: 323–325, 1934.

72. Naylor, A.: The biophysical and biochemical aspects of intervertebral disc herniation and degeneration. Ann. Roy. Col. Surg. Eng., *31*:91–114, 1962.

73. Naylor, A.: Intervertebral disk prolapse and degeneration. The biochemical and biophysical approach. Spine, *1*:108–114, 1976.

74. Naylor, A., and Smare, D. L.: Fluid content of the nucleus pulposus as a factor in the disc syndrome. Brit. Med. J., *2*:975–976, 1953.

75. Nugent, G. R.: Clinicopathologic correlations in cervical spondylosis. Neurology (Minneap.), *9*:273–281, 1959.

76. Nurick, S.: The natural history and the results of surgical treatment of the spinal cord disorder associated with cervical spondylosis. Brain, *95*:101–108, 1972.

77. O'Connell, J. E. A.: Involvement of the spinal cord by intervertebral disc protrusions. Brit. J. Surg., *43*:225–247, 1955.

78. Pallis, C., Jones, A. M., and Spillane, J. D.: Cervical spondylosis: Incidence and implications. Brain, *77*:274–289, 1954.

79. Payne, E. E., and Spillane, J. D.: The cervical spine. An anatomico-pathological study of 70 specimens (using a special technique) with particular reference to the problems of cervical spondylosis. Brain, *80*:571–596, 1957.

80. Pemberton, R.: Arthritis and Rheumatoid Conditions. Their Nature and Treatment. Philadelphia, Lea & Febiger, 1929, p. 156.

81. Penning, L.: Some aspects of plain radiography of the cervical spine in chronic myelopathy. Neurology (Minneap.), *12*:513–519, 1962.

82. Reid, J. D.: Effects of flexion-extension movements of the head and spine upon the spinal cord and nerve roots. J. Neurol. Neurosurg. Psychiat., *23*:214–221, 1960.

83. Robertson, J. T.: Anterior cervical disc removal with and without fusion. Clin. Neurosurg., *20*:259–261, 1973.

84. Robinson, R. A., and Smith, G. W.: Anterolateral cervical disc removal and interbody fusion for cervical disc syndrome. Johns Hopkins Hosp. Bull., *96*:223–224, 1955.

85. Robinson, R. A., Walker, A. E., Ferlic, D. C., et al.: The results of anterior interbody fusion of the cervical spine. J. Bone Joint Surg., *44-A*:1569–1587, 1962.

86. Rothman, R. H., and Simeone, F. A.: The Spine. Vol. 1. Philadelphia, W. B. Saunders Co., 1975, p. 428.

87. Sachs, B., and Fraenkel, J.: Progressive ankylotic rigidity of the spine (spondylose rhizomelique). J. Nerv. Ment. Dis., *27*:1–15, 1900.

88. Sarpyener, M. A.: Spina bifida aperta and congenital stricture of the spinal canal. J. Bone Joint Surg., *29*:817–821, 1947.

89. Schneider, R. C., Papo, M., and Alvarez, C. S.: The effects of chronic recurrent spinal trauma in high diving. A study of Acapulco's divers. J. Bone Joint Surg., *44-A*:648–656, 1962.

90. Schneider, R. C., Thompson, J. M., and Bevin, J.: Acute central cervical cord injury. J. Neurol. Neurosurg. Psychiat., *21*:216–227, 1958.

91. Scoville, W. B.: Cervical spondylosis treated by bilateral facetectomy and laminectomy. J. Neurosurg., *18*:423–428, 1961.

92. Scoville, W. B., Dohrmann, G. J., and Corkill, G.: Late results of cervical disc surgery. J. Neurosurg., *45*:203–210, 1976.

93. Semmes, R. E., and Murphey, F.: The syndrome of unilateral rupture of the sixth cervical intervertebral disk. J.A.M.A., *121*:1209–1214, 1943.

94. Spillane, J. D.: Localized neuritis of the shoulder girdle. Lancet, *2*:532–535, 1943.

95. Spurling, R. G.: Lesions of the Cervical Intervertebral Disc. Springfield, Ill., Charles C Thomas, 1956.

96. Spurling, R. G., and Bradford, F. K.: Neurologic aspects of herniated nucleus pulposus. J.A.M.A., *113*:2019–2022, 1939.

97. Spurling, R. G., and Scoville, W. B.: Lateral rupture of cervical intervertebral discs; common cause of shoulder and arm pain. Surg. Gynec. Obstet., *78*:350–358, 1944.

98. Spurling, R. G., Mayfield, F. H., and Rogers, J. B.: Hypertrophy of the ligamenta flava as a cause of low back pain. J.A.M.A., *109*:928–933, 1937.

99. Steinhausen, T. D., Dungan, C. E., Furst, J. B., et al.: Iodinated organic compounds as contrast media for radiographic diagnosis. III. Experimental and clinical myelography and iodophenylundecylate (Pantopaque). Radiology, *43*:230–235, 1944.

100. Stookey, B.: Compression of the spinal cord due to ventral extradural cervical chondromas: Diagnosis and surgical treatment. Arch. Neurol. Psychiat., *20*:275–291, 1928.

101. Symonds, C. P.: The interrelation of trauma and cervical spondylosis in compression of the cervical cord. Lancet, *1*:451–454, 1953.

102. Taylor, A. R.: Mechanism and treatment of spinal cord disorders associated with cervical spondylosis. Lancet *1*:717–720, 1953.

103. Taylor, A. R.: Vascular factors in the myelopathy associated with cervical spondylosis. Neurology (Minneap.), *14*:62–68, 1964.

104. Taylor, J., and Collier, J.: The occurrence of optic neuritis in lesions of the spinal cord. Injury, tumor, myelitis. (Case 5.) Brain, *24*:533–552, 1901.

105. Tew, J. M., and Mayfield, F. H.: Proceedings: Society of British Neurological Surgeons: Anterior cervical discectomy—a microsurgical approach. J. Neurol. Neurosurg. Psychiat., *38*:4413, 1975.

106. Tung, A., Reilley, K., and Albin, M. S.: Use of an air bubble illuminator as an adjunct for surgery in the sitting position. Surg. Neurol., *6*:133–134, 1976.

107. Turnbull, I. M.: Blood supply of the spinal cord. *In* Vinken, P. J., and Bruyn, G. W., eds,: Handbook of Clinical Neurology. Vol 12. New York, American Elsevier Publishing Co., 1972, pp. 478–491.

108. Turnbull, I. M., Breig, A., and Hassler, O.: Blood supply of cervical spinal cord in man; a microangiographic cadaver study. J. Neurosurg., *24*:951–955, 1966.

109. VanGelderen, C.: Ein orthotisches (lordotisches) Kaudasyndrome. Acta Psychiat. Neurol. Scand., *23*:57–68, 1948.

110. Verbiest, H.: Further experiences on the pathological influence of a developmental narrowness of the bony lumbar vertebral canal. J. Bone Joint Surg., *37-B*:576–583, 1955.

111. Verbiest, H.: A lateral approach to the cervical spine: Technique and indications. J. Neurosurg., *28*:191–203, 1968.

112. VonBechterew, W.: Steifigkeit der Wirbelsaule und ihre Verkrummung als besondere Erkrankungsform. Neurol. Zbl., *12:*426–434, 1893.

113. Wilkinson, M.: Historical introduction. *In* Cervical Spondylosis. 2nd Ed. Philadelphia, W. B. Saunders Co., 1971, pp. 1–9.

114. Wolf, B. S., Khilnani, M., and Malis, L.: Sagittal diameter of the bony cervical spinal canal and its significance in cervical spondylosis. J. Mount Sinai Hosp. N.Y., *23*:283–292, 1956.

81

ANTERIOR OPERATIVE APPROACH FOR BENIGN EXTRADURAL CERVICAL LESIONS

The introduction of the anterior approach to the cervical spine for disc disease by Robinson and Smith opened an entirely new field for the neurosurgeon.[37] Many clinical problems could be approached in a most satisfactory and direct way. The basic concept of the approach was rapidly modified and enlarged. Special instrumentation for the operative procedure was designed by Cloward, who also broadened its use to include trauma.[6] Many other individuals have made significant contributions to the use of and indications for the anterior approach. Bailey and Badgley developed precise indications for its use to obtain stability of the spine.[2] Myers popularized the technique of complete removal and replacement of a vertebral body for fractures or extensive spondylotic disease.[31] The extension of the operative exposure upward to the clivus was proposed by Stevenson, Stoney, Perkins, and Adams.[43] Recently, the disc and osteophyte without fusion has been advocated.[21,26,35] Robertson removes the entire disc. The patients develop a slight swanneck deformity, and ultimately fusion takes place spontaneously.[35] Hankinson and Wilson drill out a tunnel in the vertebral body above and the vertebral body below, which is wider posteriorly than anteriorly. They leave intervertebral disc material laterally, thus maintaining interspace height.[21] The author's experience with these two approaches indicates that they are satisfactory. As many as three levels can be done by this technique. The anterior approach without fusion is contraindicated in cases of trauma.

As originally described, the operative approach was parapharyngeal; thus, its use in the extreme upper cervical spine was difficult. Fang, Ong, and Hodgson proposed a transoral approach to the highest levels of the neck.[17] Mullan, Naunton, Hekmatpanah, and Vailati used a similar approach in a few patients.[30] More recently the use of the transoral approach for the treatment of atlantoaxial dislocation due to odontoid hypoplasia was described by Greenberg, Scoville, and Davey.[19] Verbiest has described a modification of the direct anterior approach, an approach behind the sternocleidomastoid muscle.[47] These various modifications have greatly increased the neurosurgeon's ability to deal successfully with a wide variety of cervical spine disease.

The chief virtues of the anterior approach are its technical simplicity and direct exposure of pathological conditions lying ventral to the spinal cord and roots. Patients have less postoperative discomfort than after laminectomy, hemilaminectomy, or laminotomy.[6,14,29,47]

OPERATIVE TECHNIQUE

In most instances the procedure is performed under general anesthesia and using an endotracheal tube of sufficient rigidity that it will not collapse during retraction of the trachea. Some surgeons, notably Cloward, perform the procedure under local anesthesia and find this method eminently satisfactory.[6] If the procedure is to be done transorally or transpharyngeally, a tracheostomy or cuffed endotracheal tube to prevent aspiration is mandatory.[17]

Several donor sites for the bone graft have been recommended. The iliac crest is the most common. Usually the patient's own bone is used as the graft; however, bone bank bone has been used in one large series.[6]

The patient is placed supine with a small sandbag beneath the upper dorsal spine so that the shoulders will fall backward. The head is turned approximately 15 degrees away from the side of the operative incision. Wristlets with attached cords are placed on the patient's arms to enable an assistant to pull the shoulders downward to facilitate adequate x-ray localization. A cervical halter may be fitted to use for applying traction if it becomes necessary. Either side of the neck may be used for the approach. Most surgeons prefer to make the incision on the right, as it makes the dissection easier for a right-handed surgeon. It places his dominant hand in the best rela-

tionship to the intervertebral interspace (Figs. 81–1 and 81–2).

After routine operative preparation of the skin of the neck and donor site, the incision is made, slanted slightly from the horizontal, in a prominent skin crease. The level of the incision is determined by the space to be explored; for C5 and C6 it is usually at the level of the thyroid cartilage. It is better that the skin incision be slightly high, as the platysma fibers make superior extension more difficult. The incision should extend from the midline anteriorly to the anterior border of the sternocleidomastoid muscle. The platysma is dissected free from the overlying skin and opened in the direction of its fibers. If the incision is appropriately placed for the desired level of the cervical spine, the incision in the platysma need be no more than about 3 cm in length. Dissecting the platysma from the skin and opening it in this way reduces scarring postoperatively. If the incision is not properly placed, however, the platysma may be divided to gain better access.

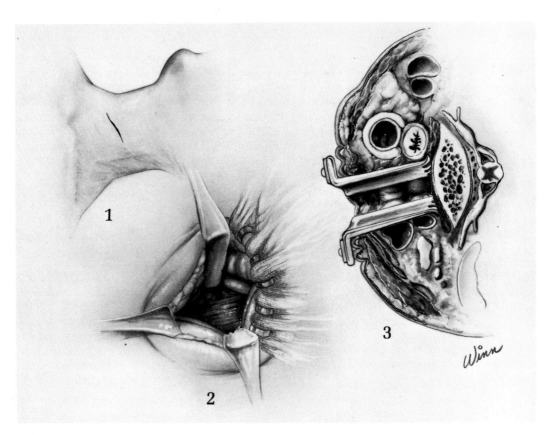

Figure 81–1 1. Location of skin incision. 2. Dissection deep to platysma. 3. Cross-section of neck showing plane of dissection.

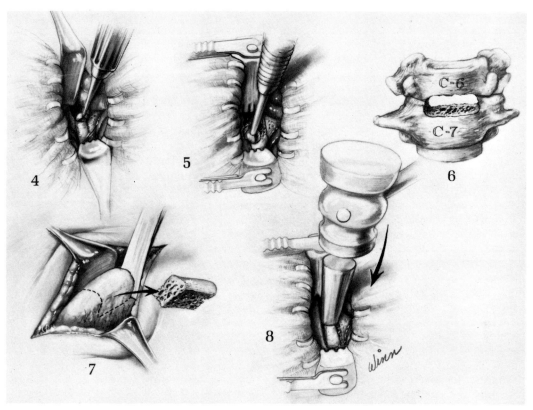

Figure 81–2 4. Removal of disc material by curet. 5. Removal of osteophyte by air drill. 6. Diagram of area of bone removed from vertebral bodies. 7. Removal of bone graft from iliac crest. 8. Impacting bone graft into the prepared intervertebral disc space.

The fascial plane between the cervical strap muscles, trachea, and esophagus medially, and the carotid sheath and sternocleidomastoid muscle laterally, is identified. This plane is opened by using combined sharp and blunt dissection. Crossing the operative field are several structures that must be dealt with safely. The superior thyroid artery may cross the fascial plane. If it compromises the exposure, it should be doubly ligated and divided. Occasionally, the external jugular vein or veins from the thyroid passing to the internal jugular vein are in the way and should be ligated. Ligation with fine silk rather than cautery is recommended for vessels of this size. An enlarged thyroid gland may intrude into the operative field. If the surgeon accidentally enters the substance of the gland, vigorous bleeding may be provoked. This bleeding can best be controlled by suture ligatures. With dissection too far laterally, the carotid sheath may

be opened, requiring increased care to avoid damage to the carotid artery, internal jugular vein, or vagus nerve.

Once the retroesophageal space is clearly identified, the esophagus is dissected off the prevertebral fascia. It is displaced laterally across from the midline. The surgeon should avoid retraction on the carotid sheath, which lies lateral to the dissection and the proposed operative field and need not be disturbed.

Perforation of the esophagus or hypopharynx may occur during dissection in the prevertebral space. Gentle dissection is necessary to avoid this complication. In the esophagus, the lateral or posterolateral aspect is the most likely place to look for the rent. Perforation of the hypopharynx is more likely, however, as the structure is much thinner and less muscular than the esophagus. In operations on the upper cervical spine, the surgeon must take special care to avoid the problem; a good way is to enter the prevertebral space caudal to the operative level and then dissect cephalad to the appropriate level.

It is important to gain adequate exposure of the anterior surface of the vertebral column. Both longus colli muscles should be visualized and clearly identified, but it is not necessary to strip them from the vertebral bodies. To do so simply causes troublesome bleeding. The midline, of course, lies between them and is used as a guide for opening the interspace. If the interspace is opened laterally, damage to the vertebral artery, sympathetic chain, or nerve root may occur. A needle is placed in an intervertebral disc, and a single lateral x-ray is obtained for localization. This provides a permanent, accurate, and satisfactory method of identifying the interspace. Injection of dye to mark the disc space has been advocated, but this is not as satisfactory as x-ray.[6]

While the x-ray film is being developed, the donor site is exposed and the bone graft obtained. The anterior superior part of the iliac crest is usually used. (Positioning the patient with a sandbag placed under one hip makes access to the crest of the ilium easy.) A curvilinear incision is made just below the level of the crest and carried down to the periosteum. Depending on the type of bone graft to be fashioned, the muscles around the iliac crest are dissected free subperiosteally. For the Cloward technique, it is necessary only to dissect those muscles free from the outer side of the ilium. The circular Wiltberger plug cutter is then passed transversely through the ilium, leaving the crest undisturbed. This will obtain a suitably sized dowel of bone with cortical bone on two sides. If the graft is removed across the ilium, the patient has much less postoperative discomfort than when there is dissection of the iliacus muscle or removal of the crest.

If, however, a Smith-Robinson fusion is planned, or if a large piece of bone is required, as for the bread-loaf graft of Myers, the crest of the ilium itself must be stripped of its muscle attachments. The lateral and medial surfaces of the ilium are cleaned of their muscular attachments subperiosteally. A bone graft of appropriate size is cut from the crest of the ilium. This graft has cortical bone on three of its four surfaces.

Occasionally it is necessary to use pure cortical bone for the graft. Either an onlay or an inlay technique may be used.[2] The author's experience indicates that the onlay method is easier and perfectly satisfactory. Tibial bone is usually used as the graft. It is obtained through a linear incision along the medial posterior surface of the tibia. This is carried down to the periosteum, and the posterior surface of the tibia is stripped of its periosteal attachment for the appropriate distance. Parallel cuts in the posterior surface of the tibia are made with either the Stryker rotating saw or an osteotome. This usually produces no structural weakness of the tibia, but the patient should be cautioned against vigorous exercise for several months, as a fracture of the tibia may occur.

Closure of the donor site incision includes closure of the periosteum and the muscles overlying it, the subcutaneous tissue, and the skin. Wounds are closed without drainage and with nonabsorbable interrupted sutures. Careful hemostasis is essential, as the resultant reduction in hematoma formation will reduce postoperative pain.

After the graft has been obtained attention is returned to the operative exposure in the neck. The appropriate interspace having been identified by x-ray localization, retractors are inserted and engaged beneath the longus colli muscles. Either hand-held retractors or self-retaining ones may be used. Additional retractors are placed as needed, either superiorly or inferiorly. The surgeon should feel for carotid artery pulsations above the retractor blades after they have been positioned.

The anterior longitudinal ligament is sharply incised and a piece is removed from it. This excision should extend completely across the exposed interspace. The disc material is removed with a curet and pituitary forceps. Curettage is done with great care to avoid pushing disc material posteriorly toward the spinal cord or spinal roots. Once curettage has been carried most of the way through the interspace, a vertebra spreader is used to widen the interspace, providing improved visualization of the remaining disc material. Careful inspection of the posterior ligament is done in all cases to check the integrity of the structure. A hole in it will indicate the location of a free fragment of disc material. If necessary for retrieval of a fragment, the ligament may be opened. If the posterior longitudinal ligament is opened laterally, the nerve root sleeve may be visualized for a distance of 2 to 3 mm.[33]

If the pathological process is spondylotic in nature, the surgeon must remove the osteophyte. This may be done with a curet or by using the high-speed air drill and a diamond burr. The curets must be small and sharp. Angled or "hooked" ones are helpful in removing osteophytes from the foraminal area. Thorough, careful curettage is done. It is usually easy to tell when the osteophyte has been removed, as the feel of the curet against normal bone is considerably different from that against the osteophyte. The latter is harder, cuts with a sharper sound, and feels smoother and more polished. The operating microscope is helpful in providing light and magnification.

If no fusion is contemplated, the wound is drained with a small Penrose drain, and closed in layers.

The operative procedure after disc or osteophyte removal varies depending on the precise technique employed. If the Smith-Robinson technique is used, the cartilaginous plates that lie between the two contiguous vertebral bodies are thoroughly curetted, insuring that raw bone will be present for contact with the graft. A small high-speed air-driven burr is quite helpful in removing the cartilaginous plates. It may also be used to shape the bone graft for a snug fit. The interspace is distracted by the vertebral body spreaders. Supplemental head traction may be used if needed. An appropriately fitted bone graft is then inserted into the interspace. This should be countersunk beneath the anterior longitudinal ligament to insure that it will remain in position.

If the Cloward technique is used, the next step is careful measurement of the depth of the interspace. The drill guide is then set to the measured depth and attached across the intervertebral space. The drill is fitted into the drill guide and the drilling of the interspace done. For successful use of this technique, several points are crucial. First, no intervertebral disc material should remain in the interspace prior to drilling. The drill may not cut disc material in a satisfactory manner and may push it through the interspace and against the spinal cord. Second, careful measurement of the depth to be drilled is essential;

the appropriate devices for this crucial measurement are an integral part of the operative armamentarium. The depth drilled should leave the posterior cortex of the vertebral bodies intact. These may be removed with a sharp curet, if desired, after the drilling procedure. Third, the drilling of the interspace should be done with a single use of the drill. Once seated, the drill guide should not be removed and repositioned. If the guide is repositioned, the hole in the intervertebral space will be of varying shape, size, and direction, which in turn will produce problems with graft insertion and fixation.

If the Cloward technique is used at adjacent interspaces, the drill holes must be placed to insure that adequate vertebral body remains between them. This is done by putting them slightly off the midline, alternately to the left and right, so they are staggered. The smallest drill available is the best one to use in this situation.

Once the interspace has been drilled, further curettage of remaining osteophytes may be required. Once the surgeon is satisfied with their removal, the graft is inserted. The interspace is distracted by the vertebral body spreaders supplemented by head traction. The bone dowel is cut to an appropriate length and is impacted into the shaped drill hole. The anterior surface should be countersunk below the anterior surface of the vertebral bodies.

If the vertebral body is to be resected, removal is accomplished by using double-action bone rongeurs or a high-speed air drill. It is usually easier to do this by rongeuring the body away, using the air drill to remove the last remaining bit of the vertebral body. Removal need not extend far laterally. The posterior longitudinal ligament should be preserved. After bone removal is complete, the bone graft is fashioned to the appropriate size. The cervical spine should be distracted by halter traction and the graft inserted. Occasionally it will be necessary to fasten the graft with either heavy silk or wire sutures. These are placed through drill holes in the adjacent vertebral bodies and the graft.

Wound closure begins by placing a ⅜-inch Penrose drain down to the bone graft. It is led out through the skin incision. Closure of the platysma and the skin is done in layers with interrupted nonabsorbable fine sutures.

Operations through the pharynx for upper cervical spine disease involve the routine use of preoperative antibiotics and thorough oral cleansing for several days prior to operation. The routine performance of tracheostomy has been advocated by most of the proponents of this technique. The mouth is held open by a special retractor. The incision is made through the mucosa in the midline of the oral pharynx and is carried either upward or downward, depending on the direction desired. If the odontoid process is the target, the soft palate should be split in the midline and sutured laterally to gain access. The retropharyngeal space and the prevertebral space are dissected and retracted laterally, and by careful subperiosteal dissection the diseased area is exposed. Identification by x-ray is used to confirm the location, and the appropriate procedure is carried out. This is usually the removal of the odontoid, but bone grafting can be done safely.[16,19] If the odontoid is removed, a posterior fusion of C1, C2, and C3 is required.[19] The wound is closed with absorbable sutures through the mucosa only, and no drainage is employed. Antibiotic therapy of a broad-spectrum type is employed routinely in all cases of a transpharyngeal approach to the upper cervical spine.

POSTOPERATIVE CARE

The patient is kept in bed for the first 12 to 24 hours. Unless the procedure has been done transorally, no antibiotics are used. Analgesics are given to control pain; usually, only codeine is required. Postoperative x-rays are taken to check the position of the bone graft. After assurance that the graft is in place, and if the patient's condition otherwise warrants, ambulation is begun. Routine use of a cervical brace or cervical collar is not required unless multiple levels have been operated upon or there is some question regarding the stability of the neck. If it is known that there is instability of the neck, as after removal of vertebral bodies, the patient is kept in skeletal traction until secure union has occurred. Most such cases involve trauma rather than elective operations and, therefore, are rarely encountered in benign disease.

The operative drain is removed at 24 hours, the skin sutures at 3 days from the neck incision and at 7 to 10 days from the donor site. The patient, in cases of single-level fusion, is usually discharged from the hospital around the fourth to the eighth postoperative day. Instructions to the patient include the avoidance of long automobile trips, violent exercise, or physical labor for a period of eight weeks. The follow-up examination is done between the eighth and ninth weeks. X-rays of the neck are taken. If solid bony fusion is present, the patient is released to full activity. If there is persistence of the interspace, an additional period of limited activity for another eight weeks with collar support is suggested. Repeat x-rays are obtained until firm union can be demonstrated.

The patient should be re-evaluated by the operating surgeon at eight weeks, four months, and one year after the procedure. These examinations should document the disappearance of old symptoms and the development of new ones. Examination of the range of motion of the neck is important. Significant loss of mobility is rare in single-level fusions and should alert the surgeon to possible trouble. Neurological status should be evaluated and compared with the preoperative one.

USE OF ANTERIOR APPROACH IN SPECIFIC DISEASES

While the potential for treating any or all diseases of the cervical spine and spinal cord by an anterior approach exists, there are certain definite indications and contraindications to its use. Beyond these virtually absolute conditions, the individual surgeon must recognize his own limitations and be guided by his past experience or lack of it. Occasionally, the choice of procedure is dictated by the availability of supporting professional personnel or equipment. The surgeon must consider these individualized aspects of caring for his patient, as they override mere technical feasibility.

Spinal Cord Tumors

Occasionally, an extrinsic extra-axial spinal cord tumor, such as a meningioma, may lie directly anterior to the cervical cord.[30] The surgeon may elect an anterior approach, but in general, this problem is best handled by a laminectomy. To reach such lesions requires the removal of a considerable portion of several vertebral bodies, and this seems more of an undertaking than necessary. In the case of neurofibromas involving the vertebral body, however, the anterior approach affords the advantage of direct access to the lesion in its entirety. The involved bone as well as the intradural tumor can be removed.

For the patient with an intrinsic spinal cord tumor, the anterior approach is contraindicated. Adequate visualization of the lesion is difficult, and myelotomy is hazardous because the anterior spinal artery is in the way.

Infections of Cervical Vertebrae

The most common bone infections found in the United States are tuberculosis, brucellosis, and hematogenous osteomyelitis. These rarely involve the cervical vertebrae. The principles of management are simple.

Adequate drainage and removal of all infected bone must be accomplished. In most circumstances these maneuvers are best done from the anterior approach, as the infection involves the vertebral body. The patient is kept in skeletal traction until stability of the spine is assured by a sound fusion. Primary bone grafting should not be done in pyogenic osteomyelitis. Reconstitution of bone is prompt, and satisfactory fusion occurs spontaneously. In tubercular osteomyelitis, however, primary bone grafting can be employed and will hasten the fusion process.[17] In all cases the use of appropriate antibiotic therapy is routine and of maximum importance.

Tumors of Cervical Vertebrae

Patients occasionally present with giant cell tumors of the cervical vertebral bodies. Other forms of benign bone tumors, chondromas, or osteomas are rarely seen involving this area. Such tumors produce difficulty of either a neurological or a mechanical nature; they may cause partial obstruction to swallowing. If symptomatic in any way, or if there is doubt as to the nature of the lesion, they should be removed through an anterior approach because of

the distinct advantages of dealing directly with the lesion. Stability of the neck is assured by appropriate grafting.

The use of the anterior approach with attempted resection of all involved bone in metastatic tumors has been advocated by Mullan and co-workers.[30] Experience with this procedure indicates its usefulness in the occasional case of limited vertebral body involvement. Resection and successful grafting can be accomplished and decompression of the spinal cord is adequate and feasible from this approach. The problem is to maintain stability of the neck after removal of the tumor, as in the usual case the cervical vertebral bodies are rather extensively involved before spinal cord compression occurs. It is a race between the disseminated cancer growth rate and the progress of the fusion toward stability of the neck.

Hypoplasia of Odontoid Process

This rare entity causes neurological symptoms and signs because the spinal cord is compressed between the rim of the foramen magnum and the ring of C1. Occasionally it is associated with other anomalies about the occipitoatlantic joint.[12,19] Decompression of the spinal cord from the posterior can be quite hazardous, as stability of the spine is further endangered.[19] Secondary fusion is difficult after laminectomy and suboccipital craniectomy, which compounds the problem.

It seems clear from the literature that transoral decompression followed by posterior stabilization is the current procedure of choice.[19] Transoral fusion is feasible, but more neurosurgical experience seems required before its routine use can be recommended.

Compression of Vertebral Artery by Osteophytes

Again, this is a rare disease. The patient presents with symptoms of vertebral-basilar artery insufficiency, the crucial point being that such symptoms occur only with certain head and neck movements or postures. Angiography with the head placed in the symptomatic position will demonstrate extraluminal compression or occlusion of the vertebral artery in the neck.

Removal of the offending osteophyte may be done by either an anterior or a lateral approach.[3,22,47] The anterior one is the simplest and most direct.

Intervertebral Disc Disease

The two related entities that occur with disc degeneration, herniation and spondylosis, are the most common afflictions of the cervical spine. The anterior approach was designed to improve the results of operative treatment of these common diseases. In discussing its use, a distinction should be made between the types of disc disease, such as "soft" or "hard," and the location of the protrusion, either central, paracentral, or lateral.

In a masterful paper in 1928, Stookey recognized three types of protrusions: the central disc protrusion, producing signs of total spinal cord compression; a paracentral extrusion, with evidence of compression of half the spinal cord plus radicular signs at the appropriate level; and the lateral protrusion with only radicular signs.[44]

In considering an operative approach for cervical disc disease, one should recall these three types. The patient with a midline extrusion and signs of spinal cord compression is the rarest, statistically, of the three.[4] Many large series report the incidence to be about 4 to 6 per cent.[7,10,20,29,32,46] But, this patient is the one for whom the anterior approach is most appropriate, as it is difficult to reach the lesion through a posterior laminectomy with the spinal cord lying between it and the operating surgeon. In fact, it has been recommended that in the presence of a bony midline protuberance, only a laminectomy and dentate ligament section be done.[24] An alternate procedure has been laminectomy and foraminotomy without opening the dura.[40,45] Removal of the osteophyte by curettage extradurally has been suggested by Mayfield and by Epstein and co-workers.[15,28] Scoville has reported increased neurological deficit after such procedures.[40] "Soft" discs, or true herniation of the disc material, can be removed from the posterior, usually, after a transdural approach that displaces the spinal cord laterally by dentate ligament section.[4] Neurological disaster has resulted from this maneuver.

Results obtained by the posterior approach, either with or without opening the dura, cover a wide range, with anywhere from 6 to 71 per cent excellent results being reported.[17,20,29,32] The anterior approach has an equally wide range of excellent results, running from 17 to 100 per cent.* The usual problem of assessing any clinical procedure exists: disagreement between reported series as to criteria for selection of patients or for improvement achieved, inclusion of patients with radiculopathy or other causes of cervical myelopathy, differences in patient populations, differences in patient follow-up time, and bias on the part of the reporting surgeon. Crandall and Batzdorf reported their experience with patients from a single clinic treated by both approaches.[11] Their data on 62 patients managed by laminectomy (23), laminectomy plus dural graft (11), anterior discectomy and fusion (21), and both an anterior and a posterior approach (7) indicate clear superiority of the anterior approach.

Galera and Tovi, however, report a much less optimistic outlook.[18] In 51 patients, 33 with signs of spinal cord compression, only 17 per cent showed a satisfactory result.

Mayfield has reported an extensive experience with both approaches for cervical spondylotic disease.[29] His data suggest that the end-results are essentially the same: 11 of 27 patients achieving a good result with the laminectomy and foraminotomy, and 17 of 25 having a good result with an anterior discectomy and fusion.

In summary of the treatment of cervical myelopathy due to spondylosis, it must be concluded that if operation is indicated the anterior route affords several advantages: direct access to the pathological process, restoration of the ventral contour of the spinal canal to normal, extradural procedure, and no interference with stability of the neck. The secret of success lies in proper patient selection.

Patients who are under 50 years of age and who have significant narrowing of the sagittal diameter of the cervical spinal canal, one or two levels of segmental compression, rapid progression, and not too severe neurological deficit are prime candidates for the anterior operation. In patients who are older, who have multiple levels of involvement or slow progression, or in whom the diagnosis is in doubt, exploration

---

* See references 7, 18, 29, 36, 38, 39, 46.

should be performed posteriorly, and the dura opened and grafted to enlarge that compartment.

The treatment of the paracentral disc and ridge can be summed up quite succinctly. Since the problem is always at one level and the anterior approach offers so many distinct and clear-cut advantages, it is the treatment of choice.

Treatment of patients with radiculopathy is more controversial. The issue is again clouded by many of the same factors that beset the management of the more serious problem of myelopathy. The only additional factors influencing the choice of procedure in radiculopathy patients are the type of disc problem and the incidence of complications from the anterior as compared with the posterior approach.

Some concern has been expressed regarding the relation of the choice of approach and handling of the problem to the nature of the compressing mass. If the operation is via a posterior approach for a "soft" disc, removal of the offending fragment is routinely advised. For a "hard" disc or osteophyte, however, the usual advice is to leave it alone and be content with a foraminotomy. When operating from the anterior, it has been felt, finding the offending fragment might be difficult. The addition of a fusion may render adjacent discs subject to additional strain. Aronson, Bagan, and Filtzer reported 44 patients with soft disc extrusions.[1] All were successfully found and removed from the anterior. This experience parallels the author's personal experience.

The other problem, potential danger to adjacent disc levels, is more troublesome. The exact incidence is difficult to assay, as it requires exquisite long-term follow-up studies. That it does occur is unequivocal. Cloward reported that of 200 patients, there were 7 who required a second operation for an "unrecognized disc lesion adjacent to the one previously treated or who developed another disc injury."[7] Experience at the Southwestern Medical School in over 600 anterior cervical operations has shown a very low incidence of this problem. Fewer than 10 patients have been known to develop difficulty at another level. Most of the patients were operated on less than 10 years ago, however, and most are still under 60 years of age. The true incidence and clinical significance of this potential problem remain to be identified.

Results of treating cervical disc disease with radiculopathy by a posterior hemilaminectomy approach have been reported by Odom, Finney, and Woodhall, by Haft and Shenkin, and by Stoops and King.[20,32,45] Their results are quite impressive. Odom and his associates reported 90 per cent and 96 per cent improvement rates for hard and soft disc disease operated on from the posterior.[32] Stoops and King reported that 57 per cent of their series of 49 patients with spondylosis were significantly improved, with an additional 16 per cent showing lesser degrees of improvement.[45]

The only series comparable in size to that of Odom and co-workers are Cloward's of 200 patients and Stuck's of 151 patients.[7,32,46] Cloward reported that 90 per cent of his patients had complete relief of all preoperative pain, with only 6 patients gaining no relief, and no patient being worse as far as pain was concerned.[7] He reported that 88 per cent had disappearance of objective neurological deficit, with only 6 patients being unchanged, and only one being worse. Stuck reported that 142 patients out of 151 operated upon were improved.[46] Stuck's results have been corroborated by Connolly, Seymour, and Adams, who found that, on analysis, his figures were close to their own smaller series.[10] They reported a 60 per cent improvement rate in soft disc disease and a 65 per cent rate in osteophytic disease.

COMPLICATIONS

Like any other procedure, the anterior approach has its complications. These can be reduced by careful evaluation of the patient and of the operative procedure. The complication list is long and appears formidable, but in reality, many are of minor or little consequence. Their relationship to patient morbidity is negligible in some instances. Nonetheless, it appears that the incidence of complications may be significantly higher for this approach than for hemilaminectomy.

This increased incidence is probably of little or no importance in certain diseases. For example, comparison between laminectomy and the anterior approach for a midline cervical disc is spurious. The reason is obvious; most of the complications of the anterior approach involve remedial problems, while the major complication of laminectomy is added neurological deficit. This outweighs the other less devastating complications.

Wound infection, delayed postoperative hemorrhage, operative hemorrhage, and anesthetic complications may occur, as in any operation. Operative hemorrhage is usually from a major artery or vein, particularly the vertebral ones. It is, in that circumstance, the result of the operative exposure being made too far laterally. Control of the hemorrhage may be accomplished by packing with gauze. Care should be taken to insure that packing is not placed against the nerve root, sympathetic chain, or spinal cord. Operative exposure of the vertebral artery and vein can be accomplished by removing the bony arch of the foramen transversarium through an anterior or lateral approach.[5,47] The possibility of arteriovenous fistula formation when only packing is used for control must be considered. Vertebral angiography should be done routinely in such cases. If a fistula is demonstrated, it should be repaired promptly.

Postoperative hemorrhage may be severe enough to produce airway obstruction. Evacuation of the clot should afford relief. After this, the offending vessel should be searched for and ligated. Tracheostomy is to be avoided, as it may lead to infection of the bone graft. Oral or nasal intubation is adequate.

Wound infection is a potential major catastrophe. If it extends deep, the bone graft may become involved. When this happens, removal of the graft is mandatory; if it is not done promptly an epidural abscess may result. The patient should be kept in bed, skull traction should be used if any suspicion of instability of the spine exists, and appropriate antibiotics should be administered. Sound bony fusion usually occurs in 8 to 10 weeks. Cloward reported one bone graft infection in his series of 200 cases.[7] Connolly and his associates had three infections in 63 patients.[10] Infection of the donor site may also occur. Riley and co-workers report one case, and the author has had a similar case.[34]

Specific complications of the anterior approach include injuries to soft tissues of the neck such as the esophagus, trachea, and carotid artery. These should be avoidable by attention to operative technique. Their management is clear. Repair or reconstruction of the damaged structure must be done immediately.

If perforation of the pharynx or esophagus occurs, the rent should be repaired with absorbable interrupted sutures. A single-layer closure is sufficient. The procedure should then be terminated, the wound drained for five to six days, and oral feedings prohibited for a similar period of time.

Injuries to the nervous tissue are the most devastating operative complications. Only one patient has been reported who suffered a spinal cord injury; this case report should be required reading for every surgeon doing the procedure.[8] Damage to a nerve root usually results from making the exposure too far laterally, or from too vigorous curettage in the lateral recesses of the exposure. The root may be damaged without injury to the vertebral artery, so absence of bleeding is no assurance.

Damage to the cervical sympathetic chain is rare, but can occur. Robinson and Smith reported two cases of transient Horner's syndrome.[36] Unless the exposure is made quite lateral, it is likely that such damage is really to the rami communicantes at the root level rather than to the sympathetic chain.

Pneumothorax due to perforation of the pleura is a rare complication, but potentially disastrous if unrecognized. Cloward reports one case, as do Connolly and co-workers.[7,10] Treatment is with closed-chest thoracotomy and underwater suction.

Damage to nerves to the larynx is likely to occur, as they lie in the area of the dissection. The superior laryngeal nerve is located on the lateral side of the pharynx and may be damaged by retraction or by dissection. This nerve is in particular danger if the exposure is a high cervical one. It supplies sensory fibers to the larynx and motor fibers to the pharyngeal constrictors. When it is injured, the patient has a husky, fuzzy sound to the voice, and the tone of the voice is lowered. Since the vocal cords move well, laryngoscopy does not help in the diagnosis. Only sensory examination of the larynx is positive, other than the complaint and the finding of a change in the voice. When the nerve is damaged, no return of function can be expected. One patient in the author's series, followed for over 10 years, has shown no evidence of return of function.

The recurrent laryngeal nerve ascends in the sulcus between the trachea and the esophagus and is more likely to be damaged in exposures of the lower cervical levels.

Hoarseness has been reported in 4 patients by Robinson and Smith, and in 20 patients by Cloward.[7,37] Both authors indicate that it was transient. Indirect laryngoscopy should be done prior to operation to determine the integrity of laryngeal function. When damage occurs to this nerve, paralysis of the intrinsic laryngeal muscles results. The patient has a low, hoarse, brassy speech. If no recovery ensues, silicone rubber injection into the arytenoid cartilage may result in some symptomatic improvement.

Bony complications include bone graft infections, extrusion of the graft, avascular necrosis, and pseudarthrosis. Graft infections have been mentioned. If the bone graft slips out of place, it should be replaced by open operation. During this procedure careful inspection of the graft and its bed may reveal the cause for the extrusion. Correction may require a new graft of a more appropriate size, or wires or screws may be used to fix the graft securely in place.

Extrusion of the graft occurred "in a few cases" in Cloward's series, twice in Riley, Robinson, Johnson, and Walker's series of 93 cases, and once in Aronson, Bagan and Filtzer's series (Fig. 81–3).[1,7,34]

Avascular necrosis or graft absorption is more likely to occur if several adjacent spaces are fused. Only a slender remnant of a vertebral body may be left, and, if the blood supply is inadequate, progressive collapse occurs. The graft depends on the vertebral body for its blood supply. If the body becomes avascular, the graft is resorbed, along with the avascular part of the vertebral body.

The patient may complain of increasing neck pain, and angulation of the neck will be apparent on examination. X-rays have a characteristic appearance (Figs. 81–4 and 81–5). Treatment consists of applying traction with the patient recumbent until the length of the cervical spine is restored. Then the avascular area should be resected and the bone graft replaced with either an onlay graft or a bread-loaf graft.

The incidence of avascular necrosis or graft resorption is low. Cloward mentions a 3 to 5 per cent figure.[7] Mayfield reported three cases in a series of 300 joint fusions.[29]

Pseudarthrosis is a complication whose incidence is difficult to define. If the patient has no symptoms, and no motion is shown to be present, it may be discounted

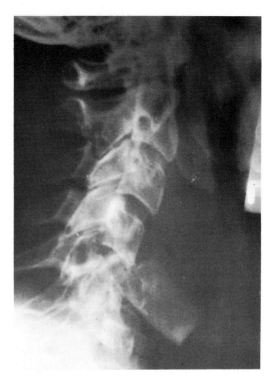

Figure 81–3 Extrusion of a bone graft.

(Figs. 81–6 and 81–7). Cloward reported a 2 per cent incidence and Stuck a 5 per cent one.[7,46] Dereymaeker, Ghosez, and Henkes had a 26 per cent incidence.[13] Connolly and his associates defined the presence of pseudarthrosis as being the absence of radiographic evidence of fusion.[10] It occurred in 21 per cent of their patients. Riley and coworkers found a 14 per cent incidence of pseudarthrosis.[34] Robinson, Walker, Ferlic, and Wiecking could not correlate the fact of fusion failure with the clinical result obtained.[38] This observation must mean that fusion is not a critical part of the operation, or that some form of fibrous non-bony union has occurred. Nonetheless, it is disturbing to find such a potentially high incidence of pseudarthrosis reported.

EVALUATION OF PATIENTS FOR ANTERIOR CERVICAL OPERATION FOR CERVICAL DISC DISEASE

This category of patients presents the greatest challenge as well as the greatest numbers. Generally, only patients with objective neurological deficit should be cho-

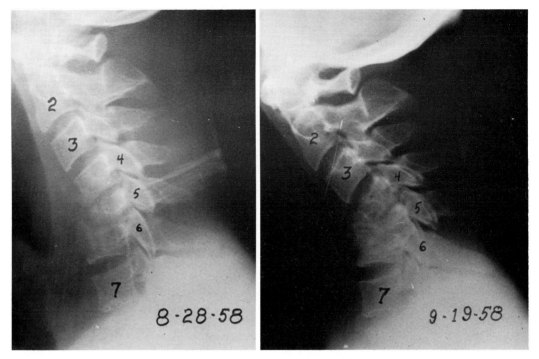

Figure 81–4   Avascular necrosis and bone graft resorption.

sen. Progress of the deficit is of some importance in the decision to operate, rapid progression being associated with greater improvement. A trial of conservative therapy is warranted in all cases.

The greatest problem is management of patients with purely subjective complaints of neck pain, arm pain, and headache. Riley and co-workers have reported a large series of patients, many with only subjective symptoms, in whom they had gratifying results.[34] They stress the need for careful and painstaking understanding of such patients.

The patient should have x-rays of the cervical spine, including motion studies of the spine, either simple flexion and extension films, or using cinefluorography. It is important that the patient perform the motion actively, as passive manipulation of the head may lead to disastrous results if instability is present.

Electromyography, of both the suspected area and adjacent and remote areas, is helpful in patients who have signs and symptoms suggestive of cervical myelopathy secondary to cervical osteoarthritis. Such patients may well have intrinsic degenerative disease of the spinal cord with no compressive component being present. Electro-

myography may reveal widespread fasciculations, indicating anterior horn cell disease of a diffuse type. In patients with monoradicular syndromes, electromyography is helpful and confirms the extent and location of the neurological lesion.

The contrast study of choice is myelography, as this gives the best possible information regarding the level of the lesion, its extent, its nature, and perhaps something about prognosis. The routine use of myelography will avoid the major diagnostic error of overlooking intradural causes of root or spinal cord compression. Since the anterior approach affords the surgeon no opportunity to inspect these structures, he must rely on myelographic evidence that no disease is present in areas beyond the proposed operative exposure.

If a limited procedure is planned, the exact level must be known. Similarly, the number of levels involved is important in planning the procedure. The surgeon should not leave significant disease at adjoining spaces, as future difficulty from them seems likely.

The myelogram is helpful in prognosis as well. Connolly and co-workers found a preoperative myelographic identification of the

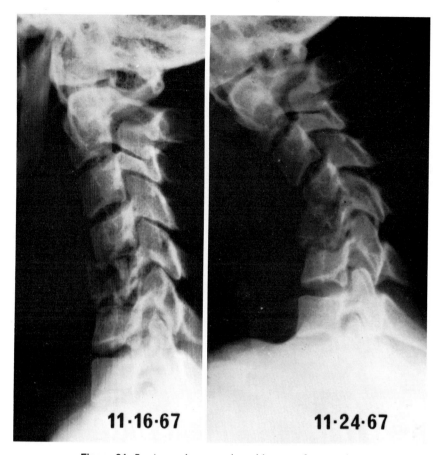

Figure 81–5   Avascular necrosis and bone graft resorption.

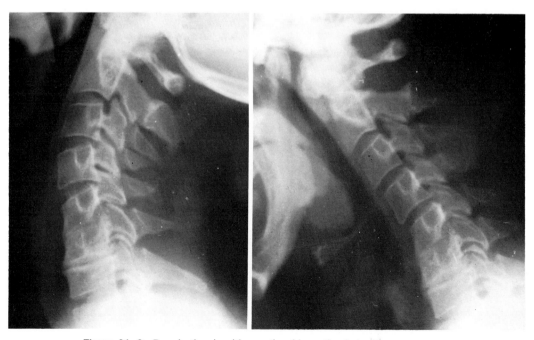

Figure 81–6   Pseudarthrosis with questionable motion but without symptoms.

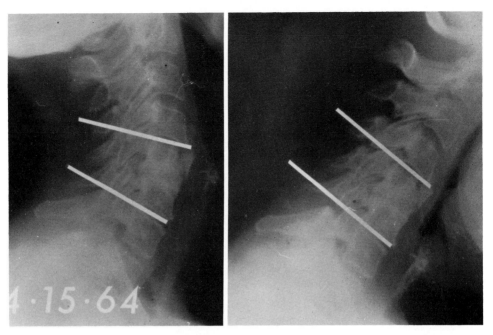

Figure 81–7 Pseudarthrosis with motion. Symptoms of pain and crepitus were present.

defect to be correlated with a good or excellent result in 80 per cent of their cases.[10] If the myelogram demonstrates multiple level involvement, the results are not likely to be so good. Riley and associates found that a satisfactory result could be expected in 75 per cent of the patients undergoing single- or double-level fusions.[34] This figure fell to 58 per cent if three or more levels were involved.

The use of discography should almost always be avoided in making decisions regarding operation for disc disease. There are numerous objections to this procedure. Discography relies heavily on subjectively evoked pain as part of the test. Injection of a hypertonic solution around joints routinely produces various forms of referred pain; in fact, this is the classic method of studying referred pain.[25,48] Because of this aspect of the technique, the test results are only questionably valid.

Holt's study of discography on asymptomatic volunteer patients demonstrated a high incidence of findings indicative of disease.[23] His report provides ample evidence that the appearance of the injected disc has little relationship to clinical disease. Riley's group used discography in a very high percentage of cases and found it quite useful.[34] The discrepancy between their findings and

Holt's is more apparent than real, however, as they employed discography after the decision to operate had been made and on the operating table. They relied on the clinical findings, plain x-ray changes, and knowledge of the course under conservative therapy to make the decision to operate. Thus, they confirm Holt's findings. Discography alone is of little value unless the clinical state is strongly indicative of degenerative disc disease.

All these ancillary tests must be considered as only confirmatory of the diagnosis, and the decision for operation must never depend on findings from them. All tests have the potential for misleading the unwary. For instance, 31 of 113 cases were "abnormal" when cervical myelography was done for other reasons in patients who had no signs or symptoms referable to the neck. More striking was the finding from the same series of a "positive" myelogram in 62 per cent of patients over 50 years of age.[27] Again, the need for careful evaluation of the patient, not the x-ray, is underscored.

Obviously, if no positive evidence of disease can be found by these tests, no operation should be contemplated. For instance, if the myelogram is completely normal, no operation should be carried out. If this happens often, the surgeon should carefully review his personal indications for myelography. A careful history, physical examination, and plain x-rays of the neck should give a firm concept of the disease process and its location. No patient, unless he has fulminating neurological deficit, should undergo operation without a trial of conservative treatment for cervical disc disease or spondylosis. The extent and type of nonoperative therapy will depend on the patient, his disease, and its response.

In summary, the anterior approach is a very useful one for benign disease of the cervical spine. The rapidity of adoption of the anterior approach by neurosurgeons throughout the world indicates its degree of superiority in managing the common benign diseases of the cervical spine. Neurosurgery owes a debt of gratitude to the individuals who developed this approach.

Careful evaluation of the patient is of prime importance. The surgeon must be sure that the symptoms are real, are caused by the suspected disorder, and are of sufficient severity to warrant operation. Failure to do so will lead to unhappiness with the procedure and the results obtained.

REFERENCES

1. Aronson, N., Bagan, M., and Filtzer, D. L.: Results of using the Smith-Robinson approach for herniated and extruded cervical discs. Technical Note. J. Neurosurg., 32:721–722, 1970.
2. Bailey, R. W., and Badgley, C. E.: Stabilization of the cervical spine by anterior fusion. J. Bone Joint Surg., 42-A:565–594, 1960.
3. Bakey, L., and Leslie, E. V.: Surgical treatment of vertebral artery insufficiency caused by cervical spondylosis. J. Neurosurg., 23:596–602, 1965.
4. Bucy, P. C., Heimburger, R. F., and Oberhill, H. R.: Compression of the cervical spinal cord by herniated intervertebral discs. J. Neurosurg., 5:471–492, 1948.
5. Clark, K., and Perry, M. O.: Carotid vertebral anastomosis: An alternate technique for repair of the subclavian steal syndrome. Ann. Surg., 163:414–416, 1966.
6. Cloward, R. B.: The anterior approach for removal of ruptured cervical discs. J. Neurosurg., 15:602–617, 1958.
7. Cloward, R. B.: New method of diagnosis and treatment of cervical disc disease. Clin. Neurosurg., 8:93–127, 1962.
8. Cloward, R. B.: Questions and answers. Clin. Neurosurg., 8:129–130, 1962.
9. Cloward, R. B.: Lesions of the intervertebral discs and their treatment by interbody fusion methods. The painful disc. Clin. Orthop., 27:51–77, 1963.
10. Connolly, E. A., Seymour, R. J., and Adams, J. E.: Clinical evaluation of anterior cervical fusion for degenerative cervical disc disease. J. Neurosurg., 23:431–437, 1965.
11. Crandall, P. H., and Batzdorf, U.: Cervical spondylotic myelopathy. J. Neurosurg., 25:57–66, 1966.
12. Dastur, D. K., Wadia, N. H., Desai, A. D., and Sinh, G.: Medullospinal compression due to atlanto-axial dislocation and sudden haematomyelia during decompression. Brain, 88:897–924, 1965.
13. Dereymaeker, A., Ghosez, J. P., and Henkes, R.: Le traitement chirurgical de la discopathie cervicale. Résultats comparés de l'abord postérieur (laminectomie) et de l'abord ventral (fusion corporeal) dans une cinquantaine de cas personnels. Neurochirurgie, 9:13–20, 1963.
14. Dohn, D. F.: Anterior interbody fusion for the treatment of cervical disc disease. J.A.M.A., 197:897–900, 1966.
15. Epstein, J. A., Epstein, B. S., and Lavine, L. S.: Cervical spondylotic myelopathy. Arch. Neurol., 8:307–317, 1963.
16. Estridge, M. N., and Smith, R. A.: Transoral fusion of odontoid fracture. J. Neurosurg., 27:462–465, 1967.
17. Fang, H. S. Y., Ong, G. B., and Hodgson, A. R.: Anterior spinal fusion: The operative approaches. Clin. Orthop., 35:16–33, 1964.
18. Galera, G. R., and Tovi, D.: Anterior disc excision with interbody fusion in cervical spondylotic myelopathy and rhizopathy. J. Neurosurg., 28:305–310, 1968.
19. Greenberg, A. D., Scoville, W. B., and Davey, L. M.: Transoral decompression of atlantoaxial dislocation due to odontoid hypoplasia. Report of two cases. J. Neurosurg., 28:266–269, 1968.
20. Haft, H., and Shenkin, H. A.: Surgical end results of cervical ridge and disc problems. J.A.M.A., 186:312–315, 1963.
21. Hankinson, H. L., and Wilson, C. B.: Use of the operating microscope in anterior cervical discectomy without fusion. J. Neurosurg., 43:452–456, 1975.
22. Hardin, C. A., Williamson, W. P., and Steegmann, A. T.: Vertebral artery insufficiency produced by cervical osteoarthritic spurs. Neurology, 10:855–858, 1960.
23. Holt, E. P., Jr.: Fallacy of cervical discography. Report of 50 cases in normal subjects. J.A.M.A., 188:799–801, 1964.
24. Kahn, E. A.: The role of the dentate ligaments in spinal cord compression and the syndrome of lateral sclerosis. J. Neurosurg., 4:191–199, 1947.
25. Kellgren, J. H.: On the distribution of pain arising from deep somatic structures with charts of segmental pain areas. Clin. Sci., 4:35–46, 1939.
26. Martins, A. N.: Anterior cervical discectomy with and without interbody bone graft. J. Neurosurg., 44:290–295, 1976.
27. Martins, A. N., Kempe, L. G., Pitkethly, D. T., and Ferry, D. J.: Reappraisal of the cervical myelogram. J. Neurosurg., 27:27–31, 1967.
28. Mayfield, F. H.: New instrument. J. Neurosurg., 14:469, 1957.

29. Mayfield, F. H.: Cervical spondylosis: A comparison of the anterior and posterior approaches. Clin. Neurosurg., *13*:181–188, 1965.

30. Mullan, S., Naunton, R., Hekmatpanah, J., and Vailati, G.: The use of an anterior approach to ventrally placed tumors in the foramen magnum and vertebral column. J. Neurosurg., *24*:536–543, 1966.

31. Myers, P. W.: Anterior spinal fusion. Minn. Med., *52*:391–408, 1969.

32. Odom, G. L., Finney, W., and Woodhall, B.: Cervical disc lesions. J.A.M.A., *166*:23–28, 1958.

33. Raynor, R. B., and Kingman, A. F., Jr.: Decompression of a cervical root sleeve by the anterior approach. A laboratory study. J. Neurosurg., *21*:378–380, 1964.

34. Riley, L. H., Jr., Robinson, R. A., Johnson, K. A., and Walker, A. E.: The results of anterior interbody fusion of the cervical spine. J. Neurosurg., *30*:127–133, 1969.

35. Robertson, J. T.: Anterior removal of cervical disc without fusion. Clin. Neurosurg., *20*:259–261, 1973.

36. Robinson, R. A.: Anterior and posterior cervical spine fusions. Clin. Orthop., *35*:34–62, 1964.

37. Robinson, R. A., and Smith, G. W.: Anterolateral cervical disc removal and interbody fusion for cervical disc syndrome. Bull. Johns Hopk. Hosp., *96*:223–224, 1955.

38. Robinson, R. A., Walker, A. E., Ferlic, D. C., and Wiecking, D. K.: The results of anterior interbody fusion of the cervical spine. J. Bone Joint Surg., *44-A*:1569–1587, 1962.

39. Rosomoff, H. L., and Rossman, F.: Treatment of cervical spondylosis by anterior diskectomy and fusion. Arch. Neurol., *14*:392–398, 1966.

40. Scoville, W. B.: Cervical spondylosis treated by bilateral facetectomy and laminectomy. J. Neurosurg., *18*:423–428, 1961.

41. Smith, B. H.: Cervical Spondylosis and Its Neurological Complications. Springfield, Ill., Charles C Thomas, 1968.

42. Southwick, W. O., and Robinson, R. A.: Surgical approaches to the vertebral bodies in the cervical and lumbar regions. J. Bone Joint Surg., *39-A*:631–644, 1957.

43. Stevenson, G. C., Stoney, R. J., Perkins, R. K., and Adams, J. E.: A transcervical transclival approach to the ventral surface of the brain stem for removal of a clivus chordoma. J. Neurosurg., *24*:544–551, 1966.

44. Stookey, B.: Compression of the spinal cord due to ventral extradural cervical chondromas. Diagnosis and surgical treatment. Arch. Neurol. Psychiat., *20*:275–291, 1928.

45. Stoops, W. L., and King, R. B.: Neural complications of cervical spondylosis. Their response to laminectomy and foramenotomy. J. Neurosurg., *19*:986–999, 1962.

46. Stuck, R. M.: Anterior cervical disc excision and fusion. Report of 200 consecutive cases. Rocky Mountain Med. J., *60*:25–30, 1963.

47. Verbiest, H.: A lateral approach to the cervical spine. Technique and indications. J. Neurosurg., *28*:191–203, 1968.

48. Weddell, G., Sinclair, D. C., Feindel, W. H., and Falconer, M. A.: The intervertebral ligaments as a source of segmental pain. J. Bone Joint Surg., *30-B*:515–521, 1948

82

SCOLIOSIS, KYPHOSIS, AND LORDOSIS

Deformities of the spine are a common problem. When severe, they may lead to grotesque cosmetic deformities as well as serious alterations of body function. Any curvature significantly involving the thoracic spine may alter lung function. As the curvature progresses, lung function decreases, and eventually death may occur. Deformities of the lumbar spine, because of the increased motion and stresses in the lumbar spine, often lead to disc degeneration and painful arthritic conditions. Untreated kyphotic deformities, particularly if sharp and angular, may produce paraplegia. Thus, curvature of the spine may have profound physical as well as psychological implications. Like headache, spinal deformity is a symptom, not a disease. Prudent management is based upon sound diagnosis and sound application of basic principles.

Table 82–1 gives the official glossary of the Scoliosis Research Society. In this glossary several terms are used to describe curves. These terms have often been used interchangeably when they should not have been. Therefore it seems desirable to comment further at this time in order to avoid confusion later in this chapter. The terms that cause confusion are: "primary curves," "secondary curves," "compensatory curves," "major curves," "minor curves," "structural curves," and "nonstructural curves."

A structural curve is "a segment of the spine with a *fixed* lateral curvature. Radiographically, it is identified in supine lateral side-bending films by the failure to correct." The key word here is "fixed." There is a segment or area of the spine that does

not have normal segmental mobility. By definition, then, a nonstructural curve has normal flexibility. A good example of a nonstructural curve is the one seen in the lumbar spine of a patient with inequality of leg length. With the leg length corrected by a lift, the curve disappears. In the sitting or supine position, the curve disappears. As demonstrated on bending films, the spine bends equally to right and left, with no area of fixation. Leg length inequality, even if it exists for many years, does not cause a structural curve.

A compensatory curve is "a curve above or below a major curve that tends to maintain normal body alignment. It may be structural or nonstructural." When a patient has a single structural curve, regardless of etiology, there must be a curve above or below that curve (or both) in order to maintain an erect posture with reference to gravity. At first, the compensatory curve is fully flexible, thus nonstructural. Over the course of time, however, the tissues become "fixed" in this curved position, and the compensatory curve becomes structural. Even though it develops structural qualities, it is still a compensatory curve.

"Secondary curve" is another name for a compensatory curve. The word "secondary" is used by those physicians who like to use the term "primary curve" to describe the original structural curve of the patient.

A "primary curve" is "the first or earliest of several curves to appear, if identifiable." Often the patient comes to the physician at the age of sixteen with two structural curves, both quite significant,

R. WINTER, J. LONSTEIN, AND S. CHOU

TABLE 82–1 TERMINOLOGY FROM OFFICIAL GLOSSARY OF THE SCOLIOSIS RESEARCH SOCIETY*

Adolescent scoliosis	Spinal curvature presenting at or about the onset of puberty and before maturity	Iliac epiphysis (iliac apophysis)	The epiphysis along the wing of an ilium
Adult scoliosis	Spinal curvature existing after skeletal maturity	Infantile scoliosis	Spinal curvature developing during the first 3 years of life
Apical vertebra	The most rotated vertebra in a curve; the most deviated vertebra from the vertical axis of the patient	Juvenile scoliosis	Spinal curvature developing between skeletal age of 3 years and the onset of puberty
Body alignment, balance, compensation	The alignment of the midpoint of the occiput over the sacrum in the same vertical plane as the shoulders over the hips	Kyphos	A change in the alignment of a segment of the spine in the sagittal plane that increases the posterior convex angulation beyond normal
Café au lait spots	Light brow irregular areas of skin pigmentation. If sufficient in number and with smooth margins, they suggest neurofibromatosis	Kyphoscoliosis	Lateral curvature of the spine associated with either increased posterior or decreased anterior angulation in the sagittal plane in excess of the accepted norm for that region
Compensatory curve	A curve above or below a major curve that tends to maintain normal body alignment. It may be structural or nonstructural	Lordoscoliosis	Lateral curvature of the spine associated with an increase in the anterior curvature or a decrease in posterior angulation in the sagittal plane in excess of normal for that region
Congenital scoliosis	Scoliosis due to congenitally anomalous vertebral development		
Curve measurement	Cobb method: Select the upper and lower end vertebrae. Erect perpendiculars to their transverse axis.	Major curve	Term used to designate the larger(est) curve(s), usually structural
	They intersect to form the angle of the curve. If the vertebral end plates are poorly visualized, a line through the bottom or top of the pedicles may be used	Minor curve	Term used to refer to the smaller(est) curve(s), which may be structural or nonstructural.
		Pelvic obliquity	Deviation of the pelvis from the horizontal in the frontal plane
Double major scoliosis	A scoliosis with two structural curves	Primary curve	The first or earliest of several curves to appear, if identifiable
End vertebra	The most cephalad vertebra of a curve whose superior surface, or the most caudad one whose inferior surface tilts maximally toward the concavity of the curve	Rib hump	The prominence of the ribs on the convexity of a spinal curvature, usually due to vertebral rotation best exhibited on forward bending
Nonstructural curve, functional curve	A curve which has no structural component and which corrects or overcorrects on recumbent side-bending roentgenograms	Skeletal age, bone age	The age obtained by comparing an anteroposterior roentgenogram of the left hand and wrist with the standards of the Gruelich and Pyle Atlas
Gibbus	A sharply angular kyphos	Structural curve	A segment of the spine with a fixed lateral curvature. Radiographically, it is identified in supine lateral side-bending films by the failure to correct. They may be multiple
Hysterical scoliosis	A nonstructural deformity of the spine that develops as a manifestation of a conversion reaction		
Idiopathic scoliosis	A structural spinal curvature for which no cause is established		

* From Moe, J. H., Winter, R. B., Bradford, D. S., and Lonstein, J. E.: Scoliosis and Other Spinal Deformities. Philadelphia, W. B. Saunders Co., 1978, pp. 9–10. Reprinted by permission.

both about equal in magnitude, and both having structural qualities. In this case, it can be quite difficult or even impossible to know whether the patient has one primary curve and one secondary curve with highly structural qualities, or two primary curves.

Double or even triple primary curves are well recognized.

Because of the frequent difficulty of defining a "primary" curve, many physicians abandoned that term and used instead the word "major." A major curve is "the

TABLE 82–2 CLASSIFICATION OF SCOLIOSIS

STRUCTURAL SCOLIOSIS
Idiopathic
  Infantile
    Resolving
    Progressive
  Juvenile
  Adolescent
Neuromuscular
  Neuropathic
    Upper motor neuron
      Cerebral palsy
      Spinocerebellar degeneration
        Friedreich's
        Charcot-Marie Tooth
        Roussy-Lévy
      Syringomyelia
      Spinal cord tumor
      Spinal cord trauma
      Other
    Lower motor neuron
      Poliomyelitis
      Other viral myelitides
      Traumatic
      Spinal muscular atrophy
        Werdnig-Hoffmann
        Kugelberg-Welander
      Myelomeningocele (paralytic)
    Dysautonomia (Riley-Day)
    Other
  Myopathic
    Arthrogryposis
    Muscular dystrophy
      Duchenne (pseudohypertrophic)
      Limb-girdle
      Facioscapulohumeral
    Fiber-type disproportion
    Congenital hypotonia
    Myotonia dystrophica
    Other
Congenital
  Failure of formation
    Wedge vertebra
    Hemivertebra
  Failure of segmentation
    Unilateral (unsegmented bar)
    Bilateral
  Mixed
Neurofibromatosis

Mesenchymal disorders
  Marfan's syndrome
  Ehlers-Danlos syndrome
  Others
Rheumatoid disease
Trauma
  Fracture
  Operative
    Postlaminectomy
    Postthoracoplasty
  Irradiation
Extraspinal contractures
  Postempyema
  Post burns
Osteochondrodystrophies
  Diastrophic dwarfism
  Mucopolysaccharidoses (e.g., Morquio's)
  Spondyloepiphyseal dysplasia
  Multiple epiphyseal dysplasia
  Other
Infection of bone
  Acute
  Chronic
Metabolic disorders
  Rickets
  Osteogenesis imperfecta
  Homocystinuria
  Others
Related to lumbosacral joint
  Spondylolysis and spondylolisthesis
  Congenital anomalies of lumbosacral region
Tumors
  Vertebral column
    Osteoid osteoma
    Histiocytosis X
    Other
  Spinal cord (see neuromuscular)
NONSTRUCTURAL SCOLIOSIS
Postural scoliosis
Hysterical scoliosis
Nerve root irritation
  Herniation of nucleus pulposis
  Tumors
Inflammatory (e.g., appendicitis)
Related to leg length discrepancy
Related to contractures about the hip

larger curve, usually structural," as distinguished from a minor curve, "the smaller curve, which may be structural or nonstructural."

Thus, the patient presenting with two curves, both large and both structural, would have what might be called a "double primary curve pattern" by one physician and a "double major curve pattern" by another.

ETIOLOGY

As can be seen in Tables 82–2, 82–3, and 82–4, there are many causes for spinal deformity. At the turn of the century, most patients from North America presenting with deformity of the spine had tuberculosis. Later, there were large numbers of patients with spinal deformity due to poliomyelitis, particularly in the great epidemics of the 1940's and 1950's. With the eradication of poliomyelitis, it might have been assumed that the number of patients with curvature of the spine would significantly diminish, but it has not.

The most common cause of spinal deformity now is idiopathic scoliosis. The etiology of this condition is unknown. It accounts, however, for about 70 per cent of the patients coming to any spinal deformity clinic.[29] It is a genetically related disease. Although in the population at the age of nine or ten the sex incidence of idiopathic

TABLE 82-3   CLASSIFICATION OF KYPHOSIS

Postural
Scheuermann's disease
Congenital
   Defect of formation
   Defect of segmentation
   Mixed
Neuromuscular
Myelomeningocele
   Developmental (late paralytic)
   Congenital (present at birth)
Inflammatory
   Due to bone or ligament damage without cord injury
   Due to bone or ligament damage with cord injury
Postoperative
   Postlaminectomy
   Post excision of vertebral body
Postirradiation
Metabolic
   Osteoporosis
     Senile
     Juvenile
   Osteomalacia
   Osteogenesis imperfecta
   Other
Skeletal dysplasias
   Achondroplasia
   Mucopolysaccharidoses
   Neurofibromatosis
   Other
Collagen disease
   Marie-Strümpell disease
   Other
Tumor
   Benign
   Malignant
     Primary
     Metastatic

scoliosis with very mild curves is nearly equal, it is the female who is most likely to have a progressive curve, a curve requiring treatment. In the authors' experience, about 80 per cent of those being treated by operation or braces are girls. No definite abnormality of the bones, muscles, nervous system, or connective tissue system has been demonstrated in idiopathic scoliosis. These children are born with a straight spine, which at some point during growth begins to bend and deform, tending to get progressively worse until the end of growth. Recent experiences with large school screening projects demonstrated

TABLE 82-4   CLASSIFICATION OF LORDOSIS

Postural
Congenital
Neuromuscular
Postlaminectomy
Secondary to hip flexion contracture
Other

nearly 5 per cent of the North American population has a slight curve by the age of 12.[23] Only about three children per thousand require treatment, however. Thus, a large number of mild curvatures exist in the population but are nonprogressive and nonpathological. These minor curves, which cause little concern other than the fear that they might become progressive, are not discussed in this chapter. It is the progressively deforming curvatures that demand treatment and that are discussed.

The second most common deformity presenting to the authors' clinic is Scheuermann's disease, or adolescent kyphosis. Following in frequency are congenital spinal deformities (curvatures due to congenital abnormal bone development). These are seen fairly frequently by neurosurgeons and are discussed at some length later. Next in frequency are paralytic curves due to any type of paralyzing condition in the growing child. An uncommon, but very troublesome, cause of deformity of the spine is von Recklinghausen's neurofibromatosis. Although the incidence of these curvatures is low, the curvatures themselves are very difficult to manage and are fraught with problems both in the untreated and treated patients.

The many other causes of spinal deformity are seen less frequently. Generally, the more unusual the cause of the deformity, the more difficult it is to treat.

NATURAL HISTORY

Spinal deformity is more than a cosmetic problem. It deserves serious study and may need treatment.

When studying the natural history of any disease process, it is of utmost importance to locate large numbers of patients who have never had any treatment and to study their condition in its undisturbed state. Fortunately, several studies have been made of scoliosis in the untreated individual. The best are those by Nachemson and Nilsonne and Lundgren.[34,37] These two studies from Scandinavia showed that the mortality rate of untreated scoliotics was twice that of the normal population, and for thoracic curvatures alone, the mortality rate was four times that in the normal population. In addition, in Nilsonne and Lundgren's study, 76 per cent of the females were unmarried, and there frequently were psychosomatic disorders related to poor body image. Nilsonne and Lundgren's study dealt only with idiopathic scoliosis. Nachemson's study examined scoliosis from many different causes, and he showed that the patient with congential thoracic scoliosis was particularly at risk for cor pulmonale. The study by Collis and Ponseti is of considerable interest in that they demonstrated that curvatures tended to progress throughout life rather than to stop progressing at the end of growth (Fig. 82–1).[10]

Pain in Adult Scoliosis

Scoliosis frequently is seen in adults. Most centers for correction of spinal deformities are seeing an increasing number of adults as treatment methods are improved and more patients seek correction of their problems. The most frequent complaint in the adult is pain. This complaint is most commonly associated with primary lumbar curves, second with the thoracolumbar curves, and a little less commonly with the purely thoracic curves. The pain is caused by degenerative disc disease and degenerative facet joint disease in the curvature itself and sometimes in the compensatory curve below the primary curve. Seldom radicular in character, the pain usually is of a mechanical type, absent at night and with rest, not very bothersome early in the day, but progressive through the day. When severe, the pain significantly hampers the activity of the patient, and may force him to bed for varying periods of the day. The manual laborer may be totally incapacitated and need reeducation for other employment if the problem is not corrected. In the housewife, the condition may hamper her ability to carry on the normal activities of the house (cf. Fig. 82–1).

Loss of Pulmonary Function

The loss of pulmonary function is of critical importance and is the compelling reason for treatment of most patients with scoliosis.* In general, curvatures above 60 degrees, as measured by the Cobb technique, tend to produce diminution of pulmonary

---

* See references 1, 14, 15, 27, 46, 48.

function with greater loss of function with greater curvature.[32] If the patient is slightly kyphotic, the lung can increase its anteroposterior diameter when the lateral diameter is impaired and thus may maintain normal pulmonary function despite a significant lateral curvature. Severe kyphosis, however, will result in such loss of vertical height of the thorax that pulmonary function may be seriously impaired.

Lordotic problems, particularly in the thoracic spine, produce the most serious impairment of pulmonary function owing to the squeezing of the lung between the spine posteriorly and the sternum and ribs anteriorly.[48] Since this loss of pulmonary function is virtually impossible to correct to any great extent once it has occurred, it is of the utmost importance that curvatures be treated early enough to prevent any significant loss of pulmonary function. Individuals with paralytic diseases such as poliomyelitis already may have impaired pulmonary function due to intercostal paralysis and are thus unable to tolerate even a small additional diminution due to the curvature. Patients seldom die of cor pulmonale during their growing years and relatively infrequently during the 20's, but among those with quite severe curvatures, the death rate begins to increase in their 30's and 40's and increases precipitously after the age of 45.[37] Thus, the best treatment for the 45-year-old patient with cor pulmonale due to spinal deformity would be to have prevented the condition by adequate correction when the person was a growing child.

Psychological Impact

Psychological impairment of the patient can be significant with ugly deformities. As is true with many problems, some patients react strongly to even a mild deformity, whereas others may tolerate a hideous or grotesque deformity. Nevertheless, the psychological aspects of the person's self-image cannot be ignored and enter strongly into the need for treatment.

Paralysis Due to Curvature

Of particular concern to the neurosurgeon is the problem of paralysis *caused by*

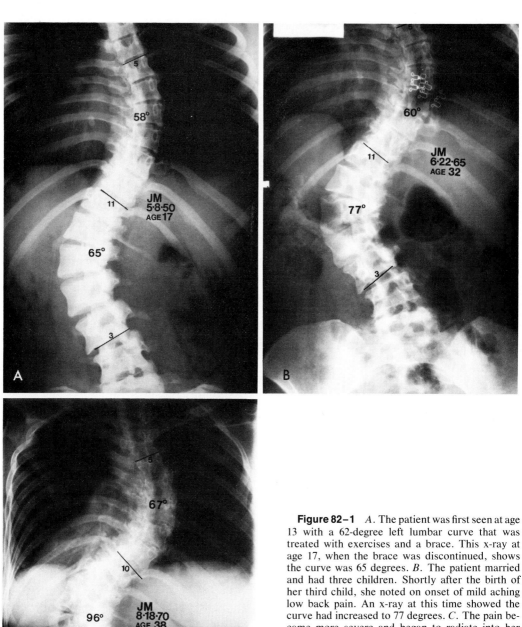

Figure 82–1 *A.* The patient was first seen at age 13 with a 62-degree left lumbar curve that was treated with exercises and a brace. This x-ray at age 17, when the brace was discontinued, shows the curve was 65 degrees. *B.* The patient married and had three children. Shortly after the birth of her third child, she noted on onset of mild aching low back pain. An x-ray at this time showed the curve had increased to 77 degrees. The pain became more severe and began to radiate into her legs. At age 38, the curve had increased to 96 degrees.

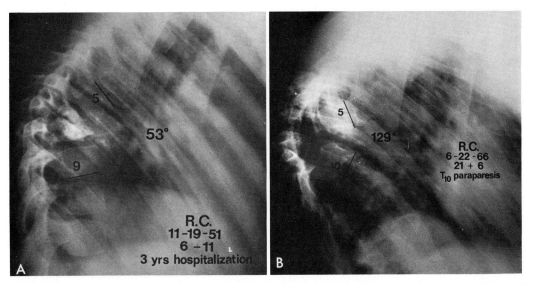

Figure 82–2   *A*. This boy contracted tuberculosis at age 4. After three years of hospitalization, he was discharged with a thoracic kyphosis of 53 degrees. *B*. The kyphosis progressed, and he presented at age 21 years and 6 months with a sharp angular kyphosis of 129 degrees and a T10 level paraparesis.

the curvature. Scoliosis alone, no matter how severe, does not cause paraparesis or paraplegia. The authors have seen curvatures as great as 200 degrees without paralysis. A patient who develops paralysis due to the curve has either pure kyphosis or kyphoscoliosis. It is usually a sharply angulated spinal deformity and is most commonly a congenital kyphosis. The patient with congential kyphosis is particularly prone to a sharp angular deformity owing to absence of the vertebral body anteriorly and may also have a tethered cord leading to paralysis sooner than would be expected with the amount of deformity present. The second most common sharply angulated kyphoscoliosis causing paralysis is that of neurofibromatosis. Another paralysis-causing curve is found in acute tuberculosis with both abscess and the kyphotic deformity. Late tuberculosis in which the infection is dormant but a sharply angulated residual kyphus remains may cause pressure on the spinal cord. Any sharply angulated kyphosis, particularly if it is in the thoracic spine and especially if it is at the "watershed area" at T4 through T8, may cause paraplegia.[25] The treatment of this is discussed later (Fig. 82–2).

NONOPERATIVE TREATMENT

When confronted with a patient with an abnormal curvature of the spine, the treating physician has three choices: (1) observation of the problem without active medical treatment, (2) treatment by nonoperative methods, and (3) treatment by operative methods. For minimal curvatures that are producing no complaints, mere observation of the patient is indicated. For example, a 25-year-old woman with a 25-degree thoracic scoliosis without any symptoms does not require any treatment. She has a minimally deforming curvature, not sufficient to cause impairment of pulmonary function, not painful, and not altering her life style. The quantity of visible deformity is so minimal that psychological impairment does not occur. A 25-degree thoracic curve in an 11-year-old girl is totally different. Because of the patient's age and the natural history of this condition, she should be treated. If she is not, she will probably develop a progressive deformity and any or all of the problems listed earlier. A 10-degree curve in this 11-year-old child would not require treatment but should be carefully watched at frequent intervals. If the curvature shows any tendency toward progression, treatment should begin.

Nonoperative treatment is essentially treatment with braces. Exercises alone do not correct any deformities except those such as sway back and round back that are due to purely postural causes. In these situations, it is really not the exercises that correct the curvature but rather the awareness of their own body contours that patients derive from the exercise that is therapeutic. Exercises are frequently combined with brace treatment to produce an optimal curve correction as well as to maintain good muscle tone while the patient is wearing the brace.

Treatment with braces has become a widely used and well-refined art. There are many different styles of braces, but the two basic types are the Milwaukee brace and the lumbar brace (Fig. 82–3). Considerable experience has been gained with the Milwaukee brace and its use has proved highly reliable in preventing curves from progressing in the growing child.[2,8,28,30] It has, however, not proved of great value in permanently transforming large curves into small curves. It has been used successfully to prevent an increase of the curve and the need for operation in a large number of patients with adolescent idiopathic scoliosis. The second greatest benefit of the brace has been its application to young children with serious curvature problems that eventually require fusion. Use of the brace allows the spine to grow so that when the fusion is done, it does not cause stunting of trunk height. This feature is particularly valuable in patients with paralytic and congenital spine disorders.[7,50]

The Milwaukee brace is even more effective for Scheuermann's disease than it is for the usual scoliosis problems for which it was designed. Scheuermann's disease, being a midthoracic deformity, does not respond to lumbar braces or braces that only come up to the sternum. Virtually all cases of Scheuermann's disease in growing children can be successfully treated with braces and do not require operative treatment.[3] A few symptomatic and advanced cases of Scheuermann's disease in young adults do require an operation.[4]

Curvatures involving the lumbar spine do not require treatment with the Milwaukee brace. These can be managed with a molded plastic brace designed specifically for lumbar curves. Like the Milwaukee

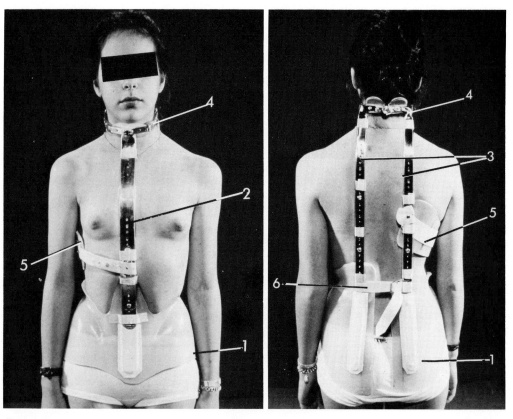

Figure 82–3 Anterior and posterior view of a patient in a Milwaukee brace. The brace consists of a molded plastic pelvic section (1) with a single anterior upright (2) and two posterior uprights (3), which connect to the neck ring (4). A corrective thoracic pad (5) and a lumbar pad (6) help control the scoliotic curves. (Brace designed by Blount and Schmidt.)

brace, these must be individually designed to fit the patient and the particular curve problem, and cannot be obtained "off the shelf" from a brace supplier.

Stiff and rigid deformities do not respond to bracing and usually require an operation. Braces will not correct adult curvatures and thus are applicable only to growing children. They can be used in the adult for relief of pain due to curvatures but not for correction of the curve or prevention of increase in it.

OPERATIVE TREATMENT

Hibbs performed the first spinal fusion for the treatment of kyphosis in 1911.[19] Since then thousands of fusions have been performed in the treatment of spinal deformity, particularly scoliosis. At first these posterior fusions were done merely to stop further progression, with no attempt at correction of the problem.

In the 1920's and 1930's corrective casts were designed, which not only held the spine still while the fusion was solidifying but also placed the spine in a corrected position so that the patient actually had some improvement of the deformity by the time the fusion was solid. In those years, without good blood banking and with precarious anesthetic techniques, the risks of operation for scoliosis were rather grave, and this was not a widely used technique.

In the 1940's and 1950's, with the advent of good anesthesia and good transfusion capability, a vast improvement in the operative treatment of scoliosis evolved. At this time posterior spinal fusion was still the only operation available, but it was done with increasingly better results and smaller risks. By the late 1950's the posterior spinal fusion with cast correction had become a highly polished operative technique that, when applied with reasonable care and to curvatures of reasonable degree, was extremely successful in correcting the curve and maintaining that correction for life.

About 1960 enormous changes emerged in the operative treatment for spinal deformity. Hodgson and co-workers worked with patients with tuberculosis to devise the anterior approach to the spine.[20] About the same time, Harrington invented the rods that were the first truly effective method of internal fixation of the spine

(Fig. 82–4).[12,16–18] Meanwhile, Perry and associates developed the halo mechanism, an adaptation of a device originally designed for treatment of maxillofacial injuries (Fig. 82–5).[36] Finally in the late 1960's, Dwyer invented an anterior device for not only fusion but also correction from the anterior approach.[13] These advanced methods, in terms of both correction and internal stabilization, brought marvelous improvements in the ability of surgeons to treat spinal deformity, as shown in Figures 82–4 and 82–6, but unfortunately, they have also brought an increased number of complications, particularly neurological.

Posterior Fusion

Posterior fusion requires a careful subperiosteal exposure of the area to be fused, including the capsules of the facet joints. The ligamentum flavum is left intact. The articular joints are carefully excised with sharp gouges and osteotomes, and all cartilage is removed from them. Small plugs of autogenous iliac cancellous bone are packed into the spaces from which the joints have been excised. The entire exposed bone surface is then decorticated, a sharp gouge lifting up chips and slivers of bone throughout the proposed fusion area. These chips and slivers are scattered up and down in a longitudinal fashion, and on top of these are layered further slivers and chips of autogenous iliac bone removed from the posterior iliac crest area through a separate incision. Once all these bone chips have been inserted, the muscles are laid back over the fusion mass and sutured in place along the midline. Subcutaneous and skin closure follow. About five to seven days postoperatively the patient is placed in a corrective cast, usually a Risser localizer cast, which gives a good correction of the deformity and holds the spine in the corrected position while the bone knits. The usual healing time for such a spinal fusion is nine months (Fig. 82–7).

Anterior Fusion

For certain problems, both anterior and posterior fusion are necessary. Anterior fusion has been found vital for the fusion of kyphotic deformity, whereas posterior fu-

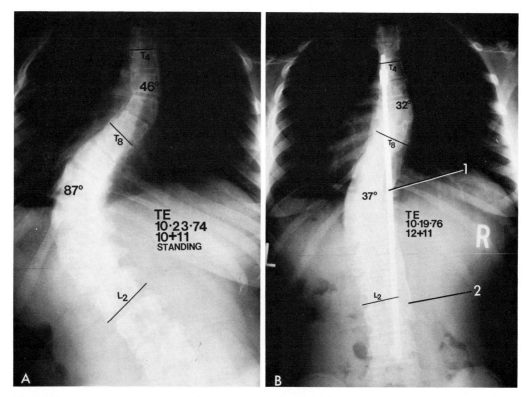

Figure 82–4   *A.* Initial standing x-ray of a 10-year-and-11-month-old girl with a T4–T8 right thoracic curve of 46 degrees and a T8–L2 left thoracolumbar curve of 87 degrees. *B.* Approximately two years after spinal fusion with instrumentation with a Harrington rod (1) the curves measure 32 degrees and 37 degrees. The lumbar fusion mass is well seen (2).

sion alone usually suffices for purely scoliotic deformities. In the performance of an anterior fusion, the spine is exposed through an anterior incision, which for T1 to T12 is a thoracotomy, or if the fusion has to be extended below T12, a combined thoracotomy and retroperitoneal dissection. For purely lumbar curves, a sympathectomy-type incision is utilized. Once the area to be fused has been properly identified, the segmental vessels along the lateral aspect of the vertebral body are ligated and the vertebral bodies exposed subperiosteally. The discs are thoroughly excised back to the posterior longitudinal ligament and the posterior annulus, but it is not necessary to enter the spinal canal. In certain cases, strong struts of bone are necessary. For these struts, cortical iliac bone, a piece of rib, or in some cases a segment of fibula may be used. For other situations, it is only necessary to clean out the disc spaces and pack them with small chips of bone obtained from the rib and iliac crest. In either case, fusion takes about nine months to so-

lidify to the point of being able to support the patient without any cast or brace. In most circumstances in which anterior fusion is performed, a posterior fusion of the same area is usually done about two weeks later.

Harrington Instrumentation

Harrington instruments were devised as a method of posterior internal correction and stabilization of the spine.[12,16–18] These consist of two types of metal rods and hooks, the most commonly used being the distraction rod, which is a solid bar of stainless steel ratcheted at one end, each end fitting into hooks of the same metal. With a distractor, the rod is gradually elongated on the hook, and the curve is corrected. When the appropriate correction has been obtained, the rod is wired into place on the hook so that it will not loosen. Then the same type of fusion is performed as described earlier. Fusion must *always* be per-

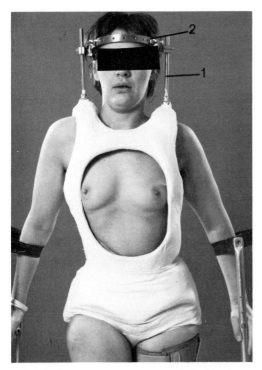

Figure 82–5   A postpoliomyelitis patient in a halo and cast. The pelvic area is well molded above the iliac crests, and there is a large chest window to allow full chest expansion. Two ''lo profile'' halo uprights (1) connect the cast to the halo (2).

formed in conjunction with instrumentation, since the instruments are only temporary holding devices and do not substitute for a fusion (see Fig. 82–4). The second type of Harrington instrument is called a contracting rod and consists of a thin ⅛-inch threaded metal rod with hooks that fit over the transverse processes in the thoracic spine and under the edge of the lamina in the lumbar spine. These cause a shortening of the convex side of the curve and correct kyphosis quite well (Fig. 82–8). Contracting rods are quite often used in conjunction with a distraction rod, compressing and shortening the convex side of the curve while the concave side is lengthened and distracted. For purely kyphotic deformities, two contracting rods with several hooks are usually used.

Dwyer Instrumentation

The Dwyer instrument is a device that provides internal correction and fixation for anterior spinal fusions.[13] It is most applicable to curves with the major portion between T10 and L4, since anatomical exposure below this level is difficult and above this level the discs are so narrow that very little correction can be obtained. The Dwyer screw and staple unit is inserted after the discs have been removed, a cable is then threaded through a hole in the eye of the screw, and the screw heads are pulled together. The screw heads are then crimped on the cable, preventing them from spreading apart again (Fig. 82–9). This procedure corrects a curve by shortening the convex side. Because the discs are removed and the bodies are pulled together, this apparatus is excellent for correcting lordosis but has a great disadvantage in that if the patient has a normal lumbar lordosis it tends to pull the spine into an abnormal lumbar kyphosis. This device is also useful for long curvatures that result from paralysis. In these patients it is combined with a Harrington instrumentation posteriorly at a separate stage (see Fig. 82–6). The Dwyer procedure is performed far less commonly than the Harrington procedure. The four foregoing procedures constitute the majority of operations performed for the treatment of spinal deformity. Other operations are worth mention, however, since they too may have potential neurological complications.

Osteotomy of the Fusion Mass

Patients who were operated upon many years ago often had a fusion performed without correction and thus were locked into a pathological position. For many years there was no adequate answer for this problem. Recently it has been found that one can osteotomize the posterior fusion mass, re-creating the normal amount of mobility of the spine.[31,43] Since the discs remain virtually normal anteriorly, even though a posterior fusion has been performed several years before, once the posterior fusion mass is divided, mobility is created again. Most centers doing a significant number of reconstructive and salvage procedures on the spine have found this osteotomy to be extremely useful. Most often several osteotomies of the old fusion mass are performed, and the patient is then placed in skeletal traction for two weeks for

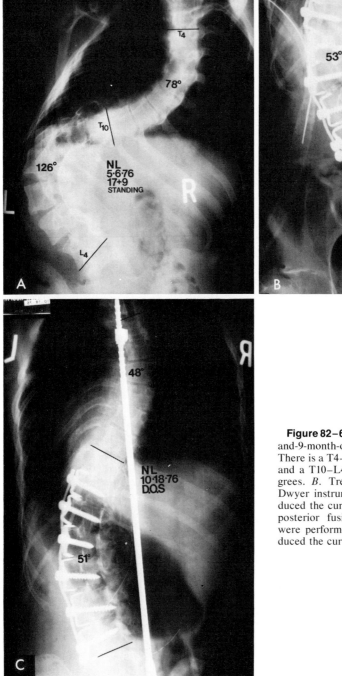

Figure 82–6 *A*. Initial standing x-ray of a 17-year-and-9-month-old boy with cerebral palsy scoliosis. There is a T4–T10 right thoracic curve of 78 degrees and a T10–L4 left thoracolumbar curve of 126 degrees. *B*. Treatment was by anterior fusion and Dwyer instrumentation from T11 to L4, which reduced the curve to 53 degrees. *C*. Two weeks later posterior fusion and Harrington instrumentation were performed from T4 to the sacrum, which reduced the curves to 48 degrees and 51 degrees.

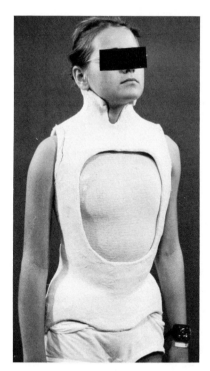

Figure 18–7 A patient in a postoperative Risser-Cotrel body cast. Note the well-molded pelvic section with careful molding over the iliac crests. There is a large thoracic window to allow full chest expansion. The cast fits snugly around the neck and under the occiput and mandible to help control the spine.

a slow correction of the deformity while awake. After an adequate correction is obtained, the wound is reopened, the rod is inserted to maintain the correction, and bone graft is added to obtain fusion of the corrected position (Fig. 82–10).

Osteotomy of the Ankylosed Spine

Patients with ankylosing spondylitis (Marie-Strümpell disease) often present with severe kyphotic deformity. Osteotomy of the posterior elements can be made, preferably at the L2–L3 level below the conus, and Harrington compression rods inserted and the osteotomy site closed.[41] The ossified anterior longitudinal ligament will give way, permitting 30 or 40 degrees of correction at one level. This is then maintained in a cast until the osteotomy site is solidly healed, usually requiring six to nine months. These patients are usually grateful for the increased view of the world that they obtain. Since it is a closing wedge pos-

teriorly, care must be taken to insure adequate foraminal space for the exiting nerve roots (Fig. 82–11).

Excision of Hemivertebra

A hemivertebra, particularly if located low in the lumbar spine, may cause a severe and progressive deformity of the spine with marked decompensation.[42] The deformity is rigid, and there is no opportunity for compensation of the spine below the area of deformity, since it is so close to the pelvis. In these cases, and seldom for any other indication, excision of the hemivertebra is performed. The excision is done in two stages. First the body of the hemivertebra is resected; it must be removed back to the epidural space. The base of the pedicle is

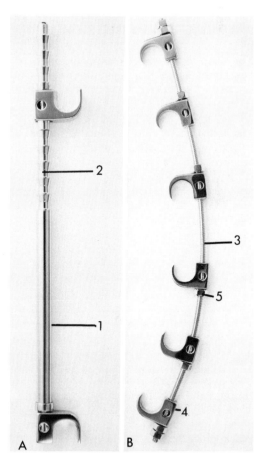

Figure 82–8 *A.* The Harrington distraction rod (1) has two hooks and an area with ratchets (2) to allow distraction. *B.* The compression apparatus consists of a threaded rod (3) with hooks (4) and nuts (5) placed in a manner to apply a compressive force.

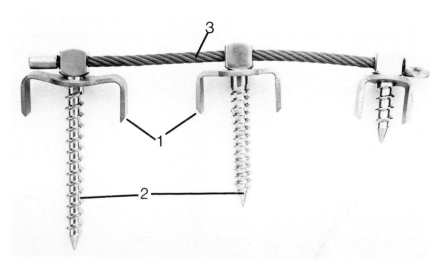

Figure 82–9 Dwyer instrumentation. The staple (1) fits over the vertebral body, and the screw (2) penetrates the vertebral body. A cable (3) fits through a hole in the screw heads. By approximating the screws (the intervertebral discs have been removed), a compressive force is applied to the convexity of the curve. The screw heads can be crimped onto the cable, thus maintaining the correction obtained.

also removed at that time. Usually the only problem encountered is epidural bleeding. Ten days to two weeks later, the posterior components of the hemivertebra are removed, including the lamina, pedicle, facet joints, and transverse process. The wedge-shaped area left by the excision of the hemivertebra must then be pulled together, preferably by using Harrington compression instruments on the convexity of the curve, sometimes assisted by lifting up the other side with a short Harrington distraction instrument.[19,37] This area is then fused to maintain the corrected position. Hemivertebra excision must always be accompanied by fusion of the curve in which the hemivertebra exists. The procedure is merely a closing wedge osteotomy, both anteriorly and posteriorly, of a congenital scoliosis in which the hemivertebra is the apical segment of the curve. It is done to achieve correction and proper body alignment when no other technique is available for that particular patient. When done carefully in two stages, it has had a low complication rate. In the authors' experience, transient mild root symptoms in 3 of 20 patients so treated have been the only complication (Fig. 82–12).

The Halo

The halo, originally designed by Nickel and Perry and their associates for the treatment of severe paralytic curvatures, has become widely utilized for many spinal deformity problems.[36] It is, in essence, an excellent method of grasping the skull in a secure but uncomplicated manner. Because the pins are applied at or below the maximal circumference of the skull, the fixation is adequate and pin dislocation or slippage is rare, even though the patients may be ambulatory in a halo cast for six to nine months. Second, the four-pin fixation provides far greater stability than previous types of skull fixation devices having only two points. The technique of application is simple, does not require an incision in the skin or any tool that is more complicated than a simple screwdriver. Except in small children, it can be applied under local anesthesia. Owing to the thinness of the child's cranium, it is not recommended for children under the age of 3 or for children with thin skulls due to hydrocephalus or osteogenesis imperfecta. Although brain abscess as well as cranial osteomyelitis has been reported, considering the number of applications, these complications are extraordinarily rare.[45]

The halo is used for two purposes: first, as a method of grasping the skull in order to obtain correction of a curvature by traction, and second, to be incorporated into a cast as a method of immobilizing the spine either for a fracture or following spinal fusion.

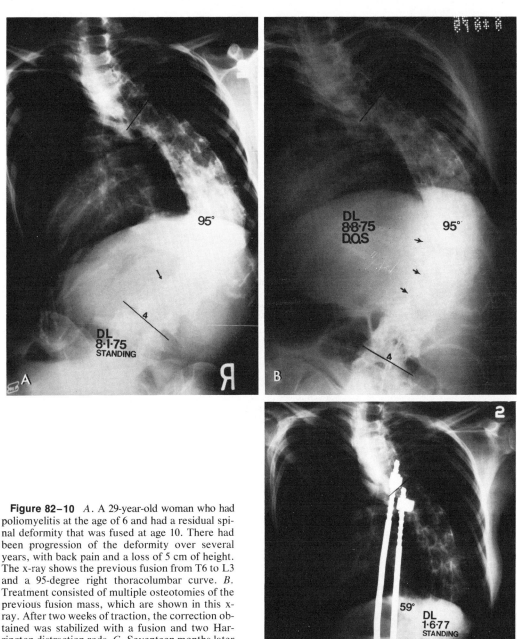

Figure 82–10 *A*. A 29-year-old woman who had poliomyelitis at the age of 6 and had a residual spinal deformity that was fused at age 10. There had been progression of the deformity over several years, with back pain and a loss of 5 cm of height. The x-ray shows the previous fusion from T6 to L3 and a 95-degree right thoracolumbar curve. *B*. Treatment consisted of multiple osteotomies of the previous fusion mass, which are shown in this x-ray. After two weeks of traction, the correction obtained was stabilized with a fusion and two Harrington distraction rods. *C*. Seventeen months later this x-ray shows a solid fusion with the curve measuring 59 degrees. The patient is pain-free and the spine is stable.

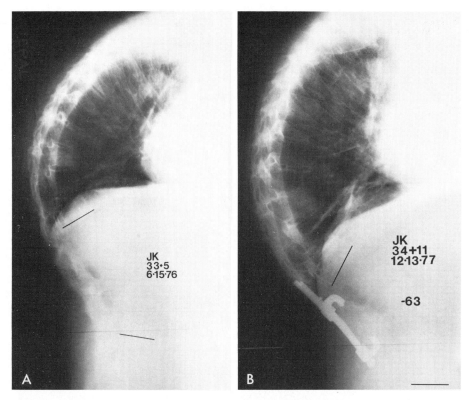

Figure 82–11 *A*. This 33-year-old man with ankylosing spondylitis presented with kyphosis of his whole spine. He had difficulty seeing ahead of himself and back pain due to his efforts to hold himself upright. *B*. Treatment consisted of a closing wedge lumbar osteotomy to increase the lumbar lordosis and thus lift his head up. The osteotomy was closed by means of two Harrington compression rods, well seen in this x-ray taken 18 months postoperatively.

Halo-Femoral Traction

Halo-femoral traction has become a standard method throughout the world for the preoperative correction of severe spinal deformities, regardless of their cause. Although it is possible to apply skeletal traction to the pelvis, it is difficult to apply and cumbersome to maintain. Similarly, skeletal traction through a pin in the tibia, although easy to accomplish, requires pulling through both the knee joint and hip joint to correct the spine, whereas a distal femoral pin pulls only through the hip joint. When reasonable weights, i.e., 20 to 25 per cent of body weight, are used for a reasonably short period, i.e., two to six weeks, no damage to the hip joint occurs. When dealing with pelvic obliquity, as frequently seen in paralytic curves, asymmetrical weights can be applied, thus pulling down the "high" side of the pelvis. The importance of halo-femoral traction lies in the slow and gradual correction of a severe curve with

the patient fully awake and able to indicate any neurological complications. At operation, one merely inserts rods to *maintain* correction already *obtained* by the halo-femoral traction. Thus, sudden stretching of the entire curve in the operating room can be avoided.

Halo-femoral traction is not without its own complications.[23] The most frequent is paralysis of the sixth cranial nerve (abducens). Paralysis of other cranial nerves, brachial plexus, and bladder as well as total paraplegia have been reported.[26] Traction weights should be added slowly and the neurological situation monitored very carefully, and at the first hint of difficulty, the weights should be sharply reduced or eliminated. It has been amply demonstrated that total weight on head and legs of no more than 30 per cent of body weight is adequate for the correction of almost all curvatures. Correction can usually be obtained in about two to three weeks. Weights greater than this or periods of time longer than three

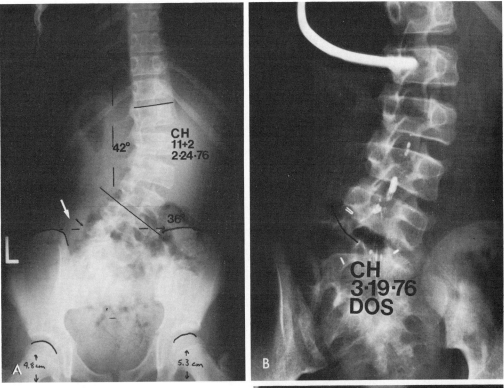

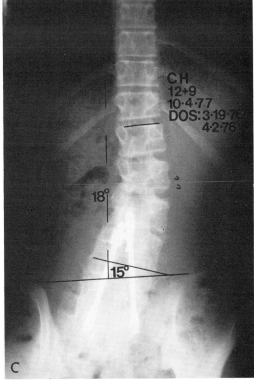

Figure 82–12 *A*. Hemivertebra excision. This 11-year-old girl presented with decompensation to the right and inability to stand erect without bending her left leg. The standing x-ray shows a hemivertebra at L5 on the left with a tilt of L4 of 36 degrees and a right lumbar compensatory curve or 42 degrees. *B*. Treatment consisted of excision of the hemivertebra anteriorly via a sympathectomy approach. The x-ray on the day of operation shows the body removed and three clips marking the limits of the anterior excision. *C*. Two weeks later a posterior excision and fusion were performed utilizing compression and distraction Harrington instrumentation. The x-ray 18 months later shows the correction and a solid fusion. The patient is only slightly decompensated to the right and can now stand upright with both knees extended.

weeks have not yielded improved correction. There is only so much "slack" in a curvature, and it is highly dangerous to attempt correction beyond this amount by traction. If one wishes a greater amount of correction, it is necessary to shorten the long side of the curve by a closing wedge osteotomy rather than trying to elongate the concavity of the curve and risking paraplegia.

Halo-Pelvic Traction

Halo-pelvic traction was an outgrowth of the skeletal traction with the halo and femoral pins. It was obvious that it would be ideal to have some fixation on the pelvis, avoiding the need to pull through the hip joints and also allowing the patient to remain ambulatory. DeWald and Ray are largely credited with devising the most effective method of pelvic fixation.[11] O'Brien and co-workers further extended and modified its use.[38,39] Although sounding ideal, the halo-pelvic device has a large number of problems, including osteomyelitis of the pelvis, bowel perforation, and a high incidence of neurological defects.[38] In addition, once the device is in place, it is virtually impossible to obtain adequate fusion to the sacrum for long paralytic curves, and it is difficult to obtain an adequate bone graft from the iliac crest because of the presence of the pins and pin tract. For these reasons, use of the halo-pelvic device has remained limited to only special circumstances (Fig. 82–13).

Complications of Operative Treatment

As in any major operative procedure, complications can occur in operations for spinal deformity. Of particular interest to the neurosurgeon are the neurological complications following operations for scoliosis.

The most feared complication of operative procedures for scoliosis is paraplegia. Prior to 1960, when the only method of curve correction was cast application, paralysis was very rare. The ability of the skin to tolerate cast pressure limited the amount of correction so the spinal cord was not compromised. Although the use of a cast was excellent with regard to the freedom

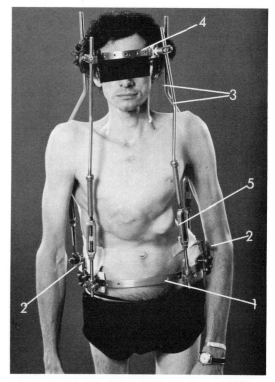

Figure 82–13　Halo-pelvic apparatus. The pelvic hoop (1) is secured to the pelvis by two pins, which pass through the iliac wings (2). Four uprights (3) connect the pelvic hoop to the halo (4). A turnbuckle (5) in each upright allows for distraction to be applied.

from paraplegia, it was not satisfactory because of the poor quality of correction of the spinal deformity.

With the advent of powerful distraction devices such as the Harrington rod, halo-femoral traction, and halo-pelvic traction, paraplegia, unfortunately, was more frequently reported.[26] This is not to say that paralysis did not occur with earlier types of treatment. Several cases were reported in which paralysis occurred following simple spinal fusion, even when instruments did not inadvertently enter the spinal canal.[40] These patients usually had a sharp kyphosis for which a posterior fusion was done in an area where the spinal cord was stretched tightly over the kyphus. Even though the cord was not stretched in any way, the reaction to the operative procedure apparently caused sufficient regional swelling to obliterate the blood flow in the anterior spinal artery and thus cause paraplegia.

Paraplegia can occur either intraoperatively, from the distraction with Harrington rods, or postoperatively, when the patient may awake from the procedure with perfectly normal neurological function and become paraplegic a few hours later. Both these situations appear to be due to compromise of the blood supply of the spinal cord. For this reason, when a patient awakens neurologically normal but develops paraplegia a few hours later, he must be returned immediately to the operating room, and the rods must be removed. Removing the rods is all that is necessary. Laminectomy, opening of the dura, and similar maneuvers have not proved of any value. It is simply the removal of the distracting force that is critical. If the rods are removed within four hours of the onset of the first signs of paralysis, total recovery is the rule.[26] If, however, the patient has gone to a level of complete paraplegia and has remained so for more than eight hours, recovery virtually never occurs. Thus, the prompt recognition of the problem and prompt removal of the rods is critical.

For the patient who awakens from operation with a paraplegia following instrumentation, the prognosis is not good. Most of these patients, despite prompt rod removal, have not recovered.[26] For this reason, methods of monitoring the neurological function during operation have evoked great interest. In a few sophisticated centers, cortical evoked potentials are being utilized for intraoperative neurological monitoring.[35] In most areas, this technology and equipment is not available and the Stagnara "wake-up" test is used.[44] For this test, the anesthesia is sufficiently lightened immediately following the rod insertion so that, on verbal command, the patient can voluntarily move his feet first right and then left, demonstrating intact neurological function. The authors have used this technique extensively and have found it to be reliable. Of 700 patients in whom rods were inserted, 4 demonstrated inability to move their feet with this test; and with removal of the rods or merely lessening of the traction on them, the ability to move the feet returned within a few minutes. These patients did not have postoperative neurological difficulty. Further, they do not remember anything about the problem.

In the operative treatment of spinal deformity, paraplegia is most likely to occur in the patient with sharply angular kyphosis, particularly congenital kyphosis and particularly when that kyphosis is in the mid to upper thoracic spine at the "watershed" area of the blood supply to the spinal cord. Three such catastrophes have occurred in the authors' series of 3000 spinal fusions for curvatures of all types. Two of these patients had congenital kyphosis, and the third had a severe kyphosis secondary to diastrophic dwarfism. All three patients were operated on while in halo-femoral traction, which probably stretched the spinal cord more tightly over the apex of the kyphosis, thus decreasing the precarious blood flow to the spinal cord. In one of these patients, an anterior vertebral body resection was done. The patient awakened from operation with an anterior spinal artery syndrome and never recovered. The second patient had an anterior and posterior hemivertebra excision while in halo-femoral traction and awoke neurologically normal, but subsequently developed paralysis on the third postoperative day and progressed to a severe paraparesis that, on removal of traction and partial correction of the curve, gradually resolved and eventually recovered totally.[47] The third patient had a severe high thoracic congenital kyphosis and had merely a posterior spine fusion performed. She was in halo-femoral traction, and despite a delicately performed posterior spinal fusion, she awoke neurologically normal but developed paraplegia on the fourth postoperative day. She never recovered from the paralysis and eventually died of pyelonephritis secondary to her paraplegia.

It is tempting to think orthopedic correction should not have been done in these patients, thus avoiding these tragic complications. Unfortunately, the natural history in all three of these patients was such that they were inevitably headed for spontaneous paraplegia due to the evolution of their curves. Thus, paraplegia must be feared both as a complication of treatment and as a complication of nontreatment. In all three cases, severe deformities existed on presentation for treatment. In all three cases, paraplegia could easily have been prevented by adequate early spinal fusion many years earlier. These cases represent failure of adequate treatment of the growing child more than failures of operative treatment.

For the neurosurgeon, especially when called in consultation by an orthopedic surgeon when paraplegia has occurred, it is important to know what orthopedic procedures have been done, what are their potential neurological complications, and what corrective steps need to be taken. If the patient awakes from a Harrington instrumentation procedure with total and complete paraplegia, the rods should be removed immediately. Exploration of the spinal canal is not necessary unless there has been a fracture at the site of hook insertion, indicating a possible epidural hematoma that could be removed. If the patient has had a normal awakening from the instrumentation procedure and subsequently develops deteriorating paraparesis, the treatment of choice is immediate removal of the rods. Procrastination with steroid treatment should not be done. A myelogram is not indicated. It will accomplish nothing, and the time necessary to perform it should be used in getting the patient back to the operating room and removing the rods.

If paralysis or paresis occurs during skeletal traction, as with halo-femoral traction or halo-pelvic traction, the treatment of choice is marked reduction or elimination of the traction. This alone suffices for treatment. Steroids have not been found to improve the rate of recovery. Myelography could be useful to rule out a diastematomyelia, tight filum terminale, or other cause for tethering of the spinal cord.

Many neurosurgeons mistakenly believe that removal of the diastematomyelia or other tethering structure will alleviate the patient's curvature problem. This is not true. The curvature is due to the congenitally anomalous bone development and not to paralytic causes.[49] Thus, the neurosurgeon removing a spur from a patient with a curvature should seek adequate consultation with the scoliosis physician in order to manage both components of the patient's condition properly.

SPECIAL PROBLEMS OF NEUROSURGICAL AND ORTHOPEDIC INTEREST

Dysraphism and Deformity

Diastematomyelia and other forms of spinal dysraphism are well known to the neurosurgeon (see Chapter 35). These lesions are frequently seen in association with congenital spinal deformity, particularly congenital scoliosis.[49] Thus, difficulty in management can arise in the treatment of the curvature when a tethered spinal cord is found. The diastematomyelia may be within the area of the curvature or may be in a different area, either proximally or distally. Particularly when the diastematomyelia is in the area of the curvature, the deformity and warping of the spine due to the curvature may obscure the standard roentgenological findings. For example, widening of the interpedicular distance cannot be appreciated if there is torsion of the spine in the area of the lesion. The orthopedic surgeon must maintain a high index of suspicion of spinal dysraphism whenever congenital deformities of the spine are to be subjected to either distractive treatment modalities or Harrington instrumentation. The patient must have a myelogram prior to the beginning of treatment. If diastematomyelia or other tethering structure is identified, then the neurosurgeon must remove the tethering structure prior to the institution of any orthopedic treatment of the curvature. With this regimen, the authors have avoided causing paraplegia when such a lesion has been identified.[49]

Harrington rods are particularly dangerous in congenital spinal deformities because of the high incidence of tethered cords, some of which can be detected on myelography and others of which cannot. Therefore, it is preferable to obtain correction by other means and insert rods only as internal stabilizers, or to go back to old-fashioned methods of spinal fusion without the rods.

The neurosurgeon treating the patient under such circumstances must remember that a spinal fusion is necessary for the treatment of the patient's curvature problem, and if a laminectomy is necessary for the removal of the spur, then that laminectomy must be minimal, must be kept specifically to the area of the anomaly, and should not destroy the facet joints laterally.

The spinal fusion should not be performed at the same operative procedure as the laminectomy, but should, rather, be done during the same hospitalization about 10 days after the laminectomy. By this time the dural suture has become healed, but the exposure remains easy, since dense scar tissue has not formed yet. The neurosurgeon and orthopedic surgeon should collaborate, particularly in the placement of the skin incision for the laminectomy, since it should coincide with the line of the incision that will be used later for the spinal fusion.

If the laminectomy is to be done in an area that is not to be included in the fusion, then there is no particular problem, and the two procedures can be done independently. The spur removal must always precede the correction of the curvature and the fusion of the spine.

What if a laminectomy for spur removal is necessary in an area of the spine that has already been fused for scoliosis? Although this is a rare occurrence, it constitutes no severe problem, since the area of the spur can be identified by needle markers placed in the fusion mass. A window can then be made in the fusion and the spur removed without destroying the stability of the fusion. This should be done as a combined procedure with both the neurosurgeon and the scoliosis surgeon taking part.

Paraplegia Related to Curves

There are three situations in which combined curvature and paralysis may occur: (1) there may be a curve due to the paralytic problem, (2) there may be a paraplegia due to the curve, and (3) there may be coexistent but unrelated paralysis and scoliosis.

Thus, the patient presenting with a combination of paralysis and curvature deserves very careful evaluation. Any child having a paralytic problem will develop a curvature of the spine. If the paralysis is total and complete, a collapsing type of spine develops, quite flexible at first, but subsequently becoming quite structural. In a series of 250 children under the age of 18 presenting at Rancho Los Amigos Hospital with paraplegia secondary to spinal cord injury, all girls under age 12 and all boys under age 14 developed significant curvature of the spine. Individuals who become paraplegic or quadraplegic after the completion of growth do not develop curvatures.[6] Such curvatures demand very early bracing and usually require stabilization of the spine at the time of the growth spurt. Operative stabilization of these children's spines gives them a vast improvement in sitting stability and considerably enhances their rehabilitation (Fig. 82–14).

As stated previously, paralysis due to the curvature itself does not occur in pure scoliosis but only in patients with kyphosis or kyphoscoliosis, particularly when the kyphosis is in the mid to upper thoracic spine. The most common causes of such paralyses are, first, congenital kyphosis, second, kyphoscoliosis due to neurofibromatosis, and third, old tuberculosis.

Such patients require careful management to alleviate the paralysis and also to correct and stabilize the curve problems so that the paralysis will not recur.

Laminectomy is absolutely contraindicated for such paralysis problems. The paralysis is due to pressure of the vertebral bodies pushing back against the anterior part of the spinal cord. There is usually a great deal of room between the dura and the laminae, and removal of the laminae only weakens the spine, allowing further angulation of the kyphosis, and usually results in increased paraplegia.[9,25]

Satisfactory treatment depends upon anterior removal of the vertebral body bone that is pressing against the spinal cord. This can be accomplished either via costotransversectomy (Capener approach) or, preferrably, via the transthoracic route, which permits better control of bleeding and allows simultaneous anterior spinal fusion (Fig. 82–15).[33]

It is useless to decompress the cord by vertebral body removal in the growing child unless, either at the same time or subsequently, the spine is fused to stabilize the deformity. Otherwise, both the deformity and the pinching of the spinal cord will recur (Fig. 82–16).

Evaluation of these patients prior to operation must include a myelogram, but the standard prone myelogram with 6 to 12 ml of Hypaque is inadequate. These patients require either large-volume myelography or supine myelography. Of 43 patients who presented because of paralysis related to spinal deformity, all had a kyphotic problem. Of those treated by laminectomy, none were improved, 4 had no change, and 6 showed deterioration. Of those treated by anterior spinal cord decompression and spinal fusion, 16 were improved, 7 remain unchanged, none showed deterioration, and 2

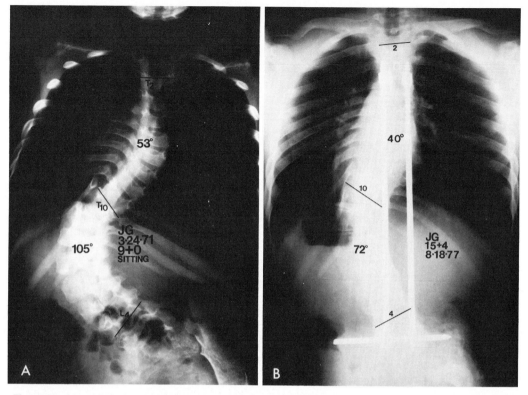

Figure 82–14 *A*. This 9-year-old-boy suffered paraplegia as a result of an exchange transfusion at birth. A sitting x-ray shows a 105-degree left thoracic lumbar curve with a 53-degree upper left thoracic curve and extreme pelvic obliquity. He had difficulty sitting because of the severe curve and pelvic obliquity. *B*. Treatment was by fusion and instrumentation utilizing two distraction rods and a transverse sacral bar. Six months later a pseudarthrosis at L2–L3 required repair. This x-ray taken six years later shows a level pelvis, the head centered over the pelvis, and curves of 40 degrees and 72 degrees.

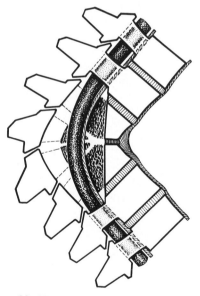

Figure 82–15 Technique of anterior transthoracic spinal cord decompression. The spinal cord is compressed at the apex of the kyphosis. The wedge of bone at the apex of the kyphos is removed, leaving bone anteriorly and at the far cortex. Once the dural sac moves into the space created and dural pulsations return, the discs are removed and an anterior strut fusion is performed.

died in the immediate postoperative period.[25]

Coexistent But Unrelated Paralysis in Scoliosis

An interesting patient is the one presenting with progressive paralysis and scoliosis in whom it is tempting to think that the curvature is causing the paralysis, whereas in fact, some other lesion is causing the paralysis and the scoliosis is merely a "red herring." One such patient presented to the authors with a severe thoracic scoliosis, but she did not have any kyphosis, and the level of paralysis did not correspond to the apex of the curvature. On myelography, it was demonstrated that she had a space-occupying intramedullary tumor, and on exploration it proved to be an intramedullary arteriovenous malformation that was totally unrelated to her curvature. A second patient presented with a thoracolumbar kyphoscoliosis and progressive paraparesis at the age of 57. His curvature was due to poliomyelitis; his paralysis to an aneurysm of

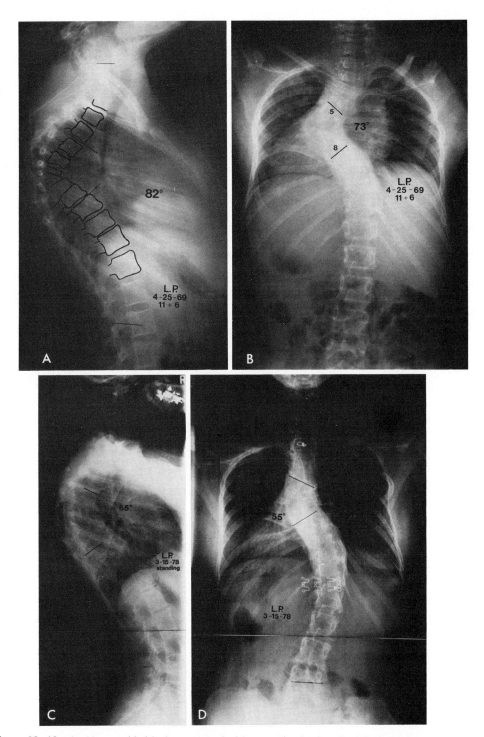

Figure 82–16   An 11-year-old girl who presented with severe kyphosis and scoliosis due to neurofibromatosis and a two-month history of progressive T8 paraparesis. *A*. Presenting lateral x-ray shows a sharp angular midthoracic kyphosis of 82 degrees. *B*. The anteroposterior view shows a short sharp scoliotic curve in the same area of 73 degrees. Treatment was by an anterior transthoracic spinal cord decompression and anterior fusion followed by posterior fusion. Neurological improvement occurred, but the fusion was not solid and repeat posterior and anterior fusions were necessary to stabilize the spine. *C*. Nine years after initial presentation there is residual hyperreflexia in the lower extremities with no weakness. The fusion is solid, and the kyphosis is 55 degrees. *D*. The scoliosis 55 degrees. The lateral x-ray shows well the multiple struts of rib crossing the kyphosis.

the abdominal aorta that caused impairment of the blood flow to the spinal cord. A third patient presented with an increasing paraparesis and a very mild 25-degree thoracic scoliosis due to a hemivertebra with no kyphosis. A myelogram revealed an extensive syringomyelia involving the thoracic spinal cord—totally unrelated to the hemivertebra.

Postlaminectomy Spinal Deformity

One of the most serious causes of kyphosis is a laminectomy in a growing child. It is pointed out by Lonstein and co-workers that kyphosis occurs in a large percentage of patients on whom a laminectomy has been performed during the childhood years.[22,24] This is particularly true if the laminectomy includes the facet joints. With the ever-improving survival rate following treatment of spinal cord tumors in the child, this problem of postlaminectomy kyphosis has rapidly become of paramount importance (Fig. 82–17).

Every child having a laminectomy for any reason should have orthopedic consultation. Baseline upright anteroposterior and

lateral x-rays of the spine should be obtained prior to the laminectomy, and detailed anteroposterior and lateral spine x-rays obtained immediately following the laminectomy to document the area and quantity of bone removal. Preferably the orthopedic surgeon should scrub in at the time of the laminectomy to know precisely and exactly which tissues have been removed and to encourage the neurosurgeon to remove as little bone as possible, especially the facet joints. No facet excision is required for tumor removal or biopsy of virtually all intramedullary tumors such as gliomas. The only patients requiring facet removal are usually those with dumbbell tumors of neurofibroma or neuroblastoma.

If bilateral facet excision has been necessary as part of the tumor removal, then the child should be fitted with an appropriate brace for the spine prior to the assumption of upright activities. This is true regardless of the child's state of general paralysis. If the child survives the tumor, and develops a progressive kyphosis, then spinal fusion should be performed before the deformity becomes severe. If the child has an extremely malignant tumor and is likely to die

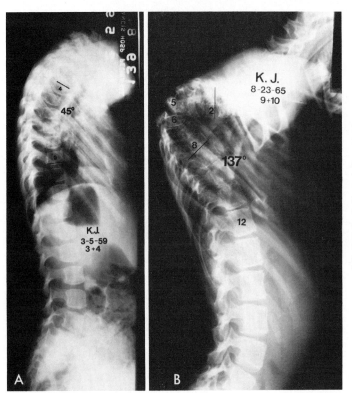

Figure 82–17 This girl had a laminectomy from T3 to T6 at age 20 months for a neuroblastoma of the spinal cord. *A.* Lateral x-ray at the age of 3 years and 4 months shows a thoracic kyphosis of 45 degrees. *B.* Standing lateral x-ray at age 9 years and 10 months, six years later, shows a sharp thoracic kyphosis of 137 degrees. Note that the apex of the deformity is in the area of the laminectomy. The facets had been removed completely on both sides at the T5–T6 level.

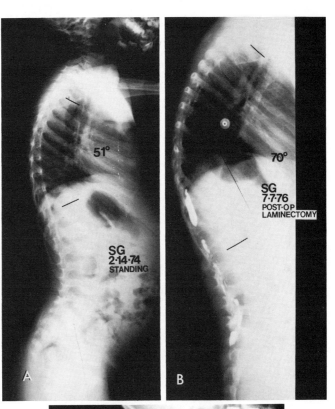

Figure 82–18 This 2-year-and-3-month-old girl presented with atypical-appearing 31-degree thoracic scoliosis. *A.* The lateral x-ray on presentation showed a 51-degree thoracic kyphosis. Because of the unusual appearance of the curve, neurological consultation was obtained, but no abnormality was found. A Milwaukee brace was fitted and excellent curve correction was achieved. After the brace had been worn for two years, an abnormal gait was noted. There was weakness of the quadriceps and anterior tibial muscles on the right. A myelogram showed a complete block at the conus, and the spinal fluid protein was 1200 mg per 100 mil. Laminectomy and myelotomy revealed an intramedullary cyst but no tumor. The gait became normal, but two weeks later the patient gradually became paraplegic. A myelogram showed a block at T8–L1. The laminectomy was extended from T3 to L3, and a grade II astrocytoma was found and subtotally resected. Postoperatively the tumor was irradiated. *B.* A lateral x-ray at the time of the laminectomy showed the kyphosis to be 70 degrees. *C.* Use of the Milwaukee brace was continued to control the kyphosis, and this lateral view 18 months later shows good control. If brace control is lost or when the patient reaches her growth spurt, an anterior fusion will be performed to stabilize the spine.

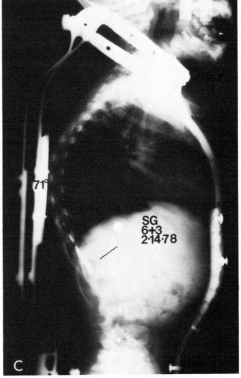

within one or at the most two years, then fusion is not indicated. If the tumor prognosis, i.e., a neuroblastoma in a child over age 3, so indicates, then fusion of the spine can be considered in the same hospitalization as the laminectomy procedure. This would require close cooperation with the radiotherapist and onconologist (Fig. 82–18)

SUMMARY

The field of spinal deformity is of considerable interest to the neurosurgeon because of his natural interest in the spine and spinal cord. This chapter has delineated the problems of spinal deformity, including scoliosis, lordosis, and kyphosis. The causes are many and the problems are varied. Many patients have mild curvatures that cause no functional disability and do not require medical attention or treatment. Others have mild but increasing deformities that demand treatment early to prevent development of severe deformities. Severe deformities produce many problems for the patient including cor pulmonale, arthritis, even spinal cord compression. Such dire complications are far better prevented than treated after their development.

Of particular interest to the neurosurgeon are: (1) neurological complications of the orthopedic treatment of spinal deformity, (2) the correlated problems of neurospinal dysraphism and spinal deformity, and (3) the problem of paraplegia caused by curvatures. Cooperation between neurosurgeon and orthopedic surgeon in the management of these difficult and complex problems is strongly urged.

REFERENCES

1. Bergofsky, E. H., Turino, G. M., and Fishman, A. P.: Cardiorespiratory failure in kyphosis. Medicine (Balt.), 38:263, 1959.
2. Blount, W. P., and Moe, J. H.: The Milwaukee Brace. Baltimore, Williams & Wilkins Co., 1973.
3. Bradford, D. S., Moe, J. H., Montalvo, F. J., and Winter, R. B.: Scheuermann's kyphosis and roundback deformity—results of Milwaukee brace treatment. J. Bone Joint Surg., 56-A:740–758, 1954.
4. Bradford, D. S., Moe, J. H., Montalvo, F. J., and Winter, R. B.: Scheuermann's kyphosis: Results of surgical treatment by posterior spine

5. arthrodesis in twenty-two patients. J. Bone Joint Surg., 57A:439–448, 1975.
5. Brown, H. P.: Spine Deformity Subsequent to Spinal Cord Injury. Orthop. Seminar Rancho Los Amigos Hospital, 5:41, 1972.
6. Brown, H. P., and Bonnett, C. C.: Spine deformity subsequent to spinal cord injury. J. Bone Joint Surg., 55-A:441, 1973.
7. Bunch, W. H.: The Milwaukee brace in paralytic scoliosis. Clin. Orthop., 110:63, 1975.
8. Carr, W. A., Moe, J. H., Winter, R. B., and Lonstein, J. E.: Treatment of idiopathic scoliosis in the Milwaukee brace, long term results. J. Bone Joint Surg., 62-A:599–612, 1980.
9. Chou, S. N.: The treatment of paralysis associated with kyphosis: Role of anterior decompression. Clin. Orthop., 128:149, 1977.
10. Collis, D. K., and Ponseti, I. V.: Long-term followup of patients with idiopathic scoliosis not treated surgically. J. Bone Joint Surg., 51-A: 425–445, 1969.
11. DeWald, R. L., and Ray, R. D.: Skeletal traction for treatment of severe scoliosis. The University of Illinois halo-hoop apparatus. J. Bone Joint Surg., 52-A:233–238, 1970.
12. Dickson, J. H., and Harrington, P. R.: The evolution of the Harrington Instrumentation technique in sediosis. J. Bone Joint Surg., 55-A:993–1002, 1973.
13. Dwyer, A.: An anterior approach to scoliosis. A preliminary report. Clin. Orthop., 62:192–202, 1969.
14. Fishman, A. P.: Pulmonary aspects of scoliosis. In Zorab, P. A., ed.: Proceedings of a Symposium on Scoliosis. National Fund for Research into Poliomyelitis and Other Crippling Diseases. London, Vincent House, 1966.
15. Gazioglu, K., Goldstein, L. A., Femi-Pearse, D., and Yu, P. N.: Pulmonary function in idiopathic scoliosis. J. Bone Joint Surg., 50-A:1391, 1968.
16. Harrington, P. R.: Treatment of scoliosis—correction and internal fixation by spine instrumentation. J. Bone Joint Surg., 44-A:591, 1962.
17. Harrington, P. R.,: The management of scoliosis by spine instrumentation: An evaluation of more than 200 cases. Southern Med. J., 56: 1367–1377, 1963.
18. Harrington, P. R., and Dickson, J. H.: An eleven-year clinical investigation of Harrington Instrumentation, a preliminary report on 578 cases. Clin. Orthop., 93:113–130, 1973.
19. Hibbs, R. A.: An operation for progressive spinal deformities. New York Med. J., 93:1013, 1911.
20. Hodgson, A. R., Stock, R. E., Fang, H. S. Y., and Ong, G. B.: Anterior spinal fusion. The operative approach and pathological findings in 412 patients with Pott's disease of the spine. Brit. J. Surg., 48:172, 1960.
21. Leatherman, K. C.: The management of rigid spinal curves. Clin. Orthop., 93:215, 1973.
22. Lonstein, J. E., Winter, R. B., Bradford, D. S., Moe, J. H., and Bianco, A. J.: Post-laminectomy spine deformity. J. Bone Joint Surg., 58-A:727, 1976.
23. Lonstein, J. E.: Screening for spine deformities in Minnesota schools. Clin. Orthop., 126:33, 1977.
24. Lonstein, J. E.: Post-laminectomy kyphosis. Clin. Orthop., 128:93, 1977.
25. Lonstein, J. E., Moe, J. H., Winter, R. B., Chou,

S., and Pinto, W.: Spinal deformity and cord compression. J. Bone Joint Surg., *56-A*:1304, 1974.

26. MacEwen, G. D.: Acute neurologic complications in the treatment of scoliosis (a report of the Scoliosis Research Society). J. Bone Joint Surg., *57-A*:404, 1975.

27. Makley, J. T., Herndon, C. H., Inkley, S., Doershuk, C., Matthews, L. W., Post, R. H., and Littell, A. S.: Pulmonary function in paralytic and non-paralytic scoliosis before and after treatment: A study of sixty-three cases. J. Bone Joint Surg., *50-A*:1379, 1968.

28. Mellencamp, D., Blount, W. P., and Anderson, A. J.: Milwaukee brace treatment of idiopathic scoliosis: Late results. Clin. Orthop., *126*:47–57, 1977.

29. Moe, J. H.,: Management of idiopathic scoliosis. Clin. Orthop., *53*:21–30, 1967.

30. Moe, J. H., and Kettleson, D. N.: Idiopathic scoliosis—analysis of curve patterns and the preliminary results of Milwaukee brace treatment in 196 patients. J. Bone Joint Surg., *52-A*:1509–1533, 1970.

31. Moe, J. H., and Welch, J. A.: Post-fusion spinal osteotomy. Presented at Gillette Children's Hospital, Dec. 18, 1971.

32. Moe, J. H., Winter, R. B., Bradford, D. S., and Lonstein, J. E.: Scoliosis and other spinal deformities. Philadelphia, W. B. Saunders Co., 1978, p. 31–33.

33. Ibid, p. 517.

34. Nachemson, A.: A long-term follow-up study of non-treated scoliosis. Acta Orthop. Scand., *39*:466–576, 1968.

35. Nash, C. L., Schatzinger, L., and Lorine, R.: Intraoperative monitoring of spinal cord function during scoliosis surgery. J. Bone Joint Surg., *56-A*:1765, 1974.

36. Nickel, V. L., Perry, J., Garrett, A., and Heppenstall, M.: The halo. J. Bone Joint Surg., *50-A*:1400–1409, 1968.

37. Nilsonne, U., and Lundgren, K. D.: Long-term prognosis in idiopathic scoliosis. Acta. Orthop. Scand., *39*:456–465, 1968.

38. O'Brien, J. P.: The halo-pelvic apparatus. Acta Orthop. Scand. (suppl.), *163*:79, 1975.

39. O'Brien, J. P., Yau, A. C., and Hodgson, A. R.: Halo pelvic traction: A technic for severe spinal deformities. Clin. Orthop., *93*:179–190, 1973.

40. Risser, J. C., and Norquist, D. M.: A followup study of the treatment of scoliosis. J. Bone Joint Surg., *40-A*:555–569, 1958.

41. Simmons, E. H., Kyphotic deformity of the spine in ankylosing spondylitis. Clin. Orthop., *128*:65, 1977.

42. Slabaugh, P. B., Lonstein, J. E., Winter, R. B., Moe, J. H., and Bradford, D. S.: Management of lumbosacral hemivertebra. Presented at annual meeting of Scoliosis Research Society, Hong Kong, Oct. 25, 1977.

43. Smith-Peterson, M. N., Larson, C. B., and Aufranc, O. E.: Osteotomy of the spine for correction of flexion deformity in rheumatoid arthritis. J. Bone Joint Surg., *27*:1, 1945.

44. Vauzelle, C., Stagnara, P., and Jouvinroux, P.: Functional monitoring of spinal cord during spinal surgery. Clin. Orthop., *93*:173, 1973.

45. Weisl, H.: Unusual complications of skull caliper traction. J. Bone Joint Surg., 54-B:143, 1972.

46. Westgate, H. D.: Pulmonary function in thoracic scoliosis: Before and after corrective surgery. Minn. Med., *53*:839, 1970.

47. Winter, R. B.: Congenital Kyphoscoliosis with Paralysis Following Hemivertebra Excision. Clin. Orthop., *119*:116, 1976.

48. Winter, R. B., Lovell, W. W., and Moe, J. H.: Excessive thoracic lordosis and loss of pulmonary function in patients with idiopathic scoliosis. J. Bone Joint Surg., *57-A*:972, 1974.

49. Winter, R. B., Haven, J., Moe, J. H., and Lagaard, S.: Diastematomyelia and congenital spine deformities. J. Bone Joint Surg., *56-A*:27, 1974.

50. Winter, R. B., Moe, J. H., MacEwen, G. C., and Peon-Vidales, H.: The Milwaukee brace in the non-operative treatment of congenital scoliosis. Spine, *1*:85, 1976.

Index

In this index page numbers set in *italics* indicate illustrations. Page numbers followed by (t) refer to tabular material. Drugs are indexed under their generic names when dosage or action or special use is given. The abbreviation vs. is used to indicate differential diagnosis.

INDEX

INDEX

Encephalomyelitis (*Continued*)
  cerebrospinal fluid in, 470
Encephalopathy, alcoholic, cerebral blood flow in, 828, *829*
  electroencephalography in, 222–226, *223, 225*
  hepatic, glutamine levels in, 451
  hypertensive, 1547–1548
    pathophysiology of, 3180(t)
  metabolic, coma in, 72
    pupillary abnormalities in, 67
  post-traumatic, cerebral blood flow in, 828, *829*
  spongiform, brain biopsy in, 386(t)
  transient, postoperative radiotherapy and, 3081
Endarterectomy, carotid, contraindications to, 1569–1571
Endocrine function, 931–988
  evaluation of, 1056
  hypothermia and, 1129
  in empty sella syndrome, 3175
  in pineal tumors, 2864
  in supratentorial tumors, in children, 2706
  multiple, adenomatosis and, 947
  pseudotumor cerebri and, 3185, *3186*
Energy, impaired substrate for, in diffuse cerebral ischemia, 1541–1543, 1543(t)
  production and use of in brain, 766–770, *766,* 766(t), *767, 769, 770*
Enflurane, as general anesthetic, 1122
  in increased intracranial pressure, 901
Engelmann's disease, osteopetrosis vs., 3255
Enterostomy, feeding, in multiple trauma, 2526–2528
Environment, genetics and, in neural tube malformations, 1242–1243
Enzymes, lysosomal, in brain tumors, 2691
  in ischemia, 781
Eosinophilic granuloma, of spine, *515*
  ultrasound scanning in, *730*
Eosinophilic meningitis, 3395
  ventricular, anatomy of, 428
Eosinophils, in cerebrospinal fluid, 440
Ependymal cyst, arachnoid cyst vs., 1436
Ependymal veins, 282, *283*
Ependymitis, pneumoencephalography in, *368*
Ependymoblastoma, cerebral hemisphere, in children, 2712, *2713*
Ependymoma, adult, 2792–2797, *2793–2796*
  brain scanning in, 150(t), 152, 162(t)
  cauda equina, angiography in, *608,* 609
  cerebral hemisphere, in children, 2712
  computed tomography in, 116, 2795, *2795, 2796*
  conus, myelography in, *533*
  exophytic, headache and, 3551, *3551*
  high-pressure hydrocephalus and, 1433
  intracranial, radiation therapy of, 3101, 3101(t)–3102(t)
  locations of, 395(t)
  lumbar vertebrae scalloping in, *3201*
  posterior fossa, in children, 2750–2751
  recurrent, chemotherapy for, 3090(t)
  spinal, *3197,* 3197(t), 3205–3206, *3206*
    chemotherapy for, 3213
    fusiform defect in, *3204*
    in children, *3216*
    operative treatment of, 3211
    radiation therapy for, 3212, 3223(t)
Ephedrine, cerebral blood flow and, 808(t)
  in atonic urinary sphincter, 1046
Epidermoid cyst(s), 2914
  cerebrospinal fluid in, 463
  incidence of, 2915
  locations of, 395(t)
  parasellar, 3154
  posterior fossa, in children, 2753–2754
  spinal, 3208
    myelography in, *535*
Epidermoid tumor, of cranium, 3232, *3233*
Epidural abscess, 3333
  in head injury, 1915
  spinal, cerebrospinal fluid in, 465

Epidural anesthesia, 3648, 3650
  diagnostic, in somatic pain, 3645
  in stereotaxic cordotomy, 3676, *3676*
  therapeutic, for pain, 3652
Epidural fibrosis, pain in, 3614, *3614*
Epidural hematoma. See *Hematoma, epidural.*
Epilepsia partialis continua, 3878
Epilepsy, 3858–3925
  alcoholic, cerebral blood flow in, 828, *829*
  behavioral aspects of, 3880–3883, 3895
  brain abscess and, 3355
  causes of, 3865–3867, 3865(t)
  deterioration from, 3881
  early, 3866
  electroencephalography in, *209,* 210, 215, 217–220, 3868–3871, *3868,* 3911
  in posterior fossa tumors in children, 2736
  Lafora familial myoclonic, 384(t)
  late, 3866
    preventive treatment of, 3875
  localization of focus in, 3867. See also *Epileptogenic focus.*
  myoclonus with, 3852
  pediatric, causes of, 3865, 3865(t)
    clinical diagnosis of, 3867
    cortical resections in, 3879–3897
    medical treatment of, 3874–3879, 3876(t), 3877(t)
      complications of, 3878
    operative treatment of, 3879-3898
      cortical resections in, 3896
      hemicorticectomy in, 3892, *3892, 3894*
      temporal lobectomy in, 3883, *3885, 3888*
    prognosis in, 3878
  post-traumatic, 2166, 2167(t), 2188–2194
  pupils in, 651
  secondary brain damage from, in head injury, 1928
  seizures in, cerebral blood flow in, 828, *829*
    cerebral metabolism during, 770
    classification of, 3864, 3865, 3865(t)
  spina bifida aperta and, 1274
  sympathectomy for, 3720
  temporal lobe, cortical excision in, 3891
    depth electrode localization in, 3917
    stereotaxic management of, 3924
  vertiginous, 687
Epileptic neurons, 3861
Epileptic psychosis, 3882
Epileptogenic focus, chemistry of, 3863, *3864*
  excision of, 3912–3923
  localization of, in adults, electrocorticography in, 3912–3923
    in children, 3867–3871
  morphology of, 3859
  physiology of, 3861
  viral encephalitis and, 3363
Epinephrine, anesthesia and, general, 1123
    local, 1120
  cerebral blood flow and, 808(t')
  in temporal lobectomy, 3884
Epiphyses, costochondral, in acromegaly, 955
Epipodophyllotoxin, in tumor chemotherapy, 3087
Episodic syndromes, altered consciousness in, 72
  clinical diagnosis in, 38
Epsilon-aminocaproic acid, in intraoperative bleeding, 1070
Erb's palsy, in newborn infant, 49
Ergot alkaloids, cerebral blood flow and, 809(t)
Erythrocytes, in cerebrospinal fluid, 436
Esthesioneuroblastoma, 3275, *3276*
Estrogens, in anterior pituitary failure, 950
Ethacrynic acid, inner ear damage and, 691, 691(t)
Ethanolism, electromyographic studies in, 633
Ethinyl estradiol, in anterior pituitary failure, 950
Ethmoid block, *3271*
Ethmoid sinus, anatomy of, 3269, *3270, 3271*
  carcinoma of, 3279, *3279*
Ethmoidectomy, in esthesioneuroblastoma, 3276
Ethosuximide, dosages of, 3877(t)

INDEX

Knee (*Continued*)
  tibial nerve injury at, 2404–2405
Krabbe disease, 385(t)
Krause's corpuscles, 3461
Kuru, cerebrospinal fluid in, 465
Kyphoscoliosis, spinal osteomyelitis and, 3454
Kyphosis, 2629–2655
  congenital, 1258
  etiology of, 2631, 2632(t)
  natural history of, 2633–2635, *2634, 2635*
  neurosurgical problems in, 2648
  nonoperative treatment of, 2635, *2636*
  operative treatment of, 2637, *2638–2646*
  orthopedic problems in, 2648
  thoracolumbar myelomeningocele, and, 1252, *1252, 1253*

Laboratory tests, in anterior pituitary hyperfunction, 953–955
  in anterior pituitary failure, 946–947, 946(t)
  in cerebral death, 751
  in metastatic tumors, of brain, 2875
    of leptomeninges, 2891
  of cerebrospinal fluid, 457–459
Labyrinth, acoustic, sound transmission in, 693
  vestibular, anatomy of, *677, 678–680, 680–682*
    toxic injury to, 691, 691(t)
Labyrinthine fistula test, in vertigo, 686
Labyrinthitis, 690
Laceration, brain, in head injury, 2033
  peripheral nerve, 2365
  scalp, 2301, *2301–2303*
Lacrimal gland tumors, 3058–3059
Lacrimal nerve, in orbit, 3027
Lactate, tissue concentrations of, in ischemia, 777, *778*
Lactotropic microadenoma, 3125
Lacunar infarcts, carotid, 1529
Lacunar skull, of newborn, 1219
Lamaze technique, 3481
Lambdoid suture, synostosis of, 1447, *1450, 1453,* 1461
Lamina terminalis, cistern of, *352*
Laminagraphy, in acoustic neuroma, 2975, *2977, 2989–2991*
Laminectomy, for cervical myelopathy, 2602–2604
  in thoracic spinal cord injuries, 2350
  infections in, 1089
Language, ventrolateral thalamus and, 3835
Larsen syndrome, characteristics of, 1214
Lateral femoral cutaneous nerve, entrapment of, 2463–2464, *2464*
Lead poisoning, intracranial hypertension in, 3180(t)
Leber, optic atrophy of, 667
LeFort fractures, 2279, *2282, 2283*
Leg. See *Extremities, lower.*
Leiomyosarcoma, hypophysectomy in, 3953
Leksell anterior capsulotomy, 3931, *3931, 3932*
Leksell stereotaxic instrument, 3805, *3806*
Leptomeninges, arteries of, in collateral circulatory system, 797
  cyst of, in children, 3245, *3249*
  development of, *1437*
  metastases to, 2888–2894, *2892, 2893,* 2893(t)
Leptomeningitis, brain abscess and, 3344
  diagnosis of, 3324
Leptospiral meningitis, cerebrospinal fluid in, 462
Lethargy, 63, 3834
Letterer-Siwe disease, skull in, 3258
Leucoencephalopathy, progressive multifocal, cerebrospinal fluid in, 465
Leucotomy, bimedial, 3928
  prefrontal, 3927
Leukemia, calvarial lesions in, 3244
  cerebrospinal fluid in, 467
  orbital, 3058
  radiation therapy in, 3104
  spinal cord tumors and, in children, *3216*
Leukodystrophy, metachromatic, cerebrospinal fluid in, 468

Leukodystrophy (*Continued*)
  metachromatic, diagnosis of, 385(t)
  sudanophilic, brain biopsy in, 386(t)
Leukoencephalitis, hemorrhagic, 3358, 3361, 3363
Leukotome, 3806
Levodopa, in Parkinson's disease, 3841
Levothyroxine sodium, in anterior pituitary failure, 949
Lévy-Roussy syndrome, cerebrospinal fluid in, 468
Lidocaine, in cerebral vasospasm, 820
Ligament of Struthers, electromyography of, 631
Lighting, for operating microscope, *1165,* 1171, *1171*
Limb, deformities of, spina bifida aperta and, 1257–1259, 1259(t)
Limbic system, 3730, *3731,* 3929
  lesions of, clinical examination in, 14–15, *15*
Lindstrom's ultrasonic radiation procedure, in psychiatric disorders, 3938, *3939*
Linear pressure regression, of cerebrospinal fluid, technique for, 455
Link's IgG index, 444
Lipid(s), in brain tumors, 2692
  in cerebrospinal fluid, 449
Lipidosis, electroencephalography in, 216, *216,* 222
Lipogranulomatosis, Farber, 385(t)
Lipoma, corpus callosum, 2713–2714, *2714*
  intracranial, 2928, *2928*
  lumbosacral, 1333–1339, *1334, 1335, 1337*
  spinal, 3208, *3208, 3216*
    computed tomography in, 139
    myelographic appearance of, *535*
Lithium carbonate, in inappropriate antidiuretic hormone secretion, 982, 1101
Litigation, chronic pain and, 3528–3529
Liver, See also *Hepatic.*
  disease of, glutamine levels in, 451
  hypothermia and, 1129
  necrosis of, postoperative, 1107
Lobectomy, temporal, in adult epilepsy, 3917, *3919–3922*
  in children and adolescents, 3883, *3885, 3888*
Lobotomy, frontal, for pain, 3732
Locked-in syndrome, 63
  rehabilitation in, 4000
Lombroso-Erba Pentothal activation test, 3896
Long thoracic nerve, entrapment of, 2462
Lordosis, 2629–2655
  development of, 1258
  etiology of, 2631, 2631(t), 2632(t)
  natural history of, 2633–2635, *2634, 2635*
  neurosurgical problems in, 2648
  nonoperative treatment of, 2635, *2636*
  operative treatment of, 2637, *2638–2646*
  orthopedic problems in, 2648
Lower motor neuron, paralysis of, clinical diagnosis of, 7–8
Lückenschädel skull deformity, in myelomeningocele, 1259
Lumbar canal, narrow, *508, 509*
Lumbar disc, failed, dorsal rhizotomy in, 3668
Lumbar drainage, in craniotomy, 1143
Lumbar paravertebral nerve block, 3646, *3647*
Lumbar puncture, 452–457
  alternatives to, 457
  cerebrospinal fluid response to, 472
  complications of, 456
  contraindications for, 452
  in brain abscess, 3346
  in cerebral infarction, 1535
  in hydrocephalus, 1426
  in intracranial hypertension, 850
  in post-traumatic meningitis, 3341
  in pseudotumor cerebri, 3188, 3191
  in spinal cord tumors, 3200
  in subdural empyema, 3335
  indications for, 452
  technique of, 453
Lumbar subarachnoid pressure, intracranial pressure and, 858
Lumbosacral lipoma, 1333–1339, *1334, 1335, 1337*
Lumbosacral plexus, pelvic metastasis to, 3629, 3629(t)